R. Denis Giblin
2/81

MEDICAL NEUROLOGY

Third Edition

Macmillan Publishing Co., Inc.
NEW YORK

Collier Macmillan Canada, Ltd.
TORONTO

Baillière Tindall
LONDON

Macmillan Publishing Co., Inc.
866 Third Avenue, New York, New York 10022

Collier Macmillan Canada, Ltd.
Baillière Tindall • London

Library of Congress Cataloging in Publication Data

Gilroy, John (date)
  Medical neurology.

    Includes bibliographies and index.
    1. Neurology. 2. Nervous system—Diseases.
I. Meyer, John Stirling, joint author. II. Title.
[DNLM: 1. Nervous system diseases. WL100.3 G489m]
RC346.G54 1979   616.8   78–26218
ISBN 0–02–343640–9

Printing: 1 2 3 4 5 6 7 8   Year: 9 0 1 2 3 4 5

PREFACE TO THE THIRD EDITION

The increasing momentum of acquisition of new knowledge in neurology is reflected by the remarkable increase in the number of journals, articles, and books related to neurology in the last few years. It is a source of satisfaction that this burgeoning knowledge is evenly divided between the neurosciences and clinical neurology, since proper care of the neurologic patient can only advance on a firm foundation of the neurosciences. However, such a rapid increase in knowledge and publications places considerable demands on the authors of a textbook of clinical neurology in an effort to maintain a practical and equitable balance of the contents. This has been the prime consideration in the preparation of the third edition of *Medical Neurology,* which remains a pragmatic textbook for the clinical practice of neurology, placing particular emphasis on newer diagnostic and therapeutic developments in the specialty.

The neurologic history and clinical examination still remain the keystone to the practice of neurology, and some practical refinements have been added to the chapter dealing with the neurologic examination (Chap. 1). However, correlation of neurologic symptoms with neuroanatomic localization of the lesion continues to be stressed.

Many recent changes in pediatric neurology are reflected in the addition of much new material in Chapter 2. The section on mental retardation has been expanded, since there is a growing need for greater involvement by the neurologist in this important subject. A method of obtaining an accurate history and the performance of an adequate neurologic examination are outlined, followed by the rational selection of diagnostic procedures for the child with mental retardation. The develop-

mental defects and metabolic disorders have been extensively revised in light of the many advances made in these areas in the last few years. There have also been major advances in the understanding of the childhood encephalopathies, which is reflected in a completely new section on Reye's syndrome.

The demyelinating diseases have been reclassified in Chapter 3 to correlate the hereditary leukodystrophies and lipidoses with underlying biochemical abnormalities. Much new material recently published concerning multiple sclerosis has been considered in the section dealing with this disease. Regrettably, the cause of multiple sclerosis still remains enigmatic despite impressive advances in the epidemiology and immunology of this disease. Nevertheless, much can be done to alleviate the suffering of patients with multiple sclerosis, and treatment is covered in its broadest concept. Newer techniques of diagnosis in the demyelinating diseases are now available, and the role of computed tomography and evoked potentials is illustrated in this chapter.

The value of computed tomography is also emphasized in the diagnosis of the degenerative diseases, which are described in Chapter 4. The increasing recognition of new and remediable causes of dementia illustrates the need for full evaluation and correct diagnosis of this increasingly common complaint seen in an aging population. The suggestion that a multidisciplinary approach to diagnosis and treatment of the dementias is desirable and the outline of the methods used in the evaluation and treatment of disorders of higher cortical function in modern neurologic practice are incorporated in this chapter. The clearer understanding of the biochemistry of neurotransmitters and the role of dopamine depletion in Parkinson's disease are reflected in the considerably revised sections on the etiology and treatment of this disease.

Chapter 5 has been extensively revised to incorporate recent advances in the understanding of the toxic and metabolic disorders affecting the nervous system. The increasing use of potent pharmacologic agents and the exposure to chemical and toxic substances in the modern environment have resulted in recognition of a number of new neurologic disorders, such as toluene encephalopathy, dementia during quinidine therapy, bismuth encephalopathy, disulfiram encephalopathy, and the fetal alcohol syndrome, which have been added to this chapter. New and improved concepts of disorders such as hepatic coma, hepatic encephalopathy, uremic encephalopathy, and dialysis encephalopathy and their treatment have now been defined, and this has required considerable revision of these subjects.

In Chapter 6, headache, migraine, epilepsy, and syncope are considered together since they so often occur as paroxysmal disorders and are frequently interrelated. Improvement in the understanding of the mechanisms involved in the various types of headache and migraine has produced a more rational therapeutic approach to these disorders. Increasing emphasis nowadays on the prophylactic management of migraine is stressed in this chapter. The treatment of seizures has been revised, incorporating a more rational approach to therapy that utilizes determinations of serum levels of anticonvulsant drugs to ensure adequate dosage. The use of established anticonvulsants and a number of newer and important drugs to obtain optimum control of seizures is discussed in depth.

Although bacterial infections of the nervous system are usually sensitive to antibiotic therapy, many remain life-threatening, and treatment is often complicated by the development of antibiotic-resistant organisms. Chapter 7 has been revised to conform to modern practice in the treatment of bacterial infection and its complications, including brain abscess, edema, and bacterial meningitis. Advances in the diagnosis and treatment of the viral encephalitides have also been added in this chapter. The success of adenine arabinoside in the treatment of herpes simplex encephalitis, it is hoped, heralds a new era in the chemotherapeutic treatment of the viral diseases of the nervous system. The concept of more

chronic viral encephalitides has been expanded beyond subacute sclerosing panencephalitis and now includes the chronic forms of rubella and Russian spring-summer panencephalitis.

Chapter 8 has been extensively changed to include modern concepts of brain trauma. The recognition of diffuse brain damage offers a logical and useful concept of brain injury following head trauma. In addition, the mechanisms of head injury described in past editions of this textbook have been revised. New ideas and newer techniques, including computed tomography, have radically altered the diagnostic approach to the head-injured patient and are described in logical order. The latest concepts of treatment of head injury and brain damage are also described, concepts that should reduce the morbidity and mortality of conditions which are so frequently encountered in modern society.

In Chapter 9 the problem of cerebrovascular disease has been revised, with emphasis on the prophylaxis of cerebrovascular insufficiency. Much can be done for the patient with transient ischemic attacks by treating those conditions that contribute to accelerated atherosclerosis. Accordingly, this chapter emphasizes the treatment of hypertension and associated heart disease, as well as the control of metabolic abnormalities and other health hazards by the elimination of smoking. In addition, there is an established place for surgical treatment in cerebrovascular insufficiency, and both conventional and newer innovations in surgical techniques have been included in this chapter. The section on subarachnoid hemorrhage has been extensively revised to reflect the attitudes of most neurosurgeons and their approach to this problem. The section on the cerebral arteritides was also changed to reflect recent publications on this fascinating subject.

The advent of computed tomography has resulted in a profound change in the early diagnosis of brain tumors. These changes are reflected in Chapter 10, where there are extensive revisions of diagnostic procedures, reflecting the importance of computed tomography and other newer diagnostic tests, and much less emphasis on older diagnostic procedures such as lumbar puncture and pneumoencephalography. The opportunity for earlier and more accurate diagnosis of brain tumors will inevitably improve treatment and prognosis, but the advent of computed tomography in no way decreases the importance of the neurologic history and physical examination. The combination of these techniques offers a major step forward in neurologic practice.

A number of additions have been made in Chapter 11 to reflect better understanding of entrapment neuropathies, which have assumed increasing importance in neurologic practice. The classification of some of the familial neuropathies adds to the understanding of these conditions.

Chapter 12 has been extensively rewritten to cover the many advances in the diagnosis and treatment of muscle diseases. The increasing importance of muscle biopsy and staining by histochemical techniques is stressed, and a number of recently described myopathies have been included in the text. Improvements in the understanding of the pathogenesis of myasthenia gravis have led to a more rational approach to treatment of this disorder.

There are many new illustrations in this third edition, reflecting the changes in emphasis on diagnostic procedures following the introduction of computed tomography into neurologic practice. There is no doubt that computed tomography has produced the most radical change in the practice of neurology in decades; however, this fact should not permit neglect of other newer techniques such as evoked potential recordings, which complement computed tomography and increase the accuracy of diagnosis in many conditions. The new emphasis on modern techniques, coupled with continued emphasis on traditional neurologic practice of care in history taking and precision in examination, has been stressed throughout this edition, reflecting a modern approach to neurology.

J. G.
J. S. M.

ACKNOWLEDGMENTS FOR THE THIRD EDITION

The authors wish to acknowledge the contribution of the medical illustration departments of both Wayne State University and Baylor College of Medicine, particularly of the late Mrs. Geraldine E. Fockler, medical illustrator, Wayne State University, who drew many of the original line illustrations. Some of Mrs. Fockler's illustrations were revised for the second edition by Dr. Robert Schwyn, and further revisions were carried out by the Department of Graphic Arts, Wayne State University, for the third edition. Illustrations of CT scans were prepared by the Medical Photography Department, Harper-Grace Hospitals, Detroit.

The extensive revision and insertion of new material in the third edition would not have been possible without the dedication and expertise of Patti L. Holliday, B.Sc., year III medical student, Wayne State University. Mrs. Holliday spent many long hours locating the hundreds of new articles and references in this edition, editing new material in the text, and preparing the index. The authors are also indebted to Mrs. Lucille Thompson, Department of Neurology, Wayne State University, and Mrs. Kathleen Whitsitt, Department of Neurology, Baylor College of Medicine, for preparation of the manuscript. Ms. Joan C. Zulch of Macmillan Publishing Co., Inc., continued to give the same enthusiastic support, as with the development of the previous edition, to the task of producing the third edition.

In addition, grateful acknowledgment is extended to the following physicians and colleagues who gave valued advice in their areas of special interest:

Bernard A. Bast, Ph.D., Assistant Professor of Neurology, Wayne State University

David Benjamins, M.D., Assistant Professor of Neurology, Wayne State University

Joyce A. Benjamins, Ph.D., Associate Professor of Neurology, Wayne State University

Y. Harati, M.D., Assistant Professor of Neurology, Baylor College of Medicine

Garron L. Klepach, M.D., Assistant Professor of Ophthalmology, Wayne State University

A. Martin Lerner, M.D., Professor of Medicine, Wayne State University

George E. Lynn, Ph.D., Professor of Audiology, Wayne State University

M. Zafar Mahmud, M.D., Assistant Professor of Neurology, Wayne State University

Robert L. Maulsby, M.D., Professor of Neurology, Wayne State University

Harvey I. Wilner, M.D., Clinical Assistant Professor of Radiology, Wayne State University

Additional reference material was obtained from the medical libraries of Harper-Grace Hospitals, Detroit; the Shiffman Medical Library, Wayne State University; and the Jesse Jones Library of the Texas Medical Center, Baylor College of Medicine, Houston.

The authors also acknowledge the following for their able assistance:

Ms. Wendy Gilroy
Mr. Ian Gilroy
Mr. Robin Gilroy
Ms. Judy Groth
Mr. John Holliday
Ms. Linda Patanis
Ms. Barbara Reeves
Ms. Suzanne Wasmundt

CONTENTS

MEDICAL NEUROLOGY

1 THE NEUROLOGIC EXAMINATION AND FUNCTIONAL NEUROANATOMY

Neurologic History Taking

The importance of the history in the evaluation of a neurologic problem can be gauged from the fact that, in the majority of cases, the history alone will provide the diagnosis or a confident differential diagnosis. Under these circumstances the remainder of the neurologic examination adds further support to the diagnosis or clarifies the differential diagnosis. Ancillary studies are confirmative acts in a logical process beginning with the history. The physician thinks in terms of anatomic localization and disturbance of physiologic processes as the history unfolds. The first consideration is "Where is the lesion?"; the second consideration is "What is the lesion?"

The history should be obtained in a relaxed atmosphere, and ample time should be taken in recording the evolution of neurologic symptoms experienced by the patient and, if possible, observed by those in close contact with the patient. When it is apparent that the patient is unable to supply an adequate history because of dysphasia or memory failure, or because there have been episodes of loss or clouding of consciousness, a close relative who is aware of the problem should be questioned. Whether the patient supplies the history, or whether it is obtained or augmented by others, the information should be recorded systematically with identification of the chief complaint and the evolution of the symptoms from the beginning of the illness.

Since the physician is analyzing historic data obtained from the patient and/or relative, it is pertinent to move into a neurologic review as soon as the history is completed. This review consists of a series of direct questions covering the range of common neurologic symptoms (Table 1–1).

TABLE 1–1

The Neurologic Review

The neurologic review is a series of direct questions posed to the patient and/or relative immediately following the neurologic history. Simple lay terms should be used.

Inquiry	Remarks
Headache	Response is likely to be affirmative
	Pursue further if of recent onset or if there is recent change in pattern of chronic headaches
Visual symptoms	Ask about *sudden* changes in ability to see, sudden blurring, dimness, or blacking out of vision
Diplopia	—
Hearing	—
Tinnitus	—
Vertigo	Do not use term "dizziness." See text
Ataxia	—
Focal weakness	—
Focal numbness	—
Sphincter control	Urgency, frequency, or incontinence
Speech	—
Writing	—
Swallowing	—
Memory	—
Loss or impairment of consciousness	Try to obtain a description from a reliable observer. See text

These questions should be posed in simple language, and a positive response should prompt more detailed inquiry until all relevant information has been recorded.

Headache, which is the first item in the neurologic review, is a very common complaint. Once the physician has decided that the complaint is pertinent, further questioning will define the seriousness of the headache. The following questions should be asked:

When did the headaches start?

When or how frequently do they occur?

Is there any warning of an attack (scotomas, paresthesias)?

What part of the head is involved?

Has the headache undergone any change recently?

Describe the pain (dull ache, throbbing, stabbing, bursting).

Does it occur at any particular time of day?

How long before it reaches maximum intensity?

Are there associated symptoms (nausea, vomiting, lacrimation, nasal obstruction, conjunctival injection, flushing, pallor, sweating)?

Does medication produce relief?

List all medications used in the past for treatment.

In a similar fashion, a series of questions should be asked regarding other positive symptoms reported during the neurologic history or neurologic review. One of the most frequent complaints is "dizziness." This is a nonspecific symptom used by patients to describe vertigo, ataxia, lightheadedness, and occasionally minor seizures. The patient with "dizziness" should be asked:

Do you feel that the room is spinning or that you are moving?

If the answer to this is "no," ask:

Are you unsteady when you walk?

Do you have a feeling of unsteadiness in your head?

When a history of syncope or seizures is obtained, the patient should be questioned about events that occur during the last several minutes preceding the loss of consciousness. This often reveals a focal component of a generalized seizure. The patient is then asked to relate all events following the episode until there was a feeling of well-being. This information is augmented by a detailed description from an observer of the events preceding the ictus, what occurred during the patient's loss of consciousness, and what was observed after the patient regained consciousness. The combination of information from two sources should give a complete picture of the event to the physician and facilitate precise diagnosis of the syncopal episode.

The neurologic review is followed by recording of the past history, family history, and social history, completing the narrative part of the examination.

The examination of the patient begins with a complete general medical examination of all organs and systems, including measurements of pulse, respiratory rate, rhythm, and depth. The blood pressure should be measured in both arms with the patient supine, immediately followed by measurement with the patient standing to detect any postural hypotension.

Neurologic disorders are often a complication of a systemic disease, or a systemic disorder may arise as a complication of a neurologic disease.

Examples of the neurologic disorders arising from systemic disease are:

1. Hemiplegia (paralysis of one side of the body) may arise from a septic cerebral embolus due to subacute bacterial endocarditis.
2. Paraplegia (paralysis of both legs) may be due to a spinal cord metastatic tumor arising from carcinoma of the lung.
3. Coma may occur in diabetes mellitus, uremia, or drug intoxication.

The commonest systemic disorders arising during the course of a neurologic disease are pulmonary and urinary tract infections. These infections should always be suspected in debilitated neurologic patients when unexplained fever occurs.

The Neurologic Examination

The neurologic examination also requires a systematic approach, and each neurologist should develop a personal method of examination. This seldom requires longer than 30 minutes in the average case.

The outline of examination presented in Table 1–2 is adequate for most neurologic disorders. The examination is modified, however, according to the special problems in each case. It is of the utmost importance in carrying out the examination to maintain an orderly approach. It has been found useful to memorize and examine the functions of the nervous system under the headings and in the order outlined in Table 1–2. If such a system is not followed, some vital sign, such as papilledema, may be overlooked.

The instruments used in the neurologic examination need not be numerous or complicated. Standard neurologic instruments include a sphygmomanometer; stethoscope; flashlight; ophthalmoscope; otoscope; material for examining the sense of smell such as tobacco, coffee, and perfume; a red glass for checking double vision; a reflex hammer; two corsage pins with white heads; cotton pledget sticks; a tuning fork (128 cps); and thin-walled containers for ice and for hot water, to test temperature sensation.

Many of these instruments have several applications. The white-headed pins are used for mapping out the visual fields and for testing pain sensation, localization of pin pricks, bilateral simultaneous stimulation, and two-point discrimination. The sphygmomanometer, in addition to its designed function in measuring blood pressure, may be used as a dynamometer to measure strength of muscle contraction. For example, the subject may be asked to repeatedly squeeze the rolled and inflated cuff held in one hand to a recorded pressure of 130 mm every second. In myasthenia gravis, progressive weakness rapidly occurs, and the recorded pressure gradually falls with each squeeze of the hand.

Mentation

The neurologic examination logically begins with assessment of the mental status or "mentation." This actually begins as soon as the patient is interviewed, but a detailed evaluation of the mental status should not be overlooked as it may reveal important signs of impairment of brain function. Examination of mental status may be divided into two parts: tests to determine general cerebral integrity and tests that indicate focal disorders of cerebral function.

Awareness

Orientation. The degree of alertness and awareness of the environment is indicated by the patient's orientation to time, place, and person. He is asked "Do you know what date it is?" "What is the name of this place?" and "Who is that man standing over there?" or "Who am I?"

Levels of Consciousness. When alertness is impaired, the patient's condition can be accurately described, using the following terms and definitions:

OBTUNDITY. The subject can be aroused by stimuli and will then respond to questions or commands. The subject remains aroused as long as the stimuli are applied. During arousal, the subject responds but may be confused.

STUPOR. Spontaneous movements occur, accompanied by groaning, in response to numerous stimuli such as pain, bright light, loud noise, and manipulation of a body part. Repeated stimulation may lead to brief intervals of responsiveness to questions.

SEMICOMA. Withdrawal of a body part in response to painful stimuli is the only response observed.

COMA. There is absence of any observed response to painful stimuli.

In general, disorders of consciousness are usually associated with diffuse cerebral injury. However, two rare conditions should be recognized. Both are due to discrete brainstem lesions. In

TABLE 1–2

The Neurologic Examination

Mentation

Awareness
Orientation (oriented to time, place, and person);
level of consciousness (obtunded, stuporous, semicomatose, comatose)

Speech
Normal, dysphasia, dysarthria, dysphonia

General knowledge
Knowledge of current events, vocabulary

Memory
Intact, recent memory impaired, remote memory impaired

Retention and recall
Recall of objects, digits forward and reversed

Reasoning
Judgment, insight, abstraction (interpretation of proverbs, similarities, and differences)

Use of symbols
Calculation, reading, writing

Object recognition
Normal, agnosia

Praxis
Ideational, ideomotor, motor, and constructional apraxias

Perception
Delusions, illusions, hallucinations

Mood
Normal, euphoric, depressed, anxious, agitated

Affect
Normal, flat, inappropriate

Gait, station
Hemiplegic, ataxic, spastic, festinating, hyperkinetic, waddling, apraxia of gait, hysterical gait, steppage gait,
Romberg test

Cranial nerves

Motor system
Atrophy, fasciculations, tremor, dystonia, involuntary movements, palpation, tone, strength

Coordination
Finger-to-nose, heel-to-shin tests, rapid alternating movements

Reflexes
Superficial reflexes, tendon reflexes

Sensation
Touch, pain, temperature, vibration and position sense, tactile localization, two-point discrimination, bilateral
simultaneous stimulation, stereognosis, barognosis, skin writing

Head and neck
Bruits over head and neck, scalp and skull tenderness and deformity, signs of head trauma, CSF drainage
from ears and nose

Spine, skin
Nuchal rigidity, hairline, shortness of neck, spinal deformity, spinal tenderness, limitation of movement of
spine, paravertebral spasm, limitation of straight leg raising, palpation for cervical ribs, pes cavus, peripheral
nerve enlargement, adenoma sebaceum, café-au-lait spots, trigeminal hemangioma

akinetic mutism the patient is comatose; however, in the "locked-in" syndrome the patient is nonresponsive due to complete paralysis.

1. *Akinetic Mutism (Coma Vigil).* This is a state of unconsciousness in which a quadriplegic patient may open the eyelids and show primitive reflex activity such as sucking, chewing, and swallowing. Akinetic mutism may occur in lesions of the mesencephalon that involve the cerebral peduncles and the reticular activating system.
2. *"Locked-in" Syndrome.* This is a state of consciousness in which the patient is totally quadriplegic due to a lesion involving the ventral pons. Afferent pathways in the pons and the reticular activating system are intact. The patient is aware of the environment and shows periods of wakefulness and sleep. Communication is possible through eye blinking.

Speech

Any disorder of speech must be accurately described if the subject is sufficiently alert to respond. If comprehension of spoken words, or the concept of words as symbols, or their motor execution is impaired owing to disordered brain function, the patient is termed "dysphasic."

Dysphasia

Dysphasia may be more briefly defined as a difficulty with comprehension or production of language due to disease of the central nervous system. When the cerebral lesion is so severe that the ability to speak is totally lost, the condition would then be correctly termed "aphasia."

There are two broad categories of dysphasia: *sensory (fluent) dysphasia,* where the difficulty lies in comprehension of language, and *motor (nonfluent) dysphasia,* where there is difficulty in the production of language. In practice the two frequently occur together, but one type usually predominates. The differentiation between these two broad categories of dysphasia is usually not difficult.

The patient with sensory dysphasia fails to comprehend simple questions or requests; he is often voluble and may converse inappropriately and talk in jargon. He may appear to be unaware of his disability since he can comprehend neither his own speech nor that of others. The patient with motor dysphasia understands simple questions or requests but finds difficulty in replying.

His vocabulary is reduced, and the speech is slow, broken, and hesitant. He may become exasperated with his efforts to communicate and shows relief when the examiner recognizes his difficulty.

In more than 90 per cent of the population the centers for speech are located in the left cerebral hemisphere; in the remainder, where the speech centers are in the right hemisphere, the individual is usually left-handed. Centers for speech are in the vicinity of the sylvian fissure (opercular area). Motor dysphasia correlates well with anteriorly located lesions (frontal lobe, Broca's area) and sensory dysphasia with posteriorly placed lesions (temporal, parietal lobes).

Dysarthria

Dysarthria is a defect in articulation of speech. Defects in articulation are due to a disorder of neuromuscular control of the muscles involved in articulation and may be classified as lingual, labial, pharyngeal, laryngeal, or cerebellar. The defect may be accentuated by asking the patient to repeat certain phrases, such as "West Register Street," "Fifty-first Artillery Brigade," and "Methodist Episcopal." When there are jerkiness and irregularity in volume and rhythm of speech as occur in cerebellar lesions, this may be brought out by asking the patient to repeat rhythmic sounds such as me-me-me or la-la-la. This type of speech is often called "scanning speech."

Dysphonia

Dysphonia is a condition of disturbed sound, rhythm, or tonal quality of speech. Paralysis of one or both vocal cords may produce hoarseness or reduce the level of speech to a whisper. Tonal quality is disturbed in paralysis agitans in which the speech is characteristically monotonous and the volume is reduced, often to a whisper.

Assuming that the patient is alert and that there is no evidence of dysphasia, the following tests of mentation should be carried out in full.

General Knowledge

More complex intellectual functions are tested by asking questions of general knowledge such as the name of the president of the United States, the governor of the state, or the mayor of the city and a description of a recent outstanding world event. This latter question will also serve as a test of recent memory and supplement any impression already gained of intellectual function during history taking.

Reduction of general mental capacity usually implies diffuse damage to the cerebral cortex. If the damage has been present since birth or early childhood, the term "amentia" (developmental retardation, etc.) is used. If the damage occurs after learning processes and speech are well established, the term "dementia" is used to define the reduction of general mental capacity.

Vocabulary

Vocabulary is the best indicator of a patient's overall premorbid intellectual capacity when compared with any other single test of mentation. Although it may be diminished in dysphasia, it is relatively refractory to the effects of many cerebral disorders. Testing the patient's vocabulary affords some assessment of his general knowledge prior to any dementia. The patient is asked to define the meaning of words that are presented at increasing levels of difficulty, e.g., winter, assemble, regulate, consume, reluctant, tangible, plagiarize.

Memory

Recent Memory

In organic disease of the temporal lobes, recent memory usually fails before memory for remote events. The degree of impairment may be gauged by specific inquiry about the events of the last two days, preceding the hospital admission.

Remote Memory

Remote memory is tested by asking questions about the patient's birthplace, parents, schooling, and any important event known to the examiner that may have occurred many years ago. More severe disease of both temporal lobes may be suspected when remote memory is disordered.

Retention and Recall

Recent memory is dependent on the patient's ability to retain information. If this faculty is impaired or lost, no "new" memories will be formed. This process may be tested by having the patient repeat a number of digits beginning with three digits and increasing until a limit is reached. The test is then repeated with the patient reversing the digits, again beginning with three digits. The patient of average intelligence can repeat six digits forward and five digits reversed.

Another test of retention consists of asking the patient to remember the names of three objects, two similar and the third dissimilar (apple, orange, umbrella). The examination continues, and three minutes later the patient is asked to repeat the three objects. Failure to do so should lead to repetition of the test with another three objects. In this case, the request to repeat them should be made at two and a half minutes. With reduction of the time span by 30 seconds after every failure, a limit of retention can be defined in seconds. In Korsakoff's psychosis, retention span may be less than 30 seconds.

A measure of language recall can be obtained if the examiner reads a small paragraph of concrete narrative to the patient. The patient is then asked to recall the specifics of the material. Assessment of retention and recall is dependent upon the patient's ability to attend to the task. A patient with intact retention and recall should be able to recall the major part of the material read to him.

Reasoning

In general, disorders of judgment, insight, and abstraction correlate well with disordered function of the frontal lobes.

Judgment

This may be defined as the ability to form an assessment of a situation and is commonly tested by asking the patient his interpretation of a simple test story involving judgment.

"What would you do if you were walking along a street and saw a sealed envelope lying on the sidewalk which had an address and an unused stamp on it?" A typical reply showing impaired judgment would be "Throw it away."

"What would you do if you were sitting in a crowded theater and you were the first person to notice a fire?" A reply of "Run for the exits yelling, 'Fire, Fire!' " would be considered to show poor judgment.

Insight

The ability to understand the reason for a given situation may be tested by asking the patient why he is in the hospital or why he is undergoing medical examination. If the answer is "I don't know; there is nothing wrong with me," insight may be considered suspect.

Abstraction

This requires understanding and judgment of a fairly high intellectual order and should be used only when the patient has had a grade 7 education or higher. Three proverbs are given: "A rolling stone gathers no moss." "People in glass houses should not throw stones." "The grass is always greener on the other side of the fence." The patient is asked what the proverb means and will usually supply an answer illustrating normal ability for abstract thinking, or his answer will be concrete, or he will fail to answer. An answer to the first proverb such as "Rolling stones don't pick up moss" may be considered concrete. Proverb interpretation can then be scored as so many points out of three, a score of 1 being awarded for each abstraction of a proverb. Concrete interpretation and failure to answer are given negative scores.

An additional test of abstraction may be given by asking the patient to assess similarities and differences between objects. A question such as "How are an apple and an orange the same and how are they different?" or, similarly, "How is a table like a chair and how are they different?" is presented.

Use of Symbols

Calculation

The recognition and use of mathematical symbols are associated with normal functioning of the angular gyrus of the parietal lobe in the dominant hemisphere. Tests of calculation are usually given by asking the patient to subtract 7 from 100, subtract 7 from the result, and keep on subtracting 7 (subtracting serial 7s). If the patient is unable to subtract, simple addition is next tested, e.g., "What is 5 plus 4?" Sometimes a more familiar situation will lead to success if subtraction is impaired. "If you had a dollar and you gave me seven cents how much would you have left?"

Reading

The recognition of symbols used in reading is a function of the parietal, temporal, and occipital zone of the dominant hemisphere near and in the angular gyrus. The patient should be given a simple sentence to read aloud; a newspaper headline is usually satisfactory. Three responses may be encountered: He may fail to read the headline; he may read the headline but fail to show any comprehension; or he may read and understand what he has read. The first two responses are examples of a reading defect (alexia, dyslexia).

Writing

Two types of writing defects are usually encountered: The patient may be unable to express himself by volitional writing; he cannot write spontaneously, is unable to write a reply to a question, and cannot write the name of an object. The ability to copy a printed or written word and to write to dictation is retained. This type of dysgraphia, which is frequently associated with a reading defect, is due to an inability to communicate in writing symbols and is often associated with a lesion in the region of the angular gyrus.

The second type of dysgraphia is a defect in writing or copying to dictation and is usually due to an apraxia of the hand and is associated with a lesion of the middle frontal convolution (Exner's writing center). This type of dysgraphia is frequently associated with motor dysphasia.

Object Recognition

The defect of recognition of simple objects is called agnosia. This may be defined as the inability to recognize simple objects in the presence of adequate primary sensory perception.

In theory there should be five categories of agnosia, but in practice three are of importance, i.e., visual, auditory, and tactile.

Visual Agnosia

Testing for visual agnosia is carried out by showing the patient simple objects and asking him to name them. The patient with motor aphasia may be asked to match an object with a similar one from a group of objects. Failure of object recognition is due to a lesion in the visual association area (that area adjacent to the calcarine occipital cortex.) More extensive lesions involving the visual association area give rise to a more severe defect in which the patient is unable to recognize simple objects or his surroundings. In addition, he cannot revisualize familiar places such as his home and cannot maintain orientation in a previously known environment (visuospatial agnosia).

A particular type of visual agnosia, *finger agnosia,* is also recognized. The patient shows an inability to identify his own fingers on request and, in severe cases, even when they are presented to him. For example, he may be asked "Show me your index finger and now your ring finger." This disability is due to a lesion of the angular gyrus and frequently forms a part of Gerstmann's syndrome, which may be defined as finger agnosia, right-left disorientation (allochiria), agraphia, and acalculia.

Tactile Agnosia

Tactile agnosia, commonly called astereognosis, is the inability to recognize a simple object by palpation in the absence of a primary sensory deficit. It is due to a lesion of the posterior parietal lobe and will be discussed below under tests for sensation.

Two forms of agnosia (autotopagnosia and anosognosia), which probably represent a combination of both visual-tactile deficits, are also recognized.

Autotopagnosia

Autotopagnosia is a loss of appreciation or identification of a body part in which the patient may fail to identify his own limb or even one side of the body. This usually occurs in lesions of the parietal lobe and generally can be demonstrated by the willingness of the patient to accept the examiner's hand or arm as his own.

Anosognosia

Anosognosia implies denial of disease and is due to loss of perception of the affected part, usually a paralyzed limb. The patient may deny that the affected limbs are paralyzed when there is an obvious hemiplegia. Such a defect is more commonly encountered in disease involving the frontal and parietal lobes of the nondominant hemisphere. While all these deficits are readily recognized in lesions of the nondominant hemisphere, they are probably present in dominant hemisphere lesions but are disguised by the presence of aphasia as well.

Auditory Agnosia

Auditory agnosia is the inability to perceive the meaning of sound despite the absence of deafness. This is normally considered to be a part of the picture of a sensory aphasia previously discussed.

Praxis

Apraxia is defined as the inability to execute a planned motor act in the absence of paralysis of the muscles normally used in the performance of the act.

Three stages may be considered in the development of a skilled act: the development of the idea of the movement, the formulation of the plan of its execution, and finally the motor performance of the plan. According to these three stages, three types of apraxia may be recognized.

Ideational Apraxia

Ideational apraxia is often due to a lesion in the supramarginal gyrus of the parietal lobe. The patient is unable to comprehend or formulate a plan of movement in response to a request. The condition resembles extreme absentmindedness. As an example, when requested to light a cigarette the patient may fail to take the cigarette out of the package or, having done so and put it in his mouth, may be unable to take a match out of a box or folder. Given a match, he may attempt to strike it on the cigarette pack or on the smooth surface of the matchbox. There is no impairment of motor movement; the idea of the movement is confused.

Ideomotor Apraxia

Ideomotor apraxia occurs when there is interference with the transmission of the appropriate impulses transcortically to the motor centers to convert the idea into coordinated motor action. This is commonly seen in diffuse cortical disease.

At a given request the patient has no difficulty in grasping the idea and in understanding the request. He is, however, unable to carry out the desired action. The patient may be unable to protrude the tongue on request yet may be observed to lick his lips spontaneously during the examination. Similarly, he will be unable to comb his hair, button his clothes, or tie his shoelaces on request, although the actions may be performed automatically.

Motor Apraxia

Motor apraxia is a failure to perform a series of finer skilled movements on request, in the absence of weakness or paralysis in the affected limbs. Planned movement involving the limbs as a whole is intact. The lesion is located in the premotor frontal cortex on the opposite side to the affected limb. There is a loss of dexterity in handling small objects and in performing rapid finger movements such as opposing one finger after another to the thumb of the same hand.

Constructional Apraxia

The ability to construct simple models or copy geometric designs depends on visual perception, revisualization, and the ability to transmit the concept into motor action. When these abilities are lost, the patient cannot copy simple models or designs, and the condition is called "constructional apraxia." The patient cannot revisualize his given task or, if he is asked to copy a model, cannot revisualize it once his gaze leaves the model. The defect lies in the visual association areas 18 and 19 of Brodmann and in the posterior parietal cortex and tends to be worse in lesions of the nondominant rather than the dominant hemisphere. Testing can be carried out by asking the patient to draw simple geometric figures such as a square, triangle, circle, or a composite figure incorporating these figures. He may be asked to copy simple designs drawn by the examiner, such as a house, a flower, or a watch, or to copy designs using Koh's blocks (blocks painted with various colors such that they may be manipulated into various designs).

Perception

Delusions, Illusions, and Hallucinations

Misconstrued perceptions and ideations are encountered in neurologic practice and should be assessed by the patient's responses during the examination. Direct questioning, particularly concerning delusions and hallucinations, requires tact if the examiner is not to arouse hostility and defensiveness on the part of the patient. Such questions as "Have you had any unusual experiences lately?" "Do you ever get the feeling that you have been in a place before or been through an experience before?" (the *déjà vu* phenomenon) may be asked. It is particularly important to inquire about unusual thoughts, dreamy states, and unusual experiences, sights, tastes, sounds, or smells in the patient suspected of having psychomotor seizures (seizures presumed to arise in the temporal lobes) since these phenomena may form an integral part or the only indication of the seizure pattern.

The following simple definitions of these terms should prove helpful:

Delusion: A false belief.
Illusion: False interpretation of a sensory perception.
Hallucination: A false sensory perception, which has no external stimulus, resulting from an ideational distortion.

Although a rigid concept of "centers" in the brain subserving highly compartmentalized functions is no longer feasible, certain areas of the brain have been found to be associated with certain functions. Impairment of these functions consequently provides information regarding localization of a disease process to certain parts of the brain. Patients with illusions and hallucinations due to organically demonstrable disease are usually found to have lesions located in the temporal, parietal, and occasionally occipital lobes.

Mood

At this stage the examiner has taken a full history from the patient and asked him a number of questions regarding the mental status examination. He should now be in a position to assess the patient's mood. Is he depressed? Elated? Fearful? Nervous? Irritable? Labile? He may also be questioned directly about mood, whether he feels happy or sad, worried, anxious, or irritable. Patients with neurologic disorders frequently show changes in mood that may be of help in the final diagnosis; e.g., depression is frequently present in early dementia.

Affect

Affect is the emotional response to a given situation. The patient's response to questions may be accompanied by inappropriate laughter suggesting euphoria, often seen in frontal lobe lesions. He may fail to show any change in emotional response throughout—a flat affect. This is commonly seen in disorders of the basal ganglia. There may be loss of emotional control resulting in pathologic laughing and crying. This is usually associated with pseudobulbar palsy, which indicates bilateral cerebral hemisphere or upper midbrain damage.

Gait and Station

It is usually convenient to examine the gait and station of the ambulatory patient before proceeding to a more complete examination of the nervous system. Gait, which is the act of walking, and station, which is the ability to stand, depend on the integration of a series of reflexes. On the sensory or afferent side, there is a continuous input of information from the peripheral nerves regarding the position of muscles, tendons, and joints, as well as from the tonic neck receptors, the labyrinths, and the visual centers. The afferent stimuli give rise to impulses that ultimately affect the anterior horn cells, modify tone, and initiate movement. These impulses arise from reflexes in the spinal cord, from labyrinthine centers in the medulla and pons, from areas of the midbrain mediating tonic neck reflexes, from visual reflexes, from complex relays involving the basal ganglia and cerebellum, and finally from the cerebral cortex.

In examination of the gait, the observer should watch the patient as he walks across the examining room. Associated movements of one upper limb are lost at an early stage in abnormalities involving the pyramidal or extrapyramidal systems. This loss of associated movements may be subtle, the patient being unaware of the loss.

Note should be made of the ability to turn since this often may reveal slight unsteadiness or ataxia. The patient is then asked to walk heel to toe along a straight line, the so-called "tandem gait," which will exaggerate ataxia. The examination is completed by having the patient walk across the room on his heels and return on his toes, followed by hopping on each foot. These last three tests, while valuable in the demonstration of ataxia, can be performed only in the presence of considerable strength in the lower limbs. Thus, a patient with weakness of the dorsiflexors of the feet cannot walk on his heels, and a patient with weakness of the calf muscles is unable to walk on his toes. Hopping may be impaired by weakness of any of the proximal muscles supporting the limb.

Certain abnormalities of gait are readily recognized.

The Hemiplegic Gait

The hemiplegic gait is the result of a lesion involving the corticospinal connections to one half of the body. This results in a spasticity of all muscle groups of the limbs on that side of the body, which is more marked in certain muscle groups. The result is a spastic extension of the lower limb with plantar flexion and inversion of the foot and a characteristic adduction and triple flexion of the ipsilateral upper limb (flexion of elbow, wrist, and hand). When the patient is walking, his foot tends to rake the ground, and he may tilt the pelvis to the opposite side and abduct the lower limb during forward motion of that limb. This results in a stiff-legged rotary motion of the limb when it is moved forward—a circumduction of the limb. Hemiplegics frequently make a rhythmic scraping sound as the toes rake the ground on the affected side. This sound and the absence of associated swinging movements of the

arm on that side may be pronounced even in the presence of mild hemiparesis. (The hemiplegic posture is really a hemidecorticate posture.)

The Spastic Gait

Spastic gait refers to the gait seen when there is bilateral involvement of the corticospinal tracts. The disability often affects the lower limbs to a much greater degree than the upper. The upper limbs may show loss of associated movements. The patient with spastic gait has difficulty in flexion movements on both sides and walks with a bilateral circumduction so that one lower limb tends to cross in front of the other. This characteristic walking pattern is sometimes called a "scissors" gait.

Festination of Gait

Parkinson's disease and certain other extrapyramidal diseases are associated with this type of gait. The patient is usually somewhat stooped with flexion of the spine, elbow, and metacarpophalangeal joints. He has difficulty in initiating movements (bradykinesis) and walks with short shuffling steps that quicken progressively as though he were attempting to chase his center of gravity (propulsion). More rarely, lateropulsion or retropulsion of gait may be seen. There is lack of associated arm movements as he walks, and the characteristic picture is completed by the lack of facial expression and infrequent blinking.

Involuntary Movements of Gait

Patients with disorders of the basal ganglia, e.g., Huntington's disease, Wilson's disease, ballism, or dystonia musculorum deformans, may show sudden flinging movements, distorted postures, or writhing motions of the limbs when walking or initiating walking movements.

The Ataxic Gait

The ataxic gait occurs under two conditions:

1. Ataxic gait may occur when there is lack of proprioceptive input to higher centers as occurs in peripheral neuropathies or diseases involving the posterior columns of the spinal cord. Under these circumstances the gait is unsteady; the patient walks with a wide base in an attempt to overcome unsteadiness; he lurches; and he slaps his feet on the ground (locomotor ataxia). When walking, he watches his feet and the ground closely since he can

compensate visually to a certain degree for the lack of proprioceptive information. Such patients are helpless in the dark or on closing their eyes and will fall.

2. Disorders of the cerebellum or cerebellar connections also produce incoordination and ataxic gait. The patient will walk with a wide base and lurch or stagger but does not use his eyes to compensate. In midline lesions involving the vermis of the cerebellum the patient is ataxic in all directions and the ataxia involves the trunk as well as the limbs (truncal ataxia). Hemispheric lesions of the cerebellum tend to produce ataxia and falling toward the side of the lesion.

The Steppage Gait

In the presence of a foot drop, the affected foot must be lifted higher than usual when walking to avoid catching the ground. The increased flexion at the knee and the hip produces the so-called steppage gait (as though stepping over an object).

The Waddling Gait

In patients with muscular dystrophy of the Duchenne or limb girdle type and in cases of polymyositis, weakness of the muscles of the pelvic girdle results in a waddling gait. A similar gait is also seen in children with bilateral congenital dislocation of the hip.

Apraxia of Gait

Apraxia of gait occurs in patients with degenerative diseases of the central nervous system such as presenile or senile dementia and cerebral arteriosclerosis. It may also occur in tumors or infarction of the frontal lobe. There is an apparent inability to walk. If the patient is helped out of bed and supported in a standing position, he is unable to initiate walking movements, despite absence of paralysis in the lower limbs. If an attempt is made to walk the patient (by moving forward and supporting his arms), the body angulates forward from the feet, which appear to be "glued" to the floor. Eventually the patient may begin walking by a series of short shuffling movements and may progress into steps resembling a normal gait. Each time the patient stops walking, he can only resume once again after the characteristic "shuffle." The latter has been termed the "slipping clutch" syndrome.

Limping

There are a number of causes of limping, with pain in the affected limb probably the most frequently encountered. However, shortening of a limb and ankylosis of joints or deformities may also produce abnormal gaits.

Hysterical Gait

The hysterical gait may take on many forms, but it is characterized by a number of consistent findings. It is always bizarre and often accompanied by certain movements of the body that could only be accomplished with intact coordination. Further neurologic examination will fail to disclose any neurologic basis for the apparent disability.

Station

The observation of the stance of the patient may reveal important abnormalities. The head may be flexed with the occiput toward the shoulder in ipsilateral disease of a cerebellar hemisphere or in early herniation of a cerebellar tonsil. Spasmodic torticollis or dystonic posturing of the head may also occur in disease of the midbrain and basal ganglia. Scoliosis is seen following poliomyelitis and syringomyelia and as an associated sign of the spinocerebellar degenerations. A pronounced lumbar lordosis may occur in muscular dystrophy or polymyositis. The patient with Parkinson's disease shows a typical stooped stance, flexed head, rounded shoulders, and flexion of the spine and at the hips, accompanied by a characteristically expressionless face, infrequent blinking, and a "pill rolling" tremor of the fingers.

Examination of station is concluded with the Romberg test. The patient stands with his feet together and eyes open, and any ataxia is noted. If he manages to maintain this stance, he is then instructed to close his eyes and maintain his position. If the patient sways so that he has to move his feet to maintain balance, the Romberg test is said to be positive. The examiner should stand close enough to the patient with his arms outstretched on either side of him to prevent sudden falls and possible injury in cases where the Romberg test is strongly positive. A positive result in this test is indicative of lack of proprioceptive impulses from the lower limbs and trunk owing to disease of the peripheral nerves or posterior columns of the spinal cord.

Cranial Nerve Examination

Examination of the cranial nerves 1 through 12 should be performed individually and in consecutive order. Detection of some abnormalities requires a certain amount of skill; consequently a routine approach should be developed that is applied to all patients. This ensures that all the cranial nerves are examined and that the examiner becomes familiar with the normal response.

First Cranial Nerve (Olfactory)

The olfactory nerve is tested by asking the patient to sniff test substances separately in each nostril. The best substances for testing are perfumes and aromatic substances such as coffee and tobacco. The volatile oils such as wintergreen, camphor, turpentine, and peppermint may be used, but irritants such as ammonia should be avoided since they stimulate the sensory endings of the fifth cranial nerve. Unilateral *anosmia* is more significant than bilateral loss of smell since the latter may be caused by sinusitis, colds, and heavy smoking.

Second Cranial Nerve (Optic)

Visual Acuity. Vision is tested at 20 ft using the Snellen test chart. Each eye is tested separately with a well-illuminated chart. The smallest type read correctly is noted, and the number printed at the side is recorded as the denominator of a fraction of the distant visual acuity. The numerator of this expression is the distance at which the type is read, i.e., 20 ft. The denominator is the maximum distance at which a subject with normal vision can clearly read the type. Thus normal distant visual acuity might be recorded as 20/20, and impaired distant acuity might be recorded as 20/40; i.e., the patient has impaired vision and sees at 20 feet what a normal individual would see at 40 feet.

A number of test cards are available for the testing of near vision; some of them use standard types of print used in books, newspapers, and magazines such as the Jaeger test type. The reading card published by the American Medical Association to be read at 14 in. from the eye is designed to give a fractional reading similar to the Snellen type and an index of near visual acuity. Visual acuity is the single most important function of the eye, and it is essential to obtain an accurate measurement of both distant and near visual acuity if preliminary testing indicates some

impairment. A documented impaired visual acuity may indicate:

1. A refractory error where the object being viewed is not projected through the cornea and lens sharply onto the fovea of the retina.
2. A structural lesion in the visual pathways—retina, optic disk, optic nerve.
3. Amblyopia.
   a. Squint.
   b. Refractory asymmetry between the eyes.
4. Conversion reaction (hysterical blindness).

A correlation between visual acuity and other findings on neuro-ophthalmologic examination may localize the lesion.

1. Good visual acuity is a function of the fovea, which is represented by the central five degrees of the visual field. Poor visual acuity without loss of this small central field suggests that a structural lesion is not present.
2. Documented 20/20 vision can be present with homonymous hemianopia associated with occipital lobe infarction when the entire central-five-degree field is preserved or when only a small segment of this same field is preserved as in homonymous hemianopia that "splits the macula."
3. An afferent pupil defect may be present and persist after recovery from an optic nerve injury when there is only a minimal deficit in visual acuity. This is tested by swinging a bright light from one eye to the other in a dimly lit room and noting a paradoxic pupillary dilatation when the light is presented to the affected eye.
4. Good visual acuity should be consistent with other visual functions.
   a. Color vision is a macular function, and red color desaturation is the earliest and most sensitive indication of loss of visual acuity.
   b. Stereopsis requires good binocular visual acuity. If stereopsis is present without good visual acuity in one or both eyes, the visual loss is likely to be nonorganic.
   c. Optokinetic nystagmus depends upon accurate pursuit of moving stripes on a rotating drum. Visual acuity is directly related to the thickness of the stripes, and the presence of optokinetic nystagmus may give some indication of visual acuity in an aphasic patient or in patients with visual loss due to a conversion reaction.

Optic Fundi and Disks: General Considerations. When the eye is examined with an ophthalmoscope, the patient is asked to fix his gaze on a distant object. The examination should begin with the light from the ophthalmoscope turned onto the cornea. This is usually accomplished with a 10+ lens, which allows examination for corneal opacities or abrasions. With the movement of lenses of decreasing power between the light source and the patient's eye, the aqueous humor, lens, and vitreous humor may be examined as the light is focused inward toward the retina. When a clear outline of the retinal vessels is obtained, both the retina and the optic disk can be examined in detail. The macula is examined by asking the patient to look directly at the light of the ophthalmoscope, and the peripheral retina can be seen by asking the patient to gaze into the quadrant that the examiner wishes to observe.

The Retina. Many neurologic diseases are accompanied by changes in the retina that fall into three categories (Table 1–3).

ABNORMALITIES OF BLOOD VESSELS. *Hypertensive Changes.* Hypertensive changes in the retinal vessels are usually graded as follows:

Grade 1: Alteration of the ratio in diameter of the arteries and veins. There is narrowing of the arteries from the normal A]V ratio of 3:4 to 2:4 or less.

Grade 2: Changes as described in grade 1 with the addition of constriction or nicking of the veins where they are crossed by the arteries.

Grade 3: Changes as described in grade 2 with the presence of exudates and/or hemorrhages in the retina.

Grade 4: Changes as described in grade 3 and the presence of papilledema.

Arteriolar Sclerosis. Although there is a close relationship between arteriosclerotic changes in the retinal vessels and hypertension, such changes may occur in normotensive individuals, particularly those with diabetes mellitus and the familial hyperlipidemias. Arteriolar sclerosis is a hyalinization of the retinal arteries and should not be confused with atheromatous changes seen in larger vessels. There are four categories of change:

Grade I: Minimal increase in light reflex and slight compression of veins.

Grade II: Moderate increase in light reflex and compression of veins.

Grade III: Marked increase in light reflex producing the "copper wire" effect.

Grade IV: Severe sclerosis with "silver wire" arteries.

Arterial Occlusion. Thrombosis or embolism with occlusion of the ophthalmic artery or the central retinal artery produces a pale retina with thin white threadlike vessels that may contain no blood or small segments of a trapped blood column producing a beaded or "box car" appearance. Branch occlusion of one of the retinal arteries may produce a segmental change of similar

TABLE 1–3

Retinal Abnormalities in Neurologic Diseases

1. Abnormalities of blood vessels
   a. Hypertensive changes
   b. Arteriolar sclerosis
   c. Arterial occlusion
   d. Arterial emboli
   e. Arterial insufficiency
   f. Arterial spasm
   g. Arteritis
   h. Venous occlusion
   i. Venous cuffing or perivenous exudation

2. Presence of exudates and hemorrhages in hypertension, toxemia of pregnancy, eclampsia, diabetes mellitus, raised intracranial pressure, subarachnoid hemorrhage, blood dyscrasias, venous obstruction

3. Abnormalities in the structure of the retina or underlying choroid
   a. Retinitis pigmentosa
   b. Cherry-red spot
   c. Chorioretinitis
   d. Angiomatous malformations

nature. The retinal pallor contrasts sharply with the redness of the macula, which receives its blood supply from the choroidal circulation producing a "cherry-red spot." Visual loss is severe, and only light perception may be retained.

Arterial Emboli. Occasionally emboli are seen in the retinal vessels following ulceration of or embolism from an atherosclerotic plaque in the neck. Cholesterol emboli are multiple highly refractile bodies that tend to move toward the periphery of the retina with the passage of time. Platelet emboli from a carotid plaque appear as white bodies in the arteriole that move slowly to the periphery. The flow of blood in the arteries proximal to the emboli is impaired, and as in central retinal artery occlusion, the column of blood is broken by segmentation of red cells producing a box car effect.*

Multiple emboli may also occur in subacute bacterial endocarditis with the production of Roth's spots—small white spots in the center of a small hemorrhage.

Arterial Insufficiency. Patients with occlusion or severe stenosis of the internal carotid artery in the neck may complain of transient monocular blindness or amaurosis affecting one eye. Ophthalmodynamometry usually shows decreased arterial pressure in the ophthalmic artery on the affected side.

Arterial Spasm. Spasm of the retinal arteries may be seen in a number of systemic diseases affecting the nervous system. The narrowing of the arteries in chronic hypertension, whether uniform or segmental, is probably due to structural changes in the vessel walls secondary to hypertension. However, spasm or narrowing may occur in acute hypertension owing to pheochromocytoma, toxemia of pregnancy, eclampsia, or acute porphyria and during malignant hypertension or hypertensive encephalopathy.

Spasm of the cerebral vessels is regularly observed arteriographically following subarachnoid hemorrhage due to rupture of a congenital saccular aneurysm. A sudden fall in intraluminal pressure owing to shock, low blood pressure, and occlusion of the internal carotid or central retinal arteries may be accompanied by collapse of the retinal arteries, which may superficially resemble spasm.

Venous Occlusion. Thrombosis of the central retinal vein may occur without apparent cause or in association with polycythemia vera. In contrast to the profound, sudden visual loss of central retinal artery occlusion, the visual loss is usually slow in onset and mild in central retinal vein occlusion. Ophthalmoscopic examination shows a profound degree of venous engorgement with numerous hemorrhages. The optic disk is swollen and the margins are indistinct.

PRESENCE OF OTHER EXUDATES OR HEMORRHAGES. The exudates and hemorrhages associated with severe hypertension are first seen in the region of the macula but may occur in any part of the retina in the later stages. In contrast to papilledema from increased intracranial pressure, the entire retina as well as the disk is edematous in severe hypertensive encephalopathy. Similar changes occur in toxemia of pregnancy and eclampsia.

Raised intracranial pressure produces venous engorgement due to impairment of venous return through the central retinal vein followed by hemorrhage and papilledema. Retinal hemorrhages are not uncommon after subarachnoid hemorrhage and may be large and plaquelike with a sharp margin. This is the subhyaloid hemorrhage, which some consider almost pathognomonic of ruptured aneurysm. Blood dyscrasias, leukemias, purpura, or a bleeding diathesis induced by anticoagulant therapy may also produce retinal hemorrhages.

ABNORMALITIES IN THE STRUCTURE OF THE RETINA OR UNDERLYING CHOROID. *Pigmentary Degeneration of the Retina.* Retinitis pigmentosa is the most common cause of pigmentary degeneration of the retina. In 90 per cent of cases it is inherited as an autosomal recessive trait, in 6 per cent as an autosomal dominant, and in 4 per cent as a sex-linked recessive trait. Those afflicted with retinitis pigmentosa show progressive constriction of the visual fields or a ring scotoma with progression to complete blindness. The retina shows degenerative changes, with striations of pigment described as crow's-feet, distributed in all areas. Pigmentary degeneration of the retina has also been described in the spinocerebellar degenerations, Refsum's

---

* Once this diagnosis is made the physician should:

1. Massage the globe to move the emboli to the periphery.
2. The patient should inspire carbon dioxide by rebreathing into a paper bag.

The immediate application of these two steps is essential to later preservation of vision.

syndrome, hypobetalipoproteinemia, juvenile cerebromacular degeneration, Hallervorden-Spatz disease, Laurence-Moon-Biedl syndrome, and Hurler's syndrome. Pigmentary degeneration is seen in certain rare pediatric syndromes including Usher's syndrome (pigmentary degeneration and deaf mutism), Hallgren's syndrome (pigmentary degeneration, congenital deafness, ataxia, and mental retardation), Cockayne's syndrome (pigmentary degeneration, dwarfism, deafness), and Kearn-Sayre syndrome (pigmentary degeneration, heart block, and progressive ophthalmoplegia).

Cherry-Red Spot. A characteristic "cherry-red spot" may be seen in the macula of children suffering from the infantile form of amaurotic familial idiocy (Tay-Sachs disease). These children are blind, severely retarded, and have an accumulation of gangliosides in their nerve cells including the ganglion cells of the retina. The presence of the ganglioside gives rise to the gray color in the retina, particularly in the area of the macula rich in ganglion cells. The fovea centralis, however, is devoid of ganglion cells, and the normal choroidal blush of the fovea appears in bright "cherry-red" contrast to the surrounding abnormal retina on ophthalmoscopic examination in Tay-Sachs disease.

Chorioretinitis. Inflammation of the retina and of the underlying choroid leads to destruction of the tissues and healing by gliosis and fibrosis. Areas of old chorioretinitis are usually creamy-white in appearance and streaked with residual pigment. Such changes may be seen in healed syphilitic chorioretinitis. Chorioretinitis is also found in mentally retarded children who suffered infection with toxoplasmosis or cytomegalic inclusion disease in utero. Occasionally, tubercles may be seen in the retina as discrete creamy-white areas in tuberculous meningitis or miliary tuberculosis.

Angiomatous Malformations. These may occur in any part of the retina and usually present as a reddish, round lobulated mass. A dilated artery and vein are attached to the mass, and the blood in the vein is redder than in the normal veins of the retina. There may be a surrounding exudate. When the angiomatous malformation occurs as an isolated abnormality, it is known as von Hippel's disease, which may be masked by a retinal detachment. When it occurs in association with hemangiomas of the cerebellum, a condition first described by Lindau, the combined defects receive the name von Hippel-Lindau disease. Cysts of the kidney, pancreas, and liver and carcinoma of the kidney and adrenal gland may also be associated with von Hippel-Lindau disease.

The Optic Disks. The healthy optic disk is yellowish-white in color with a whiter central depression known as the optic cup, from which the arteries enter and the veins leave the eye. In the majority of cases, venous pulsation may be seen where the veins enter the optic cup. When spontaneously present, venous pulsations indicate an intracranial pressure less than 200 mm water. However, when absent, the sign is of no value unless previously well-documented as observed. The production of venous pulsations by compression of the globe is of no neurologic significance.

PAPILLEDEMA. Papilledema is defined as edema of the optic disk. The edema may be noninflammatory or inflammatory, and the differential diagnosis of papilledema cannot be made by the appearance of the disk. When papilledema is known to be the result of inflammation of the optic nerve, the condition is termed "optic neuritis."

Causes. The causes of papilledema are:

1. Noninflammatory causes
   a. Central retinal artery occlusion
   b. Optic nerve tumors
      (1) Intrinsic tumors (glioma)
      (2) Sheath tumors (meningioma) usually associated with opticociliary shunt vessels.
   c. Obstruction of venous return
      (1) Thrombosis of central retinal vein
      (2) Obstruction in the orbit; this may be caused by orbital cellulitis, abscess, tumor, aneurysm of the ophthalmic artery, angioneurotic edema, or ophthalmoplegia in thyroid disease.
      (3) Obstruction in the cavernous sinus; this obstruction is most commonly caused by cavernous sinus thrombosis and traumatic internal carotid-cavernous fistula.
      (4) Mediastinal obstruction; this is seen in thrombosis of the superior vena cava, compression due to neoplasm, and aneurysm of the ascending aorta.
      (5) Intrathoracic obstruction; this occurs in emphysema and heart failure.

d. Increased intracranial pressure; this may be caused by hydrocephalus, oxycephaly, cerebral trauma, congenital arteriovenous malformation, meningitis, subarachnoid hemorrhage, cerebral abscess, cerebral tumor, brainstem tumor, intracranial sinus thrombosis, benign intracranial hypertension (pseudotumor cerebri), vascular hypertension (hypertensive encephalopathy), metallic poisoning (lead, arsenic), or carbon dioxide retention (pickwickian syndrome), and following steroid therapy, particularly in children.

e. Systemic diseases that can produce papilledema are:

(1) Severe hypertension and edema from optic and retinal arteriopathy; this occurs in acute glomerulonephritis, malignant hypertension, pheochromocytoma, and other causes of hypertension.

(2) Blood dyscrasias; papilledema may result from severe anemia, thrombocytopenic purpura, leukemia, or polycythemia, although this group is comparatively rare.

f. Elevated cerebrospinal fluid protein; papilledema has been reported in infectious polyradiculoneuropathy and spinal cord tumor with levels of protein in the spinal fluid in excess of 1,000 mg per cubic milliter.

2. Inflammatory causes (optic neuritis)

a. Multiple sclerosis and allied demyelinating diseases

b. Infections of the optic nerve; meningitis, tuberculosis, sarcoidosis, syphilis, brucellosis, cryptococcosis, infectious mononucleosis, and tularemia

c. Vascular disease and ischemic optic neuropathy; microembolism, sickle cell disease, diffuse intravascular coagulation, giant cell arteritis

d. Toxic metabolic causes; diabetes mellitus, uremia, gout, hyperemesis gravidarum, vitamin B_1 deficiency, vitamin B_{12} deficiency, and poisonings such as those due to methyl alcohol and arsenic

e. Parasitic infections; malaria, toxoplasmosis

Whatever the cause, papilledema occurs as a result of obstruction of lymph drainage in the perivascular space or due to swelling of the vessel-bearing portion of the optic nerve. The latter situation may be the result of local morbid conditions in the optic nerve, generalized brain swelling, or local or remote obstruction to venous outflow.

Clinical Features. The symptoms associated with papilledema will vary according to the cause (see Table 1–4). The classic symptoms of raised intracranial pressure, i.e., headache, nausea, vomiting, diplopia, and impairment of consciousness, are all late manifestations. The diagnosis may depend upon changes observed over a period of time, i.e., repeated examination. The early signs of papilledema include:

1. Hyperemia and increased capillarity of the disk

2. Venous dilatation and absence of venous pulsation

3. Blurring and elevation of the disk margins and absence of the physiologic cup and lamina cribrosa

4. Splinter hemorrhages at the disk margin

5. Elevation of the optic disk and enlargement of the blind spot

Further development of papilledema leads to

6. An umbilicated or "doughnut"-shaped protrusion of the disk

TABLE 1–4

Differential Diagnosis of Papilledema

Symptom	Noninflammatory Papilledema	Optic Neuritis
Visual acuity	Minimal or no visual loss	Sudden, abrupt, severe loss or blindness
Pain on eye movement	No	Yes
Unilateral or bilateral	Usually bilateral	Usually unilateral
Field defects	Enlarged blind spot and constriction of the peripheral field	Central, paracentral, or cecocentral scotoma

7. Distention and tortuosity of veins with obscuration of the arteries
8. Increased hemorrhagic changes including subhyaloid and blot hemorrhages
9. Appearance of folds and striations in the retina
10. Appearance of soft white exudates

The usual history reported by a patient suffering from inflammatory optic neuritis is the abrupt onset of diminished visual acuity or complete blindness in one eye. There is pain on eye movement, presumably due to inflammation of the meninges around the optic nerve that are stretched on eye movement, and occasionally this symptom may antedate the visual symptoms. Examination of visual fields will reveal a scotoma ("blind spot") or defect usually within the central or centrocecal visual field. However, almost any visual field defect may be found with inflammatory optic neuritis.

When the inflammatory change in the optic nerve is confined to the retrobulbar region, the inflammatory edema does not extend into the nerve head. This condition is referred to as retrobulbar neuritis. The symptoms are the same as those of optic neuritis except the optic nerve head appears normal.

Certain conditions may be mistaken for papilledema. The presence of hyaline bodies called drüsen, which appear as yellowish-white raised elevations on the nerve head, may obscure the cup and the disk margin and lead to an erroneous impression of papilledema. Similarly, a sheath of medullated nerve fibers spreading out from the disk onto the retina is another possible source of error.

OPTIC ATROPHY. Following the removal of the cause of papilledema or the resolution of the inflammation in optic neuritis or retrobulbar neuritis, the disk becomes gray or white in appearance, and optic atrophy develops. There are other causes of optic atrophy, all of which are due to degeneration of axons with demyelination of the optic nerve. The diagnosis of optic atrophy is aided by the use of a bright–red-free light (the green light on the ophthalmoscope). The peripapillary layers where there is loss of retinal nerve fibers secondary to optic atrophy appear as dark lines when compared to the glistening green of the preserved retina. There are two basic classifications of optic atrophy:

1. Primary optic atrophy: Optic atrophy occurring without prior evidence of edema or inflammation of the disk.
2. Secondary optic atrophy: Optic atrophy that follows papilledema or optic neuritis.

These arbitrary divisions are based on the ophthalmoscopic appearance and are somewhat ambiguous. For example, an optic neuritis is followed by "secondary optic atrophy," while retrobulbar neuritis, which is the same condition confined to the retrobulbar area, is followed by primary optic atrophy.

In primary optic atrophy the disk is gray or white in appearance, with sharp margins, a physiologic cup, and a distinct lamina cribrosa. In secondary optic atrophy, the disk is also gray or white, but the margins are indistinct, there is absence of the physiologic cup, and the lamina cribrosa cannot be seen.

Causes. Causes of optic atrophy are as follows:

1. Optic atrophy may follow papilledema.
2. Optic atrophy may follow optic neuritis or retrobulbar neuritis.
3. Consecutive optic atrophy follows disease of the retina with destruction of the ganglion cells such as follows pigmentary degeneration of the retina, cerebromacular degeneration, and severe chorioretinitis.
4. Occlusion of central retinal artery may cause optic atrophy.
5. Pressure on the optic nerve may cause optic atrophy.
   a. The pressure may be intraocular as in long-standing glaucoma.
   b. The pressure may be extraocular as results from pressure on the optic nerve from an aneurysm of the internal carotid or ophthalmic arteries, from pressure at the optic foramen due to osteitis deformans, osteoma, tumors of the optic nerve, compression of the optic sheath, and compression by tumors of the orbit. Pituitary tumors, sphenoid wing meningiomas, and olfactory groove meningiomas characteristically compress the optic nerves and chiasm.
6. Optic atrophy may be due to toxic and metabolic conditions such as diabetes mellitus, anemia, carcinoma elsewhere in the body, lead, arsenic, methyl alcohol, tobacco, thallium, qui-

nine, carbon disulfide, and aspidium (a fern extract used as an anthelmintic).

7. Optic atrophy may be secondary to trauma and usually follows skull fracture involving the orbit.

8. Optic atrophy may be hereditary, as in Leber's disease, the hereditary ataxias, and spinocerebellar degenerations.

Examination of the Visual Fields. F U N C - T I O N A L   N E U R O A N A T O M Y . Light from the temporal half of the visual field impinges on the nasal half of the retina, and light from the nasal half of the visual field impinges on the temporal half of the retina and all images are inverted.

The rods and cones of the retina are stimulated by light, giving rise to impulses that pass to the more superficial ganglion cells of the retina. The axons of the ganglion cells converge in centripetal fashion toward the optic nerve head at the optic disk and pass through the lamina cribrosa in the sclera to enter the retrobulbar portion of the optic nerve. The optic disk is situated on the nasal side of the macula or central fixation point of vision, and since it is devoid of rods and cones, this zone is responsible for the blind spot present in all normal visual fields.

The optic nerve leaves the orbit through the optic foramen and almost immediately joins the opposite optic nerve to form the optic chiasm.

There is a partial decussation of fibers in the optic chiasm, and the fibers from the temporal halves of the retinas enter the optic tract on the same side (Fig. 1–1). Nasal fibers inferiorly placed within the optic nerve decussate in the anterior chiasm looping just into the inferior nasal segment of the contralateral optic nerve as it joins the chiasm before continuing into the contralateral optic tract. Compression of the optic nerve in this junctional zone produces a severe ipsilateral visual loss and temporal field defect, while a wedge defect in the contralateral superior temporal field is known as a junctional scotoma. Superior nasal fibers loop into the ipsilateral optic tract before decussating in the posterior chiasm and entering the contralateral optic tract. The optic tract carries fibers from the nasal half of the contralateral retina and the temporal half of the ipsilateral retina to the lateral geniculate body located on the pulvinar of the dorsal thalamus. The fibers concerned with pupillary reflexes then pass through the lateral geniculate body and end in the pretectal nucleus of the midbrain. The majority of fibers in the optic tract terminate in a distinct pattern in relationship to the cells of the lateral geniculate body (Fig. 1–2). The axons of these cells leave the lateral geniculate body and pass as the optic radiation to both lips of the calcarine fissure on the medial aspect of the occipital lobe. The more lateral fibers, however, are

FIGURE 1–1. Distribution of nasal and temporal visual pathways.

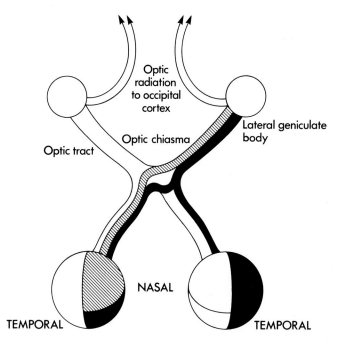

Optic radiation to occipital cortex

Optic chiasma

Lateral geniculate body

Optic tract

NASAL

TEMPORAL

TEMPORAL

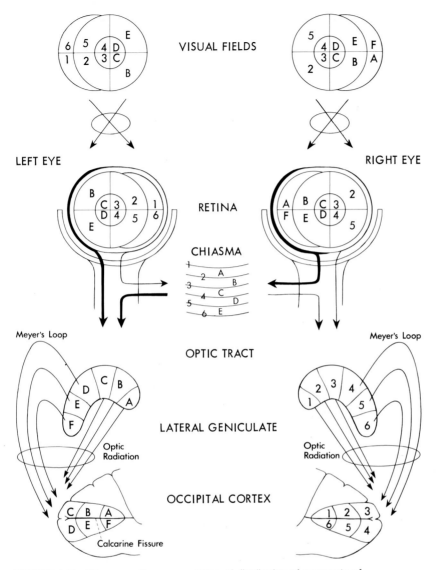

FIGURE 1–2. Diagrammatic representation of distribution of segments of visual fields.

carried forward into the temporal lobe for a variable distance (forming Meyer's loop) before passing posteriorly into the occipital lobe.

Lesions at certain points in the optic pathway may produce characteristic visual field defects. It should be noted, however, that lesions involving the optic chiasm and the optic tracts frequently produce incongruent field defects with more marked involvement of one monocular field. In contrast, the field defects seen in lesions involving the optic radiation of the occipital cortex are usually symmetric and congruent.

USEFUL CLINICAL APHORISMS. These include:

1. *Complete destruction of an optic nerve* will result in blindness in that eye and loss of pupillary reflexes.
2. *Complete division of the optic chiasm in the midline* will produce a bitemporal hemianopia.
3. *Pressure on the optic chiasm from below*, e.g., due to a pituitary tumor, will produce an upper bitemporal quadrantanopia.

4. *Pressure on the optic chiasm from above,* e.g., due to a suprasellar meningioma, will result in a lower bitemporal quadrantanopia.
5. *Pressure at the junction between optic nerve and optic tract,* which is a rare condition, will produce a nasal field defect on the same side.
6. *A destructive lesion involving the optic tract* produces a homonymous hemianopia.
7. *A lesion involving Meyer's loop in the temporal lobe* will result in an upper homonymous quadrantanopia.
8. *A lesion involving the medial part of the optic radiation in the parietal lobe* will produce a lower homonymous quadrantanopia.
9. *A total involvement of the optic radiation or the calcarine cortex* will produce a homonymous hemianopia.
10. *Destruction of both occipital lobes will produce cortical blindness* with preservation of the pupillary light reflex; bilateral destruction of areas 18 and 19 will produce anosognosia of blindness or denial of blindness (Anton's syndrome).

CLINICAL EXAMINATION OF VISUAL FIELDS BY CONFRONTATION. The routine employed at the bedside is examination by *confrontation.* The examiner and the patient face each other and the patient is instructed to place one hand over one eye. If he is unable to do this, he may close the eye or it may be covered by the hand of an assistant. The examiner then closes the opposite eye, instructing the patient to maintain gaze with the open eye into the examiner's eye. The process of confrontation is essentially a comparison between the examiner's field of vision and that of the patient. The examiner brings a small bright object, e.g., a white-headed corsage pin, in from the periphery on all sides of the visual field. The patient is instructed to report as soon as he sees the object while the examiner notes when he sees the object in his own peripheral visual field. Any discrepancy between the examiner's visual field and that of the patient should be noted and the site, upper or lower nasal or temporal quadrants, should be recorded. The examiner should also carry the test object across the visual field laterally, vertically, and diagonally, and the patient should report if at any point there is a disappearance of the object or if it appears blurred. The test object briefly disappears from view in the physiologic blind spot, at which point the object should also disappear from the

examiner's field. Disappearance at any other time implies the presence of a *scotoma.* A scotoma may be *central,* which is a defect in the central part of the visual field, or *paracentral,* an irregular defect near the central part of the visual field, or *cecocentral,* a defect involving both the central portion of the visual field and the blind spot.

The clinical demonstration of a visual field defect or a scotoma by confrontation should be confirmed by perimetry and by testing the patient with a tangent screen. Confrontation tests of the integrity of the visual field have some limitations, and the use of perimetry and the tangent screen is also advised where there are retinal or optic disk abnormalities. This will allow the detection of minor defects that are not always apparent at the bedside.

Nevertheless, confrontation tests of the visual fields will often reveal a scotoma and should not be overlooked as part of the routine examination.

Third, Fourth, and Sixth Cranial Nerves

Functional Neuroanatomy. The third nerve contains:

1. Motor fibers to the extraocular muscles of the eye
2. Motor (parasympathetic) fibers to the intrinsic muscles of the eye controlling accommodation and pupilloconstriction
3. Sensory fibers from proprioceptive receptors in the extraocular muscles

The motor fibers to the extraocular muscles of the eye supply the levator of the eyelid, superior medial and inferior rectus, and the inferior oblique muscles. The fibers arise from motor neurons in the somatic portion of the third nerve nucleus, which lies in the midbrain ventral to the aqueduct of Sylvius, and close to the medial longitudinal fasciculus, which lies on its ventrolateral aspect. There is topographic localization of the neurons supplying extraocular muscles in the nucleus, which extends from the superior aspect of the midbrain down to the level of the fourth-nerve nucleus.

The motor fibers emerge from the nucleus and sweep through the tegmentum of the midbrain and the medial aspect of the basic peduncle to emerge in a series of rootlets in the sulcus oculomotorius on the medial aspect of the cerebral peduncle. The rootlets converge to form the oculomotor nerve, which lies between the superior cerebellar artery and the posterior cerebral artery

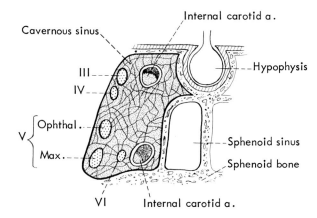

and then passes forward over the free edge of the tentorium lateral to the posterior clinoid process to pierce the dura mater and enter the lateral wall of the cavernous sinus.

The nerve continues forward in the lateral wall of the cavernous sinus (Fig. 1–3) to enter the orbit through the superior orbital fissure where it divides into superior and inferior divisions, which supply the extraocular muscles already discussed.

The motor parasympathetic fibers of the oculomotor nerve arise from neurons in the most superior portion of the oculomotor nucleus (Edinger-Westphal nucleus) and follow the same course as the other motor fibers to the orbit. The parasympathetic fibers are contained in the inferior branch of the oculomotor nerve within the orbit and enter the ciliary ganglion, which is attached to the nerve supplying the inferior oblique muscle. The preganglionic fibers synapse with cells within the ganglion, and the postganglion fibers pass as a series of short ciliary nerves to the intrinsic muscles of the eye (ciliary and sphincter pupillae muscles).

The fourth (trochlear) nerve supplies the superior oblique muscle of the eye. The fibers arise in the nucleus, which lies ventral to the cerebral aqueduct at the level of the inferior colliculus. They emerge from the dorsal aspect of the nucleus and pass dorsally to decussate in the anterior medullary velum immediately below the inferior colliculus. The nerves then run ventrally around the cerebral peduncle to pierce the dura dorsal to the posterior clinoid process and pass along the lateral wall of the cavernous sinus. The nerves enter the superior orbital fissure and innervate the superior oblique muscle proximally at its origin in the orbit.

The sixth (abducens) nerve supplies the lateral rectus muscle. It arises from motor neurons of the abducens nucleus lying in the upper pons immediately ventral to the floor of the fourth ventricle. The fibers pass ventrally and caudally to emerge near the midline in the sulcus between the pons and medulla. The nerves then pass up the ventral surface of the pons to enter the cavernous sinus immediately below the posterior clinoid process. After passing within the cavernous sinus in close approximation to the intracavernous segment of the carotid artery, the abducens nerve enters the orbit through the superior orbital fissure and ends in the lateral rectus muscle.

ACTIONS OF THE MOTOR (SOMATIC) COMPONENTS. The actions of the extraocular muscles supplied by these nerves are illustrated diagrammatically in Figure 1–4. (See also Table 1–5.) The superior and inferior oblique muscles are inserted behind the equator of the globe; consequently the superior oblique acts as a depressor while the inferior oblique acts as an elevator of the eye during adduction. During abduction of the eye the superior oblique acts to internally rotate while the inferior oblique externally rotates the globe. Elevation of the eyelid is controlled by two muscles, the levator of the eyelid supplied

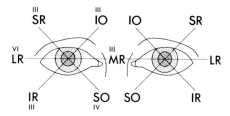

FIGURE 1–4. Action and innervation of individual ocular muscles.

TABLE 1–5

Actions of Extraocular Muscles

Cranial Nerve	Extraocular Muscle	Action on Globe	Horizontal Position of Globe
III	Medial rectus	Adducts only	
III	Superior rectus	Elevates Intorts	Abduction Adduction
III	Inferior rectus	Depresses Extorts	Abduction Adduction
III	Inferior oblique	Elevates Extorts	Adduction Abduction
IV	Superior oblique	Depresses Intorts	Abduction Abduction
VI	Lateral rectus	Abducts only	

by the third nerve and Müller's muscle supplied by the sympathetic. The levator palpebrae has the same common tendon sheath as the superior rectus muscle. Consequently, a lesion of the superior division of the oculomotor nerve involving the superior rectus is nearly always associated with ptosis. Closure of the eye is a function of the orbicularis oculi supplied by a branch of the seventh (facial) nerve.

Since the actions of the muscles supplied by these nerves are closely integrated, clinical examination is directed toward evaluating the function of the three nerves together rather than testing each one separately.

The Pupillary Light and Pupillary Near-Vision Reflexes

The pupillary light reflex is initiated by light stimulation of rods and cones in the retina, which in turn stimulate the bipolar cells of the retina. The bipolar cell axons converge on the multiple dendrites of a single ganglion cell, and as many as 130 rods and/or cones (there tends to be more of a one-to-one relationship between cones and ganglion cells) may channel their activity into one ganglion cell. The ganglion cell axons form the fibers of the optic nerve that enter the optic tract on both sides, since some fibers pass to the opposite side through the optic chiasm. Fibers subserving the light reflex pass in uninterrupted fashion from the optic tract via the superior brachium to the pretectal area of the midbrain. The fibers from the optic tract synapse in the pretectal area of the midbrain. Axons of the central neurons in the pretectal area pass directly to or cross

through the posterior commissure to the Edinger-Westphal nucleus of the oculomotor complex on both sides. The axons of the motor neurons in the Edinger-Westphal nucleus are carried in the oculomotor nerve to the ciliary ganglion. Postganglionic fibers from the ciliary ganglion innervate the iris and ciliary muscles (Fig. 1–5).

The reflex pathway for near vision follows the visual pathway to the occipital cortex. Stimulation of occipital cortical neurons initiates a series of impulses that pass through the corticotectal tract to the pretectal area of the midbrain. The axons from the occipital cortex synapse with neurons in the pretectal area, and the axons from the pretectal neurons pass to the Edinger-Westphal nucleus on both sides. Fibers subserving the near vision pupillary reflex run in a more ventral position than the fibers serving the light reflex in passing from the pretectal area to the Edinger-Westphal nucleus. The remainder of the reflex arc for near vision follows the same anatomic pathway as the pathway serving the light reflex.

Examination of the Pupil

The pupils should be equal in size, round, and centrally placed at rest. A condition of unequal pupils is referred to as anisocoria. Occasionally one pupil may be somewhat larger than the other, but this is not invariably abnormal when discovered as an isolated finding.

The pupillary reaction to light is determined by flashing a bright light into each eye separately. The response in the eye tested (direct response) is noted as well as the response in the opposite pupil (consensual response). Under normal condi-

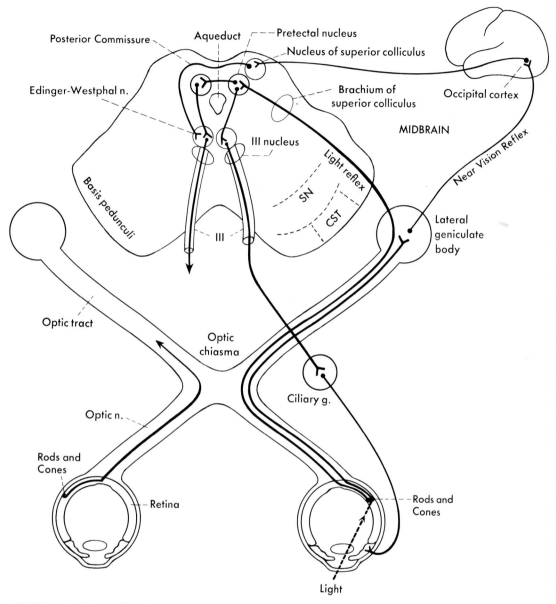

FIGURE 1–5. The pupillary light and near-vision reflexes.

tions, the pupil reacts briskly both directly and consensually to a light stimulus. Occasionally the pupil contracts briskly then shows a rhythmic relaxation and contraction called hippus. This is found in some normal individuals but is regularly found in severe barbiturate poisoning.

The pupillary reaction to light or pupilloconstrictor reflex to a bright light may be absent in the following conditions:

1. In local disease of the eye, e.g., iridocyclitis with adhesions preventing pupillary change.
2. In diseases of the eye that prevent the light stimulus from reaching the retina, e.g., corneal opacities, cataract.
3. In degenerative diseases involving the retina.
4. After destruction of the optic nerve, optic chiasm, or optic tracts.
5. After destruction of the afferent fibers to or

the efferent fibers from the pretectal nucleus.

6. After destruction of the third-nerve nucleus or the fibers in the third nerve.
7. After destruction of the ciliary ganglion or the efferent fibers to the sphincter pupillae.

The Argyll Robertson Pupil

The frequently accepted concept of the pupillary abnormality described by Argyll Robertson as a miotic pupil that fails completely to react to light but reacts "better than normal" to near vision needs to be modified. The Argyll Robertson syndrome may include:

1. Absence of response to light is noted with preservation of pupillary contraction to near vision.
2. In early cases the response to light may still be present but the response is reduced. The pupillary response to near vision is always much better than the response to light in such cases.
3. Miosis may not be marked, but the pupil tends to be smaller than normal, especially in long-standing cases. The miosis is more noticeable in dim than in bright light, because the Argyll Robertson pupil fails to dilate in darkness.
4. The condition is usually bilateral, about 10 per cent unilateral.
5. The pupils are often but not always irregular and they may be unequal (anisocoria).

Although the Argyll Robertson syndrome is usually associated with syphilis of the central nervous system (tabes dorsalis, general paresis, meningovascular syphilis), the syndrome has been seen in other conditions. It is not uncommon in advanced cases of cerebrovascular disease associated with diabetes mellitus, but the syndrome is rare in multiple sclerosis. Similarly, the Argyll Robertson syndrome may be seen as an unusual phenomenon in or following viral encephalitis, Wernicke's encephalopathy, tumors and cysts of the rostral midbrain, and as a late finding in chronic degenerative diseases of the nervous system, including peroneal muscular atrophy and chronic hypertrophic interstitial neuropathy.

Since the pupillary reaction to near vision is preserved in the Argyll Robertson syndrome, the lesion responsible for this phenomenon can only be located at a point where the pathways for the light and near-vision reflexes do not coincide. There is now conclusive pathologic evidence that the lesion in the Argyll Robertson syndrome is located immediately rostral to the Edinger-Westphal nucleus of the oculomotor nuclear complex. This lesion interrupts both crossed and uncrossed fibers proceeding from the pretectal area to the Edinger-Westphal nucleus and abolishes the light reflex. The fibers subserving the near-vision reflex are located in a more ventral position and are spared.

The Spastic Miotic Pupil (Complete or Incomplete Pupillary Rigidity)

Miotic pupils with poor or absent contractions to light and to near vision are at least as common as Argyll Robertson pupils. They develop when the lesion extends further ventrally on one or both sides. The pathologic significance of spastic miotic pupils is the same as that of Argyll Robertson pupils. In fact, patients with an Argyll Robertson pupil in one eye and a spastic miotic pupil in the other are not rare, and Argyll Robertson pupils have been observed to develop further to small, fixed pupils.

The Tonic Pupil

The tonic pupil (sometimes called Adie's syndrome) should not be confused with the Argyll Robertson pupil. The tonic pupil is large. It fails to contract or shows minimal response to light, but it does contract to near vision. This response is usually delayed, and the pupil remains small for some time at the end of near-vision effort, but returns to normal size with a slow, even movement. There is an abnormally sensitive response to the conjunctival instillation of a 2.5 per cent solution of mecholyl chloride. The tonic pupil constricts, whereas the normal pupil remains unaffected.

The tonic pupil occurs in both sexes, at all ages, and is usually unilateral. The ocular signs may be accompanied by diminished, absent, or asymmetric tendon reflexes, particularly in the lower limbs. The condition is benign and shows little change once the syndrome has been established.

The tonic pupil is believed to be the result of injury, from mechanical, infectious, or toxic causes, to some of the cells of the ciliary ganglion or pre- or postganglionic fibers. Surviving ganglion cells then reinnervate the muscle cells of the ciliary muscle and iris sphincter in such a way that the majority of regenerated fibers serve the function of accommodation.

Wernicke's Hemianopic Pupil

Wernicke's hemianopic pupil reaction is a failure of pupillary constriction when a beam of light is directed onto one half of the retina in a patient with hemianopia. This would imply that the hemianopia was due to a lesion in the optic pathway interfering with the light reflex, i.e., anterior to the lateral geniculate body. The test is of theoretic rather than practical importance since it is almost impossible at the bedside to direct a beam of light exclusively onto one half of the retina because of diffusion of light by the optic media or movement of the eye.

Examination of Eye Movements. Disorders of ocular movement are tested by instructing the patient to look upward, downward, and to each side by commands. This is repeated, having the patient's eyes follow the examiner's finger passively in eight directions. The directions tested are for lateral and medial gaze in a horizontal plane, upward and downward in a vertical plane, and at 45 degrees between the horizontal and vertical planes.

In general, three types of eye movement disorder may be recognized: disturbance of conjugate eye movements, nystagmus, and paralysis of individual extraocular muscles.

DISTURBANCE OF CONJUGATE EYE MOVEMENT. Conjugate movements of the eyes may be voluntary or purely reflex in character. Disturbance of voluntary conjugate movement occurs when the patient cannot direct his gaze toward an object on command. The patient must be conscious and cooperative to demonstrate disorders of voluntary movement of the eyes.

Disturbances of reflex conjugate eye movements may be demonstrated as an inability to follow a moving object presented to a conscious patient who understands the request, or as an impairment or absence of reflex conjugate eye movement on rotation, flexion, and extension of the head in the stuporous or comatose patient (absence of "doll's eye movements").

It is currently believed that conjugate gaze is initiated from the paramedian pontine reticular formation (PPRF) at a level between the trochlear and abducens nuclei that acts as the confluence point for visual-oculomotor (occipital-frontal), vestibular, and cerebellar pathways. Although areas outside of the pons may influence the type of eye movement performed, their coordinated

mechanism of action remains unknown. The frontal eye fields are now known to fire after the eye movement is initiated, and although influencing the saccade, are no longer thought responsible for initiating voluntary eye movements. From the PPRF, fibers are distributed to the ipsilateral abducens nucleus containing two cell types identical in appearance: (1) cells whose axons terminate in the lateral rectus muscle, and (2) interneurons whose axons leave the abducens nucleus, cross the midline, and ascend in the contralateral medial longitudinal fasciculus (MLF) to the oculomotor nucleus (Fig. 1–6).

Conjugate Deviation of the Eyes at Rest. Abnormalities of conjugate gaze with conjugate deviation of the eyes at rest result from destructive or irritative lesions involving supranuclear pathways.

1. A *destructive* lesion involving one hemisphere produces an imbalance due to uninhibited supranuclear activity arising from the intact contralateral hemisphere. This produces a conjugate deviation of the eyes toward the side of the destructive lesion.
2. An *irritative* lesion involving one hemisphere produces an imbalance with tonic activity arising in the affected hemisphere. This produces a conjugate deviation of the eyes away from the side of the irritative lesion.
3. A *destructive* lesion involving supranuclear fibers below the decussation in the brainstem produces conjugate ocular deviation of the eyes away from the side of the lesion.

Dysconjugate Position of the Eyes at Rest. Lesions involving the oculomotor nuclei or internuclear and infranuclear pathways may result in a dysconjugate position of the eyes at rest.

1. A lesion of one oculomotor nucleus or oculomotor nerve produces outward deviation of the eye on the affected side.
2. A lesion of one abducens nucleus or nerve produces inward deviation of the affected eye. In bilateral abducens involvement there is bilateral convergence of the eyes at rest.
3. Resting vertical dysconjugate gaze occurs with lesions involving the midbrain producing interruption of the tecto-oculomotor pathways on one side.
4. Skew deviation of the eyes with one eye elevated and the other eye depressed usually results from a pontine lesion affecting the medial

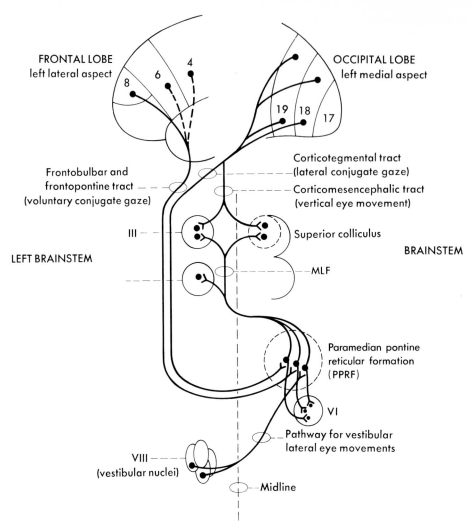

FIGURE 1–6. Diagrammatic representation of central control of conjugate eye movements.

longitudinal fasciculus on the side of the elevated eye.

Voluntary Conjugate Eye Movements. Paralysis of voluntary conjugate gaze may be seen, for example, in traumatic lesions such as contusions or lacerations, in vascular lesions such as hemorrhage or infarctions, or in tumors involving the frontal lobe. The patient is unable to direct his gaze toward the side opposite the lesion on command, but reflex deviation of the eyes may be preserved. In more diffuse disease of the frontal lobes such as general paresis or in the dementias, smooth pursuit conjugate eye movements are lost, and the patient shows coarse interrupted conju-

gate movements when asked to look at an object moving horizontally in either direction. This loss of smooth conjugate movements may be accompanied by ocular impersistence in which the patient is unable to sustain gaze on the object once movement ceases.

An irritative epileptogenic lesion within the frontal eye fields produces fixed deviation of the eyes toward the side opposite the lesion. This may occur from a localized traumatic scar causing seizures or other irritative conditions.

Destruction of the corticobulbar fibers in their descent from the frontal eye fields to the brainstem may also produce impaired voluntary eye movements or deviation of the eyes. Since the corticobulbar fibers decussate in the upper midbrain area, brainstem lesions will have the opposite effect to cortical or immediately subcortical lesions with deviation of the eyes away from the side of the destructive lesion.

Rarely, a lesion in the upper midbrain may involve the descending fibers from both frontal lobes. Under such circumstances, voluntary eye movements are grossly impaired and may be absent in all directions of gaze. The eyes are, however, parallel, and there is no strabismus or diplopia. Reflex eye movements elicited by head turning or vestibular stimulation (doll's eye response) are intact, as is the pupillary reaction to light.

Disorders of Eye Movement Arising from Pontine Lesions. Lesions of the pons commonly cause disorders of eye movement. Depending on their location, they may:

1. Affect the sixth nerve as it traverses the substance of the pons. This will result in an internal strabismus at rest owing to paralysis of the lateral rectus muscle and to diplopia at rest, which increases on any attempt to gaze toward the side of the lesion.
2. Destroy the sixth nerve nucleus. Lesions of the sixth-nerve nucleus produce conjugate gaze paralysis to the ipsilateral side. Bilateral lesions result in loss of horizontal gaze. There may be an associated seventh-nerve paralysis on the same side owing to the close association of the seventh-nerve fibers to the sixth-nerve nucleus in the pons.
3. Lesion of the medial longitudinal fasciculus in the pons. There may be complaints of double vision or oscillopsia, and there is paralysis of the opposite medial rectus muscle on attempted adduction. The abducting eye usually shows nystagmus, and there may be a slight degree of skew deviation. When convergence is preserved as in pontine lesions, the eye movement disorder is an anterior internuclear ophthalmoplegia (INO). Failure of convergence occurs if the lesion is higher in the midbrain and is occasionally described as a posterior INO. The laterality of the INO is defined clinically by the side on which the medial longitudinal fasciculus is affected or the side of the adduction weakness.

Disturbance of Reflex Conjugate Eye Movements. Reflex conjugate movements of the eyes may be considered to be of two general types:

1. Conjugate eye movements that occur when following a moving object in the visual field.
2. Conjugate eye movements that occur in response to vestibular stimuli.

Conjugate Eye Movements and Visual Stimuli. The ability to carry out reflex conjugate eye movements in following an object depends on visual perception. The afferent stimuli are visual and reach the occipital cortex via the optic nerve, tracts, and radiation. The primary center for visual impulses is area 17, which is that portion of the cortex forming the lips of the posterior calcarine fissure on the medial aspect of the occipital lobes. Fibers from area 17 pass anteriorly to area 18 of the visual cortex. The visual association areas have transcortical connections in point-to-point fashion. Stimulation of area 17 produces a predictable pattern of eye movements, which are similar to those resulting from stimulation of corresponding zones in area 18. The pattern of eye movement in area 19 is reversed so that fibers pass from the superior part of area 18 to the inferior part of area 19 and from the inferior part of area 18 to the superior part of area 19.

The projection pathways from areas 18 and 19 to the brainstem consist of two anatomically distinct tracts. Internal corticotectal fibers controlling upward gaze bypass the superior colliculi to the tectum of the midbrain, while fibers concerned with horizontal gaze bypass the superior colliculi in the corticotegmental tract and terminate in the PPRF. There are connections from the rostral tectum to the oculomotor nuclei by tecto-oculomotor fibers. The PPRF is connected directly with the ipsilateral abducens nucleus and to the third- and fourth-nerve nuclei via the medial longitudinal fasciculus, as described previously (p. 25).

Impairment of upward gaze may result from a lesion involving the pathway from areas 18 and 19 to the oculomotor nuclei at any level. The most common site is a lesion compressing the superior colliculus and pretectum due to a tumor of the pineal gland (Parinaud's syndrome) (Fig. 1–7). Vascular insufficiency, infarction, multiple sclerosis, Wernicke's encephalopathy, and encephalitic lesions of the midbrain may also produce paralysis of upward gaze. Impairment of reflex following movements of lateral gaze will occur in lesions involving the brainstem, which, of course, also impair voluntary lateral gaze.

Conjugate Eye Movements and Vestibular Stimuli. In the unconscious patient, reflex conjugate

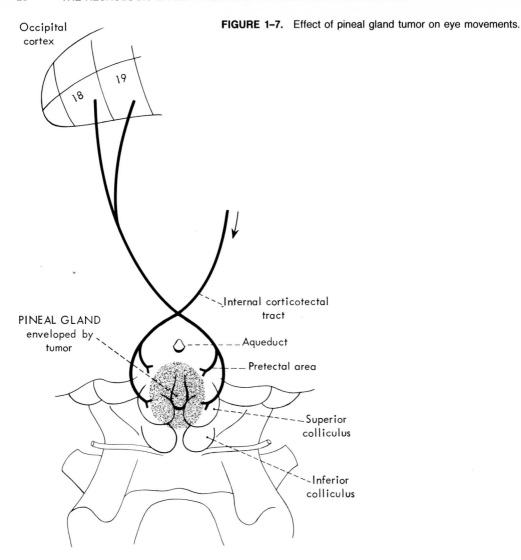

FIGURE 1-7. Effect of pineal gland tumor on eye movements.

Occipital cortex

18   19

Internal corticotectal tract

PINEAL GLAND enveloped by tumor

Aqueduct

Pretectal area

Superior colliculus

Inferior colliculus

eye movements may be tested by moving the head. This is a vestibular reflex mechanism and depends on the integrity of the vestibular apparatus and its brainstem connections with the mechanisms for conjugate eye movements already listed. When the head is turned from side to side, the eyes move laterally in conjugate fashion in the opposite direction to the head movement. Similarly, when the head is flexed and extended, the eyes appear to move in the upward and downward gaze. These movements, sometimes called "doll's eye movements," are lost in destruction of the vestibular apparatus or its central connections. In the unconscious patient, loss of doll's eye movements usually implies bilateral and extensive

involvement of these brainstem connections and is a grave prognostic sign.

NYSTAGMUS. Nystagmus may be defined as an involuntary rhythmic movement of the eyes that may be present at rest or induced by eye movement but persists for an interval after eye movement has ceased. It is usually bilateral but may occasionally be unilateral and may occur in any direction of gaze. Nystagmus may be

1. Pendular
2. Jerk, with a slow phase in one direction and an opposing quick phase. The direction is conventionally described as being in the direction of the quick component.

Congenital Nystagmus. This is a pendular type of nystagmus that is inherited as a sex-linked recessive characteristic or an autosomal dominant. It appears with birth, persists throughout life, and is occasionally accompanied by compensatory head movements. The nystagmus is rapid, bilateral, and usually horizontal, but vertical nystagmus has been described.

Spasmus Nutans. Spasmus nutans may be confused with congenital nystagmus since it appears in the infant usually between 4 and 12 months. There may be a history of confinement to a poorly illuminated dwelling, and the condition was said to be more common in children with rickets. There are three essential features: (1) pendular nystagmus, usually horizontal but occasionally vertical and monocular, (2) head nodding, which is rhythmic but apparently independent of the nystagmus, and (3) head tilting.

The condition usually disappears spontaneously around two years of age.

Ocular Nystagmus. This is also a rapid, pendular type of nystagmus that develops shortly after birth in persons with defective vision and may represent an attempt to project an image on the retina outside the macula. Ocular nystagmus is seen in patients with obstruction of macular vision such as central corneal opacities, congenital cataracts, or chorioretinitis affecting both maculae. Occupational nystagmus or "miners' " nystagmus is a variety of ocular nystagmus that develops later in life in those whose occupation keeps them in poor lighting conditions for many hours. It probably represents the projection of an image on areas of the retina other than the macula, containing a higher proportion of rods. The condition is frequently associated with head tremor and spasm of the levator palpebrae muscles.

Nystagmoid or Paretic Jerks. Transient jerking movements of the eyes may be seen in normal individuals at the extremes of lateral gaze, particularly during fatigue, and are of no importance. Similar jerking movements may, however, occur in paresis of an extraocular muscle in which case the condition is usually unilateral or in paresis of conjugate gaze when both eyes are affected. Under these circumstances, the jerking movement is sustained and may increase in amplitude. In some patients with myasthenia gravis, paretic jerks are seen briefly followed by progressive diplopia and ocular weakness in attempts at sustained vertical or lateral gaze.

Vestibular Nystagmus. Vestibular nystagmus occurs as a response to some factor that disturbs the synergistic action of the two vestibular organs or their central connections (Fig. 1–8). Labyrinthitis is a common cause. Consequently, nystagmus may occur due either to an abnormal stimulus arising in one labyrinth or to acute loss of function of a labyrinth. The nystagmus is always phasic. When the slow phase is induced by vestibular stimulation, it is always in the direction of the movement of the endolymph and has a rapid phase of recovery. Vestibular nystagmus is always associated with vertigo and is increased on turning the head or eyes in the direction of the quick phase.

Vestibular nystagmus may be induced by stimulation of the vestibular apparatus by rotating the patient using a Barany chair or employing a weak galvanic stimulation to one side. At the bedside or in the office, caloric testing is particularly useful. It is carried out by irrigating a few milliliters of cold water into the external auditory meatus with a syringe. The following responses may be seen on caloric stimulation:

1. Absence of response if there is total destruction of the vestibular apparatus or vestibular division of the eighth nerve
2. Tonic deviation of the eyes without nystagmus if there is a lesion affecting the supranuclear connections controlling eye movements
3. Increase of nystagmus in the presence of an irritative lesion of the vestibular apparatus or the vestibular nerve

Cerebellar Nystagmus. Cerebellar nystagmus probably represents dysfunction of cerebellar connections in the brainstem rather than involvement of the cerebellum in the majority of cases. There may, in fact, be widespread degeneration of the cerebellar hemisphere without the appearance of nystagmus. The condition may occur in any direction of gaze and appears as a phasic nystagmus with the rapid component in the direction of gaze and the slow phase toward the position of rest. The amplitude is increased and the movements are slower toward the side of the lesion.

Nystagmus and the Medial Longitudinal Fasciculus. A dissociated nystagmus confined to one eye may occur in the nonabducting eye with an internuclear ophthalmoplegia. The medial longitudinal fasciculus may also be involved at its lower extent by lesions of the upper part of the cervical cord. Hence nystagmus may occa-

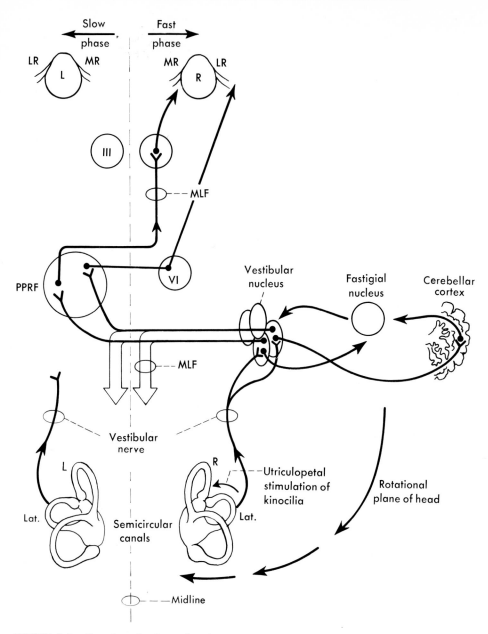

FIGURE 1–8.   Neural mechanisms of nystagmus.

sionally occur in syringobulbia and cervical cord tumors involving the cervicomedullary junction.

Drug-Induced Nystagmus. Nystagmus may be induced by a wide variety of drugs, often in therapeutic dosage, without manifestations of toxicity. This is frequently seen during the use of anticonvulsant medication, particularly phenyl-hydantoin (Dilantin), barbiturates such as sodium phenobarbital, and closely related drugs such as primidone. It may also be seen in alcoholic intoxication. The nystagmus is phasic with the quick component in the direction of the gaze and the slow phase toward the position of rest.

Seesaw nystagmus is the involuntary eye movement with opposite vertical displacement and identical torsional rotation in each eye. It is usually associated with parasellar lesions and bitemporal hemianopia or abnormalities of the vestibular mechanism.

Retraction nystagmus occurs in tectal and pretectal midbrain syndromes and is best seen by observing the patient from the side view. A sudden rapid jerking movement of both eyes back into the orbit occurs simultaneous with an adduction movement of both globes (convergence nystagmus). This can be demonstrated by an upward saccade from down gaze to the primary position or by slow downward rotation of the opticokinetic drum.

Vertical nystagmus is of useful localizing value when it is upbeat in the primary position, suggesting a lesion in the anterior vermis of the cerebellum. Small-amplitude, fine-upbeat nystagmus in the primary position may indicate a lesion of the medulla. Downbeat nystagmus exaggerated on downgaze suggests a foramen magnum or cervical medullary junction lesion.

Optokinetic nystagmus is the normal physiologic response elicited by gazing at objects that are rapidly moving across the visual field. It is the type of nystagmus induced by looking out of the window of a car or train at passing objects. There is a slow movement in the direction of the object, then a quick movement back to the position of rest. Optokinetic nystagmus may be induced by having the patient look at a rotating drum containing alternating vertical black and white stripes. The response should be symmetric on rotation to either side. Although asymmetric optokinetic nystagmus can occur in brainstem lesions, it is also depressed or absent on rotation of the drum toward the side of a parietal lobe lesion. The impaired optokinetic nystagmus indicates a lesion of the optic radiations but may be present or absent with homonymous hemianopsia.

Other Abnormal Involuntary Eye Movements. Ocular bobbing consists of brisk downward conjugate movements of both eyes followed by a slow return to the position of rest. These bobbing eye movements are seen in severe destructive lesions of the caudal pons and cerebellar hemorrhage.

Ocular flutter consists of rapid rhythmic eye movements, of decreasing amplitude, around a point of fixation following eye movement. This phenomenon of ocular flutter is usually seen in cerebellar disease and is similar to ocular dysmetria in which the eyes move past the point of fixation, then make one or more fixation saccades.

Nystagmoid jerking of one eye in a comatose patient is a rare phenomenon occurring in lateral, vertical, or rotational directions and is indicative of a severe pontine lesion.

Opsoclonus is a rare condition in which there are totally random clonic conjugate movements of the eyes in any direction. Opsoclonus is indicative of diffuse bilateral brainstem disease.

VERTIGO. Vertigo is a false sense of rotary movement of self or surrounding objects (oscillopsia). It is an unpleasant sensation associated with sympathetic overactivity producing nausea, vomiting, tachycardia, and diarrhea. Since equilibrium is impaired, ataxia, falling, and dysmetria (past pointing) will occur. Vertigo may be associated with excessive stimulation of the primary end organs concerned with the maintenance of equilibrium or with interference of their central connections.

A suitable classification is as follows:

1. Optic
   a. Due to incorrect corrective lenses
   b. Diplopia due to paralysis of extraocular muscles
   c. Due to looking down from heights with confusion of optic reference points
   d. During blind flying—conflict between information from instruments and vestibular and proprioceptive impulses
2. Vestibular—labyrinthine causes; see Vestibular Nystagmus
3. Central
   a. Cerebral hemisphere—epileptic discharge
   b. Brainstem—which may be caused by inflammation (viral encephalitis), infarction (lateral medullary syndrome), or demyelination (multiple sclerosis)
4. Toxic—due to effects of drugs; see Drug-Induced Nystagmus

PARALYSIS OF INDIVIDUAL EXTRAOCULAR MUSCLES. In testing eye movements to determine the presence of paralysis or paresis involving individual extraocular muscles, a number of simple rules should be considered:

1. There will be diplopia at rest unless there is complete external ophthalmoplegia involving the extraocular muscles in both eyes.
2. The diplopia may only be present or will be increased with attempted gaze in the direction of the pull of the paralyzed muscle.
3. A paralytic squint will be present when the

eyes are moved in the field of action of the paralyzed muscle.

4. If the paretic eye is directed to an object in the field of action of the paralyzed muscle, there will be a secondary deviation of the sound eye, owing to reciprocal innervation of the extraocular muscles. This is due to the fact that the impulse to the paretic muscle is stronger than would be necessary under normal conditions. The stronger impulse is, however, directed to the nonparalyzed muscles serving reciprocal movement in the other eye, producing a stronger contraction of the muscle involved. In paralytic squint, the secondary deviation is always greater than the primary deviation in contrast to a concomitant (nonparalytic) squint where the deviation remains the same in all directions of gaze.

5. In the attempt to fix an object in the field of a paralyzed muscle using the affected eye, the image is projected onto the retina outside of the macula. The incorrect projection of the image causes false projection of the image and past pointing by the patient.

6. If a hand is placed over the eye with a paretic muscle and then quickly removed, the eye will be found to have deviated in a direction opposite to the pull of the paretic muscle.

7. If a hand is placed over the sound eye and the paretic eye is made to fix on an object in the field of the paretic muscle, the sound eye will deviate excessively in the same direction (secondary deviation).

Paralysis of the Lateral Rectus, Supplied by the Sixth Nerve. This type of paralysis is characterized by the following:

1. There may be inward deviation of the paralyzed eye at rest.
2. There is limitation in abduction of the paralyzed eye.
3. Diplopia increases on attempted abduction and fixation on a distant target. The images are uncrossed with the false image lateral to the true image.
4. Covering the paralyzed eye produces an inward deviation of that eye. When the good eye is covered, there is a marked inward deviation (secondary deviation).
5. The face may be turned toward the affected side.

Paralysis of Muscles Supplied by the Third Nerve. In total paralysis:

1. There is outward deviation of the eye at rest.
2. The pupil is dilated and does not react to light directly or consensually.
3. Ptosis is present.
4. Abduction is the only movement present with some internal rotation if the superior oblique (fourth nerve) is intact.

Paralysis of the Superior Rectus Muscle. In paralysis of this muscle one finds:

1. There is limitation of elevation of the abducted eye.
2. Diplopia occurs on an attempted elevation with the false image above and medial to the true image.
3. The obliquity of the false image increases on adduction of the affected eye, while vertical diplopia increases on abduction.
4. There is a downward deviation of the paralyzed eye when covered and a marked upward deviation of the sound eye when covered.
5. There is an associated ptosis.

Paralysis of the Medial Rectus Muscle. This type of paralysis is characterized by the following:

1. There is an outward deviation of the affected eye at rest.
2. There is limitation of adduction of the paralyzed eye.
3. Diplopia increases on attempted adduction, with wide separation of the images (which are crossed), and the false image lies lateral to the true image.
4. There is an outward deviation of the paralyzed eye and a sharp outward deviation of the good eye when covered.

Paralysis of the Inferior Rectus Muscle. This condition is manifested by the following:

1. There is limitation in depression of the affected eye.
2. Diplopia occurs in attempted depression with the false image below and medial to the true image.
3. The obliquity of the false image increases on adduction of the affected eye, while vertical diplopia increases on abduction.
4. There is an upward and inward movement of the affected eye when covered and a marked downward and outward movement of the sound eye when covered.

Paralysis of the Inferior Oblique Muscle. In paralysis of this muscle one finds:

1. There is limitation in elevation of the affected eye when adducted.
2. Diplopia occurs on attempted elevation with the false image above and lateral to the true image.
3. On elevation and adduction of the affected eye, the separation of the images increases.
4. There is a downward and very slight outward deviation of the affected eye when covered.

Paralysis of the Superior Oblique Muscle, Supplied by the Fourth Nerve. In this paralysis one observes the following:

1. There is limitation of depression of the affected eye in adduction.
2. Diplopia occurs on attempted depression with the false image below and lateral to the true image.
3. The separation of the images increases on attempted adduction.
4. When covered, the paralyzed eye deviates upward, and covering the good eye produces a marked deviation downward and inward.
5. The head is tilted toward the sound side.

Fifth Cranial Nerve (Trigeminal)

The trigeminal (gasserian) ganglion is invaginated in dura (cavum trigeminale) and lies in a shallow depression on the anterosuperior aspect of the apex of the petrous temporal bone. The ganglion is separated from the foramen lacerum anteroinferiorly by the motor root of the trigeminal nerve. A thin plate of bone separates the ganglion and the internal carotid artery as the artery passes through the carotid canal.

The three divisions of the trigeminal nerve also have important anatomic relations. The ophthalmic division passes forward from the anteromedial aspect of the gasserian ganglion through the dura to enter the lateral wall of the cavernous sinus where it lies below the third and fourth cranial nerves. The ophthalmic division then divides into lacrimal, frontal, and nasociliary nerves, which enter the orbit through the superior orbital fissure. The frontal nerve passes forward deep to the levator palpebrae superioris and divides into supratrochlear and supraorbital nerves, which ascend over the superior edge of the orbit onto the forehead.

The maxillary division arises from the gasserian ganglion between the ophthalmic and mandibular divisions. After piercing the dura, the maxillary nerve travels along the inferior aspect of the lateral wall of the cavernous sinus, then leaves the skull through the foramen rotundum. The nerve then crosses the pterygopalatine fossa, enters the orbit through the inferior orbital fissure, and traverses the floor of the orbit in the infraorbital canal to emerge as the infraorbital nerve at the infraorbital foramen just below the orbit.

The mandibular division arises from the anterolateral aspect of the gasserian ganglion, pierces the dura, and leaves the skull through the foramen ovale where it unites with the motor root. The mandibular nerve has a number of important branches. These include the auriculotemporal nerve, which supplies sensation to the external auditory meatus, the tympanic membrane, and the face anterior and superior to the external auditory meatus; the lingual nerve, which supplies sensation to the anterior two thirds of the tongue; and the inferior dental nerve, which supplies sensation to the teeth, gums, mucosa of the lower jaw, lower lip, and chin.

The sensory root of the trigeminal nerve passes posterior and medial from the gasserian ganglion to enter the pons at the junction of the pons and middle cerebellar peduncle.

Fibers subserving tactile sensations pass to the chief sensory nucleus, which lies in the midportion of the pons. Fibers carrying pain and temperature sensation enter the descending tract or root of the trigeminal nerve and pass downward in the cord as low as the fourth cervical segment. This tract is laminated such that the mandibular fibers lie dorsal, maxillary fibers are in the middle, and the ophthalmic fibers are placed ventrally. There is further segmentation as the fibers pass downward through the pons and medulla so that the fibers carrying pain and temperature from around the mouth enter the spinal nucleus of the trigeminal nerve at medullary levels. Fibers carrying sensation further out on the face enter the nucleus at progressively lower levels down to the termination of the tract at the level of the fourth cervical segment. This concentric arrangement of pain and temperature fibers from the face as they are arranged in the brainstem and cord has been appropriately described as an "onionskin" distribution of sensation and is of value in localizing lesions in the upper cervical cord and brainstem.

Fibers carrying proprioceptive impulses enter the pons and ascend to the mesencephalic nucleus of the trigeminal nerve.

The trigeminal nerve also carries secretomotor (parasympathetic) fibers from

1. The sphenopalatine ganglion via the maxillary division of the trigeminal nerve to the mucous membrane of the nose, palate, tonsils, and uvula and to the lacrimal gland. These secretomotor fibers reach the sphenopalatine ganglion via the greater superficial petrossal nerve, which is a branch of the facial nerve.
2. The otic ganglion, which supplies secretomotor fibers to the parotid gland. These fibers originate in the glossopharyngeal nerve and pass by the tympanic plexus to the otic ganglion. The secondary relay then passes via the mandibular division of the trigeminal nerve and the auriculotemporal nerve to the parotid gland.
3. The submandibular ganglion, which supplies secretomotor fibers to the submandibular and sublingual glands. These fibers originate in the superior salivary nucleus of the seventh nerve but leave the seventh nerve in the chorda tympani to join the lingual division of the mandibular division of the fifth nerve to reach the submandibular ganglion. The lingual nerve also carries fibers of sensation and taste over the anterior two thirds of the tongue. These fibers, however, leave the lingual nerve via the chorda tympani and pass back to the pons via the seventh cranial nerve. Taste will be discussed as a function of the seventh cranial nerve.

Clinical Examination. The functions of the trigeminal nerve are recorded by testing the corneal reflex, sensation over the face, and the motor strength in the masseters, temporal and pterygoid muscles, and the jaw jerk.

THE CORNEAL REFLEX. The afferent portion of this reflex runs in the trigeminal nerve. The efferent portion producing the blink response runs in the facial nerve. The reflex is elicited by gently stroking the cornea with a wisp of cotton. The patient is asked to look up and the examiner approaches the eye from the lateral aspect. Under normal circumstances, application of the cotton produces an immediate blink response bilaterally. If there is impairment of sensation in the cornea, the direct and consensual blink response will be absent or diminished. In the presence of seventh-nerve paralysis, blinking will occur only on the nonparalyzed side when either cornea is stimulated. The corneal reflex is an extremely sensitive response, and its absence in an unconscious patient indicates a deep level of coma.

SENSATION OVER THE FACE. Touch and pinprick should be tested over both sides of the face. The patient is asked to close his eyes and to respond when touched with a wisp of cotton. He is then asked if he feels pinprick over both sides of the face and if there is any difference between the two sides. Bilateral simultaneous stimulation using touch and pinprick should then be carried out over both sides of the face.

MOTOR FUNCTION. The patient is asked to clench the jaws tightly, and the masseters and temporal muscles are palpated on both sides. As the patient clenches the teeth and exerts pressure, the muscles should contract bilaterally. The functions of the pterygoids can be tested by asking the patient to move the jaw laterally and to hold it there against pressure.

THE JAW JERK. Both the afferent and efferent portions of the jaw jerk reflex are located in the trigeminal nerve. The jaw jerk is a stretch response, and like any other reflex of this type, it is affected by upper motor neuron projections to the motor neurons of the motor nucleus of the trigeminal nerve in the pons. The jaw jerk will therefore be increased in laterally placed lesions of the motor cortex and lesions of the corticobulbar tracts as they descend to the level of the pons.

Seventh Cranial Nerve (Facial)

The seventh nerve supplies:

1. Motor (special visceral efferent) fibers to the muscles of facial expression and the posterior belly of the digastric muscle. The cells of origin of the muscles of facial expression are located in the motor nucleus of the facial nerve, which is found in the lower part of the pons just medial to the spinal tract and nucleus of the fifth nerve. Fibers emerge from the nucleus and pass dorsomedially immediately beneath the abducens nucleus and then swing around the abducens nucleus and, having almost circled it, pass between the seventh-nerve nucleus and the spinal tract of the fifth nerve to emerge between the pons and medulla. The nerve leaves the brainstem just medial to the eighth nerve in the cerebellopontine angle and enters the internal auditory canal accompanied by the eighth nerve and the internal auditory artery and passes to the geniculate ganglion (Fig. 1–9). At the level of the geniculate ganglion the greater superficial petrosal nerve leaves the

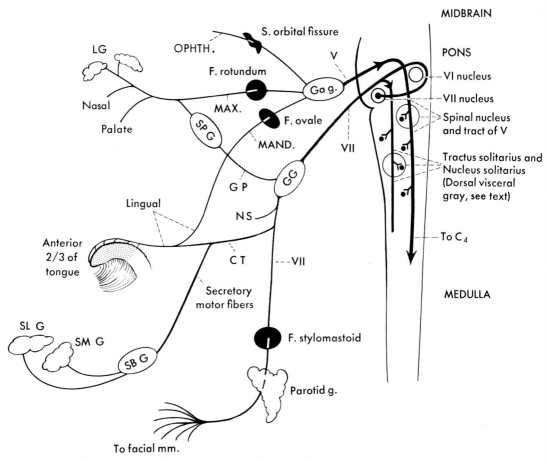

FIGURE 1–9. Central and peripheral connections of the seventh nerve.

CT. Chorda tympani	*MAND.* Mandibular division of fifth
GG. Geniculate ganglion	*SP G.* Sphenopalatine ganglion
Ga G. Gasserian ganglion (semilunar ganglion)	*NS.* Nerve to stapedius
GP. Greater superficial petrosal nerve	*SB G.* Submandibular ganglion
LG. Lacrimal gland	*SM G.* Submandibular gland
MAX. Maxillary division of fifth	*SL G.* Sublingual gland

facial nerve and passes to the sphenopalatine ganglion. The main part of the facial nerve enters the facial canal where it gives off two branches, the chorda tympani and the nerve to the stapedius. The seventh nerve leaves the temporal bone at the stylomastoid foramen and almost immediately divides into a number of branches to supply the muscles of facial expression.

2. Secretomotor (general visceral efferent) fibers.
   a. Some pass to the sphenopalatine ganglia via the greater superficial petrosal nerve and then to the lacrimal gland and the mucous membrane of the nose, nasopharynx, palate, and pharynx.
   b. Others pass to the chorda tympani and thence via the lingual nerve to the submandibular ganglion, which distributes secretomotor fibers to the submandibular and sublingual glands.

The cells of origin of the secretomotor fibers lie lateral to the main facial nucleus in the pons. The fibers join the facial nerve after it has passed around the sixth-nerve nucleus and emerge within the facial nerve at the junction of the pons and medulla, often as a separate bundle called the intermediate nerve of Wrisberg. Some fibers of the intermediate nerve leave the facial nerve at the level of the geniculate ganglion and join the greater superficial petrosal nerve. The remaining fibers enter the facial canal and leave as the chorda tympani, which passes in a canal through the petrous temporal bone. It emerges at the base of the skull and joins the lingual nerve, which carries the secretomotor fibers to the submandibular ganglion for distribution to the submandibular and sublingual salivary glands.

3. Taste (special visceral afferent) fibers. These fibers arise from the taste buds on the anterior two thirds of the tongue and pass through the lingual nerve and the chorda tympani to the facial nerve in the facial canal. The cells of origin lie in the geniculate ganglion and the axons pass back to the pons in the facial nerve to enter the tractus solitarius. After descending a short distance, these fibers synapse with cells of the dorsal visceral gray or gustatory nucleus. Fibers from the dorsal visceral gray cross the midline and ascend on the medial aspect of the medial lemniscus to both the thalamus and hypothalamus.

Clinical Examination. If there is marked weakness of the facial muscles, the patient may present with loss of the nasolabial fold, sagging of the lower eyelid, and inability to close the eye on blinking. Minor degrees of facial paralysis or palsy can be detected only by clinical examination. The patient is asked to smile and to show his teeth. The facial movements should be symmetric. He should be asked to close his eyes firmly while the examiner attempts to open the upper lids. He should be asked to frown or to furl the forehead or raise the eyebrows.

Facial weaknesses may be of two types:

1. Upper motor neuron. In this condition there is damage to the lateral cortical neurons or to the corticobulbar tract projecting from them to the contralateral seventh-nerve nucleus. The resulting facial palsy is characterized by loss of function in the lower part of the face with preservation of the function of the muscles of the forehead or upper part of the face. These are bilateral corticobulbar projections to neurons of the seventh-nerve nucleus supplying the muscles of the forehead. The projection is unilateral to neurons supplying the lower face (Fig. 1–10).

2. Lower motor neuron. Damage to the motor nucleus in the pons or to the facial nerve anywhere in its course will produce ipsilateral weakness of the muscles of facial expression.

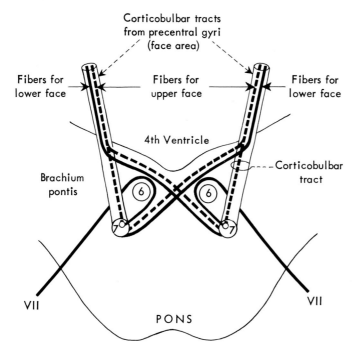

FIGURE 1–10. Supranuclear connections, seventh-nerve nucleus. There is bilateral corticobulbar innervation to the seventh-nerve nucleus for control of muscular movements of the upper face, and there is unilateral corticobulbar innervation to the seventh-nerve nucleus for muscular movement of the lower face. A unilateral lesion of the corticobulbar tract causes weakness of the lower contralateral face only.

This condition is sometimes called Bell's palsy, although this term should be reserved for an isolated paralysis of peripheral facial nerve function of unknown etiology.

Segmental damage to the facial nerve can be recognized clinically as follows:

1. Injury to the nerve peripheral to the stylomastoid foramen produces paralysis or paresis of the muscles of facial expression on the side of injury with preservation of all other functions of the facial nerve (taste, secretomotor, stapedius).
2. Injury to the nerve in the facial canal proximal to its junction with the chorda tympani produces paralysis or paresis of the muscles of facial expression plus loss of taste over the anterior two thirds of the tongue.
3. Injury to the nerve in the facial canal proximal to the origin of the nerve to the stapedius produces total loss of function of the muscles of facial expression plus loss of taste on the anterior two thirds of the tongue. In addition, there is an increase of hearing (hyperacusis) on the ipsilateral side owing to paralysis of the function of the stapedius, which acts as a damper to the stapes of the middle ear.
4. Injury to the nerve proximal to the geniculate ganglion produces total paralysis of the muscles of facial expression plus loss of taste over the anterior two thirds of the tongue and hyperacusis on the same side plus absence of lacrimation on the same side owing to involvement of the greater superficial petrosal nerve.
5. Damage to the facial nerve in the pons is frequently associated with involvement of the abducens nucleus so that the combination of facial paralysis plus paralysis of external rotation of the ipsilateral eye suggests a central or pontine lesion.

In suspected lesions of the seventh nerve the function of taste of the anterior two thirds of the tongue should always be tested. The patient is asked to protrude the tongue, which is then held by the examiner at its tip between two pieces of gauze. The surface of the tongue is dried, and a cotton applicator dipped in the test solution is applied to each side of the tongue. The patient raises his hand as soon as he tastes the solution and is then allowed to withdraw the tongue and identify the solution. Solutions used are designed to test three different types of taste. These are (1) sweet—sugar solution, (2) sour—vinegar, (3) bitter—quinine. Test solutions may be carried in small screw-top plastic containers in the examiner's bag.

ADDITIONAL MEANS OF TESTING FACIAL NERVE FUNCTION. In the unconscious patient, weakness on one side of the face may be detected by observing the tendency for that side of the face to droop more than the other side. In addition, there will be a tendency for it to "blow out" more than the opposite side during expiration. In the stuporous or semicomatose patient, pressure on the supraorbital notch with the thumb produces pain and grimacing, which will be absent or weaker on the paralyzed side.

In patients with conditions such as myasthenia gravis or postinfectious polyneuropathy (Fig. 1–11) or certain forms of muscular dystrophy that produce bilateral facial weakness, attempts at smiling or showing the teeth result in a linear movement in the angle of the mouth of small amplitude. These patients are also unable to purse the lips or to whistle on request. When the patient attempts to close his eyes, he is unable to do so and looks upward so that his lids cover his eyes. This is called Bell's phenomenon (see Fig. 1–11).

Eighth Cranial Nerve

This cranial nerve consists of two sensory nerves carrying impulses subserving the special sense of hearing (cochlear nerve) and the sensory nerve of equilibration (vestibular nerve). The cochlear nerve subserving hearing arises in ganglion cells within the spiral ganglion that innervate the hair cells of the sensory organ of Corti, while the axons pass through the internal auditory canal to the upper medulla at its junction with the inferior cerebellar peduncle. In the medulla, the auditory fibers bifurcate and pass to both dorsal and ventral cochlear nuclei. The secondary fibers from the ventral cochlear nucleus cross the midline as the trapezoid body decussates with fibers from the opposite side and enter the lateral lemniscus on the opposite side. Some fibers leave the trapezoid body and pass to the superior olivary nucleus on the same side. A connection is believed to exist between the superior olivary nucleus and the abducens nuclei that presumably serves the function of reflex eye turning in response to sound.

The secondary fibers from the dorsal cochlear nucleus cross the midline immediately beneath the floor of the fourth ventricle and enter the

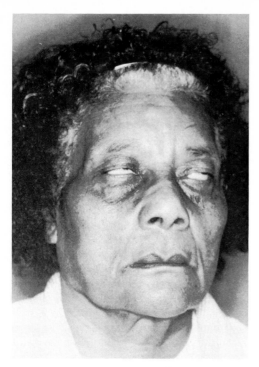

FIGURE 1-11. Bilateral facial paralysis due to postinfectious polyneuritis. The patient is trying to close her eyes and shows Bell's phenomenon (i.e., the eyes move upward under the lids since closing the eyelids is impossible).

lateral lemniscus on the opposite side. The fibers of the lateral lemniscus ascend through the pons to terminate in the inferior colliculus. There are synapses in the gray matter of the lateral lemniscus from which arise commissural connections to the opposite side. The major one of these is the commissure of Probst at the level of the superior cerebellar peduncle. The majority of fibers of the lateral lemniscus terminate in the inferior colliculus, although a few pass through the structure without synapsing and enter the brachium of the medial geniculate with fibers from the inferior colliculus to the medial geniculate body.

Fibers from the medial geniculate pass as the auditory radiation through the sublenticular portion of the posterior limb of the internal capsule to the superior transverse temporal gyri (areas 41 and 42), which are the primary auditory receptive areas of the cortex lying on the opercular surface of the superior temporal gyrus. Since there are numerous bilateral connections in the two cochlear nuclei at various levels from cochlear nuclei to the temporal cortex, unilateral lesions of the temporal cortex, of the subtemporal white matter, and of the brainstem above the cochlear nucleus do not produce a unilateral loss of hearing. Bilateral cerebral lesions may produce cortical deafness, and unilateral lesions of the cochlear nucleus or the eighth nerve will produce unilateral deafness.

Clinical Examination of the Auditory Division. The following tests are designed to evaluate the function of the auditory apparatus and the auditory division of the eighth nerve.

HEARING. (1) The examiner rubs the thumb and index finger together just outside the external auditory meatus. The sound should be instantly heard by the patient. (2) The examiner stands at the side of the patient. The patient is asked to place a finger in the opposite ear and the examiner whispers single words or numbers. The patient should reply when he hears the whispered voice. The distance of perception of the faint whisper should be noted and comparison may be made between the two sides. (3) The patient's ability to hear a tuning fork of 128 and 256 vibrations per second is compared with that of the examiner.

TESTS OF CONDUCTION. In a normal individual, air conduction is more sensitive than bone conduction. This can be tested by placing a tuning fork over the mastoid process with the patient indicating when the sound is no longer heard. The fork is then placed immediately over the external auditory meatus, and the patient is asked to indicate whether he hears the sound. Under normal circumstances, since air conduction is better than bone conduction, the patient will hear the sound at the external auditory meatus despite the fact that the tuning fork is no longer heard over the mastoid process. Under these circumstances the Rinné test is said to be positive. When air conduction is impaired, the patient will not be able to hear the sound from the external auditory meatus when it is still present over the mastoid process. Under these circumstances, bone conduction is better than air conduction and the Rinné test is said to be negative. Air conduction may be impaired owing to obstruction of the external auditory meatus by wax and foreign bodies or to disease of the middle ear that impairs the function of the drum or the ossicles. In neurologic disorders affecting the nerve supply to the cochlea or disease of the auditory nerve, *both air and bone conduction are di-*

minished although the Rinné test will remain positive.

The vibrating tuning fork is then placed in the center of the forehead and the patient is asked to indicate where he hears the sound. Under normal circumstances the sound appears to originate in the midline. When there is impairment of air conduction, however, the sound is referred to the involved side and the Weber test is said to be positive. In disease of the cochlea or in nerve deafness the sound is lateralized to the opposite side and the Weber test is said to be negative.

The initial impression of impairment of hearing may be confirmed and the deficiency plotted in graphic form using an audiometer. Audiometry may be particularly useful when there are partial lesions involving the auditory division of the acoustic nerve and only certain tones of hearing are affected.

Vestibular Division: General Considerations. The vestibular portion of the eighth nerve is also sensory and carries impulses from the vestibular apparatus to the brainstem.

The vestibular apparatus consists of the utricle, the saccule, and three semicircular canals, each lying in a plane at right angles to one another. The membranous labyrinth is contained within the bony canals lying within the petrous temporal bones and separated from the bony wall by perilymph. This membranous system contains fluid called endolymph. Each semicircular canal has a dilated portion called the ampulla with a fold of specialized epithelium—the crista—which is sensitive to movement of the endolymph. The utricle and saccule contain epithelial folds of specialized sensory cells with hair processes called the maculae. Lying in the hair processes of the maculae are crystals of calcium carbonate in an organic matrix forming the otoliths.

The macula of the utricle lies in a horizontal plane, while the macula of the saccule lies in a sagittal plane. Linear acceleration in either of these planes will produce bending of the hair processes owing to inertia. Thus, the semicircular canals record angular acceleration, while the utricle and saccule record linear acceleration.

The ganglion cells of the vestibular division of the eighth nerve lie in the internal auditory meatus, and the dendrites terminate in the specialized epithelium of the hair cells. The axons pass back to the upper medulla in association with the auditory division of the eighth nerve. On entering the medulla the fibers pass directly to the flocculonodular lobe of the cerebellum and to the four vestibular nuclei. These are named the medial or principal nucleus (Schwalbe), the superior nucleus (von Bechterew), the lateral nucleus (Deiter), and the inferior or spinal nucleus.

All four vestibular nuclei communicate with the cerebellum and with the medial longitudinal fasciculus, which brings them into communication with the third-, fourth-, and sixth-nerve nuclei and the nuclei of the accessory and upper cervical nerves. These connections permit vestibular influence on movements of the eyes and head and neck. The lateral vestibulospinal tract arises from the lateral nucleus and carries impulses to the spinal cord by synapsing with the anterior horn cells.

The pathway for communication between the vestibular nuclei and the cerebral cortex is not known but probably exists since vertigo has resulted from cortical stimulation of the posterior aspects of the temporal lobe. Furthermore, vertigo is not uncommonly one of the initial manifestations of psychomotor epilepsy or partial seizures arising from the temporal lobe.

Clinical Examination of the Vestibular Division. Disturbances of function involving the vestibular apparatus and/or the vestibular division of the eighth nerve are usually accompanied by vertigo. Vertigo may be defined as an illusion of movement that may be rotatory and objective (external objects seem to be rotating while the individual is stationary) or subjective (the individual seems to be rotating in relation to the external environment). While rotation is the most common complaint, occasionally there is a sensation of falling to one side or of horizontal or vertical movement. Abnormalities of the vestibular apparatus or vestibular division of the eighth nerve are regularly accompanied by nystagmus of a type already described under the examination of the eye movements.

Clinical tests of vestibular function are necessary when symptoms are intermittent. These tests are designed to provoke normal responses by stimulating vestibular function. The patient may be rotated for 20 seconds in a Bárány chair and then the movement is stopped abruptly.

The head should be placed in position so that one of the semicircular canals is in the horizontal plane, thus producing maximal stimulation to that canal. This is accomplished by tilting the head

30 degrees forward to test the lateral canal or 60 degrees backward to test the anterior canal with the patient seated in the chair.

Rotation of the patient is accompanied by inertia of the endolymph and stimulation of the cristae. When the movement is stopped, however, inertia of the endolymph produces stimulation of the cristae in the opposite direction. This is accompanied by a sensation of vertigo in the opposite direction from the previous rotation. Nystagmus, past pointing, and deviation of the eyes in the direction of the flow of endolymph occur in the direction of the completed rotation. The sensation of vertigo and the accompanying signs usually last about 35 seconds in a normal individual. It will be reduced or absent in disease of the stimulated canal or its vestibular nerve. It may be prolonged in patients with an unduly sensitive vestibular response either due to infection or as a personal idiosyncrasy.

Labyrinthine function may also be tested by irrigating the external auditory canal with hot or cold water by means of a syringe. The resulting temperature changes in the middle ear cause convection currents in the endolymph of the semicircular canal. Testing is usually carried out with the patient lying down and the head flexed to 30 degrees for maximal stimulation of the lateral semicircular canal and with the patient seated and the head extended 60 degrees for stimulation of the anterior canal.

The external auditory meatus on one side is first injected with a small volume of iced water (5 to 10 ml). This has the effect of producing nystagmus, past pointing, and deviation of the eyes toward the injected side and a sensation of vertigo to the opposite side. Nystagmus may persist for 60 to 90 seconds in the normal individual. When there is loss of function of the horizontal canal or damage to the vestibular division of the eighth nerve, there will be absence of any of these responses on the affected side. A partial lesion will produce a correspondingly shorter response depending on the degree of damage.

Ninth Cranial Nerve (Glossopharyngeal)

The glossopharyngeal nerve supplies (1) motor (special visceral efferent) fibers to the stylopharyngeus muscle, (2) secretomotor (general visceral efferent) fibers to the parotid gland, (3) sensory (general visceral afferent) fibers from the back of the tongue and pharynx, carotid sinus, and carotid body, and (4) taste (special visceral affer-

ent) fibers from the posterior third of the tongue.

The nuclei of the glossopharyngeal complex lie in the upper medulla. The inferior salivary nucleus, which is a rostral continuation of the dorsal nucleus of the vagus, gives origin to secretomotor fibers. The sensory fibers from the back of the tongue and pharynx, carotid sinus, and carotid body arise from ganglion cells in the petrosal ganglion and enter the fasciculus solitarius in the brainstem to terminate in the nucleus solitarius.

The fibers from the taste buds in the posterior third of the tongue also have their cell bodies in the petrosal ganglion, and their central connections run through the fasciculus solitarius to end in the dorsal visceral gray (gustatory nucleus). This complex of afferent and efferent fibers forms the glossopharyngeal nerve, which then arises as a series of rootlets in the groove between the inferior olive and the inferior cerebellar peduncle and leaves the skull through the jugular foramen, where the petrosal ganglion is located. It passes forward in the neck between the internal jugular vein and internal carotid artery, supplying fibers to both, and terminates in the pharynx.

The tympanic nerve, which supplies parasympathetic fibers to the parotid gland and sensory fibers to the middle ear, arises from the glossopharyngeal nerve just below the petrosal ganglion and passes into the middle ear to form the tympanic plexus. The lesser superficial petrosal nerve carries secretomotor fibers from the tympanic plexus to the otic ganglion, and the postganglionic fibers pass via the auricular temporal branch of the fifth cranial nerve to the parotid gland.

The carotid branches of the glossopharyngeal nerve are also important since they carry the impulses from both the chemoreceptors and pressoreceptors of the carotid body and sinus responsible for the reflex control of respiratory rate, heart rate, and blood pressure.

Clinical Examination. Sensation over the posterior third of the tongue and the pharyngeal wall may be tested by touching these areas with a cotton applicator or by gentle application of a pin.

The gag reflex consists of elevation of the palate and retraction of the tongue with contraction of the pharyngeal muscles when the posterior pharyngeal wall is stimulated. The afferent loop of the reflex runs in the glossopharyngeal nerve, while the efferent loop runs in the vagus nerve. Loss or diminution of the gag reflex is usually seen in lesions involving the glossopharyngeal nerve rather than the vagus nerve. Absence of the gag reflex may also occur in hysteria, and diminution of it may be seen in alcoholics and heavy smokers.

The gag reflex is part of a more complex reflex involved in vomiting. Repeated stimulation of the glossopharyngeal wall may produce vomiting in susceptible individuals. Under these circumstances, the afferent impulses pass through the glossopharyngeal nerve to the medulla to the nucleus solitarius. From this nucleus there is a secondary relay to the reticular substance immediately beneath the floor of the fourth ventricle, which is believed to represent the "vomiting center." This center may be excited by impulses not only from the glossopharyngeal nerve but also from cortical centers (emotion), by vestibular impulses (motion sickness, labyrinthitis), through the vagus nerve (distention and inflammatory conditions of the viscera and intestinal tract), and from the spinothalamic tract owing to painful somatic conditions.

The mechanism of vomiting is a graphic and meaningful example of the extraordinarily complex yet efficient interaction of the nervous system. The "vomiting center" has central projections (1) to the nucleus ambiguus resulting in reflex elevation of the palate, closure of the pharynx, and closure of the epiglottis, (2) to the twelfth-nerve nucleus resulting in reflex retraction of the tongue, (3) to the dorsal nucleus of the vagus resulting in increased peristalsis, (4) to the inferior and superior salivatory nuclei producing excessive salivation, (5) to the reticulospinal tracts and the anterior horn cells in the cervical cord producing contraction of the diaphragm and abdominal muscles, and (6) via descending spinal tracts synapsing with the intermediate gray matter in the thoracic spinal cord to the sympathetic ganglion resulting in sympathetic stimulation with closure of the pylorus, sweating, pallor, and tachycardia.

The increased peristalsis, closure of the pyloric sphincter, and regular spasmodic contractions of the diaphragm and abdominal muscles result in expulsion of the stomach contents and vomiting.

Tenth Cranial Nerve (Vagus)

The vagus (wandering) nerve supplies:

1. Motor (general visceral efferent) preganglionic fibers to the thoracic and abdominal viscera.

2. Motor (special visceral efferent) fibers that supply the cricothyroid muscle and the intrinsic muscles of the larynx.

3. Sensory (general visceral afferent) impulses arising from the thoracic and abdominal viscera.

4. Sensory (general somatic afferent) sensation from the external ear. This latter is a relatively unimportant function of the vagus nerve and is also shared by the glossopharyngeal and facial nerves.

The motor fibers of the vagus arise from the dorsal nucleus (parasympathetic) and the nucleus ambiguus (pharyngeal musculature) and leave the medulla between the inferior olive and the restiform body by a series of rootlets in line with the glossopharyngeal nerve. These rootlets unite, and the nerve leaves the posterior fossa through the jugular foramen. The ganglion nodosum, which contains the cell bodies for fibers supplying visceral sensation, as well as the jugular ganglion, containing the cell bodies for cutaneous sensation, are both within the jugular foramen. Centropedal fibers from these sensory cells pass from the ganglion nodosum via the tractus solitarius to the nucleus solitarius and from the jugular ganglion to the spinal tract of the trigeminal nerve.

After passing through the jugular foramen the vagus nerve enters the carotid sheath and passes down the neck supplying branches to the tympanic plexus, pharynx, and larynx and enters the thorax where it contributes branches to the cardiac, pulmonary, and esophageal plexuses. The vagus then enters the abdomen, passing through the diaphragm next to the esophagus, and is distributed to the abdominal viscera.

During its passage through the neck the vagus gives off the superior pharyngeal nerve, which passes deep to the internal carotid artery to divide into external and internal pharyngeal branches. The external pharyngeal branch supplies the cricothyroid muscle, and the internal pharyngeal branch pierces the constrictors of the pharynx to supply sensation to the pharyngeal wall, the epiglottis, the base of the tongue, and the larynx as far as the vocal cords.

The recurrent laryngeal nerve arises in relation to the anterior aspect of the subclavian artery on the right side. After winding around the artery, it ascends between the esophagus and the trachea to enter the larynx. On the left side, the left recurrent laryngeal nerve arises at the level of the arch of the aorta, winding below the arch, and ascends between the esophagus and the trachea to the larynx. The recurrent laryngeal nerve supplies all the muscles of the larynx except the cricothyroid.

Clinical Examination. Evaluation of the functions of the vagus nerve begins with observation of the quality of the voice and articulation. To understand the clinical differentiation of speech disorders arising from vagus nerve involvement, other types of speech disorders must also be recognized.

DYSARTHRIA. Difficulty in articulation, or dysarthria, may occur in lesions involving the vagus nerve but may also be seen with involvement of the seventh or twelfth cranial nerve. Dysarthria is also seen in disorders involving coordination of the muscles of articulation produced by cerebellar lesions or bilateral corticobulbar lesions (pseudobulbar palsy).

COMPARISON OF VAGAL DYSARTHRIA WITH OTHER TYPES. The following points are of major importance:

1. Involvement of the seventh cranial nerve produces paresis or paralysis of the facial muscles resulting in difficulty with lip movements; this is described as a labial dysarthria, which is most noticeable in pronunciation of the consonants *b* and *p*.
2. Weakness involving the twelfth cranial nerve produces difficulty in tongue movements and is described as a lingual dysarthria, with difficulty in the use of consonants such as *d* and *t*.
3. Palatal paralysis due to unilateral vagal paralysis results in a nasal quality to the voice owing to the inability to elevate the palate and close the nasal pharynx in articulation. The increase in this nasal quality in bilateral vagal paralysis results in special difficulty in pronunciation of *k*, *q*, and *ch*.
4. Laryngeal and vocal cord paralysis due to a lesion of the recurrent laryngeal nerve results in a brassy quality or hoarseness of the voice with loss of volume.
5. A cerebellar lesion produces scanning speech with an explosive dysrhythmic quality.
6. Pseudobulbar speech is slow, spastic, and grunting.

TESTING MOTOR FUNCTIONS OF THE SOFT PALATE. Under normal circumstances the uvula is suspended in the midline while the palate arches evenly to both sides. During inspection of the pharynx with a tongue depressor and flashlight, the patient is asked to say "Ah." While the patient is doing this, the uvula should remain in the midline and the palate should elevate evenly to both sides. When the vagus nerve is paralyzed on one side, arching of the palate is absent on that side; hence it and the uvula are drawn to the opposite side. In bilateral vagal paralysis, palatal movement is absent.

TESTING PHARYNGEAL FUNCTION. Paralysis of the pharynx is usually associated with difficulties in swallowing (dysphagia), regurgitation of liquids through the nose, and choking and aspiration of food and fluid into the lung. In testing for pharyngeal function, the examiner should note the degree of contraction of the pharyngeal muscles on both sides while testing the gag reflex, during swallowing, as well as during phonation. If the patient is severely dysphagic, nasogastric intubation for feeding may be necessary.

TESTING MOTOR FUNCTIONS OF THE LARYNX. Abnormalities of laryngeal function are usually suspected if there are hoarseness of the voice and some degree of laryngeal stridor during deep breathing. Suspicion of laryngeal paralysis should be confirmed by laryngoscopic examination. Paralysis of the superior laryngeal nerve produces hoarseness of the voice and loss of higher tones in speaking and singing. There may be loss of tension and abduction of the vocal cord on the same side when saying "Eee!" In recurrent laryngeal nerve paralysis, the loss of function frequently occurs in stages. The first manifestation is failure of abduction of the vocal cord on the affected side producing hoarseness of the voice and mild inspiratory stridor. This may be followed by complete paralysis when the cord assumes a cadaveric position midway between adduction and abduction. The vocal cord on the uninvolved side crosses the midline to meet the paralyzed cord during phonation. The voice is husky and the patient loses the ability to sing. In bilateral recurrent laryngeal nerve paralysis, loss of abduction produces stridor and dyspnea, and tracheotomy may be necessary.

Eleventh Cranial Nerve (Spinal Accessory)

The spinal accessory nerve distributes motor (general somatic efferent) fibers to the sternocleidomastoid and trapezius muscles. The motor cells lie immediately lateral to the anterior horn cells in the upper five segments of the cervical cord. These fibers pass dorsolaterally and emerge from the spinal cord midway between the anterior and posterior roots and unite to form a single trunk, which passes rostrally through the foramen magnum into the posterior fossa. The spinal accessory nerve then joins the bulbar accessory nerve, which is a lower portion of the vagus nerve, and leaves the posterior fossa through the jugular foramen accompanied by the glossopharyngeal and the vagus nerves.

The spinal accessory fibers leave the bulbar portion of the accessory nerve. The bulbar portion joins the vagus while the spinal portion descends in the neck to supply the sternocleidomastoid and trapezius muscles on the same side. It is believed that the cells giving rise to the spinal accessory fibers show segmentation in the cervical cord. The more rostral cells supply the sternocleidomastoid while the caudal cells supply the trapezius. This may be helpful in localizing a high cervical cord lesion.

Clinical Examination. The sternocleidomastoid muscles function together to flex the head and independently to turn the head to the opposite side. The patient is asked to flex his head against resistance while both sternocleidomastoids are palpated and should be felt to contract. He is then asked to turn the head to one side against resistance while the examiner palpates the opposite sternocleidomastoid muscle to feel for contraction or wasting. The trapezius elevates the shoulder on each side and is tested by asking the patient to elevate or shrug his shoulders against the resistance of the examiner's hands. Unilateral paralysis of the trapezius tends to produce drooping of the shoulder on that side, and in lower motor neuron lesions with wasting, there is loss of the normal muscular contour between shoulder and neck. The shoulder cannot be elevated or is shrugged weakly. The edge of the contracting trapezius is not seen or is felt to be weak and flabby. The patient will also have difficulty in tilting the head to the same side.

Twelfth Cranial Nerve (Hypoglossal)

The hypoglossal nerve supplies motor (general somatic efferent) fibers to the muscles of the tongue.

The motor cells of the hypoglossal nucleus lie in the dorsal medulla near the midline. The fibers traverse the substance of the medulla to emerge between the pyramid and the inferior olive in a series of rootlets that unite to form a single trunk, which passes out of the posterior fossa through the anterior condyloid foramen. The nerve then passes anteriorly across the neck, deep to the bifurcation of the carotid artery. The nerve terminates by supplying branches to the ipsilateral muscles of the tongue.

Clinical Examination of the Tongue. A great deal of useful clinical information, in addition to its motor functions, can be gained from examination of the tongue. Some other considerations will be mentioned at this time.

MOTOR FUNCTION. The patient is asked to protrude the tongue, which should lie in the midline. In lower motor neuron lesions involving the hypoglossal nucleus, or in lesions of the hypoglossal nerve, the tongue is deviated toward the side of the lesion when the patient is asked to protrude the tongue. Since the hypoglossal nucleus is bilaterally innervated by both cortical areas, upper motor lesions do not usually produce deviation of the tongue. However, some deviation is occasionally seen for a few days following an acute and severe upper motor neuron lesion, in which case the tongue deviates to the side opposite the lesion. Presumably this is due to transient transsynaptic paralysis or diaschisis.

The strength of the tongue muscles may also be checked by asking the patient to push out the cheek against the resistance of the examiner's hand. The protruded tongue should also be examined for signs of atrophy, which produces increased wrinkling and some loss of bulk on the side of a lower motor neuron lesion. Careful examination in a good light—with the tongue at rest on the floor of the mouth—may disclose fasciculations in lower motor neuron lesions. Good judgment may be necessary to distinguish fasciculations from tremor of the tongue, which is present in a large percentage of normal people. Tremor is rhythmic, while fasciculations are random contractions of individual motor units within the tongue.

STATE OF MUCOUS MEMBRANE. The state of the mucous membrane of the tongue should be noted since changes may indicate underlying systemic disease. For example, a fiery-red "beefy" tongue (magenta tongue) may be seen in patients suffering from vitamin B deficiency (often associated with Wernicke's and Korsakoff's syndrome or polyneuropathy). A smooth, atrophic tongue may occur in patients with long-standing pernicious (addisonian) anemia, which may be associated with subacute combined degeneration of the cord. Scarring or laceration of the tongue due to biting may be seen following epileptic seizures.

RAPID ALTERNATING MOVEMENTS. The patient is asked to move the tongue as rapidly as possible from side to side after it has been protruded. In patients with bilateral upper motor neuron lesions, the tongue may be slow and spastic while making such movements. Patients with cerebellar dysfunction will show dysrhythmia of such movements, which are irregular in both timing and amplitude. When rhythmic movements of the tongue are impaired, resulting dysrhythmia and incoordination are easily recognized as explosive, thick, or "hot potato in the mouth" speech.

The Motor System: General Considerations

Functional Anatomy of the Major Motor Pathways

The motor unit is the basic functional unit of the motor system, and all movement depends on the integrated action of these motor units. The motor unit is composed of the anterior horn cell or the equivalent neuron of the motor cranial nuclei in the brainstem, their axon, and the muscle fibers supplied by the axon. The number of muscle fibers innervated by a single motor neuron varies from a few in the small extraocular muscles to a large number in large muscles such as the quadriceps.

The anterior horn cell is constantly subjected to a barrage of impulses, the majority of which are inhibitory either directly or through internuncial neurons. These impulses are:

1. *Segmental*—e.g., the simple stretch reflex, such as the monosynaptic patellar jerk.
2. *Intersegmental*—through connections between different segments of the spinal cord, each able to influence the other.
3. *Suprasegmental*—through the connections from the higher centers and including, in ascending order, olivary, vestibular, cerebellar, nigral, rubral, reticular, striatal, and cortical, the latter being the highest level.

The anterior horn cell has consequently been termed the "final common pathway," for inhibitory and excitatory impulses influence it from many levels in the spinal cord, brainstem, cerebellum, basal ganglia, and cortex. These variable influences on the anterior horn cell result in a variety of changes in the innervation of the muscles. This can be demonstrated by experimental lesions in animals and is frequently seen in man as a result of disease of these structures.

Tone or Resistance to Passive Movement

In the resting state, there is a steady state of muscle contraction that is normally more marked in the extensors of the lower limbs and the flexors of the upper limbs. Tone is reflex in origin and is influenced by a constant stream of efferent impulses of segmental, intersegmental, and suprasegmental origin. Destruction of the corticospinal tract results in spasticity with the "clasp-knife response": the limb resists passive motion and then suddenly gives way like the blade of a penknife. Lesions of the substantia nigra and basal ganglia give rise to cogwheel rigidity in which passive movement of the joint feels like a ratchet or cogwheel.

Posture

The inequality of tone in muscle groups results in the posture of the limbs. This tends to produce extension in all limbs and provides a background of activity against which more dynamic activities may occur. The maintenance of an abnormal posture due to disease of the nervous system is called dystonia.

The main reflex systems governing tone and posture, which have been worked out using experimental animals, include the following:

The Stretch Reflex. This is the most important single factor controlling postural mechanisms. Stretching of muscle spindles in the antigravity (extensor) muscles produces an increase in extensor tonus and inhibition of tone in the flexor muscles in all limbs. The application of pressure to the feet results in an extensor thrust, owing to stretching of muscle spindles, and the spread of afferent impulses to anterior horn cells supplying other extensor muscles by intersegmental connections.

The Flexion Reflex. Contact with painful stimuli results in reflex withdrawal of a limb owing to inhibition of extensor and stimulation of flexor mechanisms through segmental and intersegmental connections. At the same time, there is an increase in contralateral extensor tone—*the crossed extensor response*—which is a primitive mechanism attempting to maintain posture.

The Shortening Reaction. Any reduction of tension in a muscle produces contraction of intrafusal fibers and activity of muscle spindles with maintenance of tone in the muscle.

The Lengthening Reaction. When any force is applied to a limb, there is a progressive increase in tone and resistance. Eventually there is a sudden "give" to prevent damage to muscle fibers. This becomes exaggerated as the "clasp-knife phenomenon" in corticospinal tract lesions.

The Positive Supporting Reaction. Extensor thrust reflexes are integrated at lower brainstem levels in response to cutaneous stimulation of the palms of the hands or the soles of the feet.

The Negative Supporting Reaction. The positive supporting reaction described above may be inhibited by flexion of the digits, which reduces extensor tone in the limbs.

Reflex Standing. This reflex was described in animals and consists of integration of the positive supporting reaction with tonic rigidity of the trunk muscles. The equivalent in man is seen in either decerebrate or decorticate rigidity and in states of spasticity of all four limbs.

Tonic Neck Reflexes. These reflexes are well developed in both man and animals. They can be demonstrated incompletely in infants until a few weeks after birth and are readily elicited in decorticate states in man. They include flexion of the forelimbs in response to flexion of the neck and extension of the forelimbs and flexion of the hindlegs on extension of the neck. Pressure on the dorsal surface of the neck inhibits the positive supporting reaction, and there is flexion of all four limbs, i.e., a crawling position. Turning the head increases the extensor thrust on the side to which the jaw is pointing, so that the hand and arm are extended in the position of a fencer. These reflexes appear to be integrated in the upper cervical cord and brainstem.

Righting Reflexes. The body is oriented in space by the righting reflexes. These include optical and labyrinthine reflexes at the highest level. The more primitive righting reflexes are the body-on-head reflex in which the head assumes the correct position in space when the body is turned on its side. There are also truncal reflexes mediated by unequal tactile stimuli from the two sides of the trunk. Turning the head, for example, produces torsion of the neck, which initiates the neck on body-righting reflex with the body assuming the correct position in relation to the head.

Many of these reflexes, which can be readily demonstrated in animals, are observed in various disease states in man. In man, they undergo some modification, because of the assumption of an upright posture or stance and in the initiation and maintenance of a biped gait. However, they are seen in the decerebrate state in man with severe injury to the brain and brainstem down to the level of the inferior colliculi.

The essential features of decerebrate rigidity are an augmentation of postural righting and vestibular reflexes. The patient shows increased tone in antigravity (extensor) muscles and in the trunk muscles with active tonic neck reflexes. With the head in the neutral position, all four limbs are rigidly extended, although the fingers are usually clenched. This activity is, however, dependent on intact vestibular connections and may be modified by cerebellar lesions.

Voluntary Movement. The term "voluntary movement" implies purposeful movement, which may be volitional but is not always initiated at a conscious level. It is the result of modification of reflex activity through the final common pathway (the anterior horn cell) and from impulses originating at cortical levels. These impulses are initiated in response to various afferent stimuli from other cortical or subcortical areas and are relayed to the anterior horn cells or cranial nerve neurons via corticobular or corticospinal pathways (the pyramidal tracts).

The cells of origin of the pyramidal tracts are predominantly from area 4 of the cortex, but fibers have also been traced to areas 6, 3, 2, 5, and 7. Probably 60 per cent of the fibers originate in area 4, the remaining 40 per cent from other areas in the frontal and parietal lobes. A specific pattern of fine motor movement may be obtained by stimulation of area 4. The cells controlling movement of the foot and leg are situated in the anterior portion of the paracentral lobule in the medial aspect of the hemisphere and those controlling movements of the thigh at the upper portion of the motor strip on the lateral surface.

Trunk and arm movements are represented by cells farther down the motor strip with a relatively large area for the hand, fingers, and thumb at the middle of area 4. Cells governing facial movements lie immediately below the thumb area, with those supplying neck, tongue, and laryngeal movement lying below the face area and immediately above the lateral fissure. The axons from area 4 pass through the corona radiata to the genu and anterior third of the posterior limb of the internal capsule where they are arranged in segmental form. Corticobulbar fibers are placed anteriorly followed by upper extremity, trunk, and lower extremity fibers.

The corticospinal tract then rotates 90 degrees to pass through the middle third of the basis pedunculi of the midbrain. The fibers supplying the lower extremities lie laterally and those to the upper extremities medially. As the fibers pass through the basilar portion of the pons, they are separated into bundles by the pontine nuclei and transverse pontine fibers. The two tracts form prominent pyramids on the ventral surface of the medulla, and 80 per cent of the fibers decussate in interlacing bundles in the caudal portion. The upper extremity fibers cross rostrally and the lower extremity fibers caudally.

From the pyramid, the fibers descend as the lateral corticospinal tracts of the spinal cord. Some 20 per cent of the fibers do not decussate but continue as the anterior corticospinal tracts in the ventral portion of the spinal cord. Somatotropic arrangement of fibers is maintained in the lateral corticospinal tract with the upper extremity fibers lying medially and the lower extremity fibers laterally. There is a progressive termination of fibers in relation to anterior horn cells or intercalated neurons throughout the spinal cord. The fibers from the anterior corticospinal tract undergo decussation through the ventral white commissure prior to termination.

Functions of the Corticospinal Tracts

Although it is possible that impulses arising from area 4 may produce discrete movement by stimulation of anterior horn cells, the function of this system is probably to modify reflex stimulation of the anterior horn cell from other segmental and suprasegmental levels. The end result is the production of fine coordinated movement.

Lesions of the Corticospinal Tracts

Experimental section of the medullary pyramids in animals produces a flaccid paralysis for two to three weeks. Chronic preparations are difficult to maintain for more prolonged observation. Lesions in man are always accompanied by damage to neurons or fibers of other "extrapyramidal" pathways.

Acute lesions of the corticospinal tract from the cortex through the capsule, medullary pyramids, and spinal cord result in flaccidity for two to three weeks, followed by spasticity. Lesions of area 4 result in loss of fine, coordinated movements, particularly in the fingers. Voluntary movement, if present at all, is slow and stiff. The tone of the limb is increased, and the clasp-knife reflex is elicited.

The Extrapyramidal System

This system includes a variety of interconnected nuclei that are involved in motor activity. It gives rise to the tracts that, in general, are not presumed to pass through the medullary pyramids (hence the term "extrapyramidal"). The extrapyramidal system has connections with the reticular, olivary, rubral, and cerebellar nuclei, as well as the functionally important substantia nigra of the brainstem. Diencephalic and telencephalic connections include the thalamus and subthalamic and caudate nuclei. There are also cortical connections to and from these nuclear groups, rich internuclear connections, and short-chain, polysynaptic connections between the various components and the tegmentospinal, rubrospinal, reticulospinal, and possibly other descending pathways acting on the anterior horn cells (as the final common pathway).

The terminal connections on the anterior horn cell are usually polysynaptic and influence both the internuncial neurons and the anterior horn cells, or, in functional terms, both the alpha and gamma systems. This complex relationship between the anterior horn cell and the influence of the state of tonus of the muscle is shown in Figures 1–12.

The first state of muscular contraction is initiated by the alpha system. The gamma system apparently is needed to set the state of bias in contraction by exerting afferent discharges via the gamma fibers. These impulses either inhibit or facilitate the alpha neuron, depending on such factors as the central excitatory state of the alpha neuron and suprasegmental influences mainly derived from the pyramidal and extrapyramidal systems. For example, when a muscle is strongly contracted, there tends to be stretching of the muscle spindle, with an increased afferent dis-

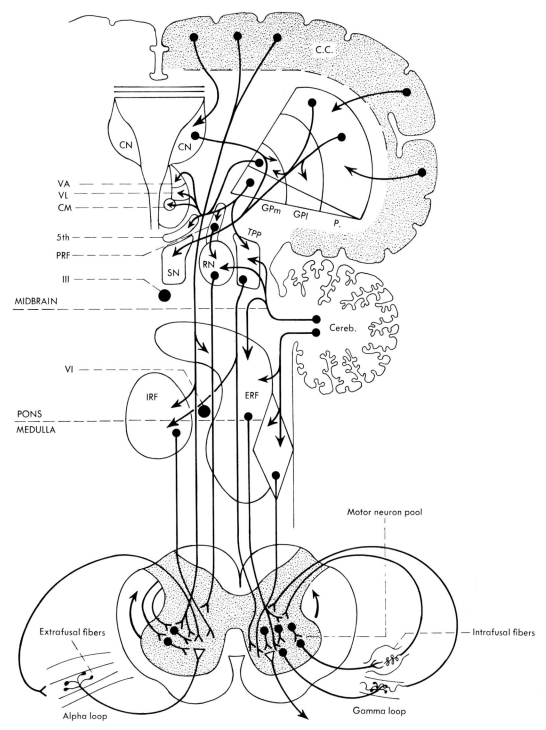

FIGURE 1–12. Cortical, subcortical, and cerebellar connections of the alpha and gamma systems. Actually, projections from the red nucleus to the spinal cord cross to the opposite side.

charge via the gamma system, which tends to decrease the central excitatory state of the neuron. Conversely, when the muscle is relaxed, the gamma afferent volley is minimal, and the central excitatory state of the alpha neuron or anterior horn cell tends to be increased.

The function of the extrapyramidal system, like that of the gamma system, is to exert either an inhibiting or an excitatory influence on the anterior horn cells. The reflex activity of the final common pathway depends on the combined influence of the various components of the extrapyramidal system integrated with discharges from the corticospinal tracts. It is not surprising, therefore, that lesions of the various components of this motor system give rise to gross disorders of movement. The effects of destructive lesions of the central nervous system frequently are "positive" in the sense that movements or muscular contractions formerly inhibited are now released.

Examination of the Motor System

Examination of the motor system involves the same principles of examination used in other clinical disciplines, particularly inspection and palpation. The neurologist, unlike other specialists, evaluates the motor system by having the patient perform certain tasks in order to test coordination, skilled movements, and motor strength (see Table 1–2, p. 4). These should be evaluated in a systematic manner, otherwise certain parts of the examination are likely to be forgotten or overlooked. The following description of the motor examination has been found useful. The patient is disrobed and wears shorts (male) or a short hospital gown (female).

Inspection, Palpation, and Percussion

The muscle groups are observed in detail. These include the trunk, chest, and abdominal muscles, including movement of the diaphragm and intercostal muscles as well as the limb muscles. In long-standing unilateral cerebral disease dating back to childhood, there is disuse atrophy of the entire hemiparetic side. The hands and fingers are smaller on the affected side, the limbs are shorter, and the muscular development is smaller.

Fasciculations may be evident in various muscle groups and are best seen with the light source placed behind the muscles to be examined. The light beam should pass across the muscle belly toward the examiner's eyes. All muscle groups are watched for several minutes. Fasciculations appear as rapid flickers and jerks of muscle contraction involving several motor units. They commonly involve more numerous motor units at the onset of voluntary contraction and hence appear as coarse fasciculations at the onset of motor movement (contraction fasciculations). When they involve the muscles of the hands and feet, the fingers and toes may jerk with each fasciculation, presenting as one form of myoclonic jerks (see p. 50).

Fasciculations should also be searched for in the tongue. The tongue should be at rest in the floor of the mouth and the mouth well lighted with a large flashlight or examining room light. Fasciculations are evidence of damage to either the anterior horn cell or the motor axon in its course to the motor unit. Sometimes generalized fasciculations are present as a rare but benign familial disorder of muscle known as benign fasciculations. In amyotrophic lateral sclerosis the fasciculations tend to be generalized. Fibrillations are spontaneous discharges of single motor units and are not visible to the naked eye but appear as short, transient, low-voltage spike discharges in the electromyograph, which have shorter duration and lower amplitude than normal action potentials.

Disease of either the anterior horn cells, the anterior roots, or the motor nerves will result in visible wasting of the muscle groups supplied by that nerve or spinal segments, and on palpation, the muscles have a flabby or jelly-like consistency.

Injury to the cervical cord at $C_{3,4,5}$ above the thoracic segments supplying the intercostal muscles will cause paralysis of the diaphragm, and in spinal shock there may be paralysis or weakness of the intercostal muscles. Inspection will reveal either respiratory paralysis, diminished respiratory excursion, or failure of intercostal movement on one or both sides. Percussion during forced inspiration and expiration may reveal that the diaphragm is paralyzed on one or both sides. The patient is asked to cough, and this will be diminished or weak in paralysis of the respiratory muscles. The ability to blow out a match held 4 in. away from the wide-open mouth is lost if the vital capacity is seriously reduced. In such cases, these rough estimates should be checked by actual measurements of vital capacity with a respirometer. If there is serious or progressive respiratory paralysis, the patient requires assisted respiration with a mechanical respirator.

Any abnormal postures or movements of the limbs such as tremors, dystonia, involuntary movements, clonus, spasms, myoclonus, and seizures should be noted.

Tremor. Tremor is a rhythmic oscillatory movement due to regular contraction of opposing groups of muscles. There are a number of types of tremor, each having some particular characteristic that facilitates recognition.

PARKINSONIAN TREMOR. Parkinsonian tremor has a frequency of 6 to 10 cps and an amplitude of a few centimeters. It involves principally the metacarpophalangeal and wrist joints. The rhythmic opposition of the pad of the index finger on the thumb has given rise to the term "pill-rolling tremor."

CEREBELLAR TREMOR. Cerebellar tremor occurs in disease of the dentate nucleus and the superior cerebellar peduncle. It is initiated by movement and tends to be maximal toward the termination of movement. The term "action" or "intention" tremor has been applied to cerebellar tremor.

RUBRAL TREMOR. Rubral tremor results from lesions involving the dentatorubrothalamic tract and is characterized by a rhythmic tremor of the limbs that is proximal in origin. Rubral tremor resembles cerebellar tremor in that it is accentuated by movement.

TREMOR OF HEPATIC ENCEPHALOPATHY. This type of tremor, also called asterixis, occurs in patients with acute or chronic liver failure and occasionally in chronic pulmonary insufficiency. It consists of an irregular flapping movement of the hands which is accentuated when the arms are outstretched.

METABOLIC TREMOR. Metabolic tremor occurs in conditions associated with disturbed metabolism or toxicity. It is a rapid rhythmic tremor affecting the fingers, lips, and tongue, occurring in hyperthyroidism, in alcoholism, and in chronic users of barbiturates.

ESSENTIAL OR FAMILIAL TREMOR. This type of tremor is absent at rest but occurs on movement and is accentuated by stress. It is not associated with any other neurologic abnormality and muscle tone is normal. It is often relieved by alcohol and mild tranquilizers.

PHYSIOLOGIC TREMOR. It should not be forgotten that tremor of the fingers, hands, and feet may occur in nervous and tense individuals during the stress of a medical examination.

Physiologic tremors may occur as a transient phenomenon after prolonged muscular activity.

Dystonia. Dystonia may be defined as "the prolonged maintenance of an abnormal posture" and occurs from lesions at several levels in the extrapyramidal system. It is seen characteristically in dystonia musculorum deformans and spasmodic torticollis.

Hemiplegic Posture. Chronic lesions involving the corticospinal tracts produce a triple flexion and adduction posture of the upper limb, which is held against the anterior surface of the thorax.

Involuntary Movements. Several forms of involuntary movements are recognized.

CHOREA. The movements of chorea are brief, irregular, and asymmetric and are present at rest but accentuated by movement. They affect any part of the body, producing grimacing in the face and jerking of the trunk and shoulders. When they first appear, they may be mistaken for restlessness or fidgeting in a child.

ATHETOSIS. The movements of athetosis have a slower, more fluid quality than those of chorea and usually consist of flexion and extension of the fingers, wrist, and elbow and abduction and adduction of the arm. These involuntary movements may be caused by release of primitive reflex movements. In athetosis, there is alternation from flexion of the hand (grasp reflex) to extension of the fingers (avoiding reaction), and the movements of the arm and head involve complex alternation between labyrinthine reflex postures and hemiplegic postures. Hence, athetosis may be considered as "dystonia in motion." The grimacing movements of the face appear to involve chewing movements (reflex chewing and biting) and sucking (reflex sucking) and swallowing movements.

CHOREOATHETOSIS. It is not unusual to see a combination of chorea and athetosis, particularly in patients with Huntington's disease. The term "choreoathetosis" is appropriate in such cases.

TARDIVE DYSKINESIA. This term was first applied to a rare state of restlessness of the limbs observed in patients with Parkinson's disease. It is now used to describe involuntary movements of the face, trunk, and extremities usually occurring after prolonged phenothiazine therapy (Chap. 5).

PSEUDOATHETOSIS.   Athetotic-like movements may be observed in a limb when there is a major impairment of sensation. This loss can occur at any level but is most likely to produce this picture with impairment of cortical position sense in parietal lobe lesions.

BALLISM.   Ballism consists of continuous irregular contraction of proximal limb girdle and axial muscles, producing complex asynergic movements with violent flinging of the extremities. These movements are augmented by physical effort or excitement, diminish at rest, and disappear during sleep. The term "hemiballism" denotes involvement of one side of the body.

Clonus.   Clonus is a repetitive, sustained stretch reflex. It is usually obtained in a severely spastic limb and may be obtained in any muscle. In practice, it is generally observed at the ankle and knee. To elicit ankle clonus, the patient is asked to relax and the examiner slowly dorsiflexes the foot, then maintains pressure upward. Rhythmic plantar flexion occurs as long as the stretching of the gastrocnemius and soleus muscles is maintained. Patellar clonus is obtained by grasping the patella between the thumb and index finger and jerking it toward the foot. Rhythmic movements of the patella occur as long as pressure is maintained due to stretching of the quadriceps.

Myoclonus.   Myoclonic jerks are lightning-like throwing movements of a limb or part of a limb. They tend to occur in diseases causing lesions within the neuron such as Tay-Sachs disease, inclusion body encephalitis, herpes simplex encephalitis, and Unverricht-Lafora type of myoclonus epilepsy. They have occasionally been seen in ischemic lesions of the brainstem reticular formation. These rapid, lightning-like movements are occasionally brought on by loud noises, flashing lights, and tapping or touching the limb (stimulus-sensitive myoclonus).

Myoclonic epilepsy is occasionally seen in epileptics with generalized seizures due to instability of cerebral neurons when they wake up in the morning. As a result, they may suffer from frequent excessive jerks of the limb when a movement is made, so that when they raise the hairbrush to brush the hair, the myoclonic response throws the hairbrush across the room.

Spasms.   This term is applied to many forms of muscular contraction arising locally in muscles or at any level in the nervous system.

MUSCLE CRAMPS.   Muscle cramps are painful spasms. There are many causes, which are discussed in Chapter 12.

HEMIFACIAL SPASM.   This condition is associated with irregular contraction of the facial muscles on one side of the face owing to irritative lesions of the facial nerve. A similar condition may occur after Bell's palsy.

BLEPHAROSPASM.   Apart from the blepharospasm that occurs with painful conditions of the eyes, reflex spasm is normally present in the newborn. The condition may recur in degenerative diseases of the brain as a release phenomenon sometimes associated with dementia.

OCULOGYRIC CRISIS.   This phenomenon occurs in the postencephalitic type of Parkinson's disease and may be seen occasionally in acute encephalitis. It consists of a tonic contraction of extraocular muscles with deviation of the eyes that may last from several minutes to several hours. The visual movement is upward but it can occur in any direction.

PALATAL MYOCLONUS OR NYSTAGMUS.   This is discussed in Chapter 6.

HICCUP.   Although hiccup is often produced by irritation of sensory nerves in the stomach or diaphragm, it can be produced by lesions in the medulla. Hiccup may be a feature of tumors infiltrating or exerting pressure on the medulla, rhomboencephalitis, infarction, vascular insufficiency, or toxic conditions such as uremia.

Seizures.   Any seizures witnessed by the examiner should be noted with care. Occasionally, epilepsia partialis continua may be mistaken for a tremor. Such continual partial epilepsy may appear monotonously for hours and days and be characterized by repetitive jerks of a finger or hand or part of the lower limb or face every two or three seconds. Simultaneous records of the EMG and EEG may show a cortical spike immediately preceding the muscular contraction. Partial or jacksonian seizures should be recorded in detail. Patterns of progression (e.g., twitching of the left side of the mouth or the left thumb or left hand followed by deviation of the head and eyes to the left and a left-sided convulsion consisting of clonic jerks of the left limbs) should be noted.

Tone.   Palpation of the muscles may reveal not only flabbiness or spasm but a peculiar, doughy consistency in muscular dystrophy, tenderness and firmness in myositis, and a cardboard consistency in type 5 glycogen storage disease of muscle (McArdle's disease).

The limbs and neck are then moved passively through full range of motion, comparing the two sides and palpating the muscle undergoing passive movement with one hand. This allows an estimate of the muscle tone or tonus, which is the result of the many reflex influences affecting the anterior horn cells. When the tone is normal, there is a slight resistance to passive movement. This is smooth, constant, and equal throughout the full range of motion. Tone is increased in spasticity and rigidity. In spasticity, the resistance to passive movement increases then suddenly decreases, producing the "clasp-knife" phenomenon. In rigidity, there is a steady increase in resistance to passive movement in both flexion and extension, and the muscle is felt to move like a ratchet, the so-called "cogwheel rigidity," which is a characteristic finding in extrapyramidal rigidity. In Parkinson's disease, rigidity appears first in the neck so that there is resistance to flexion and extension in the neck first, appearing later in the limbs.

In some cases of frontal lobe disease, the limb may be moved to counteract any movement made by the examiner. This is called paratonia or *gegenhalten*. In the acute stroke with hemiplegia, there is an initial period of hypotonia, and the limbs may be moved with great ease. There is little or no resistance to rapid passive movements. This is usually followed by a gradual increase in muscle tone resulting in a final state of spasticity.

Examination of Muscle Strength

Muscle strength may be quantitatively evaluated from 0 to 4+, where 4+ is normal and 0 indicates inability of the muscle to move a limb against gravity or to perform in a functionally useful manner. In myasthenia gravis, repeated contractions or prolonged muscular contraction will reveal progressive weakness.

Each muscle has its own segmental level of innervation in the spinal cord or brainstem (Table 1–6). Certain aphorisms are useful in deciding whether the muscle weakness is due to primary muscle disease (myopathy) or a peripheral neuropathy.

1. In peripheral neuropathy the weakness is usually distal and symmetric, whereas the weakness is generally proximal in myopathies.
2. When a patient presents with unilateral proximal weakness involving the shoulder girdle, the clinician should suspect the presence of a lesion in the brachial plexus.
3. If there is weakness of more than one muscle supplied by the same nerve, the lesion involves the nerve.
4. If there is weakness of more than one muscle, and the affected muscles are supplied by two different nerves arising from a single nerve root, the lesion involves a spinal nerve root. For example, weakness of the interossei supplied by the ulnar nerve (C_8T_1) and the abductor pollicis brevis supplied by the median nerve (C_8T_1), suggests a spinal nerve root lesion at C_8, T_1.
5. Some peripheral nerves have a pure motor function. Involvement of such a nerve will produce muscle weakness without sensory loss. For example, a lesion of the anterior interosseus branch of the median nerve results in weakness of the flexors of the fingers without any sensory loss.

More detailed examination of the hand and forearm should be performed in patients with suspected lesions of the medial, ulnar, or radial nerves. A scheme of examination by testing individual action of muscles is outlined in Table 1–7.

It is possible to test for the integrity of the three major nerves (median, ulnar, and radial) by testing movements of the thumb against resistance, i.e.

Flexion of the terminal phalanx of the thumb—flexor pollicis longus—median nerve
Extension of the terminal phalanx of the thumb—extensor pollicis longus—radial nerve
Adduction of the thumb—adductor pollicis—ulnar nerve

Evaluation of muscle strength is carried out by asking the patient to contract the muscle or muscle groups examined against manual resistance supplied by the examiner.

The patient is asked to flex and extend the neck against resistance offered by the examiner's hand (sternocleidomastoid, splenius capitis, and paravertebral cervical muscles). Elevation or shrugging of the shoulders against resistance tests the upper part of the trapezius, and bracing the shoulders backward tests chiefly the middle portion. In isolated trapezius palsy, with the shoulder girdle at rest, the scapula is displaced downward and laterally owing to the unopposed action of the serratus anterior. This is accented by abduct-

TABLE 1–6

Segmental Levels for Innervation of Muscles

Muscles	Level
Neck flexors	C_{1-6}
Neck extensors	C_1-T_1
Diaphragm	$C_{3,4,5}$
Levator scapulae	$C_{3,4,5}$
Rhomboids	$C_{4,5}$
Serratus anterior	$C_{5,6,7}$
Supraspinatus	$C_{4,5,6}$
Infraspinatus	$C_{4,5,6}$
Pectoralis major (clavicular)	$C_{5,6,7}$
Pectoralis major (sternal)	$C_{6,7,8},T_1$
Subscapularis	$C_{5,6,7}$
Latissimus dorsi	$C_{6,7,8}$
Teres major	$C_{5,6,7}$
Deltoids	$C_{5,6}$
Biceps brachii	$C_{5,6}$
Radial nerve	
Triceps	$C_{6,7,8}$
Brachioradialis	$C_{5,6}$
Extensor carpi radialis lg. and br.	$C_{6,7,8}$
Supinator	$C_{5,6,7}$
Extensor digitorum	$C_{6,7,8}$
Extensor carpi ulnaris	$C_{7,8}$
Abductor pollicis longus	$C_{7,8}$
Extensor pollicis lg. and br.	$C_{7,8}$
Extensor indicis	$C_{7,8}$
Median nerve	
Pronator teres	$C_{6,7}$
Flexor carpi radialis	$C_{6,7}$
Flexor digitorum sublimis	$C_{7,8},T_1$
Flexor dig. prof. II, III	$C_{7,8},T_1$
Flexor pollicis longus	$C_{7,8},T_1$
Abductor pollicis brevis	C_8,T_1
Opponens pollicis	C_8,T_1
Flexor pollicis brevis (superficial)	C_8,T_1
Ulnar nerve	
Flexor carpi ulnaris	$C_{7,8},T_1$
Flexor dig. prof. IV, V	$C_{7,8},T_1$
Hypothenar muscles	C_8,T_1
Interossei	C_8,T_1
Flexor pollicis brevis (deep)	C_8,T_1
Adductor pollicis	C_8,T_1
Upper abdominal	T_{6-9}
Lower abdominal	T_{10},L_1
Iliopsoas	$L_{1,2,3,4}$
Adductors of thigh	$L_{2,3,4}$
Abductors of thigh	$L_{4,5},S_1$
Medial rotators of thigh	$L_{4,5},S_1$
Lateral rotators of thigh	$L_{4,5},S_{1,2}$
Gluteus maximus	$L_5,S_{1,2}$
Quadriceps femoris	$L_{2,3,4}$
Hamstring (internal)	$L_{4,5},S_{1,2}$
Biceps femoris	$L_5,S_{1,2}$
Peroneal nerve	
Tibialis anterior	$L_{4,5},S_1$
Extensors of toes	$L_{4,5},S_1$
Peroneals	$L_{4,5},S_1$

TABLE 1–6 *(Continued)*

Segmental Levels for Innervation of Muscles

Muscles	Level
Tibial nerve	
Gastrocnemii	$L_5,S_{1,2}$
Soleus	$L_5,S_{1,2}$
Tibialis posterior	L_5,S_1
Flexors of toes	$L_5,S_{1,2}$
Intrinsic muscles of foot	$L_5,S_{1,2}$

ing the arm against resistance. The vertebral border especially at the inferior angle is *flared,* but this virtually disappears on flexion of the arm. These features help to differentiate winging of the scapula due to trapezius weakness from winging due to weakness of the serratus anterior. The serratus anterior is tested by asking the patient to push his outstretched arms against the wall or against resistance offered by the examiner. This will produce marked winging of the scapula in serratus anterior palsy, whereas abduction of the arm will produce little, if any, winging. Strength of abduction of the shoulders is now tested by having the examiner hold the patient's arm against his body while he attempts to abduct it. The movement cannot be initiated if the supraspinatus is paralyzed. The arm is then abducted to a horizontal position, and the patient resists the examiner's attempt to depress the limb. This function is impaired or lost in weakness or paralysis of the deltoid. The activity of the chief adductor of the upper limb, the pectoralis major, is tested by having the examiner place his hand on the medial aspect of the elbow and resist the patient's efforts to squeeze the hand between the elbow and thorax. The pectoralis major can be felt to contract during this maneuver if the anterior fold of the axilla is palpated between the fingers and thumb of the examiner's other hand.

The strength of the biceps and triceps muscles is evaluated by holding the wrist while the patient attempts to flex and extend the elbow. Next, strength of flexion and extension of the wrists is measured by having the examiner attempt to flex the patient's stiffly extended wrist. Pronation and supination of the wrist are examined in a comparable manner. Similarly, flexion and extension of the fingers are tested. Abduction and adduction of the fingers (important functions of the interosseus muscles) are tested by having the examiner hold the patient's extended fingers together while

TABLE 1–7

Actions of Muscles of the Forearm and Hand

Action	Muscle	Nerve
Pronation of forearm	Pronator teres	$M.C_6C_7$
Supination of forearm	Supinator ⎫	$R.C_5C_6$
	Brachioradialis ⎭	
Ulnar flexion of hand	Flexor carpi ulnaris	$U.C_1T_1$
Radial flexion of hand	Flexor carpi radialis	$M.C_6C_7$
Flexion of terminal phalanx		
Little finger ⎫	Flexor digitorum profundus	$U.C_8T_1$
Ring finger ⎬	Flexor digitorum profundus	$M.C_8T_1$
Middle finger ⎭	Flexor pollicis longus	$M.C_8T_1$
Thumb	Flexor digitorum sublimus	$M.C_7T_1$
Flexion of middle phalanx		
Flexion of proximal phalanx		
Little finger ⎫		
Ring finger ⎪		
Middle finger ⎬	Lumbricals	$M.C_8T_1$
Index finger ⎪		
Thumb	Flexor pollicis longus	$M.C_8T_1$
Flexion of little finger	Flexor digiti quinti brevis	$U.C_8T_1$
Abduction and adduction, of fingers	Interossei	$U.C_8T_1$
Abduction of thumb	Abductor pollicis brevis	$M.C_8T_1$
Adduction of thumb	Adductor pollicis brevis	$U.C_8T_1$
Abduction of little finger	Abductor digiti quinti	$U.C_8T_1$
Opposition of thumb	Opponens pollicis	$M.C_6C_7$
Opposition of little finger	Opponens digiti minimi	$U.C_8T_1$
Extension of hand	Extensor digitorum	$R.C_6C_8$
Radial extension of hand	Extensor carpi radialis	$R.C_5C_7$
Ulnar extension of hand	Extensor carpi ulnaris	$R.C_6C_8$
Extension of fingers	Extensor digitorum	$R.C_6C_8$
Extension of thumb	Extensor pollicis brevis and longus	$R.C_6C_8$
Extension of index finger	Extensor indicis	$R.C_6C_8$

the patient attempts to abduct the fingers. The examiner then interlaces his extended fingers with those of the patient, who attempts to hold them in place by adducting the fingers while the examiner draws his hand away.

Grip is tested by asking the patient to squeeze the examiner's fingers. In a normal person, maximal strength is attained immediately, whereas there is an appreciable delay in attaining maximal strength in patients with Eaton-Lambert syndrome, sometimes seen in association with carcinoma of the lung. After the patient has squeezed the examiner's fingers for a few seconds, he is told to release the grasp quickly. A persistence of contraction while trying to release the grasp is typically seen in myotonia. A sharp percussion of the thenar eminence, the deltoid, or the tongue results in a prolonged contraction in myotonic disorders. The ulnar nerve should be palpated in the ulnar groove for displacement, traumatic injury, or enlargement (as encountered in chronic interstitial hypertrophic neuropathy). If palpation

of the nerve gives rise to an "electric sensation" or paresthesias radiating to the fourth and fifth fingers (Tinel's sign), injury to the nerve may be assumed.

In cases of carpal tunnel syndrome, tapping the median nerve gives rise to paresthesias in median nerve distribution in the fingers.

To examine the abdominal muscles, the patient is asked to flex his neck or sit up from the lying position. If the upper recti are weak, the umbilicus will descend; if the lower are weak, the umbilicus will rise (Beevor's sign). The patient is asked to tense his abdomen, and the transversus and rectus abdominis can then be felt to contract. If the patient is paralyzed, the abdomen tends to protrude and the abdominal muscles cannot be contracted.

The strength of the muscles in the lower limbs is tested by manual manipulation in a similar manner. The patient flexes his hip in the sitting position while the examiner pushes the knee downward. If the hip flexors are weak (particularly the iliopsoas muscle), the examiner can overcome the patient's attempt at flexion. To test the extension of the hip, the patient, in the prone position with the knee flexed, tries to extend the hip against resistance offered by the examiner. Abduction and adduction of the hips are conveniently tested in the sitting position while the examiner resists these movements with the hand. Strength in the quadriceps femoris is tested by having the patient extend his leg while the examiner attempts to flex the knee. Conversely, the biceps femoris is tested by having the patient flex his knee while the examiner attempts to maintain it extended.

The strength of the anterior tibial muscles may be tested by everting and dorsiflexing the foot and toes against resistance.

The posterior tibial muscle is tested by asking the patient to invert the foot against resistance, with the foot in complete plantar flexion. This will eliminate the participation of the anterior tibial in inversion. To test the toe flexors, the foot is kept in neutral position, and the patient flexes the toes against resistance applied to the distal phalanges. In a patient with foot drop, weakness of inversion and toe flexion will rule out an isolated peroneal nerve lesion and direct attention to a more proximal lesion.

The gastrocnemius and soleus are tested by asking the patient to stand on one foot and raise himself up on his toes. These muscles can also be tested by plantar flexion of the foot against resistance. Minor degrees of weakness cannot be detected by this method.

The strength of the intrinsic muscles of the foot is tested during flexion, abduction, and adduction of the toes in much the same way as the corresponding muscles of the hand are tested.

Examination of Coordination

The patient is observed while sitting facing the examiner. In truncal ataxia (due to disease in the midline of the cerebellum), the patient has difficulty maintaining balance of the trunk, even in the sitting position, and tends to fall to one side. In muscular dystrophy there may be difficulty sitting up owing to weakness of the muscles.

In Parkinson's disease, the patient frequently has difficulty rising to the standing position from the sitting position because of truncal rigidity and difficulty in initiating movement. The patient tends to remain glued to the chair and keeps falling back into it, or at other times he tends to fall forward out of the chair in a stooped position.

In polymyositis, an inflammatory condition that has a predilection for the iliopsoas and limb girdle muscles, the patient has difficulty rising from a chair because of weakness of the extensors and fixators of the hips.

The patient is asked to hold the arms extended and supinated with the fingers extended and abducted and the eyes closed. The limbs and fingers should remain symmetric. Any abnormalities of posture such as dystonia should be noted and the presence of tremor recorded. Minimum weakness, undetected by testing of muscle strength, or impairment of position sense produces pronation and "drifting" of the affected limbs away from the original extended position.

The patient now opens his eyes and is asked to rapidly supinate and pronate the arms, pat the back of one hand with the palm of the other hand, and finally pat the back of one hand alternately with the palm and back of the other hand. These rapid alternating movements should be smoothly performed and symmetric in amplitude and rate. Rapid rhythmic movements are disturbed in cerebellar disorders with slowness, irregularity of rhythm, and overflinging of limbs. Frontal lobe lesions also produce slowing and loss of dexterity, but the movement is impaired, in such cases, due to motor dyspraxia.

Performance of rapid alternating movements is followed by finger-to-nose testing in which the patient is asked to alternately touch his nose and the examiner's outstretched index finger. This may bring out dysmetria (past pointing) or intention tremor of the upper limb seen in cerebellar disease. However, even slight weakness of the limb may profoundly affect this test, and interpretation of findings should be guarded if weakness is present.

When resting tremor is present, the patient should be requested to write his name and draw a spiral circle and straight line. This test produces a graphic record of tremor and is particularly useful when following patients receiving specific treatment to reduce tremor (e.g., in Parkinson's disease or benign essential tremor).

A record of the patient's handwriting is also useful in patients with tremor. The handwriting tends to be small and cramped in Parkinson's disease (micrographic) and large and clumsy in cerebellar disease.

Incoordination of the lower limbs has already been mentioned in testing gait. Additional tests of coordination useful in bedridden patients include the heel-to-shin test where the heel is run rapidly up and down the shin of each leg, rapid kicking movements of the feet, and wiggling of the toes. In disorders of the sensory peripheral nerves, the dorsal roots, and the dorsal columns, and in cerebellar ataxia, the heel-to-shin test is clumsily performed, rapid kicking movements are slow, and fine movements of the toes are difficult or impossible.

Examination of the Reflexes

It is customary to examine the reflexes from the head downward. Each reflex has a segmental level or levels of innervation within the neuraxis (Table 1–8).

TABLE 1–8
Segmental Levels for Innervation of the Reflex

Reflex	Level
Glabella	Corticopontine
Snout reflex	Corticopontine
Sucking reflex	Frontal cortex
Chewing reflex	Frontotemporal cortex
Jaw jerk	Pons, cranial nerve V
Grasp reflex	Frontal cortex
Pectoral	$C_{5,6}$
Biceps	$C_{5,6}$
Brachioradialis	$C_{5,6}$
Triceps	$C_{7,8}$
Finger jerk	$C_{7,8}T_1$
Abdominals	Upper T_{6-9}
	Middle T_{9-11}
	Lower $T_{11}-L_1$
Knee jerk	$L_{2,3,4}$
Ankle jerk	$L_5S_{1,2}$
Plantar reflex	Corticospinal tract
Cremasteric	L_1L_2
Anal reflex	$S_{3,4,5}$

Reflexes may be defined as involuntary motor responses to sensory stimuli. They are generally classified into the muscle stretch or tendon jerk type and the superficial type. In eliciting the muscle stretch reflex, the tendon or insertion of the muscle is briskly tapped with a rubber reflex hammer, and the resulting contraction is graded from 0 (no response) to 4+ (maximal or clonus response). In order to elicit the muscle stretch reflexes, the patient should be relaxed and limbs arranged so that the muscle to be tested is slightly stretched. The superficial reflexes are elicited by various types of tactile and cutaneous stimulation.

The Glabella Reflex

The glabella reflex is a superficial reflex elicited by lightly tapping the forehead between the eyebrows with the finger. If there is persistent blepharospasm and closing of the eyes, the reflex is positive, and this is evidence of damage to the connections between the frontal cortex and the facial nerve nucleus in the pons. This is frequently increased in Parkinson's disease, dementia, and diffuse tumors affecting the frontal lobe.

The Snout Reflex

The snout reflex is elicited by tapping the nose. If it is positive, there is an excessive grimace of the face. The anatomic significance is similar to that of the glabella reflex, but the snout reflex is most frequently elicited in pseudobulbar syndromes due to bilateral corticopontine lesions.

The Sucking Reflex

The sucking reflex is elicited by stroking the lip with the finger or a tongue depressor. The lips then pout and make sucking movements. This reflex is normally present in the infant but disappears after weaning. It reappears in diffuse lesions of the frontal lobe and is commonly noted in the dementias.

The Chewing Reflex

The chewing reflex is elicited by placing a tongue depressor in the mouth. If the reflex is present, reflex chewing movements of the teeth and jaws on the tongue depressor occur. Occasionally the jaw is clenched so tightly that the blade of the tongue depressor is removed with difficulty ("bulldog response"). Reflex chewing is seen in diffuse bilateral cortical lesions affecting the frontotemporal cortex (such as dementia, general paresis, and anoxic encephalopathy).

The Jaw Jerk

The jaw jerk is elicited by tapping each half of the mandible with a rubber hammer when the jaw is half open. This stretches the masseter and pterygoid muscles. If there is damage to the cortical innervation of the motor portion of the fifth cranial nerve, the jaw snaps or jerks closed. In unilateral frontal lobe lesions, the jaw jerk may be increased on the opposite side only.

The Grasp Reflex

The grasp reflex is elicited by stroking the palm of the patient's hand with the fingers of the examiner's hand. If the test is positive, there is flexion of the fingers of the patient's hand, and the examiner's fingers maintain traction on the patient's now flexed fingers. The patient may be unable to release the examiner's hand. At this point, if the examiner strokes the dorsum of the patient's fingers with his other hand, the reflex is immediately inhibited, and the patient's hand releases the examiner's hand. The reflex is normally present in the infant but usually disappears around three to nine months of age. The reflex is released in unilateral (on the opposite side) or bilateral lesions of the frontal lobe. If the lesions are diffuse, forced grasping and groping may result, in which case the patient is unable to refrain from grasping and groping at any object proffered to his visual field or touched by the palm of his hand. This is also seen in terminal congestive heart failure and anoxic or severe toxic states and indicates frontal lobe disorder.

The Pectoral Reflex

The pectoral reflex (C_5C_6) is elicited by having the examiner place his index finger over the anterior fold of the axilla containing the pectoral muscle and tap it with the reflex hammer. Usually there is little or no response, but in cortical spinal tract lesions above the fifth cervical segment, the resulting contraction is brisk and excessive.

The Biceps Reflex

The biceps reflex (C_5C_6) is elicited with the arm flexed. The tendon of the biceps is palpated in the antecubital fossa by the examiner's finger, and the finger is then briskly tapped. Normally, there is contraction of the biceps muscle with a jerk of the forearm. In corticospinal tract lesions, the reflex is brisk and excessive. In lesions of the peripheral reflex arc or in damage to $C_{5,6}$ segments of cord on the side being tested, the reflex will be absent or depressed.

The Brachioradialis Reflex

The brachioradialis reflex (C_5C_6) is elicited with the arm flexed and the forearm in the neutral position between supination and pronation. The tendon, just above its insertion at the wrist joint, is tapped with the reflex hammer.

The Triceps Reflex

The triceps reflex (C_6C_7) is elicited with the arms flexed or akimbo on the hips. The short tendon of insertion above the elbow is tapped

smartly and the belly of the muscle is observed for contraction.

The Finger Jerk

The finger jerk ($C_{7,8}T_1$) is elicited by asking the patient to flex the fingers. These are then grasped by the examiner's fingers and tapped with the reflex hammer so that the patient's fingers tend to be extended by the blow. Normally, there is little or no response, but in corticospinal tract lesions, there may be brisk and even violent contraction of the fingers. The Hoffmann reflex is another means of obtaining the same stretch reflex. The middle phalanx of the middle finger is supported by the examiner, and suddenly the terminal phalanx is snapped into flexion and released. After release, the phalanx rebounds into extension, evoking a stretch reflex of the flexors of the fingers, resulting in flexion of the fingers and thumb.

The Abdominal Reflexes

The abdominal reflexes are tested in six quadrants by stroking the skin of the abdomen with a pin toward the midline on both sides from above the umbilicus, parallel with the umbilicus, and below the umbilicus. Normally, the abdominal muscles contract below the skin touched, and the umbilicus moves toward the area stroked. In corticospinal tract lesions, the abdominal reflexes are lost on the ipsilateral side, and in segmental lesions of the cord, the abdominal reflexes may be lost only in the quadrant innervated by that segment. The abdominal reflexes are difficult to elicit in obese subjects.

The Knee Jerk (Patellar Reflex)

The knee jerk ($L_{2,3,4}$) (patellar reflex) is a stretch reflex of the quadriceps femoris muscle. The reflex is elicited with the patient in a sitting position and the knees flexed to 90 degrees over the edge of the examining couch or in the dorsal decubitus position with the examiner's hand lifting the knee from the bed. The patellar tendons of each side are then briskly struck with the reflex hammer.

The Ankle Jerk (Achilles Reflex)

The ankle jerk (L_5S_1) (Achilles reflex) is a stretch reflex of the gastrocnemius and soleus muscles. The reflex can be examined in the sitting or dorsal decubitus position by supporting the foot in the dorsi flexed position and striking the

Achilles tendon with the hammer. The reflex can be better elicited with the patient kneeling in the prone position with the knees flexed.

The Plantar Reflex

The plantar reflex is elicited in the sitting or lying position with one leg crossed over the other. The outer aspect of the sole of the foot is then stroked from the heel toward the small toe with a key or a blunt object. In normal individuals, the response is flexion of the foot and toes, which should be the same on both sides. An extensor plantar response (the sign of Babinski) is dorsiflexion of the great toe, fanning of the toes, and usually withdrawal of the foot. The extensor plantar response indicates damage to the corticospinal tract. In minor corticospinal injury, the response may consist only of a failure of the great toe to flex or flexion movement followed by extension.

The Cremasteric Reflex

The cremasteric reflex (L_1L_2) is elicited in the male by stroking the inside of the thigh with a pin. In normal individuals the testis rises on the ipsilateral side. The reflex is lost in injury to the corticospinal tract at or above the first or second lumbar segments of the spinal cord.

The Anal Reflex

The anal reflex is elicited by stroking the skin about the anal ring and perineum with a pin, which causes contraction of the sphincter. This is lost in lesions of the lower sacral segments.

The Sensory Examination

Sensation may be divided into primary or secondary types. In the primary type the impulses pass to the thalamus as simple sensations of touch, pain, temperature, and vibration. They are then projected to the cortex where the impulses are interpreted at the cortical level as secondary or discriminative sensation. For example, pinpricks will be felt at a thalamic level, but the number, location, size, and pressure of multiple simultaneous pinpricks will be interpreted as a function of the parietal cortex.

To some degree the examiner must rely on the subjective interpretation of the patient. If all patients were objective, alert, cooperative, intelligent, and not suggestible, there would be few difficulties. Unfortunately, this is not always the case, and sensory examination may be difficult and of questionable reliability. The testing should, therefore, be made as objective as possible and the reliability of the observations should be noted.

In general, a sensory chart should be completed (see Fig. 1–13) on all patients in whom sensory abnormalities are found so that the pattern of sensory abnormality can become a permanent part of the patient's record. Areas of loss of pain are mapped by vertical cross-hatching, touch by horizontal lines, and temperature by diagonal lines. The spinal segmental dermatomes are also shown in Figure 1–13. In peripheral nerve lesions, the sensory loss will be in the cutaneous distribution of that nerve, as shown in Figure 1–14.

Examination is carried out first in the dorsal decubitus position and then in the prone position so that back and front are recorded, as shown in Figure 1–13. The sensory examination is less satisfactory if carried out with the patient in the sitting position. In children and uncooperative adults, tests of pinprick and pain sensation should be left to the last.

Tests of Primary Sensation

Touch Sensation. Light touch is examined first using a wisp of cotton. The patient is asked to close the eyes, and the cotton is touched lightly over all parts of the limbs and trunk. The patient is requested to say "Yes" whenever a light touch is felt. The rhythm of touching and the areas examined should be varied to make the test as objective as possible. The patient should also be asked to identify where the touch was felt (tactile localization), which is a test of discriminatory (parietal lobe) function.

Temperature Sensation. Temperature sensation is tested with two large, dry test tubes containing ice water in one and hot water in the other. With the eyes closed, the patient is asked to identify whether the stimulus is hot or cold. The bodily sensation for temperature is explored in a similar manner to that used for touch. It is important not to alternate hot and cold but to vary the stimuli in a random manner.

Pain Sensation. Pain sensation is evaluated with a corsage pin held lightly by the shaft between thumb and forefinger. This tends to ensure equal light pressure over all areas tested as the pin will slide through the grip if too much pressure is applied. The test may be made objective by holding another pin with the head down, and the patient, with the eyes closed, is asked to report

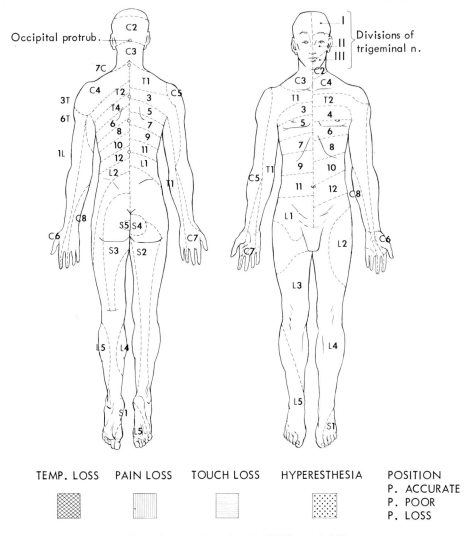

FIGURE 1–13. Sensory chart according to dermatomes.

whether the stimulus is sharp or dull. In uncooperative patients, a reflex withdrawal or grimace of the face will indicate whether the painful stimulus is felt. In general, primary sensation of pain, touch, and temperature should be tested from below up so that sensory levels and sensory loss in the distribution of roots and peripheral spinal nerves can be mapped out. Superficial pain and temperature are conducted in the medium-sized and small medullated fibers of the peripheral nerves to the spinothalamic tracts. Deep pain is tested by squeezing the Achilles tendon and the finger joints between thumb and forefinger. It ap-

pears, from clinical experience, that deep pain is conveyed by slowly conducting fibers, probably the small unmedullated fibers of the peripheral nerve via the dorsal columns, rather than the lateral spinothalamic tracts. Deep pain is lost or decreased in lesions of the dorsal columns and dorsal roots such as tabetic neurosyphilis, diabetic pseudotabes, and some tumors involving this region. Bilateral simultaneous stimulation with two pins may reveal sensory extinction (see p. 60).

Vibratory Sensation. Vibratory sensation (pallesthesia) is tested with a tuning fork (128

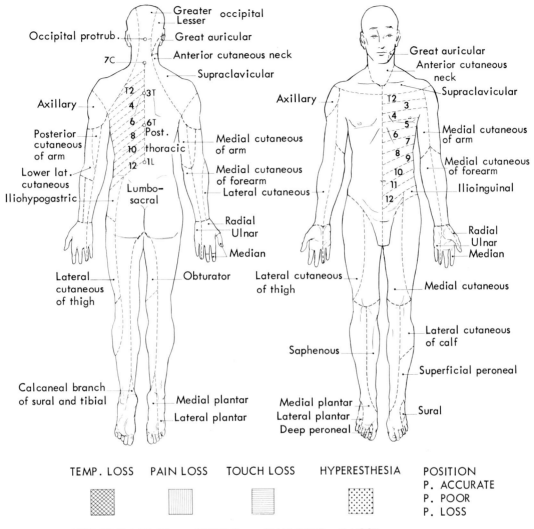

FIGURE 1-14. Sensory chart showing distribution of peripheral nerves.

cps). This is struck sharply on the examiner's knee and applied to the patient's toes, ankles, knees, anterior iliac spines, spinous processes of all vertebrae, the fingers, wrists, elbows, and sternum. In order to make the test objective, the vibration of the fork must be obliterated from time to time by grasping the prongs of the fork with the hand. The patient is asked to report whether vibration is felt and when it ceases. If the vibration sense is impaired, the vibration of the tuning fork will still be felt in the examiner's hand when the patient no longer appreciates the sensation. The base of the fork should always be firmly applied to bony prominences. The spi-

nous process of the vertebrae should be tested from below upward as a level of transection of the dorsal columns of the spinal cord can sometimes be localized in this manner.

Joint Position Sense. Joint position sense is tested by passive movements of the joints with the eyes closed. Normally, patients will identify small movements as small as 1 or 2 mm in a joint. In disorders of the peripheral nerve and dorsal columns, this ability will be lost. Since there are also discriminatory aspects to assessing joint position sense, it is also lost in the limbs opposite a lesion of the parietal cortex. The joints are usually tested from below upward, e.g., the toes, ankles, knees, fingers, wrists, elbows, and shoulders. The most severe loss of joint position sense is found in tabetic neurosyphilis, diabetic pseudotabes, and postinfectious polyneuritis.

Tests of Cortical Sensation

The ability to discern two-point stimulation, double simultaneous stimulation, numbers written on the skin (graphism), stereognosis, the position of a limb in space, joint position sense, and the weight of test objects placed in the hand (baresthesia) is an important function of the parietal cortex. These methods of testing parietal function will be valid only if primary sensation of touch and pain is preserved. Stereognosis is defined as the ability to identify objects by palpation.

Two-Point Discrimination. Two-point discrimination is tested with a pair of calipers or two pins. Different regions of the body vary widely in the capacity to discern two separate points of stimulation applied simultaneously at various degrees of separation. On the fingertips and lips, points within 0.5 cm of each other may be correctly identified, whereas on the trunk, two stimuli as far apart as 4 cm may be felt as one. Usually, the fingertips and pads of the toes are tested. After the nature of the test is explained, the patient is asked to close the eyes, and single and double stimulation are tested in a random manner, the stimulus being identified by the patient by the replies "one" or "two."

Double Simultaneous Stimulation. Double simultaneous stimulation should be tested with two wisps of cotton or two pins. One side of the body is stimulated, accompanied by a stimulus to the opposite side simultaneously. Usually homologous areas are stimulated, although this is not necessary. In parietal lobe disturbances, a single stimulus may be identified in the contralateral limb, but this will be extinguished during bilateral simultaneous stimulation (the phenomenon of "sensory extinction"). Sensory extinction may be demonstrated only in the arm, leg, or face. In such cases, this helps to further identify the lesion (e.g., medial parietal cortex for extinction of the leg, laterally placed lesion for extinction in the arm and face).

Identification of Figures Traced on the Skin. Identification of figures traced on the skin, or skin writing, is tested by writing numbers on the palm of the hands or fingertips with a sharp pencil. The digits, 1 to 9, are usually used and are tested in a random order, while the patient keeps the eyes closed. Ability to recognize digit writing is lost in the contralateral hand in parietal lobe lesions.

Stereognosis. Stereognosis is tested by placing small test objects in the supinated hands and requesting the patient to identify them. Commonly used objects are a nickel, dime, quarter, penknife, key, and pencil. Ability to identify objects by touch is lost in the contralateral hand in parietal lobe lesions.

Orientation in Space. Orientation in space is tested by asking the patient to hold a stick vertically, horizontally, and 45 degrees from the horizontal. The patient is also asked to find his way around the ward or to describe or draw how he would find his way to his home or some other well-known place. In lesions of the dominant parieto-occipital cortex, orientation in space is frequently lost. Cerebral dominance for orientation in space does not necessarily reside in the same hemisphere as cerebral dominance for speech.

Baresthesia. Baresthesia is the ability to discriminate the weight of objects held in the extended hands. A set of chemical balance weights is ideal for this purpose. The patient is asked to identify which is heavier. Most people can distinguish differences of the weights of 1 to 2 gm when two weights are held in each hand with the eyes closed. This ability to discern weights is lost in the contralateral limb in parietal lobe lesions.

Tactile Localization. Tactile localization is the ability to identify the part of the body touched by a piece of cotton or a pin. Most people localize accurately within 2 to 3 cm with the eyes closed. In parietal lesions, tactile localization is lost in the contralateral limbs, the stimulus usually being misplaced proximally to the site stimulated.

Allochiria. Allochiria is a confusion of sides (i.e., left from right). This is rarely seen in otherwise normal individuals as a congenital abnormality. There are frequent errors when the patient is asked to hold up the left hand or to identify the left side of a doll or picture of a man. This is a form of agnosia seen in lesions in or near the dominant angular gyrus as part of the Gerstmann syndrome (p. 7).

Identification of Body Parts.   Identification of body parts is tested by asking the patient to hold up or point to his ring, middle, and index fingers. Finger agnosia or inability to identify the fingers is also a part of the Gerstmann syndrome. The lesion has to be extensive before the ability to identify the thumb is lost. In severe lesions of the dominant parietal lobe, identification of all parts of the body may be lost, such as the hand and leg and face. The ultimate in such agnosia of parts of the body is seen in denial of a hemiplegia or anosognosia. In severe lesions of the parietal lobe, the examiner's hand is placed on the patient's affected limb, and when he is asked to lift up his limb, he may lift up the examiner's hand, under the impression that it is his own (autotopagnosia and anosognosia, see p. 8).

Imitation Synkinesia.   Imitation synkinesia may be observed in areas of the body where position sense and vibration sense are lost or severely impaired. Voluntary movements such as flexion and extension of a foot may be associated with flexion and extension movements of the ipsilateral hand. The abnormality is unilateral when position and vibration sense are lost on one side. It may occur on the opposite side when these sensory modalities are lost on both sides of the body. Affected individuals always show severe signs of sensory impairment seen in parietal lobe lesions (i.e., loss of two-point discrimination, etc.). However, imitation dyskinesia is not confined to parietal lobe or thalamic lesions but may be seen when there is severe loss of position sense and vibration due to lesions in the posterior column, brainstem, or higher centers.

Examination of Spine and Peripheral Nerves

While the patient is lying down, the neck is flexed to examine for nuchal rigidity such as is seen in meningitis and subarachnoid hemorrhage. In these conditions the neck is limited in flexion, while in the nuchal rigidity of Parkinson's disease, rigidity is present in all movements including extension as well as flexion.

In meningeal irritation, Brudzinski's sign may be present in which flexion of the knees occurs when the neck is flexed. Kernig's sign may also be present in spinal meningeal irritation. This sign is characterized by limitation of straightening of the legs with the hip flexed. In herniation of a lumbosacral disk, straight leg raising with flexion of the hip may be limited on the affected side owing to nerve root compression and irritation. The neck and hairline should be examined. The neck is short and the hairline low in bony malformations of the cervical spine. Limitation of movement of the spine may be present in degenerative conditions such as cervical spondylosis, when there is pain due to nerve root compression and when there may be an associated paravertebral muscle spasm. Nerve root compression in the lumbar region is usually associated with limitation in straight leg raising—Lasegue's sign. In certain conditions affecting the spinal cord, the paravertebral muscles are paralyzed, resulting in lordosis, scoliosis, and kyphoscoliosis of the spine. This is seen in conditions such as syringomyelia and poliomyelitis. Kyphoscoliosis of the lumbosacral spine is an important diagnostic sign in the spinocerebellar degenerations; however, it does not appear to be secondary to paralysis of the erector spinal muscles. Pes cavus is also seen in these conditions.

The examiner should palpate for enlarged peripheral nerves behind the elbow in the ulnar groove, in the neck, and over the neck of the fibula. Enlargement occurs in chronic interstitial hypertrophic neuropathy, Refsum's disease, and acromegaly.

Auscultation for the Presence of Arterial Murmurs (Bruits)

The neurologic examination is concluded by auscultation over the major vessels and the eye. Auscultation for murmurs is facilitated by the use of a bell stethoscope. The examiner listens over the carotid bifurcation on both sides and at the root of the neck just above the clavicles for subclavian artery murmurs. It is useful to auscultate the femoral arteries bilaterally when the peripheral pulses are absent at the ankles and in the feet. Stenotic lesions involving the lower aorta, iliac vessels, and femoral vessels often produce murmurs that can be heard at the level of the inguinal ligament with the stethoscope placed over the femoral artery.

Auscultation over the eye is performed by asking the patient to close the eyelids and placing the bell of the stethoscope over one eye. The patient is then asked to open the other lid, which immediately eliminates the roar of muscle contraction transmitted from the other eyelid. The examiner can then literally listen into the cranial cavity and may hear murmurs generated by arteriovenous malformations or a carotid cavernous sinus fistula.

2 PEDIATRIC NEUROLOGY

This chapter contains topics in pediatric neurology that are not discussed in other sections of this book. There are many neurologic problems common to both the pediatric and adult population. The conditions discussed in this chapter are always encountered in or begin in the pediatric age group and are not readily categorized with diseases discussed elsewhere.

Mental Retardation

Definition

Mental retardation may be defined as a state of arrested, incomplete, or retarded development of intellectual functioning characterized by inadequate adaptive behavior.

Approximately 5 million people in the United States can be classified as mentally retarded. Al-

most 3 per cent of newborn infants, some 126,000 per year, are mentally retarded. However, due to the increased mortality among retarded children, the overall prevalence in the population is about 2 per cent. The problem, of course, is not confined to children, but manifests itself in different ways according to age. The preschool child shows a lag in reaching the recognized milestones, particularly in retarded development of motor skills, locomotion, self-help, eating, and language. The severely retarded child is usually recognized at an early stage and frequently presents with an abnormal appearance recognized by the family and pediatrician. On the other hand, the mildly retarded child is often identified in school because development in the home has usually been satisfactory, and the child generally presents with a normal physical appearance. The adult who is mentally retarded has difficulty in remaining inde-

TABLE 2–1

Classification of Levels of Mental Retardation by Intellectual and Adaptive Criteria

Standard Deviations Below Mean IQ = 100*	Binet IQ†	Wechsler IQ‡	Designation	Adaptive Behavior
1–2	68–83	70–85	Borderline	Slow learner, may be emotionally normal
2–3	52–67	55–69	Mild	Educable to perhaps 4–5 grades, rarely more, sometimes employable
3–4	36–51	40–54	Moderate	Trainable in routine tasks and self-help skills, usually custodial
4–5	20–35	25–39	Severe	May learn minimal self-help skills; institutionalization required
5+	<20	<25	Profound	Vegetative state

* Classification of American Association of Mental Deficiency, 1960.
† SD = 16 IQ points.
‡ SD = 15 IQ points.

pendent and in meeting employment requirements.

For the purposes of description, investigation, and treatment, the mentally retarded may be divided into five groups according to the severity of the intellectual and adaptive disorder (Table 2–1).

Etiology and Pathology

There is gradual and continuing progress in the identification of etiologic factors associated with the syndrome of mental retardation. Currently, it is possible to make a suggested diagnosis in about 75 per cent of cases of moderate or severe mental retardation.[271]* These cases fall into four groups.

1. Genetically Determined. Chromosomal abnormalities make a significant contribution to this group with Down's syndrome resulting in the largest number of cases.[165] Autosomal[251] deletions (e.g., *cri du chat*), supernumerary chromosomes, and sex chromosomal abnormalities are also encountered in smaller numbers.[257]

In mentally retarded children with normal karyotypes, a number of conditions that are inherited as an autosomal dominant trait may be recog-

nized. This group includes tuberous sclerosis, Noonan syndrome, and neurofibromatosis.

There are many more conditions that may be inherited as an autosomal recessive trait, most of which are included in the aminoacidurias and mucopolysaccharidoses.

The sex-linked recessively inherited diseases form a small group and include the Lesch Nyhan and Renpenning syndromes.[229]

2. Prenatal Abnormalities. A majority of cases in this group exhibit one or more developmental defects involving the central nervous system.

Fetal infection by rubella virus, cytomegalovirus, and possibly other viruses, infection by *Toxoplasma gondii,* irradiation, certain drugs, maternal alcoholism,[135] and an active immune process in the mother have been identified as additional responsible factors in the prenatal period.

3. Perinatal Conditions. The commonest causes of mental retardation occurring around the time of birth include cerebral hemorrhage, subdural hemorrhage, hydrocephalus, kernicterus, and hypothyroidism.

4. Postnatal Conditions. Infections including meningitis and encephalitis produce the largest number of cases in this group. Head trauma, ele-

* Superscript numbers refer to references cited at the end of the chapter.

vated blood lead levels,[54] exposure to other toxins, and poisoning make a significant contribution to the total. There is evidence that inadequate nutrition can affect the physiologic development of the brain.[137] The nutritional status of the mother during pregnancy and the child during the first few years of life may affect mental development, since the immature brain is vulnerable to malnutrition during this period.[80]

The effect of environmental deprivation must also be considered in the postnatal causes of mental retardation. A child may be severely handicapped by early experiences, particularly if he is already of borderline intelligence or retarded. The main factors affecting early development may be classified as (1) maternal, (2) institutional, and (3) familial, social, cultural, and economic.

MATERNAL FACTORS. The earliest stimuli to an infant's development are provided by contact with the mother. This should be warm, rewarding, nourishing, supportive, and responsive to exploratory attempts at learning and development. The normal maternal response is often modified by factors such as guilt, hostility, and rejection. The inability of the unwed and immature mother to care for her child or the fragmentary contact provided by the working or alcoholic mother may also influence the normal maternal response. A mother with psychiatric illness, a broken home, or debilitating disease may be unable to provide affectionate care, and a substitute mother may be totally inadequate.

INSTITUTIONAL FACTORS. The quality of surrogate maternal attention given to children in an institutional setting varies enormously, but the child is virtually certain to be deprived to some degree of maternal love. Certain institutions provide planned environmental activity and stimulation, which is essential to developing children, yet this is often inadequate. The situation may be virtually one of sensory deprivation, and such environmental inadequacy may contribute to the development of mental retardation.

On the other hand, there is some evidence that preinstitutional deprivation may be an important factor in determining whether a child will show a normal course of development regardless of the institution in which he resides.[17]

FAMILY, SOCIAL, CULTURAL, AND ECONOMIC FACTORS. During childhood the family environment provides the greatest stimulus for normal development. Lack of environmental stimulation depends on many factors.

Parents of low intelligence and low economic status tend to provide less intellectual stimulation. Such families also tend to live in a restricted social, cultural, and economic environment, which tends to further restrict these children.

There is evidence that the identification of culturally deprived children and their exposure to a structured nursery and preschool program may reduce mental retardation in this group, particularly in children with mild degrees of mental retardation.

Despite impressive advances, the etiology of mental retardation is obscure or unknown in many cases, particularly in children with mild or borderline retardation. Many individuals in this group have brains of normal gross and microscopic appearance. However, some severely retarded children show abnormalities in cortical dendritic morphology. In some cases there is dendritic spine loss with the presence of long thin spines resembling the developing spines of primitive neurons.[208] These dendritic abnormalities are nonspecific in that they have been described in children with and without chromosomal abnormalities. The dendritic changes suggest the presence of an as-yet-unidentified factor in the immature brain that profoundly affects neuronal morphology and neuronal function. The abnormalities in dendritic development may be the basic pathologic process in some cases of mental retardation.[121, 209]

Another approach to the study of mental retardation is the identification of biochemical defects affecting neurotransmission. It has been demonstrated, for example, that blood serotonin levels are in some way related to severe mental retardation, but the significance of these findings is not yet clear.[196]

Diagnostic Procedures

The adequate evaluation of a patient with mental retardation is still largely dependent on the clinical examination.[76]

The history is particularly important. The following scheme is a suggested approach to the problem but may also be of value in the clinical examination of any child with a neurologic problem.

History

A. PRENATAL FACTORS
Unexplained maternal fevers suggesting viral infection

Exposure to known viruses that might damage the fetal brain, e.g., rubella

Medication taken by the mother during pregnancy, e.g., diphenylhydantoin

Maternal exposure to alcohol

Character of fetal movements

Maternal nutrition during pregnancy

Maternal diabetes mellitus

Toxemia of pregnancy

Threatened miscarriage

Placenta previa

B. PERINATAL FACTORS

Prematurity

Polyhydramnios

Breech presentation

Multiple pregnancy

Prolonged labor

Hypoxia or anoxia at birth

Need for resuscitation at birth

Need for incubator at birth

Presence of jaundice

Head circumference at birth

Birth weight

Apgar score

C. POSTNATAL FACTORS

Development milestones

1. *Smiling.* Children with IQ above 84 are smiling by 5 mo of age[227]
2. *Rolling over.* Present by 4 mo
3. *Reaching for objects.* Present by 5 mo
4. *Sitting.* Wide variation—may not occur until 14 mo
5. *Standing.* Present by 9 mo
6. *Walking.* Abnormal if not present by 18 mo
7. *Single words.* Present by 1 yr
8. *Sentences.* Present by 2 yr

D. PAST HISTORY

Head trauma

Subdural hematoma

Severe infections and electrolyte disturbances

Encephalitis

Meningitis

Hypoglycemia

Convulsions

Lead encephalopathy

E. FAMILY HISTORY

Other family members who appear to have similar problems or show slow development

Convulsions or seizures

Birthmarks

Café-au-lait spots

Consanguinity

Birthweight of all siblings, and maternal age when born

Siblings with problems in school

Gait difficulties or tremors in family members

Emotional problems in family members

F. SOCIAL HISTORY

Parental intelligence

Parental occupation

Socioeconomic status

Maternal deprivation

Schooling

G. GENERAL PHYSICAL EXAMINATION

H. NEUROLOGIC EXAMINATION. The neurologic examination must be modified according to the age and cooperation shown by the child. Children under 7 years should be examined in the presence of the mother. The examination begins with the child sitting on the examining table facing the examiner, with the lower limbs dangling over the table edge. As a minimum, the examiner should assess:

Behavioral state—whether alert, quiet, crying, or yelling

Social responsiveness—whether cooperative, reluctant, struggling

Sitting posture—presence of head tilt, dystonia, scoliosis, abduction or adduction of feet, involuntary movements

Movements while sitting—child sits quietly, is restless, hyperactive

Measurement of head circumference

Transillumination of skull

Shape of the cranium

Direction of the scalp hair—aberrant scalp hair patterns may be due to an early fetal problem and brain maldevelopment

Funduscopy

Visual fields

Pupillary reaction

Eye movements—strabismus, ataxia, nystagmus

Hearing—if dubious or impaired, request pure tone audiometry or auditory evoked potentials

Facial asymmetry, facial movements

Limb muscle tone and strength

Coordination—taking hold of offered objects, rapid alternating movements, finger-to-nose test

Standing—changes in posture, involuntary movements
Walking
Reflexes
Auscultation of the head for bruits

I. NEUROPSYCHOLOGIC EVALUATION. The spectrum of mental retardation can be divided at about IQ 50. When the IQ is above 50, the cause of mental retardation is likely to be familial or environmental. If the IQ is below 50, the child is likely to have a definite neurologic disease or acquired brain damage.

The neuropsychologist plays a critical role in the evaluation and treatment of mental retardation. Adequate neuropsychologic testing goes beyond assessment of intelligence scores and measures mental age, verbal skills, reading ability, and visual motor function. In addition, the neuropsychologist may be able to diagnose specific disabilities that correlate with brain dysfunction. It is equally important to clarify any emotional problem that may hinder the child in school. The advice of the neuropsychologist is essential in planning the education of the mentally retarded child.

Use of Ancillary Diagnostic Studies

There is a tendency to subject children to unnecessary diagnostic procedures. The neurologist should always feel that his logical assessment of the results of the history, examination, and any completed studies justifies a contemplated diagnostic procedure. Nontraumatic studies should be used whenever possible.

The choice of diagnostic studies for the child with mental retardation begins with a determination of the probable cause and the choice of one of four groups:[247] prenatal group, perinatal group, postnatal group, and undecided group.

Prenatal Group
A. Evidence of a single developmental defect
 1. CT Scan
B. Evidence of multiple congenital abnormalities
 1. Chromosomal studies of parents and child
 2. CT scan
C. Presence of seizures
 1. As for A or B above
 2. Electroencephalogram
 3. Check for hypoglycemia and hypocalcemia

Perinatal Group
1. Studies are indicated by the history and physical findings.
2. Electroencephalography and tests for hypoglycemia and hypocalcemia are necessary if seizures are present.

Postnatal Group
1. Studies are indicated by history and physical examination but should include the following:
 Serum phenylalanine level
 Serum and urinary amino acids
 Fasting blood glucose level
 Thyroid function tests
 Electroencephalography

Undecided Group
1. Buccal smear for X chromatin
2. Serum phenylalanine level
3. Electroencephalogram

Additional Studies

Skull Roentgenography. Skull roentgenograms are indicated in children with clinical evidence of craniosynostosis, hydrocephalus, increased intracranial pressure, cutaneous signs of tuberous sclerosis or Sturge-Weber disease, and evidence of prenatal infection by *Toxoplasma* or cytomegalovirus.

Long Bone or Spine Roentgenography. Patients with skeletal abnormalities or suspected mucopolysaccharidoses are candidates for this type of study.

Electroencephalography. The EEG is indicated in all cases with overt or suspected seizures.

Fasting Blood Glucose Levels. These should be obtained whenever the history suggests hypoglycemia.

Thyroid Function Tests. Congenital hypothyroidism may occur in the prenatal, perinatal, or postnatal group. Persistent indirect hypobilirubinemia and poor feeding warrant investigation for hypothyroidism.

Treatment

From the foregoing it is apparent that the problem of mental retardation requires a multifaceted as well as a multidisciplinary approach.

Prevention

A number of conditions associated with mental retardation can now be recognized before birth by use of amniocentesis. This group includes Tay-Sachs disease and Down's syndrome.

Cytomegalovirus infection in utero that produces macrocephaly and mental retardation can be prevented by vaccination of adolescent girls with a live tissue culture adapted strain of the virus.[68]

Phenylketonuria, which accounts for 1 per cent of the mentally retarded, can be diagnosed at birth before the development of brain damage by a relatively simple blood test. The early use of dietary treatment is successful in averting mental retardation in phenylketonuria. Biochemical screening at birth may be extended to detect other potentially treatable biochemical disorders.

Adequate medical and surgical treatment should be provided for the correction or palliation of developmental defects such as hydrocephalus, metabolic abnormalities, thyroid deficiency, and neonatal syphilis. Adequacy of medical and surgical treatment also assumes carefully planned and supervised prenatal, natal, and postnatal care of mother and child.

Family Support. Parents with a retarded child usually undergo profound emotional reactions as they learn to adapt to a situation that will produce a major change in their lives. The family physician or neurologist should act as long-term counselor and provide explanation, friendly encouragement, help, and understanding.

Social Services. There are usually services available in most communities to assist the retarded. These should cover all stages of development from infancy through preschool, adolescence, and adult life. The physician should be aware of the types of service available in the community and the methods of referral.

Education

There has been a tendency to reject the total segregation of mentally retarded children in meeting the special education needs of the group. This is particularly beneficial in the borderline or mildly retarded group, many of whom may benefit from being in the regular classroom with only occasional instruction in a special "resource classroom." This approach assumes that the school authorities have adequate facilities for the individual testing of children and the establishment of a "resource" or "learning" center.[79] Such programs are, however, available in only relatively few school districts, and screening with group intelligence tests is less satisfactory. However, educators are aware of the problem of education of the mentally retarded, and there will be increasing development of programs based on frequent movement between regular and special classes.

Speech and Hearing Clinics. The mildly retarded child usually has language defects or difficulties in hearing or reception of speech. The majority will benefit from evaluation and treatment in speech and hearing centers. This is particularly applicable to children with cerebral injury. A mildly retarded child with a speech or hearing impairment is often erroneously regarded as severely retarded by the untrained observer and incorrectly placed under institutional care. This results in severe emotional disruption and the development of anxiety and feelings of rejection. Such unjustified referral of patients to institutions leads to deterioration of the patient and overcrowding of institutional facilities so that the whole framework of the health program suffers.

The Multidisciplinary Approach. Adequate care of the mentally retarded may require the services of a pediatrician, neurologist, neurosurgeon, psychologist, psychiatrist, physiatrist, social worker, speech therapist, teacher, and family physician. There should be some common community center for treatment, education, exchange of ideas, research, and referral whether it be a hospital clinic, voluntary organization, or local, state, or federal agency. Experience teaches, however, that whenever there are several medical and paramedical persons involved in care of a single person, the physician (or other specialist) must provide the continuity of care.

Institutional Care. The more severely retarded child usually requires institutional care. In general, however, any child who can be adequately managed in the home is probably best cared for by parents in this environment. The physician's task is to advise the parents of the best available local institutions and private facilities and expedite referral and placement when the parents indicate that they believe such care is necessary. Just when this is achieved varies from family to family. Some parents with great ingenuity provide adequate care even for severely retarded children for many years and make adequate adjustment to the situation; others are unable to do so and their children require institutional care at an early stage. Attempts by the physician to provide more than advice and counsel on the question of institutional care may easily provoke resentment by the parents, and this should be avoided.

Developmental Defects

The most rapid changes in development of the central nervous system occur in the first three months of intrauterine life, and gross anomalies are likely to occur during this period. A number of agents have been implicated in maldevelopment of the nervous system. All of these act early in pregnancy. Fetal infection by the rubella virus and irradiation are two of the more common causes, while other virus infections, certain drugs, and genetic factors are often responsible factors.

The central nervous system is differentiated initially as an ectodermal thickening on the dorsal aspect of the embryo. At a very early stage, folding occurs with the formation of the neural tube. From that point in development the central nervous system remains a tubular structure, which undergoes many transformations in the process of maturation.

The important stages of development may be summarized as follows:

1. Closure of the neural tube
2. Development of the spinal cord
3. Development of the spinal ganglia and spinal nerves
4. Development of the brainstem and cerebellum
5. Development of the thalamus
6. Formation of the cerebral hemispheres and basal ganglia
7. Development of the eye
8. Formation of commissural projections and association fiber tracts
9. Formation of blood vessels
10. Development of the skull and vertebrae
11. Development of the autonomic nervous system

Stage 8 nears completion about the third month of intrauterine life. It is possible to recognize embryologic defects resulting from failure of or ab-

normality in development at any one of these stages. However, each stage should not be regarded as an independent process, since there is a great deal of overlap. A fault in development at any stage in cerebral morphogenesis may profoundly modify later development of the nervous system as a whole and its integrative action in terms of mental, motor, and sensory development.

Failure of Fusion of the Neural Tube

Family and epidemiologic studies indicate that the neural tube malformations of meningocele, encephalocele, iniencephaly, and anencephaly form an etiologically related group.[38] There is evidence that both genetic predisposition and intrauterine environmental factors are important elements in the development of neural tube defects. However, further identification of the genetic abnormalities and the environmental factors is still needed. The etiology of neural tube malformations remains obscure.

Types of Anomalies Involving the Spinal Cord

Meningocele. This is a defect in the posterior spinal canal with protrusion of dura and arachnoid and the formation of a cystlike structure containing cerebrospinal fluid.

Myelomeningocele. The defect is similar to meningocele except that in this case the sac contains spinal cord and/or nerve roots.

Complete Rachischisis. In this defect there is failure of fusion of the posterior spinal canal, the meninges, and the spinal cord.

Clinical Features

Meningoceles with absence of involvement of nervous tissue are rare and present with little or no neurologic deficit. The clinical presentation of the myelomeningocele varies from one with little neurologic involvement to one with severe neurologic deficits. The newborn infant with myelomeningocele may have paresis or flaccid paralysis of the lower extremities. Complete paralysis is more likely to occur in neonates with a thoracolumbar myelomeningocele. Sensory loss is difficult to demonstrate but can often be recognized by absence of response to pinprick. Hydrocephalus is occasionally present at birth but will eventually develop in 80 per cent of cases of myelomeningocele.[11] Hydranencephaly and severe malformation of the brain are contraindication to surgical treatment of myelomeningocele.

Children who survive with or without surgical treatment may show mild to severe paraparesis, loss of bladder and rectal sphincter contraction, sensory deficits in the lower limbs, and several types of orthopedic problems affecting the lower limbs.

Treatment and Prevention

Parents who have children with neural tube malformations have an increased risk of having further children born with similar malformations. The most promising method for antenatal diagnosis is amniocentesis at 14 weeks of pregnancy and analysis of the amniotic fluid for alpha fetoprotein content.[31, 164, 185] The levels of alpha fetoprotein are increased two- to tenfold in the amniotic fluid when the fetus has a neural tube defect. Corroboration of the suspected diagnosis may be obtained by ultrasonography in some cases.[77]

The surgical treatment of spinal meningocele and myelomeningocele has improved dramatically in the last decade.[10]

There is no doubt that the surgical treatment of a meningocele should be performed within 48 hours of birth. This minimizes the risk of meningitis, and the results are excellent in centers specializing in the treatment of this condition.[182, 254] Approximately 50 per cent of these children need further treatment for hydrocephalus, which usually develops by three months of age. The high risk of hydrocephalus requires careful follow-up of children with surgically treated meningocele. If the child shows clinical signs of increased intracranial pressure or the head circumference exceeds the ninety-seventh percentile line for age, a CT scan should be performed to detect ventricular dilatation due to hydrocephalus. A ventriculoatrial or similar shunting procedure is required to correct the hydrocephalus.[192]

There has been a recent change in attitude toward the treatment of infants with myelomeningocele with a shift in emphasis toward selection of cases for operation. Selection is based on the experience that many children with myelomeningocele have severe neurologic, urologic, and orthopedic defects and are unlikely to survive. Criteria have now been established to divide newly born babies with myelomeningocele into those who have a good chance of survival without severe handicap and those who are likely to either die within a few months or survive with a severe handicap.[61, 158] It has been recommended that surgery should not be performed in neonates with myelomeningocele and

1. Gross congenital anomalies such as microcephaly, severe cardiac deficits, ectopia of the bladder, or Down's syndrome
2. Roentgenograms of the skull indicating lacunar skull deformity
3. Gross hydrocephalus ⎫
4. Complete paraplegia ⎬ Two or more of
5. Severe kyphosis ⎭ these criteria
6. Thoracolumbar meningomyelocele

Some patients with paraparesis and paralysis of bladder and rectal sphincters require additional surgical treatment by orthopedic surgeons and urologists followed by an active physical therapy program.[212, 235] The ileal loop procedure is indicated in children with complete paralysis of bladder function, and surgical correction of deformities of the hips, knees, and feet improves lower limb function.

Spina Bifida Occulta

This is the most common defect involving the spinal canal and consists of a failure of fusion of the laminae, although the skin and superficial tissues are intact. The spinal cord and spinal nerves are usually intact, and spina bifida occulta is rarely associated with neurologic abnormalities. The asymptomatic spina bifida is not uncommon and does not require treatment.

Dermal Cysts and Sinuses

Dermal cysts and sinuses should be excised whether or not they are the cause of meningitis, since the sinus tract always terminates in the central nervous system.[168]

Lumbosacral Lipoma

Subcutaneous lipomas may or may not occur with a spina bifida. There is often extradural and intradural extension of these tumors, and children present with weakness in the lower extremities, gait disturbances, and abnormalities of bowel and bladder function. Roentgenograms of the spine usually reveal an underlying bony defect, and myelography is used to demonstrate the extent of the lesion and the involvement of the spinal cord. If possible, lumbosacral lipomas should be removed before the occurrence of neurologic deficits.

Involving the Cranium

Types of Anomalies. These include the following:

MENINGOCELE. The defect usually occurs posteriorly in the midline but occasionally develops in the frontal, nasal, and nasopharyngeal regions. This latter type of defect is particularly common in Southeast Asia.[256] The sac consists of dura and arachnoid containing cerebrospinal fluid.

MENINGOENCEPHALOCELE. This is a condition comparable to the spinal myelomeningocele with some brain tissue lying in the sac.

INIENCEPHALY. This is a rare malformation consisting of a defect in the occiput involving the foramen magnum, spina bifida of many vertebrae, retroflexion of the head on the spine,[152] and malformation of the brain, skull, and many other organs.[138]

COMPLETE RACHISCHISIS. The cranial bones completely fail to fuse, and this is often associated with a failure in development of the rostral portion of the neural tube and absence of the cerebral hemispheres (anencephaly). The forebrain may occasionally be represented by a small mass of undifferentiated neural tissue.

CRANIUM BIFIDUM OCCULTUM. Although this is considered the mildest form of defect in this area and may consist only of a small bony defect in the midline in the parieto-occipital area, there are occasionally some associated developmental defects in the brain.

DERMAL SINUS. A dermal sinus in the parietal or occipital and suboccipital regions may be the cause of recurrent meningitis (p. 467) since it affords a pathway for infection to enter the subarachnoid space. A preferred site of this rare condition, which may cause cerebellar abscess, is in the midline overlying the cerebellum. The sinus may also communicate with an extradural dermoid or a dermoid cyst within the substance of the brain. Periodic discharge of sebaceous material may cause a sterile meningeal reaction.

Diagnostic Procedures. The prenatal diagnosis of cranial neural tube defects is now possible by amniocentesis and determination of alpha fetoprotein in the amniotic fluid. This test should be performed when the mother is 14 weeks' pregnant in all cases where there is a previous history of a child with a neural tube malformation or where the child has been born with severe anoma-lies of the vertebral column. The value of increased maternal serum values of alpha fetoprotein in the early diagnosis of neural tube defects[32] needs further evaluation. It is possible that determination of serum alpha fetoprotein could be employed as a mass screening test with confirmation of suspected cases by amniocentesis or ultrasonography.

Treatment. Cranial meningocele and meningoencephalocele should be treated surgically as soon as possible with closure of the defect. There is no effective treatment for complete cranial rachischisis, which is rarely compatible with life for more than a few days' duration.

Anomalies of Development of the Spinal Cord

Duplication of the spinal cord (dystomyelia) and cleft of the spinal cord (diastematomyelia) are two rare congenital anomalies of the spinal cord. In diastematomyelia the spinal cord is divided anteroposteriorly by a deep cleft of fibrous or cartilaginous tissue, which may be attached to a bony septum arising in the midline from the spinal canal. The cleft may occur at any level but is most common in the dorsal and lumbar areas.

Clinical Features. Diastematomyelia may be associated with meningocele, congenital dermal sinus or dimpling, and pigmentation of the skin in the lumbar area. A heavy growth of coarse, dark or soft, downy hair rarely occurs in the midline over the defect. Neurologic findings include atrophy and weakness of muscles in a lower limb[157] and foot deformity.[131] There are, however, occasional extensor plantar responses. Sensory impairment may lead to joint deformities or ulceration of the feet. Sphincter control is usually impaired or lost. Patients are often seen first by orthopedic surgeons because of kyphoscoliosis.

Diagnostic Procedures

1. Roentgenograms of the spine may reveal a midline bony septum and widening of the spinal canal at the level of the defect. Bony abnormalities such as hemivertebrae or defects in the posterior arches, at the same level as the diastematomyelia, are common.
2. Myelography is characteristically abnormal with splitting of the dye column by a central

septum and widening of the dye column at the levels of the defect.

Treatment. Surgical removal of the midline septum may lead to some improvement in the neurologic defect.

Developmental Abnormalities of the Spinal Ganglia

The spinal ganglia are derived from a migration of neuroblasts from the neural crest during the closure of the neural groove to form the neural tube.

Congenital Indifference to Pain

Congenital insensibility to pain is a rare genetically determined condition inherited as an autosomal recessive trait.

Etiology and Pathology. Some cases do not have any demonstrative structural change in the peripheral or central nervous system and may represent an inborn error of metabolism affecting central pain receptors.[150] Other cases may be due to absence of the small primary neurons in the posterior root ganglia. Absence of these neurons is associated with absence of the small fibers in the peripheral nerves and reduction of Lissauer's tract in the spinal cord.[259]

Clinical Features. Pain sensation is absent from birth and affects the entire body. Since pain provides a protective reflex, the child suffers repeated injuries. There are numerous scars, chronic ulcerated wounds, and loss of tissue. Osteomyelitis, fractures and dislocations, and joint deformities (Charcot joints) may occur. There is loss of phalanges and the ala nasi. Corneal opacities may occur from repeated trauma to the eye. In some cases the child learns to avoid situations that may lead to injury. All other sensory modalities are intact, and the remainder of the neurologic examination is normal. There may be an associated anhidrosis in some cases.[169] Congenital indifference to pain must be distinguished from familial dysautonomia (p. 82) and hereditary sensory radicular neuropathy (p. 686).

Developmental Abnormalities of the Brainstem and Cerebellum

Dysgenesis of the Brainstem
Möbius's Syndrome

There is disagreement concerning the definition of this syndrome and consequently difficulty in defining the associated pathologic changes. The most satisfactory definition appears to be a condition in which there is a bilateral facial weakness usually associated with inability to abduct the eyes beyond the midline.

Etiology and Pathology. The condition is congenital and occasionally familial,[167] and the pathologic abnormality consists of:

1. A dysplasia of the seventh cranial nerve and sometimes other brainstem nuclei.
2. A primary dysplasia of facial and extraocular muscles.

Clinical Features. The essential features are bilateral facial weakness with wasting or absence of facial muscles. Usually there is absence of abduction of the eyes, and there may be an associated palsy of lateral gaze or even complete external ophthalmoplegia (due to either nucleus aplasia or absence of the external eye muscles). There may also be paralysis and wasting of the pharynx or tongue or involvement of other cranial nerves, absence of the pectorals, syndactyly, and, occasionally, associated mental retardation.

Dysgenesis of the Cerebellum

A variety of intrauterine developmental defects of the cerebellum have been described. The organ may be rudimentary with absence of the vermis and both hemispheres associated with the absence of the inferior olives and a small basis pontis. Other abnormalities include a small cerebellum, cerebellar microgyria, localized absence of the vermis, absence of one hemisphere, and absence of one hemisphere plus the vermis.

Clinical Features. The child may present with an ataxic form of "cerebral palsy" from birth or may show varying degrees of cerebellar dysfunction at age two or three when coordinated activity is in a stage of active development. The history usually reveals retardation in learning to sit, stand, and walk. The gait may be wide-based and ataxic and the lower limbs flaccid with decreased tendon reflexes. The upper limbs usually show dysmetria and intention tremor, and the speech is dysarthric. There is usually a tendency toward spontaneous improvement with advancing age. Familial agenesis of the vermis with episodic hyperpnea, abnormal eye movements, ataxia, and mental retardation has been described.[136]

Well-documented cases of congenital cerebellar defects have been reported without known clinical abnormality. The anomaly is then described as an incidental defect at necropsy.

The Optic Nerve and Retina

The causes of optic atrophy are discussed in Chapter 11.

The most frequent abnormality of the optic nerve is the presence of ectopic myelinated nerve fibers extending into the retina from the edge of the disk. They appear as a white triangular-shaped area extending out from the optic nerve. The condition is asymptomatic but may be associated with a scotoma corresponding to the site of the myelinated fibers.

Failure of fusion of the optic vesicle will produce a midline coloboma or retinal defect. This appears as a white midline cleft in the retina, which may extend to include the optic nerve head and the iris.

In congenital absence of the rods and cones, there is complete blindness with a normal appearance of the optic nerve head and retina. The appearance of the fundus is also normal in congenital night blindness.

Retinitis pigmentosa is discussed under neuronal degenerations (p. 185).

Septo-optic Dysplasia

Abnormal development of the optic nerves, optic chiasm, and optic tracts with anomalies of the midline structures of the anterior part of the brain has been recognized as septo-optic dysplasia. The condition is probably not rare and should be considered in blind children who show growth retardation.

Pathology. There is a failure in the full development of midline structures at any early stage of fetal development. This results in agenesis of the septum pellucidum, hypoplasia of the optic nerves, optic chiasm, and optic tracts, and maldevelopment of the hypothalamus, infundibulum, or pituitary.[109]

Clinical Features. Affected children are blind or have severely restricted vision and nystagmus from birth. Intelligence is normal but growth is retarded.[171] The pupillary reaction to light is sluggish, and the optic disk is hypoplastic with a characteristic "double-disk" appearance.

Diagnostic Procedures

1. The electroretinogram is normal.
2. Visual evoked potentials are abnormal.

3. There is severe depletion of growth hormone.[33]
4. Patients with panhypopituitarism may have hypoglycemia, hypothyroidism, and hypoadrenalism.
5. Absence of the septum pellucidum and dilatation of the chiasmatic cistern are readily demonstrated by pneumoencephalography. The abnormalities should also be demonstrated by CT scan.

Treatment. Endocrine hypofunction should be corrected by appropriate substitution therapy.

Developmental Disorders of Eye Movement

Congenital Nystagmus

Congenital nystagmus is a familial condition inherited as a sex-linked recessive or an autosomal dominant trait. The etiology is unknown. Some patients may have impairment of sensory input owing to cataract, optic atrophy, macular dystrophy, or congenital cone dysfunction, while others have abnormalities in the motor fixation system. However, these abnormalities are probably incidental, and there is evidence that the sensory input and peripheral motor systems are not involved in congenital nystagmus. The abnormality may be induced by faulty vestibular reflex activity or other malfunction of central reflex mechanisms concerned with the generation of saccadic movements.[57, 58]

The clinical features include:

1. Nystagmus described as either "pendular" or "jerk" nystagmus. Pendular nystagmus shows equal amplitude and velocity in both directions, whereas jerk nystagmus has a slow and quick component.[289]
2. The nystagmus is usually present at rest and increased in amplitude on lateral gaze.
3. The nystagmus is present at birth or appears in infancy.
4. Congenital nystagmus of both pendular and jerk type may present in latent form in which there are absence of nystagmus at rest and appearance of nystagmus on lateral gaze or on convergence only.[234]
5. There is often a positive family history.
6. There may be associated oscillatory movements of the head.
7. There is a significantly higher incidence of neurologic abnormalities, electroencephalographic abnormalities, and strabismus in patients and their families.

Treatment. Prisms may be prescribed to produce convergence when nystagmus increases on lateral gaze. This increases visual acuity and reduces eye fatigue.

Duane's Snydrome

Duane's syndrome is a not uncommon congenital disorder of ocular movement. The syndrome is inherited as an autosomal dominant trait in approximately 10 per cent of cases.

This condition is probably syndromic, and a number of different pathologic changes have been described. These include a central supranuclear abnormality, a central motor neuron disorder, a disorder of peripheral nervous innervation of the extraocular muscles, and a myopathy affecting the external rectus muscles.

Clinical Features. The abnormality is seen on eye movement and is characterized by

1. Limitation of abduction with widening of the palpebral fissure and protrusion of the eye on attempted abduction.
2. Narrowing of the palpebral fissure and retraction of the eye into the orbit on adduction. A downward and inward deviation of the eye may accompany adduction.

Duane's syndrome is often associated with one or more congenital abnormalities. These include oculoauriculo-vertebral dysplasia (Goldenhar syndrome), associated sensineural deafness and Klippel-Feil anomaly (Wildervank syndrome), spina bifida, cleft palate, paroxysmal gustatory lacrimal reflex, facial palsy, syringomyelia, and nerve deafness.[189] A familial abnormality transmitted as an autosomal dominant trait consists of Duane's syndrome, congenital heart disease, and congenital musculoskeletal defects of the upper limbs and hands (co-occurrence of the Duane and Holt-Oram syndromes).[74]

Spasmus Nutans

Spasmus nutans is an uncommon condition and may be a variant of congenital nystagmus.[134] Spasmus nutans occurs in both sexes and is said to be common in children who have spent most of their time indoors or in dark or dimly lit surroundings. There are three major symptoms.

1. Nystagmus is either horizontal, vertical, rotary, or mixed. It may be restricted to one eye and begins between the ages of 6 and 18 months. The nystagmus is abolished by head nodding.[98]
2. Head nodding is usually intermittent and is believed to be an operant conditioning response that has the effect of abolishing the nystagmus.
3. Head tilting occurs in about 50 per cent of cases. The neurologic examination is otherwise normal.

Treatment. The condition usually resolves within six months to one year after onset. It may occasionally present for three years.[113]

Maldevelopment of the Cerebral Hemispheres

Complete absence of the cerebral hemispheres (anencephaly) is associated with absence of the vault of the skull. The forebrain and midbrain are usually represented by a mass of neural tissue lying in the base of the skull. Less severe defects include absence of the forebrain and partial formation of the cerebral hemispheres, part of which may lie outside the skull (exencephaly). If these conditions are associated with an intact skull, there is an accumulation of cerebrospinal fluid, which transilluminates on examination (hydranencephaly). Children with hydranencephaly may appear to be normal at birth and exhibit reflex movements and sucking. There is a failure to thrive, and it is soon apparent that the infant is abnormal. Death used to occur within a few weeks of birth, but survival for many years is possible with modern medical care.

Forebrain malformations include alobar, semilobar, and lobar prosencephaly. In alobar prosencephaly the forebrain is represented by an undivided mass with a single ventricle. There are associated abnormalities of the basal ganglia, thalamus, and spinal cord. The condition is accompanied by facial anomalies including cyclopia,[141] ethmocephaly, and median cleft lip without philtrum[197] and may be familial.[140]

Less severe defects in the cerebral hemisphere occur as bilateral clefts that communicate with the ventricular system (schizencephaly) and in malformation of the gyri. Occasionally the surface of the hemisphere is completely smooth with absence of gyri (lissencephaly). In other cases, there may be numerous small gyri (microgyria) or wide gyri associated with a thick cerebral cortex (pachygyria).[105] Gyral abnormalities are associated with mental retardation and seizures.

One hemisphere may fail to develop normally with formation of a porencephalic cyst (Fig. 2–1) and mental and motor retardation.

Subcortical inclusion of gray matter (heterotopias) is not uncommon and may be asymptomatic, but the children are usually retarded and have associated epilepsy.

A developmental anomaly that is usually of no clinical significance is the persistence of a central cavity in the septum pellucidum (cavum septi pellucidi). The more posterior midline cavity (cavum virgii) is less common.

The majority of cerebral hemisphere abnormalities can be demonstrated by computed tomography.[84a]

Abnormalities in Commissural Projection and Association Fiber Formation

Although absence of specific fiber tracts such as the pyramidal tract has been described, the commonest example of this type of malformation is agenesis of the corpus callosum.

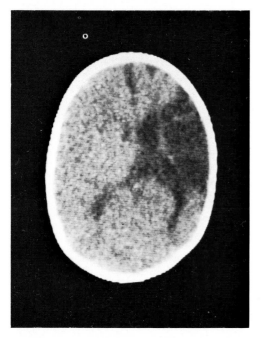

FIGURE 2–1. Computed tomography in a child with mental and motor retardation. There is an area of decreased density in the right hemisphere corresponding to a large porencephalic cyst. The frontal lobe is atrophic, and the right hemisphere is considerably smaller than the left hemisphere with dilatation and displacement of the ventricular system to the right side.

Agenesis of the Corpus Callosum

The causes of agenesis of the corpus callosum are unknown although there is some evidence that they may be genetically determined. Some possible etiologic factors are (1) deficiency in embryonic blood supply, and (2) impaired metabolism due to such factors as anoxia, intrauterine infection, and toxemia of pregnancy. There may be complete or partial absence of the corpus callosum and an association of other defects such as dilated ventricles, absence of the cingulate gyrus, microgyria, cerebral heterotopias, absent cranial nerves, and hydrocephalus.[157]

Clinical Features. This condition usually occurs as an isolated phenomenon. It may be asymptomatic if there is no associated cortical defect[71] and is frequently an incidental discovery at autopsy or an unexpected finding at pneumography. In cases with associated abnormalities of the brain, there are varying degrees of mental retardation and seizures. In a few infants there may be a rapid rise in intracranial pressure and hydrocephalus with tense fontanel and papilledema. The obstruction of the cerebrospinal fluid is usually caused by some associated anomaly.

The syndrome of agenesis of the corpus callosum, seizures, mental retardation, and areas of depigmentation of the pigmented epithelium of the choroid of the eye has been described. Affected children with this condition (Alcardi's syndrome) are all female and have a poor life expectancy.[55]

Agenesis of the corpus callosum may be associated with spontaneous recurrent hypothermia. The hypothermia is believed to be due to hypothalamic dysfunction, and selective gliosis of the hypothalamus has been described in some of the affected cases.[221]

Diagnostic Procedures

1. Diagnosis may be established by computerized tomography, which shows:[217]
   a. Wide separation of the lateral ventricles.
   b. A high third ventricle between widely separated lateral ventricles.
   c. Dilatation of the occipital horns of the lateral ventricles.
2. Neuropsychologic testing in agenesis of the corpus callosum, which is designed to evaluate interhemispheric transfer of information, may reveal subtle deficits in bimanual coordination, spatial orientation, transfer of kinesthetic

learning, and complex visual motor associations. Patients with agenesis of the corpus callosum do not show deficits in interhemispheric transfer of primary unilaterally represented stimuli, suggesting that there are alternative or compensatory mechanisms in affected individuals.[59, 70, 75]

Treatment. Seizures should be controlled with anticonvulsant medication, although control may be difficult in those with marked developmental abnormalities of the brain. Some children may require special schooling because of mental retardation. Surgical treatment may be necessary for hydrocephalus.

Abnormal Development of Blood Vessels

Arteriovenous as well as venous malformations of the brain and spinal cord and tumors of blood vessels will be considered elsewhere. Many conditions involving abnormalities of major cerebral vessels do not cause symptoms in early childhood because of adequate collateral circulation.[207] Aneurysm of the great vein of Galen may cause hydrocephalus and is often symptomatic during infancy. Patients may develop congestive heart failure. In such patients the mortality rate is high even if the condition is treated surgically.

Aneurysmal Malformation of the Great Vein of Galen

Extracranial arteriovenous aneurysms (arteriovenous shunting) occasionally attain sufficient size to produce cardiac failure of the high-output type at an early age. However, if cardiac hypertrophy and failure are due to an intracranial arteriovenous communication, this symptom usually appears in infancy.[92] Almost all recorded cases are examples of aneurysm of the vein of Galen, a rare condition that carries a high mortality rate. Heart failure can be reduced if the malformation is recognized early and treated surgically.

Etiology. The arteriovenous communication is believed to represent persistent embryonic communications between primitive vessels that develop on the surface of the neural tube. Aneurysmal dilatation of the vein of Galen is the result of shunting a large volume of rapidly flowing arterial blood through veins that lack the resistance of a vascular bed. This causes an enormous increase in cerebral blood flow, which often accounts for more than half of the total cardiac output.

Pathology. The vein of Galen is enormously dilated and may develop into a huge saccular aneurysm lined by thrombus (Fig. 2–2*A*). The dural sinuses are dilated, and the enlarged arteries feeding the anomaly are derived from the posterior communicating arteries. The aneurysm extends caudally to exert pressure on the quadrigeminal plate and aqueduct, causing hydrocephalus and ventricular dilatation. There may be ischemic or hemorrhagic infarction of the brain in areas drained by the vein of Galen.

The heart shows gross dilatation and hypertrophy, which involves predominantly the right atrium and right ventricle (Fig. 2–2*B*).

Clinical Features. The manifestations of aneurysmal malformation of the great vein of Galen are as follows:

1. The majority of cases present in infancy within a few hours or days following birth. The infants fail to thrive and develop cyanosis, dyspnea, and signs of congestive heart failure.[178]
2. In children who do not develop heart failure, there may be signs of hydrocephalus, progressive increase in size of the skull, and separation of the sutures.
3. At times this malformation may be asymptomatic during childhood yet may result in hydrocephalus in adult life. Subarachnoid hemorrhage, seizures, and chronic headaches are less frequent symptoms in children who survive without cardiac involvement.
4. Auscultation of the skull usually reveals the presence of a loud intracranial murmur.

Diagnostic Procedures.

1. The malformation is readily recognized by iodine-enhanced computed tomography.[123a]
2. The arteriovenous malformation is supplied by the vertebral basilar system and may be visualized by retrograde brachial arteriography or transfemoral catheterization of the aortic arch and selective arteriography of the vertebral basilar system.

Treatment. If the diagnosis is established before the development of heart failure, the aneurysm may be resected by intracranial approach. Patients in heart failure should be treated with

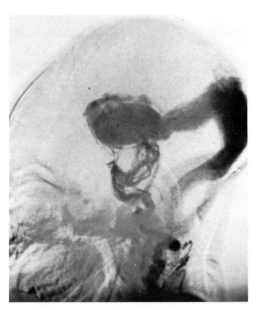
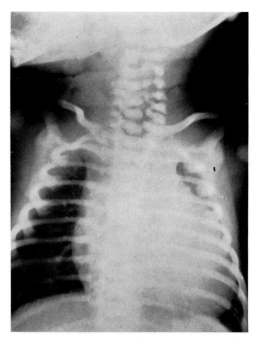

A   B

FIGURE 2–2. *A.* Selective vertebral arteriogram showing a large aneurysm of the great vein of Galen with abnormal arterial supply from the vertebral, basilar, and posterior cerebral arteries. The straight sinus and sigmoid sinus are dilated and filled rapidly by the shunting of blood through the aneurysm.

B. Same case showing cardiac enlargement due to the marked increase in cardiac output in response to the arteriovenous shunt.

digitalis, diuretics, and oxygen until they are in condition for surgery. The feeding vessels in the neck should be ligated as soon as the infant will tolerate the procedure. This will reduce both the cardiac output and the work load.

The mortality following surgical treatment is about 50 per cent.

Maldevelopment of the Skull and Vertebrae

Abnormalities in development involving the skull or vertebral column may affect the development of the brain and spinal cord. A considerable number of such abnormalities have been described, but only those regularly encountered in clinical practice will be considered here.

Craniosynostosis

Craniosynostosis is a nonspecific abnormality in which there is premature fusion of one or more of the cranial sutures.

Etiology and Pathology. The hypothesis that premature closure of a cranial suture is a primary event is no longer tenable. The developing calvarium is dependent on mechanical forces transmitted by dural fiber tracts running from the base of the skull to the calvarium. An abnormality in the development of the base of the skull produces abnormal forces that are transmitted through the dura to the calvarium and may produce premature cranial synostosis.[180]

Clinical Features. Three forms of craniosynostosis may be recognized:

1. PRIMARY CRANIOSYNOSTOSIS. There is synostosis of one or more of the cranial sutures producing an abnormal shape to the skull. There are no neurologic abnormalities, and intelligence is normal.
2. SECONDARY CRANIOSYNOSTOSIS. Craniosynostosis occurs as a secondary phenomenon in

such conditions as rickets, vitamin D–resistant rickets, and hypophosphatasia, and following excessive replacement of thyroid hormone in infantile cretinism.[204]

3. CRANIOSYNOSTOSIS SYNDROME. A large number of syndromes have been described in which craniosynostosis is associated with other congenital abnormalities. These syndromes, which are all eponymic, are inherited as autosomal dominant or autosomal recessive traits. Mental retardation, increased intracranial pressure, and seizures may occur in some cases.

The most frequently encountered condition in this group is the Crouzon syndrome. This syndrome presents with craniosynostosis, which is dependent on the order and rate of sutural synostosis. The cranial deformity may present as scaphocephaly, brachycephaly, or trigonocephaly. The orbits are shallow, and there are proptosis, strabismus, and hypertelorism. Optic atrophy occurs in most cases. Maxillary hypoplasia is prominent, and there is relative mandibular prognathism with drooping lower lip and a parrot beaked nose.[44]

Treatment. Surgical treatment of craniosynostosis should be directed toward the relief of increased intracranial pressure and the restoration of normal cosmetic appearance of the face and skull. The formation of artificial sutures in the calvarium has not been uniformly satisfactory, and modern surgery is now directed toward correction of abnormalities in the base of the skull.[78, 115] Hydrocephalus may be treated by a shunting procedure such as a ventriculoatrial shunt.

Craniocleidodysostosis

Partial failure of development of membranous bones may be associated with a variety of defects of the cranial vault, facial bones, and clavicles. This results in a highly characteristic appearance in roentgenograms (Fig. 2–3). There may be incomplete ossification of bones of the skull, particularly the frontal, parietal, and occipital bones. Persistence of anterior and posterior fontanels gives the skull a "hot cross bun" appearance. The bones of the face are small, the nasal bridge depressed, the palate highly arched, and the middle third or more of the clavicles fails to develop (Fig. 2–3). Children with craniocleidodysostosis are frequently retarded and suffer from epileptic seizures due to underlying maldevelopment of the

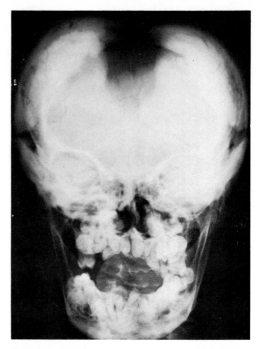

A

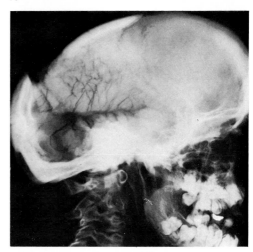

B

FIGURE 2–3.   Anteroposterior *(A)* and lateral *(B)* views of the skull in a case of craniocleidodysostosis showing bony defects in membranous bone.

brain. This includes dysplasia of the frontal lobes and anterior portion of the corpus callosum.

Microcrania and Microcephaly

A small skull (microcrania) associated with a small brain (microcephaly) is a common feature in mentally retarded children. Primary microcephaly may be genetically determined, probably as an autosomal recessive condition, or it may occur in chromosomal abnormalities, particularly Down's syndrome.[249] (Low levels of growth hormone suggest an associated pituitary hypofunction in primary microcephaly.[53]) Secondary microcephaly results from intrauterine infection by rubella or cytomegalovirus, asphyxia neonatorum, or neonatal trauma including the "battered baby,"[190] or following meningitis or encephalitis. Microencephaly occurs in about 2 per cent of the normal school population and is not uniformly associated with mental retardation.[232]

Macrocrania (Macrocephaly)

An unduly enlarged skull (macrocephaly) may be caused by increased sagittal sinus venous pressure and benign intracranial hypertension.[206a] Other cases occur in retarded children in whom there is an overgrowth of neuroglial tissue in the brain. The brain is morphologically normal but enlarged and weighs more than 1,900 gm.

Hypertelorism

Hypertelorism is a disproportionate enlargement of the lesser wings of the sphenoid bone associated with small greater wings of the sphenoid. This produces an excessive distance between the orbits and a flattening of the bridge of the nose. Hypertelorism is commonly seen in mentally retarded children and is characterized by a wide separation of the pupils (interpupillary distance) and an unusually broad junction of the base of the nose with the forehead.

Platybasia

Flattening of the base of the skull with invagination of the foramen magnum (platybasia) reduces the capacity of the posterior fossa and may exert pressure on and distortion of the upper cervical spinal cord, medulla, and cerebellum. The condition may present as a developmental anomaly, or it may be acquired later in life owing to rickets, osteomalacia, or Paget's disease in which case symptoms are much rarer. In either condition symptoms may not appear until adult life.

Clinical Features. Pressure on the spinal cord and medulla produces a progressive spastic quadriparesis sometimes accompanied by pseudobulbar signs and wasting of the tongue. Cerebellar ataxia and nystagmus may occur, and interference with the circulation of the cerebrospinal fluid may produce hydrocephalus.

Diagnostic Procedures. A roentgenogram of the skull should be made with laminography to demonstrate the foramen magnum. In the normal skull the angle formed by a line drawn from the glabella to the midpoint of the pituitary fossa and from this point to the anterior margin of the foramen magnum should be less than 140 degrees. This angle is increased in platybasia.

Basilar Invagination

Basilar invagination is an upward extension of the odontoid process, which projects into the spinal canal and compresses the spinal cord. It may be associated with platybasia or occur as an isolated abnormality. Progressive spastic quadriparesis and cerebellar signs similar to those seen in platybasia are often associated with this anomaly. This is believed to be due to compression of the brainstem and its blood supply by the odontoid process.[173]

Diagnostic Procedures. A lateral roentgenogram of the upper cervical region and foramen magnum shows that the odontoid process projects above a line drawn from the posterior aspect of the hard palate to the posterior margin of the foramen magnum (Chamberlain's line).

Treatment of Platybasia and Basilar Invagination. Removal of the posterior lip of the foramen magnum, laminectomy, and decompression of the spinal cord in the upper cervical level will relieve the pressure on neural structures and any associated hydrocephalus. Most surgeons advise opening the dura to ensure adequate decompression of the lower brainstem. Basilar invagination may be relieved by removal of the odontoid process through an anterior approach and subsequent fusion of the upper two cervical vertebrae.

Arnold-Chiari Malformation

The term "Arnold-Chiari malformation" is generally used for the syndromes due to congenital anomalies of the hindbrain. There are caudal displacement of the pons, the medulla, and the vermis of the cerebellum and elongation of the fourth ventricle.[263] The vermis and medulla lie within the upper cervical canal, and there is nearly always an associated myelomeningocele.[200]

Etiology and Pathology. The theory that this condition arises because of an "anchoring" of the filum terminale to the sacrum and downward traction of the spinal cord and brainstem due to the disproportionate growth of the spinal column and spinal cord is generally not accepted at the present time. The exact cause of the malformation is not known, but the early onset of hydrocephalus and indication of a hindbrain disorder suggest an abnormality in development involving the brainstem, posterior fossa, and upper cervical areas.

The vermis of the cerebellum usually extends downward into the upper cervical canal and may extend caudally for several inches. The medulla and fourth ventricle are also lengthened and lie within the cervical canal, and the medulla may be folded upon itself in an S-shaped fashion. There is usually a meningocele or myelomeningocele in the lumbosacral area and occasionally in the cervical area. Hydrocephalus, with dilatation of the lateral and third ventricles, is commonly associated with this condition. There may be associated aqueductal stenosis, or the herniation of the hindbrain may be responsible for the obstruction of flow of cerebrospinal fluid. There may be many associated congenital anomalies of the central nervous system including microgyria, fusion of the corpora quadrigemina, cysts of the foramen of Magendie, upward herniation of the cerebellum through an abnormally large tentorial notch, enlargement of the massa intermedia, fusion of the thalami, hydromyelia, and syringomyelia.

Clinical Features. The Arnold-Chiari malformation is manifested by the following:

1. There is usually progressive enlargement of the head in infants due to the hydrocephalus. Older children many complain of headache.
2. Malformation or compression of lower brainstem structures produces weakness and atrophy of the tongue and sternocleidomastoid and trapezius muscles with dysphagia due to weakness of the palate and pharynx. Venous congestion may produce discrete medullary hemorrhages with laryngeal stridor or respiratory obstruction which may be fatal.[179]
3. Cerebellar involvement leads to ataxia of all limbs, which particularly affects the gait when the symptoms are delayed until later in childhood.
4. Involvement of the descending corticospinal tracts, which may be secondary to hydrocephalus, produces spasticity, increased deep tendon reflexes, and extensor plantar responses.
5. Older children and adults have a somewhat different constellation of symptoms.[222] Pain in the suboccipital area, neck, and upper extremities is present in most cases and is often aggravated by neck movement. Headache occurs in the suboccipital area and is clearly precipitated by exertion. Weakness of the hands, spastic paraparesis, numbness, and paresthesias in the upper limbs occur in most cases.[88a] There are progressive ataxia of gait and dysphagia. Increasing numbers of cases of Arnold-Chiari malformation in adults have been described in association with syringomyelia.[18]

Diagnostic Procedures. These include the following:

1. Myelography reveals a defect in the upper cervical area corresponding to the "tongue" of cerebellar vermis projecting below the foramen magnum (Fig. 2–4).
2. Angiography shows abnormalities in the posterior inferior cerebellar artery. There are caudal displacement and deformity of the tonsillar hemisphere branches, visualization of the small tonsillar branches below the foramen magnum, and a caudal loop of the posterior inferior cerebellar artery below the foramen magnum. Films obtained during the venous phase will occasionally show the vermian veins lying on the surface of the cerebellar extension into the spinal canal.[84]

Treatment. In infancy, associated hydrocephalus should be treated by a ventriculoatrial shunt. Some children may develop signs of progressive brainstem compression with stridor, apneic spells, loss of gag reflex, and facial and arm weakness progressing to quadriplegia which requires suboccipital decompression and laminectomy.[114]

Chiari Type I Malformation

Herniation of the cerebellar tonsils below the foramen magnum without elongation of the medulla or fourth ventricle and without any associated form of spina bifida should be referred to as a Chiari type I malformation.[200]

The condition may be asymptomatic or may cause cerebellar signs and a progressive spastic quadriparesis, which can begin at any time during life. Syncope may occur due to transient increase in intracranial pressure induced by exertion.[60a]

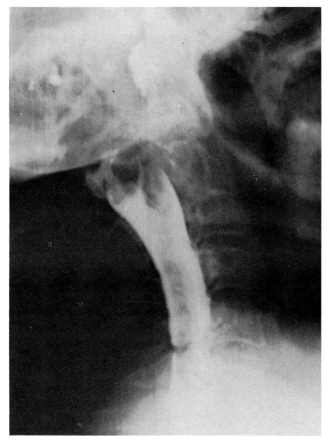
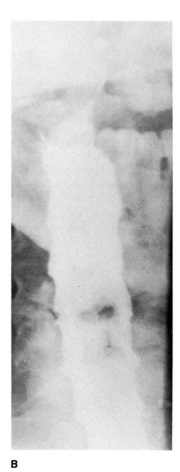

A   B

FIGURE 2–4. Myelogram in a patient with Arnold-Chiari malformation showing the characteristic downward herniation of the cerebellum and medulla. *A.* Lateral myelogram. *B.* Anteroposterior myelogram.

Diagnostic Procedures. Myelography shows a typical concave deformity of the column of dye immediately below the foramen magnum in both anteroposterior and lateral views.

Treatment. High cervical laminectomy and suboccipital decompression are indicated in cases with spastic quadriparesis.

The Klippel-Feil Syndrome

The Klippel-Feil syndrome is a condition in which there is fusion of one or more cervical vertebrae with reduction in the length of the cervical spine. The cervical spine may consist of a series of fused vertebrae including the atlas and axis with no more than three or four levels in which intervertebral disks are present. Other anomalies

of the cervical vertebrae such as hemivertebra and incomplete closure of the dorsal arch are frequent.

Clinical Features. The neck is short and the hairline low so that the head seems to rest on the shoulders. There may be folds of skin running from the ears to the shoulders. Head movements are reduced, and there may be an associated kyphoscoliosis or Sprengel's deformity (congenital elevation of the scapula). Neurologic findings include:

1. Synkinetic or mirror movements of limbs owing to failure of adequate decussation of the pyramidal tracts.[25]
2. Progressive spastic quadriparesis, which may rarely occur due to defective development of

the cervical cord with cervical spina bifida or associated Arnold-Chiari malformation.

3. The development of an associated syringomyelia later in life.
4. Deafness occurs in about 30 per cent of cases owing to malformation of the middle or inner ear.[200, 252]
5. Patients with Klippel-Feil syndrome have a high risk of associated deformities, including Sprengel's deformity, scoliosis, congenital heart disease, and renal abnormalities such as absence of a kidney, horseshoe kidneys, and hydronephrosis.[112]

Treatment.   Laminectomy and decompression are indicated when there is evidence of progressive compression of the spinal cord.

Sacrococcygeal Dystrophy

This is a defect in the development of the sacrum and coccyx usually associated with a developmental abnormality in the lumbosacral segments of the spinal cord.

Clinical Features.   Absence of the sacrum and coccyx produces a narrow pelvis and the iliac bones close the gap posteriorly. The normal contour of the buttocks is lost and dislocation of the hips may be present. Neurologic findings include flaccid paralysis of the muscles of the pelvic girdle and lower limbs, sensory loss in the lower limbs and sacral segments, and impaired sphincter control. The condition may be associated with arthrogryposis multiplex congenita involving the joints of the lower limbs. The same or a similar condition is sometimes found in diabetic families and is referred to as the caudal regression syndrome.

Maldevelopment of the Autonomic System

Familial Dysautonomia

A familial condition inherited as an autosomal recessive trait in which the predominant findings are due to autonomic disturbances has been described under the term "familial dysautonomia" (Riley-Day syndrome).

Etiology and Pathology.   There is evidence for a qualitative or quantitative abnormality in nerve growth factor in familial dysautonomia.[238] The abnormality is reflected in the pathologic changes

reported in the disease. The dorsal root ganglia, sympathetic ganglia, and parasympathetic ganglia show depletion of neurons with degenerative changes in surviving neurons and evidence of neuronophagia.[203, 213] Peripheral nerves show absence of large myelinated fibers and a marked decrease in the numbers of small unmyelinated fibers.[2] The abnormalities described in the autonomic ganglia are associated with failure of autonomic function.[202] There is absence of an increase in plasma norepinephrine and plasma dopamine beta hydroxylase activity on assumption of an upright posture after lying recumbent.[291]

Clinical Features.   Affected children are usually full-term, but breech delivery and low birth weight are common.[14] There may be difficulty in initiating respiration, and infants have episodic cyanosis, vomiting, unexplained fever, and difficulties in sucking. Death may occur in infancy or early childhood from aspiration pneumonia, and survivors show delay in physical and motor development. Absence of overflow tears is usually noticed at about three months of age, but corneal ulceration may have already occurred in some cases. Excessive sweating and blotchy erythema are often seen at mealtimes, while breath-holding spells with syncope are frequent up to the age of five years. Trauma produces little discomfort, and tongue ulceration occurs due to constant rubbing of the tongue against the teeth. Older children with familial dysautonomia are small with a nasal dysarthria, generalized hyporeflexia, and an unsteady gait. Surviving children often have a delayed puberty, limited exercise tolerance, and periodic lightheadedness on change in posture.

Diagnostic Procedures

1. Patients show miosis following instillation of a 2.5 per cent solution of methacholine into the conjunctival sac.
2. There is absence of fungiform papillae on the tip and sides of the tongue.
3. There is an elevated urinary homovanillic acid/vanillylmandelic acid ratio in the urine.
4. The cold pressor test fails to produce elevation of blood pressure. Postural hypotension is easily induced on a tilt table, and there is no rebound elevation of blood pressure with the Valsalva maneuver.
5. Intradermal injection of 0.1 ml of 1:10,000

histamine sulfate produces a wheal but no spreading flare.

Treatment. Bethanechol (urecholine), a parasympathomimetic agent, 0.2 to 0.4 mg/kg/day subcutaneously in four divided doses, has been used in this condition,[13] and some improvement has resulted. There is improvement in esophageal and gastric mobility, decreased abdominal distension, and less nausea and vomiting. Tear production and taste are restored to normal, and bladder control is improved with relief of enuresis.

Hereditary Diseases of Connective Tissue

Neurologic abnormalities occur in a number of hereditary diseases of connective tissue.

Chondrodysplasia Punctata

This rare congenital malformation has received considerable attention in the last decade because of a possible relationship to the use of anticoagulants during pregnancy.[151]

Etiology and Pathology. The etiology is unknown, but both genetic and environmental factors may be involved in this syndrome.[47] Pathologic changes consist of punctate proliferation of chondrocytes with calcification of the matrix in the epiphyses of long bones, vertebral bodies, and the sacrum.

Clinical Features. The condition is apparent at birth in infants presenting with hypoplasia of the nose, hypertelorism, frontal bossing, high arched palate, short neck, and short stature. Other less consistent features include mental retardation, cataracts, optic atrophy, congenital heart disease, renal anomalies, flexion contractures, and congenital dislocation of the hip.[260] A severe rhizomelic type has been recognized. This type is believed to be inherited as an autosomal recessive trait. The lesions are symmetric, and the prognosis is poor with death in the first year. The milder form of chondrodysplasia punctata (Conradi-Hunermann type) carries a good prognosis. This milder form has been linked to maternal hypothyroidism and the ingestion of phenacetin or warfarin sodium during pregnancy.

Diagnostic Procedures. The diagnosis of chondrodysplasia punctata is established by roentgenograms showing a characteristic stippling in cartilage throughout the body.

Treatment. Periodic respiratory distress in the first few weeks of life should be relieved by insertion of oral airway.

The Mucopolysaccharidoses

The mucopolysaccharidoses are a heterogeneous group of rare phenotypically similar, genetically distinct, inborn errors of acid mucopolysaccharide metabolism. There are currently several known types of mucopolysaccharidoses, and each is caused by a deficiency in a specific degradative enzyme. Enzymatic deficiency results in tissue storage and urinary excretion of various acid mucopolysaccharides.

Etiology and Pathology. The mucopolysaccharidoses are inherited as an autosomal recessive trait with the exception of type II, which is a sex-linked recessive condition. There is widespread accumulation of mucopolysaccharides in the tissues, including the neurons of the brain, spinal cord, and peripheral ganglia, which may be distended with stored material. There is also an accumulation of mucopolysaccharides in peripheral nerves, which interferes with myelin metabolism leading to accumulation of gangliosides in Schwann cells.[260] The various mucopolysaccharidoses and their enzymatic defects are listed in Table 2–2.

The effect of lysozyme uptakes of mucopolysaccharides in the neurons is unknown, but the following hypotheses should be considered.

1. The stored mucopolysaccharides are partially degraded by nonspecific endoglycosidases in the lysozymes. The accumulation of degraded material may interfere with the normal physiologic action of mucopolysaccharides.[47]
2. It is possible that degraded mucopolysaccharides may interfere with neuronal function by binding to receptor sites.
3. The presence of abnormal mucopolysaccharides may interfere with lysozomal enzymatic activity and affect the metabolism of sphingolysins.

Clinical Features. The various mucopolysaccharidoses are readily distinguishable clinically. The main clinical features are outlined in Table 2–2.

Features common to some of the mucopolysaccharidoses include:

1. Occular changes with corneal opacities, retinal degeneration, and optic atrophy.

TABLE 2–2

The Mucopolysaccharidoses

Type	Eponym	Enzyme Defect	Urinary Mucopolysaccharide	Mental Retardation
IH	Hurler	α-L-Iduronidase	Dermatan sulfate Heparan sulfate	Yes
IS	Scheie	α-L-Iduronidase	Dermatan sulfate Heparan sulfate	No
IH/S	Hurler/Scheie	α-L-Iduronidase	Dermatan sulfate Heparan sulfate	Yes—mild
IIA	Hunter severe	Iduronate Sulfatase	Dermatan sulfate Heparan sulfate	Yes
IIB	Hunter mild			No
IIIA	Sanfilippo	Heparan-N-sulfatase	Heparan sulfate	Yes
IIIB	Sanfilippo	N-Acetyl-glucosaminidase		
IIIC	Sanfilippo	α-Glucosaminidase		
IVA	Morquio	Chondroitin sulfate	Keratan sulfate	No
IVB	Morquio	N-Acetyl-Hexosamine-6-sulfate	Chondroitin sulfate complex	No

Type	Clinical Features	Roentgenographic Appearance	Diagnosis
IH	Inguinal and umbilical hernias at birth. Repeated respiratory tract infections. Hepatosplenomegaly. Marked mental retardation with language limited to a few words. Older children show large head, prominent forehead, root of nose broad and flat, eyebrows meet in midline. Lips full, tongue large, delayed dentition and teeth broad. Gingival hypertrophy. Neck short, chest broad. Congenital heart disease common. Hands broad, fingers short. Stiffness of interphalangeal, elbow, shoulder, knee, and hip joints. Vision impaired by corneal opacities, retinal degeneration, and optic atrophy. Quiet, cooperative children	Marked expansion of metacarpal shafts with pointed proximal ends of metacarpals. Distal ends of ulna and radius U-shaped. Lower thoracic and lumbar vertebrae egg-shaped with concave anterior and posterior borders. Acetabular cavity shallow, iliac wings widened, and pubic ramus lengthened. Skull scaphoid, sella tursica enlarged and J-shaped. Mandible broad and thick, clavicles short and thick. Ribs have spatulate appearance. Scapulae small, glenoid cavity shallow. Humerus broad and short	Demonstration of alpha-L-iduronidase deficiency in cultured skin fibroblasts or in leukocytes
IS	Mild disease. Dwarfism and mental retardation not features of this type. Corneal opacities and joint contractures occur later	Nonspecific	As for type IH
IH/S	Dwarfed individuals with similar facial appearance to type IH but mildly retarded	As for type IH	As for type IH
IIA IIB	As for type IH—with greater muscular strength, hyperactivity, and aggressive behavior. Corneas clear	As for type IH	Exclude type I by demonstrating normal alpha-L-iduronidase activity on cultured fibroblasts
IIIA IIIB IIIC	Growth and development normal until age 3 years. Gradual mental and neurologic deterioration with developmental features of type IH but normal growth maintained	Oval vertebral bodies. Spatulate ribs. Thick cranial vault	Type IIIA deficiency of heparan-N-sulfatase in leukocyte or fibroblast culture. Type IIIB deficiency of N-acetyl-alpha-glucosaminidase in skin fibroblast culture
IVA IVB	Mentally normal individuals with features of type IH	Anterocentral tonguing of thoracolumbar vertebral bodies. Hypoplasia of odontoid process. Delayed maturation of carpal bones. Short, broad metacarpals Marked U-shaped distal radius and ulna. Flaring of iliac wings, pelvic fossa shaped like a wineglass, shallow acetabular fossa, severe coxa valga	Characteristic appearance of roentgenograms. Demonstration of keratan sulfate mucopolysacchariduria

TABLE 2–2 *(Continued)*

Type	Eponym	Enzyme Defect	Urinary Mucopolysaccharide	Mental Retardation
VIA	Maroteaux classic	Aryl sulfatase B	Dermatan sulfate	No
VIB	Maroteaux mild	Aryl sulfatase B	Dermatan sulfate	No
VII	Sly	B-Glucuronidase	Dermatan sulfate Chondroitin 4,6 sulfate	Yes

2. Roentgenologic changes seen on complete survey of the skeleton.
3. Mucopolysacchariduria.
4. Hematologic findings with oval or round metachromatic inclusions in the lymphocytes in types 1H, 1S, and III. Coarse, closely packed, granular inclusions have been demonstrated in the neutrophils and eosinophils in types VI and VII. Reticular cells in the bone marrow show dense, round basophilic inclusions in type I and type II diseases. Plasma cells with polymorphic inclusions and large vacuoles are features of type III disease.
5. The presence of stored material or large cytoplasmic vacuoles in fixed biopsied material from many sites.

Treatment. It is not possible to supply specific purified enzymes to patients with mucopolysaccharidoses at this time. Replacement therapy is possible in the future but will be necessary at birth, since storage of abnormal mucopolysaccharides is already present at birth.

Family counseling should be directed toward care of the affected child and genetic counseling when parents desire further children.

Intrauterine diagnosis followed by abortion of an affected fetus is possible in the mucopolysaccharidoses after examination of cultured amniotic fluid cells.

Achondroplasia

Defective development of cartilaginous bone is responsible for the characteristic achondroplastic dwarf.

Clinical Features

The base of the skull shows defective development and is short, while the cranium shows an increased circumference with bulging of the forehead. The face is small, and the bridge of the nose is depressed. The extremities are extremely short, but the trunk has normal dimensions, although there is a marked lumbar lordosis due to anterior flaring of the sacrum.[184]

The condition is of interest to the neurologist because:

1. It may be associated with mild degrees of mental retardation.
2. Hydrocephalus is said to be common in achondroplasia, but the increased head size should not be misdiagnosed as hydrocephalus. Hydrocephalus with increased intracranial pressure and disturbance of cerebrospinal fluid circulation can be diagnosed by radioactive cisternography, which will demonstrate a cisternoventricular reflux.[60]
3. Some cases develop progressive spastic paraparesis due to platybasia or due to spinal cord compression in the small spinal canal. Compression in the spinal canal may be due to

Type	Clinical Features	Roentgenographic Appearance	Diagnosis
VIA	As for type IH but mentally normal	As for type IH	Presence of coarse packed granular inclusions in peripheral and bone marrow neurtrophils and eosinophils. Absence of aryl sulfatase B in skin fibroblast cultures
VII	As for type IH	As for type IH	Presence of coarse packed granular inclusions in peripheral or bone marrow neutrophils and eosinophils. Absence of beta glucuronidase activity in skin fibroblast cultures

herniation of one or more intervertebral disks, degenerative spondylosis, or anterior wedging of vertebral bodies in the thoracolumbar area.[162]

Treatment

The hydrocephalus, if present, may be nonprogressive and may not require treatment. It is possible that some cases may, however, require a ventriculoatrial shunt procedure.

Surgical correction of platybasia or cord compression by decompression may be necessary in cases with progressive spastic paraparesis.

The Chromosomal Abnormalities

1. Down's syndrome (mongolism)
2. Trisomy 13–15 (trisomy D) syndrome
3. Trisomy 17–18 (trisomy E) syndrome
4. Partial deletion of the short arms of chromosome 4 or 5 (B chromosome, cri-du-chat syndrome)
5. Aneuploid mosaicism
6. Sex chromosomal anomalies

There is a tendency for trisomies, monosomies, and aneuploidies to involve the progeny of older women, but no age group is free from risk.[125]

Down's Syndrome (Mongolism)

The production of a gamete with an abnormal number of chromosomes may occur during meiosis. The event is uncommon and the result is an abnormal fetus should fertilization occur. The best-known example of a chromosomal abnormality producing developmental defects is seen in Down's syndrome (mongolism), which occurs in about 1.6 per 1,000 live births. The condition is worldwide, affecting all races, and accounts for about 12 per cent of children who are mentally retarded.

Etiology

A number of genetic abnormalities have been recognized in Down's syndrome.

1. Trisomy 21. The total number of chromosomes is increased to 47 owing to the presence of an extra chromosome 21 (Denver classification). This accounts for 95 per cent of cases of Down's syndrome.

   There appears to be a linear relationship between increasing maternal and paternal age and the evidence of trisomy 21.[255]
2. Translocation 21 (13–15). These individuals have 46 chromosomes with translocation of a portion of a 21 chromosome to a chromosome in the 13–15 group.
3. Translocation 21 to 22.
4. Translocation 21 to 21 or isochromosome 21.
5. Trisomy 21—normal mosaic. There are varying proportions of 21 trisomic and normal cells.

In the case of translocation, the chances are high that one of the parents is a carrier of the translocation chromosome. Under these circumstances, all siblings and progeny of this carrier have a high risk of being carriers.

Pathology

The brain is usually underweight and the cerebellum and brainstem are particularly small. The superior temporal gyrus is also small and thin when compared to the other temporal lobe gyri. Microscopy is said by some to show some decrease in the neuronal population in the cortical gray matter although this is controversial.

Clinical Features

1. Children with Down's syndrome are small in stature and gain weight slowly in infancy and early childhood. Kyphosis and umbilical hernia are usually present.
2. The head is brachycephalic with a flattened occiput, and the ear is folded.
3. The face shows roughening and redness of the cheeks and a flat nasal bridge.
4. The eyes have prominent epicanthic folds and an oblique, slanting palpebral fissure. The iris may show spotty depigmentation (Brushfield spots). Nystagmus is usually present on lateral gaze.
5. The mouth is small and the tongue protruding but not enlarged. The teeth are also small. The lips are thickened and may show transverse fissures.

   The palate is narrow and has a high arch. Cleft lip and palate occur in 20 per cent of cases.
6. The muscles are hypotonic and the joints exhibit an unusual degree of mobility. If signs of bilateral cortical spinal tract involvement are seen, this should suggest the possibility of subluxation of the upper cervical vertebrae with spinal cord compression.
7. The hands are short and broad with shortened or tapered fingers. The fifth finger is curved and relatively shorter than the others. There is a prominent transverse palmar crease. The palmar dermatoglyphics are altered. The axial triradix, which usually begins at the wrist, is displaced forward into the palm.
8. The feet have an abnormal gap between the first and second toes. The soles show an absence of normal whorls or loops in the skin proximal to the hallux.
9. The neck is usually short and broad.
10. The abdomen shows some protrusion and diastasis recti.
11. The heart is abnormal in 40 per cent. The commonest congenital abnormalities are ventricular septal defects and patent ductus arteriosus. If hemiparesis is present, it may be the result of cerebral embolism in patients with congenital heart disease. Cerebral embolism may also lead to focal cerebral seizures.
12. The genitalia are small and puberty is delayed.
13. The bones show many abnormalities. The centers of ossification are greatly delayed in the wrist. The iliac wings are wide and flat, and the acetabular angle is narrow.
14. Intellectual function is usually severely impaired with an IQ of between 30 and 60. There is also a marked delay in the training of mental and motor functions. The patients are usually docile. Progressive organic dementia with neuronal changes similar to Alzheimer's disease may appear with increasing age (see Chap. 4).
15. The ten most discriminating signs of Down's syndrome are brachycephaly, oblique eye fissures, nystagmus, flat nasal bridge, narrow palate, folded ear, short neck, incurved fifth finger, gap between first and second toes, and muscular hypotonia.[130]
16. Life expectancy is reduced considerably and the cause of death is usually a respiratory tract infection or congenital heart disease. Some 30 per cent of children with Down's syndrome are dead by one month of age, 50 per cent by one year, and 60 per cent by the age of 16 years.[170]

Diagnostic Procedures

1. Roentgenographic confirmation of bony abnormalities may be obtained. The skull films show some degree of microcephaly. There is hypoplasia of the middle and terminal phalanges of the fifth fingers.
2. The neutrophils have a high alkaline phosphatase content and a reduction in the number of nuclear lobes. The neutrophils also have a decreased ability to combat pathogenic organisms,[51] which may account for the higher inci-

dence of infection in patients with Down's syndrome.

3. There is a dysgammaglobulinemia, which increases with age, characterized by increase in IgG and IgA and decrease in IgM. This may reflect a premature aging of the thymus-dependent immune system (which results in persistent antigenic stimulation)[231] or a genetically determined condition.[41]

Treatment

Prophylactic. Since 98 per cent of parents of children with Down's syndrome have normal chromosomes, diagnostic chromosome studies should begin with the patient. If there are 47 chromosomes present and trisomy 21, both parents may be presumed to be normal and further studies are not indicated.

If the patient has other than 47 chromosomes, a definite diagnosis should be made by repeated chromosome studies if necessary and studies of the parents performed to detect a carrier. All living blood relatives of any carrier should also be studied to detect other carriers. Genetic counseling must be based on the results of these studies.

X-Linked Mental Retardation Without Physical Abnormality (Renpenning Syndrome)

Approximately 10 per cent of moderately mentally retarded males of normal appearance have a family history of similarly affected male members. This suggests that mental retardation may be inherited as a sex-linked recessive trait in some families. All affected males have a normal neurologic and general physical examination. It has not been possible to identify any biochemical abnormalities in affected individuals at this time. The recognition of sex-linked mental retardation without physical abnormalities may account for the male preponderance of moderately mentally retarded individuals.[272, 273]

Trisomy 13–15 (Trisomy D) Syndrome

The trisomy D syndrome is rare, occurring in about 1 in 4,600 births. The infants are born a week or so before term and show gross developmental and mental retardation. The majority are microcephalic and apparently deaf and exhibit periods of apnea and frequent seizures. Harelip and cleft palate are usually present, the ears are

deformed, and there may be microphthalmos and coloboma of the iris. The hands show polydactyly, flexion deformity of the fingers with long, hyperconvex fingernails, and distal displacement of the axial triradix into the palm.[175] Males have undescended testes.

Congenital lesions of both heart and kidney are usually found in this condition. The brain may show holencephaly or other defects such as absence of the olfactory bulbs and tracts or may appear to be normal.[262]

Trisomy 17–18 (Trisomy E) Syndrome

It has been estimated that this condition occurs in 1 in 6,500 births. Because of marked developmental retardation and failure to thrive, the majority of infants die in the first weeks of life. These children have characteristic features with elongation of the skull, low-set, malformed ears, micrognathia, extra skin at the nape of the neck, or a webbed neck. There is a generalized hypertonia with limited hip abduction and a calcaneovalgus deformity of the feet. The chest is described as "shieldlike" with a short sternum. The fingers show a flexion deformity and the presence of three or more simple arches on the fingertips on dermatoglyphic examination. Nearly all children with trisomy E syndrome have congenital heart disease and may have congenital renal lesions.[244]

Partial Deletion of the Short Arms of Chromosome 4 or 5 (B Chromosome, Cri-du-Chat Syndrome)

The term "cri-du-chat syndrome" originates from the characteristic mewing cry that has been described in children with this condition. These infants are born at or near term but show a developmental and mental retardation. They are microcephalic with ocular hypertelorism, epicanthic folds, and micrognathia. The extremities tend to be hypotonic, and the hands show transverse palmar creases. Survivors lose the abnormal cry and show great variation in the severity of physical abnormalities and mental retardation.[46]

Aneuploid Mosaicism

A variety of clinically abnormal children have been described in whom there appear to be a mixture of at least two different cell populations. The commonest mixture is an autosomal trisomy/normal (47/46) mosaicism. This is usually a trisomy 21/normal mosaicism. Children with this type of mosaicism show stigmata of Down's syndrome with varying degrees of intelligence between normal intellect and mental retardation.

Sex Chromosomal Anomalies

At least ten examples of anomalies of the sex chromosomes have been recognized, many of which are associated with some degree of mental retardation. In the case of the X chromosome anomalies, it appears that the higher the number of X chromosomes in the nucleus, the greater the degree of mental retardation.[174] In the XO anomaly (Turner's syndrome), the defect is somatic, and the intelligence is frequently normal. Patients with the XXX anomaly are normal or mildly retarded, but those with XXXX or XXXXX defects are retarded, the latter showing a severe degree of retardation. In Turner's syndrome girls have absence of the ovaries, and this may be associated with Möbius's syndrome.

The most common anomaly of male genotype is the XXY anomaly, or Klinefelter's syndrome. While there is an increased frequency of XXY anomalies in the high-grade mentally retarded population,[251] many children with Klinefelter's syndrome show normal development, and the XXY karyotype is not necessarily associated with intellectual or emotional difficulties.[95] Other anomalies described in males include the XYY karyotype. Children with the XYY anomaly are also normal in appearance, intellect, and emotional development in the majority of cases. The association of the XYY karyotype with aggressive and antisocial behavior has not been confirmed in recent studies.[86]

Noonan's Syndrome

Children with Noonan's syndrome have a striking resemblance to females with Turner's syndrome. Noonan's syndrome occurs in both sexes and is inherited as an autosomal dominant trait.[15] It is possible, however, that the syndrome is not solely a genetic problem, and the Noonan phenotype may occur in offspring of alcoholic mothers.[103]

Children with Noonan's syndrome present with short stature, web neck, low posterior hairline, cryptorchism, small penis, increased carrying angle at the elbow, pectus excavatum, epicanthic folds, low-set or malformed ears, and mild mental retardation. Congenital heart disease, anomalies of the systemic arterial and venous systems, capillary hemangiomas, and lymphangectasia have been reported in about 50 per cent of cases.

Cardiac surgery carries an increased risk of complications in this syndrome due to the frequent multiplicity of congenital cardiac and vascular abnormalities and a reported higher risk of malignant hyperpyrexia during general anesthesia.[201]

The Aminoacidurias

Since the first report of the association of urinary phenylpyruvic acid with mental retardation in 1934 and the establishment of phenylketonuria (PKU) as a hereditary disorder of metabolism associated with progressive cerebral disorder, more than 30 aminoacidurias have been described, and undoubtedly more will follow. The aminoacidurias are uncommon and some are distinctly rare, but many resemble phenylketonuria in that they are associated with mental retardation and can be *prevented* or *minimized* by *adequate treatment.* To be effective, prevention requires early detection by screening procedures; otherwise, in neglected or unidentified cases damage to the central nervous system may become irreversible.

Classification

Transient Aminoacidurias of the Newborn. A number of amino acids may appear in the urine of newborn, particularly premature, children. Such transient aminoacidurias, tyrosine in particular, which occur within the first two or three months of life, are probably due to inefficiency of renal tubular reabsorption. These occur as a temporary phenomenon and are of no clinical significance except they make evaluation of aminoaciduria difficult during this early postnatal period.

Primary Aminoacidurias. In these conditions an enzymatic defect results in the blocking or modification of normal metabolic pathways usually of protein metabolism so that one or more amino acids exceed the renal threshold and are excreted in the urine. Primary aminoacidurias are all inherited as autosomal recessive characteristics.[67]

Secondary Aminoacidurias. Aminoaciduria may occur in a number of diseases producing liver damage that interferes with amino acid metabolism. It is not unusual to find aminoacidemia in severe acute hepatitis and cirrhosis including the cirrhosis of Wilson's disease. Other causes are heavy metal poisoning and exposure to hepatotoxic agents such as carbon tetrachloride. Interference with renal tubular reabsorption may also result in secondary aminoaciduria. This may be due to inherited conditions such as galactosemia, Fanconi syndrome, or oculocerebrorenal syndrome or to tubular damage following exposure to heavy metals (particularly lead) in children. Secondard aminoaciduria has also occurred following ingestion of aged tetracycline or following severe trauma or burns.

The primary aminoacidurias are of three types:

THRESHOLD AMINOACIDURIAS. In these conditions a metabolic block produces a hyperaminoacidemia and aminoaciduria when the concentration of the amino acid exceeds the renal threshold. These conditions exhibit elevated blood and urinary levels of the amino acid.

NONTHRESHOLD AMINOACIDURIAS. The metabolic block produces a substrate that is not concentrated in the blood but is immediately excreted in the urine because of the lack of active tubular reabsorption. Under these circumstances the blood levels of the amino acid are not increased and the diagnosis depends on detection of abnormal amounts in the urine.

RENAL AMINOACIDURIAS. In this type of aminoaciduria the metabolism of amino acids is intact, but there is a failure of the mechanism for reabsorption of one or more amino acids in the renal tubules. The blood levels of the amino acids are normal, and diagnosis depends on the detection of abnormal amounts in the urine.

Pathogenesis of Damage to the Nervous System in the Aminoacidurias

The hypothesis that changes in the central nervous system are due to toxic effects of high concentrations of one or more amino acids in the serum appears to be no longer feasible. In phenylketonuria, for example, there are occasional reports of individuals of normal intelligence who are entirely asymptomatic yet have maintained abnormally high serum phenylalanine levels for some time. Thus, the beneficial effect of low phenylalanine diets in babies with phenylketonuria is not believed to be due primarily to lowering the toxic effect of phenylalanine concentrations in the blood. The following points deserve consideration:

1. The hypothesis that abnormal concentrations of amino acids in the serum are neurotoxic may apply in some but not all cases.
2. If the amino acid is nontoxic, abnormal metabolites resulting from abnormal metabolic pathways of the amino acid may be neurotoxic.
3. High concentrations of the amino acid or its abnormal metabolic substrates may compete for nonspecific intracellular enzyme systems and cause a metabolic block in other amino acid systems.
4. The metabolic block leading to high concentrations of a particular amino acid prevents the formation of normal metabolic substrates. The deficiency of these substrates may lead to damage to the central nervous system.

Clinical Features

The majority of aminoacidurias are associated with some degree of mental retardation, and many of the children suffer from seizures. When either of these conditions is encountered in an infant or young child and the cause is obscure, screening tests for aminoacidemia and aminoaciduria are indicated.

Diagnostic Procedures

1. Screening tests for phenylketonuria in the newborn are mandatory in most states and may be performed with the Guthrie bacterial inhibition test or chromatographic methods.
2. In testing for a possible aminoaciduria, both blood and urine samples should be tested to reduce the risk of missing nonthreshold and renal aminoacidurias.
3. A positive ferric chloride test is unreliable in the early detection of phenylketonuria. The test is nonspecific and may be positive in phenylketonuria, tyrosinosis, maple syrup urine disease, histidinemia, oast-house urine disease, and alkaptonuria but may be useful in screening large groups of children for these abnormalities. All positive cases should have chromatographic examination of blood and urine.

Phenylketonuria (PKU)

This condition was one of the first of the aminoacidurias to be described and is the most frequent metabolic abnormality of this type associated with mental deficiency and neurologic disorder. The incidence may be as high as 1 per 10,000 to 1 per 12,000 according to screening tests.

Etiology

The absence of phenylalanine hydroxylase blocks the conversion of phenylalanine to tyrosine and results in an abnormally high concentration of phenylalanine in the blood. The normal and abnormal metabolic pathways of phenylalanine are shown in Figure 2–5.

Pathogenesis

The following abnormalities are theoretically possible in phenylketonuria. One or more may be responsible for the neurologic changes.[172]

1. High concentrations of phenylalanine may saturate the transport system that transports large neutral amino acids across the blood-brain barrier. This would result in an intracerebral deficiency of these amino acids and depressed protein and lipoprotein synthesis in in the brain.[6]
2. The damage may be due to an accumulation of abnormal metabolites, particularly phenylethylamine, which is believed to possess neurotoxic properties.
3. There may be inhibition of 5-hydroxytryptamine (serotonin) synthesis by competitive enzymatic inhibition of tryptophan hydroxylase by phenylalanine or its metabolites. The lack of serotonin may contribute to the cerebral dysfunction.
4. It is possible that there is inhibition of cerebral glutamic acid decarboxylase by hydroxyphenylpyruvic acid and lack of gamma amino butyric acid (GABA).
5. Tyrosine metabolism may be inhibited by high concentrations of phenylalanine resulting in low norepinephrine levels.
6. There may be an alteration in myelin synthesis or breakdown owing to interference with either protein or glycolipid synthesis by high levels of phenylalanine or its abnormal metabolites.

Pathology

The brain is normal in appearance but is usually underweight. The gray matter appears to be normal with normal neuronal content. There is a varying degree of pallor of the white matter owing to progressive demyelination, which may be severe in untreated adult cases. In most severe cases the white matter has a spongy appearance because of loss of myelin and reactive gliosis. Some sudanophilic breakdown products may be present, and the cerebroside content is reduced.

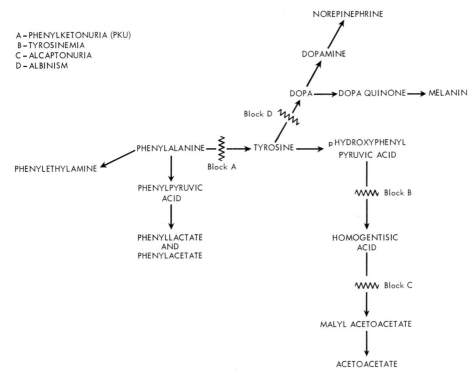

A – PHENYLKETONURIA (PKU)
B – TYROSINEMIA
C – ALCAPTONURIA
D – ALBINISM

FIGURE 2–5. The metabolism of phenylalanine.

Myelin deficiency suggests that there may be some abnormality in the metabolism of the oligodendrocytes, which show intracytoplasmic inclusions (PKU bodies) on electron microscopic examination.[191]

Clinical Features

There is some disagreement whether a child with PKU may be normal at birth. In all cases, signs of retarded development appear early and the child is often described as listless and feeds poorly. There is a lag in achieving the normal developmental milestones, and it is usually obvious that the child is retarded by six months of age. Sitting, standing, crawling, and walking are all delayed. Speech is late in development and is often severely limited. About 60 per cent of children with PKU are severly retarded, and the majority have an IQ level below 60. Seizures occur in about 30 per cent of infants with PKU but have usually disappeared by early adolescence. Some 30 per cent have eczema. The "typical" patient with PKU is said to have fair hair and blue eyes, but this is not always the case. Examination usually reveals a restless, hyperirritable child with a measured head circumference below normal for age. Apart from the mental retardation and developmental retardation described, gross neurologic abnormalities are infrequent. There may be some mild ataxia and incoordination, but the deep tendon reflexes are normal and the plantar responses are flexor.

Diagnostic Procedures

1. The Guthrie bacterial inhibition test is positive for elevated blood levels of phenylalanine. This is a useful test requiring a small drop of blood on filter paper.
2. Chromatographic methods are used in many centers as screening tests and may also reveal elevated blood phenylalanine levels.
3. Quantitative tests will reveal serum phenylalanine about 15 mg per cent with normal serum tyrosine levels (less than 5 mg per cent); urinary phenylalanine will be greater than 100 μg per milliliter, and urinary orthohydroxyphenylpyruvic acid will be greater than 10 μg per milliliter.
4. The electroencephalogram shows minor abnormalities until the age of six months, when more severe changes occur. About 15 to 25 per cent of patients show a pattern of hypsarrhythmia. Others show high-voltage sharp and slow waves or paroxysmal delta discharges.[280] Fifty per cent of the patients exhibit seizure patterns even though there is no clinical evidence of seizures. There is improvement on a phenylalanine-restricted diet, but spike activity and a hypsarrhythmic pattern may persist.

Treatment

The treatment of PKU is based on providing sufficient phenylalanine in the diet to meet the nutritional needs of the patient but not to exceed the limited capacity of the patient to metabolize it.

As soon as the diagnosis is established in the infant, the formula should be changed to contain about one sixth of the phenylalanine given to normal infants. The serum phenylalanine levels are measured frequently and maintained between 3 and 8 mg per cent. As the child grows older, changes in the diet are necessary and an expert dietitian is required in order to maintain a low dietary intake of phenylalanine.

The benefits of a low phenylalanine diet are less obvious in children with PKU detected after the age of three months. However, there may be slow improvement in intellectual capacity in some cases, which justifies the use of dietary treatment in all these children.

One of the diagnostic problems lies in the identification of children with hyperphenylalaninemia at birth who do not have PKU. Several types of phenylalaninemias have now been recognized that do not require treatment.[23] The differentiation of PKU and the phenylalaninemias can be made by giving phenylalaninemic subjects challenge diets and determining the serum phenylalanine levels and the urinary excretion of phenylalanine and its metabolites.

Prognosis

Many children have experienced normal mental development on the low phenylalanine diet. The treatment is generally accepted to be of value in early cases of PKU.[106] The question whether it is possible to abandon the diet in older children is not yet settled.

Patients with PKU who have normal intelligence and survive into adult life pose problems of marriage and genetic counseling.

Mothers with PKU may give birth to mentally retarded children due to the harmful effects of maternal phenylalaninemia on the developing fetal brain.[8] This type of problem in genetic coun-

TABLE 2–3

Primary Aminoacidurias

Disease	Amino Acid Increase	Type	Clinical Features	Treatment
A. *Phenylalanine tyrosine system disorders*				
Phenylketonuria	Phenylalanine	Threshold	Mental retardation, seizures, eczema, fair skin	Diet low in phenylalanine
Phenylalaninemia	Phenylalanine	Threshold	None—diagnose by diet challenge	None
Dihydropteridine reductase deficiency	Phenylalanine	Threshold	Severe progressive neurologic deficits	? biopterin or 6,7 dimethylpterin[246]
Tyrosinemia	Tyrosine	Threshold	Liver failure	Diet low in tyrosine
Neonatal tyrosinemia	Tyrosine	Threshold	Premature infants rarely last more than 1 month	High doses of ascorbic acid, 60 mg daily
Oasthouse urine disease	Phenylalanine, tyrosine, methionine, valine, leucine, isoleucine	Threshold	Mental retardation, white hair, seizures	Not known
B. *Sulfur amino acid disorders*				
Homocystinuria	Homocystine methionine	Threshold	Mental retardation, dislocated lens, seizures, thromboembolic phenomena	Some cases benefit from pyridoxine, 500 mg daily; others need diet low in methionine, high in cystine
Cystathioninuria	Cystathionine	Threshold	Mental retardation, congenital anomalies	Possibly large doses of pyridoxine
Sulfite oxidase deficiency	Sulfocysteine	Nonthreshold	Mental retardation, dislocated lenses	None
C. *Branched-chain amino acid disorders*				
Maple syrup urine disease	Valine Isoleucine Leucine	Threshold	Myoclonus epilepsy, mental retardation, spasticity, early death	Diet low in valine, isoleucine, leucine
Hypervalinemia	Valine	Threshold	Mental retardation	Diet low in valine
Isovalericacidemia	Isovaleric acid	Threshold	Offensive odor, mental retardation	Possibly diet limited in leucine
Hydroxyisovaleric aciduria	Leucine (plasma)	—	Spinal muscular atrophy, peculiar odor of urine	Diet low in leucine
Methylmalonic aciduria	Methylmalonic acid	Nonthreshold	Failure to thrive, acidosis	Large doses of vitamin B_{12}, 1,000 μg daily
D. *Disorders of urea cycle*				
Citrullinemia	Citrulline	Nonthreshold	Mental retardation, episodic vomiting, ammonic intoxication	Low-protein diet
Argininosuccinic aciduria	Argininosuccinic acid Citrulline	Nonthreshold	Mental retardation, seizures, abnormal hair, "trichorrhexis nodosa"	None
Arginase deficiency	Argininine	Threshold	Mental retardation, seizures, spastic paraparesis	Low-protein diet

TABLE 2–3 *(Continued)*

Disease	Amino Acid Increase	Type	Clinical Features	Treatment
Hyperlysinemia	Lysine	Threshold	Mental retardation, periodic coma, hyperammonemia	None
Saccharopinuria	Saccharopine	Nonthreshold	Mental retardation	None
Histidinemia	Histidine	Threshold	Mental retardation, language defects	Possibly diet low in histidine
E. *Miscellaneous aminoacidurias* Hyperprolinemia	Proline	Threshold	Type 1: mental retardation, seizures, deafness, renal disease; type 2: mental retardation, seizures	None
Ketotic hyperglycinemia	Glycine	Threshold	Severe ketosis, coma, death, newborns	None
Nonketotic hyperglycinemia	Glycine	—	Mental retardation, seizures	None
Hyper-β-alaninemia	β-Alanine aminobutyric acid	Threshold	Seizures	Seizures respond to pyridoxine
Carnosinemia	Carnosine	Threshold	Seizures, mental retardation	None
Hypersarcosinemia	Sarcosine	Threshold	Mental retardation	None
Hartnup disease	Tryptophan	Nonthreshold	Pellagra-like rash, cerebellar ataxia, photosensitivity	Nicotinic acid

seling is likely to become more frequent since there are now a number of aminoacidurias in which treatment is possible.

Other Aminoacidurias

The other aminoacidurias associated with neurologic abnormalities, usually seizures and mental retardation, are rare. A list of most of them described in the literature is given in Table 2–3.

Hypophosphatasia

This condition is a familial disease that is believed to be inherited as an autosomal recessive trait.

Etiology and Pathology

The disease is believed to be due to the lack of alkaline phosphatase activity in bone. There is failure to lay down apatite.

Clinical Features

The condition is indistinguishable from rickets. Premature synostosis of the cranial sutures may produce increased intracranial pressure and exophthalmus. Three types are recognized: (1) infants with lesions present at birth, (2) children who develop lesions after six months of age, and (3) a more benign childhood form of the disease. Children in this latter group show premature loss of deciduous teeth and development of dysplasic, discolored hypoplastic secondary dentition.

Diagnostic Procedures

1. The roentgenographic appearances are somewhat different from those of classic untreated rickets. There is a failure of epiphysial calcification with "notching" of the ends of the long bones, unlike the "cupping" seen in rickets.
2. Serum calcium and phosphorus levels are normal. Alkaline phosphatase activity is decreased in serum and leukocytes.[258]
3. Phosphorylethanolamine may be demonstrated in the plasma and urine in excessive amounts in hypophosphatasia.[210]
4. The prenatal diagnosis of hypophosphatemia is suggested by failure to demonstrate a fetal head by ultrasonography. The diagnosis is con-

firmed by the absence of alkaline phosphate in the amniotic fluid obtained by amniocentesis.[21, 219]

Treatment

There is no adequate treatment for this condition; vitamin D supplements have no apparent effect. Premature synostosis should be treated surgically.

Disturbances of Carbohydrate Metabolism: Hypoglycemia in Childhood

The effect of hypoglycemia on the infant brain may be severe,[42] resulting in repeated seizures, episodic stupor or coma, mental retardation, and ataxia.[127] All infants who develop seizures and retardation should be investigated for hypoglycemia. Early detection and treatment are important since they may prevent cerebral damage. These children are normal at birth.

The most frequent causes of hypoglycemia in childhood are listed in Table 2–4.

Disturbances of Glycogen Metabolism

Four of the glycogen storage diseases (types 1, 2, 3, and 6) may be associated with episodic hypoglycemia. The condition is most severe in type 1. It is milder and tends to be provoked by infection in types 2, 3, and 6.

Type 1

Etiology. A deficiency of glucose-6-phosphatase in the hepatic parenchyma results in decreased or absent release of glucose from the liver into the general circulation (Fig. 2–6).

Clinical Features. The disease is usually detected in the first year of life because of massive liver enlargement and retardation of growth and development. Fifty per cent of cases die in early childhood. Surviving children and adults develop seizures. Their skin has a yellow hue, and xanthomas develop on their elbows and knees. Older patients develop gout due to chronic elevation of serum uric acid. Some patients have a bleeding tendency because of platelet dysfunction.[120] A lipid storage myopathy with proximal muscle weakness and hypotonia has been reported.[287a]

TABLE 2–4

Hypoglycemia in Infancy and Childhood

1. *Disturbances of glycogen metabolism*
   a. Glycogen storage disease
   b. Deficiency of glycogen synthetase
2. *Galactosemia*
3. *Spontaneous hypoglycemia*
   a. Postprandial hypoglycemia
   b. Leucine-sensitive hypoglycemia
   c. Hereditary intolerance to fructose
   d. Functional failure of adrenal medulla
   e. Ketotic hypoglycemia
   f. Early manifestation of familial diabetes mellitus
   g. Idiopathic infantile hypoglycemia
4. *Neonatal hypoglycemia*
   a. Infants of diabetic mothers
   b. Infants of toxemic mothers
   c. Prematurity
5. *Islet cell disturbance (organic hyperinsulinism)*
   a. Hyperplasia of the islet cells
   b. Islet cell tumor
6. *Other endocrine disturbances*
   a. Adrenal insufficiency
   b. Pituitary insufficiency
7. *Hepatic disturbances*
   a. Viral hepatitis
   b. Bacterial cholangitis
   c. Toxins—carbon tetrachloride, chloroform, etc.
   d. Cirrhosis of liver
8. *Cerebral dysgenesis and hydrocephalus*
   a. Cerebrohepatorenal syndrome

Diagnostic Procedures

1. There is severe hypoglycemia.
2. Serum phosphate and serum alkaline phosphatase are decreased.
3. Serum lactate and pyruvate levels may be elevated.
4. Serum lipid levels are elevated.
5. Liver function tests are abnormal.
6. Impairment of renal tubular absorption results in glycosuria and aminoaciduria.
7. Epinephrine or glucagon injections produce little response because of inability to convert liver glycogen to glucose.[161]
8. The oral fructose tolerance test (0.5 gm/kg) fails to produce a rise in blood glucose due to a block in the conversion of fructose to glucose at glucose-6-phosphate.

Treatment. Frequent glucose feedings are given at intervals of three to four hours (night and day) to maintain normal cerebral develop-

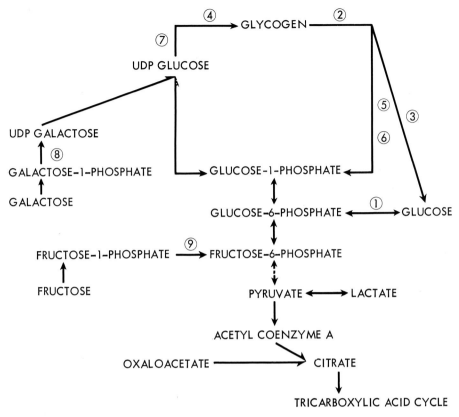

FIGURE 2-6. Pathway of glucose and glycogen metabolism (Embden-Myerhof pathway).

Number	Enzyme Deficiency	Disease
1	Glucose-6-phosphatase	Type 1 Glycogen storage
2	Alpha 1:4 glucosidase	Type 2 Glycogen storage
3	Amylo 1:6 glucosidase	Type 3 Glycogen storage
4	Amylo 1:4–1:6 transglucosidase	Type 4 Glycogen storage
5	Muscle phosphorylase	Type 5 Glycogen storage
6	Liver phosphorylase	Type 6 Glycogen storage
7	Glycogen synthetase	Glycogen synthetase deficiency
8	Galactose-1-phosphate uridyl transferase	Galactosemia
9	Fructose-1-phosphate splitting hepatic aldolase	Hereditary fructose intolerance

ment and minimize hypoglycemia and metabolic acidosis. Administration of diazoxide and surgical construction of a portacaval shunt (as a last resort) have also been advocated.

Type 2

Etiology and Pathology. The enzymatic defect producing generalized glycogenosis is alpha 1,4 glucosidase. This is a lysosomal storage disease with failure to degrade glycogen in lysosomes. Subsequently, the lysosomes enlarge. Glycogen metabolism outside the lysosome is normal. There is accumulation of glycogen in lysosomes in many organs, including the heart, liver, kidneys, adrenals, muscle, and central nervous system.

Clinical Features. There are several variants of alpha glucosidase deficiency, and infantile, juvenile, and adult forms have been recognized. The infant is usually normal at birth and well until the third month. Symptoms of vomiting, anorexia, failure to thrive, easy fatigue, weakness, dyspnea, and cyanosis appear at this time. There is evidence of cardiac enlargement and an apical systolic murmur. The muscles have a "doughy" feeling on palpation, and there is progressive weakness with hypotonia. There may be enlargment of the tongue and hepatomegaly in some cases. Hypoglycemic episodes have occurred during infections. Children who survive to the age of one year may show evidence of mental retardation. Death is due to heart failure or intercurrent infection. The condition may be confused with Werdnig-Hoffman disease (p. 128), but the absence of fasciculations of the tongue and differences felt on palpation of muscles help distinguish the two conditions. Juvenile and adult variants of alpha glucosidase usually present with chronic muscle weakness and wasting and are frequently misdiagnosed as muscular dystrophy.[69, 226]

Diagnostic Procedures. The fasting blood sugar, glucose tolerance test, and galactose and fructose tolerance tests are usually normal. Glucagon and epinephrine tests also show a normal response. The diagnosis may be established by the demonstration of decreased alpha 1,4 glucosidase activity in the tissues.

The leukocytes contain glycogen deposits, which can be demonstrated by suitable staining methods.

Prenatal diagnosis of generalized glycogenosis can be accomplished by electron microscopic demonstration of abnormal lysosomes within uncultured aminiotic cells.[19]

Treatment. The usual treatment for heart failure may produce temporary improvement, but there is no specific treatment for this disease.

Type 3 (Limit Dextrinosis)

This is a rare condition caused by the absence of the debranching enzyme amylo 1,6 glucosidase.[73] Glycogen synthesis is normal.

During degradation, the external branches of the molecule are polymerized by phosphorylase, leaving a residue that accumulates in the tissues. Further metabolic breakdown cannot occur in the absence of amylo 1,6 glucosidase. The abnormal glycogen is deposited in the liver, heart, and skeletal muscle.

The clinical picture is similar to type 1 glycogen storage disease with episodic hypoglycemia and retarded development. There is a low fasting blood sugar, acetonuria, and a diminished hyperglycemic response to epinephrine. Treatment is similar to that of the type 1 form.

Type 4 (Amylopectinosis)

Glycogen synthesis is abnormal in this condition. Molecules with long chains resembling plant starch are formed due to the absence of the enzyme amylo 1,4–1,6 transglucosidase.[19, 72] The abnormal glycogen accumulates in the liver, spleen, and intestinal mucosa, and there is progressive enlargement of the liver and spleen with ascites and death during the second year. Since 50 per cent of the molecules can be degraded by phosphorylase, there is a diminished response to epinephrine. Hypoglycemic episodes have not been recorded.

Type 5 (Absence of Muscle Phosphorylase, McArdle's Disease) and Type 7 (Muscle Phosphofructokinase Deficiency)

Hypoglycemic episodes do not occur in these conditions (see Chap. 12).

Type 6 (Defect in the Liver Phosphorylase System)

There are three variants of this condition: a true liver phosphorylase deficiency, a sex-linked recessive phosphorylase kinase deficiency, and an autosomal recessive phosphorylase kinase deficiency. The disease is mild, and affected individuals show asymptomatic liver enlargement and mild growth retardation. Treatment should be directed toward the prevention of hypoglycemia, which may accompany febrile illnesses in childhood.

Deficiency of Glycogen Synthetase

The enzyme glycogen synthetase is necessary for the conversion of uridyl-diphosphate (UDP) glucose to glycogen, and its deficiency produces a failure of glycogen synthesis in the body.[193] The condition cannot be referred to as glycogen storage disease since there is a marked absence of glycogen in the tissues, but it is related to this group of metabolic abnormalities.

Clinical Features. Children with glycogen synthetase deficiency present with profound hypoglycemia shortly after birth with seizures and retarded mental development.

Diagnostic Procedures. Since there is a lack of glycogen, none of the tests that promote conversion of glycogen to glucose (epinephrine and glucagon stimulation) will be positive. The diagnosis depends on the demonstration of the absence of glycogen synthetase in liver biopsy material.[154]

Treatment. A diet that is high in carbohydrate should be prescribed and should include extra feedings at midnight. This prevents profound hypoglycemia in these children.

Galactosemia

Etiology

This disorder of childhood is caused by either absence of galactose-1-phosphate uridyl transferase[230] or galactokinase deficiency.[117] High blood levels of galactose may stimulate insulin production and produce episodic hypoglycemia.

Clinical Features

Symptoms usually appear in the immediate postnatal period or during the first few weeks of life. The infant develops vomiting and diarrhea with failure to thrive. Hepatomegaly is a constant feature, and some infants are jaundiced with ascites and anemia. Hypoglycemic episodes are sometimes accompanied by epileptic seizures.

There is delay in growth and development in childhood with severe mental retardation in untreated cases.[132] Bilateral cataracts are occasionally seen in the neonatal period and are usually present by three months of age.

Diagnostic Procedures

1. The urine is positive on testing for reducing substances but is negative for glucose. The blood also shows elevation of total reducing substances with a low blood glucose.
2. The diagnosis can be confirmed by demonstration of deficiency of galactose-1-phosphate uridyl transferase or galactokinase deficiency.

Treatment

Infants should be given a galactose-free formula, which is substituted for the regular milk formula. Galactose must be avoided in the diet. In later life milk can usually be tolerated.

Spontaneous Hypoglycemia

Postprandial Hypoglycemia

Some older children occasionally develop signs of hypoglycemia between one and two hours after a meal, particularly after a high-carbohydrate meal. The symptoms usually consist of weakness, sweating, palpitation, and lightheadedness. These symptoms may be provoked by factors causing epinephrine release, and it is possible that this type of hypoglycemia is a factor in some children with seizures. The diagnosis can be established by the glucose tolerance test, which must be preceded by at least a two-day diet high in carbohydrate.

Treatment. Prescribing a high-protein and low-carbohydrate diet is effective in preventing hypoglycemia attacks in this condition.

Leucine-Sensitive Hypoglycemia

Severe episodic hypoglycemia (which can be precipitated by ingestion of leucine) has been described in infants and children. It may also occur in adults with some types of insulin-secreting neoplastic tumors, particularly adenoma or carcinoma of the islet cells.[133]

Etiology. Dietary intake of 1-leucine is followed by an increase in circulating insulin since leucine and related amino acids in the diet promote the release of insulin from the beta cells of the pancreas. Dietary administration of 1-isoleucine, 1-valine, and the keto acid derivative of leucine-2-keto-isocaproic acid also produces hypoglycemia in leucine-sensitive cases.

Clinical Features. Infants with leucine-sensitive hypoglycemia develop seizures within a few months of birth. The attacks are frequent, usually occurring about one hour after meals, and are refractory to the usual anticonvulsant medication. There is retardation of both mental and motor development unless treatment is instituted at an early age. The motor signs are a mixture of hypotonia with mild cerebral cortical and cerebellar involvement.

Diagnostic Procedures.   These are as follows:

1. The fasting blood glucose is low and the oral glucose tolerance test shows an initial rise and rapid fall to hypoglycemic levels.
2. Subcutaneous epinephrine and intramuscular glucagon produce a rapid rise in blood sugar levels owing to mobilization of glycogen reserve.
3. Oral 1-leucine, 150 mg/kg, produces a prompt hypoglycemic response.
4. The electroencephalogram varies with the effects of the hypoglycemia on the brain. One of the earliest changes is an increased sensitivity to hyperventilation with the appearance of bursts of bilaterally synchronous frontal dominant slow activity. Further lowering of the blood glucose level leads to a diffuse dysrhythmia with increased theta activity and then further slowing into the delta range. If the patient recovers from lasting hypoglycemia, permanent slowing of the basic rhythm to 6 to 7 cps may be noted.

Treatment.   ACTH or glucocorticosteroids may be effective in elevating the blood sugar in some cases. Subcutaneous injections of 1 mg of glucagon may be given to abolish hypoglycemic attacks. The diet should be low in protein with carbohydrate supplements. Diazoxide given orally once or twice a day is effective in maintaining blood glucose at satisfactory levels in most cases. Sodium glutamate added to the diet may reduce hypoglycemic episodes.[90]

Hereditary Intolerance to Fructose

This condition is inherited as an autosomal recessive trait and is due to a deficiency of fructose-1-phosphate splitting hepatic aldolase. The fructose-1-phosphate produces a competitive inhibition of phosphoglucomutase, which blocks glycogenolysis and results in hypoglycemia.[83]

Clinical Features.   Symptoms commonly begin in infancy after the child has been placed

on cow's milk and consist of attacks of vomiting and diarrhea. The infants develop hepatomegaly and fail to thrive. A number of children show episodic seizures, stupor, and coma. Older children and adults tend to suffer attacks of sweating, trembling, and dizziness during hypoglycemia and learn to avoid sweet foods containing fructose.

Diagnostic Procedures.   The intravenous fructose tolerance test (0.25 gm/kg) or oral test (0.5 gm/kg) produces a prompt fall in blood glucose and inorganic phosphorus levels.

Treatment.   Severe restriction of fructose in the diet is effective in preventing hypoglycemic episodes in these children.

Functional Failure of the Adrenal Medulla

A number of children with seizures secondary to hypoglycemia have been shown to have a lack of epinephrine secretion during insulin-induced hypoglycemia.[29, 30] There may be mental retardation and some degree of growth retardation. None of the patients show epinephrine-like symptoms of sweating, palpitation, or hypertension during hypoglycemia. The epinephrine tolerance test is normal.

The condition is believed to be due to either a primary failure of the adrenal medulla or a developmental anomaly of the autonomic nervous system.[29]

Treatment.   A diet should be prescribed that is low in carbohydrate and high in protein, and there should be frequent feedings. This reduces the stimulus to insulin secretion and the tendency to hypoglycemia. Treatment with ACTH or glucocorticosteroids may also be beneficial. In some cases hypoglycemic episodes may also be prevented by ephedrine.

Hypoglycemia in Hypopituitarism

Children of short stature who have hypopituitarism or growth factor deficiency occasionally develop symptomatic hypoglycemia.[116] The hypoglycemia usually presents as recurrent seizures or occasionally as lethargy or coma. The hypopituitarism is often idiopathic but also accompanies craniopharyngioma, pituitary adenoma, histiocytosis, septo-optic dysplasia, and arachnoiditis. The first attack of hypoglycemia occurs before the age of four years.

Diagnostic Procedures

1. The glucose tolerance test, arginine tolerance test, and intravenous insulin tolerance test result in hypoglycemia in symptomatic children.
2. Anterior pituitary hormone deficiencies can be demonstrated.

Treatment. Administration of human growth hormone abolishes the hypoglycemia. The basic cause of the pituitary dysfunction should be treated.

Ketotic Hypoglycemia

The occurrence of periodic hypoglycemia preceded by the sudden development of ketosis has been described in some children after the age of 18 months. It is probably inherited as an autosomal recessive trait and appears to be due to a failure of secretion of insulin necessary to preserve liver glycogen.[147]

Clinical Features. The attacks are rare before 18 months of age and are usually infrequent. The hypoglycemia is associated with lethargy, stupor, coma, and seizures, which follows a period of starvation or ingestion of a ketogenic diet. The attacks are infrequent, and the child is perfectly normal in the interval between attacks.[45]

Diagnostic Procedures. These are as follows:

1. The urine is positive for acetone during an attack.
2. There is hypoglycemia following ketosis but the fasting blood glucose and glucose tolerance test are normal at other times.
3. The epinephrine, glucagon, and leucine tests are all normal between attacks but the epinephrine and glucagon response is poor during ketosis.

Treatment. There is a prompt response to intravenous glucose during an attack.

Prevention depends on the early detection of ketosis. The urine should be checked for acetone at bedtime and each morning, and the carbohydrate intake should be increased at the first sign of acetonuria.

Early Manifestation of Familial Diabetes Mellitus

A number of infants and young children with episodic hypoglycemia and seizures have a family history of diabetes mellitus.[156] These children show abnormally elevated blood glucose curves during the glucose tolerance test signifying impaired glucose tolerance.[215] The cause of the fasting hypoglycemia in these children is unknown at this time.

Idiopathic Infantile Hypoglycemia

Despite improved understanding of hypoglycemia in infants, there still remain a number of children who are classified as suffering from idiopathic hypoglycemia. Pancreatectomy with removal of 80 to 90 per cent of the pancreas will eliminate hypoglycemia in some cases when there is failure to control the condition by medical treatment.[108] It is possible that some of these children have a disturbed relationship between blood glucose levels and the quantity of circulating serum insulin. Elevated levels of serum immunoreactive insulin have been described in some cases of hypoglycemia in the absence of pancreatic tumor.[243]

Neonatal Hypoglycemia

The occurrence of hypoglycemia in the neonatal period may be:

1. Symptomless and transient
2. Transient but symptomatic
3. The early manifestation of one of the metabolic abnormalities causing hypoglycemia.

Certain infants run a higher risk of hypoglycemia and include those of diabetic mothers, infants of toxemic mothers, and premature infants.

Clinical Features

The blood glucose levels may fall to hypoglycemic levels during the first two weeks of life without symptoms. The immature brain shows a remarkable tolerance of hypoglycemia during this period, and there is no apparent damage or subsequent delay in development.

The symptomatic hypoglycemic infant is often listless and difficult to arouse. There may be periods of pallor, trembling, sweating, and myoclonic jerks, which are presumably a response to excess epinephrine secretion secondary to hypoglycemia. Seizures followed by long periods of coma may occur, and after a few months, there is a definite retardation of development.[7, 110, 123]

Diagnostic Procedures

All infants with symptomatic hypoglycemia should receive complete diagnostic evaluation

TABLE 2–5

Diagnostic Tests in Infantile Hypoglycemia

1. Fasting blood glucose
2. Glucose tolerance test
3. Epinephrine response (0.03 mg/kg after 12-hour fast; total dose not to exceed 0.5 mg)
4. Glucagon response (0.010 mg/kg after 12-hour fast by subcutaneous injection)
5. Leucine response (150 mg 1 kg orally)
6. Fructose response (0.25 gm/kg IV or 0.5 gm/kg orally)
7. Tolbutamide tolerance test (abnormal in insulin-secreting tumors or islet hyperplasia)
8. Pituitary function tests
9. Adrenocortical function tests
10. Thyroid function tests
11. Serum and urinary amino acids by chromatography
12. Erythrocyte content of galactose-1-phosphate-uridyl-transferase
13. Liver biopsy for enzyme deficiencies

(Table 2–5). A definite diagnosis is mandatory before instituting more than symptomatic treatment since the metabolic abnormalities require specific therapy and empiric treatment may make the hypoglycemia worse. The use of a high-protein diet, for example, which is effective in postprandial hypoglycemia, would provoke low blood glucose levels in a child with leucine-sensitive hypoglycemia.

Treatment

Infants with symptomatic hypoglycemia should receive emergency treatment with 0.5 ml of 50 per cent dextrose per kilogram of body weight. Attempts should be made to raise the blood sugar level to normal or above-normal levels. If possible, the blood sugar level should be maintained with a continuous intravenous infusion of 10 per cent dextrose.

Once a definite diagnosis has been made, specific therapy as already outlined should be instituted.

Hypoglycemia and Organic Hyperinsulinism

A number of infants with persistent or recurrent hypoglycemia episodes have been described with hyperinsulinism due to islet cell hyperplasia or islet cell adenoma of the pancreas.[20] Every effort should be made to identify these children by appropriate screening tests (Table 2–5) before brain damage occurs since the condition can be alleviated by surgery. Serum insulin levels obtained during hypoglycemia are usually but not invariably elevated, and repeated determinations may be necessary. The tolbutamide tolerance test is often helpful in adults but is less reliable in infants.[99]

Treatment

The failure to maintain adequate blood glucose levels after an adequate trial of medical treatment is an indication for laparotomy and subtotal pancreatectomy. The majority of, but not all, infants have a good response following surgery.

Cerebrohepatorenal Syndrome

This rare condition is a congenital abnormality with cerebral, hepatic, and renal anomalies.

Children are severely mentally retarded with severe hypotonic external ear defects, high forehead, large fontanels, flat occiput, epicanthic folds, and cataracts. There is liver dysfunction with hypoprothrombinemia, hypoglycemia, and elevated serum iron levels. Roentgenograms show changes similar to those seen in chondrodysplasia calcificous punctata.[88] There is no therapy for this disease, and death occurs within six months.[198]

Congenital Hypothyroidism

Thyroid function has a fundamental influence on mental development in the infant, and hypothyroidism is a potential cause of severe mental retardation. Substitution therapy, if started early in life, minimizes the threat to mental development although evidence suggests that significant irreversible damage to the brain may occur during fetal life.

Etiology and Pathology

The thyroid gland may fail to develop, or congenital hypothyroidism may occur endemically, owing to low concentrations of iodine in the diet. Both sporadic and familial hypothyroidism may be due to deficiency or absence of one or more enzymes regulating iodine metabolism or synthesis or transport of thyroid hormones.[12] Congenital hypothyroidism can also occur in the offspring of pregnant women who have received antithyroid drugs for hyperthyroidism during pregnancy.[124]

Untreated cases of congenital hypothyroidism have small brains with reduction in the number of cortical neurons.

Clinical Features

Signs of hypothyroidism are seldom present in the newborn. A goiter may be present in infants born to mothers who have ingested large amounts of iodine in cough medicines during pregnancy.[104] Early signs of hypothyroidism include edema of the genitalia or extremities, umbilical hernia, lethargy, feeding problems, poor weight gain, constipation, prolonged physiologic jaundice,[144] hoarseness, and a persistent nasal discharge. There is a large posterior fontanel, mottling of the skin, retarded linear growth, hypothermia, bradycardia, episodic cyanosis, and respiratory difficulties. Undetected cases of neonatal hypothyroidism progress to the full clinical picture of cretinism with dry scaly skin, supraclavicular and axillary pads of fat, and a large head and thick calvarium. The facial appearance is characteristic with strabismus, depressed nasion, wrinkled forehead, thickened eyelids and lips, and an open mouth with a large, protruding tongue. There is severe mental retardation, particularly when treatment is delayed for more than three months after birth.[65] Children with endemic hypothyroidism may develop mental retardation, deaf mutism, ataxia, and spasticity.

Diagnostic Procedures

1. Serum thyroid-stimulating hormone TSH is elevated, and serum thyroxine (T4) and triiodothyronine (T3) are depressed in primary hypothyroidism. Low levels of TSH, T3, and T4 occur in hypothyroidism due to hypothalamic or pituitary disease (secondary hypothyroidism).[102, 163]
2. Roentgenographic examination will reveal absence of ossification in the lower femoral and upper femoral epiphyses in neonatal hypothyroidism. Both epiphyses should show ossification in normal, full-term infants.

Treatment

Thyroid replacement should be started as soon as the diagnosis of hypothyroidism is made. Therapy consists of desiccated thyroid (10 mg/kg/day) or L-thyroxine (15 μg/kg/day). The dose is adjusted according to serum TSH and T4 levels.[28]

Hypothyroidism in Children

Occasionally the onset of hypothyroidism is delayed until children have passed through the stage of infancy in apparently normal fashion. The onset is heralded by failure of normal development and cessation of growth. The clinical picture is one of apathy and slowness rather than mental retardation. One of the earliest signs of hypothyroidism is thickening of the retropharyngeal soft tissue. This thickening can be demonstrated roentgenographically.[99] Some children develop hypothyroid myopathy (p. 739).

The diagnosis and treatment have been discussed under congenital hypothyroidism.

Pseudohypoparathyroidism and Pseudopseudohypoparathyroidism

It is probable that these two conditions represent a complete and incomplete variant of a single syndrome. Pseudohypoparathyroidism is a condition in which there are clinical and biochemical abnormalities of hypoparathyroidism, but unlike hypoparathyroidism, there is no response to parathyroid extract (see p. 256). In pseudopseudohypoparathyroidism clinical findings are similar to those of pseudohypoparathyroidism without any signs of hypoparathyroidism.

Both conditions are inherited as a sex-linked recessive trait.

Clinical Features

Abnormalities of Parathyroid Function (Pseudohypoparathyroidism Only). The low serum calcium and elevated serum phosphorus levels are associated with tetany, carpopedal spasm, laryngeal stridor, pharyngeal weakness with dysphagia, choreiform movements, epileptic seizures, hypoplasia of the dental enamel, and brittle nails.

Features Common to Pseudo- and Pseudopseudohypoparathyroidism. Patients are usually short in stature with a round face, cataracts, and a masklike expression. They tend to be overweight or frankly obese. The hands are reminiscent of those seen in Down's syndrome with short fourth and fifth metacarpal bones, continuous palmar creases, and a central triradix. The majority of cases show a mild degree of mental retardation.

Diagnostic Procedures

1. In pseudohypoparathyroidism there is elevation of the serum phosphorus levels, and calcium levels are abnormally low. There is occasional elevation of serum alkaline phosphate levels and prolongation of the Q-T interval in the electrocardiogram.

2. Calcification of the basal ganglia may occur in both conditions.
3. Roentgenograms of the long bones may reveal a coarse fasciculation or evidence of osteitis fibrosa cystica in a few cases of pseudohypoparathyroidism. The metacarpals are unusually short, and there may be numerous exostoses of long bones. The radius shows a varying degree of curvature.
4. There is a high incidence of a diabetic type of response to the glucose tolerance test in both conditions.

Treatment

If osteitis fibrosa cystica is present in pseudohypoparathyroidism, it will respond to high doses of vitamin D and calcium.

Hyperaldosteronism and Ophthalmoplegia

A number of children have been described with hyperaldosteronism and progressive external ophthalmoplegia.

Etiology and Pathology

The primary abnormality appears to be a hyperaldosteronism in which there is hyperplasia of the juxtaglomerular apparatus in the kidney and hyperplasia of the zona glomerulosa in the adrenals. This would be compatible with hyperactivity of the renin-angiotensin-aldosterone system.[241]

Clinical Features

These children are normal at birth, but are retarded in growth and physical development, although there is no mental retardation. There is progressive ophthalmoplegia with pigmentary degeneration of the retina and a progressive proximal muscle weakness involving the limbs.

Diagnostic Procedures

1. The cerebrospinal fluid is under normal pressure but shows elevation of protein content.
2. There is periodic hypokalemia and possibly hypomagnesemia.
3. Aldosterone secretion is elevated and plasma renin levels are high.
4. Muscle biopsy shows abnormalities that have been described as "ragged red fibers."
5. The EMG is compatible with a myopathy.

Treatment

The use of spironolactone may return the serum potassium levels to normal in some patients. This can be supplemented by an increase of potassium intake.

The Kleine-Levin Syndrome

Although specific endocrinologic disturbances have not been described in this syndrome, it is believed by some to represent an intermittent disturbance of hypothalamic function and as such can be classified with the endocrine abnormalities in children.

The etiology and pathology are unknown. The suggestion that the intermittent hypothalamic disturbance may be due to seizure discharges in that area has not been proven by scalp or depth recording. However, markedly abnormal electroencephalograms have been obtained during episodes of hypersomnolence.[96] The condition usually begins in the second decade of life and is more common in males. There is some relationship to the menstrual period in female patients.

Clinical Features

The initial sympton is usually a change in personality. The patient appears withdrawn and introverted. He ceases to show interest in friends, parents, and hobbies, and in some instances behavior is frankly bizarre. This is followed by excessive periods of sleeping during the day, coupled with restlessness at night. When awake, the patient eats and drinks excessively and may show considerable weight gain. There may be periods of repetitive tuneless singing or humming and expressions or actions suggesting fear of assault. Adolescent males may exhibit aberrant sexual behavior.[85] The condition may last from several days to four weeks in some cases with gradual improvement and full recovery.[52]

Treatment

Dextroamphetamine or Ritalin is said to alleviate or prevent the attacks in some cases.

Disorders of Purine Metabolism

Lesch-Nyhan Syndrome

The Lesch-Nyhan syndrome is a disorder of purine metabolism inherited as a sex-linked recessive trait.

Etiology and Pathology

Affected males have a deficiency in all tissues of the enzyme hypoxanthine-guanine phosphoribosyltransferase, which is essential in the metabolic breakdown of the purine base hypoxanthene to inosenic acid.[285]

There are scattered areas of perivascular demyelination in the cerebral hemispheres and cerebellum. The blood vessels show a variety of changes including ball hemorrhages, chronic thickening of the vessel walls, and sometimes obliteration of the lumen by hyaline material in some cases. Similar changes have been described in chronic uremia. There is a marked degeneration of the granular cells of the cerebellum.[224] The kidneys show interstitial nephritis and focal glomerulosclerosis with granulomas containing uric acid crystals in the medulla.

Clinical Features

Infants are sometimes hypotonic at birth, but all cases have hypertonia within one year. Self-mutilation begins with the eruption of the teeth with marked loss of tissues around the mouth. In addition, there are severe mental retardation, choreoathetosis, generalized spasticity, and acute arthritis. Hematuria, crystalluria, and tophi appear later.[187]

Diagnostic Procedures

1. The serum uric acid is usually elevated above 10 mg/100 ml.
2. Erythrocytes and cultured fibroblasts show a marked deficiency of hypoxanthine-guanine phosphoribosyltransferase (HGPRT).
3. Prenatal diagnosis of Lesch-Nyhan syndrome can be made following amniocentesis. Cultivated amniotic cells show marked reduction in HGPRT enzyme activity.[242]

Treatment

1. Custom-designed seating devices that control arm movement and prevent self-mutilation should be used. These devices prevent self-injury but allow the child to participate in many activities of daily living.[153]
2. Allopurinal (10 mg/kg/day), which decreases uric acid synthesis, is reported to benefit some patients.
3. 5-Hydroxytryptophan, 100 mg/day, reduces involuntary movements but does not alter the patient's mood or reduce self-mutilation.[82]

Disorders of Copper Metabolism

1. Hepatolenticular degeneration (Wilson's disease) (p. 296)
2. Kinky hair disease (Menke's disease)

Kinky Hair Disease

Kinky hair or steely hair syndrome is inherited as an autosomal recessive trait and is an example of abnormal copper metabolism.

Etiology and Pathology

There are deficient absorption of copper from the intestinal tract, low serum copper levels, low ceruloplasmin levels, prolonged retention of copper in the liver, and slow excretion of copper in the urine and stools.[56]

The brain shows diffuse atrophy with neuronal loss, astroglial proliferation, and cystic degeneration.[283a] There is tortuosity and elongation of the cerebral arteries with marked thickening of the walls and fragmentation of the internal elastic lamina and thickening of the intima. The changes in the brain may be the end result of vascular insufficiency.

Clinical Features

These children are usually lethargic at birth and show progressive deterioration. The maximum development seems to be some control of the head. There is severe spasticity of all muscles, and spontaneous movement is reduced. Drowsiness, lethargy, and hypothermia are striking features. Seizures and myoclonic jerks are usually present.

The appearance is said to be quite characteristic in these children with a lack of expression and somewhat pudgy appearance to the face. The hair is stubby, white, and stiff with an appearance resembling steel wool.[93] Microscopically, the hair is twisted around its longitudinal axis (pile torte).

Diagnostic Procedures

Roentgenograms of the bones show widening of the metaphyses with the formation of lateral spurs and subperiosteal calcification along the shafts of long bones. Serum copper and serum ceruloplasmin levels are low.

Computed tomography is abnormal in later stages of the disease with diffuse cortical atrophy, evidence of subdural effusion, and the presence of multiple areas of ischemic infarction in some cases.[229a]

Treatment

Oral copper administration is followed by increased copper absorption, but this copper is not used in the synthesis of ceruloplasmin.[159] Intravenous or intramuscular copper will produce a satisfactory increase in ceruloplasmin levels, but the results of parenteral administration of copper have been equivocal.[283]

The Phakomatoses

This term applies to conditions in which neurologic lesions are combined with either ocular or cutaneous lesions. Apart from this feature, the five conditions usually grouped under this heading have little in common.

This group consists of:

1. Neurofibromatosis (von Recklinghausen's disease) (p. 660)
2. Von-Hippell-Lindau disease (p. 634)
3. Tuberous sclerosis
4. Sturge-Weber disease (p. 108)
5. Ataxia telangiectasia (p. 110)

Tuberous Sclerosis

A certain number of children with chronic seizures and mental retardation are suffering from tuberous sclerosis. The recognition of tuberous sclerosis in a child presenting with seizures may be quite difficult prior to the development of the characteristic adenoma sebaceum of the face. Early in life depigmented spots of "leaflike" lesions of the skin may be noted. Well-developed facial lesions are illustrated in an adult case in Figure 2–7.

Etiology and Pathology

The condition is believed to be genetically determined and probably represents an autosomal dominant trait with incomplete penetration and high mutation rate.

The changes are essentially due to hamartoma-

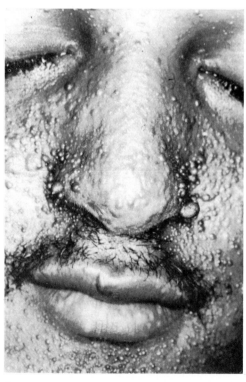

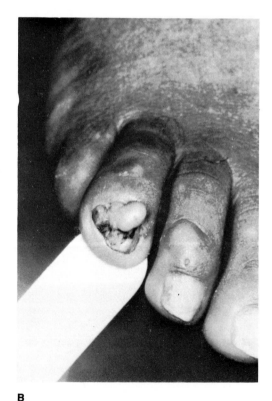

A   B

FIGURE 2–7. *A.* Photograph of typical advanced adenoma sebaceum in an adult case of tuberous sclerosis with seizures and mental retardation. *B.* Subungual fibroma from the same case.

tous growths, which may be present in many organs.

The Brain. The tubers (or nodules in the brain) may be found in any part of the cerebrum and project outward from the cortical surface and into the ventricles from the ependymal lining. They slowly increase in size, and a tuber situated at a critical site may produce hydrocephalus by obstruction of the foramen of Monro or of the cerebral aqueduct. The nodules are composed of abnormal astrocytes and glial fibers and contain some nerve cells, which are often abnormal or bizarre in appearance. An increase in the rate of growth with histologic changes assuming those of an astrocytoma and frank malignancy are not infrequent.[199]

The Retina. Phakomas of the retina may be seen as flat or elevated grayish areas of glial fibers or as mulberry-like tumors near the optic nerve head. Drüsen bodies near and on the optic disk are also quite common in tuberous sclerosis.

The Skin. The characteristic adenoma sebaceum develops in the nasolabial folds and later involves the cheeks, nose, and rarely the chin below the lip. These tumors consist of adenomatous sweat glands suspended in a fibrous stroma containing pigment cells and capillary telangiectasia. Café-au-lait spots may also be seen in any part of the body. "Shagreen areas" (from the French *peau chagrin*) of wrinkled, roughened leathery skin usually occur in the lumbar and pelvic areas. Subungual fibromas composed of proliferating fibrous tissue and capillaries often occur beneath the nails. Areas of vitiligo, in the shape of a leaf, are also characteristic of this condition.

The Heart. Rhabdomyomas occasionally occur in tuberous sclerosis. These tumors composed of malignant muscle cells have a high glycogen content and a loose "spiderweb" appearance histologically. They may cause heart murmurs and heart failure.

The Kidney. Spindle cell tumors and leiomyofibromas of the kidney occur but rarely undergo malignant change, although they may cause death from uremia. These tumors may be demonstrated by intravenous pyelogram.

The Lung. Fibrous overgrowth in the lungs in the region of the terminal bronchioles produces a typical "honeycomb appearance" on roentgenogram of the chest. This finding is rather infrequent.

Bones. Both cysts and areas of sclerosis may be found in any of the bones.

Clinical Features

The striking features are the association of mental retardation and seizures with skin lesions over the face and phakomas elsewhere. Some of these children with seizures are of normal intellect. A few patients suffer from congestive heart failure and heart murmurs in infancy because of the presence of rhabdomyomas in the heart. Renal tumors also occur and are a rare cause of death in tuberous sclerosis. Children with tuberous sclerosis may develop seizures, including infantile spasms, when hypopigmented macules may be the only manifestation of tuberous sclerosis.[216] The characteristic adenomata sebaceum appear at about four years of age or sometimes later. Under some circumstances the diagnosis can be made by observing subungual fibromas, "shagreen" areas, café-au-lait spots, or phakomas of the retina. While some patients have average intelligence, the majority show mild to severe mental retardation.

Diagnostic Procedures

1. Roentgenograms of the skull may show evidence of intracranial calcification in the tubers.
2. Serum protein levels and alkaline phosphatase are elevated in some cases. There may be a deficiency in IgG and elevation of IgM on immunoelectrophoresis.[220]
3. Electroencephalographic abnormalities occur in most cases. Hypsarrhythmia has been described in infants. The EEG may show progressive slowing over many years.
4. Computerized axial tomography has replaced pneumoencephalography in the diagnosis of tuberous sclerosis by identification of subependymal calcification[91] (Fig. 2–8). CT scanning may also identify tubers in asymptomatic relatives.[181]

Treatment

Seizures are controlled by anticonvulsants (p. 361). Hydrocephalus may be treated by removal of the tuber, if this is feasible, or by a ventriculoatrial shunt procedure. Removal of tumors of the heart, kidney, and brain may be necessary if there

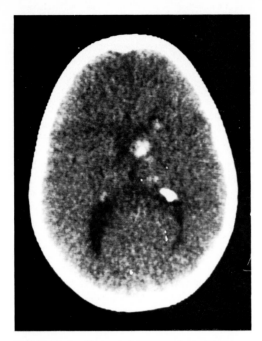

FIGURE 2–8. Computed tomography in tuberous sclerosis. There are irregular areas of increased density in the walls of the ventricles corresponding to the subependymal nodular tubers found in tuberous sclerosis.

is malignant change. Some patients require institutional care because of severe mental retardation.

Sturge-Weber Disease

The symptoms of seizures and hemiparesis occurring in a patient with a facial nevus and buphthalmos were first described by Sturge in 1879. The eponym Sturge-Weber disease arose after the radiologic description of cerebral calcification in this disease by Weber in 1929. Similar changes had already been described by Dimitri in 1923, and the condition is sometimes called Sturge-Weber-Dimitri disease.

The complete syndrome is characterized by[3]:

1. Cutaneous angiomatosis of the face and other parts of the body
2. Seizures
3. Mental retardation
4. Angiomatosis of the choroid in the eye with buphthalmos and/or glaucoma
5. Hemiparesis on the side opposite the facial nevus
6. Homonymous hemianopia

Pathogenesis

The condition is believed to be due to persistence of primitive blood vessels that appear over the brain and facial regions at an early stage in embryonic development.

The pathologic findings in the complete syndrome include the following:

Cutaneous Angiomatosis. This involves the face and scalp and occasionally extends onto the neck and thorax. The angioma consists of endothelial-lined vessels surrounded by a thin layer of collagen lying in the dermis. There is no particular direction of flow in these vessels, the pressure is low, and the oxygen content is that of venous blood.

Meningeal Angiomatosis. Similar thin-walled vessels are found in the meninges and subarachnoid space over the parieto-occipital areas of one hemisphere. They may be closely packed and many layers thick, but they do not penetrate the surface of the cerebral cortex.

Intracranial Calcification. This develops beneath the area of meningeal angiomatosis. The calcium salts, consisting of calcium phosphate and carbonate in an acid mucopolysaccharide matrix, are laid down in all layers of the cortex but are particularly dense in layers 4 and 6. Calcification apparently begins around capillaries, but as the condition develops, the areas of calcification coalesce and form larger deposits. In addition, calcium salts may be laid down in random fashion beneath the angiomatosis without relationship to capillaries, particularly in areas of marked neuronal loss.

Loss of Neurons. This is quite marked and appears to be progressive in the cortex beneath the meningeal angiomatosis. The destruction of neurons is probably due to progressive obliteration of the capillary bed by calcium deposits and is also secondary to the hypoxia induced by seizures. Such lowering of oxygen tension may have a profound effect on a cortex already damaged by the hypoxia induced by the meningeal angiomatosis.

Loss of Myelin. This is found in the cerebral white matter beneath the meningeal angiomatosis and is presumably a secondary effect due to progressive neuronal degeneration.

Angiomatosis of the Choroid. This may result in excessive secretion of aqueous humor, a rise in intraocular tension, and the development of an enlarged eye (buphthalmos) or glaucoma.

Clinical Features

The facial angiomatosis is apparent at birth. This condition is, however, not uncommon in many people who are apparently normal and who do not have Sturge-Weber disease. The essential feature in cases of Sturge-Weber disease is the presence of the angiomatosis in the area supplied by the ophthalmic division of the trigeminal nerve. The diagnosis of Sturge-Weber disease cannot be made unless the nevus involves the skin above the lateral angle of the eye. The first symptom that brings the patient to the physician is the early onset of epilepsy. Seizures, either partial or generalized, may occur in the limbs on the opposite side of the body to the facial lesion. They are frequently followed by slowing of intellectual development and mental retardation of varying degree. The majority of children with Sturge-Weber disease reported to date have been mentally retarded. Progressive deterioration may occur in patients with frequent uncontrolled seizures, particularly in those who have episodes of status epilepticus. If the seizures are controlled, mental retardation does not necessarily occur.

There is usually a hemiparesis on the side opposite the facial angiomatosis, and the limbs on that side develop poorly and are measurably smaller because of disuse atrophy.

The development of buphthalmos or glaucoma occurs in about 30 per cent of cases of Sturge-Weber disease.

The presence of homonymous hemianopia is quite frequent in this condition, and it occurs in patients with involvement of the occipital lobes.

Diagnostic Procedures

1. The roentgenographic appearance of the skull is characteristic. A double contour of gyriform calcifications is seen over one hemisphere, usually in the parieto-occipital area.
2. The electroencephalogram may show low-voltage activity or appear isoelectric over the area of meningeal angiomatosis. Activity, if present, is slower than that recorded over the opposite hemisphere, and there may be irregular spike wave discharges in the interictal period.
3. Computerized axial tomography will detect the intracranial calcifications at an early stage

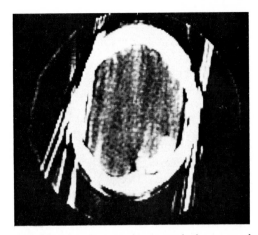

FIGURE 2-9. Computed tomography in a case of Sturge-Weber disease. The area of increased density in the right parieto-occipital area corresponds to the intracranial calcification seen in Sturge-Weber disease.

(Fig. 2–9). Bilateral hemispheric calcifications occur in about 15 per cent of cases.[27]

Treatment

1. Every effort should be made to control seizures at an early stage since these may be the cause of retarded intellectual development.
2. Status epilepticus in children requires prompt and adequate treatment (p. 367).
3. Cosmetic creams may be used to cover the facial nevus.
4. Special schooling or institutional care may be necessary for the severely retarded.
5. After adequate trial of anticonvulsants, hemispherectomy should be considered, but only as a last resort and only in patients with poor seizure control. This procedure is particularly beneficial in those with marked slowing or flattening of electroencephalographic activity over the affected area or in those with homonymous hemianopia. There may be improvement in intellect following removal of what is essentially a nonfunctioning but epileptogenic area of the brain.

Children with Sturge-Weber disease may enter a normal educational program if the epilepsy is controlled at an early stage. In the majority of cases that have been reported, however, special schooling or institutional care has frequently been necessary owing to uncontrolled seizures and progressive intellectual deterioration. There is a tendency for seizure activity to decrease in the third and fourth decades with improvement of mental status.

Ataxia Telangiectasia

This condition, first described in 1941, has also been called the Madame Louis Bar syndrome after the French author of the original paper.

Etiology and Pathology

The etiology is not known. A number of cases have been described in families, suggesting an autosomal recessive pattern of inheritance. There are marked degenerative changes in the cerebellum with widespread loss of Purkinje and granular cells and reduction in the number of basket cells. There is also a neuronal loss in the cerebral cortex, basal ganglia, brainstem nuclei, and the anterior horns of the spinal cord. Enlarged venules have been described in the cerebellar meninges.

A number of abnormalities occur outside the nervous system, including absence or poor development of the thymus, gonadal hypoplasia, chronic pulmonary fibrosis, and bronchiectasis.

Clinical Features

General Features.   Children with this affliction have a typical facial appearance described as a "sad expression." Many have strabismus. The development of ataxia is followed by the appearance

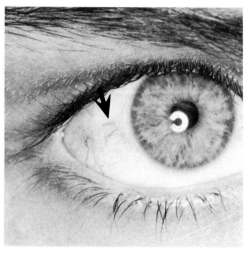

FIGURE 2–10.   Photograph of the sclera and eye of a patient suffering from ataxia-telangiectasia of the scleral vessels.

of oculocutaneous telangiectasia between three and six years of age. The dilated blood vessels usually appear in the more peripheral parts of the exposed conjunctiva first and fade as they approach the cornea (Fig. 2–10). Eventually the dilated vessels spread to the butterfly area of the face, the eyelids, and the pinnae. Occasionally, telangiectasia may occur in the neck, antecubital and popliteal fossae, and on the dorsum of the hands and feet.

The majority of children have a history of repeated attacks of sinusitis and pneumonia, and many eventually develop bronchiectasis. Lymphoreticular tumors, including lymphoma, lymphosarcoma, and Hodgkin's disease, are a feature of ataxia telangiectasia. Disturbances of endocrine function, including hypogonadism, delayed development of secondary sex characteristics, and insulin-resistant diabetes mellitus, have also been described in ataxia telangiectasia.

Neurologic Features.   Mental retardation of mild degree is not uncommon, and there usually is some arrest of intellectual development after the age of ten years. There may also be some retardation in body growth beginning at about the same time.[87] These children have an unusually equitable disposition, but the speech may be dysarthric and further impaired by drooling.

Eye movements are accompanied by ocular dysmetria and a coarse nystagmus in all directions of gaze.[17a] Choreoathetosis is present in most cases, particularly in older children. Coordination becomes progressively impaired with intention tremor and dysmetria in the upper limbs. Gait is ataxic, and there is progressive truncal and limb ataxia with eventual dependence on a wheelchair. The reflexes are hypoactive and the plantar responses are normal. The Romberg test is negative. The sensory examination is intact.

Diagnostic Procedures

1. Low serum immunoglobulin levels (IgA and IgE) have been described and may account for the increased susceptibility to infection and malignancy. Serum alpha fetoprotein levels are significantly elevated suggesting that liver function is not fully developed in ataxia telangiectasia.[276]
2. Roentgenograms of the chest often reveal evidence of infections and may occasionally show a mediastinal lymphoma. Roentgenograms of the skull may show absence of adenoid and

tonsillar tissue and chronic paranasal sinusitis.

3. Abnormal amino acids have been described in the urine.
4. Computerized axial tomography shows cerebellar atrophy in the early stages of the disease and a diffuse cerebrocerebellar atrophy in advanced cases.

Treatment

Repeated infections may be controlled by appropriate antibiotic therapy, and bronchiectasis may be helped by postural drainage.

Every effort should be made to keep these children ambulatory, and intermittent courses of physical therapy are helpful. The use of antibiotics extends the life-span of these children, and many now reach adulthood. This means that the syndrome will be recognized with increasing frequency in the future. Complicating systemic neoplasia probably related to the immunoglobulin deficiency is common in this disorder, and such complications should be watched for and treated.[101]

Other Neuroectodermal Disorders

Congenital Ichthyosis and Mental Retardation

There are a number of other neuroectodermal disorders. Two distinct syndromes, both rare and characterized by congenital ichthyosis and mental retardation, are known.

The association of congenital ichthyosis with mental retardation and spasticity is known as the *Sjögren-Larsson syndrome*. The disease is inherited as an autosomal recessive trait. There is marked loss of myelin in the central nervous system in the adult brain.[171] The salient features are congenital ichthyosis, mental retardation, speech defects, spastic diplegia, kyphoscoliosis, hypertelorism, tooth abnormalities, and dermatoglyphic abnormalities. Optic atrophy, pigmentary degeneration of the retina, and basilar compression may occur. Children with Sjögren-Larsson syndrome reach their maximal potential before the age of ten years and then experience a chronic decline in neurologic function.

Rud Syndrome

The association of ichthyosis, hypogonadism, and mental retardation is a sex-linked recessive trait[205] sometimes referred to as the Rud syndrome. Affected children have cryptorchism and a small penis; anosmia has been described in some cases. The production of follicle-stimulating hormone, luteinizing hormone, and growth hormone is reduced, and there is a decrease in ACTH response to metyrapone.[1]

Incontinentia Pigmentia (Block-Sulzberger Syndrome)

Children with this condition have mental retardation and neurologic signs associated with dermatologic, ocular, and dental abnormalities. The etiology is unknown, but the herpes simplex virus has been isolated from the skin vesicles, seen in the early stage of the disease. The condition usually occurs in female infants.

The dermatologic changes consist of a papular rash followed by the formation of vesicles and occasionally bullae. This stage is remittent and the vesicles fade, leaving areas of pigmented skin. The second stage consists of verrucous lesions, which also disappear leaving pigmented skin areas.

The neurologic changes include deformity of the skull (small in the bifrontal plane), seizures (partial or generalized), progressive spastic paraparesis, and mental retardation.[240] The ocular changes include strabismus, cataracts, papillitis, chorioretinitis, and optic atrophy. Development of the teeth may be delayed, and when they appear, they may be pegged in appearance.

Prenatal Infections

Toxoplasmosis

Etiology

Toxoplasma gondii is a protozoan organism found in a number of small mammals and birds. Human infection may be congenital owing to the passage of the organism transplacentally from mother to fetus or may be acquired in childhood and occasionally in adult life. The mode of transmission from animals to human beings is unknown.

Pathology

Congenital Form. The *Toxoplasma* organisms enter the neurons, glial cells, and endothelium of the blood vessels. Severe infection produces an acute inflammatory response throughout the brain. In other cases, collections of epithelioid cells produce miliary granulomas, some of which develop into pseudocysts and later calcify. Hydrocephalus may result from aqueductal stenosis and ependymitis. Retarded brain development produces microcephaly, mental retardation, and seizures. Chorioretinitis is usually a prominent feature in the congenital form of toxoplasmosis.

Acquired Form. More acute forms of acquired toxoplasmosis may occur in children and adults producing a meningoencephalitis similar to the congenital form. Subacute or chronic meningoencephalitis may also occur, but calcification is uncommon. In the adult cases an associated myositis may occur. A rare form of a large, solitary granuloma resembling a brain tumor has also been described.

Clinical Features

Congenital Toxoplasmosis. Many children are stillborn. Those who survive may show signs of generalized infection in the first few months of life with skin rash, jaundice, hepatomegaly, splenomegaly, and ascites. Death usually occurs within a few weeks. In the more chronic infections, the children are often premature and show retarded development, epilepsy, hydrocephalus, or microcephaly.[22] A few children are asymptomatic and are found to have an isolated, circumscribed area of chorioretinitis during retinoscopy later in life.

Acquired Toxoplasmosis. An acute form has been described with a typhus-like illness and rash resembling Rocky Mountain spotted fever. Occasionally acquired toxoplasmosis presents as an acute meningoencephalitis. Subacute or chronic toxoplasmic meningoencephalitis can produce seizures, ataxia, and progressive intellectual deterioration.[146] Large solitary granulomas, producing progressive focal neurologic signs and suggesting a brain tumor, are rare.

Diagnostic Procedures

1. The cerebrospinal fluid may show signs of meningeal inflammation with a lymphocytic pleocytosis and increased protein content in some cases. The organisms may be isolated by inoculation of guinea pigs.
2. Complement-fixation tests and dye tests may indicate toxoplasmosis.
3. Computed tomography of the brain may show calcification in the congenital form of toxoplasmosis (Fig. 2–11).

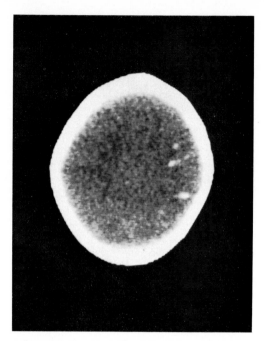

FIGURE 2–11. Computed tomography in a case of congenital toxoplasmosis. The discrete areas of increased density correspond to intracranial calcifications.

Treatment

Both sulfonamides and pyrimethamine have been used in the treatment of human toxoplasmosis with little evidence of benefit.

The Neurologic Syndromes of Congenital Rubella

Between 10 and 40 per cent of women who develop clinical signs of rubella during the first trimester of pregnancy give birth to infants with congenital defects. The risk of giving birth to a child with congenital abnormalities is at least five times greater than in women who have not had rubella during this period of gestation.[111]

Etiology and Pathogenesis

Infection by rubella virus in nonimmune women during the early months of pregnancy results in a viremia and transplacental infection of the fetus.

The fetal infection is chronic and interferes with certain stages of development of the nervous system. Virus excretion continues for as long as two years after birth, suggesting that some infants may suffer the effects of a chronic panencephalitis after birth. A defect in the immune system with inhibition of specific antibody formation has been demonstrated in congenital rubella infection.[250]

Clinical Features

Maternal. The rash of rubella is nonspecific and may be confused with other exanthemas or rashes due to allergy, drugs, or toxins. Many cases of maternal infection appear to occur without the development of any rash, making the clinical diagnosis of rubella difficult if not impossible. Infection in suspected cases can now be confirmed by demonstrating a fourfold or greater increase in maternal antibodies to rubella virus occurring within a three-week period. Even so, gamma globulin should be given to all exposed or suspected cases during the first trimester of pregnancy. The development of a method to detect antibodies means that infection may be confirmed or excluded in women who have been exposed to rubella during the first trimester of pregnancy.

Newborn. CENTRAL NERVOUS SYSTEM. These children frequently show mental retardation, microcephaly, and possibly meningocele with or without hydrocephalus. Deafness is common. Involvement of the central nervous system is frequently associated with microphthalmia, cataracts, and chorioretinitis. There may be a variety of defects of cardiac development, the commonest being a persistent patent ductus arteriosus and septal defects. The birth weight may be low owing to intrauterine retardation of growth. Liver function is often abnormal owing to hepatitis with hepatosplenomegaly and thrombocytopenic purpura. Roentgenograms of the bones may show multiple radiolucent defects.

Treatment

Prophylaxis. All pregnant women who are known to have been exposed to rubella during the first trimester of pregnancy should be given injections of gamma globulin to reduce the incidence of fetal infection.

Immunization of young women with rubella vaccine is a safe procedure. This vaccine contains live attenuated virus, but there is no evidence that it is transmitted to the fetus in an undetected pregnancy.[128]

Therapeutic Abortion. The added risk of bearing a child with multiple congenital defects following exposure to rubella during the first trimester has been cited by some physicians as a justification for therapeutic abortion. Other physicians believe that the fivefold increase in the risk factor does not warrant such intervention. In addition to such arguments, social, religious, and psychologic factors must be taken into consideration since each case presents different problems.

Cytomegalic Inclusion Disease

Cytomegaloviruses, which were first isolated in 1956, have proved to be responsible for a chronic intrauterine encephalitis.[183] While frequently compatible with survival, the disease results in a variety of developmental defects of the central nervous system.[107]

The virus is ubiquitous, and approximately 80 per cent of adults have serologic evidence indicating previous subclinical infection. Transmission is probably by droplet infection via the nasopharynx or by ingestion. Mothers who give birth to infected infants have been infected during pregnancy and may continue to excrete the virus in the urine for many months. They also develop antibodies against cytomegaloviruses so that it is highly unlikely that congenital infection will occur in subsequent pregnancies.[288]

Cytomegalovirus is the most common viral cause of mental retardation and is responsible for severe mental retardation with microcephaly, as well as more subtle mental defects in some infected children.[166] Affected children may show some degree of chorioretinitis, and there may be optic atrophy with serious visual impairment or blindness. Motor involvement includes hypertonia and spastic diplegia. Cerebral calcification with some degree of mental retardation may be the only evidence of intrauterine infection. About one third of those infected in utero suffer central nervous system damage.[277]

Infection in infancy and in the first years of life does not usually result in central nervous system involvement, although isolated examples of cytomegalic virus encephalitis have been reported during this period. Older children may be infected during a debilitating disease such as acute leukemia, lymphoma, or Hodgkin's disease and show evidence of hepatic involvement, but the central nervous system is spared.

Encephalopathies of Infancy and Childhood

Benign Paroxysmal Vertigo of Childhood

The condition of benign paroxysmal vertigo is not uncommon in pediatric practice but may give rise to some difficulty in diagnosis.[145]

Clinical Features

The symptoms consist of brief episodic vertigo lasting from a few seconds to a few minutes, during which time the child is incapacitated and may fall to the ground. There is no loss of consciousness. All attacks occur abruptly without warning. The children are pale, nauseated, and may vomit. They are usually frightened and unable to maintain their normal posture. They may search for support and clutch an object or their parents. The frequency of attacks varies from several per week to one every two or three months. These children have normal neurologic examinations, and all laboratory investigations are essentially negative. Caloric testing shows hypofunction of the vestibular system, which is said to be characteristic of this condition.

Treatment

The symptoms of benign paroxysmal vertigo tend to disappear over a period of several months to several years. The use of dimenhydrinate may provide dramatic relief in some patients.

Reye's Syndrome

More than 1,000 cases of Reye's syndrome (acute encephalopathy with fatty infiltration of the viscera) have been reported in the medical literature since this condition was first described in 1963. A possibility exists that there is an increase in the incidence of this dramatic and dangerous disease.

Etiology and Pathology

The association of virus infections, including influenza A and B, varicella, and mixed viral infections by herpes virus and paramyxovirus, with Reye's syndrome has been determined.[37, 155, 218, 253, 261] Exposure to other potentially toxic substances, such as antiemetics, aspirin, acetaminophen, and agricultural pesticides, has been reported in some cases.[211, 239] A disease resembling Reye's syndrome has been reported as an endemic condition in Thailand during the rainy season when contamination of food stuffs with aflatoxin is high.[225] A similar condition, Jamaican vomiting sickness, is produced by hypoglycin, a toxic substance found in the unripe fruit of the akee tree. At the present time it seems that there may be multiple etiologic factors, including viral, environmental, and genetic factors, which predispose certain children to Reye's syndrome.[265]

The pathologic changes in Reye's syndrome are distinct and consist of a noninflammatory encephalopathy with cerebral edema and a characteristic fatty infiltration of the viscera, particularly the liver. The cerebral edema is cytogenic with marked intracellular edema affecting neurons and astrocytes. The neurons show mitochondrial injury with marked disruption and swelling. Some neurons show thickening of the endoplasmic reticulum and nuclear damage.[195] There is fatty infiltration in a panlobular fashion in the liver, and the mitochondria of the liver cells are damaged in a manner resembling the mitochondrial damage in neurons. This finding suggests that there may be simultaneous damage to mitochondria in neurons, brain capillaries,[110a] and liver cells by a toxic substance as yet unidentified,[194] possibly endotoxin derived from anaerobic intestinal flora.[9, 50]

Whether the mitochondrial damage in Reye's syndrome is a direct result of virus infection, endotoxins, or other factors, the result is a profound disturbance of ammonia metabolism. However, it is possible that there is also an inherited defect in ammonia metabolism in the mitochondria in some children with Reye's syndrome.[28, 248] A deficiency in ornithine transcarbamylase and carbamyl phosphate synthetase has been demonstrated in some children recovering from Reye's syndrome,[264] while the deficiency is transient in others.[34]

There is early and sustained hyperammoniuria in Reye's syndrome, and the rapid development of encephalopathy is compatible with neurotoxicity from ammonia. Ammonia derived from protein metabolism is metabolized in the urea cycle in a series of reactions in liver cells. Ammonia is converted to carbamyl phosphate by the mitochondrial enzyme carbamyl phosphate synthetase, and the carbamyl phosphate interacts with ornithine to enter the urea cycle as citrulline (see Fig. 2–12). This reaction is catalyzed by the enzyme ornithine transcarbamylase. Failure of the enzyme carbamyl phosphate synthetase will lead to a rapid buildup of ammonia and hyperam-

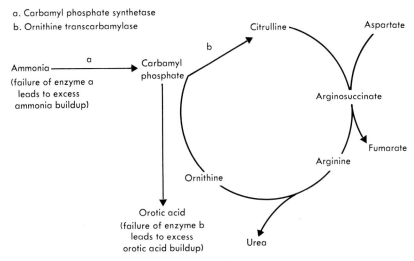

a. Carbamyl phosphate synthetase
b. Ornithine transcarbamylase

FIGURE 2–12. Possible metabolic abnormalities in Reye's syndrome.

monemia. However, the reduced amounts of carbamyl phosphate are unable to enter the urea cycle because of failure of the enzyme ornithine transcarbamylase, and the carbamyl phosphate is converted to orotic acid by an alternative pathway. Orotic acid is believed to inhibit the release of triglycerides from the liver, producing the fatty liver of Reye's syndrome.

The hyperammonemia of Reye's syndrome produces a marked change in cerebral metabolism in a brain where mitochondrial activity may have been impaired at the onset of the illness. There is failure to detoxify ammonia in the brain, followed by a failure of oxidative metabolism and increased lactic acid formation. The hyperammonemia also leads to marked hyperventilation, while the combination of preexisting mitochondrial damage and hyperammonemia may account for the cytogenic cerebral edema of Reye's syndrome.[233]

Clinical Features

The onset of Reye's syndrome is extremely acute, and early recognition of the syndrome may save the life of the child. There is usually a history of a upper respiratory tract infection that seems to be resolving when the child suddenly begins to vomit and appears lethargic. There is rapid progression to delirium, stupor, and coma within 24 hours. The syndrome presents in five stages.[160]

Stage 1. Vomiting, lethargy, little interest in surrounding stimuli, early evidence of liver dysfunction.

Stage 2. Disorientation, combativeness, seizures, hallucinations, hyperventilation, increased deep-tendon reflexes, extensor plantar responses, marked evidence of liver dysfunction.

Stage 3. Coma, decerebrate rigidity, which may be spontaneous or occur on stimulation, pupillary reaction to light and reflex eye movements still present.

Stage 4. Deep coma, hyperventilation, decerebration and painful stimulation, pupils fail to react to light, absence of reflex eye movements with head movement.

Stage 5. Deep coma, no response on painful stimulation, respiratory failure leading to respiratory arrest.

The majority of children who survive do not show neurologic abnormalities. However, signs of permanent brain damage, including hemiparesis, dystonia, involuntary movements, and seizures, have been reported in some cases.[36] Recurrence of Reye's syndrome is unusual.

Diagnostic Procedures

1. The serum venous ammonia level is elevated above 50 mg/100 ml.
2. Liver enzyme activity is abnormally high.
   a. Serum glutamic oxalacetic acid transaminase (SGOT) is elevated beyond 36 units.
   b. Serum glutamic pyruvic transaminase (SGPT) is elevated beyond 35 units.
3. Plasma prothrombin time is increased at least three times beyond control levels.

4. There is occasional occurrence of hypoglycemia, free fatty acidemia, and hypolypoproteinemia.

5. The cerebrospinal fluid is clear and may show increased pressure. The cellular content and protein content are normal. Glucose levels may be reduced if there is hypoglycemia. Lumbar puncture should not be performed when there is obvious increase in intracranial pressure.

6. Computed tomography shows diffuse cerebral edema with increased density in the deep white matter and increased gray-white matter contrast.[220a]

7. Serial electroencephalography provides an accurate graphic record of deterioration or improvement.[40, 269]

8. Liver biopsy is regarded as a safe procedure for confirmation of diagnosis in some centers.[194]

9. Serum creatine phosphokinase (CPK) is elevated in severely affected children. Studies of isoenzymes show that this elevation of CPK is mainly from the muscle fractions. A progressive rise in CPK is reported to indicate a poor prognosis.[4]

Treatment

The treatment of Reye's syndrome is under constant review, and modification can be expected with improvement in the understanding of the pathophysiology of the disease. The following methods have been suggested.

A. Mild cases should be treated with intravenous fluids to correct dehydration, electrolyte imbalance, and any tendency toward hypoglycemia. Aspirin, antiemetics, and acetaminophen should be avoided.

B. Severe cases (stages 2 through 5)
   1. Constant monitoring of intracranial pressure and maintenance of intracranial pressure below 20 mm of mercury.[269a] This may be accomplished by hyperventilation to induce hypocapnia, constant serum hyperosmolality (approximately 320 mOsm), and sedation. Acute elevation of intracranial pressure should be treated with intravenous mannitol (1 gm/kg body weight).[236]
   2. Administration of ornithine, arginine, or citrulline in an attempt to correct defects in the urea cycle and reduce hyperammonemia.[188, 264, 270]
   3. Constant intracranial pressure monitoring, regulation of increased intracranial pressure with intravenous mannitol, hypothermia, and total body washout.[149]
   4. Early elective endotracheal intubation and control of cerebral edema by hyperventilation and intravenous mannitol.[142] Neomycin by nasogastric tube (50 mg/kg/day) or neomycin enemas may reduce ammonia production in the gastrointestinal tract.[160]
   5. Exchange transfusion or peritoneal dialysis has been advocated to reduce hyperammonemia.
   6. Craniotomy and cerebral decompression have been used successfully in some cases.

Myoclonus Encephalopathy of Infants

A benign condition with generalized myoclonic jerks occurring during infancy and childhood may have been described under several names in the literature.[43, 66, 143]

Clinical Features

There is an acute onset in a previously normal child often preceded by an upper respiratory tract infection. The first neurologic abnormality may be ataxia and clumsiness, but this is followed by the development of generalized myoclonus. There is an associated conjugate movement of the eyes sometimes called opsoclonus or ocular dysmetria. The myoclonic jerking in these children is often so severe that it interferes with sitting and feeding. They may be sensitive to sound and light, but myoclonus disappears during sleep. Although the child may be unable to speak because of the frequency of involuntary movement, there is no mental retardation.

Treatment

The disease runs a protracted course, but the response to corticosteroids has been gratifying in some cases. Those who respond may require a prolonged maintenance dose of corticosteroids.

Infantile Neuroaxonal Dystrophy

This rare disease appears to be inherited as an autosomal recessive trait.

Etiology and Pathology

The etiology is unknown. There is a progressive neuronal loss throughout the central nervous system with the presence of spheroid bodies and axonal swellings throughout the central and peripheral nervous system.[287] These changes are accompanied by defective myelination. The spheroids and axonal swellings contain mitochondria and glycogen-like material, suggesting a metabolic abnormality affecting carbohydrate metabolism in the axons.[237]

Clinical Features

Affected children show normal development for several months after birth. This is followed by progressive mental deterioration with gradual loss of motor skills. Seizures may occur in some cases. Death occurs in some cases three to seven years after onset.[286]

Diagnostic Procedures

The characteristic axonal swellings can be demonstrated by peripheral nerve biopsy.

Treatment

There is no specific treatment for this disease.

Encephalopathy Associated with Burns

Transient neurologic abnormalities are not uncommon in children with relatively minor burns. Most abnormalities resolve completely, but occasionally rapid fatal encephalopathy occurs. This is possibly due to cerebral edema, but the cause is obscure.[278]

Clinical Features

Neurologic symptoms, such as vomiting, clouding of consciousness, seizures, generalized muscle twitching, and respiratory arrest, appear 15 to 40 hours after relatively minor burns. The electroencephalogram shows increased generalized delta activity, which diminishes with clinical improvement.

Treatment

1. It is most important to maintain adequate blood oxygenation and to assist respiration if necessary.
2. Measures to reduce cerebral edema such as the use of 50 per cent glucose solution intravenously may be helpful.

Acute Hemiplegia in Children

Acute hemiplegia in infants or children is a postnatally acquired condition that develops in a child who is apparently neurologically normal at birth. The condition is syndromic with many recognized causes (Table 2–6) and a group of unknown etiology.

TABLE 2–6

Acute Hemiplegia in Children

Congenital
Arteriovenous malformation
Cerebral microangioma
Fibromuscular hyperplasia of the carotid artery
Dissecting aneurysm of carotid artery

Traumatic
Carotid artery thrombosis
Contusion or laceration of brain, epidural hemorrhage, subdural hematoma, intracerebral hemorrhage
Fat embolism
Air embolism

Infectious
Viral encephalitis
Bacterial meningitis
Mycotic aneurysm
Cerebral venous thrombosis
Postinfectious leukoencephalopathy

Metabolic
Hypoglycemia
Homocystinuria

Neoplastic
Brain tumor
Tuberculoma

Blood dyscrasias
Sickle cell disease
Polycythemia vera
Secondary polycythemia

Toxic causes
Lead encephalopathy

Vascular
Arteritis—Takayasu's disease, polyarteritis nodosa
Migraine
Severe hypertension
Embolism

Cardiac
Thrombosis and polycythemia in congenital heart disease
Cerebral abscess in congenital heart disease
Cerebral embolism—rheumatic heart disease
Embolism—bacterial endocarditis
Embolism—myxoma of heart

Systemic diseases
Systemic lupus erythematosus, polyarteritis nodosa, thrombotic thrombocytopenic purpura

Unknown cause
Hemiconvulsion, hemiplegia, epilepsy syndrome (HHE syndrome)

Clinical Features

There are three forms of onset.[39]

1. *Abrupt with Seizures.* The affected child presents with sudden onset of seizures, coma,

hemiplegia, and an elevated temperature. The seizures are usually partial and localized to one side, and the seizure activity may last for several days. The child may remain in coma for several hours after the cessation of seizure activity. The hemiplegia is flaccid initially and affects the upper extremity more than the lower extremity. Recovery is often incomplete, particularly in the upper extremity.

2. *Acute Onset of Hemiplegia.* Some cases present with the sudden onset of hemiplegia but without seizure activity.

3. *Intermittent Hemiplegia.* The hemiplegia may present intermittently in some cases of carotid artery thrombosis.

The hemiplegia or hemiparesis is maximal at onset and flaccid. Spasticity does not usually appear for several weeks. Recovery may be rapid, or there may be slow improvement over several months. Approximately 50 per cent of affected children have residual weakness of the affected limb. Choreoathetotic movements may begin several months later. Mirror movements which are normal in childhood may persist in the paretic and nonparetic hand.[285a]

There may be additional deficits, including sensory changes in the affected limbs, homonymous hemianopia, and recurrent seizure activity. Lesions of the dominant hemisphere result in dysphasia, dyslexia, and dyspraxia.

Prognosis

The prognosis is dependent on the condition causing the acute hemiplegia. A number of children die in the acute phase of the illness, but this is often related to underlying systemic disease such as congenital heart disease. Approximately 75 per cent of the survivors have a neurologic deficit with 50 per cent of the survivors having partial, generalized, or psychomotor seizures. The majority of surviving children have some intellectual impairment, but this is usually mild and 25 per cent of the surviving children can be regarded as mentally retarded. Nevertheless, behavior and learning problems are common, occurring in 80 per cent of cases.

Diagnostic Procedures

The diagnostic evaluation is governed by the clinical evaluation of the child. An infectious process or space-occupying lesion must be excluded. Roentgenograms of the skull and chest, paranasal sinuses, and mastoid air cells, electroencephalography, and CT scan should precede cerebral arteriography whenever possible.

Treatment

Acute Phase

1. Control seizures (see status epilepticus).
2. Maintain fluids and electrolytes.
3. Reduce cerebral edema.

Chronic Phase

1. Seizures require continuing anticonvulsant therapy.
2. Motor deficits can be improved by physical therapy.
3. Language problems will require speech therapy.
4. Behavioral problems require parental counseling to establish a positive attitude and a structured environment. The effect of drugs such as methylphenidate or phenothiazines is unpredictable.
5. Schooling problems require neuropsychologic evaluation and appropriate use of learning centers in the school system.

Cerebral Palsy

Unfortunately this "catch-all" term has been used loosely in the past and has not been well defined. There is general agreement that "cerebral palsy" should indicate an abnormality in cerebral control of motor function, present at or shortly after birth. Apart from the motor handicap, many of these children show hyperkinetic behavior and limited attention spans.[274]

General Considerations

Definition

Cerebral palsy is a syndrome in which an abnormality in the cerebral control of motor function results from maldevelopment of or injury to motor centers or their connections within the central nervous system.

This definition implies that (1) the abnormalities occur in the prenatal period or in infancy and include development abnormalities, injuries, and infections in utero, at birth, and in infancy, and (2) the condition is not progressive. Active disease of the central nervous system is not present at time of diagnosis.

Incidence

About 5 per 1,000 children have a motor deficit compatible with cerebral palsy. In 50 per cent the disability is mild, while 10 per cent have severe handicaps. Some 25 per cent are of average intelligence, but 30 per cent have an intelligence quotient (IQ) below 70 and are significantly mentally retarded. Seizures occur in about 35 per cent of children with cerebral palsy, and 50 per cent have remediable disorders of speech. The incidence is higher in boys than girls (1.4:1.0).

Clinical and Anatomic Classification

The most satisfactory classification should be based on the type of neurologic deficit:[26]

1. Spastic diplegia or uncomplicated diplegia of prematurity. This is due to bilateral involvement of corticospinal tracts only, other systems being normal.
2. Hemiplegic cerebral palsy. This is due to unilateral involvement of corticospinal tracts with predominant involvement of the upper limbs.
3. Complex diplegia or spastic quadriplegia with choreoathetosis. This is due to bilateral involvement of corticospinal tracts and other systems.
4. Athetotic cerebral palsy or choreoathetosis. This is due to involvement of the extrapyramidal system.
5. Ataxic form of cerebral palsy. This is due to involvement of the cerebellum and its connections.

Etiology and Pathogenesis

The major factors associated with cerebral palsy are outlined in Table 2–7. Since this is a broad and loose term, many etiologic and pathogenetic factors have been discussed elsewhere in this text. Therapeutic irradiation to the lower abdomen during pregnancy should be avoided, since cerebral malformations, mental retardation, and cerebral palsy have been reported in children born following this procedure. Experimental irradiation of pregnant rats produces similar malformations.

The pathogenetic relationship of toxemia of pregnancy to cerebral palsy is not clear. It is possible that the toxemia produces cerebral damage in the fetus, but anoxia at birth is also increased in infants of toxemic mothers. Other common causes are postnatal infections and trauma during infancy and early childhood. If these causes are

TABLE 2–7

Etiology and Pathogenesis of Cerebral Palsy[3]

A. *Prenatal factors*
1. Developmental abnormalities
2. Infections in utero (including cytomegalovirus, rubella, toxoplasmosis, other viruses, syphilis)
3. Irradiation in utero
4. Asphyxia in utero (abruptio placentae, placenta previa, maternal anoxia, abnormalities of umbilical cord, premature separation of placenta, placental hemorrhage)
5. Toxemia of pregnancy
6. Maternal age over 35 years or less than 20 years
7. Twinning
8. Disseminated intravascular coagulation due to prenatal death of a twin

B. *Natal factors*
1. Anoxia
2. Trauma
3. Prematurity or postmaturity
4. Breech delivery
5. Prolonged or precipitous labor

excluded, there still remain those children with less well-defined cerebral palsy. These cases sometimes can be related to prematurity, kernicterus, infection in the mother, and malnourishment, but, unfortunately, in many cases the exact cause is not determined.

Uncomplicated Diplegia of Prematurity

These children present with diplegia due to corticospinal involvement affecting primarily the lower limbs, hence the term "spastic diplegia." There is impairment of motor development with delay in sitting, standing, and walking. Speech and intelligence are usually normal. Examination shows hypertonia or spasticity, which is particularly marked in the adductors of the lower limbs. The tendon jerks are hyperactive, and there are bilateral extensor plantar responses. The gait is abnormal and is traditionally described as a "scissors gait." Involvement of the upper limbs is usually less marked, but some imbalance of extraocular muscles or strabismus is not infrequent.

These children are usually premature, weighing less than 2,000 gm at birth. There is a greater weight loss in the postnatal period than occurs in prematures without cerebral spasticity. Since the cerebral damage is more or less localized to the paracentral lobule bilaterally and symmetrically, it is possible that premature infants who become severely dehydrated (and therefore lose weight) have an increased risk of thrombosis of the midline cerebral venous sinuses. Seventy per cent of babies weighing less than 1.35 kg (3 lb) at birth have corticospinal tract signs.

Hemiplegic Cerebral Palsy

In this type of cerebral palsy there is impairment of motor function on one side of the body with most marked paralysis involving the upper limb.

Etiology

Many cases of infantile hemiplegia occur in infancy or in children who, until the paralytic ictus, have developed normally. There is usually a history of an acute febrile episode followed by unilateral epileptic seizures, a period of coma, and then hemiparesis when consciousness is regained. Some cases appear to be due to encephalitis, others to thrombotic occlusion of the carotid or middle cerebral artery or to cortical venous thrombophlebitis. Some are due to developmental disorders of the carotid system, such as constricting bands or fibromuscular hyperplasia.

The perinatal-natal group of infantile hemiparesis can be divided into two groups:

Hemiplegia Without Seizures. This condition may follow cerebral embolism shortly after birth. It is possible that venous emboli arising in the placenta before the cord is severed or in the umbilical veins may pass through a patent foramen ovale in the heart and enter the arterial system. One or more may lodge in a middle cerebral artery. There is often a history in children with infantile hemiparesis of a sudden cyanotic episode and resuscitation shortly after birth, which could be related to an embolic episode of this type.

Hemiplegia with Seizures. The association of hemiplegia and seizures suggests damage to cortical gray matter, and it is possible that these cases are related to cerebral contusion during parturition. There appears to be some association between position of the head in relation to the pelvic brim at birth and the incidence of cerebral contusion, hemiplegia, and seizures.

Clinical Features

Children with hemiplegic cerebral palsy show maximum involvement of the upper limbs often with marked loss of function and flexion dystonia of fingers, wrist, and elbow. There are increased tone, hyperreflexia, and flexion deformities at the elbow, fingers, and thumbs.

The lower limb is less severely affected, but there are varying degrees of hypertonia and impairment of gait. Hemianopia, seizures, hemisensory impairment, and mental retardation occur in about 30 per cent of cases.

Diagnostic Procedures

1. Roentgenograms of the skull may show asymmetry and reduction of the size of the cranial cavity on one side with elevation of the petrous ridge and smaller air sinuses on the affected side (the so-called Davidoff-Dyke syndrome). Intracranial calcification may be present in some cases.
2. About 90 per cent of patients with hemiplegia and seizures show EEG abnormalities. The changes may be unilateral or bilateral, focal or diffuse. Combinations of slowing and spike or sharp waves may be seen, which disappear after intravenous injection of diazepam (Valium), implying that the disturbance is seizure-related. Persistent disturbance following intravenous diazepam reflects the abnormality produced by the damaged portion of the brain.
3. Cerebral atrophy can be demonstrated by computerized tomography showing atrophy of the damaged hemisphere and unilateral ventricular dilatation (Fig. 2–13).
4. A middle cerebral artery occlusion or carotid stenosis, occlusion, or irregularity may be demonstrated in some cases by arteriography.
5. A number of children have evidence of congenital heart disease, which may suggest an embolic etiology.

Complex Diplegia

The term "complex diplegia" implies the presence of other abnormalities in addition to the involvement of the corticospinal tracts. These include hypotonic ataxia, involuntary movements, seizures, or mental retardation, which indicates more widespread damage to the central nervous system (Fig. 2–12).

Etiology

A number of developmental defects (p. 69) involving the brain may produce complex diplegia including anoxia, due to asphyxia neonatorum (p. 124). Traumatic injury to the brain can occur at birth with cerebral hemorrhage. This may re-

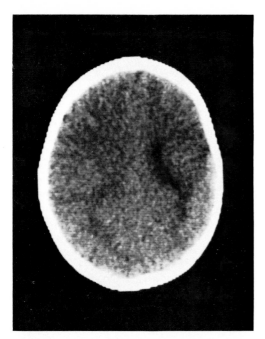

FIGURE 2-13. Computed tomography in hemiplegic cerebral palsy. There is atrophy of the right hemisphere with unilateral dilatation of the right lateral ventricle, which is displaced to the right.

sult in subarachnoid hemorrhage or multiple intracerebral perivenous hemorrhages.

Clinical Features

The disturbance of corticospinal motor function in these children is severe with hypertonia, increased reflexes, and bilateral extensor plantar responses. Usually, when seen by the neurologist, these children present with a mixed syndrome of pyramidal and extrapyramidal signs, with both spasticity and rigidity. There may be profound hypotonia in some severely affected children. Infants show a lack of spontaneous activity, and there is excessive persistence of the tonic neck reflexes.

The development of motor milestones is seriously delayed, and many of these children are never able to walk. The persistence of reflex activity, including extensor thrust, symmetric tonic neck reflexes, assymmetric tonic neck reflexes, and the absence of foot placement and parachute reflexes should be noted. Children with two or more of these abnormalities do not attain walking. On the other hand, a child who can sit at the age of two years will eventually walk.

There may be damage to the cerebellum or cerebellar connections with nystagmus and truncal and limb ataxia. Diffuse cerebral damage in some cases produces mental retardation. Many of these children are microcephalic. Damage to frontal or occipital eye fields may produce inability to follow objects with the eyes. About 50 per cent of children with complex diplegia have epilepsy. Almost all types of seizures may occur, and myoclonic jerks may occur in the interictal period.

Athetotic Cerebral Palsy (Choreoathetosis)

This type of cerebral palsy is characterized by spontaneous involuntary movements that take the form of extension and flexion of the upper limbs and fingers and grimacing of the face. Involuntary movements may involve the lower extremities. These children are usually severely hypotonic during the first year of life and develop choreoathetosis after the first year and occasionally later in childhood.

Etiology

About 50 per cent of cases are the result of kernicterus. The remaining 50 per cent of cases are believed to be due to asphyxia neonatorum.

Clinical Features

Patients with choreoathetosis due to asphyxia neonatorum tend to show signs of corticospinal tract involvement, while those with choreoathetosis due to kernicterus usually do not. Mental retardation and seizures are also more characteristic of the asphyxia neonatorum rather than the kernicterus group.

Ataxic Cerebral Palsy

This is the rarest form and least well-defined type of the cerebral palsies. Children with signs of ataxia and spasticity (ataxia diplegia) should probably be included in the complex diplegia group. The children with ataxia alone probably represent a syndrome of cerebellar dysfunction. The major causes of cerebellar ataxia in children are listed in Table 2-8.

Clinical Features

Children with ataxic cerebral palsy are hypotonic from birth and show few spontaneous movements. The motor development is delayed, and when the children begin to walk, the gait is broad-based and flat-footed. There is truncal ataxia, dys-

TABLE 2–8

Causes of Cerebellar Ataxia in Children

1. *Developmental defects*
   a. Cerebellar agenesis
   b. Cerebellar hypoplasia
   c. Vermis hypoplasia
   d. Dandy-Walker cyst or syndrome
   e. Arnold-Chiari malformation
   f. Basilar invagination
   g. Cerebellar microgyria

2. *Progressive developmental disorders*
   a. Familial spinocerebellar degeneration (Friedreich's ataxia)
   b. Ataxia telangiectasia

3. *Posttraumatic*
   a. Birth trauma and hemorrhage
   b. Head injury in childhood
   c. Cervical spine injury with damage to vertebral arteries

4. *Infections*
   a. Sequel to bacterial meningitis and high fever
   b. Sequel to viral encephalitis (particularly the ECHO group)
   c. Postinfectious leukoencephalopathy

5. *Hydrocephalus*
   a. Compensated hydrocephalus
   b. Treated hydrocephalus

6. *Cerebellar tumors*
   a. Medulloblastoma
   b. Astrocytoma
   c. Hemangioblastoma

metria, intention tremor, hypotonia, and hyporeflexia with flexor plantar responses. There is slow and often scanning speech. In the majority of patients intelligence is normal and seizures are uncommon.

The Treatment of Cerebral Palsy

The care of the child with cerebral palsy requires the full cooperation of the family and is more satisfactory if organized through the facilities of a cerebral palsy clinic. This arrangement allows access to the full range of medical and paramedical personnel who are concerned with the problem and permits a continuous assessment of progress as the child grows older.[274]

Treatment of Motor Disabilities

If indicated, a physical therapy program should be planned for children who acquired cerebral palsy at an early age. Bracing requires skill and observation as part of an expert physical therapy program. It is immaterial whether this is organized under a physiatrist, an orthopedist, or a neurologist as long as the program is effective. Some 25 per cent of children with cerebral palsy have a squint and require ophthalmologic care. A smaller number have disorders of eye movement owing to brainstem damage, which may impair reading in school.[245]

Children with speech difficulties need precise diagnosis and the services of a speech therapist. Similarly, those with poor hearing or deafness require the diagnostic services of an audiologist for possible use of a hearing aid, as well as the special skills of a corrective speech therapist.

Disturbance of the complex mechanisms of swallowing results in embarrassing drooling in children with cerebral palsy. Bilateral tympanic neurectomy and unilateral chorda tympanectomy is reported to control drooling in these cases.[81]

Surgical treatment by muscle lengthening, rerouting of tendons, wedge osteotomy of the os calcis, triple arthrodesis, and other orthopedic measures on the lower limbs may improve the gait.[16] Thalamotomy is useful in athetotic involuntary movements and dystonia.[94] Chronic cerebellar stimulation reduces spasticity and athetosis and improves speech and functional status.[48]

Education

About 50 per cent of children with cerebral palsy are mentally retarded, and many of these children must be taught in special classes at schools.[266] The staff of the social services department of a cerebral palsy clinic, familiar with the community resources, local educational facilities, and family counseling, can advise the parents regarding a suitable school. The parents should be warned that if the child is severely retarded, institutional care may be required. Until the parents agree to place the child in a special facility, he can be treated while living at home.

Children of average or superior intelligence can usually pursue normal education to and including college level but at this point find their progress hindered by motor difficulties, such as spasticity or involuntary movements. These handicaps may be compensated, to a certain extent, by drug therapy, surgery, and the use of special devices, such as electric typewriters. However, even a number of children with normal intelligence and severe motor difficulties will require education in special classes for the handicapped.[126]

The child with a severe hearing problem (which often occurs as a sequal to kernicterus) must be educated in a school for the deaf, specially equipped for this purpose.

Employment

The eventual mode of employment and placement of the patient with cerebral palsy must be decided on the basis of intelligence testing and educational attainment. Occupations requiring little motor skill or participation usually require professional or executive abilities, which emphasizes the necessity for adequate education. About 80 per cent of hemiplegic children without mental retardation are eventually self-supporting.[206] The percentage is lower when bilateral cerebral damage has occurred.

If the patient is mildly retarded or if education has been poor, training is offered in special workshops for the handicapped in many communities. Placement of these individuals requires adequate social services and is usually provided by a cerebral palsy center.

Epilepsy

Control of seizures is discussed in Chapter 6 (p. 361).

Emotional Factors

The Family. A handicapped child has a profound emotional effect on the entire family. Adjustments by parents and siblings will be helped by experienced advice and counseling by professionals either in the office or at cerebral palsy clinics. Parental feelings of guilt or resentment are commonly encountered and must be treated by counseling, listening, and advice.

The Patient. The handicapped child with cerebral damage is particularly vulnerable to frustration and emotional problems. When a child with cerebral palsy suddenly fails to do well in school, this is frequently due to some emotional problem although it is often erroneously ascribed to mental slowness and limited intelligence. Such problems require sympathy and care by social workers who are familiar with these situations. Overt psychotic behavior is occasionally seen in the teens and twenties and requires psychiatric help. The precipitating factor is often some change to a more stressful situation or environment.

Emotional difficulties may be exacerbated in adolescence by the knowledge that marriage is unlikely or impossible, by the desire to lead an independent adult life, and by related sexual problems. There is a need for continuing community facilities for cerebral palsy patients in adult life.

Medication

Muscle Relaxants. There are many preparations available that allegedly relax spastic or hypertonic muscles. Few are effective, and many produce a limited effect by sedation rather than by direct action on muscle tone. Diazepam or baclofen may benefit some cases (see also Treatment of Involuntary Movements).

Stimulants. Methylphenidate or dextroamphetamine is often effective for the hyperactive child. It should be given on awakening in the morning and again at noon to avoid any action that may prevent sleep in the evening.

Anticonvulsants. Anticonvulsants are also prescribed if the patient has seizures or evidence of seizure abnormalities in the EEG.

Phenothiazines. This group of drugs is particularly effective in the hyperactive or emotionally disturbed child who requires tranquilization without sedation.

Diazepam and Chlordiazepoxide. These two preparations have been used with some success in the treatment of involuntary movements in cerebral palsy. Diazepam is probably the most effective and can be given in 2-mg doses three times a day and increased gradually to as much as 5 mg five times a day.

Kernicterus

Prior to the development of exchange transfusion as a practical form of treatment, about 10 per cent of cerebral palsy cases were due to kernicterus. With this form of treatment the percentage has been reduced to about 1 or 2 per cent.

The condition may be defined as cerebral damage resulting from hyperbilirubinemia, which may be present at or shortly after birth. Whether bilirubin itself is the sole cause of damage to the central nervous system is by no means settled and it is possible that other factors are involved in the pathogenesis of kernicterus.

Etiology and Pathogenesis

Maternal Isoimmunization as a Hyperbilirubinemic Factor. The commonest situation is that of the Rh-positive child and the Rh-negative mother. Antibodies against the Rh factor present in the fetal erythrocytes are formed by the mother and diffuse across the placenta to enter the fetal circulation and produce hemolysis. The child may be born with hemolytic anemia and jaundice (kernicterus) or with severe anemia and edema (hydrops fetalis). High titers of maternal antibodies against the fetal erythrocytes with the Rh factor occur only when the mother has been sensitized previously to the antigen. In the case of Rh incompatibility, kernicterus does not occur in the firstborn child unless the mother has been sensitized by previous blood transfusion of Rh-incompatible blood.

Occasionally, maternal antibodies against other blood factors (A, B, Kell, etc.) may be responsible for hemolysis in the infant.

Drugs as a Cause of Hyperbilirubinemia. The administration of sulfonamides and salicylates in the neonatal period has been found to be associated with an increased incidence of kernicterus. The mechanism of action of these drugs is uncertain, but it is possible that they displace bilirubin from binding sites to serum proteins or inhibit conjugation of bilirubin in the liver.

Premature infants receiving more than adequate dosage of vitamin K have shown a rapid increase in serum bilirubin with the development of kernicterus in some cases. The mechanism is obscure, but it is possible that excess vitamin K inhibits conjugation of bilirubin in the liver.

Prematurity as a Cause of Hyperbilirubinemia. The premature infant with jaundice, especially the male, shows a higher incidence of ker-

nicterus. This is apparently due to restricted capacity of the liver to conjugate bilirubin in premature infants.

Asphyxia Neonatorum

Immediately before birth the oxygen saturation of fetal blood is only about 60 per cent. This borderline hypoxia is compensated by the ability of fetal hemoglobin to take up and release oxygen with greater facility than adult hemoglobin. The fetal brain also has mechanisms for anaerobic metabolism, which is not readily available to the adult. However, any severe reduction of oxygen supply to the fetus will be catastrophic, particularly to the brain, with the production of different degrees of irreversible damage.

The newborn infant may also suffer similar damage to the brain if respiration is not established within minutes after birth. Asphyxia neonatorum is consequently a condition of asphyxia immediately before, during, or after birth. The chief causes are listed in Table 2–9.

Pathology

Anoxia of the brain results in increased vascular permeability, cerebral edema, and both arterial and venous hemorrhages. The cerebral edema resulting from damage to vascular endothelium may not develop for a number of days after the episode of asphyxia. Direct anoxic damage to neurons may produce a neuronal atrophy.

Two basic patterns may be recognized.[186] In the mature newborn infant, anoxia produces neuronal atrophy maximal in the cortex with infarction in the depth of the gyri (ulegyria). In anoxic damage to the fetus or premature infant, the basal

TABLE 2–9

Etiology of Asphyxia Neonatorum

1. *Prenatal causes.* Any condition producing interference with placental circulation
   a. Abruptio placentae, placenta previa, maternal hemorrhage
   b. Maternal shock with reduction of blood pressure and poor perfusion pressure of the placenta

2. *During parturition*
   a. Prolonged labor
   b. Cerebral trauma due to excessive molding of the head or use of instruments for delivery
   c. Compression of cerebral arteries and veins during molding of the head

3. *Immediate postnatal period.* Failure to establish respiration
   a. Prematurity
   b. Cerebral trauma during labor
   c. Respiratory diseases—atelectasis, hyaline membrane disease
   d. Congenital heart disease
   e. Depressed respiratory center from drugs or anesthetics

ganglia show neuronal loss and gliosis with a peculiar overgrowth of myelin into the gray matter of the thalamus and basal ganglia giving them a marble-like appearance (status marmoratus, état marbré).[268, 284]

Clinical Features

Infants with moderate degrees of asphyxia neonatorum appear lethargic or obtunded at birth. The limbs are flexed and the tendon reflexes are brisk. The sucking and Moro reflexes are weak, but the oculovestibular and tonic neck reflexes are strong. There is parasympathetic overactivity with miosis, bradycardia, profuse salivation, and diarrhea. Focal or generalized seizures may occur. Resolution of these signs within a five-day period is usually followed by normal development.[223]

More severely affected infants are stuporous, flaccid with absent reflexes, and show intermittent decerebration. Approximately 50 per cent of these infants die, but about 75 per cent of the survivors are apparently normal.[228] Infants with permanent damage from anoxic encephalopathy show persistent flaccidity with absence of the Moro response, absence of grasp reflexes, and thumbs adducted and flexed into the palms (thalamic hand). The visual following responses are impaired, and the tactile placing reactions of hands and feet are absent. At about three months of age spasticity develops and the child lies with the upper limbs flexed and the lower limbs extended and adducted in a position of decortication. The tonic neck reflexes persist into the first year of life, and by six months the child may be microcephalic (by measurement of the circumference of the skull). Involuntary movements frequently appear at four months of age with the gradual development of bilateral choreoathetosis. There is marked delay in reaching the usual milestones of motor development such as holding the head up, sitting, standing, and walking. Seizures begin in about one fourth of cases, and speech development is delayed and may never become developed in severe cases. Severe mental retardation occurs in about 30 per cent of cases of complex diplegia due to asphyxia neonatorum. A further 20 per cent may show intellectual or perceptual defects of a less severe nature but, unless recognized, these will prove to be a handicap in school.

Diagnostic Procedures

1. The persistence of electroencephalographic abnormalities consisting of periodic generalized high-voltage discharges, preceded by continuous delta activity, carries a poor prognosis in terms of later neurologic impairment.
2. Visual evoked responses and somatosensory evoked responses are abnormal in asphyxia neonatorum. Persistent abnormality is indicative of cerebral damage.[118]

Treatment

1. The provision and use of adequate prenatal care will minimize the majority of prenatal factors producing asphyxia neonatorum.
2. Maintenance of adequate ventilation is essential to prevent recurrence of hypoxemia and hypercapnia.
3. Seizures should be controlled with phenobarbital (10 mg/kg administered intravenously). Maintenance doses of 5 to 10 mg/kg are used to maintain an adequate serum level of phenobarbital. This drug has the advantage of decreasing cerebral metabolic rate.
4. Hypoglycemia should be prevented using parenteral glucose.
5. Cerebral edema should be treated by avoiding fluid overloading. The use of corticosteroids is controversial in the neonate.[275]

Hypoxia as a Cause of Hyperbilirubinemia. Liver cells may be damaged by hypoxia with decreased conjugation of bilirubin by the damaged liver cells. Epidemiologic evidence suggests that perinatal and neonatal hypoxemia plays an important role in the development of kernicterus.

Sepsis as a Cause of Hyperbilirubinemia. In infants with kernicterus unrelated to maternal isoimmunization there is a high incidence of bacterial sepsis.[139] Hepatic damage by infection appears to play a major role in this latter group.

Congenital, Familial Nonhemolytic Jaundice. This rare condition is due to a genetically determined absence of the enzyme glucuronyl transferase in the liver with inability to conjugate bilirubin. The infants are jaundiced, and in some the hyperbilirubinemia has been associated with kernicterus.

Factors Influencing Susceptibility of Neurons to Damage by Hyperbilirubinemia

Hyperbilirubinemia in both Rh-sensitized and nonisosensitized infants is related to decreased glucuronyl transferase activity in the liver. Fetal bilirubin is excreted through the placenta, but at the time of birth the excretory pathway is changed suddenly and depends entirely on the glucuronyl transferase system of the neonatal liver. Excessive hemolysis and bilirubin production result in production of bilirubin exceeding the body's capacity to conjugate and remove it, with an increase in serum bilirubin levels.

There is some degree of relationship between the levels of hyperbilirubinemia and damage to the central nervous system producing kernicterus, but the relationship of kernicterus to serum bilirubin levels is not one that is absolute or threshold. Kernicterus tends to occur with lower serum bilirubin levels in premature infants, but it is known that only that fraction of bilirubin not bound to albumin can cross the blood-brain barrier. This free bilirubin is present in higher concentrations at lower total serum bilirubin levels in the sick, premature infant.[290]

The Blood-Brain Barrier. Selective staining of certain specific areas of the central nervous system by bilirubin in kernicterus indicates that the passage of bilirubin is influenced by the blood-brain barrier. Nonconjugated bilirubin is also more lipid-soluble and hence more likely to be taken up by the brain. It also seems likely that the permeability to bilirubin by the blood-brain barrier is increased in the premature infant. The increased permeability may be due to an enhanced affinity between free bilirubin and neonatal gangliosides.[281] There is less affinity between free bilirubin and adult gangliosides, and the difference may account for the marked cytotoxicity of free bilirubin for the infant brain. In any event, once high concentrations of bilirubin reach the nerve cells, it appears to have a direct toxic effect and probably interferes with enzyme systems necessary for neuronal metabolism.

Hypoxia. There is some similarity in the areas of damage produced by hypoxia in the central nervous system to those found damaged by kernicterus. Lowered oxygen tension, in addition to producing damage to neurons, also impairs the blood-brain barrier as well as damaging the liver cells.

The Role of Free Fatty Acids

The premature infant has relatively high concentrations of free fatty acids in the serum and low serum albumin concentrations. The free fatty acid serum albumin ratio is further increased in hypothermia, hypoglycemia, sepsis, starvation, acidosis, and hypoxia. It is possible that a free fatty acid bilirubin complex occurs in the serum of newborn infants and that the complex is rapidly transported into all cells in the body, including the brain, with intracellular release of bilirubin from this complex.[86]

Anemia. Rapid hemolysis of red cells increases the serum bilirubin levels and reduces the oxygen-carrying capacity of the blood. This also contributes to impairment of liver function and the efficiency of the blood-brain barrier as well as increasing blood bilirubin levels.

Other Possible Contributing Factors in Kernicterus. As has been said, kernicterus due to Rh sensitization does not occur in the firstborn unless the mother has been previously sensitized by blood transfusion. Thus, repeated pregnancies and multiple transfusions increase the liability of kernicterus. Twinning also will increase the risk of kernicterus owing to the increased liability of hypoxemia in twins.

Pathology

The meninges, choroid plexus, pituitary gland, ependyma, and certain parts of the brain all show a yellow-brown discoloration. The globus pallidus, subthalamic nucleus, Ammon's horn, induseum griseum, mammillary bodies, interstitial nucleus of Cajal, cranial nerve nuclei, inferior olivary nuclei, vermis of the cerebellum, and dentate nucleus are the parts that usually show heavy staining with bilirubin. Microscopic examination of these areas shows a loss of neurons. The globus pallidus, subthalamic nucleus, and Ammon's horn regularly show severe loss of neurons, while the other areas are less severely affected. There is relative preservation of neurons in the inferior olivary nuclei and in the vermis of the cerebellum even when those areas are stained heavily with bilirubin.

Clinical Features

Neonatal Period. After birth there is progressive jaundice beginning during the first day with edema of the face and enlargement of the liver and spleen. The urine and stool are heavily bile-stained. The child is anemic and listless and feeds poorly. Severely affected cases show progressive lethargy, stupor, and coma punctuated at intervals by convulsions and opisthotonus and, if untreated, followed by death. There is generalized rigidity with intermittent spasms and involuntary movements. Children who survive usually improve for a few months and then develop a characteristic hypotonia at about three months of age. The permanent features of kernicterus begin to appear after 18 months and include the following: There may be some degree of mental retardation, although a few children with kernicterus are apparently of normal intelligence. The majority of children develop some degree of athetosis, rigidity, or spasticity alone or in combination. Some develop a more or less pure syndrome of hypertonia and ataxia. The most common disturbance is a paralysis of upward gaze, but other forms of gaze palsy are also seen. Although many children have diminished auditory acuity, problems in speech and hearing are coupled with auditory defects, dysphasia, and dysarthria. The deciduous teeth are frequently bile-stained and show dysplasia, such as semilunar defects of the enamel, particularly in the upper incisors and canines.

Treatment

1. All Rh-negative mothers should receive antirhesus immunoglobulin at delivery. This will prevent the formation of antirhesus antibodies in response to fetal cells that might have entered the maternal circulation and protect the fetus from injury by antibodies at a subsequent pregnancy.
2. Severe cases of kernicterus should be treated by exchange transfusion.
   a. If the reserve serum albumin binding capacity falls below 50 μg/ml of serum.[279]
   b. If the child shows signs of neurologic involvement (poor motor activity, loss of the Moro reflex, or loss of a sucking reflex).
   c. If the level of free bilirubin exceeds 0.1 mg/100 ml of serum. In exchange transfusion, aliquots of 10 ml of the infants' blood are removed by umbilical catheter and replaced by an equal volume of group O Rh-negative blood until a total of 80 ml/kg body weight has been exchanged.
3. Bile pigments are rapidly broken down when exposed to light, and the water-soluble products are excreted in the bile and urine. The exposure of premature infants to light in phototherapy units appears to be an effective method of preventing hyperbilirubinemia of

prematurity and reducing the risk of kernicterus.
4. The administration of phenobarbital to the mother before delivery may be a useful adjuvant in the prevention of kernicterus. Phenobarbital stimulates the glucuronyl transferase system in the infant liver and increases the conjugation of bilirubin, thereby reducing the risk of kernicterus in the newborn infant.

The Neuronal Atrophies of Childhood

Progressive Cerebral Poliodystrophy (Alper's Disease)

It seems evident that some cases of neuronal degeneration encountered in infancy and childhood are not related to the lipidoses or to viral infection or to inclusion bodies and have a relative preservation of white matter. Unequivocal evidence that progressive cerebral poliodystrophy is a distinct disease entity rather than a syndrome has, however, not been established. It is possible that the progressive neuronal degeneration represents a nonspecific response to a number of etiologic factors.[97]

Etiology and Pathology

The study of autopsied cases suggests that one or more of the following factors may be important in this disease:

1. Anoxia at birth or in the immediate postnatal period
2. Anoxia secondary to seizures
3. Neuronal atrophy secondary to some genetically determined intracellular enzymatic defects. This concept is supported by the description of more than one case occurring in a family, suggesting a genetically determined defect.[122] The presence of cirrhosis or subacute hepatitis in some children may indicate the presence of a genetically determined metabolic error as yet unidentified.

The brain shows neuronal loss affecting the cortex and subcortical nuclei without any inflammatory response and with relative preservation of white matter.

Clinical Features

The majority of cases begin in the first year of life, but isolated cases have been reported in children up to five years of age. There is a progressive dementia, with seizures beginning early in the illness. In a few patients, the duration of the illness is short and death occurs within a few weeks. Others show a more protracted course during which they develop spasticity, myoclonic jerks, choreoathetoid movements, visual deterioration, and optic atrophy. Death may occur in status epilepticus or following a prolonged period of deterioration, usually from intercurrent infection.

Diagnostic Procedures

There are no specific diagnostic tests for the condition, and the diagnosis is usually made at autopsy.

Treatment

Life may be prolonged by good nursing care and prevention of intercurrent infection, but there is no specific treatment that will delay the neuronal degeneration.

Infantile Spinal Muscular Atrophy (Werdnig-Hoffmann Syndrome)

The diffuse motor neuron atrophy of infancy and childhood is now known to present with different degrees of severity, and cases of later onset tend to merge with the juvenile proximal spinal muscular atrophy or the Kugelberg-Welander syndrome (p. 214).

Etiology and Pathology

Infantile spinal muscular atrophy is inherited as an autosomal recessive trait. The cause of the neuronal degeneration is unknown, but it probably results from the failure of intracellular enzymatic systems and the blocking of essential metabolic pathways. There is a diffuse loss of motor neurons in the anterior horns of the spinal cord and motor nuclei of the brainstem. Surviving cells show central chromatolysis and neuronophagia, and there is a diffuse gliosis with increase in astrocytes and microglia, which is particularly marked in the areas of neuronal atrophy.

Severe cerebellar hypoplasia associated with degenerative changes in the brainstem nuclei has been reported in some cases.[282]

The loss of neurons reduces the content of motor nerve fibers in the anterior nerve roots and peripheral nerves, and there is diffuse atrophy of muscle fibers in the distribution of motor units throughout the entire musculoskeletal system.

Clinical Features

It is possible to recognize four distinct groups of patients with this condition:[35, 63]

Group I. The onset occurs in utero and the mother notices that the infant's movements become weaker later in pregnancy. The baby is inactive at birth and shows progressive weakness. This is characterized by generalized hypotonia, paucity of limb movements, and areflexia ("floppy infant syndrome"). Extraocular movements and diaphragmatic contractions are quite strong with paradoxic respiratory movements and collapse of the thoracic cage as the diaphragm descends. There is a characteristic posture when the child lies in the supine position with the arms abducted and flexed at the elbows and the lower limbs externally rotated, abducted at the hips, and flexed at the knees (the "frog" position). Death usually occurs before the first birthday from pneumonia.

Group II. Children in this group are apparently normal at birth and develop weakness after the second postnatal month. The onset is gradual with weakness beginning in the lower limbs and involving the upper limbs later. Fasciculations may be present in the tongue and limb muscles, and there is hypotonia with absent reflexes in the lower limbs. The majority of children are never able to crawl and stand, males being more severely affected than females.[201a] Death usually occurs around two years of age, but there have been occasional survivors to seven years of age.

Group III. Weakness begins at 12 months of age or later, and most of the children in this group are eventually able to stand unaided.[206b] Fasciculations of the tongue and limb muscles are present in most cases. The disease is slowly progressive but may become arrested, and the majority of children are able to attend school.[100] Patients in this group with later onset of weakness may be regarded as examples of the juvenile proximal spinal muscular atrophy of Kugelberg and Welander.[62]

Group IV. Weakness of the facial, glossopharyngeal, and extraocular muscles begins at age 12 months, and progressive bulbar paralysis occurs with death by the third year. This is known as Fazio-Londe's disease and is comparable to the bulbar form of amyotrophic lateral sclerosis of adults. At autopsy the children show atrophy of neurons of the brainstem motor nuclei.[89]

Diagnostic Procedures

1. Electromyography will usually show the presence of fasciculations and fibrillations in children in group I, but this finding may be delayed for some time in children in the other three groups.
2. The muscle biopsy is characterized by diffuse atrophy of motor units, which is typical in neurongenic muscle atrophy.

Treatment

There is no treatment known to affect the course of this disease. Life may be prolonged by prompt and adequate treatment of respiratory infections.

Patients in group III who survive into adolescence and adult life require daily respiratory therapy to prevent pneumonia and should receive realistic education and vocational training.

Cited References

1. Abe, K.; Matsuda, I.; et al. X-linked ichthyosis, bilateral cryptorchism, hypogenitalism and mental retardation in two siblings. *Clin. Genet.,* **9:**341–45, 1976.
2. Aguayo, A. J.; Nair, C.; and Bray, G. Peripheral nerve abnormalities in the Riley-Day syndrome. *Arch. Neurol.,* **24:**106–16, 1971.
3. Alexander, G. L., and Norman, R. M. *The Sturge-Weber Syndrome.* Wright, Bristol, 1960.
4. Alvita, M., and Forman, D. Biochemical abnormalities in Reye's syndrome. *Ann. Clin. Lab. Sci.,* **4:**477–83, 1974.
5. Ames, M. D., and Schut, L. Results of treatment of 171 consecutive myelomeningoceles, 1963 to 1968. *Pediatrics,* **50:**466–70, 1972.
6. Anderson, A., and Avins, L. Lowering brain phenylalnine levels by giving other large neutral aminoacids. *Arch. Neurol.,* **33:**684–86, 1976.
7. Anderson, J.; Milner, R.; and Strich, S. Effect of neonatal hypoglycemia on the nervous system. *J. Neurol. Neurosurg. Psychiatry,* **30:**295–310, 1967.
8. Angeli, E.; Denman, A.; et al. Maternal phenylketonuria: A family with seven mentally retarded siblings. *Dev. Med. Child Neurol.,* **16:**800–807, 1974.
9. Aprille, J. Reye's syndrome: Patient serum alters mitochondrial function and morphology in vitro. *Science,* **197:**908–10, 1977.
10. Archer, M., and Pate, A. An analysis of 469 children with spina bifida treated in the Richmond Hospital between 1967–1973. *Irish Med. J.,* **68:**293–99, 1975.
11. Arthur, A.; Bush, R.; Guard, F.; and Weston, H. Spina bifida cystica: Survey of 107 cases. *N.Z. Med. J.,* **75:**272–77, 1972.
12. AuRuskin, T.; Braverman, L.; and Crigler, J. Thyroxine binding globulin deficiency and associated neurological deficit. *Pediatrics,* **50:**638–45, 1972.
13. Axelrod, F.; Branom, N.; Becker, M.; Nachtigall, R.; and Dancis, J. Treatment of familial dysautonomia with bethanecol (urecholine). *J. Pediatr.,* **81:**573–78, 1972.
14. Axelrod, F.; Nachtigall, R.; and Davies, J. Familial dysautonomia: Diagnosis, pathogenesis and management. *Adv. Pediatr.,* **21:**75–96, 1974.
15. Baird, P., and DeJong, B. Noonan's syndrome (XX and XY Turner phenotype) in three generations of a family. *J. Pediatr.,* **80:**110–14, 1972.
16. Balcer, L.; Bassett, F.; and Dyas, E. Surgery in the rehabilitation of cerebral palsied patients. *Dev. Med. Child Neurol.,* **12:**330–42, 1970.
17. Balla, D.; Butterfield, E.; and Zigler, E. Effects of institutionalization on retarded children: A longitudinal cross-institutional investigation. *Am. J. Ment. Defic.,* **78:**530–49, 1974.
17a. Balsh, R. W.; Yee, R. D.; and Boder, E. Eye movements in ataxic telangiectasia. *Neurology* (Minneap.), **28:**1099–1104, 1978.
18. Banerji, N., and Millar, J. Chiari malformation presenting in adult life. Its relationship to syringomyelia. *Brain,* **97:**157–68, 1974.
19. Bannayan, G.; Dean, W.; and Howell, R. Type IV glycogen-storage disease. Light-microscopic, electron-microscopic and enzymatic study. *Am. J. Clin. Pathol.,* **66:**702–709, 1976.
20. Bell, W.; Sammaan, N.; and Langnecker, D. Hypoglycemia due to organic hyperinsulinism in infancy. *Arch. Neurol.,* **23:**330–39, 1970.
21. Benzie, R.; Doran, T.; et al. Prenatal diagnosis of hypophosphatasia. *Birth Defects,* **12:**271–82, 1976.
22. Beverly, J. K. Toxoplasmosis. *Br. Med. J.,* **2:**475–78, 1973.
23. Blaskovics, M.; Schaeffer, G.; and Hack, S. Phenylalanaemia. Differential diagnosis. *Arch. Dis. Child.,* **49:**835–43, 1974.
24. Black, E. Locomotor prognosis in cerebral palsy. *Dev. Med. Child Neurol.,* **17:**18–25, 1975.
25. Bluestone, C.; Delerme, A.; and Samuelson, G. Airway obstruction due to vocal cord paralysis in infants with hydrocephalus and meningomyelocele. *Ann. Otol. Rhinol. Laryngol.,* **81:**778–83, 1972.
26. Bobath, K. *The Motor Deficit in Patients with Cerebral Palsy.* William Heineman Medical Books, Ltd., London, 1966.
27. Bolthauser, E.; Wilson, E.; and Hoare, R. Sturge-Weber syndrome with bilateral intracranial calcification. *J. Neurol. Neurosurg. Psychiatry,* **39:**429–35, 1976.
28. Brem, A., and Haddow, J. Hypothyroidism in infancy. *J. Maine Med. Assoc.,* **67:**1–3, 1976.
29. Broberger, O.; Jurzner, I.; and Zetterstrom, R. Studies in spontaneous hypoglycemia in childhood. Failure to increase the epinephrine secretion in insulin-induced hypoglycemia. *J. Pediatr.,* **55:**713–19, 1959.

30. Broberger, O., and Zetterstrom, R. Hypoglycemia, with an inability to increase the epinephrine secretion in insulin induced hypoglycemia. *J. Pediatr.,* **59:**215–22, 1961.

31. Brock, D. J. Alpha fetoprotein and neural tube defects. *J. Clin. Pathol.,* **29** supp. 10:157–64, 1976.

32. Brock, D. J.; Bolton, A.; and Monaghan, J. Prenatal diagnosis of anencephaly through maternal serum alpha fetoprotein measurements. *Lancet,* **2:**923–24, 1973.

33. Brook, C.; Sanders, M.; and Hoore, R. Septo-optic dysplasia. *Br. Med., J.* **3:**811–13, 1972.

34. Brown, T.; Hug, G.; et al. Transiently reduced activity of carbamyl phosphate synthetase and ornithine transcarbamylase in liver of children with Reye's syndrome. *N. Engl. J. Med.,* **294:**861–67, 1976.

35. Byers, R., and Banker, B. Infantile muscular atrophy. *Arch. Neurol.,* **5:**140–64, 1961.

36. Caillie, M.; Morin, L.; et al. Reye's syndrome relapses and neurological sequelae. *Pediatrics,* **59:**244–49, 1977.

37. Carey, L.; Ruben, R.; et al. Influenza B associated Reye's syndrome: Incidence in Michigan and potential for treatment. *J. Inf. Dis.,* **135:**398–407, 1977.

38. Carter, C. O. Clues to the etiology of neural tube malformations. *Dev. Med. Child Neurol.,* **16** supp. 32:3–15, 1974.

39. Carter, S., and Gold, A. Acute infantile hemiplegia. *Pediatr. Clin. North Am.,* **14:**851–64, 1967.

40. Chavez-Carballo, E.; Gomez, M.; and Sharborough, F. Encephalopathy and fatty infiltration of the viscera. (Reye-Johnson syndrome). *Mayo Clin. Proc.,* **50:**209–15, 1975.

41. Chen, H.; Watz, D.; and Carroll, J. Immunoglobulinopathy in Down's syndrome. *Ohio State Med. J.,* **73:**27–29, 1977.

42. Childhood hypoglycemia. *Br. Med. J.,* **1:**5, 1972.

43. Christoff, N. Myoclonus encephalopathy of infants. A report of two cases and observations on related disorders. *Arch. Neurol.,* **21:**229–34, 1969.

44. Cohen, M. An etiologic and nosologic overview of craniosynostosis syndromes. *Birth Defects,* **11:**137–89, 1975.

45. Colle, E., and Ulstrom, R. Ketotic hypoglycemia. *J. Pediatr.,* **64:**632–51, 1964.

46. Colover, J.; Lucas, M.; Comley, J.; and Roe, A. Neurological abnormalities in the cri-du-chat syndrome. *J. Neurol. Neurosurg. Psychiatry,* **35:**711–19, 1972.

47. Constantopoulos, G.; McComb, R.; and Dekaban, A. Neurochemistry of the mucopolysaccharidoses: Brain glycosaminoglycans in normals and four types of mucopolysaccharidoses. *J. Neurochem.,* **26:**901–908, 1976.

48. Cooper, J.; Riklan, M.; et al. Chronic cerebellar stimulation in cerebral palsy. *Neurology* (Minneap.), **26:**744–53, 1976.

49. Cooperman, E. Acute hemiplegia in childhood. *Can. Med. Assoc. J.,* **114:**13, 1976.

50. Cooperstock, M.; Tucher, R.; and Baubles, J. Possible pathogenic role of endotoxin in Reye's syndrome. *Lancet,* **2:**1272–74, 1975.

51. Costello, C., and Webber, A. White cell function in Down's syndrome. *Clin. Genet.,* **9:**603–605, 1976.

52. Critchley, M. Periodic hypersomnia and megaphagia in adolescent males. *Brain,* **85:**627–56, 1962.

53. Dacou-Voutetakis, C.; Karpathios, T.; et al. Defective growth hormone secretion in primary microcephaly. *J. Pediatr.,* **85:**498–502, 1974.

54. David, O.; Hoffman, S.; et al. Low lead levels and mental retardation. *Lancet,* **2:**1376–79, 1976.

55. DeJong, J.; Delleman, J.; Houben, M.; et al. Agenesis of the corpus callosum, infantile spasm, ocular anomalies (Alcardi's syndrome). *Neurology* (Minneap.)., **26:**1152–58, 1976.

56. Dekaban, A.; Aamodt, R.; et al. Kinky hair disease. Study of copper metabolism with use of ^{67}Cu. *Arch. Neurol.,* **32:**672–75, 1975.

57. Dell'Osso, L.; Flynn, J.; and Daroff, R. Hereditary congenital nystagmus. *Arch. Ophthalmol.,* **92:**366–74, 1974.

58. Dell'Osso, L.; Gauthier, G.; et al. Eye movement recordings as a diagnostic tool in a case of congenital nystagmus. *Am. J. Ophthal. Am. Acad. Optom.,* **49:**4–14, 1972.

59. Dennis, M. Impaired sensory and motor differentiation with corpus callosum agenesis: A lack of collosal inhibition during ontogeny. *Neuropsychologia,* **14:**455–69, 1976.

60. Depresseux, J.; Carlier, G.; and Stevenaert, A. CSF scanning in achondroplastic children with cranial enlargement. *Dev. Med. Child Neurol.,* **17:**224–28, 1975.

60a. Dobkin, B. H. Syncope induced by adult chiari anomaly. *Neurology* (Minneap.), **28:**718–20, 1978.

61. Dougall, A.; Grant, J.; and O'Connor, J. Late follow-up in spina bifida cystica. *Scott. Med. J.,* **20:**129–32, 1975.

62. Dubowitz, V. Benign infantile spinal muscular atrophy. *Dev. Med. Child Neurol.,* **16:**672–75, 1974.

63. Dubowitz, V. Infantile muscular atrophy. Prospective study with particular reference to a slowly progressive variety. *Brain,* **87:**707–18, 1964.

64. Durkin, M.; Kaveggia, E.; et al. Analysis of etiologic factors in cerebral palsy with severe mental retardation. I. Analysis of gestations, parturitional and neonatal data. *Eur. J. Pediatr.,* **123:**67–81, 1976.

65. Dussault, J.; Coulambe, P.; et al. Preliminary report on a mass screening program for neonatal hypothyroidism. *J. Pediatr.,* **86:**670–74, 1975.

66. Dyken, P., and Kolar, O. Dancing eyes, dancing feet: Infantile polymyoclonia. *Brain,* **91:**305–19, 1968.

67. Efron, M. L. Animoacidurias. *N. Engl. J. Med.,* **272:**1058–67, 1107–13, 1965.

68. Elek, S., and Stern, H. Development of a vaccine against mental retardation caused by cytomegalovirus infection in utero. *Lancet,* **1:**1–5, 1974.

69. Engel, A. G. Acid maltase deficiency in adults. Studies in four cases of a syndrome which may mimic muscular dystrophy or other myopathies. *Brain,* **93:**599–616, 1970.

70. Ettinger, G.; Blakemore, G.; Milner, A.; and Wilson, J. Agenesis of the corpus callosum: A further behavioral investigation. *Brain,* **97:**225–34, 1974.

71. Ettinger, G.; Blakemore, G.; Milner, A.; and Wilson, J. Agenesis of the corpus callosum. A behavioral investigation. *Brain,* **95:**327–46, 1972.

72. Fernandes, J., and Huying, F. Branching enzyme deficiency glycogenosis studies in therapy. *Arch. Dis. Child.,* **43:**347–52, 1968.

73. Fernandes, J., and VandeKamer, J. Hexose and protein tolerance tests in children with liver glycogenosis caused by a deficiency of the debranching enzyme system. *Pediatrics,* **41:**935–44, 1968.

74. Ferrell, R.; Jones, B.; and Luiss, R. Simultaneous occurrence of the Holt-Oram and Duane syndromes. *J. Pediatr.,* **69:**630–34, 1966.

75. Ferris, G., and Dorsen, M. Agenesis of the corpus callosum. 1. A neuropsychological study. *Cortex,* **11:**95–122, 1974.

76. Ferry, P. Neurological evaluation of retarded children: Recent advances and new diagnostic techniques. *J. Nat. Med. Assoc.,* **68:**398–401, 1976.

77. Fishman, M. A. Recent clinical advances in the treatment of dysraphic states. *Pediatr. Clin. North Am.,* **23:**517–26, 1976.

78. Foltz, E., and Loeser, J. Craniosynostosis. *J. Neurosurg.,* **43:**48–57, 1975.

79. Forness, S. R. Education of retarded children. *Am. J. Dis. Child.,* **127:**237–42, 1974.

80. Fox, J.; Fishman, M.; Dodge, P.; and Prensky, A. The effect of malnutrition on human central nervous system myelin. *Neurology* (Minneap.), **22:**1213–16, 1972.

81. Friedman, W., and Kaplan, B. Tympanic neurectomy. Correction of drooling in cerebral palsy. *N.Y. State J. Med.,* **75:**2419–22, 1975.

82. Frith, C.; Johnstone, E.; et al. Double-blind clinical trial of 5-hydroxytryptophan in a case of Lesch-Nyhan syndrome. *J. Neurol. Neurosurg. Psychiatry,* **39:**656–62, 1976.

83. Froesch, E.; Wolf, H.; Baitsch, H.; Prater, A.; and Labhart, A. Hereditary fructose intolerance. An inborn defect of hepatic fructose-1-phosphate splitting aldolase. *Am. J. Med.,* **34:**151–67, 1963.

84. Gabrielsen, T.; Seeger, J.; and Amundsen, P. Some new angiographic observations in patients with Chiari type I and II malformations. *Radiology,* **115:**627–34, 1975.

84a. Garcia, C. A.; Dunn, D; and Trevor, R. The lissencephaly (agyra) syndrome in siblings. Computerized tomographic and neuropathologic findings. *Arch. Neurol.,* **35:**608–11, 1978.

85. Garland, H.; Sumner, D.; and Fourman, P. The Kleine-Levin syndrome. Some further observations. *Neurology* (Minneap.), **15:**1161–67, 1965.

86. Gartner, L., and Lee, K. Bilirubin binding, free fatty acids and a new concept for the pathogenesis of kernicterus. *Birth Defects,* **11:**265–74, 1976.

87. Gershenck, J., and James, V. Ataxia telangiectasia and growth failure. *Am. J. Dis. Child.,* **122:**538–40, 1971.

88. Gilchrist, K.; Gilbert, E.; et al. The evaluation on infants with the Zellweger (cerebro-hepato-renal) syndrome. *Clin. Genet.,* **7:**413–16, 1975.

88a. Gol, A., and Hellbusch, L. C. Surgical relief of progressive upper limb paralysis in Arnold-Chiari malformation. *J. Neurol. Neurosurg. Psychology,* **41:**433–37, 1978.

89. Gomez, M.; Clermont, V.; and Bernstein, J. Progressive bulbar paralysis in children (Fazio-Londe disease). *Arch. Neurol.,* **6:**317–23, 1962.

90. Gomez, M.; Gotham, J.; and Meyer, J. Effect of sodium glutamate on leucine-induced hypoglycemia: Clinical and electroencephalographic study. *Pediatrics,* **28:**935–42, 1961.

91. Gomez, M.; Mellenger, J.; and Reese, O. The use of computerized transaxial tomography in the diagnosis of tuberous sclerosis. *Mayo Clin. Assoc.,* **50:**553–56, 1975.

92. Gomez, M.; Whitten, C.; Nolke, A.; Bernstein, J.; and Meyer, J. Aneurysmal malformation of the great vein of Galen causing heart failure in early infancy. *Pediatrics,* **31:**400–11, 1963.

93. Gordon, N. Menke's kinky hair (steely hair) syndrome. *Dev. Med. Child Neurol.,* **16:**827–29, 1974.

94. Gornall, P.; Hitchcock, E.; and Kirkland, I. Stereotaxic neurosurgery in the management of cerebral palsy. *Dev. Med. Child Neurol.,* **17:**279–86, 1975.

95. Grant, W., and Hamerton, J. A cytogenic surgery of 14,069 newborn infants. II. Pulmonary clinical findings on children with sex chromosome anomalies. *Clin. Genet.,* **10:**285–302, 1976.

96. Green, L., and Cracco, R. Kleine-Levin syndrome. A case with EEG evidence of periodic brain dysfunction. *Arch. Neurol.,* **22:**166–75, 1970.

97. Greenhouse, A., and Neuberger, K. The syndrome of progressive cerebral poliodystrophy. *Arch. Neurol.,* **10:**47–59, 1964.

98. Gresty, M., et al. A study of head and eye movement in spasmus nutans. *Br. J. Ophthalmol.,* **60:**652–54

99. Grunebaum, M., and Moskowitz, G. The retropharyngeal tissues in young infants with hypothyroidism. *Am. J. Roentgenol.,* **108:**543–45, 1970.

100. Guinter, R.; Hernreid, L.; and Kaplan, A. Infantile neurogenic muscular atrophy with prolonged survival. *J. Pediatr.,* **90:**95–97, 1977.

101. Haerer, A.; Jackson, J.; and Evers, C. Ataxia telangiectasia and gastric adenocarcinoma. *J.A.M.A.,* **210:**1884–87, 1969.

102. Hahn, M. Congenital nongoitrous hypothyroidism. *Postgrad. Med.,* **57:**71–74, 1975.

103. Hall, B., and Orenstein, W. Noonan's phenotype in an offspring of an alcoholic mother. *Lancet,* **2:**680–81, 1974.

104. Hamilton, W. Sporadic cretinism. *Dev. Med. Child Neurol.,* **18:**384–86, 1976.

105. Hanaway, J.; Lee, S.; and Netsky, M. Pachygyria: Relation of findings to modern embryologic concepts. *Neurology* (Minneap.), **18:**791–99, 1968.

106. Hankey, I.; Hanley, W.; Davidson, W.; and Lindsao, L. Phenylketonuria: Mental development behavior and termination of low phenylalanine diet. *J. Pediatr.,* **72:**646–55, 1968.

107. Hanshaw, J. B. Congenital and acquired cytomegalovirus infection. *Pediatr. Clin. North Am.,* **13:**279–93, 1966.

118. Harken, A.; Filler, R.; AvRuskin, T.; and Crigler, J. The role of total pancreatectomy in the treatment of uremitting hypoglycemia of infancy. *J. Pediatr. Surg.,* **6**:284–89, 1971.

109. Harris, R., and Haas, C. Septo-optic dysplasia with growth hormone deficiency (DeMorsier syndrome). *Arch. Dis. Child.,* **47**:973–76, 1972.

110. Haworth, J., and McRae, K. The neurological and developmental effects of neonatal hypoglycemia. *Can. Med. Assoc. J.,* **92**:961–65, 1965.

110a. Haymond, M. W.; Karl, I. E.; et al. Metabolic response to hypertonic glucose administration in Reye syndrome. *Ann. Neurol.,* **3**:207–15, 1978.

111. Heggie, A. Rubella: Current concepts in epidemiology and teratology. *Pediatr. Clin. North Am.,* **13**:251–66, 1966.

112. Hensinger, R.; Lang, J.; and MacEwen, G. Klippel-Feil syndrome. A constellation of associated anomalies. *J. Bone Joint Surg.,* **56A**:1246–53, 1974.

113. Hoefnagel, D., and Biery, B. Spasmus nutans. *Dev. Med. Child Neurol.,* **10**:32–35, 1968.

114. Hoffman, H.; Hendrick, E.; and Humphreys, R. Manifestations and management of Arnold-Chiari malformation in patients with myelomeningocele. *Child's Brain,* **1**:255–59, 1975.

115. Hoffman, H., and Mohr, G. Lateral canthal advancement of the supraorbital margin. A new corrective technique in the treatment of coronol synostosis. *J. Neurosurg.,* **45**:376–81, 1976.

116. Hopwood, N.; Forsman, P.; et al. Hypoglycemia in hypopituitary children. *Am. J. Dis. Child.,* **129**:918–26, 1975.

117. Hoyt, W. F.; Kaplan, S.; et al. Septo-optic dysplasia and pituitary dwarfism. *Lancet,* **1**:893–94, 1970.

118. Hrbek, A.; Karlberg, P.; et al. Clinical application of evoked electroencephalographic responses in newborn infants. 1. Perinatal asphyxia. *Dev. Med. Child. Neurol.,* **19**:34–44, 1977.

119. Hug, G. Enzyme therapy and prenatal diagnosis in glycogenosis type I. *Am. J. Dis. Child.,* **128**:607–609, 1974.

120. Huijing, F. Glycogen metabolism and glycogen storage diseases. *Physiol. Rev.,* **55**:609–58, 1975.

121. Huttenlocher, P. R. Dendritic development in neocortex of children with mental defect and infantile spasms. *Neurology* (Minneap.), **24**:203–10, 1974.

122. Huttenlocher, P. R.; Solitaire, G.; and Adams, G. Infantile diffuse cerebral degeneration with hepatic cirrhosis. *Arch. Neurol.,* **33**:186–92, 1976.

123. Hypoglycemia in infancy and childhood. *Br. Med. J.,* **3**:130, 1971.

123a. Iannuasi, A. M.; Buonanno, F.; et al. Arteriovenous aneurysm of the vein of Galen. A clinical angiographic CT scan and neuropathological study. *J. Neurol. Sci.,* **40**:29–37, 1979.

124. Ibbertson, H.; Seddon, R.; and Croxson, M. Fetal hypothyroidism complicating medical treatment of thyrotoxicosis in pregnancy. *Clin. Endocrinol.,* **4**:521–23, 1975.

125. Ingalls, T. H. Maternal health and mongolism. *Lancet,* **3**:213–15, 1972.

126. Ingram, T.; Jameson, S.; Errington, J.; and Mitchell, R. Living with cerebral palsy. A study of school leavers suffering from cerebral palsy in eastern Scotland. *Clin. Dev. Med.,* **14**:1–20, 1964.

127. Ingram, T.; Stark, G.; and Blackburn, I. Ataxia and other neurological disorders as a sequel of severe hypoglycemia in childhood. *Brain,* **90**:851–62, 1967.

128. Isacson, P.; Kehrer, A.; Wilson, H.; and Williams, S. Comparative study of live attenuated rubella virus vaccines during the immediate puerperium. *Obstet. Gynecol.,* **37**:332–37, 1971.

129. Isler, W. *Acute hemiplegias and Hemisyndromes in Childhood.* Spastras International Medical Publication, J. B. Lippincott Co., Philadelphia, 1971.

130. Jackson, J.; North, E.; and Thomas, J. Clinical diagnosis of Down's syndrome. *Clin. Genet.,* **9**:483–87, 1976.

131. James, C., and Lassman, L. Diastematomyelia and the tight filum terminale. *J. Neurol. Sci.,* **10**:193–96, 1970.

132. Jan, J., and Wilson, R. Unusual late neurological sequelae in galactosemia. *Dev. Med. Child Neurol.,* **15**:72–74, 1973.

133. Javier, Z., and Gershberg, H. Leucine sensitive hypoglycemia. Treatment with zinc glucagon and corticosteroids. *Am. J. Med.,* **41**:638–44, 1966.

134. Jayalakshmi, P.; McNair, Scott T.; et al. Infantile nystagmus: A prospective study of spasmus nutans, congenital nystagmus and unclassified nystagmus of infancy. *J. Pediatr.,* **77**:177–87, 1970.

135. Jones, K.; Smith, D.; et al. Outcome in offspring of chronic alcoholic women. *Lancet,* **1**:1076–78, 1974.

136. Joubert, M.; Eisenring, J.; Robb, P.; and Andermann, F. Familial agenesis of the cerebellar vermis, syndrome of episodic hyperpnea, abnormal eye movements, ataxia and retardation. *Neurology* (Minneap.), **19**:813–25, 1969.

137. Kaplan, B. J. Malnutrition and mental deficiency. *Psychol. Bull.,* **78**:321–34, 1972.

138. Karch, S., and Urich, M. Occipital encephalocele. A morphological study. *J. Neurol. Sci.,* **15**:89–112, 1972.

139. Keenan, W.; Perlstein, P.; Light, I.; and Sutherland, J. Kernicterus in small sick premature infants receiving phototherapy. *Pediatrics,* **49**:652–55, 1972.

140. Khan, M.; Rozdilsky, B.; and Gerrard, J. Familial holoprosencephaly. *Dev. Med. Child Neurol.,* **12**:71–76, 1970.

141. Khudr, G., and Olding, L. Cyclopia. *Am. J. Dis. Child.,* **125**:120–22, 1973.

142. Kindt, G.; Waldman, J.; et al. Intracranial pressure in Reye's syndrome. *J.A.M.A.,* **231**:822–25, 1975.

143. Kinsbourne, M. Myoclonic encephalopathy of infants. *J. Neurol. Neurosurg. Psychiat.,* **25**:271–76, 1962.

144. Klein, A.; Foley, T.; et al. Neonatal thyroid function in congenital hypothyroidism. *J. Pediatr.,* **89**:545–49, 1976.

145. Koenigsberger, M.; Chutorian, A.; Gold, A.; and Schvey, M. Benign paroxysmal vertigo of childhood. *Neurology* (Minneap.), **20**:1108–13, 1970.

146. Koeze, T., and Klingston, G. Acquired toxoplasmosis. *Arch. Neurol.,* **11**:191–97, 1964.

147. Kogut, M.; Blaskovics, M.; and Donnell, G. Idio-

pathic hypoglycemia: Study of 26 children. *J. Pediatr.,* **74:**853–71, 1969.

148. Lagergren, J. Motor handicapped children: A study from a Swedish county. *Dev. Med. Child Neurol.,* **12:**56–63, 1970.

149. Lansky, L.; Kolavsky, S.; et al. Hypothermic total body washout and intracranial pressure monitoring in stage IV Reye's syndrome. *J. Pediatr.,* **90:**639–40, 1977.

150. Lau, T.; Schmidt, B.; and Piva, S. Pain insensibility. A metabolic disease. *Lancet,* **1:**598–99, 1977.

151. Legum, C.; Schorr, S.; and Berman, E. The genetic mucopolysaccharidoses and mucolipidoses: Review and comment. *Adv. Pediatr.,* **22:**305–47, 1976.

152. Lemire, R.; Beckwith, J.; and Shepard, T. Iniencephaly and anencephaly with spinal retroflexion. A comparative study of eight human specimens. *Teratology,* **6:**27–36, 1972.

153. Letts, R., and Hobson, D. Special devices as aids in the management of child self-mutilation in the Lesch-Nyhan syndrome. *Pediatrics,* **55:**852–55, 1975.

154. Lewis, G.; Spencer-Peet, J.; and Stewart, K. Infantile hypoglycemia due to inherited deficiency of glycogen synthetase in liver. *Arch. Dis. Child.,* **38:**40–48, 1963.

155. Linnemann, C.; Shen, L.; et al. Reye's syndrome: Epidemiologic and viral studies. 1963–1974. *Am. J. Epidemiol.,* **101:**517–26, 1975.

156. Lloyd, J. K. Diabetes mellitus presenting as spontaneous hypoglycemia in childhood. *Proc. Roy. Soc.,* **57:**1061–63, 1964.

157. Loeser, J., and Alvord, E. Clinicopathological correlations in agenesis of the corpus callosum. *Neurology* (Minneap.), **18:**745–56, 1968.

158. Lorber, J. Spina bifida cystica. Results of treatment of 270 consecutive cases with criteria for selection for the future. *Arch. Dis. Child.,* **57:**854–73, 1972.

159. Lott, I.; Dipaolo, R.; et al. Copper metabolism in the steely hair syndrome. *N. Engl. J. Med.,* **292:**197–99, 1975.

160. Lovejoy, F.; Bresnan, M.; et al. Anticerebral aedema therapy in Reye's syndrome. *Arch. Dis. Child.,* **50:**933–37, 1975.

161. Lowe, C.; Sokal, J.; Mosovick, L.; Sarcione, E.; and Doray, B. Studies in liver glycogen disease. Effect of glucagon and other agents on metabolic patterns and clinical status. *Am. J. Med.,* **33:**4–19, 1962.

162. Lutter, L., and Langer, L. Neurologic symptoms in achondroplastic dwarfs—surgical treatment. *J. Bone Joint Surg.,* **59:**87–92, 1977.

163. MacFaul, R., and Grant, D. Early detection of congenital hypothyroidism. Annotation. *Arch. Dis. Child.,* **52:**87–88, 1977.

164. Macri, J.; Weiss, R.; et al. Prenatal diagnosis of neural tube defects. *J.A.M.A.,* **236:**1251–54, 1976.

165. Magnelli, N. Cytogenetics of 50 patients with mental retardation and multiple congenital abnormalities and 50 normal subjects. *Clin. Genet.,* **9:**169–82, 1976.

166. Marx, J. L. Cytomegalovirus: A major cause of birth defects. *Science,* **190:**1184–86, 1975.

167. Masaki, S. Congenital bilateral facial paralysis. *Arch. Otolaryngol.,* **94:**260–63, 1971.

168. Matson, D., and Jerva, M. Recurrent meningitis associated with lumbosacral congenital dermal sinus tracts. *J. Neurosurg.,* **25:**288–97, 1966.

169. Mazar, A.; Herold, H.; and Vardy, P. Congenital sensory neuropathy with anhidrosis. Orthopedic complications and management. *Clin. Orthop.,* **118:**184–87, 1976.

170. McGowen, C. H. Prolonged survival in a patient with Down's syndrome. *J.A.M.A.,* **237:**673–75, 1977.

171. McLennan, J.; Gillis, F.; and Robb, R. Neuropathological correlation in Sjögren-Larsson syndrome. *Brain,* **97:**693–708, 1974.

172. Menkes, J. H. The pathogenesis of mental retardation in phenylketonuria and other inborn errors of amino acid metabolism. *Pediatrics,* **39:**297–308, 1967.

173. Michie, I., and Clark, M. Neurological syndromes associated with cervical and craniocervical abnormalities. *Arch. Neurol.,* **18:**241–47, 1968.

174. Miller, O. J. The sex chromosomal abnormalities. *Am. J. Obstet. Gynecol.,* **90:**1078–89, 1964.

175. Miyaski, K.; Murao, S.; et al. Congenital brain and facial abnormalities in the D_1 trisomy syndrome. Report of a case and a review of literature. *Acta Pathol. Jpn.,* **26:**263–72, 1976.

176. Molnar, G., and Gordon, S. Cerebral palsy: Predictive value of selected clinical signs for early prognostication of motor function. *Arch. Phys. Med. Rehab.,* **57:**153–58, 1976.

177. Monteleone, J.; Beutter, E.; Monteleone, P.; Utz, C.; and Casey, E. Cataracts, glycosuria and hypergalactosemia due to galactokinase deficiency. Studies of a kindred. *Am. J. Med.,* **50:**403–407, 1971.

178. Montoya, G.; Dohn, D.; and Mercer, R. Arteriovenous malformation of the vein of Galen as a cause of heart failure and hydrocephalus in infants. *Neurology* (Minneap.), **21:**1054–58, 1971.

179. Morley, A. R. Laryngeal stridor, Arnold-Chiari malformation and medullary hemorrhages. *Dev. Med. Child Neurol.,* **11:**471–74, 1969.

180. Moss, M. L. Functional anatomy of cranial synostosis. *Child's Brain,* **1:**22–33, 1975.

181. Murphy, J.; D'Souza, B.; and Haughton, V. CT scans and tuberous sclerosis. *J.A.M.A.,* **236:**1115, 1976.

182. Naglo, A., and Hellstrom, B. Results of treatment in myelomeningocele. *Acta Paediatr. Scand.,* **65:**565–69, 1976.

183. Navin, J., and Angevine, J. Congenital cytomegalic inclusion disease with porencephaly. *Neurology* (Minneap.), **18:**470–72, 1968.

184. Nehme, A.; Riseborough, E.; and Tredwell, S. Skeletal growth and development of the achondroplastic dwarf. *Clin. Orthop.,* **116:**8–23, 1976.

185. Nevin, N.; Thompson, W.; and Nesbit, S. Amniotic fluid alpha fetoprotein in the antenatal diagnosis of neural tube defects. *J. Obstet. Gynaecol. Br. Commonw.,* **81:**757–60, 1974.

186. Nicholson, A.; Freeland, S.; and Brierley, J. A behavioral and neuropathological study of the sequelae of profound hypoxia. *Brain Res.,* **22:**327–45, 1970.

187. Nyhan, W. L. Clinical features of the Lesch-Ny-

han syndrome. *Arch. Intern Med.,* **130:**186–72, 1972.

188. Oetgen, W. J. The use of citrulline for the treatment of Reye's syndrome: Case reports. *Milit. Med.,* **42:**162–64, 1977.

189. Okihiro, M.; Tasoki, T.; et al. Duane syndrome and congenital upper limb anomalies. A familial occurrence. *Arch. Neurol.,* **34:**174–79, 1977.

190. Oliver, J. F. Microcephaly following baby battering and shaking. *Br. Med. J.,* **2:**262–64, 1975.

191. Oteruelo, F. T. "PKU bodies": Characteristic inclusions in the brain in phenylketonuria. *Acta Neuropathol.,* **36:**295–305, 1976.

192. Page, L., and Welch, F. Neurosurgical care of the patient with spina bifida aperta. *J. Fla. Med. Assoc.,* **63:**892–94, 1976.

193. Parr, J.; Teree, T.; and Larner, J. Symptomatic hypoglycemia, visceral fatty metamorphosis and aglycognosis in an infant lacking glycogen synthetase and phosphorylase. *Pediatrics,* **35:**770–77, 1965.

194. Partin, J. C. Reye's syndrome (encephalopathy and fatty liver): Diagnosis and treatment. *Gastroenterology,* **69:**511–18, 1975.

195. Partin, J.; Partin, J.; et al. Brain ultrastructure in Reye's syndrome. *J. Neuropath. Exp. Neurol.,* **34:**425–44, 1975.

196. Partington, M.; Tu, J.; and Wong, C. Blood serotonin levels in severe mental retardation. *Dev. Med. Child Neurol.,* **15:**616–27, 1973.

197. Patel, H.; Dolman, C.; and Byrne, M. Holoprosencephaly with median cleft lip. *Am. J. Dis. Child.,* **124:**217–21, 1972.

198. Patton, R.; Christie, D.; Smith, D.; and Beckwith, J. Cerebro-hepato-renal syndrome of Zellweger. *Am. J. Dis. Child.,* **124:**840–44, 1972.

199. Paulson, G., and Lyle, C. Tuberous sclerosis. *Dev. Med. Child Neurol.,* **8:**571–86, 1966.

200. Peach, B. Arnold-Chiari malformation. Anatomic features of 20 cases. *Arch. Neurol.,* **12:**613–21, 1965.

201. Pearl, W. Cardiovascular anomalies in Noonan's syndrome. *Chest,* **71:**677–79, 1977.

201a. Pearn, J. H.: Gardner-Medwin, D.; and Wilson, J. A study of chronic childhood spinal muscular atrophy. A review of 141 cases. *J. Neurol. Sci.,* **38:**23–37, 1978.

202. Pearson, J., and Pytel, B. A. Quantitative studies of sympathetic ganglia and spinal cord intermediolateral gray columns in familial dysautonomia. *J. Neurol. Sci.,* **39:**47–59, 1978.

203. Pearson, J.; Axelrod, F.; and Dancer, J. Current concepts of dysautonomia, neuropathological defects. *Ann. N.Y. Acad. Sci.,* **228:**288–300, 1974.

204. Penfold, J., and Simpson, D. Premature craniosynostosis a complication of thyroid replacement therapy. *J. Pediatr.,* **86:**360–63, 1975.

205. Perrin, J.; Idemoto, J.; et al. X-linked syndrome of congenital ichthyosis, hypogonadism, mental retardation and anosmia. *Birth Defects,* **11:**267–74, 1976.

206. Pollock, G., and Stark, G. Long-term results in the management of 67 children with cerebral palsy. *Dev. Med. Child Neurol.,* **11:**17–34, 1969.

206a. Portnoy, H. D., and Croissant, P. D. Megalencephaly in infants and children. The possible role of increased dural sinus pressure. *Arch. Neurol.* (Chicago), **35:**306–16, 1978.

206b. Pou-Serradell, A.; Monserrant, L.; and Ugarte, A. "Intermediate" forms of infantile spinal amyotrophy. Twenty personal cases. *Rev. Neurol.,* **134:** 35–44, 1978.

207. Prensky, A., and Davis, D. Obstruction of major cerebral vessels in early childhood without neurologic signs. *Neurology* (Minneap.), **20:**945–53, 1970.

208. Purpura, D. P. Dendritic spine "dysgenesis" and mental retardation. *Science,* **186:**1126–28, 1974.

209. Purpura, D. P. Dendritic differentiation in human cerebral cortex: Normal and aberrant developmental patterns. *Adv. Neurol.,* **12:**91–134, 1975.

210. Rasmussen, K. Phosphoryethanolamine and hypophosphatasia. *Dan. Med. Bull.,* **15** supp. 2:1–112, 1968.

211. Reye's syndrome: Etiology uncertain but avoid anti-emetics in children. *FDA Drug Bull.,* **7:**40–41, 1976.

212. Ridlon, H.; Markland, C.; et al. Myelomeningocele: Suggested minimal urological evaluation and surveillance. *Pediatrics,* **56:**477–78, 1975.

213. Riley, C. M. Familial dysautonomia, clinical and pathophysiological aspects. *Ann. N.Y. Acad. Sci.,* **228:**283–87, 1974.

214. Roden, V.; Cantor, H.; et al. Acute hemiplegia of childhood associated with Coxsackie A9 viral infection. *J. Pediatr.,* **1:**56–58, 1975.

215. Rosenbloom, A., and Sherman, L. The natural history of idiopathic hypoglycemia of infancy and its relation to diabetes mellitus. *N. Engl. J. Med.,* **274:**815–20, 1966.

216. Roth, J., and Epstein, C. Infantile spasms and hypopigmented macules: Early manifestations of tuberous sclerosis. *Arch. Neurol.,* **25:**547–51, 1971.

217. Rothner, D.; Duchesneau, P.; and Weinstein, M. Agenesis of the corpus callosum revealed by computerized tomography. *Dev. Med. Child Neurol.,* **18:**160–66, 1976.

218. Ruben, F., and Mistaelis, R. Reye's syndrome with associated influenza A and B infection. *J.A.M.A.,* **234:**410–12, 1975.

219. Rudd, N.; et al. Prenatal diagnosis of hypophosphatasia. *N. Engl. J. Med.,* **295:**146–48, 1976.

220. Rundle, A.; Atkin, J.; and Dollmore, J. Serum and tissue proteins in tuberous sclerosis. II. Immunoglobulin levels. *Hum. Genet.,* **151:**147, 1975.

220a. Russell, E. J.; Zimmerman, R. D.; et al. Reye syndrome: Computed tomographic demonstration of disordered intracerebral structure. *J. Computer Ass. Tomography,* **3:**217–20, 1979.

221. Sadowsky, C., and Reeves, A. Agenesis of the corpus callosum with hypothermia. *Arch. Neurol.,* **32:**774–76, 1975.

222. Saez, R.; Onofrio, B.; and Yanagihara, T. Experience with Arnold-Chiari malformation. 1960 to 1970. *J. Neurosurg.,* **45:**M416–22, 1976.

223. Sarnat, H., and Sarnat, M. Neonatal encephalopathy following fetal distress. *Arch. Neurol.,* **38:**696–705, 1976.

224. Sass, J.; Itabashi, H.; and Dexter, R. Juvenile gout with brain involvement. *Arch. Neurol.,* **13:**639–55, 1965.

225. Schiff, G. M. Reye's syndrome. *Ann. Rev. Med.,* **27:**447–52, 1976.

226. Schlenska, G.; Heene, R.; et al. The symptomatology, morphology and biochemistry of glycogenosis type II in the adult. *J. Neurol.,* **212:**237–52, 1976.

227. Schmitt, R., and Erickson, M. Early predictors of mental retardation. *Ment. Retard.,* **11:**27–29, 1973.

228. Scott, M. Outcome of very severe birth asphyxia. *Arch. Dis. Child.,* **57:**712–16, 1976.

229. Scott, C., and Thomas, G. Genetic disorders associated with mental retardation. *Pediatr. Clin. North Am.,* **20:**121–40, 1973.

229a. Seay, A. R.; Bray, P. F.; et al. CT scans in Merke's disease. *Neurology*(Minneap.), **29:**304–12, 1979.

230. Segal, S.; Blair, A.; and Roth, H. The metabolism of galactose by patients with congenital galactosemia. *Am. J. Med.,* **38:**62–70, 1965.

231. Seger, R.; Buchinger, G.; and Stroder, J. On the influence of age on immunity in Down's syndrome. *Eur. J. Pediatr.,* **124:**77–87, 1977.

232. Sells, C. J. Microcephaly in a normal school population. *Pediatrics,* **59:**262–65, 1977.

233. Shannon, D.; DeLong, R.; et al. Studies of the pathophysiology of encephalopathy in Reye's syndrome: Hyperammonemia in Reye's syndrome. *Pediatrics,* **56:**999–1004, 1975.

234. Sharpe, J.; Hoyt, W.; and Rosenberg, M. Convergence evoked nystagmus. Congenital and acquired forms. *Arch. Neurol.,* **32:**191–94, 1975.

235. Sharrard, W. The orthopedic management of spina bifida. *Acta Orthop. Scand.,* **46:**356–63, 1975.

236. Shaywitz, B.; Leventhal, J.; et al. Prolonged continuous monitoring of intracranial pressure in severe Reye's syndrome. *Pediatrics,* **59:**595–605, 1977.

237. Shimono, M.; Ohta, M.; et al. Infantil neuroaxonal dystrophy. Ultrastructural study of peripheral nerve. *Acta Neuropathol.,* **36:**71–79, 1976.

238. Siggers, D.; Rogers, J.; et al. Increased nerve growth factor B chain cross reacting material in familial dysautonomia. *N. Engl. J. Med.,* **295:**629–34, 1976.

239. Sillanpää, M.; Makela, A.; and Koivikko, A. Acute liver failure and encephalopathy (Reye's syndrome?) during salicylate therapy. *Acta Paediatr. Scand.,* **64:**877–80, 1975.

240. Simonsson, H. Incontinentia pigmenti. Block-Stutzberger's syndrome associated with infantile spasms. *Acta Paediatr. Scand.,* **61:**612–14, 1972.

241. Simopoulos, A.; Delea, C.; and Bartter, F. Neurodegenerative disorders and hyperaldosteronism. *J. Pediatr.,* **79:**633–41, 1971.

242. Singh, S.; Willers, I.; and Goedde, H. A rapid micromethod for prenatal diagnosis of Lesch-Nyhan syndrome. *Clin. Genet.,* **10:**12–15, 1976.

243. Slone, D.; Soeldner, J.; Steinke, J.; and Crigler, J. Serum insulin measurements in children with idiopathic spontaneous hypoglycemia and in normal infants, children and adults. *N. Engl. J. Med.,* **274:**820–26, 1966.

244. Smith, D. W. Autosomal abnormalities. *Am. J. Obstet. Gynecol.,* **90:**1055–77, 1964.

245. Smith, V. Visual disorders and cerebral palsy. *Little Club Clin. Dev. Med.,* #9, 1963.

246. Smith, I.; Clayton, B.; and Wolff, O. New variant of phenylketonuria with progressive neurological illness unresponsive to phenylalanine restriction. *Lancet,* **1:**1108–11, 1975.

247. Smith, D., and Simons, E. Rational diagnostic evaluation of the child with mental deficiency. *Am. J. Dis. Child.,* **129:**1285–90, 1975.

248. Snodgrass, P., and DeLong, G. Urea-cycle enzyme deficiencies and an increased nitrogen load producing hyperammonemia in Reye's syndrome. *N. Engl. J. Med.,* **294:**855–60, 1976.

249. Somasundaram, O.; Papakumari, M.; et al. Microcephaly. *Ind. J. Pediatr.,* **43:**21–27, 1976.

250. South, M.; Montgomery, J.; and Rawls, W. Immune deficiency in congenital rubella and other viral infections. *Birth Defects,* **11:**234, 1975.

251. Speed, R.; Johnston, A.; and Evans, W. Chromosome survey of total population of mentally subnormal in north-east of Scotland. *J. Med. Genet.,* **13:**295–306, 1976.

252. Stark, E., and Barton, T. Hearing loss and the Klippel-Feil syndrome. *Am. J. Dis. Child.,* **123:**233–35, 1972.

253. Stechenberg, B.; Keating, J.; et al. Epidemiologic investigations of Reye's syndrome. *J. Pediatr.,* **87:**234–37, 1975.

254. Stein, S.; Schilt, L.; and Ames, M. Selection for early treatment of myelomeningocele: A retrospective analysis of selection procedures. *Dev. Med. Child Neurol.,* **17:**311–19, 1975.

255. Stene, J.; Fischer, G.; and Stene, E. Paternal age effect in Down's syndrome. *Ann. Hum. Genet.,* **40:**299–306, 1977.

256. Sunanwela, C., and Sunanwela, N. A morphological classification of sincipital encephalomeningoceles. *J. Neurosurg.,* **36:**201–11, 1972.

257. Sutherland, G.; Murch, A.; et al. Cytogenetic surgery of a hospital for the mentally retarded. *Hum. Genet.,* **34:**231–45, 1976.

258. Svejcar, J., and Walther, A. The diagnosis of the early infantile form of hypophosphatasia tarda. *Humangenetik,* **28:**49–56, 1975.

259. Swanson, A.; Bucher, G.; and Alvord, E. Anatomic changes in congenital insensitivity to pain. *Arch. Neurol.,* **12:**12–18, 1965.

260. Swift, T., and McDonald, F. Peripheral nerve involvement in Hunter syndrome. *Arch. Neurol.,* **33:**845–46, 1976.

261. Tang, T.; Siegesmund, K.; et al. Reye's syndrome. A correlated electron microscopic viral and biochemical observation. *J.A.M.A.,* **232:**1339–46, 1975.

262. Taylor, A. I. Patau's, Edwards', and cri du chat syndromes. A tabulated summary of current findings. *Dev. Med. Child Neurol.,* **9:**78–86, 1967.

263. Teng, P., and Papatheodorou, C. Arnold-Chiari malformation with normal spine and cranium. *Arch. Neurol.,* **12:**622–24, 1965.

264. Thaler, M. M. Pathogenesis of Reye's syndrome. A working hypothesis *Pediatrics,* **56:**1081–84, 1975.

265. Thaler, M. M. Metabolic mechanisms in Reye's syndrome. End of a mystery? *Am. J. Dis. Child.,* **130:**241–43, 1976.

266. Thelander, H. E. Prognosis of children with cerebral palsy. Reflection on a stock-taking. *Clin. Pediatr.,* **7:**294–98, 1968.

267. Tibbles, J., and Brown, B. Acute hemiplegia of childhood. *Can. Med. Assoc. J.,* **113:**309–14, 1975.

268. Towbin, A. Cerebral hypoxia. Damage in fetus and newborn: Basic patterns and their clinical significance. *Arch. Neurol.,* **20:**35–43, 1969.

269. Traurer, D.; Stockard, J.; and Sweetman, L. EEG correlation with biochemical abnormalities in Reye's syndrome. *Arch. Neurol.,* **34:**116–18, 1977.

269a. Traurer, D. A.; Brown, F.; et al. Treatment of elevated intracranial pressure in Reye's syndrome. *Ann. Neurol.,* **4:**275–78, 1978.

270. Tremblay, G. Ornithine and citrulline therapy in treatment of Reye's syndrome. *N. Engl. J. Med.,* **292:**160–61, 1975.

271. Turner, G. An etiological study of 1000 patients with an I.Q. assessment below 51. *Med. J. Aust.,* **2:**927–31, 1975.

272. Turner, G.; Engisch, B.; Lindsay, D.; and Turner, B. X-linked mental retardation without physical abnormality. (Renpenning syndrome) in sibs in an institution. *J. Med. Genet.,* **9:**324–30, 1972.

273. Turner, G.; Turner, B.; and Collins, E. X-linked mental retardation without physical abnormality: Renpenning syndrome. *Dev. Med. Child Neurol.,* **13:**71–78, 1971.

274. Vining, E.; Accardo, P.; et al. Cerebral palsy: A pediatric developmentalist's overview. *Am. J. Dis. Child.,* **130:**643–49, 1976.

275. Volpe, J. J. Perinatal hypoxic-ischemic brain injury. *Pediatr. Clin. North Am.,* **23:**383–96, 1976.

276. Waldwan, T., and McIntyre, K. Serum alpha-fetoprotein levels in patients with ataxia telangectasia. *Lancet,* **2:**1112–15, 1972.

277. Walker, G., and Tobin, J. Cytomegalovirus infection in the northwest of England. *Arch. Dis. Child.,* **45:**513–22, 1970.

278. Warlow, L., and Hinton, P. Early neurologic disturbance following relatively minor burns in children. *Lancet,* **2:**978–82, 1969.

279. Waters, W. J. The reserve albumin binding capacity as a criterion for exchange transfusion. *J. Pediatr.,* **70:**185–92, 1967.

280. Watson, C.; Nigam, M.; and Paine, R. Electroencephalographic abnormalities in phenylpyruvic oligophrenia. *Neurology* (Minneap.), **18:**203–7, 1968.

281. Weil, M., and Menkes, J. Bilirubin interaction with ganglioside: Possible mechanism in kernicterus. *Pediatr. Res.,* **9:**791–93, 1975.

282. Weinberg, A., and Kirkpatrick, J. Cerebellar hypoplasia in Werdnig-Hoffman disease. *Dev. Med. Child Neurol.,* **17:**511–16, 1975.

283. Wheeler, E., and Roberts, P. Menke's steely hair syndrome. *Arch. Dis. Child.,* **51:**269–74, 1976.

283a. Williams, R. S.; Marshall, P. C.; et al. The cellular pathology of Merke's steely hair syndrome. *Neurology* (Minneap.), **28:**575–83, 1978.

284. Windle, W. F. Brain damage at birth. Functional and structural modification with time. *J.A.M.A.,* **206:**1967–72, 1968.

285. Wood, M.; Fox, R.; Vincent, L.; Reye, C.; and O'Sullivan, W. The Lesch-Nyhan syndrome: Report of three cases. *Aust. N.Z. J. Med.,* **1:**57–64, 1972.

285a. Woods, B. T., Tauber, H. L. Mirror movements after childhood hemiparesis. *Neurology* (Minneap.), **28:**1152–58, 1978.

286. Yagishita, S., and Kimura, S. Infantile neuroaxonal dystrophy (Seitelberger's disease). *Acta Neuropathol.,* **29:**115–26, 1974.

287. Yagishita, S., and Kimura, S. Infantile neuroaxonal dystrophy (Seitelberger's disease). *Acta Neuropathol.,* **31:**191–200, 1975.

287a. Yamaguchi, K.; Santa, T.; et al. Lipid storage myopathy in von Gierke's disease. A case report. *J. Neurol. Sci.,* **38:**195–205, 1978.

288. Yeager, A.; Martin, H.; and Stewart, J. Congenital cytomegalovirus infection outcome for the subsequent sibling. *Clin. Pediatr.,* **16:**455–58, 1977.

289. Yee, R.; Wong, E.; et al. A study of congenital nystagmus waveforms. *Neurology* (Minneap.), **26:**226–33, 1976.

290. Zamet, P.; Nakamura, H.; et al. Determination of unbound bilirubin and the prevention of kernicterus. *Birth Defects,* **11:**236–44, 1976.

291. Ziegler, M.; Lake, C.; and Kopin, I. Deficient sympathetic nervous system response in familial dysautonomia *N. Engl. J. Med.,* **294:**630–33, 1976.

292. Zilka, A.; Mendelsohn, F.; and Borofsky, L. Acute hemiplegia in children complicating upper respiratory infections. *Clin. Pediatr.,* **15:**1137–42, 1976.

3 DEMYELINATING DISEASES OF THE NERVOUS SYSTEM

Demyelinating disease may be defined as a condition in which there is injury to myelin with relative preservation of axons. It has been applied somewhat loosely to the heterogenous group of diseases listed in Table 3–1. There is little difficulty in applying such a definition to the most common of these disorders, namely multiple sclerosis, particularly in the early stage of the disease, but this definition should be used with reservation in some of the demyelinative conditions generally classified in this group. For example, there is widespread involvement of neurons in the lipidoses, and some axonal degeneration is regularly seen in the leukodystrophies as well as in the postinfectious, postvaccinal, and viral leukoencephalitides. Nevertheless, the classification outlined in Table 3–1 is useful from a clinical point of view and will be utilized in the organization of this chapter. With increasing knowledge of the different causes of the demyelinating diseases, it is likely that they will all eventually be reclassified on the basis of etiology, e.g., specific viral or metabolic demyelinating disorders.

The Leukodystrophies

A number of familial conditions, which occur predominantly in infancy and childhood and are characterized by the abnormal formation of myelin, have been described under the term "leukodystrophy." Additional features are symmetric distribution of lesions with some destruction of axons, preservation of nerve cells, and absence of any inflammatory reaction.

The current belief is that the leukodystrophies represent inborn errors of metabolism or enzymatic deficiencies that result in defective catabolism of the lipid components of myelin. In some

TABLE 3-1

Classification of the Demyelinating Diseases

1. *The leukodystrophies* (genetically determined metabolic disorders with primary involvement of myelin)
   a. Metachromatic leukodystrophy
   b. Globoid cell leukodystrophy (Krabbe's disease)
   c. Spongy degeneration
   d. Adrenoleukodystrophy
   e. Leukodystrophy with diffuse Rosenthal fiber formation
   f. Pelizaeus-Merzbacher disease
2. *Lipid storage diseases often with neuronal involvement* (genetically determined metabolic disorders with secondary involvement of myelin)
   a. GM_2 gangliosidoses (Tay-Sachs disease)
   b. GM_1 gangliosidoses
   c. Ceroid-lipofuscinoses
   d. Niemann-Pick (sphingomyelin lipidosis)
   e. Gaucher's disease (cerebroside lipidosis)
   f. Cerebrotendinous xanthomatosis
   g. Fabry's disease
3. *Acquired allergic and infectious diseases resulting in breakdown of myelin*
   a. Multiple sclerosis
   b. Devic's disease (neuromyelitis optica)
   c. Postvaccinal encephalomyelitis
   d. Postinfectious encephalomyelitis (acute disseminated encephalomyelitis)
   e. Acute hemorrhagic leukoencephalitis
   f. Postinfectious polyneuritis (Landry-Guillain-Barré syndrome)
4. *The viral group*
   a. Subacute sclerosing panencephalitis (SSPE)
   b. Subacute rubella panencephalitis
   c. Russian spring-summer panencephalitis
   d. Progressive multifocal leukoencephalopathy
5. *The degenerative group*
   a. Central pontine myelinolysis
   b. Marchiafava-Bignami disease
   c. Subacute necrotizing encephalopathy
   d. Eales's disease

cases, failure of normal metabolic processes results in the accumulation of intermediate metabolic products found in macrophages. Normal catabolism of myelin leads first to the appearance of complex lipids followed by their metabolism to cholesterol esters. The complex lipids are weakly sudanophilic, and cholesterol esters are strongly sudanophilic.

The occurrence of abnormal amounts of lipid material in the brain in some cases of the leukodystrophies suggests a close relationship with the lipidoses.

In some diseases in both groups there is a deficiency of catabolic enzymes required for degradation of complex sphingolipids. A schematic diagram of the metabolism pathways is shown in Figure 3-1.

Metachromatic Leukodystrophy (Sulfatide Lipidosis)

The metachromatic form of leukodystrophy (MLD) is characterized by an accumulation of metachromatic lipids in the white matter of the central nervous system and peripheral nerves. It is probably the most common form of this group of rare diseases. MLD is so called because of metachromatic staining of the abnormal white matter when stained with cresyl violet.

Etiology and Pathology

The condition is inherited as an autosomal recessive trait and characterized by a genetically determined enzymatic defect. Late infantile, juvenile, and adult forms of the disease have been described; each form probably represents an independent autosomal recessive disorder (Table 3-2).

An abnormality in metabolism of myelin results in the accumulation of metachromatic products in several tissues including the brain. The abnormal lipids are sulfatides and the condition is due to a lack of the enzyme arylsulfatase A.

The brain is usually normal in external appearance and weight. The white matter is firm with a brownish discoloration involving the centrum semiovale but usually sparing the U fibers. Occa-

TABLE 3-2

Leukodystrophies: Age of Onset

Type	Age of Patient at Onset
1. Metachromatic leukodystrophy	Infancy, childhood, adolescence, early adult life
2. Globoid cell (Krabbe) leukodystrophy	Infancy
3. Spongy degeneration of the central nervous system	Infancy
4. Adrenoleukodystrophy	Childhood, adolescence
5. Leukodystrophy with diffuse Rosenthal fiber formation (Alexander)	Infancy, childhood, early adult life
6. Pelizaeus-Merzbacher disease	Infancy, childhood, adolescence, early adult life

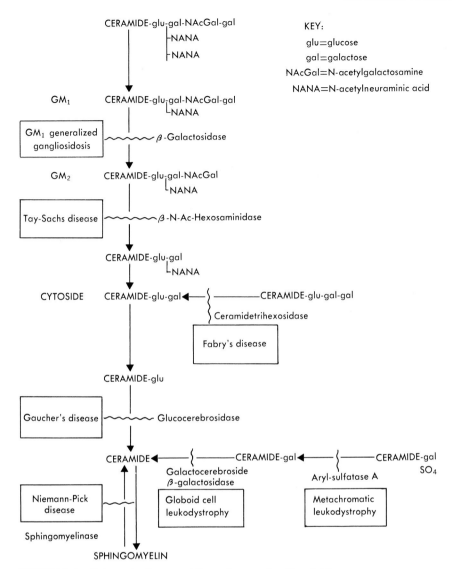

FIGURE 3–1. Schematic diagram of the pathways of sphingolipid metabolism.

sionally, some cavitation may occur, but this is not a marked feature. Cerebroside is replaced by sulfatide in the myelin, and the myelin subsequently becomes biochemically and functionally abnormal.[13, 14, 15]

Microscopic Examination

Central Nervous System. There are diffuse loss of myelin sheaths, diminution of oligodendrocytes, axonal degeneration, and an accumulation of lipid material which may lie free in the tissues or within macrophages and neurons. The neu-

ronal involvement is patchy, with maximal accumulation in neurons of the cerebral cortex, hypothalamus, basal ganglia, pons, anterior horn cells, and spinal root ganglia. In the cerebellum, the dentate nucleus is involved but the Purkinje cells are spared. There are marked loss of ganglion cells in the retina and optic atrophy.[146]

Peripheral Nerves. Similar changes of demyelination, axonal loss, and accumulation of lipid material within macrophages and Schwann cells may be seen in peripheral nerves.

Viscera. The lipid material accumulates in the cytoplasm of the epithelium of the renal tubules and has also been demonstrated in Kupffer cells and in the cells of the intrahepatic ducts in the liver and gallbladder.

Clinical Features

There are three distinct forms of this disease.

Late Infantile Form. The child develops normally until 12 to 18 months of age at which time symptoms begin to appear. The first symptom is a disturbance of gait due to weakness in the lower limbs. They may be hypotonic or spastic, and there is a progressive ataxic element wih upper limb involvement occurring later. The child shows progressive dementia and a regression of speech and intelligence. There may be visual loss with optic atrophy, and a few children may develop macular degeneration with the characteristic appearance of a "cherry-red spot." Seizures occur in about 50 per cent of cases. The progressive deterioration produces generalized hypertonia with increased deep tendon reflexes and bilateral extensor plantar responses. In the terminal stage, which occurs between two and ten years after the onset of the illness, there are decortication or decerebration and lack of response to auditory and visual stimuli.[95]

Juvenile Form. In this form of the disease the age of onset is between five and ten years with the development of progressive impairment of performance in school and progressive ataxia. The clinical course is then similar to the late infantile form but is more protracted.

Adult Form. An erroneous diagnosis of schizophrenia may be made in the adult form of metachromatic leukodystrophy.[24] The symptoms suggest psychiatric illness with gradual intellectual deterioration, beginning with an inability to continue to work for more than a short period and episodes of moodiness and withdrawal. There may be delusions of grandeur and outbursts of rage or hallucinations. The progressive dementia continues steadily until death occurs after a period of some years.

Diagnostic Procedures

1. The spinal fluid protein is elevated.
2. Metachromatic bodies may occasionally be seen on direct examination of the centrifuged urinary sediment after the addition of two drops of an aqueous solution of toluidine blue or cresyl violet. They appear as golden-brown bodies within the sediment and are seen only in this disease.
3. A more reliable method is to take the sediment from a refrigerated 24-hour specimen of urine and extract the lipids with 2:1 chloroform: methanol. An equal volume of water is added, and the lipids collect as a white fluff at the interface of the solutions. This material is applied to filter paper and stained with 0.01 per cent toluidine blue in 0.5 per cent acetic acid. If the test is positive, a red-pink metachromasia appears, which persists after rinsing with 2 per cent acetic acid.
4. The urinary lipids may be separated by paper chromatography and stained with cresyl violet.
5. Metachromatic bodies may be demonstrated in frozen sections of sural nerve biopsies. This is a relatively simple and reliable method of confirming the diagnosis.[11]
6. Nerve conduction velocities show marked reduction in patients with metachromatic leukodystrophy.[71]
7. There is a deficiency of arylsulfatase A in the urine and in leukocyte preparations from patients with MLD. Assay of this enzyme in leukocytes is a relatively simple and reliable method for the diagnosis of MLD.[61]
8. Cultures of skin fibroblasts show a deficiency of arylsulfatase A. Fibroblasts cultured in a medium containing sulfatide show numerous lipid-laden lysosomes.[134]
9. Computed tomography of the brain shows the presence of diffuse cortical atrophy and scattered areas of decreased density in the central white matter representing areas of demyelination (Fig. 3–2).

Treatment

Arylsulfatase A has been administered in this condition as an intravenous or intrathecal injection with no obvious beneficial effects. Prenatal diagnosis can be made by measurement of arylsulfatase A in the amniotic fluid.

Globoid Cell (Krabbe) Leukodystrophy

This disorder affects infants and young children. The descriptive term "globoid leukodystrophy" is derived from the presence of distended epithelioid (globoid) cells and collections of multinucleated cells (globoid bodies) in the white mat-

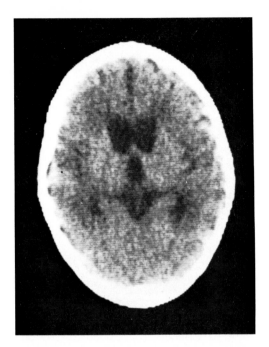

FIGURE 3–2. Computed tomography in a case of metachromatic leukodystrophy showing dilatation of the third, fourth, and lateral ventricles and scattered areas of decreased density in the central white matter. There is some degree of cortical atrophy.

ter of the brain and spinal cord. The condition is inherited as an autosomal recessive trait. The metabolic abnormality is a deficiency of galacto-cerebroside β-galactosidase (Fig. 3–1).

Pathology

The brain is small and shows diffuse loss of myelin in the cerebellum and spinal cord. The arcuate fibers may be spared, and a few small lacunae may be scattered throughout the centrum semiovale. The characteristic distended and mul-tinucleated epithelioid or globoid cells may be seen scattered throughout the parenchyma. Glo-boid bodies consisting of collections of multinu-cleated cells are also seen in the devastated white matter. These cells contain weakly sudanophilic and nonmetachromatic material believed to be cerebrosides. The epithelioid and globoid cells show tubular inclusions when examined with the electron microscope.[173] They contain increased galactocerebrosides, apparently resulting from the deficiency of galactocerebroside β-galactosidase, and an accumulation of mucopolysaccharides. Total lipid, phospholipid, and galactolipid frac-

tions are reduced in white matter reflecting the paucity of myelin. Although the ratio of cerebro-side to sulfatide is abnormally high in the brain, the composition of myelin is normal.[65]

Clinical Features

Symptoms usually begin between the ages of three and five months. The infant ceases to de-velop and loses the ability to sit and hold up the head, smile, and coo. The infant also becomes extremely irritable and suffers prolonged crying spells. This is followed by the gradual develop-ment of generalized hypotonia or, occasionally, generalized spasticity. Nystagmus develops at an early stage and optic atrophy occurs later. Gener-alized seizures may occur, and there may be sound or tactile-sensitive myoclonic jerks and an exag-gerated startle response. In the terminal stages, the head is reduced in size when compared to normal values for this age and the child shows decerebrate rigidity or decerebrate spasms. Death usually occurs within one year of the onset of the disease.

Diagnostic Procedures

1. The cerebrospinal fluid protein is elevated.
2. The EEG is normal in the early stages of the disease. Progressive disorganization of back-ground activity with addition of diffuse theta and delta activity may be noted as the disease progresses. The absence of periodic discharges and a paucity of the spike slow-wave complexes differentiates this condition from Tay-Sachs disease.
3. Computerized tomography of the brain shows cerebral atrophy and ventricular dilatation.
4. There is slowing of nerve conduction velocities in peripheral nerves.[60]
5. The diagnosis is established by measurement of the activity of galactocerebroside β-galacto-sidase in leukocytes or fibroblasts.[73]
6. Antenatal diagnosis may be established by demonstrating galactocerebroside β-galacto-sidase deficiency in cultured amniotic fluid cells.[65a]

Treatment

There is no other treatment apart from suppor-tive care. The enzyme deficiency can also be mea-sured in amniotic fluid as well as leukocytes and fibroblasts. This allows prenatal diagnosis of an affected fetus and detection of carriers, who have lower-than-normal enzyme activity.

Spongy Degeneration of the Central Nervous System

This form of familial leukodystrophy, also called Canavan's disease, is rare and occurs almost exclusively in the descendants of Jewish immigrants having common family origins in eastern Europe who emigrated to this country bringing the genetic trait with them.[17, 161] The name is derived from the extensive spongiform degeneration of subcortical white matter found in this condition.

Etiology and Pathology

There is some disagreement as to whether spongy degeneration represents a failure of myelin maturation or a deterioration of mature myelin.[66] In this disease, the relative rarity of macrophages containing sudanophilic breakdown products tends to rule out a destructive process. The presence of hyperplastic protoplasmic astrocytes (Alzheimer type II cells) suggests a metabolic abnormality that has not been defined as yet.

The brain is megancephalic and shows widespread demyelination of cerebral white matter affecting the convolutions more than the centrum semiovale. There is intense vacuolation of tissue, which is most marked in the deeper layers of the cerebral cortex and basal ganglia. The astrocytes are deficient in ATPase, and succinic dehydrogenase and dihydronicotinamide adenosine dinucleoside diphosphorases are decreased in their mitochondria. ATPase is deficient in cerebral blood vessels.

Clinical Features

There is a close similarity between the clinical course of spongy degeneration and globoid cell leukodystrophy. Infants with spongy degeneration are apparently normal at birth and appear to thrive until the second or third month of life. They then regress, lose the ability to smile and coo, and become unable to support the head. The arms become hypertonic, and the infant develops adductor spasms of the lower limbs. As the condition progresses, intermittent decorticate or decerebrate posturing occurs, and the child no longer responds to light and develops optic atrophy. Death usually occurs from intercurrent pulmonary infection before one year of age, but some patients have survived with severe mental retardation for many years.

Diagnostic Procedures

Brain biopsy with characteristic histopathologic changes is necessary to establish the diagnosis.

Treatment

There is no known treatment for this condition at the present time. The enzymes that are deficient indicate a severe defect in cerebral energy metabolism.

Adrenoleukodystrophy (Sex-Linked Sudanophilic Leukodystrophy with Adrenocortical Atrophy)

Adrenoleukodystrophy, which is inherited as a sex-linked recessive trait, is believed to be almost as common as metachromatic leukodystrophy and more frequent than globoid cell leukodystrophy. The majority of cases previously diagnosed as Schilder's disease in boys were probably cases of adrenoleukodystrophy.

Etiology and Pathology

The inborn error of metabolism is unknown, but adrenoleukodystrophy is probably a lipid storage disease.[165] There is an extensive symmetric demyelinating process in the brain involving the subcortical white matter of the centrum semiovale with predilection for the parieto-occipital areas. Microscopic examination shows extensive demyelination, sparing of axons, and accumulation of lipid-laden sudanophilic macrophages, which are often arranged around vessels and produce perivascular cuffing.[162]

The adrenal glands are atrophic and show ballooned cells with eccentric nuclei. Electron microscopy shows adrenal cell inclusions that have a characteristic lamellar appearance.[144]

Clinical Features

Adrenoleukodystrophy occurs predominantly in school-age boys although there have been rare reports of adult cases.

The earliest symptoms are of progressive deterioration in school work which may be diagnosed as "minimal brain damage." This is followed by progressive visual failure and the development of spasticity and ataxia. There is steady deterioration with failure of hearing and increasing dysarthria. The final state is that of a blind, deaf, mute, decorticate adolescent male. Seizures may occur at any time during the illness. Death usually occurs within two years of the onset of symptoms.

Signs of adrenal failure are variable. Many cases do not have overt signs of adrenal insufficiency, whereas others show brown skin pigmentation and other stigmata of Addison's disease.

Diagnostic Procedures

1. The cerebrospinal fluid protein content may be elevated.
2. The electroencephalogram shows bilateral symmetric slowing in the posterior head regions in the early stages of the disease. This is followed by progressive bilateral generalized slowing in the later stages.
3. Computed tomography of the brain shows areas of decreased density in the parietal and occipital areas with a periventricular distribution. This corresponds to the areas of profound loss of myelin.[59]
4. An ACTH infusion test is abnormal and indicates primary adrenal insufficiency.
5. The diagnosis can be confirmed by adrenal gland biopsy.

Treatment

There is no specific treatment for adrenoleukodystrophy.

Leukodystrophy with Diffuse Rosenthal Fiber Formation

A rare form of infantile leukodystrophy, characterized by diffuse demyelination and the presence of Rosenthal fibers in the white matter, has been described under the eponym Alexander's disease.[70]

Etiology and Pathology

Rosenthal fibers are believed to represent relatively inert metabolic products that occur following degeneration of glia.[184]

The disease may be a primary metabolic derangement of astrocytes[159] or a genetically determined defect. The defect leads to a proliferation of glial elements responsible for myelin formation (oligodendrocytic spongioblasts), which then degenerate. The cellular debris is transformed into Rosenthal fibers. At the same time, a severe and diffuse failure of myelin formation occurs around the axons throughout the central nervous system.

The condition is characterized by an increase in brain volume and diffuse demyelination involving most of the white matter of the central nervous system. There are proliferation of astrocytes, preservation of axis cylinders, and diffuse Rosenthal fiber formation around the blood vessels and in the paraventricular regions.

Clinical Features

The condition is present at birth. The infant fails to develop, and progressive muscular weakness, mental failure, and enlargement of the head result. Death occurs within a few months to a few years. A rare chronic form of this disease with clinical features resembling multiple sclerosis has been described in adolescents and adults.[167]

Treatment

There is no effective treatment available at this time.

Pelizaeus-Merzbacher Disease

There is some disagreement concerning the criteria necessary for the diagnosis of Pelizaeus-Merzbacher disease, and some regard it as a variant of adrenoleukodystrophy. However, it does appear that the disease is a clinical and pathologic entity of a sex-linked recessive nature and that it is an example of a distinct form of a leukodystrophy which can be diagnosed during life.[74]

Etiology and Pathology

Chemical analyses have shown that there is a reduction in white matter lipids, particularly cerebrosides and sulfatides. This suggests that there is an arrest of myelination or hypomyelination in Pelizaeus-Merzbacher disease.

The brain is severely atrophic and usually weighs less than 600 gm. The atrophy includes the cerebellum, which becomes very small and more atrophic than the brainstem. The cerebral hemispheres contain irregular areas of concentric demyelination with islands of apparently normal myelin resulting in a tigroid appearance. The gray matter appears to be normal, and the axis cylinders are preserved.[168] There is also marked demyelination in the cerebellum with atrophy of both Purkinje cells and granular cells in the cerebellar gray matter. All areas of demyelination show a paucity of oligodendroglial cells, dense gliosis, and a few microglial cells but no inflammatory response. Fat stains show the presence of occasional sudanophilic droplets.

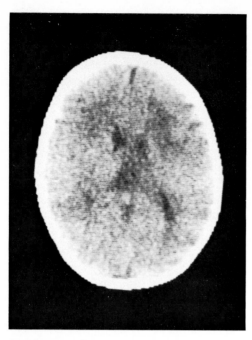

FIGURE 3–3. Computed tomography in Pelizaeus-Merzbacher disease. There are irregular areas of decreased density in the central white matter and evidence of early cortical atrophy.

Clinical Features

There is frequently a history of constant jerking of the eyes beginning within a few days after birth. This is followed by failure to achieve early milestones such as rolling over or sitting. The child may show spasticity, cerebellar ataxia, or choreoathetoid movements, and there is progressive mental retardation. The disks may show some degree of optic atrophy, and eye movements are characterized by coarse nystagmus or oscillopsia.

The degenerative course usually proceeds for a number of years, but there may be an apparent arrest of the disease with survival into adolescence or early adult life.

Diagnostic Procedures

1. The electroencephalogram shows diffuse symmetric slowing of moderate degree.
2. Visual evoked responses, auditory evoked potentials, and somatosensory evoked potentials are all abnormal.[185]
3. Computed tomography shows evidence of cortical atrophy and patchy areas of decreased density in the central white matter representing areas of demyelination (Fig. 3–3).

Lipid Storage Diseases

Historically, diseases involving neuronal storage of lipid and cerebromacular degeneration were thought to share a common etiology and were termed "amaurotic familial idiocies." Some of the diseases traditionally placed in this category are listed in Table 3–3, but they can now be organized according to the storage material and age of onset. Cerebromacular degeneration refers to the accumulation of lipid in the ganglion cells of the retina. The accumulation produces a diffuse gray appearance except at the fovea, which is normally free of ganglion cells. The fovea then appears as a dark-purple or cherry-red spot. The cherry-red spot is not pathognomonic for any specific neuronal storage disease but may be seen whenever the ganglion cells are involved. The first lipid storage disease to be described was Tay-Sachs disease, which involves a deficiency of β-hexosaminidase with accumulation of its substrate, GM_2 ganglioside. Thus, Tay-Sachs disease

TABLE 3–3

Neuronal Lipid Storage Diseases

Type	Age of Onset	Eponym
GM_2 gangliosidoses	Infantile, type 1 Infantile, type 2 Juvenile	Tay-Sachs Sandhoff's
GM_1 gangliosidoses	Infantile Juvenile	
"Ceroid lipofuscinoses"	Late infantile Juvenile Adult	Bielschowsky-Jansky Batten's or Vogt-Spielmeyer Kufs's or Hallervorden-Spatz

can be classified as a GM_2 gangliosidosis with infantile onset.

Other lipid storage diseases, previously described on the basis of clinical symptoms and pathology, are now recognized by the chemistry of the stored material and, in some instances, the enzyme deficiency. In some of these diseases, such as Niemann-Pick disease, there is neuronal storage of lipid and cerebromacular degeneration in common with the diseases listed in Table 3–3. Others show little evidence of neuronal storage but do have nervous system involvement.

Myelin is markedly involved in most of the lipid storage diseases, but the mechanisms leading to the paucity of myelin are not known. Where there is neuronal damage or degeneration, the involvement of myelin may be secondary to the faulty development or metabolism of the neurons and their axons. In those diseases where myelin has been isolated and analyzed, the composition is abnormal but similar in each case, with lowered galactocerebroside and ethanolamine phospholipid content and higher content of cholesterol. Similar changes are seen in other diseases where secondary demyelination may be occurring, such as subacute sclerosing panencephalitis. These changes suggest a common response of the oligodendroglia to insult, rather than a specific change related to the enzyme deficiency involved. It is not known whether the changes in myelin are due to decreased formation (hypomyelination), synthesis of abnormal unstable myelin that breaks down (dysmyelination), destruction of normal myelin, or some combination of events.

GM$_2$ Gangliosidoses

The most common form of this disorder is infantile type 1, or Tay-Sachs disease, which is inherited as an autosomal recessive trait. The carrier rate is high in many Jewish families whose antecedents emigrated from the Kovno and Grodno areas of Lithuania and Poland, and it is likely that some 90 per cent of cases are from this stock. The disease has also been described in many areas of the world in non-Jewish families who probably contribute about 10 per cent of cases.[174]

Etiology and Pathology

The metabolic abnormality in Tay-Sachs disease is a deficiency of the enzyme β-D-N-acetyl hexosaminidase A leading to accumulation of GM_2 ganglioside in the neurons of the retina and central nervous system.

The neuronal inclusion bodies contain the GM_2 type of ganglioside[39, 130] because in this and other forms of lipidosis there is a deficiency of the catabolic enzymes required for degradation of complex lipids (Fig. 3–1). Hexosaminidase occurs as two isozymes, A and B1, but only the A form is deficient in Tay-Sachs disease. However, a variant of the disease with deficiency of both hexosaminidase A and B has been described. The clinical and pathologic aspects of this variant, sometimes termed Sandhoff's disease, or type 2, are similar to those of Tay-Sachs disease, but also include visceral involvement.

GM_2 is normally present in the brain but does not exceed 1 per cent of total gangliosides. In the infantile form, GM_2 gangliosides are greatly increased together with abnormal aminoglucolipids in gray and white matter. In the peripheral blood the enzymes serum glutamic oxaloacetic transaminase (SGOT), serum glutamic pyruvic transaminase (SGPT), and lactic acid dehydrogenase (LDH) (types 1, 2, and 3) are increased and fructose-1,6-diphosphate aldolase and LDH-type 5 are reduced. What relation, if any, these enzyme disorders have to the cerebral manifestations is unknown, but they may be important from the point of view of genetic counseling since this pattern of enzyme disorder is also present in heterozygotes. Sphingomyelin is measurably decreased in the envelope of circulating erythrocytes, and N-acetyl-neuraminic acid and α-2 globulin fractions are both increased in the peripheral blood.

The ultrastructural abnormality consists of membranous cytoplasmic inclusion bodies in neurons and glial cells consisting of gangliosides, cholesterol, phospholipids, and other glycolipids.

The deficiency of beta-D-N-acetyl-hexosaminidase A can be measured in the amniotic fluid within the first 12 weeks of pregnancy, making possible genetic counseling and potential therapeutic abortion. Transabdominal amniocentesis carries minimal danger to either mother or fetus, and a culture of amniotic fluid cells can be used for estimation of hexosaminidase A. Genetic counseling based on prenatal screening of the amniotic fluid in families at risk should reduce the incidence of Tay-Sachs disease with its early mortality, grave morbidity, and consequent problems for the family and community.

Patients who die within a few months of onset of Tay Sachs disease have atrophic brains and also ventricular dilatation. However, patients who survive longer may have relatively enlarged brains, which are abnormally heavy, firm, and leathery in texture.

Microscopic examination shows the following:

1. The neurons in the brain and spinal cord are distended with lipid. The nucleus is pushed to the periphery of the cell, and there is loss of Nissl substance.
2. There is diffuse proliferation of astrocytes, and numerous lipid-laden microglial cells are found throughout the central nervous system.
3. There is a diffuse loss of myelin in both the central nervous system and peripheral nerves with relative preservation of axons.
4. The optic nerves show marked demyelination.

Clinical Features

Infantile Type. In the infantile form, the infant shows normal development until about six months of age when there is an insidious but progressive onset of lack of interest in the parents and surroundings. A loss of previously achieved milestones in development is noted. It is soon apparent that the child has visual impairment, which progresses to blindness. Examination of the fundus shows a striking dark-purple or cherry-red spot in the area of the fovea. Optic atrophy occurs at a later stage. There is progressive and generalized muscle weakness with increased tone, clonus, and, finally, intense spasticity and hyperactive reflexes with bilateral extensor plantar responses. Seizures and myoclonic jerks are frequent and are usually provoked by sensory stimulation such as loud sounds. They regularly occur in the early stages and persist throughout the illness. The terminal state is one of spastic quadriplegia with decerebrate rigidity and generalized wasting. Usually there is slight enlargement of the head. Death usually occurs about 24 months from the onset of the illness.

Juvenile Type. An extremely rare form of the disease has been described as the juvenile type and begins at three or four years of age. This disease pursues a chronic degenerative course with progressive dementia, seizures, myoclonic jerks, cerebellar ataxia, and visual failure. The cherry-red spot is absent in these cases, but optic atrophy is present.[119]

Diagnostic Procedures

1. In early infancy, when the vision is still intact, the EEG is likely to be normal. However, abnormalities appear with the development of neurologic deficits and the loss of vision. There is a progressive disorganization of background activity. Theta activity is at first noted in brief bursts and gradually becomes longer in duration. When the patient develops seizures, single or multiple sharp wave potentials appear and are often followed by slow wave complexes giving the sharp-slow wave complexes a pseudotriphasic configuration. High-voltage delta activity may also be seen in bursts of variable duration. In the advanced stage of the disease with myoclonus, periodic symmetric sharp and slow wave complexes may be seen followed by periodic generalized bursts of electrical suppression. After the age of three years, the EEG shows fewer epileptiform discharges, and a general decrease in amplitude is noted. Stimulation of such patients produces little or no alteration of the background activity. The EEG in the juvenile form of cerebral lipidosis has a similar evolution, except that the changes occur over a longer period of time and periodic discharges and triphasic complexes have not been described.
2. In the infantile and juvenile types, the lymphocytes in smears of the peripheral blood have been reported to contain large azurophilic granules.[158]
3. Rectal biopsy may reveal abnormal lipid material in the neurons of Auerbach's and Meissner's plexus in any of the types described.[26]
4. Computed tomography of the brain may show evidence of atrophy with ventricular enlargement and widening of the sulci.
5. Brain biopsy will show the typical neuronal changes described earlier.
6. Increased values of SGOT, SGPT, and LDH types 1, 2, and 3 have been reported in the serum and cerebrospinal fluid in the infantile type. Fructose-1,6-diphosphate aldolase activity and LDH type 5 activities are decreased in the serum.
7. Serum, skin biopsies, and tissue cultures of fibroblasts show reduced hexosaminidase A activity or reduced hexosaminidase A and B activity (Sandhoff variant).
8. Amniocentesis makes possible the measurement of the hexosaminidase deficiency during fetal life while therapeutic abortion is possible.

Treatment

Treatment includes management of seizures, myoclonus, and spasticity. Genetic counseling with the prevention of the birth of children afflicted with Tay-Sachs appears to be the best method of controlling the disorder.

GM₁ Gangliosidosis (Generalized Gangliosidosis)

This disorder, in which GM_1 ganglioside is stored in the nervous system and viscera, occurs in two distinct forms. Type 1 GM_1 gangliosidosis is present at birth and shows gross dysmorphic features and rapid progression. Type 2, or juvenile, GM_1 gangliosidosis has a later onset, a more protracted course, and less marked bony deformities.[127]

Pathology and Etiology

Both types of GM_1 gangliosidoses are inherited as an autosomal recessive inheritance trait and involve deficiency of a lysosomal β-galactosidase that utilizes GM_1 ganglioside as substrate. While GM_1 ganglioside accumulates in the nervous system, mucopolysaccharides similar to keratan sulfate are predominantly stored in the visceral organs, in a ratio of about $50:1$ relative to GM_1 ganglioside. In the infantile form, visceral histiocytosis is evident, with strongly PAS-positive, weakly metachromatic, and sudanophilic inclusions apparently due to the mucopolysaccharides. There is vacuolation of renal glomerular epithelial cells, which is not seen in any other lipid storage diseases except juvenile GM_1 gangliosidosis and Fabry's disease. Neurons throughout the cortex, brainstem, spinal cord, and Meissner's plexus show ballooning of the cytoplasm and vacuolation, with stored ganglioside that is strongly sudanophilic and weakly PAS-positive. Electron microscopy shows neuronal inclusions that appear similar to the membranous cytoplasmic bodies seen in Tay-Sachs disease. Reactive gliosis and demyelination are frequently severe. The type 1 form is associated with coarse facial features and bony abnormalities similar to those found in the mucopolysaccharidoses. In the juvenile form, visceral involvement and bony deformities are less marked or absent.

Clinical Features

Infantile-Onset (Type 1). Symptoms are generally present at birth, and death occurs within one to two years. Mental and motor development is markedly retarded with feeding difficulties, apathetic behavior, and an exaggerated startle response. Hypotonia is followed later by spastic quadriparesis. Clonic movements and seizures are an early and prominent symptom. Blindness and cerebromacular degeneration occur, with cherry-red spots observed in about half the cases.[111]

Juvenile-Onset. The child appears to be normal at birth, and the first symptoms appear at one to three years of age. There is progressive psychomotor retardation with death three to ten years after onset, generally due to recurrent respiratory tract infections. The initial symptom may be locomotor ataxia, with subsequent difficulty in hand coordination and speech. Spasticity, hyperacusis, and seizures appear within one to two years after the initial onset. Enlargement of visceral organs, cerebromacular degeneration, and blindness generally do not occur.

Diagnostic Procedures

Diagnosis can be confirmed by assay of β-galactosidase activity in serum, white cells, or skin fibroblasts. Either GM_1 ganglioside or the artificial substrate p-nitrophenyl-β-D-galactopyranoside may be used (although the two activities are not identical). The extent of deficiency is similar in both infantile and juvenile types.

Treatment

No treatment other than supportive care is known; enzyme replacement has not been attempted. Since heterozygotes can be detected and amniotic cells can be assayed for activity, genetic counseling is possible.

Neuronal Ceroid Lipofuscinoses

This group of diseases is characterized by accumulation of insoluble autofluorescent lipopigments, ceroid and lipofuscin, in the neurons of affected individuals and progressive nervous system degeneration. Since the biochemical defect(s) are not known,[181a] it is not established that these diseases have a common etiology. On the basis of clinical criteria, three different types have been described. However, even within each type there are considerable heterogeneity and variability with regard to age of onset, clinical course, and presence of lymphocytic vacuolation, suggesting that these diseases may represent a collection of different enzymatic defects.

Pathology and Etiology

Lipopigment accumulation is most prominent in neurons throughout the CNS, but is also seen in astroglia, endothelial cells, and the viscera. Depending on age of onset and duration of disease, the brain may be of normal size or markedly atrophied, with neuronal loss and relatively good preservation of white matter. Lymphocytic vacuolation is frequently present and may aid in detecting heterozygotes. Inspection of neuronal and lymphocytic inclusions by electron microscopy reveals a wide range of morphology, with the presence of irregular curvilinear bodies, fingerprint patterns, and crystalloid inclusions in contrast to the more regular membranous cytoplasmic bodies in Tay-Sachs disease. The inclusion bodies stain for acid phosphatase and other hydrolases, indicating their lysosomal origin.

Inclusion bodies have been isolated and analyzed, and the ceroid and lipofuscin pigments have been characterized as cross-linked polar and neutral lipids that have undergone peroxidation. It has been proposed that a biochemical defect, perhaps in control of peroxidation, leads to accumulation in the nondividing neurons of these compounds, which cannot be further catabolized.[191] Retinoic acid has been identified as one of the major materials stored in the inclusions from the brain of a child with Batten's disease, a finding that may provide clues to the etiology of this group of diseases if substantiated in other cases.[187]

Clinical Features

Infantile-Onset (Bielschowsky-Jansky). The age of onset is generally two to four years, with seizures as the initial symptom. The course is rapidly progressive, with early onset of dementia, seizures, optic atrophy, blindness, and death within one to six years. Macular degeneration and retinitis pigmentosa are sometimes seen in the later stages of the disease. Brain atrophy is severe.

Juvenile-Onset (Batten; Vogt-Spielmeyer or Spielmeyer-Sjögren). This form usually presents with later onset between four and eight years, with blindness as the first symptom. The course is more protracted, with an average of 11 years. Dementia is of later onset and less severe. Macular degeneration and retinitis pigmentosa are usually present at an early stage.

Adult-Onset (Kufs). Onset generally occurs after 20 years of age with mental changes and,

occasionally, seizures as the first symptoms. Blindness and fundal changes do not occur, unlike the two forms with earlier onset. The course of the disease is more protracted with a duration of 5 to 35 years, and dementia is a prominent symptom in some cases but absent in others.

Diagnostic Procedures

Aside from the clinical symptoms described, examination of the lymphocytes for inclusions has proved valuable in cases of both infantile and juvenile onset. Rectal or brain biopsy has been necessary in the past to confirm diagnosis.

Treatment

Control of seizures, supportive care, and genetic counseling are indicated. Trials of antioxidant therapy or low-vitamin A diets have so far given no conclusive results.

Niemann-Pick Disease

The sphingomyelin lipidosis called Niemann-Pick disease is a rare condition that is probably inherited as an autosomal recessive trait. It has been described in many races and in many countries.

Etiology and Pathology

There is an enzymatic defect in the catabolism of sphingomyelin with accumulation of sphingomyelin and cholesterol in large "foam" cells throughout the body.[50, 51] The enzyme sphingomyelinase, which catalyzes hydrolysis of sphingomyelin to phosphorylcholine and ceramide, is lacking in Niemann-Pick's disease.

The brain shows some evidence of atrophy with widening of the sulci but without ventricular dilatation. The macrocephaly of Tay-Sachs disease is not seen, and the weight of the brain is usually less than normal. The neurons have a similar appearance to those in Tay-Sachs disease with pale cytoplasm, an eccentric nucleus, degeneration of Nissl substance, and swelling of the dendrites. There is marked loss of myelin with many lipid-laden microglial cells and some foam cells in the brain and meninges. These changes are present throughout the brain and spinal cord but the cerebellum may be more severely affected than the cerebral hemispheres. Chemical analysis shows a marked increase in sphingomyelin content in the central nervous system. Analysis of the fatty acid content of gray and white matter of the brain in the sphingomyelin fraction shows a deficiency of long-chain fatty acids, which is also found in the liver.

The spleen, lymphoid tissue, and bone marrow show diffuse infiltration with foam cells, and the Kupffer cells of the liver contain lipid. Suppurative and xanthomatous lesions laden with foam cells may also occur in the skin as well as in the alveoli of the lung. A typical "cherry-red spot" may occur in the macula, similar to that described in Tay-Sachs disease.

Clinical Features

Infantile Form. This form occurs in 85 per cent of cases with the onset at about six months of age. Infants with this disease feed poorly, and there are frequent vomiting and gradual development of hepatosplenomegaly. There are also progressive muscular weakness and wasting of the limb muscles. Weakness of the abdominal muscle accentuates the protuberant abdomen, which is due to visceromegaly. The child loses interest in its surroundings and develops progressive dementia and blindness. A cherry-red spot is seen in the macula in about 50 per cent of cases. The terminal stage is one of complete unresponsiveness, hypotonia, and anemia.

Childhood Form. This form begins later in childhood with loss of appetite and the development of splenomegaly. There are slowly progressive dementia and cerebellar ataxia, which occur over a period of 20 years or more. In later years, there is a tendency for a decrease in the rate of progression.

Visceral Form. This form is characterized by visceral involvement with sparing of the central nervous system.

Diagnostic Procedures

1. A synthetic chromogenic analog of sphingomyelin may be used for the diagnosis of Niemann-Pick disease using tissue specimens or extracts of cultured fibroblasts as a source of enzyme.[28]
2. A deficiency of sphingomyelinase in leukocytes can be demonstrated using radioactive sphingomyelin.
3. Brain or rectal biopsy will show typical neu-

ronal involvement with sphingomyelin deposition.

Treatment

A number of treatments have been tried in Niemann-Pick disease with equivocal results. These include irradiation, the use of cytotoxic agents, vitamin E, and injections of anterior pituitary extract. Splenectomy is hazardous and should be reserved for patients with definite hypersplenism.

Gaucher's Disease (Cerebroside Lipidosis)

Cerebroside lipidosis is a relatively uncommon condition and, like other lipidoses, is inherited as an autosomal recessive trait.

Etiology and Pathology

The metabolic fault appears to be a deficiency of the enzyme glucocerebrosidase, which catabolizes glucocerebrosides. Hence they accumulate in neurons and in reticuloendothelial cells (Gaucher cells) throughout the body.[30] The spleen is enlarged and shows loss of normal architecture and widespread replacement by Gaucher cells. Hypersplenism may occur, producing anemia, thrombocytopenia, and leukopenia. There may be a generalized lymphadenopathy with infiltration by Gaucher cells, particularly marked in the abdominal and thoracic nodes. The liver is enlarged with groups of Gaucher cells compressing and destroying parenchymal cells. This may lead to considerable distortion of the liver parenchyma and compression of the portal venous system. Ascites may occur, but liver function tests are usually within normal limits.

Masses of Gaucher cells in the bone marrow and cancellous bone may lead to pathologic fracture of long bones or collapse of vertebral bodies. The skin has a yellowish tinge, although Gaucher cells have not been reported in the skin. Bilateral pingueculae presenting as yellow wedge-shaped areas on the sclera with the base on the cornea are not uncommon.

Changes in the central nervous system are non-specific, and the involvement of neurons as seen in Tay-Sachs disease or Niemann-Pick disease does not occur. There is, however, a diffuse neuronal degeneration and active microglial phagocytosis of the cellular remains. Occasional perivascular collections of Gaucher cells may occur.

Clinical Features

The infantile form occurs in about 15 per cent of patients with Gaucher's disease with the initial symptoms appearing between the first week and six months of life. This is a rapidly progressive disease with loss of any developed motor skills, anemia, wasting of muscles, either hypo- or hypertonia, and a protuberant abdomen, due to hepatic and splenic enlargement. Seizures may occur, and paralysis of extraocular muscles with strabismus is usually seen. Death usually occurs at the end of the first year preceded by a terminal stage of decerebration.

Juvenile Form. This is a very rare form and begins later in childhood. The course is chronic with some evidence of cranial nerve involvement but little evidence of diffuse cerebral involvement. Hypersplenism and anemia are the predominant findings.[85]

Chronic Noncerebral Form. This form may occur at any age with hypersplenism, anemia, skin pigmentation, and pingueculae. Patients usually survive into adult life.

Diagnostic Procedures

1. Diagnosis of homozygotes and detection of heterozygous carriers can be made by measuring lipid hydrolase activity of peripheral blood leukocytes or cultured skin fibroblasts on radioactive glucocerebroside.[29]
2. Monitoring of pregnancies at risk for Gaucher's disease can be performed by measuring enzymatic activity in fetal cell cultures obtained by amniocentesis.
3. Roentgenographic examination of the long bones, spine, and phalanges may reveal translucent areas due to the presence of masses of Gaucher cells, with collapse of vertebral bodies or pathologic fractures.
4. There is an elevation of acid phosphatase activity in the serum and splenic tissues in all forms of Gaucher's disease. The cause is not known but may be due to release of acid phosphatase from lysosomes damaged by the accumulated cerebrosides. The acid phosphatase activity is not inhibited by 1-tartrate in contrast to that found in prostatic carcinomas.

Cerebrotendinous Xanthomatosis

A rare but distinct familial disease has been described due to an inborn error of metabolism causing a derangement in cholesterol metabolism.[120, 166]

Etiology and Pathology

The essential abnormality appears to be a disturbance of cholesterol metabolism with the accumulation of cholesterol and a metabolic derivative cholestanol in a number of tissues including the cerebellum, cornea, lung, and tendons. There is an accumulation of cholesterol within granulomas in the tendons and lung. The brain shows areas of demyelination, particularly in the brainstem and cerebellum.

Clinical Features

The condition is inherited as an autosomal dominant trait. The earliest symptoms consist of enlargement of the Achilles tendons during childhood followed by the development of cataracts in the second or third decade. There are chronic progressive cerebellar ataxia and dementia, which usually begin in the sixth decade.

Diagnostic Procedures

Demonstration of cholesterol and cholestanol in biopsy material, such as tendinous xanthoma, is considered diagnostic.

Treatment

There is no specific treatment for this disease. Cataracts should be removed surgically when visual impairment is sufficiently advanced to warrant the operation.

Fabry's Disease

This is a sphingolipidosis due to an inherited metabolic disorder causing a deficiency of ceramidetrihexosidase (Fig. 3–1). As a result of this deficiency there is an accumulation of trihexose ceramide and possibly other glycolipids in vessel walls throughout the body.[30, 108]

Etiology and Pathology

The abnormal glycolipid accumulation occurs in endothelial and smooth muscle cells throughout the body, including the retina as well as the central and peripheral nervous system. Glycolipid-filled macrophages and arachnoidal cells are found throughout the CNS. Diffuse and focal ischemic changes are found in the brain parenchyma. Measurement of the lipid-bound hexose content in the microsomal fraction of the brain shows this lipid complex to be increased fivefold.

The kidney, myocardium, skin, conjunctiva, and retina contain abnormal glycolipid deposits.

Clinical Features

The condition is inherited as a sex-linked recessive trait. The course in male patients is usually dominated by deterioration of kidney function and in some by impaired cardiac function also. The skin shows pinpoint, elevated, brownish-red zones located on the trunk, thighs, and genital region. Attacks of pain in the extremities, paresthesias, headache, and fever appear. The diagnosis should be considered when the dermatologic findings are associated with vascular abnormalities of the eye and brain together with corneal opacities.

Neurologic signs and symptoms begin in the teens and consist of repeated episodes of hemiplegia, aphasia, and/or brainstem and cerebellar signs. They are transient at first.

Diagnostic Procedures

1. Deficiency of ceramidetrihexose activity may be demonstrated in rectal biopsy specimens or in cultures of skin fibroblasts.
2. The ophthalmologic picture is pathognomonic with a characteristically abnormal appearance of the retina due to infiltration with lipids. There are whorllike epithelial changes in the cornea, and the lenses show posterior cataracts with a spider-like appearance. Biopsy of the conjunctiva may be diagnostic.
3. Arteriograms in young patients with strokelike symptoms may show occlusion of the middle cerebral or other major cerebral vessels.

Treatment

Infusion of purified ceramidetrihexosidase is said to reduce levels of circulatory ceramidetrihexosidase and to benefit patients with this disorder.[30] Infusion of human plasma and renal transplantation have also been recommended.

Patients with renal and cardiac failure or acute cerebral infarction should be treated appropriately.

Acquired Allergic or Infectious Diseases Associated with Breakdown of Normal Myelin

The conditions discussed so far in this chapter have been characterized by inherited metabolic abnormalities affecting lipid metabolism with pathologic changes in white matter resulting from decreased myelination, breakdown of abnormally formed myelin, or in some instances breakdown of myelin of apparently normal composition.

The group of demyelinating diseases to be described in this section is different in that they are not usually genetically determined and are almost always associated with breakdown of normal myelin.[157] Multiple sclerosis is the most common clinical entity encountered in this group and will be the first one to be discussed in detail.

Multiple Sclerosis

Despite an ever-increasing amount of research activity, multiple sclerosis remains a disease of attractive theories and unknown cause. At the present time, it would appear that a number of factors must be involved in the etiology and pathogenesis of multiple sclerosis, but the relative importance of these factors has not been delineated. The current emphasis on the search for a viral agent has had equivocal results, but it is clear that if a viral infection is present, it must be of the "latent" or "slow" virus type. There is no generally accepted specific diagnostic test for multiple sclerosis, and the clinician is faced with a diagnostic challenge in early or mild cases. However, the development of new electrophysiologic techniques and more detailed analysis of serum and cerebrospinal fluid components may increase the ability to make a positive diagnosis of multiple sclerosis at an earlier stage.

Since the cause of the disease is unknown, treatment of multiple sclerosis is still empiric or symptomatic. There is no firm evidence that drugs including ACTH and corticosteroids affect the course of the disease during the acute phase or the reduction of the relapse rate. The disabled patient with multiple sclerosis requires the cooperative efforts of the neurologist, physiatrist, and community social worker in a program of continued association with the patient and his family for many years.

Incidence

Although multiple sclerosis, compared to many disorders, is the most common form of the demyelinating diseases, it is still uncommon. There are only 50 to 60 cases per 100,000 population reported in areas considered to have a high incidence of the disease.

Age and Sex. The incidence is extremely low prior to the age of ten years and rises to a peak at 30 to 35 years and then falls steeply in the fifth and sixth decades. Several studies have shown that the peak incidence is reached at an earlier age in the female and that the disease is more common in women. There is a female to male ratio of 1.7:1.0.

Geographic Distribution. The disease has been recognized in all countries, but there is marked variation in the incidence of multiple sclerosis that appears to be related to latitude.[8, 139]

Multiple sclerosis has a high prevalence rate in Europe between latitudes 65° and 45° north with a similar distribution in the northern United States and southern Canada. A similar prevalence rate is found in comparable latitudes in the Southern hemisphere covering New Zealand and southern Australia.[99] Since these high-risk areas occur in Europe and former European colonies, it is suggested that there is a higher risk for multiple sclerosis in Caucasians.[98] The highest prevalence rates have been reported in the inhabitants of the Orkney and Shetland Islands,[143] where studies indicate two distinct clinical and epidemiologic groups of patients with multiple sclerosis, suggesting that multiple sclerosis may not be a single disease entity.[142]

A series of studies carried out in Israel have shown a low prevalence rate for multiple sclerosis in immigrants from Afro-Asian countries and a high prevalence rate for immigrants from Northern and Central Europe. Native-born Israelis of both Afro-Asian and European ancestry have high rates similar to those of European immigrants, suggesting that the prevalence of multiple sclerosis may change with socioeconomic conditions.[104]

RACIAL DIFFERENCES. Multiple sclerosis is relatively rare in Japan and extremely rare (0.05 per 100,000) in Korea.[132] The disease also has a lower-than-expected prevalence among Japanese Americans,[56] who show a more frequent occurrence of optic nerve involvement and of acute transverse myelopathy.[170] It is possible that racial differences affect the prevalence of multiple sclerosis because of genetic factors within the racial group.[6]

DIET. There is a suggestion that the geographic distribution of multiple sclerosis is related to the increased intake of foods of animal origin or to the consumption of dairy products in the world.[9, 33, 86] However, the relationship between diet and multiple sclerosis is unproven[128] and could possibly reflect an association between socioeconomic status and the risk of multiple sclerosis.

Infection. A history of antecedent infection is not unusual in multiple sclerosis, but the relationship to the disease process is not clear.[151] There seems to be a significant increase in infections in early life with further infection in the second decade in patients with multiple sclerosis.[53]

Contact with House Dogs. It is possible to demonstrate an increased ownership of small indoor dogs in the five-year period before symptoms of multiple sclerosis appear.[45, 49, 93] There is also an increased exposure to neurologically ill dogs by multiple sclerosis patients.[46] These findings suggest that indoor dogs may be an animal vector for an infectious agent causing multiple sclerosis and question the role of the common distemper virus (a paramyxovirus) in multiple sclerosis.

Family Incidence. There is an increased frequency of second cases of multiple sclerosis in families when compared with a control population.[163, 164] The risk of contracting multiple sclerosis is about 20 times greater in siblings and about 12 times greater if the parent is affected. Some 10 per cent of patients give a positive family history, while the incidence in a second twin is about 17 per cent.

An individual who has an identical twin with multiple sclerosis has a 20 to 25 per cent chance of developing the disease, suggesting some involvement of common genetic factors. An individual who has an affected fraternal twin has a less than 15 per cent chance of developing multiple sclerosis. This rate is higher than the risk between sibs and suggests that there is some influence in sharing the same environment. When one twin is affected, there appears to be significant excess exposure to tonsillectomy, infections, and animals in the affected twin.[100]

Family studies are more suggestive of an infective process with a long incubation period rather than a genetic trait.[76]

Genetic Factors. It has been suggested that a gene predisposing to the development of multiple sclerosis is located in chromosome 6 in the histocompatibility complex region. A number of studies have shown the presence of particular

HLA haplotypes in family members with multiple sclerosis[7, 129] and a more-than-significant association of certain HLA genes in patients with chronic multiple sclerosis.[124, 178] The presence of a "complement abnormality susceptibility gene" linked to HLA genes has been proposed[181] or that an HLA-linked T cell deficiency may exist in some cases of multiple sclerosis.[133] However, some studies on histocompatibility typing in multiple sclerosis are equivocal[117] or not significant[31, 149, 133] and do not support the hypothesis that there is a genetic factor that enhances autoimmunity in multiple sclerosis.[62]

Trauma. There are probably well-documented cases of trauma preceding the onset of multiple sclerosis. Trauma usually occurs at the site of the initial symptom. All that can be said at this time is that trauma may or may not be an aggravating factor in some cases of multiple sclerosis.

Pregnancy. The impression that the relapse rate in patients with multiple sclerosis increased during pregnancy has not been substantiated by recent studies.[164] There is some increase, however, during the first three months postpartum. Still, the overall risk of relapse during a pregnancy year (nine months of pregnancy, three months postpartum) is only 50 per cent greater than in a nonpregnancy year.

Changes in Temperature. An increase in temperature may cause a temporary intensification of symptoms of multiple sclerosis, which disappears as the temperature falls. Certain patients notice the development of long-dormant symptoms if they take a hot bath or if the air temperature is high. There is, however, no evidence that exposure to high temperature predisposes to an exacerbation of multiple sclerosis.

Allergy. Studies showing a higher incidence of allergic reactions in patients with multiple sclerosis have not been substantiated. Reports of delayed reactions to skin sensitivity tests (using PPD tuberculin and other allergens) in multiple sclerosis patients have not been confirmed. However, the immune response to inoculation of standard typhoid-paratyphoid vaccine appears to be less in multiple sclerosis patients than in controls.[68]

Etiology

It is not surprising to find that a considerable number of theories have been or are presently entertained in a disease of unproved etiology.

At the present time it is postulated that multiple sclerosis is (1) a slow virus infection or (2) an autoimmune disease or (3) both.

Slow Virus Theory. The existence of agents that produce chronic degenerative diseases was first postulated and proved with kuru. Kuru is a chronic neuronal degeneration, affecting natives of eastern New Guinea, which is characterized by pseudobulbar symptoms, dementia, and ataxia. A slow virus disease is also believed to be responsible for visna, a demyelinative disease involving the central nervous system in sheep similar to multiple sclerosis. Other diseases caused by slow virus infection include subacute sclerosing panencephalitis (SSPE), progressive multifocal leukoencephalopathy, and Jakob-Creutzfeldt disease.

Evidence for a slow virus etiology in multiple sclerosis may be summarized as follows:

1. Paramyxovirus-like intranuclear inclusions have been identified by electron microscopy in autopsy material from patients who died during the acute phase of multiple sclerosis.[147, 175] Paramyxovirus has also been recovered from the jejunum in patients with chronic multiple sclerosis,[145] and measles antigen has been identified in the jejunal mucosa by immunofluorescence.[135] Parinfluenza 6/94 virus has been cultured from autopsy material after early sterile biopsy and fusion technique in acute multiple sclerosis.[18] A relationship between multiple sclerosis and virus infection is suggested by the presence of a small virus-like agent in mice innoculated with brain homogenate obtained from multiple sclerosis cases.[37]

2. An elevation of gamma globulins frequently seen in the cerebrospinal fluid of patients with multiple sclerosis also occurs in well-accepted chronic infections of the central nervous system. Immunologic studies indicate a frequent association between measles virus infection and multiple sclerosis.[81, 126] The presence of oligoclonal IgG in the cerebrospinal fluid is indicative of immunologic activity in the brain[55, 64, 176, 182, 186] and is associated with elevated measles antibody titers.[10] Part of oligoclonal IgG is a measles virus–specific IgG.

Elevated levels of IgM have been reported in the spinal fluid in some cases of multiple sclerosis,[118] and a measles-specific IgM has been demonstrated in the sera of some patients with the disease.[69]

3. Epidemiologic studies of the familial incidence of multiple sclerosis are compatible with an infectious disease with a long incubation period. If it is an infectious disease, the infection is probably acquired in early life and overt symptoms do not appear until some years later.[54]

4. The fact that there is a relapsing and remitting course could be in favor of an infective process. Known hypersensitivity reactions, such as postvaccinal leukoencephalitis, produce maximal damage to the central nervous system at the onset and rarely relapse.

Autoimmune Theory. Autoimmune mechanisms have been demonstrated in a number of diseases occurring outside the central nervous system, and the theory of antibody production and destruction of body tissues is widely accepted. In the case of multiple sclerosis, it is presumed that some agent, possibly a virus, passes through the blood-brain barrier and produces a localized destruction of myelin. The breakdown products of myelin act as antigens and stimulate immunologic systems within the brain, or, by passing through the blood-brain barrier, they stimulate the systemic immunologic mechanisms.

A local immunologic change in the brain is suggested by the demonstration of an increased number of T lymphocytes in the cerebrospinal fluid as compared to the peripheral blood.[5] T lymphocytes are relatively diminished in the peripheral blood and show decreased activity in multiple sclerosis, while the B lymphocytes are increased in the systemic circulation.[150] This is a consistent finding in known autoimmune diseases. There is evidence of altered cellular immunity in multiple sclerosis, which could be related to the destruction of myelin, and lymphocytes are present in excess at the site of the lesions during the acute phase of the disease.[97]

The concept of multiple sclerosis as an autoimmune disease has been enhanced by the development of an experimental animal model of chronic relapsing experimental allergic encephalomyelitis.[80, 148]

Combined Viral and Autoimmune Theory. It can be seen from the above that these two theories are not mutually exclusive since destruction of brain tissue by a viral infective agent may initiate an autoimmune reaction.

Pathology

The brain has a normal external appearance in acute cases of multiple sclerosis. Coronal sections show brownish gelatinous areas of demyelination scattered throughout the white and bordering gray matter but particularly marked in the periventricular area.[2] In chronic cases, there may be generalized shrinkage of the hemispheres with widening of the sulci and some ventricular dilatation. There are also irregular, depressed areas over the pons and spinal cord. Plaques of demyelination also occur in irregular fashion in the hemispheres, particularly around the ventricles. Many appear to terminate at the junction of the white and gray matter but, in fact, extend into the gray matter. Others apparently spare a thin rim of white matter immediately beneath the gray matter.

Lesions in the brainstem are most marked around the cerebral aqueduct and beneath the floor of the fourth ventricle. They may occur anywhere in the spinal cord but frequently appear as conical areas of demyelination with the broad base on the surface of the cord and the point extending inward to involve both white and gray matter. On microscopic examination, the clearly defined plaque with sharp edges proves to be a false impression, and demyelination is seen to fade away gradually into normal tissue. In such cases, there is loss of myelin with sparing of axons and an increase in microglial cells containing lipid material which is weakly sudanophilic. Perivascular cuffing by lymphocytes and plasma cells occurs as an early event in active plaques, and perivenous cuffing without demyelination occurs outside the plaque in apparently intact areas. As the myelin products are phagocytosed by microglial cells, there are a proliferation of astrocytes and an increase in glial fibers with eventual formation of a glial scar[66] and impaired regional enzymatic activity.[43]

The demyelinating process varies in intensity from an incomplete loss of myelin, the "shadow" plaque, to an intense demyelination with cyst formation. Occasionally, concentric areas of demyelination separated by normal white matter occur in patients with multiple sclerosis. If extensive, the process is sometimes referred to by the eponym "Balo's disease."

Clinical Features

Since the lesions of multiple sclerosis may occur in any part of the central nervous system, the signs and symptoms are extremely varied and protean in nature. It is, in fact, the variability of signs indicating widespread but patchy involvement of white matter that permits the diagnosis of multiple sclerosis in early cases. The diagnosis is extremely difficult and, at best, presumptive when there is only one focal sign. The two major factors in the diagnosis of multiple sclerosis are:

1. Signs and symptoms of disseminated disease
2. A tendency to relapse and remit

However, these factors are not to be construed as anything more than useful guidelines in the diagnosis. Although relapse and remission of focal signs, such as retrobulbar optic neuritis, are associated with a high degree of correlation in multiple sclerosis, it is also apparent that 10 per cent of patients do not show a well-defined relapsing course but appear to pursue one that is more or less a steadily progressive course. Furthermore, other neurologic conditions, such as brain tumor, may also show occasional remissions.

The onset of multiple sclerosis is extremely variable, and the disease may suddenly develop in otherwise healthy young adults.[183] Some patients describe a period of vague ill health with prodromas that include easy fatigue, lack of energy, intermittent and fleeting blurring of vision, headache, a vague feeling of unsteadiness of gait, and ill-defined muscle and joint pains for variable periods of time prior to the overt attack. Such patients are not infrequently regarded as psychoneurotic or as examples of conversion hysteria, which may delay the diagnosis of multiple sclerosis.[12]

Although there is a wide variation in symptomatology, certain complaints and findings are encountered more frequently than others.

The most frequent initial complaint appears to be some degree of motor weakness, while a symptom of numbness or paresthesias is almost as common. Many patients first experience visual symptoms, which include blurring of vision, impairment of vision, and diplopia. The fourth initial symptom in order of frequency is ataxia of gait, which may be due to either cerebellar incoordination or posterior column involvement or both.

Less frequent initial complaints include the sudden onset of vertigo and vomiting, urgency and incontinence of urine, and occasionally seizures.[94]

Motor Symptoms. There is marked variation in the motor symptoms in multiple sclerosis. In the mild type, the patient may notice "something wrong" with the legs during exercise, which clears rapidly with rest. At the other end of the scale, the patient with the fulminating type presents with paraparesis, progressing to paraplegia within a period of days. In the progressive nonremitting form of the disease, the patient frequently presents with a chronic mild paraparesis or hemiparesis of a slow progression.

On examination of the affected limbs, there are usually increased tone, hyperactive deep tendon reflexes, and extensor plantar responses. The abdominal reflexes are frequently, but not invariably, absent in multiple sclerosis with early motor symptoms.

Occasionally, the occurrence of a plaque near the posterior nerve root entry zone may produce depression or absence of the deep tendon reflex in the appropriate segment. This may be the explanation for occasional patients with root pain. Similarly, a plaque near the anterior nerve root exit zone may produce the rare complication of localized muscle weakness followed by wasting.

Sensory Symptoms. Fleeting localized episodes of numbness and tingling are common in multiple sclerosis but are frequently forgotten unless a direct inquiry is made at the initial examination. In fact, this suggests that sensory symptoms may be more frequent as an initial manifestation of multiple sclerosis than is usually stated.

A lesion involving the lateral spinothalamic tract sometimes results in thermal dysesthesia, a feeling of warmth, coldness, or burning in a limb or affecting the trunk on the opposite side below the level of the plaque. Another form of dysesthesia is the occurrence of a band of hyperalgesia, which may occur at the upper margin of a zone of sensory loss. In addition to the heightened intensity and unpleasant reaction to pinprick, there may be spontaneous soreness or burning in the involved area.

Interference with posterior column function produces impairment of vibration and position sense and ataxia in the affected limb. In extreme cases a "useless" hand or limb or pseudoathetosis can occur, which may be aggravated by cerebellar ataxia. A Lhermitte sign, due to involvement of the cervical spinal cord, which can develop at any time during the course of multiple sclerosis, consists of a sudden unpleasant sensation down the spine to the legs and feet on flexion of the head and neck. This form of dysesthesia is often compared by the patient to an electric shock and is believed to be due to traction on the posterior columns of the spinal cord by stretching of the nerve roots during flexion of the neck.

Visual Symptoms. A definite episode of optic neuritis or retrobulbar neuritis often occurs as the initial symptom in multiple sclerosis. About 50 per cent of patients, whether children or adults, who develop optic neuritis without any other signs will eventually develop multiple sclerosis. In many patients with a definite diagnosis of multiple sclerosis, optic neuritis is mild, and temporal pallor develops without subjective symptoms. At least 25 per cent of patients with multiple sclerosis show temporal pallor within five years of the onset of the disease, so that this is a most useful clinical sign.

The symptoms and signs of optic neuritis are presented in Table 3–4.

Patients with mild multiple sclerosis recover in a short period of time, often with no detectable visual impairment. However, pattern-reversed visual evoked responses are usually abnormal in patients with previous optic neuritis.[40] Patients with severe multiple sclerosis experience varying degrees of persistent visual loss, particularly in the central portions of the visual fields.

Visual field defects are infrequent in multiple sclerosis but may develop owing to strategically placed plaques on the optic chiasm, optic tracts, or the radiations. The sudden appearance and resolution of a homonymous field defect in a young person may be due to multiple sclerosis.[87]

"Frontal Lobe" Signs. Acute dementia or onset with an acute psychosis is occasionally seen in multiple sclerosis and suggests the presence of widespread plaques of demyelination.[189] Chronic changes involving affect are not uncommon, and at least 60 per cent of patients show some evidence of euphoria with inappropriate laughter and an exaggerated sense of well-being. While euphoria is regarded as a frequent and classic symptom of multiple sclerosis, it is not generally realized that in some patients depression may be a problem, although suicide is infrequent. The problem of depression seems to be critical in two situations. When patients learn of the diagnosis, they may anticipate a shortened life-span and dependence on others. Also, patients with the chronic form of the disease may become depressed over continuing degeneration of their condition, particularly when sphincter control is involved.

Mild chronic dementia occurs in a reasonable percentage of patients with multiple sclerosis and is similar to that seen in other forms of organic brain disease with initial loss of judgment, impaired retention, and loss of recent memory. Ventricular dilatation may be demonstrated by computerized tomography in patients with more advanced disease.

Brainstem and Cerebellar Involvement. Scattered plaques of demyelination are frequently found in the brainstem in multiple sclerosis with involvement of motor, sensory, nuclear, and internuclear tracts as well as the cerebellar connections. About 14 per cent of patients show clinical evidence of brainstem involvement at the onset and 65 per cent during the course of the disease.[96] Oculomotor signs with diplopia due to paralysis of the third, fourth, or sixth nerve, paralysis or paresis of conjugate eye movements, internal ophthalmoplegia due to involvement of the medial longitudinal fasciculus, and nystagmus are com-

TABLE 3–4

Symptoms and Signs of Optic Neuritis

Symptoms	Signs
1. Blurring of vision	1. Reduction of visual acuity
2. Impairment of color vision	2. Central, paracentral, or cecocentral scotoma
3. Pain behind the eye aggravated by eye movement	3. A sluggish pupillary reaction to light
4. Frontal headache	4. Papilledema and retinal phlebitis
5. Progression to dimness of vision and, in some cases, blindness	5. Computed tomography of the orbits may show demyelination of optic nerves[34a]
	6. Eventual appearance of temporal pallor or optic atrophy

mon in this disease. Sensory changes over the face, including numbness, hypalgesia, pain, or trigeminal neuralgia, may occur, most likely owing to plaques involving the spinal tract of the trigeminal nerve or situated at the entrance of the nerve fibers into the pons.

The reported incidence of trigeminal neuralgia in multiple sclerosis varies, but it probably occurs in 1 to 2 per cent of cases. Involvement of the intrapontine portion of the facial nerve may produce facial palsy, facial hemispasm, or loss of taste over the anterior two thirds of the tongue. Pontine demyelination may also interrupt vestibular connections with resultant nystagmus, vertigo, and vomiting. Deafness is uncommon unless there is widespread bilateral demyelination in the pons. Such demyelination also produces marked bulbar signs of dysarthria and dysphagia and occasionally pathologic laughing and crying characteristic of pseudobulbar palsy. Dysarthria is frequently "cerebellar" or "scanning" in type owing to involvement of cerebellar connections in the brainstem and incoordination of the articulatory mechanisms. Other signs of cerebellar involvement include titubation of the head, nystagmus, slowing of rapid alternating movements, dysmetria, truncal ataxia, and ataxia of gait. Bulbar involvement also affects the corticospinal tracts with varying degrees of spastic quadriparesis, increased deep tendon reflexes, and extensor plantar responses.

Spinal Cord Involvement.   Some patients with multiple sclerosis have what appears to be predominantly spinal cord involvement. Impairment of the corticospinal tracts produces spastic paraparesis, which is frequently associated with marked adductor spasm, clonus, and extensor plantar responses. Sensory involvement may occur with plaques in either posterior or lateral white funiculi or, as frequently happens, with involvement of both areas. A plaque in the posterior columns results in an ataxia of gait with a positive Romberg test. The ataxia is often compounded by cerebellar dysfunction.

Involvement of the lateral spinothalamic tracts produces a loss of pain and thermal sensation, and it is often possible to demonstrate a level of sensory loss on clinical examination. There may be unpleasant dysesthesias in the areas of sensory loss and a band of hyperalgesia at the upper border. The impairment of the descending inhibitory fibers to the sacral "bladder center" causes urgency and incontinence of urine. The anal sphincter is fortunately spared in the majority of patients, but if it is involved, this results in fecal incontinence.

If the spinal cord is involved in multiple sclerosis, the lower limbs nearly always show a greater degree of involvement than the upper limbs. Many patients are confined to wheelchairs but manage to maintain a degree of independence because of the ability to use the hands and upper limbs.

Diagnostic Procedures

1. *Cerebrospinal Fluid.*   There may be some increase in mononuclear cells in the fresh specimens of cerebrospinal fluid and an increase in total protein content (rarely more than 100 mg/dl) in some cases of multiple sclerosis. Gamma globulin levels expressed as a percentage of total protein content are abnormal in about 66 per cent of cases.

   Cerebrospinal fluid IgG is also abnormal in about two thirds of multiple sclerosis patients,[75] particularly in the acute phase of the disease,[102] but this is not a specific finding since similar changes occur in neurosyphilis, acute meningitis, and encephalitis.[92]

   Approximately 90 per cent of patients with multiple sclerosis show the presence of oligoclonal IgG bands when concentrated cerebrospinal fluid is subjected to agarose electrophoresis.[138] The pattern is unique for each patient and apparently is stable over a long period of time. Cerebrospinal fluid amino acids are abnormal in some cases during the active phase of the disease, and the CSF protein serine residue is highly correlated with CSF IgG.[140]

2. Positive C-reactive protein tests and elevated levels of C-3 proactivator ovosomucoid and serum IgM levels have been reported by study of serum proteins during the active phase of multiple sclerosis.[58]

3. There appears to be an increased capacity of lymphocytes from patients with multiple sclerosis to adhere to measles-infected human epithelial cells. This finding may form the basis for the development of an accurate blood test for multiple sclerosis.

4. *Neuropsychologic Testing.*   Neuropsychologic studies of patients with multiple sclerosis have consistently revealed deficits with primary motor functions and motor problem-solving activities.[76] There does not seem to be impairment of the use of stored verbal material, but

the processing and storage of new material are disrupted.[19] Assessment of cognitive deficits has had inconsistent results, which may be related to the variability of the tests employed, the extent and location of the lesions in the brain, and the performance of testing during periods of exacerbation or remission. However, impairment of cognitive and adaptive abilities does occur in multiple sclerosis to some degree.[152]

Neuropsychologic testing is particularly useful in assessing the rehabilitative potential in many patients. Changes observed on serial tests over several years may indicate that the disease continues to be active even though there is little apparent change in the neurologic examination. The psychologist may occasionally detect a significant depression rather than signs of exacerbation in some cases who have a sudden deterioration of function.

5. Nystagmus may be induced or enhanced by raising body temperature in clinically suspected cases of multiple sclerosis.[91]

6. Pattern reversal, visual evoked responses,[34, 63, 67, 82, 169a, 190] auditory evoked potentials,[41, 155, 156] and somatosensory evoked potentials[170a] are abnormal in a high percentage of cases of multiple sclerosis.

7. *Computed Tomography.* Areas of periventricular contrast enhancement may be seen if scanning is performed during the acute phase of the disease or during an acute exacerbation.[3, 43] These areas are seen more easily in 3-mm or 8-mm sections than in 13-mm sections. The contrast enhancement is believed to represent foci of active demyelination with extravasation of iodine contrast material through a defective blood-brain barrier.[4] Areas of decreased density are occasionally seen in the periventricular regions in nonenhanced scans in chronic multiple sclerosis and probably represent areas of sclerosis[79] (Fig. 3–4). Many patients with chronic multiple sclerosis have diffuse ventricular dilatation and evidence of cortical atrophy.

8. A number of techniques including visual

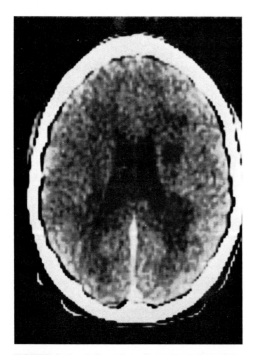 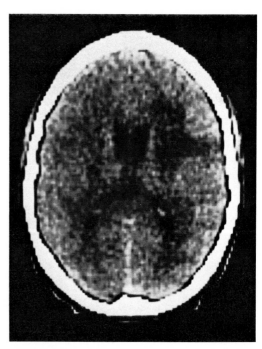

FIGURE 3–4.   Adjacent sections on computed tomography in chronic multiple sclerosis. There is marked decreased density in the central white matter, particularly in the periventricular regions. The slight degree of contrast enhancement in the periventricular area may represent active demyelination. The ventricular system is symmetrically dilated, indicating chronicity in this case, but there is no cortical atrophy.

Electrode Locations

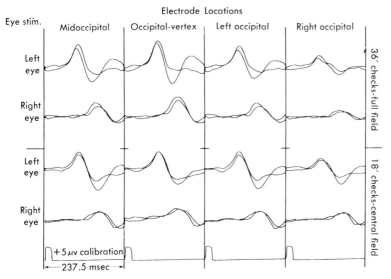

FIGURE 3–5. Pattern reversal visual evoked potentials in a case of multiple sclerosis with right optic nerve involvement. There is increased latency of response on the right side with reduced amplitude, in contrast to the normal response on the left side.

evoked responses, auditory evoked potentials, somatosensory evoked potentials, measurement of subclinical eye movement disorders,[113, 171] and computed tomography have a complementary role in the diagnosis of multiple sclerosis[112] (Figs. 3–5 and 3–6).

Treatment of Multiple Sclerosis

Adequate Rest. A patient suffering from an acute attack or exacerbation of multiple sclerosis should be treated with bed rest or limited activity until there are signs of improvement. This usually

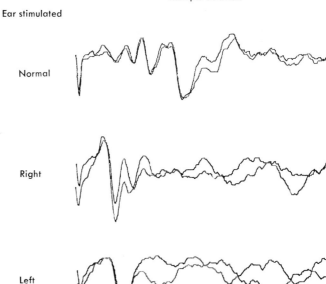

FIGURE 3–6. Auditory evoked brainstem potentials in a case of multiple sclerosis. There is increased latency in the early waves and absence of waves 4 and 5 on the right side. There are no identifiable waves after wave 1 on the left side.

means two or three weeks of rest until there is an amelioration of symptoms without the appearance of new signs. Patients may continue to deteriorate if they are placed in an active program of physical therapy in the early stages of a severe attack. In patients with ataxia and disturbances of gait, prolonged bed rest should be avoided.

Steroid Therapy. Both adrenocorticotropin (ACTH) and corticosteroids have been recommended in the treatment of acute multiple sclerosis or during exacerbations.[48, 121] This is based on the findings of a number of studies which have indicated that steroid therapy is beneficial, particularly in the remission of corticospinal, cerebellar, and bladder symptoms.[123, 180] The use of ACTH is limited because of side effects, including hypertension, edema, peptic ulceration, gastrointestinal bleeding, masked infection, osteoporosis, and electrolyte disturbances. The problem of side effects can be avoided or minimized by the use of oral glucocorticoids given in relatively large doses once every 48 hours. There is some clinical evidence that the anti-inflammatory effect of steroids given in this fashion may last longer than the metabolic effect. This program permits the patient's adrenal glands to recover from temporary suppression toward the end of the 48-hour period. When recovery occurs, side effects of steroid therapy are minimal and, if necessary, long periods of therapy are possible. The recommended dosage is 128 mg or 1.5 to 2.0 mg/kg of methyl prednisolone (or a comparable dose of other oral corticosteroids) given in a single dose once every 48 hours (q.o.d.). The dose may be reduced gradually by 8 to 16 mg every one or two weeks as improvement occurs.

There is no evidence that long-term steroid therapy reduces the risk of relapse in multiple sclerosis, and there is an increased risk of pulmonary infections during administration of corticosteroids.[169] Consequently, steroid therapy should be discontinued when the clinical condition is stable.

Increasing experience with oral steroid therapy given as a single dose once every 48 hours has shown that there is a lack of serious side effects from this form of therapy. Nevertheless, any patient who requires emergency surgery or anesthesia for any cause for one year after steroid therapy has been discontinued should probably be given steroids during the period of stress.

Intrathecal steroids should not be used in the treatment of multiple sclerosis since there is no evidence of added benefit from this form of therapy. There is also a risk of sclerosing pachymeningitis following intrathecal steroid therapy.[23, 125]

Immunosuppressive Therapy. On the hypothesis that multiple sclerosis is an autoimmune disease and that suppression of the immune process might arrest demyelination, therapeutic trials with immunosuppressive drugs have been carried out. Experience to date indicates that this form of therapy may be effective in multiple sclerosis,[78] but it is obviously difficult to administer and control. However, a combination of immunosuppressive and steroid therapy may be considered in rapidly progressive cases with severe and frequent exacerbations. If immunosuppressive therapy is instituted, complete blood counts should be repeated at intervals of approximately three weeks to ensure that suppression of the bone marrow does not result.

Dietary Therapy. On the basis that serum linoleate levels are reduced together with reports that there is relative depletion of linoleate in brain lipids, platelets, and erythrocytes in multiple sclerosis, dietary linoleate supplementation or a high polyunsaturated fat diet has been recommended as part of the treatment. In one double-blind controlled trial of patients with multiple sclerosis, those receiving vegetable oil supplement containing linoleate did better than those receiving oleate. Relapses were less frequent and significantly less severe and of shorter duration in the linoleate-supplemented group.[122] The daily linoleate supplement was 30 ml of sunflower oil emulsion containing 8.6 gm of linoleic acid.

Other Forms of Therapy. Treatment with antilymphocytic globulin has had equivocal results, and there is a high incidence of allergic reactions with this preparation.[109, 153] The use of transfer factor in multiple sclerosis has not produced any significant improvement.[21]

Treatment of Associated Conditions

Treatment of Infections. If the patient develops an acute attack of multiple sclerosis or a clinical relapse following an infection, every effort should be made to treat and eradicate the infection as soon as possible.

Consideration of Emotional and Psychologic Factors. The development of obviously disabling symptoms in a young patient frequently leads to overt anxiety and depression. The average patient is usually intelligent enough to guess or overhear the diagnosis if the treating physician attempts to withhold it.

In order to allay anxiety, prevent depression, and maintain the patient's confidence, a frank but tactful approach is advised.

The pathologic changes of demyelination can be explained in simple terms and the prognosis discussed in an optimistic vein. At the same time, the patient should be made aware of the necessity for continuing medical observation and treatment.

The question of marital advice requires tactful understanding on the part of the physician. In the case of the benign form of multiple sclerosis with good recovery, a reasonably optimistic approach is justifiable. However, in patients in whom there are already severe residual symptoms, a more cautious prognosis must be given without imparting a completely gloomy outlook for the future and destroying morale. Advice on the effects of pregnancy should point out that there is an increased risk of relapse in the puerperal period. In view of this, pregnancy should be postponed for a period of several years. During this time, the risk of relapse will be less in those with the benign forms of multiple sclerosis, while those with the more severe types may well have had an extended remission, and the situation should then be assessed once more.

Physical Therapy. As soon as there are signs of improvement after an acute attack or relapse, the patient should be placed on a graded program of physical therapy when motor symptoms are present. This is usually begun in the hospital and should be continued after discharge either on an outpatient basis or at home after the patient and the relatives are instructed concerning how the exercises should be performed. Patients with cerebellar ataxia should be ambulated early, and gait training with a walker is important.

For patients with chronic spastic paraplegia, admission to the hospital for therapy may help to maintain mobility. Many patients deteriorate slowly and fail to recognize this fact. Periodic physical therapy as an inpatient can prevent such deterioration.

Relief of Spasticity. The results of medical treatment for spasticity are equivocal. The most valuable drugs at this time appear to be diazepam

and baclofen.[105, 160] These two drugs may be tried as combined therapy in some patients. If clonus and muscle spasms in the lower limbs are troublesome, quinidine, 100 mg twice or three times daily, may help. Drugs marketed as relieving "muscle spasm" are for the most part quite ineffective in treating the paraparesis of multiple sclerosis. Diazepam should be given in doses of 5 mg at night with gradual increments of 5 to 25 mg every eight hours. Baclofen can be given in doses of 10 mg every six hours increasing to 100 mg daily if necessary.

In patients with severe adductor spasm, or flexion of the lower limbs, surgical procedures such as obturator tenotomy or obturator neurectomy may be employed. The insertion of a dorsal column stimulator is effective in reducing hypertonia in the lower limbs and improving bladder function in some cases.[1]

Care of the Bladder. Urgency of micturition and occasional incontinence can be reduced by the use of atropine, belladonna compounds, or probanthine orally. In the less frequent situation of acute retention of urine, temporary catheterization followed by oral bethanechol chloride (Urecholine) is often effective.

When sphincter control is paralyzed, a clip urinal and bag may be worn by the male. This situation requires the use of a bladder catheter in the female with the added risk of infection. The advice of a consulting urologist may be valuable in such cases. Studies should include complete evaluation of bladder function with tests of bladder sensation, cystometrogram, intravenous pyelogram, cystogram, and measurement of residual urine after attempts at voiding.

When the bladder control is totally lost, consideration should be given to the performance of an ileal loop procedure. The ileal conduit reduces the risk of bladder and kidney infections, which are so debilitating in multiple sclerosis, and the procedure is usually well accepted by patients who are no longer encumbered by urethral catheters.

Care of the Bowels. Regular use of enemas or morning suppositories may be useful in patients suffering from incontinence of feces. This trains and stimulates evacuation of the bowel at a convenient and predictable time. Patients with paraparesis and poor abdominal muscles are prone to develop fecal impaction, particularly in hot weather, or when they are dehydrated from other causes. This may be presaged by frequent passage of a small volume of liquid stool and incontinence. The condition should be treated by digital removal, enemas, and mild laxatives.

Prevention of Decubiti. Paraplegic or quadriparetic patients may develop decubiti over the sacrum, buttocks, heels, and elbows if confined to bed for any length of time. This can always be prevented by good nursing care including rotation from side to side every two or three hours, diligent changing of bed linen, and skin care in the case of the incontinent patient.

Relief of Intention Tremor. Carefully selected patients with incapacitating intention tremor may benefit from thalamotomy. This is rarely helpful except when intention tremor is the dominant disability,[47] corticospinal tract involvement is minimal, and medical therapy with drugs such as propranolol and diazepam has proved ineffective.

Clinical Variants and Prognostic Implications

The Benign Form

This occurs in about 30 per cent of cases and is characterized by (1) initial symptoms of optic neuritis, brainstem involvement, or dorsal column involvement, (2) minimal involvement of the corticospinal tracts and cerebellar connections, (3) a good recovery from the initial attack, (4) infrequent relapses, and (5) onset after age 20 years and before age 40 years.[115]

The prognosis for life is good in this group, and it includes the bulk of patients who show evidence of minor disability ten years or more after the onset of the disease. In general, the earlier the age of onset before 20 and the more severe the initial attack, the worse the prognosis, and vice versa. The exception to the latter rule is a rare group with onset of symptoms after age 40 years, who will be discussed separately.

The Chronic Relapsing Form

This affects the majority (60 per cent) of patients with multiple sclerosis. Patients in this group show classic relapses and remissions characteristic of the disease with increasing evidence of damage to the nervous system following each relapse. The longer the time interval between relapses, the better the prognosis. The relapse rate varies enormously.

Those more severely afflicted show frequent and severe relapses culminating in severe disabil-ity and early death. The opposite also appears to be true. Some cases may not relapse for 12 years or longer. The overall picture in this group is that at least 25 per cent of patients have one relapse within a year of onset and 50 per cent have relapsed within a three-year period. The prognosis for this group seems to depend on the frequency of relapses. Figures from older case series in which the patient was essentially without treatment indicate that once a relapse has occurred, some 50 per cent of patients were dead within ten years while the remaining 50 per cent were disabled. This does not mean that the mortality rate is 50 per cent in the chronic relapsing form. Many years may elapse between the initial episode and the first relapse. Furthermore, early diagnosis and the advent of newer medications, such as antibiotics and steroids, and rehabilitation programs will hopefully reduce both morbidity and mortality. Death is usually from intercurrent pulmonary and urinary tract infection.

The Chronic Progressive Form

Some 10 per cent of patients with multiple sclerosis show a chronic, progressive disability without obvious relapse and remission. This form tends to occur in older patients after the age of 40 years. Fortunately, this type is the rarest, since the overall prognosis is particularly bad. After signs of progression appear, the prognosis for the chronic progressive form is the same as that for the chronic relapsing form. The mortality is 50 per cent within ten years of onset, and the disability is usually severe.

The division of cases of multiple sclerosis into three forms is by no means a rigid classification. Patients who appear to have a benign form of the disease may develop symptoms of a severe relapse and chronic progression at any time. However, the overall outlook is better for this group.

In all three groups, age definitely affects the prognosis. Patients who develop the first symptoms before the age of 20 or in their late thirties and forties have a poorer prognosis. The prognosis is also slightly worse for males than for females. The average duration of life appears to be about 25 years from the first symptoms, and life expectancy is reduced by approximately 9.5 years for the male patient and 14.5 years for the female.

Devic's Disease (Neuromyelitis Optica)

The development of optic neuritis associated with signs and symptoms of myelitis has been described as a distinct clinical entity in the past under the eponym Devic's disease. It now seems that the condition can occur as a manifestation of two well-recognized demyelinating diseases, postinfectious leukoencephalitis and multiple sclerosis. The majority of cases occurring before the age of ten years are probably due to postinfectious leukoencephalitis. These patients sometimes show a polymorphonuclear pleocytosis and a cerebrospinal fluid protein content of more than 100 mg per cent. They usually do not experience the remissions and relapses of multiple sclerosis.

About 50 per cent of patients have cerebrospinal fluid changes similar to those found in multiple sclerosis, and the initial attack is followed by the development of further signs of multiple sclerosis.

Pathology

Two types of abnormality have been described in the central nervous system in addition to the demyelination in the optic nerves and spinal cord. Changes similar to those seen in postinfectious leukoencephalitis may be seen in some patients. Others show plaque formation in many areas of the central nervous system identical to that seen in multiple sclerosis.

Clinical Features

A history of an upper respiratory tract infection may be obtained varying from a few days to two weeks before the onset of failing vision. The visual loss is generally rapid and severe with the development of a large central scotoma and progressing, in rare instances, to complete blindness. Symptoms of myelitis begin hours, weeks, or occasionally two or three months later. The initial symptom consists of pain in the back or neck, radiating in girdle fashion into the arms or around the chest. This is followed by paresthesias in the lower extremities and abdomen, progressive weakness of the lower limbs, and retention of urine. Deep tendon reflexes are depressed initially, but there is a bilateral extensor plantar response. Sensory loss usually extends upward to the midthoracic area with a zone of hyperesthesia separating the areas of hypalgesia and normal sensation.

The course may be progressive with ascending paralysis, respiratory failure, and death. Other patients show partial or complete recovery, then develop typical remissions and relapses indistinguishable from multiple sclerosis. A number recover completely, and some show a partial recovery but do not relapse.

Treatment

The treatment of neuromyelitis optica is the same as that outlined under multiple sclerosis. Steroid therapy is particularly effective in those who are believed to have postinfectious leukoencephalitis.

Schilder's Disease (Encephalitis Paraxialis Diffusa)

The term "Schilder's disease" has been applied to a diffuse demyelinating disease resembling multiple sclerosis, to a leukodystrophy, and to subacute sclerosing leukoencephalitis in the past. There seems to be little purpose in retaining this eponym, and its use should be discontinued since it only adds to further confusion in the medical literature.

Postinfectious and Postvaccinal Encephalomyelitis (Acute Disseminated Encephalomyelitis)

Acute neurologic illness following a virus infection such as measles, smallpox, chickenpox, or influenza occasionally occurs, and the complication may result in serious damage to the central nervous system. A similar condition may occur as a complication of rabies vaccination if the older Pasteur preparations that contain myelin as well as the killed rabies virus are used. The complication is rare following smallpox vaccination.

Etiology and Pathology

There is a similarity between postinfectious and postvaccinal encephalomyelitis and experimental allergic encephalomyelitis with the development of humoral and cell-mediated responses to myelin basic protein in these conditions.[137] The consistent elevation of gamma globulin in the cerebrospinal fluid is also suggestive of antibody production within the central nervous system.

The lesions consist of scattered areas of perivenous demyelination in the brain, brainstem, cerebellum, and spinal cord. The demyelination is particularly prominent in the periventricular white matter, optic nerves, and temporal lobes. The myelin loss is intense with minimal damage to axons in the same areas. The blood vessels show a marked perivascular cuffing with lymphocytes and plasma cells.

Clinical Features

Two clinical types can be recognized in this disease, a cerebral form and a spinal form. The cerebral form begins between 4 and 14 days after the precipitating illness with an acute onset of headache, vomiting, drowsiness, and confusion. Mental symptoms are prominent and include hallucinations, delusions, and dysphasia. Visual acuity will be impaired if there is optic neuritis, and blindness sometimes results in a relatively short period of time. Lesions in the cerebral hemisphere or brainstem produce various degrees of paralysis with hemiplegia or quadriparesis, and paralysis of cranial nerves may also occur. Seizures or narcolepsy may also complicate the course in some cases.

The spinal form also begins acutely with rapid development of flaccid paraparesis, sensory loss, usually below midthoracic levels, and bladder paralysis.[42] Both cerebral and spinal forms terminate fatally in about 20 per cent of cases, while survivors usually begin recovering at about the tenth day. Many make a complete recovery, but those with the cerebral type may show some impairment of intellectual function, antisocial behavior, and emotional outbursts. Variable permanent sequelae may also affect motor function in both the cerebral and spinal types. A few cases have been described in which there are subsequent relapses with the development of a clinical and pathologic picture indistinguishable from the chronic relapsing form of multiple sclerosis.

Diagnostic Procedures

The cerebrospinal fluid often shows a moderate pleocytosis with mononuclear cells that occasionally exceed 100 per cubic millimeter. The protein content may be elevated to about 100 mg per cent, with increased gamma globulin and IgG levels.

Electroencephalography indicates nonspecific slowing and occasional focal seizure activity, but there is no specific pattern in this condition.

Treatment

Patients should be treated as outlined under multiple sclerosis. There is usually prompt and gratifying response to steroids, which should be given in large doses once every 48 hours until the acute phase has resolved. Patients with residual neurologic deficits require physical therapy, reeducation, and retraining. Since relapses are rare, the question of further disability need not be considered. This condition should be differentiated from subacute sclerosing panencephalitis.

Acute Hemorrhagic Leukoencephalitis

The pathologic changes in this fulminating condition are analogous to the pathologic features of hyperacute experimental allergic encephalitis.[20, 22]

Etiology and Pathology

Acute hemorrhagic leukoencephalitis appears to be a fulminating allergic response to a virus infection. The brain may be edematous, and there are scattered areas of perivenous or perivascular ball-like hemorrhages throughout the white matter of the central nervous system. On microscopic examination, there are prominent fresh, perivenous hemorrhages with necrosis of myelin and less intense but variable destruction of axons. The blood vessels show a fibrinoid necrosis, and there is a marked perivascular cuffing of polymorphonuclear leukocytes.

Clinical Features

The onset is acute, occurring about ten days after an upper respiratory infection, with nuchal rigidity, severe headache, and confusion, rapidly progressing to stupor and coma. Seizures of both focal and generalized types are not unusual, while focal signs of hemiplegia and temporal lobe seizures may suggest a focal structural lesion beginning in one hemisphere or one region of the brain. There is rapid increase in intracranial pressure and early papilledema.

Diagnostic Procedures

1. The cerebrospinal fluid frequently shows cloudiness and xanthochromia as well as a pleocytosis and an admixture of erythrocytes and polymorphonuclear and mononuclear cells, which may be present in the thousands. The protein content is usually elevated above 100 mg per cent. Increased intracranial pressure and papilledema are not uncommon.
2. The EEG is always abnormal and shows a loss of the basic rhythm with the appearance of high-voltage diffuse delta activity maximally in one of the temporal areas. Persistent high-voltage focal sharp waves or sharp slow-wave complexes, often resistant to intravenous diazepam (Valium), are often seen over the maximally affected lobe. If the patient survives, the abnormality tends to clear, but there is some residual focal slow activity with intermixed sharp waves in the area of maximal involve-

ment, with the return to near-normal activity in the less affected areas of the brain.

3. Computed tomography may show diffuse edema involving both hemispheres. The areas of decreased density due to edema may be asymmetric with a shift of the midline structures to one side giving a spurious impression of a focal mass lesion.

Treatment

A number of patients have received craniotomy and decompression sometimes in order to exclude a brain abscess or intracerebral hemorrhage in one hemisphere.

In suspected cases or cases proved by brain biopsy, steroid therapy should be instituted at once. This requires high doses of corticosteroids and reduction of intracranial pressure with intravenous mannitol or glycerol, which can be titrated using continuous intracranial pressure monitoring.

Degenerative Demyelinating Diseases

Certain diseases that are included under the heading "degenerative demyelinating diseases" have been recognized by neuropathologists only in relatively recent times. They are still of major interest to the pathologist and are rarely, although occasionally, diagnosed during life. The first two conditions have a common etiologic factor in that they occur in association with a systemic disease. Subacute necrotizing encephalomyelopathy is included in this section since it has features of a degenerative process.

Central Pontine Myelinolysis

Although rare, this condition has been studied in considerable detail by neuropathologists. A more general awareness of its existence may lead to clinical recognition in the future.

Etiology

The original cases were described in patients suffering from chronic alcoholism and nutritional deficiencies. However, it would appear that no factor is responsible for central pontine myelinolysis,[88] which has been reported in other conditions. These conditions include malnutrition, cerebral ischemia, cerebral edema, impaired fat metabolism, infection, liver dysfunction, inappropriate secretion of antidiuretic hormone, and electrolyte abnormalities. The majority of reported cases have shown severe hyponatremia.[32, 179]

Pathology

There is a sharply marked area of demyelination in the central portion of the basis pontis, extending on both sides of the median raphe. Microscopic examination shows a severe myelin loss with relative preservation of axons with many lipid-containing macroglial cells and astrocytic proliferation. There is some neuronal degeneration in the center with central chromatolysis of nerve cells immediately around the periphery of the lesion.

Extension of the demyelinating process into the medulla (medullary myelinolysis) has been reported.[25]

Clinical Features

So far, the condition has rarely been diagnosed during life. However, the development of cranial nerve abnormalities such as diplopia, ptosis, defective conjugate eye movements, facial weakness, dysarthria, and dysphagia in a dehydrated patient, particularly an alcoholic, should arouse suspicion of central pontine myelinolysis. Brainstem auditory evoked potentials are abnormal and have been reported to vary with the severity of the condition.[172]

Central Demyelination of the Corpus Callosum (Marchiafava-Bignami Disease)

This is another rare condition in which there is a focal demyelination within the central nervous system. A common etiologic factor shared with central pontine myelinolysis is a possibility.

Etiology and Pathology

The disease was first recognized in Italians who drank red wine, but there have been subsequent descriptions in non-Italian, non-wine-drinking alcoholics. The common factor indicates chronic alcoholism and nutritional deficiency.

The brain appears to be normal externally, but there is a central symmetric myelinolysis involving the corpus callosum. Other areas are apparently normal. Microscopic examination shows an intense demyelination in the central corpus callosum. Some axons are preserved even in the central areas, which may have a necrotic appearance. The demyelination is strictly limited to the central part of the corpus callosum.[90]

Clinical Features

The diagnosis has usually been established at autopsy, but retrospective studies have shown that the onset is frequently acute with a sudden lapse into stupor or coma. On recovery, there are marked dysphasia and dyspraxia. The condition progresses to generalized rigidity with hyperactive reflexes and extensor plantar responses. There are bilateral grasp reflexes and incontinence of urine. Seizures may occur in the course of the disease.

Signs of interhemispheric disconnection can be demonstrated in some patients who show left-handed dyspraxia, anomia, agraphia, inability to report stimuli or name pictures flashed in the left visual field, and failure to appreciate words in the left ear using dichotic listening tests.[103, 107]

Diagnostic Procedures

There are no reports of abnormalities in the cerebrospinal fluid, and electroencephalographic studies have shown nonspecific slowing without any characteristic changes.

Treatment

Treatment of this condition, which usually has a fatal termination in a period varying from days to several months, should be directed toward adequate hydration, vitamin therapy, and abstention from alcohol.

Subacute Necrotizing Encephalopathy

This condition, also known as Leigh's syndrome,[101] appears to be invariably fatal and occurs either in early childhood or in early adolescence.[154]

Etiology and Pathology

Many biochemical defects have been reported in this disease which appear to be associated with an abnormality in the Krebs tricarboxylic acid cycle. The identification of a substance in the urine that interferes with the formation of thiamine triphosphate and the finding of low thiamine triphosphate levels in the brain supports the hypothesis that thiamine triphosphate deficiency is related to subacute necrotizing encephalopathy.[137] Neuropathologic changes consist of a symmetric vacuolation of the white matter of both hemispheres, and electron microscopy shows marked axonal swelling in the region of the vacuoles.[36]

Clinical Features

The familial occurrence has been reported in some cases.

Two distinct groups have been identified. The first group consists of children who develop symptoms in early childhood and in whom the disease is fatal within a few years. In the second group, the patients are between 10 and 15 years of age and the disease tends to run a more chronic course.

The symptoms are of progressive motor weakness with signs of corticospinal tract involvement, ataxia, paresis of extraocular movements progressing to complete ophthalmoplegia, and disturbances of consciousness. The clinical picture may resemble a progressive brainstem tumor, but computed tomography shows marked wasting of the brainstem (Fig. 3–7). Death is usually due to respiratory failure.

Treatment

Treatment with thiamine (1.5 gm/day) and thiamine propyl disulfide (300 mg/day) has been

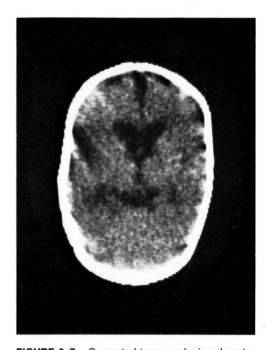

FIGURE 3–7. Computed tomography in subacute necrotizing encephalomyelopathy (Leigh). There is marked ventricular dilatation with diffuse cortical atrophy. The brainstem is atrophic, and there is dilatation of the fourth ventricle, quadrigeminal cistern, and ambiens cisterns.

associated with marked improvement[136] although CSF levels of thiamine cannot always be maintained above 50 μg/100 ml CSF. Remissions and exacerbations correlated well with the CSF levels of thiamine; the higher the levels, the greater the remission and vice versa.

Viral Demyelinating Diseases

Subacute sclerosing panencephalitis (SSPE) has all the features of a viral disease, including intranuclear inclusion bodies (see Chap. 7). Evidence that the disease is due to measles virus is strong.[77] Other viral encephalitides, including herpes virus, may be associated with demyelination.[84, 177]

In New Zealand, an outbreak of subacute sclerosing panencephalitis was related to a mass vaccination of schoolchildren with Salk vaccine. The vaccine used probably contained live SV40 virus. Killed measles virus was another possible contaminant.[15]

The possibility that multiple sclerosis is a "slow virus" disease has also been discussed.

Progressive Multifocal Leukoencephalopathy

Progressive multifocal leukoencephalopathy is a progressive papovavirus infection of the central nervous system that usually occurs in the immunologically suppressed individual. The increasing use of chemotherapy in the treatment of leukemia and cancer and the need for chronic immunosuppressive therapy after organ transplantation enhance the risk of progressive multifocal leukoencephalopathy, which may be seen with increasing frequency in neurologic practice in the future.[116]

Etiology and Pathology

Progressive multifocal leukoencephalopathy has been reported most frequently in immunosuppressed patients with impaired cell-mediated immunity[114] such as occurs in chronic leukemia, Hodgkin's disease, or the lymphomas.[35] It may also occur in association with other neoplastic conditions such as pulmonary and other carcinomas and multiple myelomatosis. Cases of a similar or related condition have also been reported to be associated with sarcoidosis, systemic lupus erythematosus, polycythemia vera, primary hypersplenism, and Whipple's disease.[110]

The viral etiology of progressive multifocal leukoencephalopathy has been established by the isolation of a papovavirus Ic virus in several cases.[131]

The brain has a normal external appearance, but there are numerous scattered areas of demyelination throughout the cerebral hemispheres, brainstem, cerebellum, and spinal cord. The microscopic appearance consists of severe myelin destruction in the affected area with relative preservation of axons and sudanophilic material in microglial cells.

There is a marked reactive astrocytosis with the presence of many bizarre and hypertrophied astrocytes in the affected area. The oligodendroglial cells are also enlarged and contain intranuclear inclusion bodies.[52] Since oligodendroglia lay down myelin in the central nervous system, their destruction leads to demyelination.

Clinical Features

The disease is manifested as a progressive, asymmetric disorder affecting many systems of the central nervous system. Men are affected about twice as commonly as women. Death usually occurs in 1 to 18 months although survival for years has been reported. Patients present with protean symptoms, some of which resemble multiple sclerosis. The most common symptoms include mental changes, confusion, progressive dementia, and clouding of consciousness. Localized motor weakness with increased reflexes may suggest the presence of a focal mass lesion in the brain. Visual impairment is an early symptom in many cases and may be due to involvement of the optic nerves or the optic radiation. Cerebellar signs are common. Other signs and symptoms include dysphagia, dysarthria, and hemisensory loss. Diplopia and gaze palsies, facial palsy, nystagmus, and dysphagia occur with involvement of the brainstem. Seizures may also occur. The course is progressively downhill.

Diagnostic Procedures

1. The spinal fluid usually shows mononuclear pleocytosis and elevation of protein levels.
2. The EEG is usually diffusely or focally slowed.
3. Computed tomography shows areas of decreased density in the central white matter of the brain with scalloped lateral borders corresponding to the contours of the subcortical gray matter–white matter junction.[38] There is no enhancement of the scan following intravenous injection of contrast material.[44]

Treatment

There is need for further evaluation of treatment for progressive multifocal leukoencephalopathy, although a trial use of steroids is worthwhile. Treatment may be directed toward the control of the primary disease, but it has not been established whether this influences the course of the neurologic condition.

There have been isolated reports of successful treatment of progressive multifocal leukoencephalopathy using cytosine arabinoside.[16] Adenine arabinoside, a potentially more powerful therapeutic agent, does not seem to have any effect in this disease.[188] It is possible that continued neurologic deterioration might be due to the development of simultaneous opportunistic bacterial and fungal infections in the brain in some cases and that these infections may be identified and treated.[110, 114]

Leukoencephalopathy of Childhood Malignancies

There have been a number of reports of leukoencephalopathy following intrathecal, intraventricular, or oral administration of chemotherapeutic agents in children with malignancies. The neurotoxicity of chemotherapeutic agents may be enhanced by concomitant irradiation.

Neuropathologic examination shows multiple areas of demyelination with axonal loss and swelling. There is a reactive astrocytosis and lipid phagocytosis in subcortical and central areas of the white matter.[57]

Clinical Features

There is an acute neurologic deterioration with confusion, somnolence, ataxia, spasticity, seizures, and progressive dementia that coincides with administration of a chemotherapeutic agent. Computed tomography shows irregular zones of decreased density in the central white matter. Serial CT scans show improvement in the abnormal areas when chemotherapy is discontinued.[72]

Cited References

1. Abbate, A. D.; Cook, A. W.; and Atallah, M. Effect of electrical stimulation on the thoracic spinal cord on the function of the bladder in multiple sclerosis. *J. Urol.,* **117:**285–88, 1977.
2. Adams, C. W. M. Pathology of multiple sclerosis. Progression of the lesion. *Br. Med. Bull.,* **33:**15–20, 1977.
3. Aita, J. F.; Bennett, D. R.; et al. Acute multiple sclerosis on cranial computerized tomography. *Neurology* (Minneap.), **27:**387, 1977.
4. Aita, J. F.; Bennett, D. R.; et al. Cranial CT appearance of acute multiple sclerosis. *Neurology* (Minneap.), **28,** 251–58, 1978.
5. Allen, J. C.; Sheremata, W.; et al. Cerebrospinal fluid T and B Lymphocyte kinetics related to exacerbations of multiple sclerosis. *Neurology* (Minneap.), **26:**579–83, 1976.
6. Alter, M., and Harshe, M. Racial predilection in multiple sclerosis. *J. Neurol.,* **210:**1–20, 1975.
7. Alter, M.; Harshe, M.; et al. Genetic association of multiple sclerosis and HL-A determinants. *Neurology* (Minneap.), **26:**31–36, 1976.
8. Alter, M., and Speer, J. Clinical evaluation of possible etiologic factors in multiple sclerosis. *Neurology* (Minneap.). **18:**109–16, 1968.
9. Alter, M.; Yamoor, M.; and Harshe, M. Multiple sclerosis and nutrition. *Arch. Neurol.,* **31:**267–22, 1974.
10. Ammitzbou, T.; Clausen, J.; and Fog, T. Oligoclonal IgG and measles antibody in CSF of multiple sclerosis patients. *Acta Neurol. Scand.,* **56:**153–58, 1977.
11. Argyrakis, A.; Pilz, H.; et al. Ultrastructural findings of peripheral nerve in a preclinical case of adult metachromatic leukodystrophy. *J. Neuropathol. Exp. Neurol.,* **36:**693–711, 1977.
12. Aring, C. D. Observation on multiple sclerosis and conversion hysteria. *Brain.* **88:**663–74, 1965.
13. Austin, J. H. Metachromic form of diffuse cerebral sclerosis. I. Diagnosis during life by urine sediment examination. *Neurology* (Minneap.), **7:**415–26, 1957.
14. Austin, J. H. Metachromic form of diffuse cerebral sclerosis. II. Diagnosis during life by isolation of metachromic lipids from urine. *Neurology* (Minneap.), **7:**716–23, 1957.
15. Austin, J. H.; Armstrong, D.; Fouch, S.; Mitchell, C.; Stumpf. O.; Shearer, L.; and Briner, O. Metachromatic leukodystrophy (MLD). *Arch. Neurol.,* **18:**225–40, 1968.
16. Backman, R., and Wilshaw, E. Progressive multifocal leukoencephalopathy treated with cytosine arabinoside. *Br. J. Haematol.,* **34:**153–55, 1976.
17. Banker, B. Q., Robertson, J. T., and Victor, M. Spongy degeneration of the central nervous system in infancy. *Neurology* (Minneap.), **14:**981–1001, 1964.
18. Bauer, H. J.; terMeulen, V.; et al. Early sterile autopsy in etiologic studies on multiple sclerosis. *Z. Neurol.,* **208:**159–74, 1975.
19. Beatty, P., and Gange, J. Neuropsychological aspects of multiple sclerosis. *J. Nerv. Ment. Dis.,* **164:**42–50, 1977.
20. Behan, P. O.; Kies, M. W.; et al. Immunologic mechanisms in experimental encephalomyelitis in non-human primates. *Arch. Neurol.,* **29:**4–9, 1973.
21. Behan, P. O.; Melville, I. D.; et al. Transfer-factor therapy in multiple sclerosis. *Lancet,* **1:**988–90, 1976.
22. Behan, P. O.; Moore, M. J.; and Lemarche, J. B. Acute necrotizing hemorrhagic encephalopathy. *Postgrad. Med.,* **54:**154–60, 1973.
23. Bernat, J. L.; Sadowsky, C. H.; et al. Sclerosing spinal pachymeningitis. A complication of intrathecal administration of depo-medrol for multiple

sclerosis. *J. Neurol. Neurosurg. Psychiat.,* **39:**1124–28, 1976.

24. Betts. T. A.; Smith, W. T.; and Kelly, R. E. Adult metachromatic leukodystrophy (sulfatide lipidosis) simulating acute schizophrenia: report of a case. *Neurology* (Minneap.), **18:**1140–42, 1968.

25. Bhagavan, B.; Wagner, J. A.; and Juanteguy, J. Central pontine myelinolysis and medullary myelinolysis. *Arch. Pathol. Lab. Med.,* **100:**246–52, 1976.

26. Bodain, M., and Lake, B. D. Rectal approach to neuropathology. *Br. J. Surg.,* **50:**702–14, 1963.

27. Boldt. H. A.; Haerer, A. F.; Tourtellotte, W. W.; Henderson, J. W.; and DeJong, R. N. Retrochiasmal visual field defects in multiple sclerosis. *Arch. Neurol.,* **8:**565–75, 1963.

28. Brady, R. O. Enzymological approaches to the lipidoses. *Ann. Clin. Lab. Sci.* **7:**105–12, 1977.

29. Brady, R. O. Heritable catabolic and anabolic disorders of lipid metabolism. *Metabolism,* **26:**329–45, 1977.

30. Brady, R. O.; Tallman, J. F.; Johnson, W. G.; Gal, A. E.; Leahy, W. R.; Quirk, J. M.; and Dekaban, A. S. Replacement therapy for inherited enzyme deficiency. Use of purified ceramidetrihexosidase in Fabry's disease. *N. Engl. J. Med.,* **289:**9–14, 1973.

31. Brautbar, C.; Latana, E.; et al. Lack of association between HLA-DW2 and multiple sclerosis in Israeli Jewish patients. *N. Engl. J. Med.,* **296:**1537–38, 1977.

32. Bursar, P. J.; Norenberg, M. D.; and Yarnell, P. R. Hyponatremia and central pontine myelinolysis. *Neurology* (Minneap.), **27:**223–26, 1977.

33. Butcher, J. The distribution of multiple sclerosis in relation to the dairy industry and milk consumption. *N. Z. Med. J.,* **83:**427–30, 1976.

34. Bynke, H.; Olsson, J.-E.; and Rosen, I. Diagnostic value of visual evoked responses, clinical eye examination and CSF analysis in chronic myelopathy. *Acta Neurol. Scand.,* **56:**55–69, 1977.

34a. Cala, L. A.; Mastaglia, F. L.; and Black, J. L. Computerized tomography of brain and optic nerves in multiple sclerosis. Observation of 100 patients including serial studies in 16. *J. Neurol. Sci.,* **36:**411–26, 1978.

35. Canning, B.; Kobayaski, C. B.; et al. Progressive multifocal leukoencephalopathy. *West. J. Med.,* **125:**364–69, 1976.

36. Carleton, C. C.; Collins, G. M.; and Schimpff, R. D. Subacute necrotizing encephalopathy (Leigh's disease): Two unusual cases. *South. Med. J.,* **69:**1301–1305, 1976.

37. Carp, R. I.; Merz, G. S.; and Licursi, P.C.: A small virus-like agent found in association with multiple sclerosis. *Neurology* (Minneap.), **26:**(Part 2)70–71, 1976.

38. Carroll, B. A.; Lane, B.; et al. Diagnosis of progressive multifocal leukoencephalopathy by computed tomography. *Radiology,* **122:**137–41, 1977.

39. Caspary, E. A. Comparison of immunological specificity of gamma globulin in the cerebrospinal fluid in normal and multiple sclerosis subjects. *J. Neurol. Neurosurg. Psychiat.,* **28:**61–64, 1965.

40. Celesia, G. G., and Daly, R. F. Visual electroencephalographic computer analysis (VECA). A new electrophysiologic test for the diagnosis of optic nerve lesions. *Neurology* (Minneap.), **27:**637–41, 1977.

41. Chiappa, K. H., and Norwood, A. E. A comparison of the clinical utility of pattern-shift visual evoked responses and brain stem auditory evoked potentials in multiple sclerosis. *Neurology* (Minneap.), **27:**397, 1977.

42. Clark, G.; Hashem, B.; and Rosenber, G. Transverse myelitis following rubeola vaccination. *Neurology* (Minneap.), **27:**360, 1977.

43. Cole, M., and Ross, R. J. Plaque of multiple sclerosis seen in computerized transaxial tomogram. *Neurology* (Minneap.), **27:**890–91, 1977.

44. Conoway, J. P.; Weinstein, M. A.; et al. Computed tomography in progressive multifocal leukoencephalopathy. *Am. J. Roentgenol.,* **27:**663–65, 1976.

45. Cook, S. D., and Dowling, P. C. A possible association between house pets and multiple sclerosis. *Lancet,* **1:**980–82, 1977.

46. Cook, S. D.,; Natelson, B. H.; et al. Further evidence of a possible association between house dogs and multiple sclerosis. *Ann. Neurol.,* **3:**141–43, 1978.

47. Cooper, I. S. Relief of intention tremor of multiple sclerosis by thalamic surgery. *J.A.M.A.,* **199:**689–94, 1967.

48. Cooperative study in the evaluation of therapy in multiple sclerosis, *Neurology* (Minneap.), Supplement 18, June, 1968.

49. Craelius, W., and Newby, N. A. Multiple sclerosis, sunlight and indoor pets. *Lancet,* **2:**565, 1977.

50. Crocker, A. C., and Farber, S. Niemann-Pick disease; review of 18 patients. *Medicine* (Baltimore), **37:**1–95, 1958.

51. Crocker, A. C., and Landing, B. H. Phosphatase studies in Gaucher's disease. *Metabolism,* **9:**341–62, 1960.

52. Cunningham, M. D.; Kishore, P. R. S.; et al. Progressive multifocal leukoencephalopathy. Presenting as focal mass lesion in the brain. *Surg. Neurol.,* **8:**448–50, 1977.

53. Currier, R. D.; Martin, E. A.; and Woolsley, P. C. Prior events in multiple sclerosis. *Neurology* (Minneap.), **24:**748–54, 1974.

54. Dean, G.; McLaughlin, H.; et al. *Br. Med. J.,* **1:**861–64, 1976.

55. Delmotte, P., and Gonsette, R. Biochemical findings in multiple sclerosis. IV. Isoelectric focusing of the CSF gamma globulins in multiple sclerosis (262 cases) and other neurological diseases (272 cases). *J. Neurol. Sci.,* **33:**27–37, 1977.

56. Detels, R.; Visscher, B. R.; et al. Evidence for lower susceptibility of multiple sclerosis in Japanese-Americans. *Am. J. Epidemiol.,* **105:**303–10, 1977.

57. Devivo, D. C.; Malas, D.; et al. Leukoencephalopathy in childhood leukemia. *Neurology* (Minneap.), **27:**609–13, 1977.

58. Dowling, P. C., and Cook, S. D. Disease markers

in acute multiple sclerosis. *Arch. Neurol.,* **33:**668–70, 1976.

59. Duda, E. E., and Hottenlocker, P. R. Computed Tomography in Adrenoleukodystrophy correlation of radiological and histological findings. *Radiology,* **120:**349–50, 1976.

60. Dunn, H. G.; Dolman, C. L; et al. Krabbe's leukodystrophy without globoid cells. *Neurology* (Minneap.), **26:**1035–41, 1976.

61. Durbois, G.; Harzer, K.; and Baumann, N. Very low arylsulphatase A and cerebroside sulphatase activities in leukocytes of healthy members of metachromatic leukodystrophy family. *J. Hum. Genet.,* **29:**191–94, 1977.

62. Eldridge, R.; McFarland, H.; et al. Familial multiple sclerosis: Clinical histocompatibility and viral serological studies. *Ann. Neurol.,* **3:**72–80, 1978.

63. Ellenberger, C., Jr., and Ziegler, S. B. Visual evoked potentials and quantitative perimetry in multiple sclerosis. *Ann. Neurol.,* **1:**561–64, 1977.

64. Esiri, M. M. Immunoglobulin-containing cells in multiple sclerosis plaques. *Lancet,* **2:**478–80, 1977.

65. Eto, Y.; Suzuki, K.; and Suzuki, K. Globoid cell leukodystrophy (Krabbe's disease): Isolation of myelin with normal glycoplipid composition. *J. Lipid Res.,* **11:**473, 1970.

65a. Farrell, D. S.; Sume, S. M.; et al. Antenatal diagnosis of Krabbe's leucodystrophy: enzymatic and morphological confirmation in an affected fetus. *J. Neurol. Neurosurg. Psychiat.,* **41:**76–82, 1978.

66. Feigin, I., and Popoff, N. Regeneration of myelin in multiple sclerosis; role of mesenchymal cells in such regeneration and in myelin formation in the peripheral nervous system. *Neurology* (Minneap.), **16:**364–72, 1966.

67. Fernsod, M.; Abramsky, O.; and Auerbach, E. Electrophysiologic Examinations of visual system in multiple sclerosis. *J. Neurol. Sci.,* **20:**161–75, 1973.

68. Field, E. J.; Green, C. A.; and Miller, N. Response of normal and multiple sclerotic patients to typhoid-paratyphoid vaccine injections. *J. Neurol. Neurosurg. Psychiat.,* **24:**78–79, 1961.

69. Fraser, K. B. Multiple sclerosis: A virus disease. *Br. Med. Bull.,* **33:**34–39, 1977.

70. Friede, R. L. Alexander's disease. *Arch. Neurol.,* **11:**414–22, 1964.

71. Fullerton, P. N. Peripheral nerve conduction in metachromatic leucodystrophy (sulphatide lipidosis). *J. Neurol. Neurosurg. Psychiat.,* **27:**100–5, 1964.

72. Fusner, J. E.; Poplak, D. G.; et al. Leukoencephalopathy following chemotherapy for rhabdomyosarcoma: Reversibility of cerebral changes demonstrated by computed tomography. *J. Pediatr.,* **91:**77–79, 1977.

73. Gal, A. E.; Brady, R. O.; et al. A practical chromogenic procedure for the diagnosis of Krabbe's disease. *Clin. Chem. Acta,* **77:**53–59, 1977.

74. Gerstl, B.; Malamud, N.; Hayman, R. B.; and Bond, P. R. Morphological and neurochemical study of Pelizaeus-Merzbacher disease. *J. Neurol. Neurosurg. Psychiat.,* **28:**540–47, 1965.

75. Glasier, H. Y globulins and cerebrospinal fluid

during various phases of multiple sclerosis. *J. Neurol.,* **206:**327–32, 1974.

76. Goldstein, G., and Shelly, C. Neuropsychological diagnosis of multiple sclerosis in a neuropsychiatric setting. *J. Nerv. Ment. Dis.,* **158:**280–90, 1974.

77. Gonatas, N. K. Subacute sclerosing leucoencephalitis: electron microscopic and cytochemical observations on a cerebral biopsy. *J. Neuropath. Exp. Neurol.* **25:**177–201, 1966.

78. Gonsette, R. E.; Demonty, L.; and Delmotte, P. Intensive immunosuppression with cyclophosphamide in multiple sclerosis. *J. Neurol.,* **214:**173–81, 1977.

79. Gyldensted, C. Computer tomography of the brain in multiple sclerosis: A radiological study of 110 patients with special reference to demonstration of cerebral plaques. *Acta Neurol. Scand.,* **53:**386–89, 1976.

80. Haerer, A. F.; Tourtellotte, W. W.; Richard, K. A.; Gustafson, G. M.; and Bryan, E. R. Study of the blood-cerebrospinal fluid-brain barrier in multiple sclerosis. I. Blood-cerebrospinal fluid barrier to sodium bromide. *Neurology* (Minneap.), **14:**345–54, 1964.

81. Haire, M.; Fraser, K. B.; and Millar, J. H. D. Measles and other virus-specific immunoglobulins in multiple sclerosis. *Br. Med. J.,* **3:**612–15, 1973.

82. Hannerisi, M.; Wenzel, D.; and Freund, H.-J. The comparison of small-size rectangle and checkerboard stimulation for the evaluation of delayed visual evoked responses in patients suspected of multiple sclerosis. *Brain,* **100:**119–36, 1977.

83. Heipertz, R.; Klauke, W.; et al. Serum fatty acids in multiple sclerosis. *J. Neurol.,* **214:**153–57, 1977.

84. Herpes simplex encephalitis. *J.A.M.A.,* **195:**1144, 1966.

85. Herrlien, K. M., and Hillborg, P. O. Neurological signs in juvenile form of Gaucher's disease. *Acta Paediatr.* (Stockholm), **51:**137–54, 1962.

86. Hussey, H. H. Multiple sclerosis: Exploration of cause. *J.A.M.A.,* **235:**2630, 1976.

87. Hutchinson, W. M. Acute optic neuritis and prognosis for multiple sclerosis. *J. Neurol. Neurosurg. Psychiat.,* **39:**283–89, 1976.

88. Iannocone, P. M.; Wright, A. W.; and Cornwall, C. C. Central Pontine Myelinolysis. *N.Y. State J. Med.,* **76:**421–24, 1976.

89. Ibrahim, M. Z. N., and Adams, C. W. M. Relationship between enzyme activity and neuroglia in plaques of multiple sclerosis. *J. Neurol. Neurosurg. Psychiat.,* **26:**101–10, 1963.

90. Ironside, R.; Bosanquet, F. D.; and McMenemy, W. H. Central demyelination of the corpus callosum (Marchiafava-Bignami disease) with report of a second case in Great Britian. *Brain,* **84:**212–30, 1961.

91. Jestico, J. V., and Ellis, P. D. M. Changes in nystagmus on raising body temperature in clinically suspected and proven multiple sclerosis. *Br. Med. J.,* **1:**970–72, 1976.

92. Johnson, K. P., and Nelson, B. J. Multiple sclerosis: Diagnostic usefulness of Cerebrospinal fluid. *Ann. Neurol.,* **2:**425–31, 1977.

93. Jotkowitz, S. Multiple sclerosis and exposure to house pets. *J.A.M.A.*, **238**:854, 1977.

94. Joynt, R. J., and Green, D. Tonic seizures as a manifestation of multiple sclerosis. *Arch. Neurol.*, **6**:293–99, 1962.

95. Kaback, M. M. and Howell, R. R. Infantile metachromatic leukodystrophy. *N. Engl. J. Med.*, **282**:1336–40, 1970.

96. Kahana, E.; Leibowitz, U.; and Alter, M. Brain stem and cranial nerve involvement in multiple sclerosis. *Acta Neurol. Scand.*, **49**:269–79, 1973.

97. Knight, S. C. Cellular immunity in multiple sclerosis. *Br. Med. Bull.*, **33**:45–49, 1977.

98. Kurtzke, J. F. Reassessment of distribution of multiple sclerosis. *Acta Neurol. Scand.*, **51**:110–36, 1975.

99. Kurtzke, J. F. Geography in multiple sclerosis. *J. Neurol.*, **215**:1–26, 1977.

100. Kurtzke, J. F.; Bobowisk, A. R.; et al. Twin studies of multiple sclerosis: An epidemiologic inquiry. *Neurology* (Minneap.), **27**:341, 1977.

101. Lakke, J. P.; Ebels, E. J; and ten Thye, O. J. Infantile necrotizing encephalomyelopathy (Leigh). *Arch. Neurol.*, **16**:227–31, 1967.

102. Lamoureux, R.; Jolicoeur, R.; et al. Cerebrospinal fluid proteins in multiple sclerosis. *Neurology* (Minneap.), **25**:537–46, 1975.

103. Lechevalier, B.; Andersson, J. C.; and Morin, P. Hemispheric disconnection syndrome with a "crossed avoiding" reaction in a case of Marchiafava-Bignami disease. *J. Neurol. Neurosurg. Psychiat.*, **40**:483–97, 1977.

104. Leibowitz, U.; Kahana, E.; and Alter, M. Changing frequency of multiple sclerosis in Israel. *Arch. Neurol.*, **29**:107–10, 1973.

105. Levine, M. C., and VanBrocklin, J. D. Lioresal^R (bactofen) treatment of spasticity: A double blind comparison study with dantrolene and diazepam. *Neurology* (Minneap.), **27**:391, 1977.

106. Levy, N. L.; Auerbach, P. S.; and Hayes, E. C. Blood test for multiple sclerosis based on adherence of lymphocytes to measles-infected cells. *N. Engl. J. Med.*, **294**:1423–27, 1976.

107. Lhermitte, F.; Marteau, R.; et al. Signs of interhemisphere disconnection in Marchiafava-Bignami disease. *Arch. Neurol.*, **34**:254, 1977.

108. Lou, H. O. C., and Reske-Nielsen, E. The central nervous system in Fabry's disease. A clinical, pathological, and biochemical investigation. *Arch. Neurol.*, **25**:351–59, 1971.

109. MacFayden, D. J.; Reeve, C. E.; et al. Failure of antilymphocytic globulin therapy in chronic progressive multiple sclerosis. *Neurology (Minneap.)*, **23**:592–98, 1973.

110. Malas, D., and Weiss, S. Progressive multifocal leukoencephalography and cryptococcal meningitis with systemic lupus erythematosus and thymoma. *Ann. Neurol.*, **1**:188–91, 1977.

111. Malone, M. J. The cerebral lipidosis. *Pediatr. Clin. North Am.*, **23**:303–26, 1976.

112. Mastaglia, F. L.; Black, J. L.; et al. Evoked potentials saccadic velocities, and computerized tomography in diagnosis of multiple sclerosis. *Br. Med. J.*, **1**:1315–17, 1977.

113. Mastaglia, F. L.; Black, J. L.; and Collins, D. W. K. Saccadic velocities in multiple sclerosis. *Lancet*, **2**:1359, 1976.

114. Mathews, T.; Wisotzkey, H.; and Moosy, J. Multiple central nervous system infections in progressive multifocal leukoencephalopathy. *Neurology* (Minneap.), **26**:9–14, 1976.

115. McAlpine, D. Benign form of multiple sclerosis. *Brain*, **84**:186–203, 1961.

116. McCormick, W. F.; Schochet, S. S.; et al. Progressive multifocal leukoencephalopathy in renal transplant recipients. *Arch. Intern. Med.*, **136**:829–34, 1976.

117. McFarlin, D. E., and McFarland, H. F. Histocompatibility studies and multiple sclerosis. *Arch. Neurol.*, **33**:395–98, 1976.

118. McFarlin, D. E.; Mingioh, E. S.; et al. Quantitation of CSF immunoglobulins in the CSF by radioimmunoassay. *Neurology* (Minneap.), **27**:342, 1977.

119. Menkes, J. H.; O'Brien, J. S.; Okada, S.; Grippo, J.; Andrews, J. M.; and Cancilla, P. A. Juvenile G_{M2} gangliosidosis. *Arch. Neurol.*, **25**:14–22, 1971.

120. Menkes, J. H.; Schimschock, J. R.; and Swanson, P. D. Cerebrotendinous xanthomatosis; storage of cholestanol within the nervous system. *Arch. Neurol.*, **19**:47–53, 1968.

121. Millar, J. H. D.; Vas, C. J.; Noronha, M. J., Leveredge, L. A.; and Rawson, M. D. Long-term treatment of multiple sclerosis with corticotrophin. *Lancet*, **2**:429–31, 1967.

122. Millar, J. H. D.; Zukha, K. J.; et al. Double blind trial of linolate supplementation of the diet in multiple sclerosis. *Br. J. Med.*, **1**:765–68, 1973.

123. Miller, H.; Newell, D. J.; Ridley, A.; and Schapira, K. Therapeutic trials in multiple sclerosis. *J. Neurol. Neurosurg. Psychiat.*, **24**:118–20, 1961.

124. Myers, L. W.; Ellison, G. W.; et al. HLA and the immune response to measles in multiple sclerosis. *Neurology* (Minneap.), **26**:54–55, 1976.

125. Nelson, D. A.; Vates, T. S., Jr.; and Thomas, R. B. Complications from intrathecal steroid therapy in patients with multiple sclerosis. *Acta Neurol. Scand.*, **49**:176–88, 1973.

126. Norrby, E.; Link, H.; and Olsson, J.-E. Measles virus antibodies on multiple sclerosis: Comparison of antibody titers in cerebrospinal fluid and serum. *Arch. Neurol.*, **30**:285–92, 1974.

127. O'Brien, J. S. GM_1 gangliosidosis. In Stanbury, J. B.; Wyngaarden, J. G.; and Fredrickson, D. S. (eds.). The *Metabolic Basis of Inherited Diseases*, 3rd ed. McGraw-Hill Book Co., New York, 1972, pp. 639–62.

128. Olson, W. H. Diet and multiple sclerosis. *Postgrad. Med.*, **59**:219–21, 1976.

129. Olsson, J. E.; Mollar, E.; and Link, H. HLA haplotypes in families with a high frequency of multiple sclerosis. *Arch. Neurol.*, **33**:808–12, 1976.

130. Padgett, B. L.; Walker, D. L.; ZuRhein, G. M.; and Eckroade, R. J. Cultivation of Papova-like virus from human brain with progressive multifocal leucoencephalopathy. *Lancet*, **1**:1257–60, 1971.

131. Padgett, B. L.; Walker, D. L.; et al. J. C. papovavi-

rus in progressive multifocal leukoencephalopathy. *J. Infect. Dis.,* **133**:686–90, 1976.

132. Park, C. S. Multiple sclerosis in Korea. *Neurology* (Minneap.), **16**:919–26, 1966.

133. Paty, D. W.; Dosseters, J. B.; et al. HLA in multiple sclerosis: Relationship to measles antibody, mitogen responsiveness and clinical course. *J. Neurol. Sci.,* **32**:371–79, 1977.

134. Percy, A. K.; Kaback, M. M.; and Herndon, R. M. Metachromatic leukodystrophy: Comparison of early and late-onset forms. *Neurology* (Minneap.), **27**:933–41, 1977.

135. Pertschuk, L. P.; Cook, A. W.; and Gupta, J. Measles antigen in multiple sclerosis: Identification in the jejunum by immunofluorescence. *Life Sci.,* **19**:1603–1608, 1976.

136. Pincus, J. H.; Cooper, J. R.; Itokawa, Y.; and Gumbinas, M. Subacute necrotizing encephalomyelopathy. Effects of thiamine and thiamine propyl disulfide. *Arch. Neurol.,* **24**:511–17, 1971.

137. Pincus, J. H.; Soutare, G. R.; and Cooper, J. R. Thiamine triphosphate levels and histopathology. Correlation in Leigh disease. *Arch. Neurol.,* **33**:759–63, 1976.

138. Porter, K. G. Oligoclonal immunoglobulin G in cerebrospinal fluid in multiple sclerosis. *Irish J. Med. Sci.,* **146**:146, 1977.

139. Poser, C. M.; Presthus, J.; and Hörsdal, O. Clinical characteristics of autopsy-proved multiple sclerosis; study of British, Norwegian and American cases. *Neurology* (Minneap.), **16**:791–98, 1966.

140. Poser, C. M., and Sylvester, D. L. Amino acid residues of serum and CSF protein in multiple sclerosis. Clinical application of statistical discriminant analysis. *Arch. Neurol.,* **32**:308–14, 1975.

141. Poskanzer, D. C.; Schapira, K.; Brack, R. A.; and Miller, H. Studies of blood groups, genetic linkage, tract association and chromosomal pattern in multiple sclerosis. *J. Neurol. Neurosurg. Psychiat.,* **28**:218–22, 1965.

142. Poskanzer, D. C.; Terasaki, P. I.; et al. Multiple sclerosis in the Orkney and Shetland Islands. 1. Prevalence and tissue antigens. *Neurology* (Minneap.), **27**:371–72, 1977.

143. Poskanzer, D. C.; Walker, A. M.; et al. Studies in the epidemiology of multiple sclerosis in the Orkney and Shetland Islands. *Neurology* (Minneap.), **26**:14–17, 1976.

144. Powell, H.; Tindall, R.; et al. Adrenoleukodystrophy—Electron microscopic findings. *Arch. Neurol.,* **32**:250–60, 1975.

145. Prasad, I.; Pertschute, L. P.; et al. Recovery of paramyxovirus from the jejunum of patients with multiple sclerosis. *Lancet,* **1**:1117–19, 1977.

146. Quigley, H. A., and Green, W. R. Clinical and ultrastructural ocular histopathologic studies of adult-onset metachromatic leukodystrophy. *Am. J. Ophthalmol.,* **82**:472–79, 1976.

147. Raine, C. S.; Powers, J. M.; and Suzuki, K. Acute multiple sclerosis: Confirmation of "paramyxovirus-like" intranuclear inclusions. *Arch. Neurol.,* **30**:39–46, 1974.

148. Raine, C. S., and Stone, S. H. Animal model for multiple sclerosis. Chronic experimental allergic encephalomyelitis in inbred guinea pigs. *N. Y. State J. Med.,* **77**:1693–96, 1977.

149. Reckers, P.; Hommes, O. R.; et al. HLA-typing and lymphocyte population studies in patients with multiple sclerosis. *J. Neurol. Sci.,* **33**:143–53, 1977.

150. Redde, M. M., and Goh, K. O. B and T lymphocytes in man: III. B - T and male lymphocytes in multiple sclerosis. *Neurology* (Minneap.), **26**:997–99, 1976.

151. Reed, D.; Sever, J.; Kurtzke, J.; and Kurland, L. Measles antibody in patients with multiple sclerosis. *Arch. Neurol.,* **10**:402–10, 1964.

152. Restan, R.; Reed, J.; and Dykes, M. Cognitive psychomotor and motor correlates of multiple sclerosis. *J. Nerv. Ment. Dis.,* **153**:218–24, 1971.

153. Ring, J.; Angstivium, H.; et al. Pilot study with antilymphocytic globulin in the treatment of multiple sclerosis. *Postgrad. Med. J.,* **52**:123–28, 1976.

154. Robinson, F.; Solicare, G. B.; Lamarche, J. B.; and Levy, L. L. Necrotizing encephalomyelopathy of childhood. *Neurology* (Minneap.), **17**:472–84, 1967.

155. Robinson, K., and Rudge, P. Abnormalities of the auditory evoked potentials in patients with multiple sclerosis. *Brain,* **100**:19–40, 1977.

156. Robinson, K., and Rudge, P. The early components of the auditory evoked potential in multiple sclerosis. *In Desmendt, J. E. (ed.). Auditory Evoked Potentials in Man. Psychopharmacology Correlates of Evoked Potentials. Progress in Clinical Neurophysiology,* Vol. 2. S. Karger, Basel, 1977, pp. 58–67.

157. Rose, A. S., and Pearson, C. M. (eds.) *Mechanisms of Demyelination* McGraw-Hill, New York, 1963.

158. Rosner, F.; Weisfogel, G.; and Feinerman, A. Infantile amaurotic familial idiocy. Leukocyte granulation and leukocyte alkaline phosphatase. *J.A.M.A.,* **205**:873–75, 1968.

159. Russo, L. S.; Axon, A.; and Anderson, P. J. Alexander's disease. A report and reappraisal. *Neurology* (Minneap.), **26**:607–14, 1976.

160. Sachias, B. A.; Logue, J. N.; and Carey, M. S. Baclofen, a new antispastic drug. A controlled multicenter trial in patients with multiple sclerosis. *Arch. Neurol.,* **34**:422–28, 1977.

161. Sacks, O.; Brown, W. J.; and Aguilar, M. J. Spongy degeneration of white matter; Canavan's sclerosis. *Neurology* (Minneap.), **15**:165–71, 1965.

162. Sanchez, J. E., and Lopez, V. F. Sex-linked sudanophilic leukodystrophy with adrenocortical atrophy (so-called Schilder's disease). *Neurology* (Minneap.), **26**:261–69, 1976.

163. Schapira, K.; Paskanzer, D. C.; and Miller, H. Familial and conjugal sclerosis. *Brain,* **86**:315–32, 1963.

164. Schapira, K.; Poskanzer, D. C.; Newell, D. J.; and Miller, H. Marriage, pregnancy and multiple sclerosis. *Brain,* **89**:419–28, 1966.

165. Schaumberg, H. H.; Powers, J. M.; et al. Adrenoluekodystrophy: Clinical and pathologic study of 17 cases. *Arch. Neurol.,* **32**:577–91, 1974.

166. Schemschock, J. R.; Alvord, E. C.; and Swanson, P. D. Cerebrotendinous xanthomatosis. Clinical

and pathological studies. *Arch. Neurol.,* **18:**688–98, 1968.

167. Seil, F. J.; Schochet, S. S., Jr.; and Earle, K. M. Alexander's disease in an adult. *Arch. Neurol.,* **19:**494–502, 1968.

168. Seitelberger, F. Histochemistry of demyelinating diseases proper including allergic encephalomyelitis and Pelizaeus-Merzbacher's disease. In Cumings, J. N. (ed.). *Modern Scientific Aspects of Neurology.* Edward Arnold, London, 1960, pp. 146–87.

169. Sexauer, J. M., and Fakety, F. R., Jr. Pulmonary infections complicating treatment of multiple sclerosis: Occurrence with administration of corticotropin or adrenal steroids. *Arch. Neurol.,* **30:**293–95, 1974.

169a. Shahrokhi, F.; Chiappa, K. H.; and Young, R. R. Pattern shift visual evoked responses. Two hundred patients with optic neuritis and/or multiple sclerosis. *Arch. Neurol.,* **35:**65–71, 1978.

170. Shebasaki, H.; Okihiro, M. M.; and Kuroiwa, Y. Multiple sclerosis among Caucasians and Orientals in Hawaii. A reappraisal. *Neurology* (Minneap.), **28:**113–18, 1978.

170a. Small, D. G.; Matthews, W. B.; and Small, M. The reversal somatosensory evoked potential (SEP) in the diagnosis of multiple sclerosis. *J. Neurol. Sci.,* **35:**211–24, 1978.

171. Solinger, L. D.; Baloh, R. W.; et al. Subclinical eye movement disorders in patients with multiple sclerosis. *Neurology* (Minneap.), **27:**614–19, 1977.

172. Stockard, J. J.; Rossiter, V. S.; et al. Brain stem auditory-evoked responses in suspected central pontine myelinolysis. *Arch. Neurol.,* **33:**726–28, 1976.

173. Suzuki, K., and Grover. W. D. Krabbe's leukodystrophy (globoidal cell leukodystrophy). *Arch. Neurol.,* **22:**385–96, 1970.

174. Symposium on the Cerebral Sphingolipidoses, Brooklyn and New York, 1961. *Cerebral Sphingolipidoses; a Symposium on Tay-Sachs Disease and Allied Disorders,* ed. by S. M. Aronson and B. W. Volk. Academic Press, New York, 1962.

175. Tanaka, R.; Iwasaki, Y.; and Koprowski, H. Paramyovirus-like structures in brains of multiple sclerosis patients. *Arch. Neurol.,* **32:**80–83, 1975.

176. Tavolata, B. F. Immunoglobulin G distribution in multiple sclerosis brain: Immunofluorescence study. *J. Neurol. Sci.,* **24:**1–11, 1975.

177. TerMeulen, V.; Koprowski, H.; Iwasaki, Y.; Käckell, Y. M., and Müller. D. Fusion of cultured multiple-sclerosis brain cells with indicator cells: Presence of nucleocapsids and virions and isolation of parainfluenza-type virus. *Lancet,* **2:**1–5, 1972.

178. Thornsby, E.; Helgesen, A.; et al. HLA antigens in multiple sclerosis. *J. Neurol. Sci.,* **32:**187–93, 1977.

179. Tomlinson, B. E.; Pierides, A. M.; and Bradley, W. G. Central pontine myelinolysis. Two cases with associated electrolyte disturbances. *Q. J. Med.,* **45:**373–86, 1976.

180. Tourtellotte, W. W., and Haerer. A. F. Use of an oral corticosteroid in the treatment of multiple sclerosis. *Arch. Neurol.,* **12:**536–45, 1965.

181. Troullas, P., and Betuel, H. Hypocomplimentemic and normo-complimentemic multiple sclerosis and association with specific HLA determinants (B18 and B7). *J. Neurol. Sci.,* **32:**425–36, 1977.

181a. Tsan, M. F.; Gale, A. N.; et al. Neuronal ceroid-lipofuscinosis. Studies of granulocyte enzyme activities. *J. Neurol. Sci.,* **36:**13–24, 1978.

182. Vandvik, B. Oligoclonal IgG and free light chains in the cerebrospinal fluid of patients with multiple sclerosis and infectious disease of the nervous system. *Scand. J. Immunol.,* **6:**913–22, 1977.

183. Veterans Administration Multiple Sclerosis Study Group: Five-year follow-up on multiple sclerosis. *Arch. Neurol.,* **11:**583–92, 1964.

184. Vogel, F. S., and Hallervorden, J. Leukodystrophy with diffuse Rosenthal fiber formation. *Acta Neuropath.* (Berlin), **2:**126–43, 1962.

185. Wilkas, R. J., and Farrell, D. F. Electrophysiologic observations in the classical form of Pelizaeus-Merzbacher disease. *Neurology* (Minneap.), **26:**1042–45, 1976.

186. Wisniewski, H. M., and Keith, A. B. Chronic relapsing experimental allergic encephalomyelitis: An experimental model of multiple sclerosis. *Ann. Neurol.,* **1:**144–48, 1977.

187. Wolfe, L. S.; NyYinkKin, M. K. W.; and Baker, R. R. Identification of retinoyl complexes as the autofluorescent component of the neuronal storage material in Batten disease. *Science,* **195:**1360–62, 1976.

188. Wolinsky, J. S.; Johnson, K. P.; et al. Progressive multifocal leukoencephalopathy: Clinical pathological correlates and failure of a drug trial in two patients. *Trans. Am. Neurol. Assoc.* **101:**81–2, 1976.

189. Young, A. C.; Sanders, J.; and Ponsford, J. R. Mental changes as an early feature of multiple sclerosis. *J. Neurol. Neurosurg. Psychiat.,* **39:**1008–13, 1976.

190. Zeese, J. A. Pattern visual evoked potentials in multiple sclerosis. *Arch. Neurol.,* **34:**314–16, 1977.

191. Zemen, W.; Donahue, S.; et al. In Vinken, P. J., and Bruyn, G. W. (eds.). *Handbook of Clinical Neurology,* Vol. 10. North-Holland Publishers, Amsterdam, 1970, pp. 588–679.

4 DEGENERATIVE DISEASES OF THE NERVOUS SYSTEM

The Dementias: General Considerations

A considerable number of diseases are associated with progressive dementia (i.e., progressive deterioration of mental functions resulting from disease of the brain), but the term is used here to denote a group of conditions in which progressive dementia is the early and predominant neurologic sign. The terms "presenile" and "senile" are arbitrary definitions which divide the dementias into those which occur after age 65 years (senile) and those occurring between the third decade and age 65 years (presenile).[134] The majority of conditions grouped under the dementias are caused by neuronal degeneration, but the etiology of the neuronal abiotrophy is unknown at the present time.

Although dementia occurs predominantly in older people and is therefore an increasing problem in our aging population, dementia is by no means an inevitable consequence of aging and should never be dismissed as such. There is increasing recognition of treatable causes of dementia, and the clinician should always attempt to make a correct diagnosis in each case rather than resort to empty terms such as "chronic brain syndrome."

The causes of dementia remain elusive in many cases. The familial occurrence of Alzheimer's and Pick's disease has been described, and it is possible that these diseases are genetically determined in some cases.[29] Dementia is also a feature of many of the familial spinocerebellar degenerations. Chronic bacterial and fungal infections have long been recognized as causes of dementia, but identification of viruses as the etiologic agents in two neuronal degenerations associated with dementia, namely kuru and Jakob-Creutzfeldt disease, has opened up a new avenue of research into related disorders. The first disease shown to be the result of chronic or "slow virus" infection was kuru, a degenerative neurologic disease limited to an isolated community in eastern New Guinea. The disease affects women and children who engage in cannibalism, but not the adult males who do not participate in this rite. The viral agent is presumably spread by the oral route, and the disease is expected to die out now that cannibalism has been abolished. Jakob-Creutzfeldt disease has been accidentally transmitted from human to human and has been transmitted through several generations of laboratory animals, and there is additional evidence from the electron microscopic appearance of the tissues that this is also a "slow-virus" disease.

Diagnostic Procedures for the Dementias

A complete neurologic and diagnostic evaluation should always be performed in patients with dementia in order to identify those who have conditions that are amenable to treatment.[183]

Patients should not be confined to chronic care facilities on the basis of a clinical diagnosis of presenile (or senile) dementia before every effort has been made to identify and treat potentially remediable causes for dementia and thereby restore patients to useful lives in the community. The evaluation of the patient with dementia includes:

1. Complete neurologic examination. Focal abnormalities suggest focal, e.g., tumor, subdural hematoma, rather than diffuse changes in the brain.
2. Neuropsychologic evaluation. This aids in diagnosis and quantitative evaluation of the course of the disease with and without treatment.
3. Complete blood count. Anemia may compound arteriosclerotic dementia. Dementia also occurs in pernicious anemia.
4. Roentgenography of skull and chest. A shift of the pineal gland or abnormal intracranial calcification may indicate the presence of a space-occupying lesion. Roentgenography of the chest aids in excluding primary and metastatic neoplasm involving the lungs.
5. Electroencephalography. Advanced dementias associated with diffuse neuronal degeneration show diffuse changes in the EEG. Focal slowing of the EEG suggests a focal lesion in the brain. In early dementia the EEG is frequently normal.
6. Computed tomography of the brain will demonstrate focal or diffuse abnormalities in most cases. An iodine-enhanced scan should be obtained since it is possible that small isodense lesions may not be visible on the nonenhanced scan. The results of the CT scan frequently dictate the choice of subsequent investigative procedures.
7. Lumbar puncture. Pleocytosis of the CSF suggests chronic infection, e.g., syphilis. Elevated CSF pressure and protein content suggest tumor or subdural hematoma.
8. Radioisotope cisternography. Scanning of the head after injection of radioactive [169]Yb into the lumbar subarachnoid space may show the presence of malabsorption of CSF with normal pressure hydrocephalus. Normally there is a characteristic flow of the radioactive material through the subarachnoid space and ventricular system of the brain, which clears within 24 hours. Obstruction to the flow of the radioactive material at various sites may occur in obstructive hydrocephalus, but in normal pressure hydrocephalus, which is frequently accompanied by dementia, the radioactive material remains in the ventricles in excess of 48 to 72 hours.
9. Cerebral arteriography and pneumoencephalography will only be needed in certain cases where clinical assessment suggests the presence of cerebrovascular disease or where the results of the CT scan are equivocal.

Alzheimer's Disease

This condition is one of the most common forms of the dementias, with a prevalence in the United States of about 500,000 in persons over 65 years of age.[135]

Etiology and Pathology

The etiology is unknown. Attributing this disorder to an abiotrophy or premature death of neurons is a crude concept of pathogenesis in terms of modern standards of molecular biology and intracellular physiology. Nevertheless, there is an accelerated neuronal loss in Alzheimer's disease that exceeds the normal aging rate by 5 per cent or more per year.[29a] It is probable that there is failure of some essential intracellular enzymatic systems, and there are reports of decreased activity of enzymes involved in the biosynthesis of neurotransmitters.[176] The reduction of enzymes involved in the synthesis of acetylcholine is the most consistent finding and gives rise to the concept of Alzheimer's disease as a cholinergic system failure.[48]

The finding of raised concentrations of aluminum[46] and manganese[10] in the brain suggests that high levels of these metals may be neurotoxic and produce the accelerated neuronal loss of Alzheimer's disease.

The brain is underweight and shows generalized atrophy with widening of the sulci and narrowing of the gyri. There is diffuse ventricular dilation with atrophy of both gray and white matter. The histologic findings are characterized by diffuse neuronal loss throughout the cortical and subcortical gray matter with the presence of senile plaques in the gray matter. These latter structures are numerous and stain readily with silver stains (argentophilic). Histochemically, senile plaques show evidence of increased mitochondrial activity with concentrations of oxidative enzymes above normal in the early stages followed by reduction in enzyme levels and the deposition of an amyloid-like material.

Another characteristic finding in Alzheimer's disease is the presence of neurofibrillary tangles in the neurons, particularly in Sommer's sector of the hippocampal gyrus. Neurofibrillary tangles are not confined to this area, and many occur in other parts of the hippocampal formation, amygdala, and adjacent temporal lobe, as well as in the anterior perforated substance, the cingulate gyrus, and to a lesser extent the substantia nigra and locus ceruleus. The eponym "Alzheimer's neurofibrillary tangles" does not mean that the change is peculiar to Alzheimer's disease since similar changes are seen in neurons in the parkinsonian dementia complex occurring on the islands of Guam, postencephalitic parkinsonism, and occasionally amyotrophic lateral sclerosis. Alzheimer's neurofibrillary tangles also occur in lesser numbers in brains of the elderly.

Clinical Features

Alzheimer's disease occurs with equal frequency in both sexes and may begin at any age after the early thirties. A number of cases are familial but hereditary factors are not obvious in the majority of patients.

The early symptoms of the disease may pass undiagnosed and usually consist of inappropriate behavior, uncritical statements, irritability, and a tendency toward grandiosity, euphoria, and deterioration in performance at work. If this is remarked upon by others, it is usually denied by the patient. Other cases present with depression and withdrawal, and the organic signs of dementia are, therefore, often overlooked.

Deterioration in operational judgment is often the first symptom to cause sufficient concern of the family or of colleagues to prompt medical consultation.

At this stage, there is usually some loss of insight, often resulting in elaborate and complex rationalization on the part of the patient. However, despite such excuses, it becomes obvious within a few minutes of examination that there is impairment of retention and recent memory. As the disease progresses, the patient may become uncommunicative and withdrawn. Paranoid ideas frequently develop, and some patients assault or harangue members of their family and those attending them. Others develop early dysphasia, which steadily progresses.

The fully developed clinical picture of Alzheimer's disease is an untidy, pathetic figure who is confused, dysphasic, and dyspraxic and has impared retention and recent memory. The facial expression is fixed, and there is infrequent blinking, although there are frequent sucking and licking movements of the tongue. The posture becomes semiflexed and movements are slow with evidence of generalized rigidity. Seizures and myoclonic jerks occur in some cases. Further deterioration leads to apraxia of gait with difficulty in walking and getting out of a chair. The patient finally becomes bedridden and incontinent and usually dies from pneumonia or infection of the urinary tract within five to six years from the onset of Alzheimer's disease.

Diagnostic Procedures

1. In the early stages, the EEG may be of low amplitude with reduction of alpha activity and disorganization of background activity. This is followed by the gradual development of generalized theta activity and total loss of alpha.[40] In the final stages, sharp bursts of frontal dominant delta activity as well as random delta waves are seen. The slowing may be asymmetric, and focal seizures may occur. Sleep activity tends to be suppressed bilaterally, and fast

activity may not appear if the patient is given barbiturates.

2. Computed tomography of the brain shows diffuse symmetric ventricular enlargement and the presence of enlarged cortical sulci indicating cortical atrophy[75] (Fig. 4–1). There may be relatively few signs of atrophy in the early stages of the disease.

3. Radioisotope cisternography shows enlarged ventricles without delay of emptying.

4. Brain biopsy shows characteristic histologic changes and is the only method of making the exact diagnosis during life.[114]

Treatment

Although the cause of the disease is unknown, much can be done to modify distressing symptoms and to advise the family concerning the tragic and difficult illness. The agitated, paranoid, combative patient may become tractable and manageable with the use of phenothiazine drugs. Many suffer from personal neglect and malnutrition, and prescribing thiamine and vitamin B complex may prevent rapid deterioration. Serum folate levels should be determined since an organic dementia simulating Alzheimer's disease has been reported in folic acid deficiency.[233] This condition could complicate the dementia in Alzheimer's disease, and a low folate level indicates the need for treatment with folic acid.

It is important to differentiate Alzheimer's disease from normal pressure hydrocephalus, since this condition improves with a ventriculoatrial shunt and experience with this form of treatment in Alzheimer's disease has been disappointing.

Although muscarinic binding sites decrease with advancing age, muscarinic binding sites are not apparently decreased in Alzheimer's disease. Thus, centrally acting anticholinesterase therapy may eventually prove beneficial in this condition, and oral lecithin, 60 gm per day (choline precursor), has been suggested.

In Alzheimer's disease, the aim of therapy should be directed toward maintaining optimum care at home, rather than admission to an institution where deterioration rapidly results from isolation and lack of family attention. In some cases special techniques of memory retraining[181] and stimulating interest in current affairs and activities may be rewarding.

In certain advanced cases, with antisocial behavior, commitment proceedings for compulsory institutional care will be necessary. Others require nursing home care in the terminal stages of the

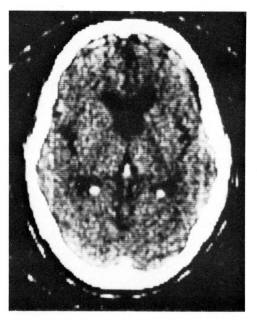 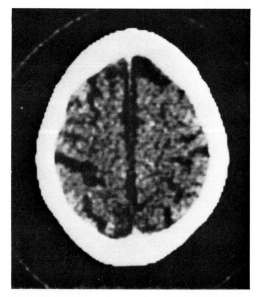

FIGURE 4–1. Computed tomography in Alzheimer's disease. There is diffuse ventricular enlargement with enlarged cortical sulci indicating cortical atrophy.

disease. When the patient shows advanced deterioration, a great deal of sympathy, tact, and understanding are required of the physician in advising the family when to admit the patient to an institution or nursing home.

Medical advice concerning the legal state of mental competence should also be considered, and provision should be made so that the patient's affairs can be managed by a guardian or trustee if mental deterioration makes this necessary.

Pick's Disease

This type of dementia is rarer than Alzheimer's disease and occasionally occurs as a familial disorder which may be inherited as an autosomal dominant trait. It occurs twice as frequently in females as in males.

Etiology and Pathology

The cause of the neuronal degeneration is unknown. Increased concentrations of zinc in the brain and increased urinary excretion of zinc have been reported in Pick's disease.[41a] The brain shows marked atrophy of the frontal and temporal lobes, which is usually symmetric. There is some variation in the degree of atrophy of the two areas. The frontal lobe shows maximal involvement in the orbital areas, including the gyrus rectus and the inferior frontal gyrus. The atrophy of the temporal lobe is maximal in the area of the temporal pole, the inferior and middle temporal gyri, and the anterior part of the superior temporal gyrus.

The areas maximally involved are those which are phylogenetically late in development. However, this pattern is not an invariable finding in Pick's disease since parietal lobe involvement has also been described. Sections of the brain show that the atrophy involves the subcortical nuclear gray matter, including the globus pallidus, caudate nucleus, putamen, and thalamus. There may be advanced cerebellar atrophy in some cases.

The affected areas of cortex show a marked loss of neurons, which is maximal in the outer three layers of the gray matter. Surviving cells are smaller with argentophilic inclusions and because of their characteristic appearance are known as Pick's cells. The pyramidal cells of Ammon's horn in the hippocampal formation show a granulovacular degeneration. All areas show a marked astroglial proliferation.

The senile plaques and neurofibrillary tangles

of Alzheimer's disease are either absent or infrequent in Pick's disease.

Clinical Features

The symptomatology of Pick's disease is essentially the same as that described under Alzheimer's disease, and the two conditions cannot be separated by the clinical signs. Patients with Pick's disease tend to survive longer than those with Alzheimer's, and the course averages about ten years from the onset to death. It may present in the third decade or, rarely, in old age.[22]

Diagnostic Procedures

1. Computed tomography shows dilatation of the frontal and temporal horns of the lateral ventricles. There is marked widening of the cortical sulci in these same areas, indicating maximal atrophic changes in the frontal and temporal lobes (Fig. 4–2).
2. The spinal fluid pressure and content are normal, although occasionally the protein content is increased.
3. The EEG changes are not as marked in Pick's disease as in Alzheimer's disease, and focal

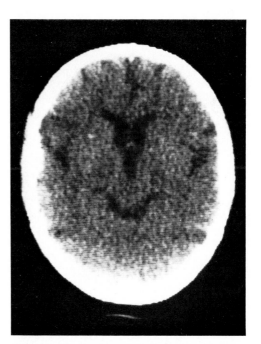

FIGURE 4–2. Computed tomography in Pick's disease. The ventricular dilation is seen predominantly in the frontotemporal regions, and the cortical atrophy is maximal in the same areas.

changes are often absent. However, in fully developed cases of Pick's disease, the EEG abnormality is similar to that encountered in Alzheimer's disease.

4. Brain biopsy with demonstration of the characteristic histologic changes is the only definitive method of making the exact diagnosis during life.

Treatment

There is no specific treatment that appears to alter the course of Pick's disease. Nutritional and palliative treatment and considerations of the general approach to the problems presented by all the dementias have been discussed under Alzheimer's disease.

Huntington's Disease

There were several independent descriptions of Huntington's disease (formerly called Huntington's chorea) in Europe and in the United States during the mid-nineteenth century. The disease takes its name from the three generations of physicians named Huntington who collected a large series of cases from families with Huntington's disease under their care in Long Island, New York State, and Ohio. The condition is seen in all races. It is not a common disease, and the reported incidence shows some geographic variation with a maximum of 6.5 cases per 100,000 population. The disease is inherited as an autosomal dominant trait with complete penetrance.

Etiology and Pathology

The disease is a genetically determined condition in which there is a deficiency of the neurotransmitter gamma-aminobutyric acid (GABA) in the basal ganglia. Considerable biochemical research has now been carried out, and GABA, homocarnosine, and glutamic acid-decarboxylase are reduced and glycerophosphoethanolamine is increased in the substantia nigra, putamen-globus pallidus, and caudate nucleus.[23, 185, 186]

The reduction of glutamic acid-decarboxylase in the basal ganglia but not in the frontal cortex accounts for the deficiency of the inhibitory neurotransmitter GABA[219] in the basal ganglia. Lack of GABA inhibition may lead to a relative overactivity of the dopaminergic systems,[66] a situation somewhat analogous to that seen in parkinsonian patients treated with an overdosage of levodopa. Dopamine concentrations are normal or moderately reduced in the rigid form of Huntington's disease. Although there is a loss of GABA neurons in the corpus striatum, depletion of GABA is not necessarily the fundamental biochemical defect in Huntington's disease and may only reflect neuron depletion. This possibility is supported by the demonstration of a marked reduction of angiotensin-converting enzyme in the corpus striatum, which suggests that the neurotransmitter angiotensin II may be deficient in Huntington's disease.[9]

Similarly, the reduction of choline acetyltransferase activity in the corpus striatum suggests that hypofunction of cholinergic neurons may have a pathophysiologic role in Huntington's disease.[6]

The cause of the neuronal loss is not known, but it has been suggested that the destruction of neurons may be a genetically determined autoimmune response based on the demonstrated abnormal activity of lymphocytes in Huntington's disease.[14, 15]

The brain shows cortical atrophy, particularly over the frontal lobes, with ventricular dilatation. The marked atrophy of the caudate nucleus and putamen accentuates the dilatation of the anterior horns of the lateral ventricles. There is a complete loss of the small neurons in the caudate nucleus and putamen, and although the larger neurons have been regarded as unaffected, many are shrunken and atrophic. There is a marked reactive gliosis, particularly in the caudate nucleus, and the astrocytes may be quite large with prominent nuclei and abundant cytoplasm. Neuronal loss also occurs in varying degrees in the cortical gray matter, thalamus, subthalamic nucleus, dentate nucleus, and cerebellar cortex.

Clinical Features

The essential features of Huntington's disease are the development of athetosis rather than chorea with progressive dementia. The condition usually occurs after the age of 30 years but has been described in children before the age of five years. The earliest symptoms, usually clumsiness of movement, slowness of finer movements, and a tendency to drop objects, may be present for some years before the development of involuntary choreoathetosis. The latter symptom begins as an apparent restlessness, which develops into an irregular athetosis with rapid jerking movements of the fingers and wrists associated with slower dystonic movements of the upper limbs.

The gait becomes ataxic with a dancing quality,

and similar movements occur in the lower limbs, neck, and trunk. There is a characteristic grimacing of the face, associated with involuntary movements of the tongue and dysarthria. The dementia usually begins after the development of athetosis but occasionally antedates its appearance.

There is a progressive loss of memory due to a failure to encode new material and to retrieve learned material.[35] This is followed by impairment of judgment and increasing social problems in relation to the family and performance at work. The writing deteriorates and the speech becomes slurred with poverty of content. Depression, hostility, anxiety, or feelings of incompetence are common. These early symptoms have led to suicides in patients with Huntington's disease.

The relentless progression of athetosis and dementia eventually leads to a bedridden state. There is often emaciation, and death usually occurs from intercurrent infection after about 10 to 15 years of the illness.

Two interesting variants of Huntington's disease have been described. In the first (Westphal) variant,[24, 37, 51, 175] the disease may begin with rigidity at an early stage. The rigidity affects the trunk and proximal limb muscles and gradually extends to involve the distal musculature. There are severe dysarthria, masklike facies, and progressive and often rapid dementia. Signs of corticospinal tract involvement are prominent with increased reflexes and bilateral extensor plantar responses. The second (juvenile) variant[37] presents as a typical Huntington's disease, or, more frequently, as the rigid variant in children and adolescents. The child appears to develop normally, then shows progressive rigidity, ataxia, dementia, and seizures. The course is more rapid than the adult form of the disease, and death occurs within a few years of onset.[88]

Both variants may exhibit marked dystonia, and seizures are more common than in the classic forms of Huntington's disease. Some atypical cases have prominent cerebellar signs.[170]

Diagnostic Procedures

1. The electroencephalogram shows progressive loss of alpha activity with generalized slowing as the disease progresses. Low-voltage records, which are unusual in other chronic neurologic disorders, occur in about 30 per cent of cases.[209]
2. Computed tomography shows ventricular dilatation, which is particularly marked in the frontal poles of the lateral ventricles (Fig. 4–3). Here, the lateral wall shows marked convexity or ballooning due to loss of the bulk of the caudate nucleus. The CT scan may be normal early in the disease.
3. Gamma aminobutyric acid is significantly reduced in the cerebrospinal fluid.[67]
4. Early diagnosis, particularly in siblings of known patients with Huntington's disease, may be obtained by psychologic tests, which are a sensitive indicator of disorders of perception, visuomotor coordination, and visual perception. The verbal intelligent quotient (IQ) is higher than the performance IQ in almost all cases of organic dementia.
5. It is believed that levodopa may produce choreiform movements in family members of patients with Huntington's disease who will develop overt signs of the disease at a later date. Levodopa does not produce choreiform movements in control subjects in doses of 2 to 5 gm daily for ten weeks or when given in doses of 800 mg daily with 200 mg peripheral dopa decarboxylase inhibitor for ten days. Choreiform movements do occur in some subjects at risk, which disappear when the drug is discontinued. These subjects may develop Huntington's disease later. However, failure to de-

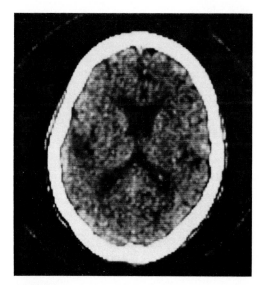

FIGURE 4–3. Computed tomography in Huntington's disease. There is slight ventricular enlargement, particularly affecting the frontal horns. The prominent sulci indicate early cortical atrophy.

velop choreiform movements does not rule out Huntington's disease.[139, 140]

Treatment

1. Depression is a common early symptom of Huntington's disease. There is risk of suicide in such patients, which requires proper precautionary and therapeutic measures. Benefit is often obtained by the use of the so-called "antidepressive" or "psychic energizer" group of drugs such as isocarboxazid, 10 mg tid, or amitriptyline, 25 mg tid.
2. Haloperidol, 3 to 6 mg daily, has been shown to be extremely effective in controlling choreoathetotic movements in advanced cases of Huntington's disease.[68, 137-139, 175]
3. The abnormal athetotic movements are considerably improved by the phenothiazine group of drugs early in the disease: chlorpromazine, in doses up to 150 mg daily; perphenazine, 10 to 16 mg tid; or trifluoperazine, 2 mg tid.
4. Reserpine is effective in controlling involuntary movements in some cases if the dose is gradually increased up to 3 to 5 gm daily.[136]
5. Tetrabenazine, 50 mg tid, is also effective in decreasing involuntary movements.[222]
6. Apomorphine hydrochloride, 1 to 4 mg IM, may produce a marked decrease in involuntary movements.[44a]
7. Administration of bromocriptine increases the choreoathetoid movements in Huntington's disease,[131] and choline is also ineffective in this disease.[100] The efficacy of drugs that inhibit GABA-degrading enzymes remains to be tested in man.[208] GABA-mimetic drugs ameliorate involuntary movements but do not improve motor or cognitive functions.[212a]

Jakob-Creutzfeldt Disease (Spongioform Encephalopathy, Spastic Pseudosclerosis)

Etiology and Pathogenesis

This condition, usually regarded as the most rapidly progressive of the neuronal degenerations, is caused by a transmissible agent that is either a virus or viroid.[17, 19] Jakob-Creutzfeldt disease can be transmitted to laboratory animals and has now been retransmitted through several generations of animals. Human-to-human transmission has been recorded in a family[34a] and in a patient who received a corneal transplant from a patient who died of Jakob-Creutzfeldt disease, and the disease has also been accidentally transmitted to a neurosurgeon.

Papovavirus-like particles have been seen in brain tissue from patients with this disease.[50]

Pathology

The brain shows evidence of cortical atrophy, particularly involving the frontal lobes with lesser involvement of other parts of cerebral hemispheres. There is generalized ventricular dilatation, but the blood vessels are healthy. There is profound loss of neurons in the cerebral cortex, the basal ganglia, thalamus, brainstem, and even in the spinal cord. Loss of nerve cells occurs in the cortex and dentate nucleus of the cerebellum in about 50 per cent of cases. Surviving neurons are swollen, with poorly staining nuclei and loss of Nissl granules. Microglial reaction is slight, but there is marked proliferation of astrocytes. In some cases numerous small lacunae occur in the gray matter (status spongiosus) and are believed to be the result of swelling of degenerated astrocytes.[160] There is some loss of white matter, which is secondary to neuronal degeneration.

Clinical Features

The condition is usually sporadic but has occasionally occurred in families. Both sexes are affected, and the disease usually begins between the ages of 40 and 70 years. It is rapidly progressive and death usually occurs some 3 to 24 months from the onset.

As would be expected with widespread involvement of the central nervous system, symptoms are protean in this disease, but it is possible to recognize five types.

The Classic Type of Jakob-Creutzfeldt Disease. The condition begins with lapses of memory and rapidly deteriorates to severe dementia. The early symptoms include dysphasia with deterioration in personal grooming. Extrapyramidal signs become evident with a fixed facial expression, stooped gait, and parkinsonian tremor. Ataxia, dysarthria, and intention tremor owing to cerebellar involvement may also appear.[33] Temper outbursts are not uncommon but are usually replaced by mumbling and perseveration. Myoclonic jerks, choreiform movements, increased startle response, and seizures may accompany the above symptoms and signs.[73] The end result is a profoundly demented, wasted, aphasic, incontinent, rigid, and bedridden patient.

The Subacute Spongiform Encephalopathic Type (Nevin-Jones). This is a rapidly progressive variant of Jakob-Creutzfeldt disease occurring in adults of both sexes.[158a,172] The initial symptoms are headache, generalized weakness, poor concentration, and episodic confusion with rapid progression to incapacitating dementia in one or two months. There are also signs of dysphasia, spasticity, rigidity, and myoclonic jerks which terminate in akinetic mutism. The myoclonus is sensitive to light and sound, and some patients have recurrent seizures. Death occurs within three months of onset.[89]

The Optic Type (Heidenhain's Type). This condition has many of the features of the classic type with the addition of prominent signs of involvement of the occipital cortex.[27] The patient may exhibit visual agnosia, poor color perception, and photopsia in the early stages of the disease, but there is rapid progression to complete cortical blindness. Additional neurologic signs of progressive dementia, dysarthria, spasticity, rigidity, myoclonic jerks, and seizures develop during the course of illness.[203]

The Cerebellar Type. A number of patients present with a progressive cerebellar ataxia that precedes the development of dementia.[90, 128] Cerebellar signs are eventually present in the majority of patients with Jakob-Creutzfeldt disease.

The Amyotrophic Type. This variant presents as a rapidly progressive amyotrophic lateral sclerosis, with progressive dementia. Signs of corticospinal tract and anterior horn cell involvement are prominent with increased tendon reflexes, fasciculations, and muscular atrophy. Progressive dysarthria, ataxia, and tremor appear as the condition progresses.

Diagnostic Procedures

1. Two types of electroencephalographic abnormality have been described.[87]
    a. Generalized progressive slowing, followed by loss of normal background activity and progression to generalized irregular delta activity, is seen in some cases.
    b. The development of distinctive 1-per-second generalized synchronous sharp waves occurs late in the disease (Fig. 4–4). Serial electroencephalography is recommended to facilitate the diagnosis of this condition.[64]
2. Computed tomography may be normal[39] or show rapidly progressive atrophic changes on serial computed tomograms of the brain.[192]
3. The diagnosis may be confirmed during life by brain biopsy. Cultures of brain biopsy tissue contain large globular cells with multiple cytoplasmic vacuoles. This finding is believed to

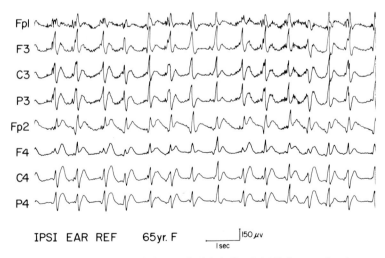

IPSI EAR REF   65yr. F $\rfloor$150 μv
_____ 1 sec

FIGURE 4–4. Electroencephalogram in Jakob-Creutzfeldt disease showing repetitive high-voltage sharp wave discharges continuously over both hemispheres and complete absence of normal background rhythms.

be a characteristic feature of Jakob-Creutzfeldt disease.[65]

Treatment

1. a. Because of the risk of human-to-human transmission, all patients with suspected Jakob-Creutzfeld disease should be nursed in isolation and all personnel must observe isolation procedures.
   b. Disposable equipment such as linens and dishes should be used whenever possible. All equipment whether disposable or non-disposable should be double-bagged and must be autoclaved for one hour at 121°C and 20 psi.
   c. Hands must be washed before and after patient contact with antimicrobial soap and dried on paper towels.
   d. Brain biopsy should be performed with septic precautions and minimal personnel involved. All disposable and nondisposable materials should be autoclaved for one hour at 121°C and 20 psi.
   e. The neuropathologist must consider all tissues from a suspected case of Jakob-Creutzfeldt disease as fully infectious even after prolonged fixation in formalin and histologic processing.
2. Therapy with antiviral agents has not been of benefit, and treatment remains symptomatic in this distressing and rapidly progressive disease.

Leber's Optic Atrophy

The descriptive term "optic atrophy" is often an artificially restricted one as applied to many of the cases with this condition reported in the literature. In many, the optic atrophy has been part of a more generalized degenerative disease affecting the central nervous system.

Etiology and Pathology

There is some evidence that Leber's optic atrophy is a hereditary metabolic disorder of cyanide metabolism.[74] It is usually inherited as an autosomal dominant trait, although sporadic cases do occur. The major abnormalities in the central nervous system include loss of ganglion cells in the retina, demyelination, and loss of axons in the optic nerves. In addition, many of the cases have shown patchy loss of myelin and axonal degeneration throughout the brain and spinal cord

with marked astroglial gliosis. Neuronal loss is variable but not severe.[146]

Clinical Features

The condition usually presents in the teens or early twenties with the rapid onset of loss of vision in one or both eyes over a few weeks. Large central scotomas develop, and the optic disk appears pale on fundoscopy. The majority of patients show progressive visual deterioration to blindness after several months or years, but approximately 20 per cent show improvement in one or both eyes. Several cases of total recovery have been reported.[34]

After an interval of several years, which may be as long as 40 years in some cases, there are signs of more diffuse involvement of the central nervous system. Associated symptoms and signs include progressive dementia, depression, signs of bulbar involvement, ataxia of both the cerebellar and spinal types, spastic paraplegia, and loss of sphincter control. There may be muscle wasting and fasciculations in some cases.

Most patients have large central scotomas or complete blindness with optic atrophy, increased tendon jerks, and extensor plantar responses. The sensory loss is usually compatible with posterior column degeneration. This disorder must be differentiated from multiple sclerosis and tumors in or near the optic chiasm.

Diagnostic Procedures

Pattern-reversal visual-evoked potentials (VEP) are normal prior to the onset of visual symptoms. Once visual symptoms appear, there is prolonged VEP latency. There is progressive prolongation of VEP latency as visual acuity declines until VEP can no longer be measured.[52]

Treatment

Tobacco smoke has been implicated as a predisposing or causative factor in this disease since tobacco smoke contains cyanide.[74] Patients with Leber's optic atrophy should be advised to cease smoking. Certain bacterial infections, particularly those due to *Pseudomonas pyocyaneus* and *Escherichia coli,* increase cyanide concentrations in body fluids. Urinary tract infections by these organisms should be treated promptly because of the possible implication of cyanide in this condition. Since hydroxycobalamin has cyanide-binding properties, massive doses given intramuscularly in doses of 2,000 μg twice weekly may have value.

Progressive Supranuclear Palsy

A variety of names have been given to this rare form of neuronal degeneration, including oculofaciocervical dystonia,[41] subcortical argyrophilic dystrophy, and heterogenerous system degeneration. None of these terms is satisfactory, and the term "progressive supranuclear palsy" has been retained because it affords a clinical method of differentiating the condition from the group of diseases usually labeled as presenile dementias.

Etiology and Pathology

The etiology is unknown, but the disease is believed to be an example of a neuronal degeneration in the presenile and senile dementia groups.[232]

The brain usually has a normal appearance, both externally and when sectioned, without evidence of ventricular dilatation. There may be some loss of pigment in the substantia nigra and locus ceruleus. The microscopic features consist of a marked loss of neurons with neurofibrillary tangles and granulovacuolar degeneration in many of the surviving cells of the basal ganglia, brainstem, and cerebellum. The changes are most marked in the globus pallidus, subthalamic nucleus, substantia nigra, red nucleus, superior colliculus, locus ceruleus, periaqueductal gray, pontine tegmentum, and the olivary, cuneate, gracile, and dentate nuclei.[124] The cerebral cortex shows similar changes with neurofibrillary tangles in the smaller neurons of the third layer of the cortex especially in the hippocampus.[123] There is some microglial proliferation with secondary gliosis in the severely affected areas together with demyelination of the connecting tracts of the basal ganglia. The corticospinal tracts and posterior columns of the spinal cord show some degree of demyelination with axonal loss and gliosis. The peripheral nerves have also been reported to show focal areas of demyelination with loss of axons and endoneural fibrosis.[220]

Clinical Features

The essential features of this condition are chronic progressive dementia of "subcortical" type 2 associated with progressive gaze palsies with predominant disturbance of vertical movements of the eyes, followed by loss of horizontal eye movements occurring later.[125, 230] There may be signs of pseudobulbar palsy with dysarthria, dysphagia, and blepharospasm.[165] The proximal limbs, neck, and trunk show a varying degree of muscular rigidity, dystonia, and occasionally tremor. The extrapyramidal signs are generally more marked in the face, neck, and upper trunk. The deep tendon reflexes are increased with bilateral extensor plantar responses, while signs of cerebellar involvement are often mild. Some involvement of the peripheral nerves and posterior columns has also been reported in some cases with distal wasting, particularly in the lower limbs, and this gives a "stork leg" appearance. There may be some peripheral loss of pinprick sensation and reduction of vibration sense at the ankle and toes.

Treatment

Levodopa or carbidopa may reduce rigidity and improve pseudobulbar symptoms in some cases. The loss of vertical eye movements prevents reading, which is distressing to many patients. The use of prism spectacles may help the patient to read material that is held comfortably in the lap.

Retinitis Pigmentosa

Retinitis pigmentosa is a hereditary degenerative disease of the retina that may be inherited as an autosomal recessive trait and rarely as an autosomal dominant or sex-linked recessive condition. It has been suggested that retinitis pigmentosa may be caused by an inborn error of copper metabolism.[78]

Pathology

The retina shows complete loss of rods with degenerative changes in the cones, and neuroglial proliferation. There is an irregular migration of pigment-containing cells into the superficial layers of the retina. The optic nerve may show some gliosis, but there is usually little evidence of atrophy even in an eye that has been completely blind for many years. Most patients develop posterior polar cataracts, and glaucoma is an occasional finding.

Clinical Features

Symptoms frequently develop in early childhood beginning with night blindness and followed by some failing of vision in the teens. There is progressive constriction of the visual fields throughout adult life, and the majority of patients are completely blind by 50 years of age. Early cases show a ring scotoma in the midportion of the visual fields, which gradually spreads peripherally and centrally. In the final stages there is a small central area of vision, which may persist for many years before showing a gradual deterioration to complete blindness.

In some cases the field defect begins centrally and extends peripherally ("inverse" retinitis pigmentosa). Associated degeneration of the auditory nerve and deafness are not infrequent.

Diagnostic Procedures

Visual-evoked potentials are abnormal[201] and show progressive increase in latency during the course of the disease.

Treatment

There is no treatment which affects or delays the degeneration in the retina.

A number of neurologic syndromes have been described that are associated with pigmentary degeneration of the retina:

1. Mental retardation
2. Epilepsy
3. The spinocerebellar degenerations including Friedreich's ataxia and cortical cerebellar atrophy
4. Hereditary spastic ataxia and spastic quadriparesis
5. Progressive ophthalmoplegia
6. Laurence-Moon-Biedl syndrome
7. Heredopathia atactica polyneuritiformis (Refsum's disease)
8. Kearns-Sayre syndrome (p. 728)
9. Homocarsinosis (familial spastic paraplegia, progressive mental deterioration, and retinal pigmentation[215]

The Laurence-Moon-Biedl Syndrome

The association of retinitis pigmentosa with mental retardation, obesity, hypogonadism, and polydactyly is inherited as an autosomal recessive trait and has been termed the Laurence-Moon-Biedl syndrome.

Clinical Features

The condition presents with mental retardation and obesity in infancy, with visual failure due to retinitis pigmentosa beginning somewhat later in childhood. Hypogonadism and polydactyly are usually but not invariably present. Other defects including syndactyly, deafness, microcephaly, shortness of stature, and kidney defects[70] may occasionally occur in this syndrome. Retinitis pigmentosa is typical in only about 20 per cent of cases and has been described as atypical with finely scattered pigment throughout the retina in the others. Optic atrophy is rarely present.

Treatment

There is no specific treatment for this condition, but replacement therapy with pituitary hormones may produce some improvement in the obesity and hypogonadism.

The Shy-Drager Syndrome (Orthostatic Hypotension with Multisystem Degeneration)

The association of orthostatic hypotension with other signs of progressive neuronal degeneration of the central nervous system particularly affecting the autonomic system is usually called the Shy-Drager syndrome. The condition is classified with the neuronal degenerations since, at necropsy, loss of the autonomic neurons in the brainstem and spinal cord, with or without neuronal atrophy in other systems, has been consistently found.[151]

Etiology and Pathology

The condition is usually sporadic but has been reported to occur in families where it appears to be inherited as an autosomal dominant trait. Neuropathologic changes consist of neuronal degeneration, neuronal loss, and gliosis. The most striking neuronal loss in the spinal cord occurs in the intermediolateral column of the spinal cord, accounting for the loss of autonomic function. Neuronal loss is also found in the hypothalamus, locus ceruleus, and substantia nigra. The peripheral autonomic ganglia show less involvement and may be normal. There may be some neuronal loss in the inferior olivary nucleus, the basal ganglia, and particularly the putamen and the Edinger-Westphal nuclei. There may be loss of nerve cells in the cerebellum, particularly the Purkinje cell layer. Cytoplasmic inclusions, similar to Lewy bodies, have been described in the substantia nigra and locus ceruleus. Changes in the anterior horns are less striking, but there is some chromatolysis and loss of neurofibrils in the neurons.[207, 227] As a result there is a central loss of autonomic function. Since cerebral autoregulation is impaired, postural syncope and other signs of orthostatic cerebral ischemia are extremely common.[166]

Clinical Features

The onset is usually in the fourth to seventh decades, and the symptoms show variations from case to case according to the site of neuronal degeneration. The presenting symptoms may be urinary urgency and frequency with progression to complete urinary incontinence. Sexual impotence is a common symptom in the male. The incapacitating symptoms which are characteristic of this syndrome are central neurogenic (orthostatic) hypotension with orthostatic syncope, ataxia, blurring of vision, and complaints of vertigo and dizziness. Part of the cerebellar signs may be due to episodes of ischemia. Some patients complain of and exhibit patchy loss of sweating. Fasciculations occur in some cases. On examination there are marked postural hypotension and dysarthria without dementia. There may be unequal pupils and, rarely, extraocular palsy and atrophy of the iris. Some cases show parkinsonian features with loss of facial expression, rigidity, and tremor. Muscle wasting and fasciculations may be present. Cerebellar ataxia involving both the trunk and limbs is evident in some patients, and in these cases the deep tendon reflexes are depressed or absent. Other cases have been reported with increased tone, hyperreflexia, and extensor plantar responses. Sensation is usually normal, but the skin is dry and areas of diminished or absent sweating may be present. The rectal sphincter may show diminished tone.

The disease runs a chronic and progressive course, and death usually occurs due to pneumonia and respiratory insufficiency about ten years after the onset of neurologic symptoms. Sporadic cases have been reported with a more chronic form of the disease. Some cases present with severe postural hypotension and clinical features resembling striatal-nigral degeneration or olivopontocerebellar degeneration. It is apparent that there are at least three variants of this spectrum of degenerative disease. All three have severe orthostatic hypotension due to central autonomic neuronal degeneration in common. These may be categorized as the extrapyramidal, amyotrophic, or olivopontocerebellar forms.

Diagnostic Procedures

1. The cerebrospinal fluid is normal.
2. Roentgenograms of the skull and chest are usually normal.
3. The sweat test (administer acetylsalicylic acid, 600 mg; 900 ml hot tea; and paint the body with 2.5 per cent iodine and starch; cover with blankets; and expose to a heat lamp for 30 minutes) usually shows patchy reduction or absence of sweating over the trunk and limbs.
4. Cystometrogram usually indicates a hypotonic or atonic bladder.
5. Slit lamp examination may reveal atrophy of the iris.
6. Electromyography may reveal diffuse fibrillations and fasciculations, and nerve conduction velocities may be prolonged in the lower limbs.
7. There is an excessive response to the injection of small doses of pressor amines (e.g., 0.2 ml, 1 : 1,000 epinephrine solution injected subcutaneously).
8. The Valsalva maneuver with recorded blood pressure shows absence of bradycardia and the usual postapneic overshoot.

Treatment

1. Efforts to overcome the postural hypotension include a high salt intake, fludrocortisone acetate in divided doses of 0.3 to 0.6 mg daily, and maintenance of good muscle tone in the lower extremities with elastic stockings or a pressure suit.
2. Levodopa provides no improvement in the parkinsonian symptoms, and it may increase the postural hypotension.[5] The use of monoamine oxidase inhibitors and tyrosine-containing foods (such as cheddar cheese) may increase the production of norepinephine.[166]

Disorders with Involuntary Movements

Parkinson's Disease

The term "Parkinson's disease" refers to what should be more accurately termed the parkinsonian syndrome, which is a variety of conditions of different etiologies that present with a similar clinical appearance. The criteria for inclusion in the syndrome are the presence of rigidity, tremor, and bradykinesis. These symptoms are known to occur in many chronic diseases of the nervous system and can be induced by certain drugs and toxins (Table 4–1).

TABLE 4–1

The Parkinsonian Syndrome

1. Paralysis agitans
2. Postencephalitic parkinsonism
3. Arteriosclerotic parkinsonism and parkinsonism following anoxia and cerebral ischemia
4. Striatonigral degeneration
5. Drug-induced parkinsonism—reserpine, phenothiazines, alpha-methyldopa
6. Infectious diseases—viral encephalitis, meningovascular syphilis
7. Toxic parkinsonism—manganese, carbon monoxide, carbon disulfide
8. Parkinsonian features in other chronic neurologic conditions—Huntington's disease; Wilson's disease; Alzheimer's disease; olivopontocerebellar degeneration; Shy-Drager syndrome; progressive supranuclear palsy; Jakob-Creutzfeldt disease; parkinsonism–dementia complex

Two most frequent causes of the parkinsonian syndrome are idiopathic parkinsonism, or paralysis agitans, and postencephalitic parkinsonism. At the present time it is estimated that 36,000 new cases of parkinsonism occur annually in the United States. The overall incidence is about 1 per cent of the population over the age of 50 years. This means that parkinsonism, in particular paralysis agitans, is a major public health problem in the older section of the population which is likely to be compounded by the increasing numbers of people aged 50 years or older in North America. On the other hand, there has been a decrease in the incidence of postencephalitic parkinsonism, the vast majority of these cases having occurred as a sequel to the pandemic of encephalitis lethargica in the years 1916 to 1926.[54, 55]

Etiology

Dopamine is produced in the neurons of the pars compacta of the substantia nigra and reaches the corpus striatum via the axons of the nigrostriatal pathway. The principal synthetic and metabolic pathways of dopamine in the CNS are summarized in Figure 4–5.

The activity of the alpha and gamma motor systems is altered by influences arising at different levels in the nervous system. One of the most active systems, which has both excitatory and inhibitory effects on motor neurons, is mediated via the corpus striatum. Biochemical analysis of the corpus striatum (caudate nucleus, putamen, and globus pallidus) in normal brain shows high concentrations of dopamine, but dopamine concentration is significantly decreased in parkinsonism. Dopamine is an important neurotransmitter since its presence is necessary for the normal functioning of the excitatory pathways to the gamma motor neurons. Loss of this action releases unrestricted inhibition of the gamma neuron, which is mediated via the corpus striatum by a cholinergic neurotransmitter system. Hence, anticholinergic drugs tend to improve the symptoms of parkinsonism.

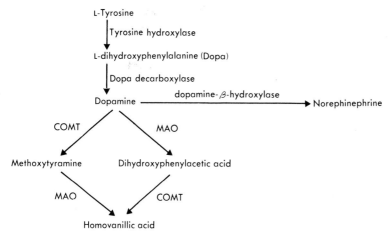

FIGURE 4–5. Synthesis and metabolism of dopamine.

The cardinal clinical features of Parkinson's syndrome include bradykinesia, rigidity, and tremor. These result from an imbalance in the activity of the alpha and gamma motor systems.[179] There appear to be depression of gamma activity and increased alpha activity.[214]

Bradykinesia. Patients show both brady-kinesia[210] and hypokinesia due to difficulty in initiating voluntary movements. Bradykinesia and hypokinesia are the result of increased inhibitory influences from the higher centers which act on the gamma neuron. One of the main inhibitory pathways projects via the ventrolateral nucleus of the thalamus, which accounts for the effectiveness of thalamotomy in parkinsonism.

Rigidity. The increased tone of both antagonist and protagonist muscle groups in parkinsonism is due to augmentation of alpha motor neuron activity. Rigidity, which occurs in animals treated with reserpine, has also been shown to result from increased alpha motor neuron activity and decreased gamma activity. Furthermore, reserpine depletes dopamine concentration in the corpus striatum, which is the characteristic biochemical abnormality in Parkinson's syndrome. The experimental production of rigidity by reserpine can be abolished by administration of levodopa with return of normal gamma efferent activity and reduction of excessive alpha motor neuron activity to normal levels.

Tremor. When the gamma motor neuron system is inhibited and the gamma circuit loses sensitivity as a servo mechanism, this loss of sensitivity decreases the fine control of motor movement and posture with the production of tremor at rest. Tremor is associated with heightened activation of the alpha motor neuron system, which is influenced by rhythmic discharges projected through the ventrolateral nucleus of the thalamus.

In summary, parkinsonism may be defined in pathophysiologic terms as an imbalance between excitatory and inhibitory striatal influences, or it may be defined in biochemical terms as an imbalance between dopamine-activated and acetylcholine-activated neurons of the corpus striatum.[53]

Pathology

The essential pathologic change in paralysis agitans is neuronal loss in the substantia nigra.[164]

The cell loss is incomplete but occurs mainly in the zona compacta. Surviving cells usually contain hyaline intracytoplasmic inclusions known as Lewy bodies, which are rich in sphingomyelin.[49] Involvement of the corpus striatum and other areas of the brain and brainstem has been described but is not considered specific for paralysis agitans.

Destruction of neurons in the substantia nigra is regularly found with lack of melanin pigmentation in this area, which may be quite striking on gross inspection of the sections of midbrain. Other pathologic changes may be diffuse, involving cerebral cortex, basal ganglia, thalamus, and brainstem with ventricular dilatation in some cases. There is marked neuronal degeneration in the locus ceruleus, oculomotor nucleus, and dorsal nucleus of the vagus. Surviving neurons in the brainstem nuclei and scattered neurons throughout other areas show neurofibrillary tangles, which are often particularly marked in Sommer's sector of the hippocampus.

The pathologic changes caused by other conditions producing the parkinsonian syndrome show considerable variation. The brain may show numerous areas of lacunar infarction of varying sizes in hypertensive arteriosclerotic and syphilitic parkinsonism, while toxic substances, such as manganese, carbon monoxide, and carbon disulfide, produce diffuse neuronal loss, usually most marked in the basal ganglia.

Clinical Features

Paralysis Agitans. The presenting symptom may be either tremor or rigidity. Tremor appears initially in the distal muscles of the limbs, often beginning with rhythmic apposition of thumb and index finger at a rate of four to eight per second. This is the characteristic "pill-rolling tremor." It is usually regular but occasionally may be irregular in amplitude. The tremor occasionally affects one limb and may be confined to this limb for months or years before affecting the opposite side. Eventually, all four limbs, lips, tongue, jaw, and neck are involved. There is some improvement of the tremor with the development of rigidity. The tremor also disappears during sleep and is increased by muscular exertion or emotional stress.

Rigidity is the most common sign of paralysis agitans and is due to an increase in tonic innervation resulting from excess reflex responses to muscle stretch. There is free movement between five and ten degrees when the affected limb is passively moved. Thereafter there is tonic contraction of the stretched muscle. The cogwheel phenomenon is due to regular contraction and relaxation of the muscle as stretching continues. Rigidity usually appears proximally in one limb and spreads distally. It is usually seen initially in the shoulder followed by involvement of the forearm and hand. This type of involvement results in early loss of swinging of the arm when walking (loss of associated movements), and this may be the first symptom of paralysis agitans. The involvement of one upper limb is almost inevitably followed by some involvement of the opposite side. Rigidity of the neck and axial muscles is responsible for the flexed attitude which is the hallmark of advanced disease. When rigidity spreads to the face, this results in the characteristic masklike facies with immobility, loss of skin creases, and infrequent smiling and blinking.

Patients with paralysis agitans complain of weakness and easy fatigue. However, there is no loss of muscle bulk or obvious weakness on testing individual muscles, and the deep tendon reflexes are normal. The bradykinesis induced by the rigidity produces slowness of finger movements with difficulty in fine motor performance such as buttoning buttons and in writing. The handwriting becomes characteristically cramped and small-formed ("micrographia"). Tremor further distorts the writing, which may be illegible in severe cases. Pseudobulbar involvement of speech results in gradual loss of amplitude as the disease progresses, and speech may become reduced to a whisper. It is slowed, monotonous, and without inflection.

The gait is characteristic with small steps as though chasing the center of gravity, a condition called festination. The general flexed posture and the tendency to fall forward result in progressive acceleration with small steps (propulsion), which may terminate in a fall. Similarly, the phenomenon of retropulsion or lateropulsion may occur if the patient is suddenly pushed backward or to one side, and in certain unusual forms of the disease these movements may occur spontaneously when the patient stands or walks.

Although paralysis agitans is usually considered to be a disease limited to the motor system, sensory symptoms are not unusual. Many patients complain of pain, which is often intermittent, cramplike, and poorly localized. Others experience paresthesias, particularly in the distal extremities. The sensory symptoms are present in early cases of paralysis agitans and apparently originate within the nervous system.[216]

Some degree of autonomic dysfunction is present in most patients with paralysis agitans, including abnormalities in sweating, excess salivation, bladder and bowel dysfunction, and orthostatic hypotension. The autonomic disturbances are due to cell loss in sympathetic ganglia, which may be progressive,[193] and orthostatic hypotension can be a major problem in the management of some patients.

Dementia occurs in about one third of patients with paralysis agitans. The dementia tends to be more marked in the more severely disabled patients, and there is a positive correlation between severity of rigidity, hypokinesia, and dementia.[115, 158]

In chronic, severe, and neglected cases the patient may become bedridden with flexion contractures of the limbs. Pain in the immobile and rigid muscles and joints is often severe. Progressive intellectual deterioration may follow with impairment of retention, recent memory, and calculation. In the majority of untreated patients, the disease progresses slowly and significantly reduces the life-span, but with medical treatment and active physical therapy, the mortality rate is significantly reduced, although it remains in excess of that in the general population.[129a]

Postencephalitic Parkinsonism. This form of the parkinsonian syndrome resulted almost exclusively from a pandemic of encephalitis lethargica that began in 1918 and lasted until 1928. Fortunately, there have been no new epidemics, so that there has been a steady decrease in the number of patients who can be classified in this group. The history of acute encephalitis usually includes an acute illness with fever, clouding of consciousness, cranial nerve palsies, and hyperkinetic behavior. A few patients developed signs of parkinsonism in the acute phase. The majority made an apparently complete clinical recovery but developed the signs of the disease months or years later. Occasionally patients in this group have been diagnosed as having postencephalitic parkinsonism because of the development of characteristic symptoms seen only in this type of disorder. In these cases it was inferred that they had suffered from a subclinical attack of encephalitis lethargica during the years of the epidemic.

Patients with postencephalitic parkinsonism

show most of the signs of paralysis agitans with certain additional features. One of the most common pathognomonic and dramatic symptoms is the oculogyric crisis. This consists of a tonic conjugate deviation of the eyes, usually in the vertical plane, which may last for a period varying from a few to 20 minutes. Some patients experience blepharospasm, while others have marked retraction of the upper lids which may result in inflammation of the eyes. Paralysis of accommodation and nystagmus may occur, and loss of smooth saccadic eye movements is common. Irregularity of respiration is also more common in the postencephalitic group, and pulmonary function may be impaired with increased risk of pneumonia.

Autonomic disturbances include sialorrhea with drooling of saliva from the corners of the mouth and almost continuous perspiration producing an oily or shiny appearance to the skin of the face. Postural hypotension and vasomotor, sudomotor, pilomotor, and bladder disturbances have all been documented in this disease.[4]

A number of patients with postencephalitic parkinsonism develop psychotic behavior and dementia.

There are still occasional reports of the rapid onset of parkinsonism following an attack of a viral encephalitis.[121, 198, 213] This suggests that there are still a small number of new cases of postencephalitic parkinsonism entering the total population of patients with Parkinson's disease.

Arteriosclerotic Parkinsonism. While coincidental paralysis agitans undoubtedly occurs in patients with cerebral arteriosclerosis, there is an additional group of patients who can be classified as having arteriosclerotic parkinsonism because of the coexistence of symptoms of parkinsonism and occlusive cerebrovascular disease. These patients are usually hypertensive with a history of transient ischemic episodes or of past focal neurologic deficits due to lacunar infarcts in the pons and basal ganglia. These "little strokes" may be frequent and are eventually associated with signs of rigidity, bradykinesis, and masklike facies. A short-steppage gait or gait à petit pas is common. "Pseudobulbar palsy," with sudden inappropriate crying, dysarthria, and dysphagia, may be prominent. Additional features include incontinence and progressive dementia. The brain shows evidence of numerous subcortical infarcts, usually of the lacunar type, distributed through the basal ganglia and brainstem.

Diagnostic Procedures

A number of recording devices have been designed to measure rigidity, tremor, and bradykinesia in Parkinson's disease. At this time, their use is limited to research centers, but a number of simple clinical tests can be given to patients periodically to assess the effectiveness of medication.

Rigidity may be accentuated if the patient extends the arm and rapidly flexes and extends the fingers while the opposite limb is moved passively by the examiner. Similarly, rigidity is increased in the lower limbs by Jendrassik's maneuver. Any minor form of stress accentuates tremor. The patient may be asked to count backward from 100 with the arms extended or may be given a rapid series of simple arithmetic problems, while the observer notes the degree of tremor. At each visit a record of tremor may be obtained by asking the patient to draw a square, a circle, and a series of concentric circles. He should also write his name, address, and a simple sentence. Serial records should be compared to note the efficacy of therapy.

A useful measurement of functional activity is shown in Figure 4–6. This scheme permits comparison of performance at each visit.

Computed tomography of the brain may show evidence of ventricular dilatation and diffuse cortical atrophy in the more advanced cases of parkinsonism, particularly in patients with dementia (Fig. 4–7).

Treatment

Untreated parkinsonism, in all its forms, is a chronic, progressive, disabling, and often depressive illness. The patient and the family should be assured that much can be done therapeutically, but this requires close cooperation between patient and physician. If the physician explains these facts to the patient, he must accept the obligation of treating the patient over a long period of time and of making himself available to discuss problems that may arise.

Medical Therapy. The principal metabolic pathways in the synthesis of dopamine from L-tyrosine, the conversion of dopamine to norepinephrine, and the catabolism of dopamine to homovanillic acid are summarized in Figure 4–5.[218]

The most important contribution to the treatment of parkinsonism is replacement therapy with levodopa,[45, 235] which passes the blood-brain bar-

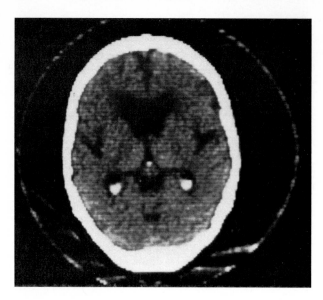

FIGURE 4–6. Computed tomography in advanced Parkinson's disease with dementia. There is ventricular enlargement with cortical atrophy.

rier. Dopamine is unable to pass the blood-brain barrier, and the levodopa is converted to dopamine in the brain, replenishing depleted dopamine stores in the brainstem and basal ganglia.[57, 76, 96] Large oral doses of levodopa may be required for adequate replacement of depleted dopamine in the brain. Administration of 6 to 9 gm daily may occasionally be necessary (see Table 4–2), but the average dose is 3.5 to 4.0 gm daily in most cases.[194] Side effects are common but are fewer when the dose is gradually increased by 250- to 500-mg increments every five days. The most common side effects are nausea and vomiting. Mental confusion may occur.[119] Improvement of symptoms usually begins to appear after one or two weeks of treatment or when the daily dose exceeds 2.5 gm daily, and further improvement occurs thereafter as the dose is increased. Overdosage results in postural hypotension, abnormal involuntary movements such as grimacing and sucking movements of the mouth, and choreoathetotic movements of the neck and extremities. These symptoms may be due to increased plasma O-methyl-dopa levels [184a] and are readily reversible once the dosage is reduced. The dosage tolerance of each patient for levodopa is unpredictable.

Combined therapy using levodopa plus drugs which block extracerebral dopa-decarboxylase activity enhances the uptake of levodopa by the brain and reduces the amount of levodopa that must be administered daily. This has the effect of decreasing toxic side effects of levodopa therapy and producing more rapid and smooth relief of symptoms.[36]

The two most commonly used dopadecarboxylase inhibitors are L-alphamethyldopahydrazine (carbidopa) and benserazide hydrochloride. Both are equally effective in double-blind trials.[92] The levodopa/carbidopa combination (Sinemet) is widely used in the United States at this time.

The advantages of treating patients with levodopa and a dopadecarboxylase inhibitor include the following:[147] (1) The optimally effective dose of levodopa can be reduced by about 75 per cent. (2) Nausea and vomiting are reduced. (3) Effective therapeutic levels can be achieved quickly. (4) Competitive antagonism of the therapeutic effect of levodopa by dietary pyridoxine is avoided. (5) The number of patients responding to treatment is increased. The incidence of side effects including orthostatic hypotension, abnormal involuntary movements, and mental confusion is unchanged.

At this time it seems that levodopa or levodopa/carbidopa is the most effective treatment of most forms of Parkinson's disease.[236]

The drugs are less effective in advanced cases where dementia, depression, or lack of motivation is present. Therapy may have to be discontinued in about 25 to 30 per cent of patients because of lack of therapeutic results or because of intolerable side effects. In general, the majority of patients show a gratifying reduction in rigidity and

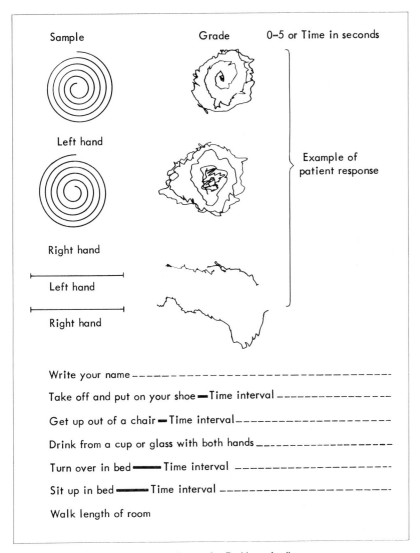

Sample   Grade   0–5 or Time in seconds

Left hand

Right hand   Example of
                                              patient response

Left hand

Right hand

Write your name _

Take off and put on your shoe ▬Time interval _ _ _ _ _ _ _ _ _ _ _ _ _ _ _ _ _

Get up out of a chair ▬Time interval _

Drink from a cup or glass with both hands _ _ _ _ _ _ _ _ _ _ _ _ _ _ _ _ _ _

Turn over in bed ▬▬▬Time interval _ _ _ _ _ _ _ _ _ _ _ _ _ _ _ _ _ _ _

Sit up in bed ▬▬▬Time interval _ _ _ _ _ _ _ _ _ _ _ _ _ _ _ _ _ _ _

Walk length of room

FIGURE 4–7. Diagram of standard tests for Parkinson's disease.

bradykinesia with improvement in mood and a temporary improvement in memory.[104] However, the patient with parkinsonism may run into problems during long-term levodopa or levodopa/carbidopa therapy. There may be an insidious loss of benefit from drug therapy, and a few patients may show progressive worsening of symptoms over a period of several years.[157] This is undoubtedly due to the steady progression in the underlying pathologic process causing parkinsonism.[11]

The majority of patients who respond to levodopa show a relatively short duration of response to the drug. This is characterized by improvement

followed by a short period of dystonia at peak plasma concentrations of L-dopa, followed by continuing clinical improvement gradually giving way to symptoms of parkinsonism (I-D-I response). A few patients with onset of parkinsonism at an unusually young age show a different response after levodopa consisting of initial dystonia followed by improvement, then a second phase of dystonia, and abrupt return of parkinsonism symptoms (D-I-D response).[168] Patients with the I-D-I response will show optimum results if the dosage of levodopa is adjusted so that few dystonic symptoms occur and if the next dose of levodopa is not given until all signs of dystonic

TABLE 4–2

Drugs Used in Therapy of Parkinson's Syndrome

Drug	How Supplied	Daily Requirements
Neurotransmitter Replacement therapy		
Levodopa	100-mg tablets or capsules 250-mg tablets or capsules 500-mg tablets or capsules	1.5–6 gm
Carbidopa/Levodopa ratio 1:10 (Sinemet)	10 mg/100 mg	Use for patients requiring up to 600 mg/day
	25 mg/250 mg	Use for patients requiring more than 600 mg/day
Benserazide/levodopa ratio 1:4 (Madopar)	25 mg/100 mg	
Receptor agonists	50 mg/200 mg	
Bromocriptine	5 mg	15 mg initially increasing slowly to therapeutic effect
Amantadine hydrochloride (Symmetrel)	100-mg tablets	100–300 mg
Anticholinergic drugs		
Trihexyphenidyl (Artane)	2-mg tablets 5-mg tablets 5-mg long-acting tablets	6–15 mg
Cycrimine hydrochloride (Pagitane)	1.25-mg tablets 2.5-mg tablets	2.5–15 mg
Biperiden (Akineton)	2-mg tablets	2–10 mg
Benztropine mesylate (Cogentin)	2-mg tablets	2–6 mg
Ethopropazine (Parsidol)	50–100-mg tablets	50–60 mg
Antihistamines		
Diphenhydramine hydrochloride (Benadryl)	50-mg tablets	50–150 mg
Chlorphenoxamine hydrochloride (Phenoxene)	50-mg tablets	150–400 mg

movements have disappeared. Patients with the D-I-D response are more difficult to treat but may respond to small doses of levodopa at frequent intervals, e.g., 50 mg of levodopa plus 5 mg of carbidopa every hour.

The most dramatic response to levodopa therapy is the so-called on-off phenomenon. This is a sudden response to levodopa administration with a rapid change from parkinsonian symptoms to dystonia, then back to the parkinsonian state as the effect of the drug decreases. The on-off phenomenon may respond to small doses of levodopa at frequent intervals, or to the addition of bromocriptine in divided doses up to 30 mg per day.[17a] But some cases are intractable and require other forms of therapy.

Additional benefit from levodopa therapy might be obtained by the concomitant administration of a monoamine oxidase inhibitor. This would delay the breakdown of newly synthesized dopamine in the brain by monoamine oxidase enzymes and potentiate the effects of dopamine. There is some indication that combined therapy using levodopa and a monoamine oxidase inhibitor produces improvement in patients with parkinsonism and reduces the on-off effects.[25, 148]

Some patients respond well to levodopa or combined levodopa/carbidopa therapy with reduction of rigidity and bradykinesia but show little reduction in tremor. The tremor can often be controlled by the use of antihistamine, or the use of the beta-adrenergic blocking agent propranolol, 10 to 40 mg three times a day, may be effective in some cases.

When selecting patients for levodopa therapy, the severity of the parkinsonism and associated diseases should be considered. Severe heart disease may be a contraindication to levodopa therapy. Elderly patients with minimal signs and symptoms of Parkinson's disease should be treated first with the anticholinergic drugs (solanaceous drugs) such as trihexyphenidyl or cycrimine (see Table 4–2). Amantadine, which stimulates release of catecholamine stores in the brain, is another alternative form of therapy, and although it is not as effective as levodopa, it has less severe side effects. In selected cases, levodopa therapy combined with amantadine or the anticholinergic group of drugs may be more effective. Amantadine also may produce side effects, which include agitation, confusion, and hallucinations.[202, 205]

Drugs of the anticholinergic group protect the patient to some degree against the gastrointestinal side effects of levodopa, but the phenothiazine group of drugs, amphetamines, and vitamin preparations containing pyridoxine are contraindicated since they interfere with the pharmacologic actions of levodopa.

There is evidence that dopamine receptor agonists may be of benefit in the treatment of Parkinson's disease as an alternative to replacement therapy with levodopa.[195] Bromocriptine, an ergot derivative that acts as a dopamine receptor agonist, reduces tremor rigidity and bradykinesia in parkinsonism.[132] Bromocriptine is well tolerated by most patients when given in doses of 2 to 5 mg three times a day, increasing the dose slowly to a therapeutic effect or until side effects develop.[91, 178] Bromocriptine is probably less effective than levodopa in the treatment of parkinsonism but should be considered as an alternative therapy in patients who fail to respond to levodopa. Side effects are similar to those observed with levodopa and include nausea, vomiting, abnormal dystonic movements, "on-off" attacks, mental disturbances, nightmares, blurred vision, drowsiness, and orthostatic hypotension. Combined therapy with levodopa and bromocriptine may be used if this seems to produce additional benefit to the patient.

Surgical Therapy. Prior to the introduction of levodopa therapy, surgical procedures were used in the treatment of parkinsonism but now these are seldom used.[105] The most satisfactory form of surgical therapy was thalamotomy in which the objective was to produce a small lesion in the ventrolateral nucleus of the thalamus without injury to the internal capsule. The operation was performed on the side opposite the limbs with greater rigidity and tremor. It is still a useful procedure in some patients who are refractory to medical treatment.

Physical Therapy. The majority of patients with Parkinson's disease benefit from physical therapy. The program can often be organized at home if the patient is well motivated, but an initial course in a department of physical medicine with instruction in the types of exercises and tasks most suited to the patient's disability is usually necessary or desirable. The program of physical medicine should be considered as a long-term one and requires periodic reassessment in view of possible changes in the degree of rigidity, tremor, and disability.

Therapy of Associated Conditions. Many patients with parkinsonism have bladder dysfunction which may be aggravated by antiparkinsonian drugs. Urinary retention, dribbling, and cystitis are not uncommon and require appropriate treatment.[217]

Postural hypotension is often compounded by levodopa therapy and is generally refractive to treatment. Ephedrine, 75 to 100 mg daily in divided doses, or fludrocortisone, 0.1 mg, or hydrocortisone, 20 mg on alternate days, may be effective in some cases.

Advanced cases of parkinsonism often develop dysphagia with a risk of aspiration pneumonia. This can be a serious complication and requires prompt treatment.

Striatonigral Degeneration

A number of cases have been described which present with symptoms of paralysis agitans but, at autopsy, show pathologic changes which can be classified as striatonigral neuronal degeneration.

Etiology and Pathology

The condition is rare and nonfamilial. There is a marked neuronal atrophy involving the putamen and substantia nigra with lesser changes in the globus pallidus, caudate nucleus, and subthalamic nucleus. Less consistent neuronal loss may occur in the cerebellar cortex, dentate nucleus, locus ceruleus, brainstem nuclei, and cerebral cortex. Lewy bodies have been described in surviving neurons in some cases.

Clinical Features

The semeiology is that of paralysis agitans which progresses to death in a six- to ten-year period. Some cases have shown additional features of cerebellar ataxia, and it is suggested that this finding with parkinsonian features should lead to the consideration of a diagnosis of striatonigral degeneration.

Treatment

Treatment is the same as described for parkinsonism.

The Parkinsonism-Dementia Complex of Guam

The occurrence of a disease in a relatively small and isolated community offers a unique opportunity for its study by the epidemiologist, geneticist, biochemist, and pathologist. This has been the case for the parkinsonism dementia complex of Guam, which has received considerable attention in the past decade.[150]

Etiology and Pathology

The disease occurs among the Chamorros of the Mariana Islands. The incidence is equal in males and females, and there is a strong familial tendency, although this does not necessarily imply a genetic trait in such a small population. There is, in fact, a possibility that the disease may result from contact with some as-yet-unidentified toxin or may even be a "slow-virus" infection.

The brain shows severe cortical atrophy, which is most marked in the frontal and temporal areas. There is loss of pigment in the substantia nigra and locus ceruleus. Histologic examination shows severe neuronal loss in the cerebral cortex, Ammon's horn, amygdala, hypothalamus, globus pallidus, thalamus, substantia nigra, periaqueductal gray, and tegmentum of the brainstem. Surviving neurons contain neurofibrillary tangles, particularly in Ammon's horn.[164]

Clinical Features

The first symptoms appear between the ages of 30 and 60 years and consist of progressive intellectual deterioration and bradykinesia. This is followed by development of generalized rigidity often associated with hostile and destructive behavior. Hallucinations and delusions occur in some cases. Examination at this stage reveals dementia, lack of judgment and insight, disorientation, poor recent memory, and acalculia. There is marked rigidity with masklike facies, bradykinesis, pill-rolling tremor, a flexed posture, and a slow gait with lack of associated arm movements. The course is one of progressive deterioration, and death usually occurs within four years.

An additional feature of considerable interest in this disease is the appearance of signs and symptoms of amyotrophic lateral sclerosis in a number of patients before they develop parkinsonism and dementia. The two conditions appear to represent different stages along a spectrum which probably represents a single disease entity.

Treatment

Clinical and biochemical results of therapeutic trials with levodopa in parkinsonism-dementia show improvement in the extrapyramidal function but not in the dementia.[32, 180, 204] The levels of the metabolic product of dopamine, homovanillic acid (Fig. 4–1), are reduced in the CSF but increase in direct proportion to the dose of levodopa administered.

Benign Familial or Hereditary (Essential) Tremor

Benign familial or hereditary (essential) tremor has been recognized for over a century. The tremor is similar to, but a gross exaggeration of, the normal physiologic tremor seen in fatigue. The disease is inherited as an autosomal dominant trait and is believed to be due to abnormal function of central, rather than peripheral, beta-adrenergic receptors.[239]

Essential tremor is not a serious disease but can be incapacitating. The major symptom is rhythmic bilaterally symmetric tremor (4 to 10 c/s) usually beginning in the fingers and then spreading to involve the hands and head and seldom affecting the legs.[108]

Mild cerebellar signs such as ataxia of finger-to-nose test may be present. Symptoms appear in youth or middle age. The disease progresses slowly, and characteristics of parkinsonism such as rigidity, hypokinesia, and bradykinesia are always absent in benign familial tremor. Nystagmus and truncal ataxia are not present, and in other respects the neurologic examination is within normal limits. The tremor is greatly exaggerated by emotion such as anger and excitement and is particularly disturbing to the patient when holding papers or a pointer in public or to those whose position requires manual dexterity. Many patients find that the tremor is temporarily relieved by alcohol.[101]

Etiology and Pathology

Neurophysiologic studies on a limited number of cases have suggested that the abnormality may be the result of degenerative changes in the corpus striatum and cerebellar systems. The pharmacologic response to therapy suggests that the disease is due to an imbalance in neurotransmitter systems with a relative hyperactivity of dopaminergic and noradrenergic systems, since the disease is made worse by levodopa and improved by the beta-adrenergic blocker propranolol.

Treatment

The tremor is relieved or significantly benefitted by the administration of propranolol,[237] 10 to 40 mg three times daily.[223] This drug should be given with caution to patients with incomplete heart block, since the heart rate may be seriously reduced in such patients. Diazepam is also useful beginning with 5 mg daily and increasing by 5-mg increments every seven days. The slow increase in dosage reduces the tendency to drowsiness, which is the main side effect of diazepam.

The Dystonias

The synonyms "torsion dystonia" and "dystonia musculorum deformans" have been used loosely in the past to indicate what are now generally termed the dystonias.[59] They are a group of neurologic disorders characterized by the preserveration of abnormal postures or sustained dystonic postures often brought about by interference with the initiation of a voluntary movement. For example, the head, neck, and trunk may become involved with extension of one arm and flexion of the other with the thumbs clenched between the fingers. Such postures may be maintained for many minutes and eventually may become irreversibly fixed due to contractures. The dystonias may result from anoxia at birth, manganese intoxication, Wilson's disease, viral encephalitis, Huntington's disease, brain trauma, cerebral infarction, Hallervorden-Spatz disease, and persistent tardive dyskinesias after prolonged use of phenothiazines.[38] However, if these conditions are excluded, there remains the "idiopathic group" in which the etiology and pathology are not well understood.

Dystonia Musculorum Deformans

Etiology and Pathology. Dystonia musculorum deformans is usually inherited as an autosomal dominant or recessive trait although sporadic cases also occur.[60, 144]

Dystonia musculorum deformans has not been associated with tangible histopathologic changes in the basal ganglia, and the pathologic substrate of the disease is unknown.[240]

Clinical Features. The first symptoms usually appear within the first two decades of life and generally before 40 years of age. Infantile, juvenile, and adult forms have been described. The onset is gradual, most commonly beginning before the age of ten years with intermittent contraction of muscles producing abnormal postures of the limbs, such as writer's cramp or torticollis.

As the condition progresses, the dystonic movements become more accentuated and consist of prolonged, slow, writhing, sustained, and contorting movements of axial and limb muscles. Tonic contractions are mainly noted in the muscles of the neck, spine, and proximal limb girdles. If the condition is primarily unilateral, it produces severe contortions of the spine resulting in grotesque postures of the trunk. Other patients develop flexion of the hips or contortions of the shoulder muscles during walking. Volitional movements become severely impaired. The spasms usually, but not invariably, disappear during sleep and under general anesthesia. A myostatic type of dystonia musculorum deformans has been described, in which there may be periodic extension movements of the spine resembling decerebrate rigidity with a marked lordosis and rigid gait.

The disease may progress slowly or become arrested. Mild cases, or forme frustes, occur in families with torsion dystonia. Untreated and advanced cases develop severe disability with persistent skeletal deformities.

Treatment. Oral haloperidol in doses of 0.5 to 2 mg three times daily in combination with amantadine hydrochloride in doses of 200 to 600 mg daily may be an effective form of therapy.[82, 83] In addition to haloperidol, diazepam in doses of 15 to 40 mg daily may be added. Some cases show improvement with levodopa,[16, 59] either alone or in combination with haloperidol.

Carbamazepine therapy has produced improvement in some cases of dystonia musculorum deformans but is not effective in others.[122] Cryothalamectomy with discrete lesions in the ventrolateral nucleus of the thalamus produces improvement in about two thirds of patients with severe dystonia.[42]

Spasmodic Torticollis

This is a limited form of dystonia and results from intermittent recurring involuntary contractions of the neck muscles which result in tonic episodes of deviation of the head to one side (laterocollis). Bilateral involvement may occur and results in retrocollis or anterocollis.

Etiology and Pathology. The cause is not always discernible and hence the condition is a syndrome rather than an etiologic diagnosis.[226] Some cases are familial,[84] while others are postencephalitic. There is no evidence that psychiatric disorders play a part. Associated emotional instability may be the result rather than the cause of the disability or the disease. Dystonic posturing of the neck may present as one of the features of Huntington's disease, Wilson's disease, double athetosis, viral encephalitis, carbon monoxide intoxication, multiple sclerosis, Jakob-Creutzfeldt disease, meningovascular syphilis, tardive dyskinesias resulting from neurotransmitter depletion after phenothiazine or haloperidol therapy, and generalized dystonias (dystonia musculorum deformans). These cases are distinguished from spasmodic torticollis by the presence of additional signs.[221]

Spasmodic torticollis is a disorder of the postural reflex mechanisms of the neck. Normal posture is the product of several tonically active antagonistic reflex mechanisms, which are in dynamic equilibrium. An increase or decrease in tonic activity of one of these mechanisms produces an imbalance with an alteration in posture. This probably accounts for the fact that lesions have been reported at various levels in the central nervous system in this disease. Analysis of the pathologic findings indicates that, most consistently, lesions are found in the neurons of the caudate nucleus, putamen, globus pallidus, and their connections. More widespread changes have been reported in the thalamus, subthalamic nuclei, substantia nigra, vestibular nuclei, and cerebellum. It is apparent that torticollis may be a sign of generalized extrapyramidal disease.[106, 226]

Clinical Features. Initial symptoms usually begin in adult life, although they have been reported to begin in adolescence. The disease occurs in both sexes but is said to be more frequent in males. Torticollis usually develops gradually with a progressive increase in the severity of the dystonia. The essential feature is intermittent contraction of the neck muscles resulting in rotation of the head to one side, often with elevation or depression of the chin and retrocollis. Rarely, these may be persistent tonic deviation, but more commonly the head movement is intermittent with jerking movements, which may be myoclonic or rhythmic. The increased muscular activity leads to hypertrophy of the neck muscles. The movement is usually aggravated by stress and emotion.

Diagnostic Procedures

1. Thyroid function should be evaluated. Some cases associated with hyperthyroidism have been reported to resolve when the patient is rendered euthyroid.
2. Electromyography shows sustained activity in the muscles of one or both sides of the neck. Others show sustained activity on one side with irregular bursts of activity on the other side. Caloric stimulation of the horizontal semicircular canal with cold water increases the tonic activity in the muscles of the same side.

Treatment. Medical treatment should be attempted first with diazepam in doses of 10 to 40 mg per day,[21] which relieves the movements in mild cases although they may not be sustained. In more severe cases, amantidine, 100 mg three times daily, and haloperidol, 0.5 mg four times daily, are recommended.[82, 83] The medical therapeutic approach is similar to that described under treatment of the dystonias, although levodopa therapy is seldom of benefit.[16] Deanol, 600 mg daily, or clonazepam, 3 to 5 mg, may be helpful.

Biofeedback techniques have been employed with some success in some cases. Thalamic surgery is only employed in severely incapacitated patients since experience has shown that bilateral lesions are required to produce alleviation of symptoms, and the operative procedure is beneficial in only 60 per cent of cases.[43]

**Blepharospasm-Oromandibular
Dystonia Syndrome
(Brueghel's Syndrome)**

This unusual and distressing dystonia syndrome is another example of a dystonia somewhat akin to spasmodic torticollis.

Etiology and Pathology. In common with other dystonic conditions, Brueghel's syndrome results from a disorder of function in the basal ganglia. The pathologic changes are unknown at this time.

Clinical Features. The condition appears in elderly patients who are apparently healthy. There is a gradual development of blepharospasm with irregular spasms of the orbicularis oculi which last as long as 60 seconds and which recur frequently with only a few seconds between episodes. Oromandibular dystonia may develop at the same time or some months after the appearance of blepharospasm and consists of opening of the jaw, retraction of the jaw, spasm of the platysma, and occasionally tongue protrusion. The patient is unable to speak clearly, and the continuous movements of the jaw cause pain in and occasional dislocation of the temporomandibular joints. This syndrome is frequently mistaken for a psychiatric illness, a misdiagnosis that is reinforced by the depression that the illness induces in the unfortunate patient.

Treatment. Many drugs have been tried in an attempt to alleviate the blepharospasm and oromandibular dystonia. There is no effective treatment, but combinations of butyrophenone and benzodiazepine may give temporary relief. Treatment of the associated depression will allow the patient to tolerate the disability more readily.[155]

Diseases Characterized by Chorea and Athetosis

Chorea and choreoathetosis are symptomatic of many diseases of the nervous system, the most important of which are listed in the accompanying table. Some of these diseases are discussed elsewhere in this book; others will be briefly reviewed here (Table 4–3).

Sydenham's Chorea

The term "Sydenham's chorea" or "chorea minor" refers to a condition almost certainly related to rheumatic fever that occurs in children and young adolescents. (The term "chorea" may be defined as involuntary, brief, and nonrepetitive dystonic movements.) The relationship between Sydenham's chorea and rheumatic fever has been established in a sizable number of cases, so that it is justifiable to reserve this term for typical

TABLE 4–3

Diseases Characterized by Chorea or Choreoathetosis

1. Sydenham's chorea
2. Athetotic cerebral palsy (double athetosis), anoxic encephalopathy at birth, kernicterus
3. Viral encephalitis
4. Postinfectious leukoencephalitis
5. Henoch-Schonlein purpura
6. Systemic lupus erythematosus
7. Hepatic encephalopathy
8. Wilson's disease
9. Familial paroxysmal choreoathetosis
10. Familial benign chorea
11. Huntington's chorea
12. As a side effect during phenothiazine therapy

cases of the clinical syndrome even when the rheumatic etiology is obscure.[8]

Chorea may be caused by other diseases in which the involuntary movements are similar to those of Sydenham's chorea. For example, choreiform movements have been described in viral encephalitis and in the postinfectious leukoencephalopathies. Chorea also occurs in other conditions including lupus erythematosus in childhood[99] and meningovascular syphilis. Similar movements have been reported as a result of metabolic disorders including hypocalcemia and hyperthyroidism. Chorea may be seen from time to time as a manifestation of anoxic encephalopathy, carbon monoxide poisoning, and brain tumors. It is also seen as a complication of therapy with the phenothiazine group of drugs and occurs in certain degenerative diseases mentioned in this chapter. Chorea occurring in pregnancy (chorea gravidarum) is thought by some to be a recurrence of Sydenham's chorea during pregnancy.

Etiology and Pathology

As mentioned previously, it is not always possible to demonstrate a relationship between chorea and rheumatic fever. A history of a recent streptococcal infection can be obtained in some cases, but it is apparently a subclinical infection in the majority. There may also be a considerable interval between the streptococcal infection and the development of chorea. The eventual development of signs of rheumatic fever in a considerable number of patients with Sydenham's chorea suggests a rheumatic etiology.

In a few cases studied at necropsy, the brain was reported to be grossly normal, but under the microscope areas of arteritis were noted with swelling of the endothelium, perivascular infiltration, and petechial hemorrhages. Occlusion of small cerebral vessels with microinfarction has also been reported. These scattered zones of vasculitis produced areas of neuronal loss dispersed throughout cortex, basal ganglia, brainstem, and cerebellum. There was no predilection for any one site, and the changes were not confined to the basal ganglia.

Clinical Features

Sydenham's chorea usually develops in children and young adolescents between the ages of 5 and 15 years and is more common in females. There is an increased prevalence in families where the incidence is ten times that of the general population. The condition is characterized by involuntary movements, incoordination, and weakness. Involuntary movements may not be obvious in the early stages, and the child may be regarded as "clumsy." However, as the disease progresses, it becomes apparent that the patient is making brief, sudden, nonrepetitive dystonic movements involving primarily the limbs and face. Eventually, these movements may be seen in any part of the body. The movements are present at rest and disappear during sleep.

On examination, the patient appears to be restless and makes frequent changes of posture. There may be dysarthria, and speech may be explosive due to irregularities of respiration. Facial grimacing is common, but the movements are irregular and tend to be nonrepetitive. If the patient is asked to protrude the tongue, it cannot be maintained immobile but is protruded and retracted in an irregular manner (the darting-tongue sign).

Examination of the upper limbs shows decreased tone on passive movement. The hands are often held in a typical posture with flexion at the wrist, hyperextension at the metacarpophalangeal joints, extension of the interphalangeal joints, and abduction of the thumb. When extended above the head, the hands tend to pronate (the pronator sign). There is usually some generalized weakness and inability to maintain contraction when the patient is asked to grasp the examiner's fingers. Similar hypotonia and weakness are usually present in the lower limbs.

The tendon jerks show considerable variation in response depending on the phase of chorea when the tendon is struck with the hammer. There may be delayed response from time to time. The knee jerks are usually pendular in type. Tests

of coordination exacerbate the involuntary movements, and the performance of rapid alternating movements is interfered with by the chorea. Sydenham's chorea occasionally involves only one side of the body (hemichorea).

Diagnostic Procedures

1. The blood count is usually within normal limits, although the erythrocyte sedimentation rate is sometimes elevated.
2. Lumbar puncture shows normal opening and closing pressures, and cerebrospinal fluid is normal.
3. Serum calcium and phosphorus levels should be obtained to rule out hypocalcemia.
4. Roentgenograms of the skull are within normal limits. Intracranial calcification, if present, suggests the possibility of hypocalcemia due to hypoparathyroidism or other disorders of calcium metabolism.
5. Electrocardiograms should be obtained since this may disclose abnormalities due to rheumatic carditis.
6. Evidence of streptococcal infection should be obtained by measuring antistreptolysin 0 titers in the blood, which are often elevated.

Treatment

Acute Phase. The patient should be treated with bed rest in a quiet room with good nursing care.

A 7-to-14-day course of corticosteroids (prednisone, 60 to 75 mg daily) may produce a dramatic improvement within a few days.[98] Haloperidol is also effective in many cases, but the danger of drug-induced dystonia means that it should be reserved for severe cases.[212] Tetrabenazine, 25 mg twice or three times a day, is reported to produce improvement in some cases.[107]

Convalescent Stage. Recurrent attacks of Sydenham's chorea do occur but are unusual. About one third of patients subsequently develop signs of rheumatic fever and rheumatic carditis. Rheumatic complications may be prevented by the long-term use of antibiotics, particularly penicillin. This is usually given as benzathine penicillin G intramuscularly, 1,200,000 units every month, or penicillin G orally, 250,000 units twice daily. Prophylactic penicillin should be continued until 21 years of age.

In addition to antibiotic therapy, all patients who have had Sydenham's chorea should be followed carefully and examined frequently for the development of subsequent heart disease. There are no neurologic complications of Sydenham's chorea other than recurrences in a small number of cases. Emotional disturbances and transient intellectual impairment[24a] have been described in patients after recovery from the acute phase. This complication can be reduced by the alert physician who detects potentially stressful situations in school or in the family environment and ensures that they are prevented or avoided.

Familial Benign Chorea

A benign form of chorea has been described in both Negro and caucasian families in the United States and appears to be transmitted as an autosomal dominant trait. The movement disorder begins between 2 and 12 years of age and varies in severity in different members of the affected family.[20] The disability is maximal at onset, nonprogressive, and nonparoxysmal and is not associated with dementia or other neurologic abnormalities. The typical choreiform movements cause little disability apart from some clumsiness.[103]

Treatment

Haloperidol, reserpine, phenothiazine, and diazepam therapy may improve the involuntary movements.

Athetotic Cerebral Palsy (Double Athetosis)

The majority of patients with this condition are probably examples of striatopallidal damage secondary to anoxic encephalopathy at or shortly after birth. This view is supported by the fact that the reported pathologic changes consist of gliosis and neuronal loss with ectopic myelination of nerve fibers in the putamen and, to a lesser extent, in the globus pallidus. This unusual pathologic picture has been termed "status marmoratus" and is generally conceded to be due to anoxic damage. Improvement in the involuntary movements occurs following medical treatment with haloperidol, reserpine, or diazepam.

Ballism

The term "ballism" refers to a particular type of involuntary movement that is a symptom rather than a disease or a diagnosis. Nevertheless, the involuntary movement is highly characteristic

of damage to a small area of the brain, a few millimeters in size.

Etiology and Pathology

Hemiballismus is the term used to describe involuntary movements of the limbs of one side of the body. It occurs after damage to the subthalamic nucleus or connections between it and the globus pallidus of the opposite side of the brain. These striking involuntary movements have occurred due to infarction of this area resulting from arteriosclerosis or meningovascular syphilis as well as destruction of these neurons and their connections as a consequence of viral encephalitis, granulomatous inflammation, multiple sclerosis, trauma, and primary or metastatic brain tumors.

Clinical Features

Hemiballism is the most dramatic of all the involuntary movements seen in clinical neurology. The movements of the affected limb look like a baseball pitcher's "windup" with irregular flinging movements of the hand, arm, and leg on the side opposite to the lesion. The movements originate predominantly in the proximal muscles, but some involvement is also discernible in the most distal muscles with a dystonic component such as flexion and extension of the hand and fingers. The movements are accentuated by any attempt at voluntary movement but disappear during sleep. Although complex, the movements tend to be repetitive and continuous, and if the condition is untreated, the limbs become bruised and swollen and the patient may die of exhaustion. Occasionally, the movements are so violent that the patient is flung from his bed to the floor. After eight weeks there is a tendency for the movements to spontaneously decrease in severity.

Treatment

The condition usually responds dramatically to intravenous diazepam (Valium), 10 mg injected slowly over a 60-second period.

Control of the movements can usually be maintained with perphenazine, 4 mg three times a day. Tetrabenazine, reserpine, and haloperidol are also effective.[129] Dimethylaminoethanol, 50 mg three times a day, is also effective and relatively free from side effects.[127]

Hallervorden-Spatz Disease

The diagnosis of Hallervorden-Spatz disease is usually made by the neuropathologist at autopsy since the clinical picture during life may vary a great deal from case to case. Indeed, the semeiology is so varied that such a condition may be regarded as the Hallervorden-Spatz syndrome rather than a single disease.[199]

Etiology and Pathology

The etiology is unknown. Familial cases have been described which affect both sexes, suggesting that some cases may be inherited as an autosomal recessive trait. Despite the demonstration of iron and calcium deposits in the globus pallidus, the systemic metabolism of both elements appears to be normal.

At autopsy, the brain and meninges are normal in appearance, but there is a rusty-brown discoloration of the globus pallidus that is best seen on coronal section. Histologically, there is a marked loss of neurons in the globus pallidus, substantia nigra, and subthalamic nucleus with lesser degrees of involvement in the caudate nucleus and cerebellum. The axons in the globus pallidus are swollen, and there is marked loss of myelin. Scattered pigmentary granules are seen in the cytoplasm of the astrocytes and lying free in the tissues.

Clinical Features

The initial symptoms occur at any time during childhood or adolescence. There is a progressive generalized rigidity and dementia. Choreoathetosis and dystonic postures occur in some cases, while others show marked cerebellar ataxia. The terminal state is one of severe rigidity, dementia, and spasticity with hyperactive tendon jerks, extensor plantar responses, dysarthria, and dysphasia. Some patients have developed visual impairment due to associated retinitis pigmentosa.

Treatment

Various drugs known to affect rigidity and tremor (see Parkinson's Disease) may be helpful. These include levodopa, amantadine, and the solanaceous drugs.

The Spinocerebellar Degenerations: General Considerations

The literature referring to spinocerebellar degeneration contains many descriptions of familial conditions that have been regarded as original diseases by the authors and were promptly dubbed with a title or eponym. It is apparent that many reports dealt with neurologic disorders that were not original but were descriptions of variants of a well-known disease. This situation produces considerable difficulty in attempting to classify the spinocerebellar degenerations. The outline in Table 4–4 is a classification in keeping with the present state of knowledge.[94]

It is possible, however, that the spinocerebellar degenerations form a spectrum of disease. Many transitional forms exist, which are classified with one of the better-known "classic" types for the purpose of convenience. Different clinical types have been described in a single family pedigree, and many of the classic forms contain additional features usually encountered in other clinical types.

The spinocerebellar degenerations generally are regarded as a premature axonal and neuronal degeneration, sometimes referred to as an "abiotrophy," which may be due to failure of intracellular enzymatic systems. It is quite possible that the degeneration may be more pronounced in one or more systems in some families, producing a fairly stereotyped clinical picture in those afflicted. A similar process affecting different systems in another family will produce an entirely different clinical picture, although the basic process is the same. If this pathogenesis is correct, it is not difficult to see how there might be some association between Friedreich's ataxia, hereditary areflexic dystasia of Roussy and Levy, hereditary spastic ataxia, and hereditary spastic paraplegia. These latter conditions are, in fact, regarded by many neurologists as variants or formes frustes of Friedreich's ataxia. There is also an obvious pathologic association between Friedreich's ataxia and olivopontocerebellar degeneration, while the latter condition has many features in common with cerebello-olivary degeneration (Holmes).

Familial Cerebellar Degenerations of Infancy and Childhood

This is a heterogeneous group of diseases of which ataxia telangiectasia is probably the most common example (p. 110). The other forms listed in Table 4–4 have been described in a small number of families. Cerebellar ataxia with retinal degeneration may be an infantile form of olivopontocerebellar degeneration. In the majority of cases,

TABLE 4–4

The Spinocerebellar Degenerations

A. *Familial cerebellar degenerations of infancy and childhood*
1. Ataxia telangiectasia
2. Cerebellar ataxia with optic atrophy
3. Cerebellar atrophy with retinal degeneration
4. Congenital granule cell hypoplasia
5. Hypoplasia of the neocerebellum with systemic degeneration
6. Spinocerebellar degeneration with congenital cataract, somatic and mental retardation (Marinesco-Sjögren syndrome)

B. *Familial spinocerebellar degenerations in adults*
1. Predominantly spinal forms
   a. Friedreich's ataxia
   b. Hereditary areflexic dystasia (Roussy-Levy)
   c. Hereditary spastic ataxia (Marie)
   d. Hereditary spastic paraplegia
   e. Peroneal muscular atrophy (Charcot-Marie-Tooth)
2. Predominantly cerebellar forms
   a. Olivopontocerebellar degeneration (Dejerine-Thomas)
   b. Cortical cerebellar degeneration (Holmes)
   c. Dyssynergia cerebellaris myoclonica (Ramsay-Hunt)
   d. Cerebrocerebellar degeneration
   e. Acute intermittent familial cerebellar ataxia
   f. Vestibulocerebellar ataxia

C. *"Toxic" cerebellar degenerations*
1. Alcoholic cerebellar degenerations
2. Subacute cerebellar degeneration in neoplasia
3. Diphenylhydantoin (Dilantin) intoxication
4. Cerebellar degeneration in myxedema

the disability is severe, and death occurs in childhood or adolescence.

Familial Spinocerebellar Degenerations in Adults

Friedreich's Ataxia

This disease is probably the most common form of the spinocerebellar degenerations and is inherited as an autosomal recessive trait. It may be secondary to a defect in the membrane transport of taurine and β-adenine or due to a modification of cell membrane structure secondary to a reduction in high-density lipoproteins.[13] A deficiency in the activity of the enzyme lipoamide dehydrogenase has been demonstrated in Friedreich's ataxia.[195a]

Pathology

The spinal cord is usually reported to be smaller than normal, and the atrophy involves the posterior columns, which is apparent on transverse section of the cord. However, under the microscope, degeneration is also seen to involve the direct and indirect spinocerebellar tracts and the corticospinal (pyramidal) tracts as well as the posterior columns. In the areas of degeneration, there is a loss of axons and myelin with some gliosis resulting in shrinkage of the affected tracts.

The degenerative changes begin in the neurons of the posterior root ganglia, and there is a "dying back" of axons in the posterior columns of the spinal cord. Similar neuronal changes eventually occur in the nucleus gracilis and cuneatus producing degenerative changes in the medial lemniscus. The ganglioneuropathy also produces involvement of the dorsal and ventral spinocerebellar tracts. The corticospinal tracts also show loss of axons with increasing involvement as they descend from the upper cervical to the lumbar segments. There is loss of Purkinje cells in the cerebellum and some degeneration of the dentate nucleus and the superior cerebellar peduncles. This latter finding provides a link with the Ramsay Hunt syndrome.

Cardiac hypertrophy with diffuse myocardial fibrosis and degeneration of cardiac muscle cells is present in all cases.[200]

Clinical Features

The first symptoms of ataxia usually begin in the early teens, although an onset before the age of ten years is not unusual. The great majority of cases have well-established signs of the disease before the age of 20 years. The ataxia presents as a clumsiness of gait and is followed by progressive dysarthria. The ataxia then progresses to involve the upper limbs.

The fully developed syndrome is characterized by a mild degree of dementia in some cases. Optic atrophy, with visual failure, has also been reported. The eye movements are jerky, and nystagmus is usually, but not always, present. Many patients show progressive loss of hearing. The speech may be described as slow, staccato, and explosive at times and may become unintelligible in the later phases of the disease. The difficulty in speech becomes compounded by respiratory irregularity. There are generalized hypotonia and muscle weakness. Tests of coordination reveal intention tremor, dysdiadochokinesia, and dysmetria or past pointing, which is accentuated when the eyes are closed.

The gait is both spastic and ataxic and becomes wide-based and reeling. The patient sways when standing owing to truncal ataxia. The Romberg test is positive. The deep tendon reflexes are always absent in the lower limbs and are depressed or absent in the upper limbs. There is a bilateral extensor plantar response within two years of onset of the ataxia.[12]

On examination of sensation, touch is usually found to be intact but there is impairment of tactile discrimination, tactile localization, and stereognosis in the hands and feet. Vibration and position sense are always decreased in the lower limbs and usually decreased in the upper limbs. A deformity of the feet, with pes cavus, extension of the metatarsophalangeal joints, and flexion of the interphalangeal joints, is present in 90 per cent of cases. It should be pointed out, however, that pes cavus is not a specific sign of this disease since it occurs in any condition in which there has been chronic involvement of the corticospinal (pyramidal) tracts since childhood. It is sometimes present in patients with Friedreich's ataxia before they develop neurologic signs of the disease. Lumbosacral kyphoscoliosis is less consistent and usually appears later. Rarely, the spinal deformity may be severe, producing impairment of respiratory movements.

The disease runs a progressive course, and most patients are unable to walk five years from the onset of symptoms. Death occurs from pulmonary or cardiac complications about 10 to 20 years later.[229]

Diagnostic Procedures

1. Clinical diabetes mellitus is present in about 20 per cent of patients, and a further 20 per cent have an abnormal glucose tolerance test. There are low fasting insulin levels.
2. Serum levels of unconjugated bilirubin are frequently elevated.
3. Pulmonary function tests show progressive impairment in parallel with progression of kyphoscoliosis.
4. The electrocardiogram is abnormal, and phonocardiograms and echocardiograms will identify patients with obstructive hypertrophic cardiomyopathy.
5. Electroencephalography shows mild nonspecific abnormalities consisting of abnormally slow or irregular background rhythms in about one third of the cases, with occasional paroxysmal discharges in some patients.
6. Motor nerve conduction studies are normal, but sensory conduction velocities and sensory-evoked potentials are absent in the lower limbs.[188]

Treatment

Administration of choline or lecithin has been proposed on the assumption that Friedreich's ataxia is associated with abnormally low serum levels of high-density lipoprotein. In established cases, long-leg braces as well as orthopedic procedures such as triple arthrodesis and special shoes for the deformities of the feet may keep the patient ambulatory for many years. Cardiac and pulmonary complications should receive prompt attention in advanced cases since they are frequently fatal.

Hereditary Areflexic Dystasia (Roussy-Levy Syndrome)

It is generally considered that this condition is a variant of Friedreich's ataxia or a mixture of Friedreich's ataxia with peroneal muscular atrophy rather than a specific form of spinocerebellar degeneration. There is now considerable evidence that it constitutes a link in the spectrum of degenerative diseases between Friedreich's ataxia and peroneal muscular atrophy. The disease runs a much more benign course than Friedreich's ataxia.

Etiology and Pathology

Both autosomal dominant and sex-linked recessive inheritance has been described in families with this disease. The pathologic changes are similar to those described under Friedreich's ataxia, but, in addition, there is neuronal loss in the anterior horn cells of the spinal cord. When examined microscopically, the peripheral nerves may show "onionskin" hypertrophy of the type seen in chronic hypertrophic interstitial neuropathy.

Clinical Features

The disease is only mildly progressive. The symptoms may develop in childhood and always occur before the age of 30 years. They consist of progressive ataxia with absence of nystagmus and dysarthria. There is marked wasting of the muscles in the distal lower limbs. The wasting spreads as high as the distal one third of the thigh and resembles peroneal muscular atrophy. Muscle wasting in the hands may produce a typical clawhand. The deep tendon reflexes are absent, and there may be bilateral extensor plantar responses (Babinski signs). Skeletal deformities, including pes cavus, are prominent, and kyphoscoliosis is usually present. The course is one of slow progression with a tendency to become stationary or regress in some cases. Electromyography may show evidence of denervation, and nerve conduction velocities are reduced, indicating a peripheral neuropathic component in this disease.

Hereditary Spastic Ataxia (Marie)

The eponym "Marie's hereditary ataxia" is often used to describe a condition characterized by progressive spastic paraparesis or quadriparesis associated with cerebellar ataxia. Some familial cases present with a gradually progressive paraparesis and little or no cerebellar signs and will be considered under the heading of Hereditary Spastic Paraplegia. The majority of cases probably represent a variant, or forme fruste, or Friedreich's ataxia or olivopontocerebellar degeneration.

Pathology

Various degrees of neuronal degeneration involving the cerebellum, brainstem, and spinal cord have been described. The cerebellum shows loss of Purkinje's cells and neuronal loss in the dentate nucleus with some secondary demyelinative changes in the superior cerebellar peduncle. Changes in the brainstem occur predominantly in the pontine nuclei and inferior olives. The posterior columns, spinocerebellar tracts, and corticospinal (pyramidal) tracts show demyelination, loss of axons, and reactive gliosis.

Clinical Features

This is a disease of adults and begins with impairment of gait followed by the gradual development of a spastic and ataxic gait. The patient walks with a broad-based and stiff-legged gait. On examination, brainstem signs are minimal, although slight dysarthria may be present. There are generalized hypertonia, increased deep tendon reflexes, and bilateral extensor plantar responses. Tests of coordination show finger-to-nose and heel-to-shin ataxia, but the Romberg test is negative. Sensation is intact or may show slight impairment, which is insufficient to account for the marked ataxia. Pes cavus is present in some cases. Optic atrophy and ocular palsies have rarely occurred in some members of affected families.

Hereditary Spastic Paraplegia (Primary Lateral Sclerosis)

Both familial and sporadic forms of primary lateral sclerosis have been recognized, although in retrospect it is probable that the condition was diagnosed too frequently in the past. The recognition of cervical spondylosis as a cause of a chronic spastic paraparesis has been followed by a decrease in the diagnosis of primary lateral sclerosis, but the latter condition undoubtedly exists as a rare clinical entity.

Etiology and Pathology

The familial forms of this rare disease may represent variants of Friedreich's ataxia, while some sporadic cases may be unusual forms of motor neuron disease (see Amyotrophic Lateral Sclerosis). One of the problems in the hereditary cases is that the disease is chronic without shortening the life-span, so that there are no reliable pathologic reports concerning this condition.

Clinical Features

The onset is insidious with a gradual stiffening and spasticity of the lower limbs. This interferes with gait, which is stiff-legged, and both limbs must be circumducted to produce forward motion. There is some unsteadiness with frequent falls due to inability to make corrective movements of the hypertonic limbs in order to adjust for sudden changes of posture. Slow progression may lead to loss of ambulation in some cases while others appear to become arrested and are able to continue walking. Examination shows marked increase in the tone of the lower limbs with ankle clonus. The deep tendon reflexes are increased in all four extremities, and the jaw jerk is hyperactive. There are bilateral extensor plantar responses. The other systems are apparently normal.

A heterogeneous group of familial forms of hereditary spastic paraplegia has been described in which there are a number of associated abnormalities. They are inherited as autosomal dominant or recessive traits. The other clinical manifestations include optic atrophy, mental retardation, and seizures. Some patients show associated kyphoscoliosis and electrocardiographic abnormalities characteristic of Friedreich's ataxia. A number of families have also been reported with spastic paraplegia, dysarthria, nystagmus, and distal muscle wasting. These families constitute a link between the characteristic forms of spastic paraplegia, the spinocerebellar degenerations, the peroneal muscular atrophies, and amyotrophic lateral sclerosis, which is occasionally encountered in families.

Peroneal Muscular Atrophy

The inclusion of peroneal muscular atrophy with spinocerebellar degenerations appears to be justified since it probably represents one type of this spectrum of degenerative disorders. Certainly, many cases of spinocerebellar degeneration have clinical or electrical evidence of peripheral nerve involvement.[18] Peroneal muscular atrophy is an example of a myeloneuropathic form of the degenerative process. When associated with evident spinocerebellar degeneration, it is called the Roussy-Levy syndrome, and some cases have signs presenting with a striking resemblance to Friedreich's ataxia and the other types of degenerative disorders already discussed in this section, including amyotrophic lateral sclerosis.

Etiology and Pathology

Peroneal muscular atrophy is another example of an "abiotrophy," the nature of which has been discussed at the beginning of this section. It usually is inherited as an autosomal dominant or recessive trait. The main changes consist of degeneration involving axons and myelin in both anterior and posterior nerve roots and peripheral nerves. A similar change occurs in the posterior columns of the spinal cord, presumably due to degeneration secondary to the atrophic process found in the posterior nerve roots. There is loss of neurons in the posterior root ganglia and some loss of anterior horn cells in the lumbar area. The affected muscles show evidence of neurogenic atrophy.

Clinical Features

The earliest symptoms usually occur at the end of the first or during the second decade of life. There is a slowly progressive atrophy of the distal limb muscles, beginning with the peroneal group in the anterior compartment of the leg. This produces weakness of dorsiflexion and eversion of the foot with a characteristic steppage type of gait. This is followed by atrophy of the calf muscles and the distal third of the quadriceps femoris. Fasciculations occasionally occur. The contrast between the atrophic areas and normal bulk of the upper thigh has led to the term "stork legs." The distal muscles in the upper limbs are involved at a later stage, which produces atrophy of the small muscles of the hands which gradually spreads to the forearms. There are rarely complaints of pain in the lower limbs, but some loss of touch and vibration sense can usually be detected in the distal parts of both upper and lower extremities. The disease runs a chronic course with slow progression, but severe disability is unusual.[206]

Diagnostic Procedures

Motor nerve conduction velocities display a binary distribution being either relatively normal or substantially reduced. This separation has a genetic basis since affected relatives tend to display similar values.[228]

Treatment

There is no specific treatment for peroneal muscular atrophy, but the use of short leg braces may assist in walking and help to maintain an ambulant state. Triple arthrodesis, tenotomies, and wedge osteotomies for hammertoes provide more stable feet. Physical therapy appears to maintain optimum strength in the affected extremities.

Olivopontocerebellar Atrophy (Dejerine-Thomas)

The term "olivopontocerebellar atrophy" describes the essential changes found in certain cases of cerebellar degeneration, which occur sporadically but which occasionally show a familial tendency. While this raises the possibility that olivopontocerebellar atrophy may be a syndrome due to two conditions that present with a similar pathologic picture, most neurologists believe that a single disease causing neuronal atrophy in these regions is more likely. There is some variation in the clinical and pathologic findings described in the case reports of olivopontocerebellar atrophy, a major variant being the association of spinal cord degeneration in several cases.

Etiology and Pathology

The condition may occur sporadically or may be inherited as an autosomal dominant or autosomal recessive trait. Although the brunt of the degenerative process falls on certain areas of the brain, it is a diffuse process and the brain may show moderate atrophy of the gyri over the frontal areas, but the most marked atrophy is found in the cerebellum, pons, and medullary olives. There is diffuse ventricular dilatation of a moderate degree.

Histologic examination shows a severe loss of neurons in the medullary olives with marked gliosis. The ventral portion of the pons is shrunken with loss of both ganglion cells and the transverse fibers, while the cerebellum shows loss of Purkinje cells and demyelination of both the middle cerebellar peduncle and the central white matter of the cerebellar hemispheres. The vermis and phylogenetically older areas of the cerebellum are spared. Degenerative changes in the spinal cord vary from case to case, but they have been described in the spinocerebellar tracts, dorsal columns, and corticospinal tracts. Less convincing losses of neurons have also been described in the substantia nigra and basal ganglia.

Clinical Features

The age of onset varies considerably from case to case. The disease may begin in adolescence or as late as the fifth decade. The earliest symptom is usually ataxia of gait followed by dysarthria, then ataxia of the upper limbs, intention tremor, and titubation of the head. There is progressive deterioration with the development of generalized rigidity and "parkinsonian" features in some cases. The dysarthria becomes so severe that the speech becomes unintelligible and the tendon jerks become hyperactive with bilateral extensor plantar responses. There is a progressive visual deterioration due to associated retinitis pigmen-

tosa in a few cases, while signs of posterior column degeneration are noted in others. Many patients develop signs of dementia as a late feature of this disease, while others show postural hypotension and other signs of autonomic disturbance due to involvement of autonomic neurons (see Shy-Drager Syndrome).

Diagnostic Procedures

1. Computed tomography shows atrophy of the brainstem with enlargement of the fourth ventricle and quadrigeminal, ambient, and prepontine cisterns.[1] The cerebellar sulci are prominent, indicating cerebellar atrophy, and there is enlargement of the cisterna magna and supracerebellar cisterns. There may be some degree of dilatation of the lateral ventricles and enlargement of the cortical sulci compatible with cortical atrophy (Fig. 4–8).
2. Auditory-evoked potentials are abnormal with increased latencies of the early waves indicating maximal involvement of the pons.[85]

Treatment

Parkinsonian features may respond to levodopa therapy, and postural hypotension may be treated with fludrocortisone acetate (see Shy-Drager Syndrome). The disease is usually slowly progressive with the expected survival averaging 20 to 25 years from the onset of symptoms. Death usually follows from aspiration pneumonitis.

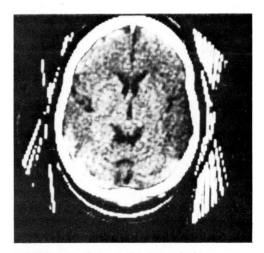

FIGURE 4–8. Computed tomography in olivopontocerebellar degeneration. There are atrophy of the brainstem, prominence of the cerebellar sulci, and early cerebral cortical atrophy.

Cortical Cerebellar
Degeneration (Holmes)

This condition has been described under a number of names including cortical or lamellar cerebellar atrophy. It is characterized by progressive degeneration of the cerebellar cortex and the main cerebellofugal pathway due to neuronal atrophy.

Etiology and Pathology

Study of involved families suggests that the disorder is transmitted by an autosomal dominant mode of inheritance. There is marked atrophy of the cerebellar hemispheres and vermis with a generalized loss of Purkinje cells and reactive gliosis. The granular layer also shows neuronal loss, and there is some neuronal loss in the dentate nucleus resulting in atrophy and demyelination of the superior cerebellar peduncle. The majority of cases show slight neuronal atrophy in the inferior olives, but the brainstem and cord are otherwise unremarkable.

Clinical Features

The earliest symptoms of ataxia appear between the ages of 30 and 60 years. Ataxia usually begins in the lower limbs with impairment of gait, but the upper limbs are soon involved and dysarthria is prominent. Clinical findings include nystagmus, dysarthria, and marked dysmetria with dysdiadochokinesia and intention tremor of the upper limbs. There may be titubation of the head, truncal ataxia, and the development of a wide-based and ataxic gait. The deep tendon reflexes are hypoactive but the plantar response is usually extensor. The sensory examination is normal.

A number of patients have been reported with a progressive dementia, and some cases are associated with seizures and myoclonus epilepsy. Thus there may be some overlap or relationship to olivopontocerebellar atrophy and dyssynergia cerebellaris myoclonica (see below). The course is chronic with an average survival of about 12 years from the onset of symptoms.

Diagnostic Procedures

Computed tomography confirms the atrophy of the folia of the cerebellum and enlargement of the fourth ventricle in all cerebellar atrophies.

Dyssynergia Cerebellaris Myoclonica (Ramsay Hunt's Disease)

There have been few references citing this condition as a distinct clinical entity,[24b] although it is extremely doubtful that it is so. The occurrence of myoclonus in the spinocerebellar degeneration seems to depend on degenerative changes involving the dentate nucleus and superior cerebellar peduncle. It has already been pointed out that such degenerative changes have been observed in Friedreich's ataxia and cortical cerebellar degeneration and that the myoclonus may be observed in patients with either of the two conditions. Under these circumstances, dyssynergia cerebellaris myclonica is a clinical syndrome that may result from spinocerebellar degeneration or cortical cerebellar degeneration, and it is questionable whether this form of Ramsay Hunt's syndrome really exists as a separate disease entity (see Familial Myoclonus and Ataxia).

Cerebrocerebellar Degeneration

Although dementia has been described in association with the cerebellar, olivopontocerebellar, and spinocerebellar degenerations, it is not unusual to see patients with a strikingly progressive dementia who also show signs of mild or moderate cerebellar dysfunction. It is possible that these changes occur in a number of neuronal degenerations including Alzheimer's disease and Huntington's chorea. It is doubtful that cerebrocerebellar degeneration exists as a distinct pathologic entity. Other cases may be examples of dementia associated with the spinocerebellar degenerations. These patients show diffuse ventricular dilation by computed tomography, indicating an atrophic process involving the cerebrum particularly in the frontal lobes and in the cerebellum.

Acute Intermittent Familial Cerebellar Ataxia

This interesting condition is inherited as an autosomal dominant trait. Although there is no evidence that the disorder is progressive, it is classified here with the cerebellar degenerations.[110]

Etiology and Pathology

The attacks have been reported to be elicited by such factors as viral infections, psychologic trauma, and infestation with *Ascaris lumbricoides*. The pathologic changes are unknown since the condition is benign.

Clinical Features

Attacks occur in both children and adults. The onset is sudden with headache, lethargy, fever, and vomiting. Others develop acute signs of cerebellar ataxia without such prodromas. There are ataxia of gait, truncal ataxia, dysarthria, nystagmus, upper limb ataxia, choreoathetosis, and, rarely, myoclonus. The attacks gradually subside within ten days and recovery is complete. Episodes tend to subside in late adolescence and adult life.

Treatment

The elimination of precipitating infections appears to hasten recovery.

Vestibulocerebellar Ataxia

An unusual form of familial ataxia has been described in which there are periodic episodes of vertigo, diplopia, and ataxia. The condition appears to be inherited as an autosomal dominant trait.[71]

Etiology and Pathology

The pathologic changes are unknown, but there appears to be a disturbance of vestibular connections in the brainstem associated with chronic degeneration of the cerebellar connections.

Clinical Features

The symptoms develop between the ages of 20 and 50 years and consist of attacks of vertigo, tinnitus, diplopia, and ataxia, lasting from a few minutes to two months. The frequency varies from recurrent daily episodes to as long as one year between attacks. The onset is sudden, and vertigo and diplopia are associated with nystagmus, which is maximal on abduction of the eye, suggesting involvement of the medial longitudinal fasciculus in the brainstem. The presence of vertical nystagmus in some cases also indicates a similar level of involvement. The ataxia occurs only during episodes of vertigo initially, but as the condition progresses, persistent cerebellar ataxia with titubation of the head and nystagmus may appear slowly over many years.

Treatment

The attacks are decreased in frequency and severity by using antihistamines such as dimenhydrinate (Dramamine).

"Toxic" Cerebellar Degeneration

A number of toxic agents can produce cerebellar degeneration, but there are three main causes seen in neurologic practice. The degenerations associated with alcohol and neoplasia are discussed elsewhere. The toxic effect of diphenylhydantoin (Dilantin) may be acute and reversible and less commonly chronic with permanent cerebellar damage. In the acute type of toxicity, due to diphenylhydantoin, the patient is obtunded and occasionally confused, with nystagmus and severe truncal and limb ataxia. This resolves within several days when the dosage of the drug is decreased. Occasionally, patients with seizures who have been receiving high doses of diphenylhydantoin for many years develop a permanent cerebellar ataxia, which may be so severe as to impair walking.[141] It is probable that there has been permanent damage to the Purkinje cells in the cerebellum in such cases, as these neurons have been shown to undergo necrosis with toxic doses of diphenylhydantoin in experimental animals.

Cerebellar degeneration and ataxia may arise on occasion as a complication of chronic myxedema. Autopsy studies have revealed a loss of Purkinje cells in the cerebellum, with mild gliosis, vacuolation, and a decrease in the number of granular cells.[191]

Motor Neuron Disease or Amyotrophic Lateral Sclerosis

This disease has been assigned a number of synonyms, including progressive muscular atrophy of Aran and Duchenne, motor neuron disease, and amyotrophic lateral sclerosis. The latter is probably the most widely used term, although motor neuron disease best describes the essential pathologic change.

In the United States it has become customary to use the term "amyotrophic lateral sclerosis" for all forms, but three clinical variants deserve special recognition.[221] These are progressive muscular atrophy, progressive bulbar palsy, and primary lateral sclerosis, described earlier.

Etiology and Pathology

There are several possible etiologies to be considered although the exact cause is not known. Amyotrophic lateral sclerosis may be a virus infection, an autoimmune disease, a toxic degeneration, or a paraneoplastic phenomenon. The demonstration of virus-like particles in anterior horn cells[182] and in muscle,[177] the presence of virus antigen in the jejunal mucosa, and evidence of immune complex[174] formation in patients with amyotrophic lateral sclerosis[187] suggest a viral etiology. However, efforts to culture a virus and to transmit the disease to animals have not been successful at this time. Histocompatibility typing shows an increased incidence of HL-A3 antigen and suggests a relationship between amyotrophic lateral sclerosis and poliovirus but would also be compatible with an autoimmune disease.

Several laboratories have shown that blood from patients with amyotrophic lateral sclerosis destroys cultures of anterior horn cells,[26, 238] which would support an autoimmune process. However, recent studies have shown no tissue culture cytotoxicity from amyotrophic lateral sclerosis sera.[117] The evidence for a toxic degeneration of anterior horn cells is supported by the demonstration of patient exposure to lead and mercury and the presence[72] and the measurement of abnormally high lead levels in the cerebrospinal fluid.[117] One form of the disease is due to the remote effects of carcinoma which would be compatible with a viral infection or autoimmune condition.

Both the brain and spinal cord are essentially normal in appearance except that there may be atrophy of the anterior roots. Microscopically, there is loss of motor neurons in layers 3 and 5 in the frontal lobes. Section of the brainstem shows degeneration in the corticospinal (pyramidal) tracts and neuronal loss in the motor cranial nerve nuclei. The direct and indirect corticospinal tracts are degenerated in the spinal cord with a striking loss of motor neurons in the anterior horns. The anterior nerve roots contain fewer motor fibers, while the atrophy of muscles is characteristic, with loss of muscle fibers in fascicles or in the distribution of motor units. There is little inflammatory response, apart from the presence of a few phagocytes surrounding recently degenerated muscle fibers.

Clinical Features

Amyotrophic lateral sclerosis is not a common disease. The prevalence is about 3 per 100,000 population, and the average annual incidence ranges from 0.4 to 1.4 per 100,000 population in different regions of the world.[130] The disease rarely occurs before the age of 35 years with maximal incidence in the fourth and fifth decades. It occurs more commonly in the male than the female, with a ratio of incidence of 2:1 among the sexes. Between 5 and 10 per cent of cases in the United States are familial. The familial form is inherited as an autosomal recessive trait, and

these cases often show atypical features such as paralysis of the bladder and, rarely, impairment of vibration sense in lower extremities associated with otherwise typical signs and symptoms of motor neuron degeneration.[112]

Many familial cases are probably formes frustes of a spinocerebellar degeneration,[116, 190, 225] and it is not unusual to find a number of different neurologic disorders in family members.[79] About 10 per cent of cases are paraneoplastic and occur in patients with overt or occult carcinoma.

The disease usually presents with atrophy, weakness, fasciculations, spasms, and cramping of the affected muscles. In 40 to 50 per cent of cases, the atrophy begins in one or both hands, and in the remainder of cases, the legs are first affected. There is gradual loss of muscle bulk in both thenar and hypothenar eminences as well as atrophy of the interossei (Fig. 4–3). The other hand soon shows signs of atrophy, usually within several months. When the legs are first involved, progressive foot drop with wasting of the anterior tibial compartment is usually noted first, with atrophy and weakness of the gastrocnemius and quadriceps being noted later. However, the disease may present with wasting and weakness with fasciculations in one shoulder girdle with later involvement of the other shoulder, suggesting a cervical cord lesion. In this type of onset, the weakness gradually spreads to the muscles of the upper limbs in a segmental fashion and reaches the hands at a later stage. The degree of muscle wasting in the shoulders may be masked by the plump, subcutaneous tissues in this area, and there may be profound weakness, particularly in women, without much visible evidence of wasting. In such patients, the shoulders usually sag to a marked degree and the normal contour of the area is lost.

Whether or not the weakness begins in the hands or shoulders, there is a relentless spread to involve other muscles. Atrophy of the intercostal muscles terminally results in reduction of respiratory reserve with dyspnea. The cough reflex is reduced so that secretions accumulate in the trachea and bronchi, with the risk of aspiration pneumonia.

There is usually marked corticospinal tract involvement by the time that atrophy and fasciculations become generalized. The combination of spasticity and wasting produces the characteristic phenomenon seen in this disease, increased deep tendon reflexes in muscles that are grossly atrophic and weak. The disease usually progresses to involve the muscles supplied by the bulbar motor nuclei, with difficulty in swallowing, coughing, and speaking. Weakness, atrophy, and fasciculations appear in the tongue, and there is progressive involvement of the pharyngeal and laryngeal muscles in the terminal stages of the disease. Chewing and swallowing become difficult, and finally only a soft diet can be handled owing to progressive weakness of the muscles of mastication and the facial muscles. In the terminal stages, secretions accumulate in the pharynx that can neither be swallowed nor expectorated. Death usually occurs from respiratory insufficiency and aspiration pneumonia.

Rarely, patients with motor neuron disease present with the form of the disease known as primary lateral sclerosis. This may occur in the familial form, the form associated with carcinoma as a remote effect, and in the idiopathic form. In this group of patients there are signs only of spasticity in all four extremities, although it may begin unilaterally. Wasting and fasciculations are not present in the early stages of the disease although they may appear late. This form runs a more benign course and may continue for ten years. Pseudobulbar signs and occasionally euphoria and dementia are present. Except in the familial forms, there is no bladder involvement or sensory loss. Late in the disease, degeneration of the corticobulbar pathways leads to emotional lability, inappropriate laughing and crying, dysarthria, and dysphagia. The movements of the tongue may be slow and spastic, and the jaw jerk, glabella, and snout reflexes may all be hyperactive.

The term "progressive bulbar palsy" is applied to the group of patients who present with wasting of the bulbar muscles, particularly of the tongue at an early stage in the disease. In these cases the disease runs a rapid course and the patient rarely survives more than 18 months from the onset of symptoms.

The five-year survival for all patients with amyotrophic lateral sclerosis is about 40 per cent.[195b] Patients who present with signs of progressive muscular atrophy with no spasticity have the best prognosis with survival exceeding ten years in some cases. Similarly, the primary lateral sclerosis form is usually slowly progressive with survival for many years. If atrophy, weakness, and fasciculations occur with spasticity, the outlook is less favorable and death usually occurs three or four years from the onset of the disease. In some cases, clear-cut remissions occur for reasons that are not yet understood.[173] Patients with progressive bulbar palsy have the worst prognosis. Once signs of bulbar paralysis occur in all forms of this disease, they indicate a poor prognosis with survival seldom exceeding 18 months.

Diagnostic Procedures

1. It is important to identify those cases due to the remote effects of carcinoma, so that chest roentgenograms, roentgenographic gastrointestinal series, and other diagnostic tests to exclude latent malignancy are indicated. It is also important to differentiate this disease from polymyositis and compressive lesions of the spinal cord that are remediable.

2. Electromyography and measurement of nerve conduction velocity aid in establishing the diagnosis. The nerve conduction velocities are normal, but electromyography usually shows widespread denervation patterns with fibrillations and fasciculations. Insertion activity is usually normal, but often prolonged discharges of diphasic spikes or larger positive waves are noted together with the characteristic fibrillations at rest. Maximal voluntary contraction yields an abnormal response with reduction in motor unit action potentials. The reduction is proportional to the degree of atrophy, and in advanced cases few motor units, if any, are found. Occasionally, giant action potentials are recorded. These may be due to selective destruction of smaller motor units or synchronous activity of remaining motor units, which may result from alteration of the excitability of motor neurons in the anterior horns by this disease. It is also likely that such abnormal activity results from undamaged motor neurons making contact and reinnervating denervated motor units through proliferation and branching of the terminal axons.

3. Myelography should be performed to exclude the possibility of cord compression in the cervical area or at the base of the skull or multiple nerve root compression (i.e., conditions that show good response to surgical treatment).

4. Measurement of serum creatine phosphokinase (CPK) usually reveals levels elevated to 1.5 to 3 times normal in the active stage of denervation atrophy.

5. Diagnosis is usually confirmed by biopsy of involved muscles, which show the characteris-

tic pattern of denervation atrophy with fascicles of intact muscle fibers adjacent and subjacent to atrophic groups of angular fibers corresponding to the pattern previously innervated by dying axons (Fig. 4–9).

6. Serial charting of the strength of the individual muscles by a trained physical therapist (manual muscle chart) remains the best method of objectively measuring the course and progression of this disease.

7. Videotape recording during the swallowing of barium is helpful in establishing pharyngeal weakness.

8. Serial pulmonary function tests are useful in establishing or estimating any impairment of pulmonary function due to intercostal or diaphragmatic paralysis although impairment of pulmonary function usually appears suddenly and is a preterminal sign. Assisted respiration with a mechanical respirator can be considered and discussed with the family (see below) if the maximum breathing capacity falls below 30 liters per minute and should be controlled by accurate estimations of the arterial partial pressure of oxygen and carbon dioxide (P_{O_2} and P_{CO_2}).

Treatment

At the present time, there is no specific treatment for amyotrophic lateral sclerosis.[169]

During the early stages, the patient should be advised to continue, if possible, his occupation and to remain as active as possible. Much depends, of course, on the nature of the patient's occupation, and those with a sedentary occupation will be able to work much longer than those engaged in manual labor. Any factors that could possibly have a deleterious effect, such as poor diet or infections, should be treated.

Lightweight plastic foot-drop braces are helpful in maintaining ambulatory those patients with wasting of the anterior tibial muscles. Postural hypotension of the central neurogenic type (similar to that described under the Shy-Drager syndrome) may occasionally be seen and require fludrocortisone therapy.

Counseling the patient and his family is important but presents certain problems in the early

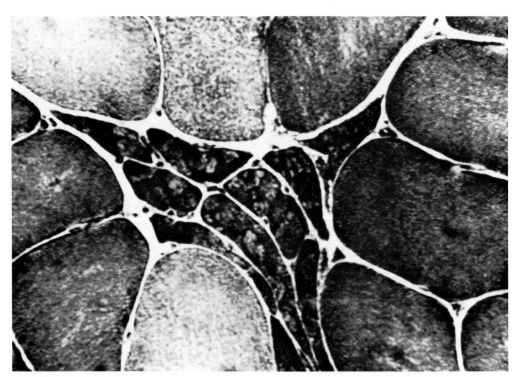

FIGURE 4–9. NADH-TR reaction showing densely staining groups of angular fibers classically seen in motor neuron disease.

stages of the disease because it is difficult to determine how much the patient should be told about his condition. Should the patient be told that he has a progressive disease, the prognosis should not be discussed in gloomy terms. Undue emphasis on the poor prognosis may create anxieties and depression. The nature of the disease and the possible outcome should be discussed frankly, however, with some responsible member of the family. This enables planning to meet the potential problems created by total disability in the terminal stages of the illness.

When weakness and atrophy have advanced to the stage of impairment of ambulation, the patient may be advised to use a wheelchair. Painful contractions and subluxation of the shoulder joint can be avoided by the use of suitable splints and slings.

During the terminal phase there is the danger of aspiration and pneumonia, which can be reduced by suctioning and early treatment with antibiotics. Difficulties in chewing and dysphagia are usually minimized by a semisolid or liquid diet. The use of a plastic nasogastric tube should be postponed as long as possible but must be resorted to if nutrition is not maintained. Gastrostomy is indicated in patients with malnutrition due to bulbar paralysis.

The decision regarding whether or not to use a respirator is difficult in the majority of cases. When respiratory insufficiency is such that assisted respiration is necessary, tracheotomy should be performed. This permits the use of a machine over a relatively long period of time and facilitates the removal of secretions. It is distressing, however, for all concerned to witness further deterioration in the patient's muscle strength on the respirator until, in some cases, virtually only movement of the eyes remains. With these considerations in mind, it is wise to discuss this possibility with the family before beginning artificial respiration. In some cases the patient or family may request that artificial respiration should not be used.

Any progressive disability is likely to produce anxiety and depression. Amyotrophic lateral sclerosis is no exception. The physician should recognize such secondary symptoms and treat the patient with tranquilizers or antidepressant drugs as required. Pain is not a problem in amyotrophic lateral sclerosis, so that the use of narcotic drugs is not indicated. However, the wise use of sedation may do much to alleviate suffering in the terminal stages of this disease.

Local anesthesia, rather than general anesthesia, for any surgery is preferred in patients with far-advanced disease, since depression of respiration may precipitate respiratory insufficiency.

Amyotrophic Lateral Sclerosis in Guam

Reference has already been made to the parkinsonism-dementia complex which occurs in the Chamorro population in the Mariana Islands. There is also an unusually high incidence of amyotrophic lateral sclerosis among the indigenous Chamorros on the island of Guam. The disease if often familial, but there is evidence that it may occur in non-Chamorro people who have lived on the island for many years. It is questionable that this form of amyotrophic lateral sclerosis is hereditary.[62, 63]

Etiology and Pathology

Two possible causes are currently under investigation. The first possibility is that the disease is caused by a slow virus infection and the second is that it may result from some exogenous or endogenous toxin.

The pathologic changes in this form of amyotrophic lateral sclerosis are similar to those described in parkinsonian-dementia complex except that the regions affected are different. There is widespread loss of motor neurons in the cerebrum, brainstem, and anterior horn cells of the spinal cord. Alzheimer's neurofibrillary tangles are found in surviving neurons in these areas of neuronal damage, particularly in Ammon's horn and the hippocampal formation.[111, 113]

Clinical Features

This form of amyotrophic lateral sclerosis, unlike that seen elsewhere, is twice as common in females and tends to occur at a somewhat earlier age than the classic form of the disease. It has other differences in that some patients develop dementia while others eventually show signs of the parkinsonism-dementia complex.

The disease tends to run a more protracted course among the Chamorro people with a longer period of survival in about one third of the cases when compared with classic amyotrophic lateral sclerosis. However, the survival period is short following the development of bulbar symptoms, a feature common to all types of the disease.

The Kugelberg-Welander Syndrome (Familial Spinal Muscular Atrophy)

An infrequent and relatively benign form of neuronal atrophy involving the anterior horn cells was described in 1954. Since then, a number of families with this condition, which is inherited either as an autosomal recessive or as an autosomal dominant trait, have been studied.[7, 231]

Clinical Features

The muscular atrophy usually begins in childhood or adolescence and is often confined to the proximal muscles of the limb girdle. The disease is commonly confused with the muscular dystrophies.[155]

The course is benign, with slow progression or apparent arrest in adult life. The bulbar muscles are occasionally involved and there may be fasciculations and hypo- or hyperreflexia.[197] Some cases show pseudohypertrophy of the calf muscles and slight elevation of serum enzymes suggesting that there may be a myopathic component in addition to the neuronal atrophy. Although the condition bears a superficial resemblance to the limb girdle form of muscular dystrophy, it can be readily distinguished by the electromyographic findings and by muscle biopsy, both of which show changes characteristic of neurogenic atrophy.

Hydrocephalus

The term "hydrocephalus" indicates the presence of excess cerebrospinal fluid (CSF) within the cranial cavity. It results from an imbalance between the production and absorption of CSF, which are normally in equilibrium.

The CSF is secreted by the choroid plexus in the lateral, third and fourth ventricles, and the direction of flow is from the lateral ventricles. The fluid leaves the third ventricle through the cerebral aqueduct (aqueduct of Sylvius). It enters the fourth ventricle and flows out into the subarachnoid space through the lateral foramina of Luschka and the medial foramen of Magendie, situated in the ependymal roof of the fourth ventricle. The subarachnoid space surrounds the brain and spinal cord, and the CSF circulates throughout the entire space.

There is evidence that the flow of CSF is active rather than passive and that the CSF is actively propelled within the subarachnoid space by the pulsation of the cerebral arteries and probably also by respiratory movements affecting the cerebral veins. The major portion of the CSF is absorbed through the arachnoid villi into the dural sinuses. However, some fluid is absorbed via the Virchow-Robin spaces within the brain substance and via radicular veins and capillaries within the subarachnoid space around the proximal roots of the spinal nerves. Under abnormal conditions, when there is obstruction to the circulation of CSF, it may also be absorbed into the brain parenchyma after passage through the ependymal wall of the ventricles.

Pathogenesis

Hydrocephalus may occur under the following circumstances:

1. Cerebral dysgenesis
2. Excessive production of CSF
3. Obstruction to the flow of CSF
4. Deficiency in absorption of CSF
5. Following cerebral atrophy (hydrocephalus ex vacuo)

Cerebral Dysgenesis. Many cerebral malformations are associated with failure or arrested development of some part of the brain with an accumulation of CSF to compensate for the absent brain tissue. The most obvious example is hydranencephaly due to failure of development of the cerebral hemispheres.

Excessive Production of CSF. This is a rare cause of hydrocephalus. Occasional examples of an actively secreting papilloma of the choroid plexus have been described, but the condition is rarely diagnosed during life. This type of hydrocephalus responds well to resection of the choroid plexus.

Obstruction to the Flow of CSF. The majority of cases of symptomatic hydrocephalus fall into this category. The obstruction may occur at any point within the ventricular system or subarachnoid space. The clinical terms "internal," "obstructive," or "noncommunicating" hydrocephalus are used to denote obstruction within the ventricular system, and "communicating" hydrocephalus is used to describe failure of absorption or diffuse obstruction in the subarachnoid space. In general, these clinical terms are unsatisfactory or confusing and should be abandoned.

Obstruction to the flow of CSF may be intermittent as with a ball-valve tumor of the ventricular system or an elongated basilar artery which intermittently obstructs the aqueduct with each arterial pulsation.[31]

Deficiency in Absorption of CSF. It is possible that there is a deficiency in absorption of CSF associated with certain malformations of the brain such as meningomyelocele, since surgical repair is often followed by hydrocephalus. Obstruction of the arachnoid villi may result as a complication of acute meningitis, following subarachnoid hemorrhage, and when the protein content of the CSF is excessively high. All of these have been reported to cause hydrocephalus.

Following Cerebral Atrophy. Hydrocephalus ex vacuo is the term given by pathologists to describe the excessive volume of CSF that compensates for cerebral atrophy. This type of hydrocephalus is asymptomatic.

Hydrocephalus may occur at any age. The majority of cases are due to obstruction of the circulation of CSF. There are two conditions that require particular consideration: infantile hydrocephalus and the so-called "normal pressure" hydrocephalus of adults.

Infantile Hydrocephalus

The prognosis of the child with infantile hydrocephalus has been radically improved by the introduction of surgical measures to divert CSF into the bloodstream (ventriculoatrial shunt) or peritoneal cavity (ventriculoperitoneal shunt). Prior to this surgical advance, infantile hydrocephalus was associated with a high mortality and usually ran a chronic and tragic course. As a result of such surgical treatment, many cases have sustained apparent cure with the development of normal intelligence, life-span, and size of the head.

Etiology and Pathology

About 46 per cent of children with infantile hydrocephalus have associated malformations of the brain. The most common types are the Arnold-Chiari malformation (p. 79) or a malformation of the aqueduct causing stenosis of this important CSF pathway. The latter group includes stenosis of the aqueduct without gliosis; "forking" of the aqueduct, in which there are two channels of greatly reduced lumen diameter; and septum formation in the aqueduct, with narrowing of the

channel. Other forms of malformation may produce hydrocephalus, and these include atresia of the foramen of Magendie in the roof of the fourth ventrical and the Dandy-Walker syndrome. This latter condition consists of atresia of the foramen of Magendie with a failure of development of the vermis of the cerebellum. The fourth ventricle is dilated to a marked degree and balloons into the posterior fossa between the cerebellar hemispheres. The posterior fossa is enlarged, and the internal occipital protuberance and torcular Herophili are elevated (Fig. 4–10).

Some 50 per cent of children with hydrocephalus develop the condition following subarachnoid hemorrhage due to trauma or meningitis. Both subarachnoid hemorrhage and infection lead to inflammation and exudation, which may block the aqueduct of Sylvius or the foramina in the roof of the fourth ventricle. The basal cisterns also may be occluded by arachnoiditis with obstruction to the flow of CSF resulting in hydrocephalus.

A posterior fossa tumor is an uncommon but remediable cause of hydrocephalus in the infant and probably accounts for about 4 per cent of cases.

The brain of the hydrocephalic child shows dilatation of the ventricular system proximal to the site of the block, and thinning of the overlying hemispheric tissue to 2 cm or less in severe cases. The central gray matter, including the basal ganglia and thalamus, do not show comparable degrees of atrophy. The progressive expansion of

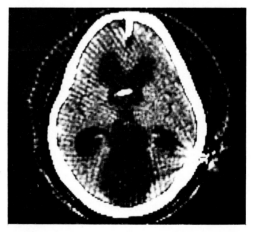

FIGURE 4–10. Computed tomography in Dandy-Walker syndrome. There are a marked degree of hydrocephalus and a huge fourth ventricle occupying most of the posterior fossa.

the ventricles results in enlargement of the skull and separation of the cranial sutures.[145]

Clinical Features

A number of children are actually born with hydrocephalus and enlargement of the head. This may be of sufficient degree to cause obstruction during labor and necessitate cesarean section. The majority of children with hydrocephalus, however, appear to be normal at birth, and symptoms of hydrocephalus are not apparent for two or three months. This group includes many of the cases with malformations.[120]

Children who develop enlargement of the head later in infancy or early childhood usually have a history of trauma to the head or meningitis.

The outstanding feature in infantile hydrocephalus is progressive enlargement of the head, the rapidity of which is proportional to the degree of increased intracranial pressure. The face, although of normal size, appears small relative to the enlarged head, and there is usually some exophthalmos and prominence of the sclera due to downward displacement of the rest of the orbit.

Severe degrees of intracranial hypertension produce a sluggish reaction of the pupils to light, absence of upward gaze, impaired lateral gaze, paralysis or spasm of convergence, nystagmus, retractions, and absence of visual fixation or response to visual threat.[61] Untreated infants with hydrocephalus fail to thrive and show retardation of motor and intellectual development. Movements of the limbs, particularly the legs, show progressive weakness and spasticity. Seizures are common.

Examination of a child with hydrocephalus reveals enlargement of the skull with prominent scalp veins, separation of the sutures, widened fontanels, and a "cracked-pot" sound on percussing the skull. There may be considerable wasting of trunk and limb muscles, spasticity, increased deep tendon reflexes, and bilateral extensor plantar responses.

The child eventually becomes unable to lift the enlarged head, and there is progressive visual loss followed by blindness with optic atrophy and paralysis. Necrosis of the scalp may eventually result with leakage of the CSF, infection, and death. The mortality rate is high, with survival of only 50 per cent of untreated cases at the age of one year and about 30 per cent at ten years of age.[152]

Rare cases that survived before surgical treatment became available are examples of arrested hydrocephalus often with various degrees of retarded mental development, spasticity of the lower limbs, and impairment of bladder function. Other cases had no neurologic deficit at all.

Diagnostic Procedures

1. In suspected cases of hydrocephalus the skull diameter should be measured at each visit and recorded for comparison with standard values for that age.
2. The fundi should be examined carefully. Papilledema is unusual in infantile hydrocephalus because of the open fontanel, but optic atrophy may be present. If papilledema occurs, it raises the possibility of a brain tumor.
3. Transillumination should be performed in all cases to exclude hydranencephaly and subdural hygroma.
4. Roentgenograms of the skull confirm enlargement due to hydrocephalus and may show separation of the sutures and increased intracranial markings due to increased intracranial pressure.
5. Computed tomography is indicated before a shunting procedure to determine the extent of the hydrocephalus, the cause of obstruction, and the presence or absence of any associated congenital abnormalities (Fig. 4–11). Pneumoencephalography with tomography may still be of value in some cases to delineate the site of obstruction, particularly in the case of posterior fossa lesions.[61]

Treatment

The use of the Spitz-Holter and similar types of ventriculoatrial valves has significantly improved the treatment of infantile hydrocephalus.[102] The mortality rate for this type of surgical treatment is low. Eighty per cent of hydrocephalic children now achieve satisfactory arrest of the hydrocephalus following this procedure. Complications, including obstruction of the catheter, infection of the catheter and valve, and thromboembolism, are infrequent risks encountered during treatment by this method. Elective revision or replacement of catheters is necessary as the child grows.

In assessing the results of surgery, it must be borne in mind that many children have brain damage because of the conditions that caused the hydrocephalus, i.e., meningitis or trauma, and that cerebral atrophy secondary to hydrocephalus may not be the most important cause of any neu-

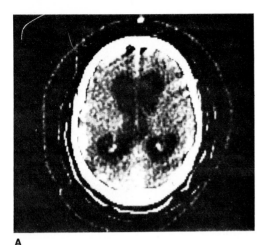
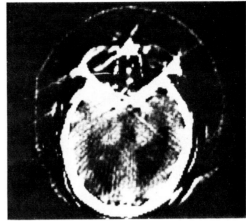

A   **B**

FIGURE 4–11. Computed tomography in infantile hydrocephalus with stenosis of the aqueduct. *A.* There is marked ventricular dilation. *B.* The fourth ventricle is not visualized, however.

rologic defect. Nevertheless, there is some general correlation between the degree of hydrocephalus before operation and the resulting impairment of intelligence. Children with less than 1 cm thickness of the cortical mantle left are likely to have persistent impairment after surgery. The presence of optic atrophy and blindness, even in long-standing cases, does not necessarily mean that the vision is irreparably lost. There is always hope for some improvement when the hydrocephalus is relieved.

Normal Pressure Hydrocephalus

This adult form of chronic hydrocephalus has only become recognized in the last decade and is of particular interest in that there may be some clinical improvement of an otherwise progressive dementia following surgical treatment by ventriculoatrial or ventriculoperitoneal shunt. It is one of the rare conditions causing dementia but is important since it may be alleviated by treatment (p. 175). For this reason continued search is justified for additional cases among patients diagnosed as having "presenile" or "senile" dementia.

Etiology and Pathology

The reported causes of this condition include aqueductal stenosis, subarachnoid hemorrhage, chronic meningoencephalitis, slowly growing tumors or cysts situated in the posterior portion of the third ventricle, elongation of the basilar artery compressing the aqueduct and third ventricle,[58] and hypertensive cerebrovascular disease.[56, 142] In some cases, however, the etiology remains obscure.

Since the majority of cases have normal CSF pressure or borderline elevation at the time of examination, it has been postulated that the hydrocephalus was initiated by an increase in CSF pressure in the past (or possibly some transient atrophic process), but the ventricles continue to enlarge owing to the action of apparently normal CSF pressure. Monitoring of the CSF pressure in these patients will usually reveal intermittent elevations of CSF pressure well above normal.[224] In addition, there is a demonstrable deficit in absorption of CSF.[153] The continued ventricular dilatation has been explained on the basis of Pascal's law, which states that the force exerted by a fluid on its surrounding medium is equal not only to the pressure of the fluid, but to the product of that pressure times the area of the surface on which its acts. Thus, once ventricular dilatation has occurred, no matter what the cause, this increases the surface area of the ventricles; hence a much lower pressure is now required to cause further hydrocephalus.

The brain shows diffuse dilatation of the ventricular system proximal to the site of obstruction, and all ventricles, including the fourth ventricle and the aqueduct, may be dilated. In contrast to other forms of dementia, there is no evidence of cortical atrophy.

Clinical Features

The essential features are a progressive dementia, dyspraxia, and spasticity of gait progressing over a period of several months. The dementia presents with lack of judgment and insight, followed by impairment of retention and recent memory. There is progressive difficulty with gait, due to a combination of dyspraxia and spasticity. Impairment or loss of sphincter control and incontinence often occur. Examination reveals signs of dementia, the tone in the lower limbs is increased, and the tendon jerks are hyperactive with extensor plantar responses.

If untreated, the disease progresses to a state where there is inability to stand, with the eventual development of akinetic rigidity and withdrawn behavior. In this state, the patient tends to sit motionless for many hours.

Diagnostic Procedures

1. The routine lumbar puncture with measurement of cerebrospinal fluid pressure is normal or slightly elevated. The serologic and chemical examinations and the cell count are normal. Monitoring the CSF pressure for 24 hours usually reveals intermittent elevation of CSF pressure above normal particularly at night.
2. The EEG is normal or shows diffuse slowing over both hemispheres, usually classified as "nonspecific slowing," and there are no focal features.
3. Computed tomography reveals diffuse enlargement of the ventricles,[47] which may persist after a shunting procedure (Fig. 4–12). In addition, the CT scan may show cortical atrophy in some cases, and the presence of cortical atrophy should not negate the diagnosis of normal pressure hydrocephalus.[126] However, there is less chance of improvement following a ventricular shunting procedure if there is significant widening of the sulci over the superior hemisphere convexity.[101a]
4. Arteriography reveals elongation of the basilar artery in some cases and enlarged ventricles with stretching of the anterior cerebral artery in its course over the lateral ventricles.
5. Intrathecal injection of radioactive ytterbium shows prolonged retention in the ventricular system. This procedure, known as radioisotope cisternography, shows enlarged ventricles with persistent radioisotope in the ventricles after 48 and 72 hours.[163] Normally, the isotope is cleared from the ventricles in 24 hours.[231]
6. Measurement of regional cerebral blood flow before lumbar puncture shows reduction of blood flow particularly in the distribution of the anterior cerebral artery. rCBF increases

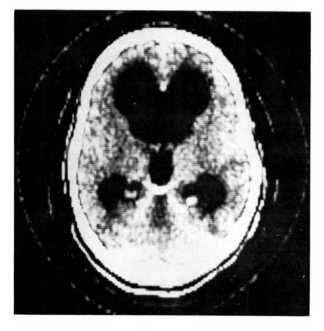

FIGURE 4–12. Computed tomography in a case of normal pressure hydrocephalus. There is diffuse enlargement of the third, fourth, and lateral ventricle, but there is no evidence of cortical atrophy in this case.

to near-normal levels when 20 ml of CSF are removed in cases of normal pressure hydrocephalus.[159]

Treatment

The response to ventricular shunting procedure may be dramatic, with reversal of symptoms of dementia and improvement in gait over a period of several days. This improvement is maintained as long as the shunt functions satisfactorily.[109] Cases of progressive dementia due to neuronal atrophy have not benefited from this operation.

Otitic Hydrocephalus

This form of hydrocephalus occurs in children with chronic otitis media and mastoiditis. It is due to thrombosis of the lateral sinus, which has been demonstrated at surgery and more recently by venography.[167]

Clinical Features

There is a history of chronic otitis media usually of three to four months' duration followed by symptoms of increased intracranial pressure, including headache, nausea, and vomiting. The child appears to be febrile and listless, usually with a perforated eardrum and purulent discharge from the ear. There may be an ipsilateral sixth-nerve paralysis, but there are few other neurologic abnormalities apart from papilledema.[95]

Diagnostic Procedures

The blood count usually shows mild leukocytosis. The cerebrospinal fluid pressure may be markedly elevated (up to 600 mm water) with an insignificant rise and fall on unilateral jugular compression on the affected side. Cell counts and sugar and protein content are normal. Clouding of the mastoid air cells can be seen by roentgenograms, and blocking of the lateral sinus may be demonstrated during the venous phase of arteriography.

Treatment

Most children show gradual improvement following mastoidectomy and removal of necrotic material around the lateral sinus. Where signs of increased intracranial pressure are present, they may be relieved by serial lumbar puncture with removal of sufficient CSF to reduce the pressure to within normal limits. Subtemporal decompression may be required in rare cases showing persistence of papilledema and the possibility of blindness from optic atrophy.

Degenerative Conditions Involving the Spinal Cord

Atlantoaxial Dislocation Due to Odontoid Hypoplasia or Dysplasia

Although odontoid dysplasia should be regarded as a congenital abnormality, the neurologic symptoms resulting from atlantoaxial dislocation are often delayed until adult life. The clinical symptoms are the result of compression with degenerative changes in the upper segments of the cervical spinal cord. The same condition may also arise from fracture of the odontoid process.

Etiology and Pathology

Odontoid dysplasia or agenesis permits dislocation at the atlantoaxial junction, with the movement of the first cervical vertebra forward on the second cervical vertebra. The spinal canal is narrowed, with compression of the spinal cord and damage by direct trauma and impairment of blood supply. The dislocation may be spontaneous or follow traumatic injury to the head or neck. The symptoms are intermittent in some cases.[77]

An autopsy, the spinal cord is narrowed and flattened in its upper segments. The cord usually shows degenerative changes involving the anterior and lateral columns with sparing of the posterior columns.

Clinical Features

Symptoms may appear in childhood, adolescence or early adult life and consist of a progressive or intermittent spastic quadriparesis. In established cases, there is generalized spasticity with clonus, hyperreflexia, and bilateral extensor plantar responses. The jaw jerk is not increased. The sensory loss is variable but usually consists of hypalgesia involving the lower limbs and trunk up to the cervical area. The functions of the posterior columns remain intact. There may be marked hypertrophy of the muscles of the neck, which act as a "splint" and attempt to induce stability at the atlantoaxial junction.

Diagnostic Procedures

Roentgenograms of the upper cervical spine show failure of fusion or fracture of the odontoid

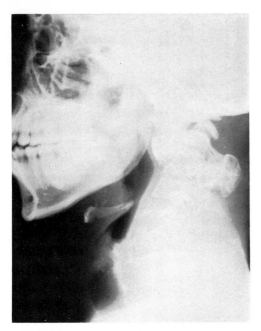

FIGURE 4–13. Lateral roentgenogram of the cervical spine showing congenital dislocation of the odontoid process in a young man with progressive spastic paraplegia.

process where it should join the body of the second cervical vertebra (Fig. 4–13). Laminograms usually show the fracture clearly. The first cervical vertebra is dislocated forward on the second during flexion of the head. The posterior displacement of the cervical cord by the odontoid process can be demonstrated by cervical myelography.

Treatment

The aim of treatment is to decompress the spinal cord and stabilize the atlantoaxial junction. This can be accomplished by transoral removal of the arch of the first cervical vertebra and removal of the odontoid process.[93] The patient is placed in Crutchfield tongs, and a posterior fusion of the first and second cervical vertebrae is usually carried out after a two-week interval.

Platybasia and Basilar Impression

Platybasia and basilar impression have also been discussed in relation to developmental disorders in children in Chapter 2. There are many clinical similarities between these two conditions and the syndrome described under odontoid hypoplasia. These conditions are usually congenital abnormalities in which symptoms may be delayed until adult life, and they are also associated with

compression of the cervical portion of the spinal cord. However, cerebellar and cervical root signs are more evident in this condition.

Etiology and Pathology

Platybasia is an invagination of the base of the skull surrounding the foramen magnum. It is usually due to a developmental abnormality and may be familial. It has also been described in conditions associated with softening of bone including Paget's disease, osteomalacia, rickets, and osteogenesis imperfecta. Basilar impression is an invagination of the odontoid process through the foramen magnum. Although it is often associated with platybasia, it may occur independently but often in association with other congenital abnormalities, such as fusion of the first cervical vertebra to the base of the skull or fusion of two or more of the upper cervical vertebrae.

Both platybasia and basilar invagination result in an abnormal angulation at the junction of the lower medulla and cervical cord. This results in pressure on the cord and degenerative changes as described under odontoid hypoplasia, plus cerebellar signs and paresthesias of the shoulder and arms due to traction on the cervical nerve roots.

Clinical Features

Chronic compression of the spinal cord produces progressive spastic quadriparesis, which may be mild in some cases. There is often some degree of involvement of the bladder with urgency of micturition. Complaints of paresthesias in the shoulders and arms with some sensory loss are not uncommon. Sensory loss is usually confined to impairment of pain sensation with preservation of function of the dorsal columns. Cerebellar signs such as ataxia and incoordination of finger-to-nose testing are not uncommon. Some patients experience sneeze syncope, which is a feeling of lightheadedness, vertigo, and nausea, lasting for several minutes after sneezing or straining at stool. There may be abrupt loss of consciousness.[44] The mechanism of sneeze syncope is unknown, but it is possible that sneezing causes mechanical percussion of the brainstem against the anterior lip of the foramen magnum or a succession of spinal fluid pressure waves into a small posterior fossa.

Diagnostic Procedures

In platybasia, the clivus lies in a more horizontal plane than normal. The abnormality can be demonstrated by roentgenograms of the skull. The basal angle between a line drawn from the glabella to the midpoint of the pituitary fossa and a line drawn from this point down to the clivus is less than 140 degrees in the normal skull but exceeds this figure in platybasia. A diagnosis of basilar impression can be made if the tip of the odontoid process lies higher than 5 mm above a line (Chamberlain's line) drawn from the posterior margin of the hard palate to the posterior superior margin of the foramen magnum. Laminograms are helpful in demonstrating the abnormalities of these structures.

The posterior displacement and angulation of the spinal cord can be demonstrated by a high cervical myelogram.

Treatment

Basilar impression may be relieved by the transoral removal of the odontoid process as described under atlantoaxial dislocation. Surgical decompression of the foramen magnum is also necessary, with section of the cervical denticulate ligaments and adhesions or fibrous bands that frequently adhere to the meninges around the medulla.

Syringomyelia and Syringobulbia

Literal translation of the Greek term "syringomyelia" means a "tube of the spinal cord." The term is used to describe a disease in which there is an abnormal cavity or cyst within the cord. The term "syringobulbia" signifies a similar cyst within the brainstem, although the cyst in the brainstem is more likely to be slitlike, rather than a cavity.

Etiology and Pathology

There have been a number of etiologies proposed for syringomyelia. The cavity may result from proliferation of embryonic cell rests that persisted in the cord during the closure of the dorsal portion of the neural tube. It may also be a result of cystic degeneration in a chronic low-grade glioma, and histologic changes reported in the wall of some syringomyelic cavities are compatible with this view.

Syringomyelia has been described in the spinal cord following meningitis, arachnoiditis, cervical spondylosis, midbrain tumors' infarction, and hematomyelia due to trauma.[184]

It has been suggested that the cavity formation is the result of a hindbrain herniation in fetal life[81] or an atresia of the rhomboencephalic roof in prenatal life.[86] In either case, this would impede the flow of cerebrospinal fluid from the fourth ventricle and lead to dilatation of the central canal of the cervical cord or dissection into the tissues of the lower medulla and cervical cord. Subsequent relief of pressure would allow the cavity to close, but it would reopen if there was a later disturbance of pressure in the posterior fossa.[234]

The syrinx usually develops in the cervical cord and may extend or be associated with another syrinx in the thoracic area. Involvement of the lumbar cord by extension or by the development of an independent syrinx also occasionally occurs. The cord is usually widened in the region of the syrinx, and transverse section shows an irregular, fluid-filled cavity. The cavity usually extends ventrally to obliterate the anterior white commissure and may protrude into the lateral white columns with destruction of the corticospinal tracts. The cavity regularly extends ventrally to produce compression and destruction of the anterior horns and their motor neurons. Microscopic examination of the walls of the cavity shows that it is surrounded by glial tissue with occasional Rosenthal fibers. The ependyma of the obliterated central canal can usually be identified in the center of the cord.

It is not unusual to see some extension of the cervical cord syrinx into the brainstem, but syringobulbia may also arise as a separate lesion. The lesion in the brainstem is usually slitlike or may have the appearance of a glial scar rather than a cavity. There are three principal sites of involvement in the medulla: in the midline with interruption of the decussating fibers of the medial lemniscus; between the pyramid and the inferior olive involving the hypoglossal nerve; and extending ventrolaterally between the inferior olive and the spinal tract of the trigeminal nerve with involvement of the vagus nerve. Extension into the pons rarely occurs with the lesion involving the tegmental area. Involvement of the midbrain by syringobulbia is extremely rare, although cases have been described in which the syrinx could be traced rostrally as high as the thalamus.

Clinical Features

Syringomyelia occurs more frequently in males than females, and the average age of onset of symptoms is usually about 30 years.[161] However, initial symptoms have been noted as early as three years of age and as late as 60. Since the syrinx usually begins in the cervical area, the most common complaint is usually loss of sensation in the hands. This is a dissociated type of sensory loss due to destruction of pain fibers as they cross in the anterior white commissure, and patients frequently complain of suffering cuts, infections, or burns of the hands without experiencing pain. When the cavity extends laterally into the corticospinal tracts, there is progressive spasticity below the level of the syrinx. This presents clinically as a progressive spastic paraparesis with ankle clonus, increased deep tendon reflexes in the lower limbs, and extensor plantar responses. Involvement of the corticospinal pathways, which apparently relay impulses to the sacral area to inhibit the bladder, results in urgency and frequency of micturition. Destruction of the anterior horn cells in the cervical area produces muscle wasting, weakness, and fasciculations in the upper limbs, usually beginning in the hands. Radicular pains of a burning type are not uncommon in the upper limbs and over the chest.

Examination of patients with syringomyelia usually reveals loss of tendon jerks in the involved segment with weakness and wasting of appropriate muscles. This is usually more obvious in the upper limbs and more marked in the hands. There are spasticity and weakness in the lower limbs with spastic gait, ankle clonus, increased reflexes, and extensor plantar responses. One of the characteristic clinical findings is sensory impairment of the dissociated type with loss of pain and temperature sensation extending over the segments involved by the syrinx with preservation of touch, vibration, and position sense. Loss of pain sensation in the joints of the upper limbs or spine may produce a syringomyelic arthropathy indistinguishable from the Charcot joints of tabes dorsalis (Fig. 4–14). A number of associated developmental abnormalities including scoliosis of the cervicothoracic spine, Sprengel's deformity, pes cavus, and neurofibromatosis are commonly present.

Syringobulbia produces symptoms of brainstem involvement and, when associated with syringomyelia, alters the clinical signs referred to above. A brainstem syrinx is often associated with a Horner's syndrome, and a pontine lesion can produce paresis of the sixth or seventh cranial nerve and loss of pain sensation over the face owing to involvement of the spinal tract of the trigeminal nerve. Interruption of the decussating fibers of the medial lemniscus in the medulla results in loss of touch, vibration, and position sense, which,

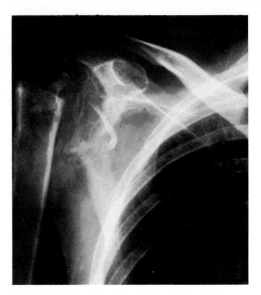

FIGURE 4–14. Roentgenogram of the right shoulder joint showing destructive changes in a painless Charcot joint due, in this case, to syringomyelia.

compounded with the loss of pain and temperature sensation due to a cervical syrinx, can produce a severe sensory loss over most of the body. Weakness of the palate leads to regurgitation of food through the nose, and syringobulbia may cause chronic laryngeal stridor.[3] The tongue commonly shows hemiatrophy with wasting and fasciculations since the hypoglossal nerve is commonly involved in the medulla (Fig. 4–15). Nystagmus has been described in some cases, presumably because of involvement of vestibular connections in the medulla. Rarely, the pupil may be ectopic, star-shaped, or irregular owing to damage to the third-nerve nucleus.

The course in syringomyelia is slow progression in most cases, but others seem to become arrested and remain stationary for many years. A few patients, possibly with associated glioma, have a more rapid course, resulting in severe disability within a period of three or four years. Sudden worsening of symptoms occasionally results from a hemorrhage into the syrinx.

Diagnostic Procedures

The spinal fluid pressure is usually normal, but the Queckenstedt test may indicate the presence of a partial block when the cord is widened due to the syrinx and the cervical canal is unusually

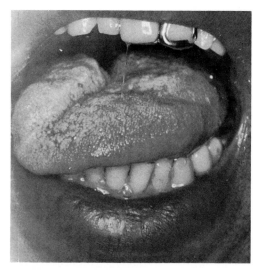

FIGURE 4–15. Wasting of the right side of the tongue in a case of syringobulbia.

narrow. It is not infrequent to find moderate elevation in the protein content of the CSF.

Roentgenographic examination of the spine may reveal additional developmental abnormalities including the Klippel-Feil syndrome, platybasia, basilar invagination, spina bifida, and cervical ribs. The widening of the cord is sometimes demonstrated by air or oil myelography, and rarely a defect in the opaque media may show an associated Chiari type I malformation.[162]

Treatment

Patients should be cautioned to avoid activities that may lead to painless cuts or burns. Any associated infection from such cuts and burns should be treated with cleansing and antibiotics. In more advanced cases, orthopedic splinting or reconstruction of Charcot joints may be indicated. Prevention of urinary and pulmonary infection is frequently required.

Some patients may benefit from irradiation of the syrinx, which appears to slow or arrest the course of the disease. The usual dose to the area of the syrinx should not exceed 5,000 roentgen units.

Surgical procedures are helpful if there is a block caused by the syrinx. These include laminectomy with decompression of the spinal cord and drainage of the cyst. Some surgeons recommend syringostomy using tantalum wire or other materials such as polyethylene tubing in an effort to maintain permanent drainage of the syrinx.

The results of this latter method are claimed to be better than nonsurgical treatment in long-term follow-up of patients with syringomyelia. Patients with an associated Chiari type I malformation should be treated by upper cervical laminectomy and suboccipital decompression.[154]

Terminal ventriculostomy, which is performed by opening the terminal portion of the central canal at the tip of the conus medullaris, has also been performed for syringomyelia. This procedure is based on the assumption that all syringomyelia is hydromyelia and that drainage of the central canal will relieve signs and symptoms of the disease.[80]

Cervical Myelopathy Associated with Rheumatoid Arthritis

Involvement of the cervical spine is quite common in rheumatoid arthritis and may ultimately lead to damage of the cervical cord.

Etiology and Pathology

The small interpeduncular joints and the synovial membrane between the odontoid process and the transverse ligament are susceptible to rheumatoid arthritis, which is accompanied by resorption of bone and destruction of ligaments. This may be followed by subluxation of the odontoid process which moves backward relative to the atlas and compresses the spinal cord. Rheumatoid arthritic changes in the other joints of the cervical spine may lead to multiple partial subluxations at lower levels in the cervical spine.[171] Both extradural and intradural compression of the spinal cord have been described at dorsal, lumbar, and sacral levels by rheumatoid nodules.[69]

Clinical Features

The symptoms usually develop after many years of severe rheumatoid arthritis.[118] Subluxation of the odontoid produces progressive spastic paraparesis with hyperreflexia and extensor plantar responses. The hands are severely disabled and show a marked sensory loss. Absence of nerve root pain is a striking feature. Many patients experience brainstem dysfunction with symptoms of dysarthria, dysphagia, vertigo, nystagmus, and diplopia due to compression of the anterior spinal or vertebral arteries by upward displacement of the odontoid process.

Compression of the spinal cord by rheumatoid nodules produces signs and symptoms similar to those of an extradural cord tumor (p. 653).

Treatment

Patients should be placed in a halo traction device followed by posterior fusion of C_1, C_2, or C_3 vertebrae to the occiput with or without laminectomy.

Cervical Spondylosis

Cervical spondylosis may be defined as a chronic, progressive degeneration of the cervical intervertebral disks. There is thickening of the annulus fibrosus associated with osteoarthritic changes in the adjacent vertebral joints and interpeduncular joints (Fig. 4–16). The resulting osteophytes encroach upon the spinal canal, compress the cervical cord and adjacent nerve roots, and compress the vertebral and segmental spinal arteries in the transverse and intervertebral foramina.[28, 30]

Degenerative arthritic changes of the cervical spine are a common radiographic finding in the middle-aged and elderly. Despite this, the majority of such patients remain symptom-free. The production of neurologic symptoms apparently depends on a number of associated factors.

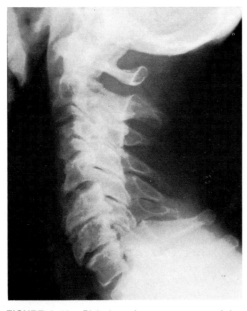

FIGURE 4–16. Plain lateral roentgenogram of the cervical spine showing degenerative changes of the vertebrae typical of cervical spondylosis. There is narrowing of the disk spaces with deformity of the vertebral bodies.

Etiology and Pathology

The intervertebral disk consists of a core of soft elastic tissue, the nucleus pulposus, surrounded by a ring of fibrous tissue called the annulus fibrosus. The nucleus pulposus has a high water content, which decreases rapidly after the fortieth year, and this loss is associated with degenerative changes in the central portion of the disk. The consequent narrowing of the disk space causes bulging and weakness of the annulus fibrosus so that the disk tends to protrude posteriorly into the spinal canal. This herniation is followed by osteoblastic reparative activity with the formation of osteophytes at the margins of the vertebral bodies. These calcified ridges or "lippings" also protrude into the spinal canal. The combination of the disk protrusion plus the surrounding osteophytes forms a bar of calcified or fibrous tissue, which narrows the diameter of the canal. Whether or not spinal cord compression will result depends on the diameter of the canal, which normally averages 17 mm in the cervical area. Patients who develop cervical spondylosis with cord compression typically have unusually narrow spinal canals, often measuring 14 mm in diameter. The encroachment on the canal is likely to compress the cord when the diameter of the canal is decreased below 12 mm.

There are a number of additional factors that may contribute to compression of the cord. The dentate ligaments, which are normally thin structures passing between the dura and the wall of the spinal canal, also may become thickened and fibrosed. This tends to anchor the spinal cord in the spinal canal, rendering it susceptible to compression by the calcified and protruded disk during movements of the neck. Loss of the substance of the nucleus pulposus results in shortening of the cervical spine with thickening and enfolding of the ligamentum flavum, which also protrudes into the posterior aspect of the spinal canal, so that it becomes even further narrowed. The degenerative changes in the disk result in malalignment of the vertebral bodies, which contributes further to disk degeneration, osteophyte formation, and narrowing of the spinal canal.

Nerve root compression within the intervertebral foramina is even more common than spinal cord compression in cervical spondylosis and is caused by similar mechanisms as outlined above. Narrowing of the disk spaces and shortening of the cervical spine produce malalignment and abnormal stresses of the interpeduncular joints. This is followed by osteophyte formation with encroachment upon the intervertebral foramina. Under normal circumstances, the nerve root occupies about one fourth of this space, but as the foramen becomes narrowed by the lateral encroachment of degenerated disks and osteophytes, the nerve root becomes thickened by fibrosis. Such changes also bind the root to the intervertebral foramen, reducing both its mobility and blood supply and increasing its susceptibility to compression as the intervertebral space is narrowed. Sudden exacerbations of nerve root compression may be caused by protrusion of the degenerated disk into the intervertebral foramen.

The vertebral and segmental arteries, which supply the spinal cord, pass through the transverse and intervertebral foramina of the cervical vertebrae and also become compressed by osteophytes in cervical spondylosis.[211] This may be exacerbated by head turning when the osteophytes compress and kink the vertebral arteries, reducing blood flow or even occluding them entirely (Fig. 4–17). Arteriosclerotic changes at the points of compression result in loss of elasticity and contribute to the kinking of the vertebral artery. Infarction of the cord may result.

Pathologic examination of the cervical cord in cervical spondylosis shows that it is flattened in the anteroposterior diameter by the posterior bars of degenerated intervertebral disks. Histologically, there is demyelination in the posterior and lateral columns and loss of neurons in the gray matter of the anterior horns with patchy infarction and cyst formation. These changes appear to be due to direct pressure or result from ischemia, owing to reduction of blood flow from the circumferential vessels arising from the anterior spinal artery. Direct pressure on the anterior spinal artery, which lies at the dorsal end of the anterior sulcus, is rare.

Compression of the cervical nerve roots produces wallerian degeneration with loss of myelin and axis cylinders. Repeated kinking and obstruction of the vertebral and segmental arteries may lead to ischemia and infarction of the brainstem and spinal cord as low as the upper thoracic segments.

Patients with cervical spondylosis are highly susceptible to trauma. This is particularly true of the common hyperextension or "whiplash" injury resulting from automobile accidents in which there is sudden hyperextension, followed by flexion of the neck. Since the spinal cord and nerve roots are anchored by fibrosis and enclosed in a narrowed space, their mobility is reduced and they are prone to compression and contusion by such violent movements of the neck. The results

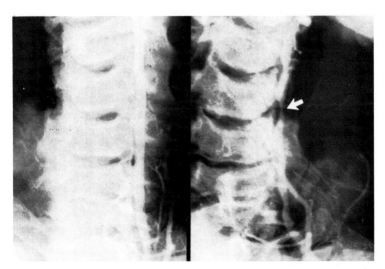

FIGURE 4–17. Left vertebral arteriograms in a patient with cervical spondylosis showing compression of the vertebral artery during rotation of the head. Arteriogram on left was made with the head in the neutral position; that on the right when the head was rotated. Arrow points to one level of compression.

of "whiplash" injuries are consequently more severe in patients with cervical spondylosis than in younger patients.

Clinical Features

Symptoms of cervical spondylosis result from combined compression and ischemia of nerve roots and spinal cord. Besides this, many patients complain of pain in the neck and headache due to the osteoarthritic changes in the cervical spine. Symptoms of vertebral-basilar arterial insufficiency (see p. 557) also occasionally occur, particularly with rotation of the neck.

Pain due to nerve root compression may begin suddenly in patients with long-standing cervical spondylosis evidenced by roentgenograms of the spine or it may begin insidiously with gradual progression. Sudden onset is usually due to an increase in disk protrusion precipitated by trauma or unaccustomed exertion. It is often severe, described as aching or stabbing, and in the distribution of the dermatomes supplied by the affected nerve root. When the sixth root is compressed, the pain may be referred to the root of the neck, and it may radiate down the anterior chest wall and over the shoulder down the lateral aspect of the upper arm and forearm to the thenar aspect of the hand and index finger. This type of pain may be mistakenly diagnosed as angina pectoris. As the pain subsides, it may become intermittent with dysesthesias or paresthesias occurring in the same area. In patients with subacute onset, the pain is usually less severe and is described as an ill-defined ache. Examination usually shows some sensory deficit in the distribution of the affected nerve root. Motor weakness is rarely prominent in the muscles innervated by the involved nerve root, but wasting of the small muscles of the hand, forearm, and shoulder is common. The deep tendon reflexes innervated by the roots are absent or depressed, which usually distinguishes the condition from amyotrophic lateral sclerosis.

Cord compression is not encountered as often as nerve root compression in cervical spondylosis and is usually accompanied by the symptoms of nerve root compression. Since multiple roots may be involved, the patient complains of pain in the neck, shoulders, and upper limbs with weakness, numbness, or paresthesias involving the hands. There is a variable amount of muscle wasting, and fasciculations may be seen in some cases due to compression of the motor roots and anterior horn cells in the affected segments of the cord.

Chronic and progressive compression of the cervical cord results in slowly developing weakness involving the lower limbs with spasticity, ankle clonus, increased deep tendon reflexes, and bilateral extensor plantar responses. Fasciculations have occasionally been reported in the lower limbs in patients with cervical spondylosis possibly due to deprivation of descending motor input to lumbar anterior horn cells.[133] Sensation is often impaired below the knees, with hypesthesia, hypalgesia, and reduction of vibration sense in the toes and ankles. The gait may be spastic or, occasionally, spastic and ataxic, in type. A number of cases present with progressive spastic paraparesis without any marked sensory involvement in the lower or upper limbs. In the past, this condition was often misdiagnosed as "primary lateral sclerosis." There is no doubt that primary lateral sclerosis is a clinical entity, and many of these patients previously diagnosed were having an unrecognized compression of the cervical cord due to cervical spondylosis, basilar impression, platybasia, or Chiari type I malformation.

Occasionally, cases of cervical spondylosis have been reported with prominent posterior column involvement. The resemblance to subacute combined degeneration of the cord may lead to some difficulty in clinical diagnosis, but blood counts, bone marrow aspiration, and the Schilling test should solve any such difficulty.

Neck pain and limitation of movement are not a common feature in cervical spondylosis. There may be acute pain following minor trauma, probably due to a sudden increase in disk protrusion. This is associated with muscle spasm and restriction of neck movement. Surprisingly, however, the majority of patients are either free of pain without limitation of neck movement or experience vague, dull aching in the neck. Movements of the neck by the examiner are usually unrestricted and full, although there may be crepitus when the neck is rotated.

A number of patients complain of suboccipital headaches, which are probably caused by associated vertebral-basilar insufficiency or compression of the nerve roots of C_2 and C_3, which supply sensation to this area of the scalp.

The association of vertebral-basilar insufficiency and cervical spondylosis has been discussed on page 225. Symptoms such as drop attacks and vertigo are usually precipitated by head turning or extension of the neck (Fig. 4–17), and these movements should be avoided. Strokes have been precipitated in such patients by manipulation of the neck and by prolonged hyperextension during anesthesia.

Diagnostic Procedures

Roentgenograms of the neck are required to make an adequate diagnosis and evaluation of the extent of the cervical spondylosis. These include anteroposterior views and lateral views taken in extension and flexion, supplemented by the two oblique views of the cervical spine. These films permit adequate visualization of the disk spaces, measurements of the anteroposterior diameter of the spinal canal, and evaluation of osteophyte formation on the vertebral bodies and around the interpeduncular joints. The oblique views are of particular value in assessing the degree of encroachment by osteophytes in the intervertebral foramina.

A definitive assessment of the extent and severity of the cervical spondylosis can be obtained by myelography. After injecting the dye, anteroposterior, lateral, and oblique views should be obtained when the radiopaque substance is concentrated in the cervical spinal canal and as high as the foramen magnum. The transverse "bars" of cervical spondylosis are well demonstrated, occurring at the level of the intervertebral disks in the anteroposterior and lateral views. A delay in the flow of dye over the "bars" can be seen on fluoroscopy as the patient is tilted in the "head-down" position. Narrowing of the spinal canal is confirmed by myelography, while pressure on the nerve roots usually produces filling defects in the nerve root sleeves, which are usually well-demonstrated during cervical myelography (Fig. 4–18).

Treatment

Medical Therapy. Patients who have a sudden onset or exacerbation of radicular pain and motor weakness following trauma or unaccustomed exertion regularly benefit from medical therapy. The acute phase requires bed rest, adequate use of analgesics, and heat to render the patient pain-free.

The use of oral "muscle relaxant" preparations is of limited value. The best drugs for this purpose are diazepam, 5 mg twice daily, and methocarbanol, 500 mg twice daily. For treatment of pain and spasm, indomethacin, 25 mg three times daily, is often effective. A short course of oral corticosteroids on a daily basis such as methyl-

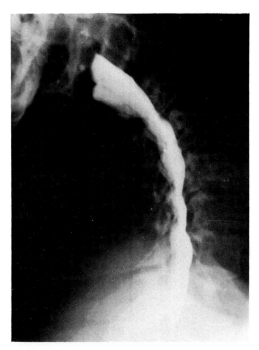

FIGURE 4–18. Cervical myelogram (lateral view) in cervical spondylosis. The "washboard" effect of the column of isophendylate (Pantopaque) is due to multiple ridges compressing the spinal cord at the intervertebral spaces.

prednisolone, 64 mg initially with reduction of dosage by 8 mg each day, is often of value.

When the pain is controlled and the patient is comfortable, neck traction, using a head halter and a pulley with 8 to 10 lb of weight attached, may be of value. The patient should be prone with the head elevated about 20 degrees above the feet and the back straight. The initial period of traction should not exceed 15 minutes. The time and weight may be increased gradually until the traction is tolerated for most of the morning and afternoon (with a break at noon) using 20 lb of weight. It should be noted that there is a marked variation of tolerance to the amount of traction by different patients. If the patient complains of traction or if there is no obvious benefit from traction within a few days, it should be discontinued and a neck collar substituted.

Many patients pass from the stage of bed rest with or without traction to an ambulant state, wearing a plastic neck collar. This serves two purposes, first by restricting neck movements which may produce pain, and second by protecting the patient from the effects of minor jolts that might cause sudden extension or flexion of the neck and exacerbate symptoms.

Certain types of physical therapy, including radiant heat, diathermy, and massage, are useful in reducing muscle spasm in the neck and alleviating pain. Patients with a poor posture or kyphoscoliosis may benefit from a gradual course of active exercises designed to strengthen the muscles of the neck and shoulder girdle.

Surgical Theapy. Surgical treatment should be considered in all patients who have persistent and disabling symptoms of nerve root compression and particularly in those who have neurologic and radiologic signs of cord compression. Some patients with vertebral basilar insufficiency clearly related to cervical spondylosis and exacerbated by head turning may also require surgery.

A number of surgical procedures have been recommended, and there are specific indications for each according to the type of disability. Some patients with nerve root compression can be treated by the anterior approach, which permits removal of degenerated disk material and osteophytes encroaching on the intervertebral foramina. This procedure is followed by an anterior interbody fusion. The postoperative course is short since immobilization and bed rest are unnecessary, and the patient may begin walking the day after surgery. Spinal cord compression is best treated by a wide laminectomy, which is essentially designed to decompress the spinal cord. This operation may be carried out at multiple levels and can be extended from the first cervical to the first thoracic vertebra if necessary.

Patients with nerve root compression alone tend to have a good prognosis and show a greater degree of improvement after surgery than patients with myelopathy. Some patients with cervical spondylitic myelopathy, particularly those with sphincter disturbances and lower limb weakness, may continue to deteriorate postoperatively.[97] The results of treatment using an anterior approach with thorough removal of projecting osteophytes and disk material are better than laminectomy or conservative management.[189]

Cited References

1. Aita, J. F. Cranial computerized tomography and Marie's ataxia. A case report. *Arch. Neurol.,* **35:**55–56, 1978.
2. Albert, M. L.; Feldman, R. G.; and Willis, A. "Subcortical dementia" of progressive supranuclear palsy. *J. Neurol. Neurosurg. Psychiat.,* **37:**121–30, 1974.
3. Alcala, H., and Dodson, W. E. Syringobulbia as a cause of laryngeal stridor in childhood. *Neurology* (Minneap.)., **25:**875–78, 1975.
4. Aminoff, M. J., and Wilcox, C. S. Assessment of autonomic function in patients with a Parkinsonian syndrome. *Br. Med. J.,* **4:**80–84, 1971.
5. Aminoff, M. J.; Wilcox, C. S.; et al. Levodopa therapy for parkinsonism in Shy-Drager syndrome. *J. Neurol. Neurosurg. Psychiat.,* **36:**350–53, 1973.
6. Aquilonius, S. M.; Eckernas, S. A.; and Sundwall, A. Regional distribution of choline acetyltransferase in the human brain: Changes in Huntington's chorea. *J. Neurol. Neurosurg. Psychiat.,* **38:**669–77, 1975.
7. Armstrong, R. M.; Fogelson, M. H.; and Silberberg, D. H. Familial proximal spinal muscular atrophy. *Arch. Neurol.,* **14:**208–12, 1966.
8. Aron, A. M.; Freeman, J. M.; and Carter, S. The natural history of Sydenham's chorea. Review of the literature and long-term evaluation with emphasis on cardiac sequelae. *Am. J. Med.,* **38:**83–94, 1965.
9. Arregui, A.; Bennett, J.; et al. Huntington's chorea: Selective depletion of activity of angiotensin converting enzyme in the corpus striatum. *Ann. Neurol.,* **2:**294–98, 1977.
10. Banta, R. G., and Markesbery, W. R. Elevated manganese levels associated with dementia and extrapyramidal signs. *Neurology* (Minneap.), **27:**213–16, 1977.
11. Barbeau, A. Six years of high level levodopa therapy in severely akinetic parkinsonian patients. *Arch. Neurol.,* **33:**333–38, 1976.
12. Barbeau, A. Friedreich's ataxia—an overview. Quebec cooperative study of Friedreich's ataxia. *Can. J. Neurol. Sci.,* **3:**389–97, 1976.
13. Barbeau, A. Friedreich's ataxia 1978—an overview. Quebec cooperative study of Friedreich's ataxia. *Can. J. Neurol. Sci.,* **5:**161–65, 1978.
14. Barkley, D. S.; Hardiwidjaja, S.; and Menkes, J. H. Huntington's disease: Delayed hypersensitivity in vitro to human central nervous system antigen. *Science,* **195:**314–16, 1977.
15. Barkley, D. S.; Hardiwidjaja, S. I.; et al. Cellular immune responses in Huntington's disease. Specificity of brain antigenicity detected with Huntington disease lymphocytes. *Neurology* (Minneap.), **28:**32–35, 1978.
16. Barrett, R. E.; Yahr, M. D.; and Duvoisen, R. C. Torsion dystonia and spasmodic torticollis: Results of treatment with L-dopa. *Neurology* (Minneap.), **20:**107–13, 1970.
17. Bass, N. H.; Hess, H. H.; and Pope, A. Altered cell membranes in Creutzfeldt-Jacob disease: Microchemical studies. *Arch. Neurol.,* **31:**174–82, 1974.
17a. Bateman, D. N.; Coxon, A.; et al. Treatment of the on-off syndrome in Parkinsonism with low dose bromocriptine in combination with levodopa. *J. Neurol. Neurosurg. Psychiat.,* **41:**1109–13, 1978.
18. Bauer, R. B.; Meyer, J. S.; and McMorrow, K.

Nerve conduction times in neurologic diagnosis. Evidence of neuropathic component in some cases of spinocerebellar degeneration. *Am. J. Phys. Med.,* **42:**166–74, 1963.

19. Becker, L. E. Slow infections of the central nervous system. *Can. J. Neurol. Sci.,* **4:**81–88, 1977.

20. Behan, P. O., and Bone, I. Hereditary chorea without dementia. *J. Neurol. Neurosurg. Psychiat.,* **40:**687–91, 1977.

21. Bianchine, J. R., and Bianchine, J. W. Treatment of spasmodic torticollis with Diazepam. *South. Med. J.,* **64:**893–94, 1971.

22. Binns, J. K., and Robertson, E. E. Pick's disease in old age, *J. Ment. Sci.,* **108:**804–10, 1962.

23. Bird, E. D.; Mackay, A. V. P.; et al. Reduced glutamic acid decarboxylase activity of postmortem brain in Huntington's chorea. *Lancet,* **1:**1090–92, 1973.

24. Bird, M. T., and Paulson, G. W. The rigid form of Huntington's chorea, *Neurology* (Minneap.), **21:**271–76, 1971.

24a. Bird, M. T.; Palkes, H.; and Prensky, A. L. A follow-up of Sydenham's chorea, *Neurology* (Minneap.), **26:**601–606, 1976.

24b. Bird, T. D., and Shaw, C. M. Progressive myoclonus and epilepsy with dentatorubral degeneration: A clinicopathological study of the Ramsay Hunt syndrome. *J. Neurol. Neurosurg. Psychiat.,* **41:**140–49, 1978.

25. Birkmayer, W.; Riederer, P.; and Ambrozi, L. Implications of combined treatment with Madopar and L-Deprenil in Parkinson's disease. *Lancet,* **1:**439–43, 1977.

26. Bornstein, M. B. A tissue culture approach to demyelinative disorders. National Cancer Society Monograph No. 11. Symposium on Organ Culture, 1962, pp. 197–214.

27. Boudouresques, J.; Toga, M.; and Roger, J. Encéphalopathie présénile d'évolution subaiguë type Heidenhain. *Rev. Neurol.* (Paris), **119:**468–76, 1968.

28. Bowder, R. E. M. Cervical spondylosis. *Proc. Roy. Soc. Med.,* **59:**1141–46, 1966.

29. Bowen, D. M.; White, P.; et al. Brain decarboxylase activities as indexes of pathologic change in senile dementia. *Lancet,* **1:**1247–49, 1974.

29a. Bowen, D. M.; Smith, C. B.; et al. Chemical pathology of the organic dementias. II. Quantitative estimation of cellular changes in post-mortem brains. *Brain,* **100:**427–53, 1977.

30. Brain, W. R., and Wilkinson, Marcia, eds. *Cervical Spondylosis and Other Disorders of the Cervical Spine.* Saunders, Philadelphia, 1967.

31. Breig, A.; Ekbom, K.; Greitz, T.; and Kugelberg, E. Hydrocephalus due to elongated basilar artery, a new clinico-radiological syndrome. *Lancet,* **1:**874–75, 1967.

32. Brody, J. A.; Hirano, A.; and Scott, R. M. Recent neuropathologic observations in amyotrophic lateral sclerosis and parkinsonism-dementia of Guam. *Neurology* (Minneap.), **21:**528–36, 1971.

33. Brownell, B., and Oppenheimer, D. R. An ataxic form of subacute presenilpolioencephalopathy (Creutzfeldt-Jakob disease). *J. Neurol. Neurosurg. Psychiat.,* **28:**350–61, 1965.

34. Brunette, J. R., and Bernier, R. G. Diagnosis and prognosis of Leber's disease. Incidence of spontaneous total recovery. *Union Med. Can.,* **99:**643–52, 1970.

34a. Buge, A.; Escourolle, R.; et al. Familial Creutzfeldt-Jakob disease: A chemical and pathological study of three cases in a family with eight affected members in three generations. *Rev. Neurol.,* **134:**165–81, 1978.

35. Caine, E. D.; Ebert, M. H.; and Weingartner, H. An outline for the analysis of dementia. *Neurology* (Minneap.), **27:**1087–92, 1977.

36. Calne, D. B.; Reid, J. L.; Vakil, S. D.; Rao, S.; Petrie, A.; Pallis, C. A.; Gawler, J.; Thomas, P. K.; and Hilson, A. Idiopathic parkinsonism treated with an extracerebral decarboxylase inhibitor in combination with levodopa. *Br. Med. J.,* **3:**729–32, 1971.

37. Campbell, A. M.; Corner, B.; Norman, R. M.; and Urich, H. The rigid form of Huntington's disease. *J. Neurol. Neurosurg. Psychiat.,* **24:**71–77, 1961.

38. Carruthers, S. G. Persistent tardive dyskinesia. *Br. Med. J.,* **3:**572, 1971.

39. Case records of the Massachusetts General Hospital. *N. Engl. J. Med.,* **297:**930–37, 1977.

40. Coblentz, J. M.; Mattis, S.; et al. Presenile dementia: Clinical aspects and evaluation of cerebrospinal fluid dynamics. *Arch. Neurol.,* **29:**299–308, 1973.

41. Constantinides, J.; Tissot, R.; and Ajuriaguerra, J. de. Dystonie oculofacio-cervicale ou paralysie progressive supranucléaire de Steele-Richardson-Olszewski. Pseudo-paralysie due regard, trouble visuospatiaux, pseudo-démence, altérations neuronales. *Rev. Neurol.* (Paris), **122:**249–62, 1970.

41a. Constantinides, J.; Richard, J.; and Tissot, R. Pick's disease and zinc metabolism. *Rev. Neurol.* (Paris), **133:**685–96, 1977.

42. Cooper, I. S. 20 year followup study of the neurosurgical treatment of dystonia musculorum deformans. In Eldridge, R., and Fahn, S. (eds.) *Advances in Neurology,* Vol. 14. Raven Press, New York, 1976, pp. 423–52.

43. Cooper, I. S. Neurosurgical treatment of the dyskinesias. *Clin. Neurosurg.,* **24:**367–90, 1976.

44. Corbett, J. J.; Butler, A. B.; and Kaufman, B. Sneeze syncope, basilar invagination and Arnold-Chiari type 1 malformation. *J. Neurol. Neurosurg. Psychiat.,* **39:**381–84, 1976.

44a. Corsini, G. U.; Onali, P. L.; et al. Apomorphine hydrochloride induced improvement in Huntington's chorea. Stimulation of dopamine receptor. *Arch. Neurol.,* **35:**27–30, 1978.

45. Cotzias, G. C.; Papavasiliou, P. S.; and Gellene, R. Modification of parkinsonism—chronic treatment with L-dopa. *N. Engl. J. Med.,* **280:**337–45, 1969.

46. Crapper, D. R.; Krishnan, S. S.; and Ouettkat, S. Aluminum neurofibrillary degeneration and Alzheimer's disease. *Brain,* **99:**67–80, 1976.

47. Crockard, H. A.; Hanlon, K.; et al. Hydrocephalus as a cause of dementia: Evaluated by computerized tomography and intracranial pressure

monitoring. *J. Neurol. Neurosurg. Psychiat.,* **40:**736–40, 1977.

48. Danes, P., and Maloney, A. J. F. Selective loss of central cholinergic neurons in Alzheimer's disease. *Lancet,* **2:**1403, 1976.

49. den Hartog Jager, W. A. Sphingomyelin in lewy inclusion bodies in Parkinson's disease. *Arch. Neurol.,* **21:**615–19, 1969.

50. deReunck, J.; deCostes, W.; et al. Papova virus like particles in a nigral type of Creutzfeldt-Jakob disease. *J. Neurol.,* **213:**179–88, 1976.

51. Dewhurst, K.; Oliver, J. E.; and McKnight, A. L. Socio-psychiatric consequences of Huntington's chorea. *Br. J. Psychiat.,* **116:**255–58, 1970.

52. Dorfman, L. J.; Nikoskelainan, E.; et al. Visual evoked potentials in Leber's hereditary optic atrophy. *Ann. Neurol.,* **1:**565–68, 1977.

53. Duvoisin, R. C. Cholinergic-anticholinergic antagonism in Parkinsonism. *Arch. Neurol.,* **17:**124–36, 1967.

54. Duvoisin, R. C., and Yahr, M. D. Encephalitis and Parkinsonism. *Arch. Neurol.,* **12:**227–39, 1965.

55. Eadie, M. J.; Sutherland, J. M.; and Doherty, R. L. Encephalitis in etiology of Parkinsonism in Australia. *Arch. Neurol.,* **12:**240–45, 1965.

56. Earnest, M. P.; Fahn, S.; et al. Normal pressure hydrocephalus and hypertensive cerebrovascular disease. *Arch. Neurol.,* **31:**262–66, 1974.

57. Editorial. Dopa and parkinsonism. *Br. Med. J.,* **276:**783, 1967.

58. Ekbom, K.; Greitz, T.; and Kugelberg, E. Hydrocephalus due to ectasia of the basilar artery. *J. Neurol. Sci.,* **8:**455–77, 1969.

59. Eldridge, R. The torsion dystonias (dystonia musculorum deformans). *Neurology* (Minneap.), **20:**1–154, 1970.

60. Eldridge, R. The torsion dystonias: Literature review and genetic and clinical studies. *Neurology* (Minneap.), **20:**1–78, 1970.

61. ElGammel, T.; Allen, M. B.; and Lott, T. Computer assisted tomography and pneumoencephalography in non-tumerous hydrocephalus in infants and children. *J. Comput. Assist. Tomogr.,* **1:**204–10, 1977.

62. Elizan, T. S.; Chen, K. M.; Mathai, K. V.; Dunn, D.; and Kurland, L. T. Amyotrophic lateral sclerosis and Parkinson-dementia complex; a study in non-Chamorros of the Mariana and Caroline Island. *Arch. Neurol.,* **14:**347–55, 1966.

63. Elizan, T. S.; Hirano, A.; Abrams, B. M.; Need, R. L.; Nuis, C. V.; and Kurland, L. T. Amyotrophic lateral sclerosis and Parkinsonism-dementia complex of Guam; neurological reevaluation. *Arch. Neurol.,* **14:**356–68, 1966.

64. Elliott, F.; Gardner-Thorpe, C.; et al. Jakob-Creutzfeldt disease. *J. Neurol. Neurosurg. Psychiat.,* **37:**879–87, 1974.

65. Ellis, W. G.; Espana, C. D.; et al. Creutzfeldt-Jakob disease; spongiform cytopathic effects in cultured human and monkey brain cells. *Neurology* (Minneap.), **26:**375, 1976.

66. Enne, S. J.; Bird, E. D.; et al. Huntington's chorea: Changes in neurotransmitter receptors in the brain. *N. Engl. J. Med.,* **294:**1305–1309, 1976.

67. Enee, S. J.; Stern, L. Z.; et al. Cerebrospinal fluid Y aminobutyric acid variations in neurological disorders. *Arch. Neurol.,* **34:**683–85, 1977.

68. Escalar, G., and Majeron, M. A. L'uso die preparati butirrofenonici nella corea di Huntington. *Minerva Med.,* **60:**2494–96, 1969.

69. Fairburn, B. Spinal cord compression by a rheumatoid nodule. *J. Neurol. Neurosurg. Psychiat.,* **38:**1056–58, 1975.

70. Falkner, B.; Langman, C.; and Katz, S. Renal histopathological changes in a child with Laurence-Moon Biedl syndrome. *J. Clin. Pathol.,* **30:**1077–81, 1977.

71. Farmer, T. W., and Mustian, V. M. Vestibulocerebellar ataxia; a newly defined hereditary syndrome with periodic manifestation. *Arch. Neurol.,* **8:**471–80, 1963.

72. Felmus, M. T.; Patten, B. M.; and Swanke, L. Antecedent events in amyotrophic lateral sclerosis. *Neurology* (Minneap.), **26:**167–72, 1976.

73. Foley, J. M., and Denny-Brown, D. Subacute progressive encephalopathy with bulbar myoclonus. *J. Neuropathol.,* **16:**133–36, 1957.

74. Foulds, W. S.; Chisholm, I. A.; and Bronte-Stewart, J. Cyanide induced optic neuropathy. *Ophthalmologica* (Basel), suppl., pp. 350–58, 1969.

75. Fox, J. H.; Topel, J. L.; and Huckman, M. S. Use of computerized tomography in senile dementia. *J. Neurol. Neurosurg. Psychiat.,* **38:**948–53, 1975.

76. Friedman, A. H., and Everett, G. M. Pharmacological aspects of Parkinsonism. *Adv. Pharmacol.,* **3:**83–127, 1964.

77. Fromm, G. H., and Pitner, S. E. Late progressive quadriparesis due to odontoid agenesis. *Arch. Neurol.,* **9:**291–96, 1963.

78. Gahlot, D. K.; Khosta, P. K.; et al. Copper metabolism in retinitis pigmentosa. *Br. J. Ophthalmol.,* **60:**770–74, 1976.

79. Gainenez-Roldan, S., and Esteban, A. Prognosis in hereditary amyotrophic lateral sclerosis. *Arch. Neurol.,* **34:**706–708, 1977.

80. Gardner, W. J.; Bell, H. S.; et al. Terminal ventriculostomy for syringomyelia. *J. Neurosurg.,* **46:**609–17, 1977.

81. Gardner, W. J., and McMurry, F. G. "Noncommunicating syringomyelia": Non-existent entity. *Surg. Neurol.,* **6:**251–56, 1976.

82. Gilbert, G. J. Spasmodic torticollis treated effectively by medical means. *N. Engl. J. Med.,* **284:**896–98, 1971.

83. Gilbert, G. J. The medical treatment of spasmodic torticollis. *Arch. Neurol.,* **27:**503–506, 1972.

84. Gilbert, G. J. Familial spasmodic torticollis. *Neurology* (Minneap.), **27:**11–13, 1977.

85. Gilroy, J., and Lynn, G. E. Computerized tomography and auditory-evoked potentials. *Arch. Neurol.,* **35:**143–47, 1978.

86. Gimencz-Roldan, S.; Esteban, A.; and Benito, C. Communicating syringomyelia following cured tuberculous meningitis. *J. Neurol. Sci.,* **23:**185–97, 1974.

87. Gloor, P.; Kalabay, O.; and Giard, N. The electroencephalogram in diffuse encephalopathies:

Electroencephalographic correlates of grey and white matter lesions. *Brain,* **91:**779–802, 1968.

88. Goebel, H. H.; Heipertz, R.; et al. Juvenile Huntington chorea: Clinical ultrastructural and biochemical studies. *Neurology* (Minneap.), **28:**23–31, 1978.

89. Goldhammer, Y.; Bubis, J. J.; Sarova-Phinas, I.; and Braham, J. Subacute spongiform encephalopathy and its relation to Jakob-Creutzfeldt disease: Report of 6 cases. *J. Neurol. Neurosurg. Psychiat.,* **35:**1–10, 1972.

90. Gomori, A. J.; Partnow, M. J.; et al. Ataxic form of Creutzfeldt-Jacob disease. *Arch. Neurol.,* **29:**318–23, 1973.

91. Goodman-Austen, R. B., and Smith, N. J. Comparison of the effects of bromocriptine and levodopa in Parkinson's disease. *J. Neurol. Neurosurg. Psychiat.,* **40:**479–82, 1977.

92. Greenaire, J. K.; Coxon, A.; et al. Comparison of levodopa with carbidopa and benserazide in Parkinsonism. *Lancet,* **2:**381–84, 1976.

93. Greenberg, A. D.; Scoville, W. B.; and Davey, L. M. Transoral decompression of atlantoaxial dislocation due to odontoid hypoplasia. *J. Neurosurg.,* **28:**266–69, 1968.

94. Greenfield, J. G. *The Spino-cerebellar Degenerations.* Blackwell, Oxford, 1954.

95. Greer, M. Benign intracranial hypertension. I. Mastoiditis and lateral sinus obstruction. *Neurology* (Minneap.), **12:**472–76, 1962.

96. Greer, M.; Collins, G. H.; and Anton, A. H. Cerebral catecholamines after levodopa therapy. *Arch. Neurol.,* **25:**461–67, 1971.

97. Gregorus, F. K.; Festrin, T.; and Crandall, P. H. Cervical spondylotic radiculopathy and myelopathy. A long term followup study. *Arch. Neurol.,* **33:**618–25, 1976.

98. Grier, L. N. Corticosteroids in the treatment of Sydenham's chorea. *Arch. Neurol.,* **35:**53–54, 1978.

99. Groothius, J. R.; Groothius, D. R.; et al. Lupus associated chorea in childhood. *Am. J. Dis. Child.,* **131:**1131–34, 1977.

100. Growdon, J. H.; Cohen, E. L.; and Wurtman, R. J. Huntington's disease: Clinical and chemical effects of choline administration. *Ann. Neurol.,* **1:**418–22, 1977.

101. Growdon, J. H.; Shatrani, B. T.; and Young, R. R. Effect of alcohol on essential tremor. *Neurology* (Minneap.), **25:**259–62, 1975.

101a. Gunasekera, L., and Richardson, A. E. Computerized axial tomography in idiopathic hydrocephalus. *Brain,* **100:**749–54, 1977.

102. Guthkelch, A. N. The treatment of infantile hydrocephalus by the holter valve. *Br. J. Surg.,* **54:**665–73, 1967.

103. Haerer, A. F.; Currier, R. D.; and Jackson, J. F. Hereditary non-progressive chorea of early onset. *N. Engl. J. Med.,* **276:**1220–24, 1967.

104. Halgin, R.; Riklan, M.; and Misiak, M. Levodopa parkinsonism and recent memory. *J. Nerv. Ment. Dis.,* **164:**268–72, 1977.

105. Hartvicksen, K., and Sem-Jacobsen, C. W. The effect of surgical and medical treatment of Parkinson's disease. *Acta Neurol. Scand.,* **39:**Suppl. 4:237–49, 1963.

106. Hassler, R., and Dieckmann, G. Die stereotaktische Behandlung des Torticollis aufgrund tierexperimenteller Erfahrungen über die richtungsbestimmten Bewegungen. *Nervenartzt,* **41:**473–87, 1970.

107. Hawkes, C. H., and Nourse, C. H. Tetrabenazine in Sydenham's chorea. *Br. Med. J.,* **1:**1391–2, 1977.

108. Herskovitz, E., and Blackwood, W. Essential (familial, hereditary) tremor: A case report. *J. Neurol. Neurosurg. Psychiat.,* **32:**509–11, 1969.

109. Hill, M. E.; Lougheed, W. M.; and Barnett, H. J. M. A treatable form of dementia due to normal-pressure, communicating hydrocephalus. *Can. Med. Assoc. J.,* **97:**1309–20, 1967.

110. Hill, W., and Sherman, H. Acute intermittent familial cerebellar ataxia. *Arch. Neurol.,* **18:**350–57, 1968.

111. Hirano, A.; Arumugasamy, N.; and Zimmerman, H. M. Amyotrophic lateral sclerosis; a comparison of Guam and classical cases. *Arch. Neurol.,* **16:**357–63, 1967.

112. Hirano, A.; Kurland, L. T.; and Sayre, G. P. Familial amyotrophic lateral sclerosis; a subgroup characterized by posterior and spinocerebellar tract involvement and hyaline inclusions in the anterior horn cells. *Arch. Neurol.,* **16:**232–43, 1967.

113. Hirano, A.; Malamud, N.; Elizan, T. S.; and Kurland, L. T. Amyotrophic lateral sclerosis and Parkinsonism-dementia complex on Guam—further pathologic studies. *Arch. Neurol.,* **15:**35–51, 1966.

114. Hirano, A., and Zimmerman, H. M. Alzheimer's neuro-fibrillary changes; a topographic study. *Arch. Neurol.,* **7:**227–42, 1962.

115. Hoehn, M. M.; Crowley, I. J.; and Rutledge, C. O. Dopamine correlates of neurological and psychological status in untreated parkinsonism. *J. Neurol. Neurosurg. Psychiat.,* **39:**941–51, 1976.

116. Horton, W. A.; Eldridge, R.; and Brody, J. A. Familial motor neuron disease: Evidence for at least three different types. *Neurology* (Minneap.), **26:**46–65, 1976.

117. Horwish, M. S.; Engel, W. K.; and Chauvin, P. B. Amyotrophic lateral sclerosis sera applied to withered motor neurons. *Arch. Neurol.,* **30:**332–33, 1974.

118. Hughes, J. T. Spinal cord involvement by C4-C5 vertebral subluxation in rheumatoid arthritis. A description of 2 cases examined at necropsy. *Ann. Neurol.,* **1:**575–82, 1977.

119. Hughes, R. C.; Polgar, J. G.; Weightman, D.; and Walton, J. N. Levodopa in Parkinsonism: The effects of withdrawal of anticholinergic drugs. *Br. Med. J.,* **2:**487–91, 1971.

120. Hydrocephalus and spina bifida, Proceedings of the Groningen meeting of the Society for Research into Hydrocephalus and Spina Bifida, 1965. *Dev. Med. Child Neurol.,* Suppl. 11, 1966.

121. Isgreen, W. P.; Chutorian, A. M.; and Fahn, S. Sequential parkinsonism and chorea following "mild" influenza. *Tr. Am. Neurol. Assoc.,* **101:**56–60, 1976.

122. Isgreen, W. P.; Fahn, S.; et al. Carbamazepine in torsion dystonia. In Eldridge, R., and Fahn, S. (eds.). *Advances in Neurology,* Vol. 14. Raven Press, New York, 1976, pp. 411–16.

123. Ishino, H., and Otsuki, S. Frequency of Alzheimer's neurofibrillary tangles in cerebral cortex in progressive supranuclear palsy (subcortical argyrophilic dystrophy). *J. Neurol. Sci.,* **28:**309–16, 1976.

124. Ishino, H.; Ikeda, H.; and Otsuki, S. Contribution to clinical pathology of progressive supranuclear palsy (subcortical argyrophilic dystrophy): Distribution of neurofibrillary tangles in basal ganglia and brain stem and its clinical significance. *J. Neurol. Sci.,* **24:**471–81, 1975.

125. Ishino, H.; Higaski, H.; et al. Motor nuclear involvement in progressive supranuclear palsy. *J. Neurol. Sci.,* **22:**233–44, 1974.

126. Jacobs, L., and Kinkel, W. Computerized tomography in normal pressure hydrocephalus. *Neurology* (Minneap.), **26:**501–507, 1976.

127. Jameson, H. D.; Braker, H. M.; and Fuchs, M. E. Hemiballismus hemichorea treated with dimethylaminoethanol. *Dis. Nerv. Syst.,* **38:**931–33, 1977.

128. Jellinger, K.; Heiss, W.-D.; and Deisenhammer, E. Ataxic (cerebellar) form of Creutzfeldt-Jakob disease. *J. Neurol.,* **207:**289–305, 1974.

129. Johnson, W. G., and Fahn, S. Treatment of vascular hemiballism and hemichorea. *Neurology* (Minneap.), **27:**634–36, 1977.

129a. Joseph, C.; Chasson, J. B.; and Koch, M. L. Levodopa in Parkinson disease: a long term appraisal of mortality. *Ann. Neurol.,* **3:**116–18, 1978.

130. Kahana, E.; Alter, M.; and Feldman, S. Amyotrophic lateral sclerosis. A population study. *J. Neurol.,* **212:**205–14, 1976.

131. Kartzinel, R.; Hunt, R. D.; and Calne, D. B. Bromocriptine in Huntington's chorea. *Arch. Neurol.,* **33:**517–18, 1976.

132. Kartzmel, R.; Perlow, M. D.; et al. Metabolic studies with bromocriptine in patients with idiopathic parkinsonism and Huntington's chorea. *Trans. Am. Neurol. Assoc.,* **101:**53–56, 1976.

133. Kasdon, D. L. Cervical spondylotic myelopathy with reversible fasciculations in the lower extremities. *Arch. Neurol.,* **34:**774–76, 1977.

134. Katzman, R. Prevalence and malignancy of Alzheimer's disease: A major killer. *Arch. Neurol.,* **33:**217–18, 1975.

135. Katzman, R. The prevalence and malignancy of Alzheimer's disease. *Arch. Neurol.,* **33:**217–18, 1976.

136. Kempinsky, W. H.; Boniface, W. R.; Morgan, P. P.; and Busch, A. K. Reserpine in Huntington's chorea. *Neurology* (Minneap.), **10:**38–42, 1960.

137. Kivalo, E., and Weckman, N. The effect of haloperidol on some dyskinetic syndromes. *Scand. J. Clin. Lab. Invest.,* **23:**suppl 108, 64, 1969 (abstract).

138. Kivalo, E., and Weckman, N. Über die Verwendung von Haloperidol zur Behandlung extrapyramidaler Zwangsbewegungen. *Nervenartzt,* **41:** 567–69, 1970.

139. Klawans, H. L., Jr. A pharmacologic analysis of Huntington's chorea. *Eur. Neurol.,* **4:**148–63, 1970.

140. Klawans, H. L., Jr.; Paulson, G. W.; Ringel, S. P.; and Barbeau, A. Use of L-Dopa in the detection of presymptomatic Huntington's chorea. *N. Engl. J. Med.,* **286:**1332–34, 1972.

141. Kokenge, R.; Kutt, H.; and McDowell, F. Neurological sequelae following Dilantin[R] overdose in a patient and in experimental animals. *Neurology* (Minneap.), **15:**823–29, 1965.

142. Koto, A.; Rosenberg, G.; et al. Syndrome of normal pressure hydrocephalus: Possible relation to hypertension and arteriosclerotic vasculopathy. *J. Neurol. Neurosurg. Psychiat.,* **40:**73–79, 1977.

143. Lapresle, J., and Salisachs, P. Onion bulbs in a nerve biopsy specimen from an original case of Roussy-Levy Disease. *Arch. Neurol.,* **29:**346–48, 1973.

144. Larsson, T., and Sjogren, T. Dystonia musculorum deformans; a genetic and clinical population study of 121 cases. *Acta Neurol. Scand.,* **42:**Suppl 17:1–232, 1966.

145. Laurence, K. M. Brain damage in hydrocephalic patients. *Proc. Roy. Soc. Med.,* **60:**1265–66, 1967.

146. Lees, F.; MacDonald, A. M. E.; and Aldren Turner, J. W. Leber's disease with symptoms resembling disseminated sclerosis. *J. Neurol. Neurosurg. Psychiat.,* **27:**415–21, 1964.

147. Lee, M. C.; Lipper, D. M.; et al. The long-term effects of combining carbidopa with levodopa for Parkinson's disease. *Trans. Am. Neurol. Assoc.,* **101:**262–64, 1976.

148. Lees, A. J.; Shaw, K. M.; et al. Deprenyl in Parkinson's disease. *Lancet,* **2:**791–95, 1977.

149. LeMay, M., and Abramowicz, A. Encephalography in the diagnosis of cerebellar atrophy. *Acta Radiol. Diag.,* **5:**667–74, 1966.

150. Lessell, S.; Hirano, A.; Torres, J.; and Kurland, L. T. Parkinsonism-dementia complex, epidemiological considerations in the Chamorros of the Mariana Islands and California. *Arch. Neurol.,* **7:**377–85, 1962.

151. Lockwood, A. H. Shy-Drager syndrome with abnormal respirations and antidiuretic hormone release. *Arch. Neurol.,* **33:**292–95, 1976.

152. Lorber, J. Recovery of vision following prolonged blindness in children with hydrocephalus or following pyogenic meningitis. *Clin. Pediatr.* (Phila.), **6:**699–703, 1967.

153. Lorenzo, A. V.; Bresnan, M. J.; and Barlow, C. F. Cerebrospinal fluid absorption deficit in normal pressure hydrocephalus. *Arch. Neurol.,* **30:**387–93, 1974.

154. Love, J. G., and Olafson, R. A. Syringomyelia; a look at surgical therapy. *J. Neurosurg.,* **24:**714–18, 1966.

155. Magee, K. R., and DeJong, R. N. Neurogenic muscular atrophy simulating muscular dystrophy. *Arch. Neurol.,* **2:**677–82, 1960.

156. Marsden, C. D. Blepharospasm-oromandibular dystonia syndrome. A variant of adult onset torsion dystonia. *J. Neurol. Neurosurg. Psychiat.,* **39:**1204–1209, 1976.

157. Marsden, C. D., and Parkes, J. D. Success and

problems of long-term levodopa therapy in Parkinson's disease. *Lancet,* **1:**345–49, 1977.

158. Marttila, R. J., and Rinne, U. K. Dementia in Parkinson's disease. *Acta Neurol. Scand.,* **54:**431–41, 1976.

158a. Masters, C. L., and Richardson, E. P., Jr. Subacute spongiform encephalopathy (Creutzfeldt-Jakob disease). The nature and progression of spongiform change. *Brain,* **101:**333–44, 1978.

159. Mathews, N. T.; Meyer, J. S.; et al. Abnormal cerebrospinal fluid-blood flow dynamics: Implications in diagnosis, treatment and prognosis in normal pressure hydrocephalus. *Arch. Neurol.,* **32:**657–64, 1975.

160. May, W. W.; Itabushi, H. H.; and DeJong, R. N. Creutzfeldt-Jakob disease. II. Clinical, pathologic and genetic study of a family. *Arch. Neurol.,* **19:**137–49, 1968.

161. McIlroy, W. J., and Richardson, J. C. Syringomyelia; a clinical review of 75 cases. *Can. Med. Assoc. J.,* **93:**731–34, 1965.

162. McRae, D. L., and Standen, J. Roentgenologic findings in syringomyelia and hydromyelia. *Am. J. Roentgenol.,* **98:**695–703, 1966.

163. Messert, B., and Wannamaker, B. B. Reappraisal of adult occult hydrocephalus syndrome. *Neurology* (Minneap.), **24:**224–31, 1974.

164. Mettler, F. A. Substantia nigra and Parkinsonism. *Arch. Neurol.,* **11:**529–42, 1964.

165. Meyer, J. S.; Perusquia, E.; and Infante, E. Blepharospasm: A rare sign of corticostriatobulbar release. *Trans. Am. Neurol. Assoc.,* **97:**311–12, 1973.

166. Meyer, J. S.; Shimazu, K.; Fukuuchi, Y.; Ohuchi, T.; Okamoto, S.; Koto, A.; and Ericsson, A. D. Cerebral dysautoregulation in central neurogenic orthostatic hypotension (Shy-Drager syndrome). *Neurology* (Minneap.), **23:**262–73, 1973.

167. Meyer, J. S.; Wiederholt, I. C.; Toyoda, M.; Ryu, T.; Shinohara, Y.; and Guiraud, B. A new method for continuous sampling of cerebral venous blood without extracranial contamination in man. Bilateral transbrachial catheterization of the cerebral venous sinuses. *Neurology* (Minneap.), **19:**353–58, 1969.

168. Muenter, M. D.; Sharples, N. S.; et al. Patterns of dystonia ("I-D-I" and "D-I-D") in response to L-dopa therapy for Parkinson's disease. *Mayo Clin. Proc.,* **52:**163–74, 1977.

169. Mulder, D. W. Treatment of anterior horn cell disease. *Mod. Treatm.,* **3:**243–49, 1966.

170. Myrianthopoulos, N. C., and Rowley, P. T. Monozygotic twins concordant for Huntington's chorea. *Neurology* (Minneap.), **10:**506–11, 1960.

171. Nakana, K. K.; Schoene, W. C.; et al. The cervical myelopathy associated with rheumatoid arthritis: Analysis of 32 patients and 2 postmortem cases. *Ann. Neurol.,* **2:**144–51, 1978.

172. Nevin, S.; McMenemey, W. M.; Behrman, S.; and Jones, D. P. Subacute spongiform encephalopathy; subacute form of encephalopathy attributable to vascular dysfunction (spongiform cerebral atrophy). *Brain,* **83:**519–64, 1960.

173. Norris, F. H., Jr. Guanidine in amyotrophic lateral sclerosis. *N. Engl. J. Med.,* **288:**690–91, 1973.

174. Oldstone, M. B. A.; Wilson, C. B.; et al. Evidence for immune-complex formation in patients with amyotrophic lateral sclerosis. *Lancet,* **2:**169–72, 1976.

175. Oliver, J., and Dewhurst, K. Childhood and adolescent forms of Huntington's disease. *J. Neurol. Neurosurg. Psychiat.,* **32:**455–59, 1969.

176. OpDenVelde, W., and Stam, F. C. Some cerebral proteins and enzyme systems in Alzheimer's presenile and senile dementia. *J. Am. Geriat. Soc.,* **24:**12–16, 1976.

177. Oshiro, L. S.; Cremer, N. E.; et al. Viruslike particles in muscle from a patient with amyotrophic lateral sclerosis. *Neurology* (Minneap.), **26:**57–60, 1976.

178. Parkes, J. D.; Debono, A. G.; and Marsden, C. D. Bromocriptine in Parkinsonism: Long-term treatment dose response and comparison with levodopa. *J. Neurol. Neurosurg. Psychiat.,* **39:**1101–1108, 1976.

179. *Parkinson's Disease. Present Status and Research Trends,* U.S. Dept. of Health, Education and Welfare. National Institutes of Neurological Diseases and Blindness. Bethesda, Md. U.S. Government Printing Office, 1966.

180. Patten, B. M. Modality specific memory disorders in man. *Acta Neurol. Scand.* **48:**69–86, 1972.

181. Patten, B. M. The ancient art of memory: Usefulness in treatment. *Arch. Neurol.,* **26:**25–31, 1972.

182. Pena, C. E. Viruslike particles in amyotrophic lateral sclerosis: Electron microscopical study of a case. *Ann. Neurol.,* **1:**290–97, 1977.

183. Perez, F. I.; Rivera, V. M.; et al. Analysis of intellectual and cognitive performance in patients with multi infarct dementia. Vertebrobasilar insufficiency with dementia and Alzheimer's disease. *J. Neurol. Neurosurg. Psychiat.,* **38:**533–40, 1975.

184. Perot, P.; Feindel, W.; and Lloyd-Smith, D. Hematomyelia as a complication of syringomyelia: Gower's syringal hemorrhage, case report. *J. Neurosurg.,* **25:**447–51, 1966.

184a. Perret, J.; Feuerstein, C.; et al. Evaluations of plasmotic methoxydopa in parkinsonian patients with or without dyskinesia induced by L-dopa. *Rev. Neurol.,* **133:**627–36, 1977.

185. Perry, T. L.; Hansen, S.; and Kloster, M. Huntington's chorea. Deficiency of gamma-aminobutyric acid in brain. *N. Engl. J. Med.,* **288:**337–42, 1973.

186. Perry, T. L.; Hansen, S.; and Lesk, D. Plasma amino acid levels in children of patients with Huntington's chorea. *Neurology* (Minneap.), **22:**68–70, 1972.

187. Pertschuk, L. P.; Cook, A. W.; et al. Jejunal immunopathology in amyotrophic lateral sclerosis and multiple sclerosis. Identification of viral antigens by immunofluorescence. *Lancet,* **1:**1119–23, 1977.

188. Peyronnard, J. M.; Lapointe, L.; et al. Nerve conduction studies and electromyography in Friedreich's ataxia. *Can. J. Neurol. Sci.,* **3:**313–17, 1976.

189. Phillips, D. G. Surgical treatment of myelopathy

with cervical spondylosis. *J. Neurol. Neurosurg. Psychiat.,* **36:**879–84, 1973.

190. Power, J. M.; Horoupian, D. S.; Schaumberg, H. H.; and Wetherbee, A. I. Documentation of a neurological disease in a Vermont family 90 years later. *Can. J. Neurol. Sci.,* **1:**134–42, 1974.

191. Price, T. R., and Netsky, M. G. Myxedema and ataxia, cerebellar alterations and "neural myxedema bodies." *Neurology* (Minneap.), **16:**957–62, 1966.

192. Rao, C. V. G. K.; Brennan, T. G.; and Garcia, J. M. Computed tomography in diagnosis of Creutzfeldt-Jakob disease. *J. Comput. Assoc. Tomogr.,* **1:**211–15, 1977.

193. Rayput, A. H., and Rozditsky, B. Dysautonomia in parkinsonism: A clinicopathological study. *J. Neurol. Neurosurg. Psychiat.,* **39:**1092–1100, 1976.

194. Reveno, W. S.; Bauer, R. B.; and Rosenbaum, H. L-Dopa for parkinsonism. *Geriatrics,* **28:**86–88, 1973.

195. Rinne, U. K.; Marttila, R. J.; and Sonninen, V. Brain dopamine turnover and the relief of parkinsonism. *Arch. Neurol.,* **34:**626–29, 1977.

195a. Rodriguez-Budelli, M., and Kark, P. Kinetic evidence for a structural abnormality of lipoamide dehydrogenase in two patients with Friedreich's ataxia. *Neurology* (Minneap.), **28:**1283–86, 1978.

195b. Rosen, A. D. Amyotrophic lateral sclerosis. Clinical features and prognosis. *Arch. Neurol.,* **35:**638–42, 1978.

196. Rosenthal, N. P.; Keesey, J.; et al. Familial neurological disease associated with spongiform encephalopathy. *Arch. Neurol.,* **33:**252–59, 1976.

197. Ross, R. T.; Simpson, C. A.; and Styles, S. Wohltart, Kugelberg, Welander syndrome. *Can. J. Neurol. Sci.,* **1:**130–31, 1974.

198. Sachdeu, K. K.; Singh, N.; and Krishnamoothy, M. S. Juvenile parkinsonism treated with levodopa. *Arch. Neurol.,* **34:**244–45, 1977.

199. Sacks, O. W.; Aguilar, M. J.; and Brown, W. J. Hallervorden Spatz disease; itpathogenesis and place among the axonal dystrophies. *Acta Neuropathol.* (Berl.), **6:**164–74, 1966.

200. Sanchez-Casis, G.; Cote, M.; and Barbeau, A. Pathology of the heart in Friedreich's ataxia. Review of the literature and report of one case. *Can. J. Neurol. Sci.,* **3:**349–54, 1976.

201. Sandberg, M. A.; Berson, E. L.; and Ariel, M. Visual evoked response testing with a stimulator-opthalmoscope. *Arch. Ophthalmol.,* **95:**1805–1808, 1977.

202. Savery, F. Amantidine and a fixed combination of levodopa and carbidopa in the treatment of Parkinson's disease. *Dis. Nerv. Syst.,* **38:**605–608, 1977.

203. Scholte, W. Subakute präsenile spongiforme encephalopathie mit occipitalem Schwerpunkt und Rindenblindheit (Heidenhain's syndrome). *Arch. Psychiatr. Nervenkr.,* **213:**345–69, 1970.

204. Schnur, J. A.; Chase, T. N.; and Brody, J. A. Parkinsonism-dementia of Guam: Treatment with L-dopa. *Neurology* (Minneap.), **21:**1236–42, 1971.

205. Schwab, R. S.; England, A. C., Jr.; Poskanzer, D. C.; and Young, R. R. Amantadine in the treatment of Parkinson's disease. *J.A.M.A.,* **208:**1168–70, 1969.

206. Schwartz, A. R. Charcot-Marie-Tooth disease; a 45-year follow-up. *Arch. Neurol.,* **9:**623–34, 1963.

207. Schwartz, G. A. The orthostatic hypotension syndrome of Shy-Drager. A clinicopathologic report. *Arch. Neurol.,* **16:**123–39, 1967.

208. Schwarcz, R.; Bennett, J. P.; and Coyle, J. T. Inhibitors of GABA metabolism: Implications for Huntington's disease. *Ann. Neurol.,* **2:**299–303, 1977.

209. Scott, D. F.; Heathfield, K. W. G.; Toone, B.; and Margerison, J. H. The EEG in Huntington's chorea: a clinical and neuropathological study. *J. Neurol. Neurosurg. Psychiat.,* **35:**97–102, 1972.

210. The second symposium on Parkinson's disease. *Neurosurg.,* **24:**suppl. Part 2, 1966.

211. Sheehan, S.; Bauer, R. B.; and Meyer, J. S. Vertebral artery compression in cervical spondylosis. An arteriographic demonstration during life of vertebral artery insufficiency due to rotation and extension of the neck. *Neurology* (Minneap.), **10:**968–92, 1961.

212. Shields, W. D., and Bray, P. F. A danger of haloperidol therapy in children. *J. Pediatr.,* **88:**301–303, 1976.

212a. Shoulsen, I.; Goldblatt, D.; et al. Huntington's disease: Treatment with muscimol, a GABA-mimetic drug, *Ann. Neurol.,* **4:**279–84, 1978.

213. Shultz, D. R.; Barthal, J. S.; and Garrett, C. Western equine encephalitis with rapid onset of parkinsonism. *Neurology,* **27:**1095–96, 1977.

214. Silverside, J. L. The Parkinsonian syndrome; prognosis and treatment. *Postgrad. Med.,* **37:**440–45, 1965.

215. Sjaastad, O.; Berstand, J.; et al. Homocarsinosis 2. A familial metabolic disorder associated with spastic paraplegia progressive mental deficiency and retinal pigmentation. *Acta Neurol. Scand.,* **53:**275–90, 1976.

216. Snider, S. R.; Fahn, S.; et al. Primary sensory symptoms in parkinsonism. *Neurology* (Minneap.), **26:**423–29, 1976.

217. Snyder, B. D. Selected aspects of parkinsonism: Therapeutics. *Minn. Med.,* **60:**284–86, 1977.

218. Sourkes, T. L. The action of alpha methyl-dopa in the brain. *Br. Med. Bull.,* **21:**66–69, 1965.

219. Stahl, W. L., and Swanson, P. D. Biochemical abnormalities in Huntington's chorea. *Neurology* (Minneap.), **24:**813–19, 1974.

220. Steele, J. C.; Richardson, J. C.; and Olszewski, J. Progressive supranuclear palsy; heterogenous degeneration involving the brain stem, basal ganglia and cerebellum with vertical gaze and pseudobulbar palsy, nuchal dystonia and dementia. *Arch. Neurol.,* **10:**333–59, 1964.

221. Svien, H. J., and Cody, D. T. R. Treatment of spasmodic torticollis by suppression of labrynthine activity: Report of a case. *Mayo Clin. Proc.,* **44:**825–27, 1969.

222. Swash, M.; Roberts, A. H.; Zakko, H.; and

Heathfield, K. W. G. Treatment of involuntary movement disorders with tetrabenazine. *J. Neurol. Neurosurg. Psychiat.,* **35:**186–91, 1972.

223. Sweet, R. D.; Blumberg, J.; et al. Propranolol treatment of essential tremor. *Neurology* (Minneap.), **24:**64–67, 1974.

224. Syman, L., and Dorsch, N. W. C. Use of long term intracranial pressure measurement to assess hydrocephalic patients prior to shunt surgery. *J. Neurosurg.,* **42:**258–73, 1975.

225. Takahashi, K.; Nakamura, H.; and Okada, E. Hereditary amyotrophic lateral sclerosis. *Arch. Neurol.,* **27:**292–99, 1972.

226. Tarlov, E. On the problem of the pathology of spasmodic torticollis in man. *J. Neurol. Neurosurg. Psychiat.,* **33:**457–63, 1970.

227. Thapedi, I. M.; Ashenhurst, E. M.; and Rozdilsky, B. Shy-Drager syndrome. Report on an autopsied case. *Neurology* (Minneap.), **21:**26–32, 1972.

228. Thomas, P. K., and Calne, D. B. Motor nerve conduction velocity in peroneal muscular atrophy and evidence for genetic heterogeneity. *J. Neurol. Neurosurg. Psychiat.,* **37:**68–75, 1974.

229. Thoren, C. Cardiomyopathy in Friedreich's ataxia. *Acta Pediat.* (Stockholm), suppl. **153:**1–136, 1964.

230. Troost, B. T., and Doroff, R. B. The ocular motor defects in progressive supranuclear palsy. *Ann. Neurol.,* **2:**397–403, 1977.

231. Tsukagoshi, H.; Sugita, H.; Furukawa, T.; Tsubaki, T.; and Ono, E. Kugelberg-Welander syndrome with dominant inheritance. *Arch. Neurol.,* **14:**378–81, 1966.

232. Verhaart, W. J. Degeneration of the brain stem reticular formation, other parts of the brain stem and the cerebellum; an example of heterogenous systemic degeneration of the central nervous system. *J. Neuropathol. Exp. Neurol.,* **17:**382–91, 1958.

233. Welch, K. M. A., and Goldberg, D. M. Serum creatine phosphokinase in motor neuron disease. *Neurology* (Minneap.), **22:**697–701, 1972.

233a. White, P.; Giley, C. R.; et al. Neocortical cholinergic neurons in elderly people. *Lancet,* **1:**668–71, 1977.

234. Williams, B., and Timperley, W. R. Three cases of communicating syringomyelia secondary to midbrain gliomas. *J. Neurol. Neurosurg. Psychiat.,* **40:**80–88, 1976.

235. Wilson, J.; Linnell, J. C.; and Matthews, D. M. Plasma-cobalamins in neuro-ophthalmological diseases. *Lancet,* **1:**259–61, 1971.

236. Winkelman, A. C. Update on drug treatment of parkinsonism. *Am. Fam. Physician,* **16:**118–20, 1977.

237. Winkler, G. F., and Young, R. R. Efficacy of chronic propranolol therapy in action tremors, familial, senile or essential varieties. *N. Engl. J. Med.,* **290:**984–88, 1974.

238. Wolfgram, F., and Myers, L. Toxicity of serum from patients with amyotrophic lateral sclerosis for anterior horn cells in vitro. *Trans. Am. Neurol. Assoc.,* **97:**19–21, 1972.

239. Young, R. R.; Growdon, J. H.; and Shakani, B. T. B adrenergic mechanisms in action tremor. *N. Engl. J. Med.,* **293:**950–53, 1975.

240. Zeman, W. Dystonia: An overview. In Eldridge, R., and Fahn, S. (eds.). *Advances in Neurology,* Vol. 14. Raven Press, New York, 1976, pp. 91–102.

5 TOXIC AND METABOLIC DISORDERS OF THE NERVOUS SYSTEM

Abnormalities of Water and Electrolytes

Neurologic Complications of Hyponatremia

Etiology

The causes of hyponatremia are given in Table 5–1. The condition occurs as a result of dilution or depletion of body sodium. Hyponatremia has been reported after excessive administration of parenteral fluids and usually occurs in infants and elderly patients, particularly during postoperative treatment.[242] Excessive water ingestion with hyponatremia has been reported in voluntarily water-intoxicated infants,[71] in adults who consume excessive amounts of water or beer,[153] and in psychiatric patients who are compulsive water drinkers.[275] Hyponatremia can also occur from excessive use of diuretics[100] and may develop in congestive heart failure, hepatic cirrhosis, adrenal insufficiency, and salt-losing nephritis, and may occasionally occur in epileptic patients receiving carbamazepine.[258a] Pregnant patients receiving large doses of oxytocin can develop hyponatremia since oxytocin preparations may have significant antidiuretic properties.[197]

The inappropriate secretion of antidiuretic hormone has been described in cases of bronchial carcinoma with ectopic production of antidiuretic hormone, in a number of neurologic and neurosurgical conditions, and in a variety of other diseases (Table 5–1). Inappropriate secretion of antidiuretic hormone may occur more frequently than is generally realized, particularly following craniocerebral trauma and neurosurgical procedures.

TABLE 5–1

Causes of Hyponatremia

1. Excessive administration of parenteral fluids
2. Excessive water ingestion
3. Excessive use of diuretics
4. Complication of a chronic disorder such as congestive heart failure, hepatic cirrhosis, Addison's disease, salt-losing nephritis
5. Use of large doses of oxytocin in pregnant patients
6. Inappropriate secretion of antidiuretic hormone[83]
   a. Bronchial carcinoma
   b. Hypothyroidism
   c. Cerebral infarction
   d. Intracerebral and subarachnoid hemorrhage
   e. Acute meningitis
   f. Craniocerebral trauma
   g. After neurosurgical procedures

Pathology

Acute hyponatremia results in cerebral edema and low intracellular concentrations of sodium. More chronic cases of hyponatremia may show minimal brain edema, and the appearance of symptoms is probably related more to the decrease in intracellular sodium and potassium than to the cerebral edema.

Clinical Features

Symptoms of acute hyponatremia (acute water intoxication) develop when the serum sodium level falls below 125 mEq/L and consist of nausea, vomiting, muscle twitching, seizures, and coma. There are a high mortality and significant morbidity due to brain damage. Chronic hyponatremia presents with thirst, impaired sensation of taste, anorexia, and muscle cramps, followed by generalized fatigue, nausea, vomiting, and abdominal colic. If the hyponatremia continues, there are profound weakness, confusion, delirium, and seizures. Since the symptoms of water intoxication are usually neurologic, they may be incorrectly attributed to a primary neurologic disorder.

Diagnostic Procedures

1. Review of intake and output records may show excessive fluid intake with insufficient output.
2. Serum electrolyte studies show low sodium, chloride, and potassium levels.
3. The urine osmolality consistently exceeds the serum osmolality.

4. The syndrome of inappropriate secretion of antidiuretic hormone can be distinguished from other causes of hyponatremia by low serum osmolality, less than maximal dilution of the urine, and persistence of sodium excretion in the urine and hyponatremia following parenteral administration of sodium.
5. The electroencephalogram shows loss of normal alpha activity with generalized slowing and irregular discharges of high-amplitude slow-wave (4 to 7 Hz) activity over both hemispheres.[253]

Treatment

Inappropriate secretion of antidiuretic hormone is treated by water restriction and treatment of the underlying disease. Other causes of hyponatremia usually respond to restricted fluid intake.[56] In severe cases, infusion of hypertonic saline solution (6 ml of 5 per cent saline solution per kilogram for adults; 3 per cent saline solution is recommended for children) produces rapid improvement.

Neurologic Complications of Hypernatremia

Neurologic signs are common in hypernatremia, particularly in children, although the neurologic damage appears to be due to a combination of the hypernatremia and the subsequent cerebral edema that frequently occurs during rehydration.[154, 234]

Etiology and Pathology

The condition most commonly occurs in febrile children with anorexia who are not given parenteral fluids and suffer severe dehydration. It also occurs in adults and may be seen following vomiting and diarrhea with dehydration or excessive intake of sodium, particularly by the intravenous route. Hypernatremia has been reported as a rare complication of intra-amniotic infusion of hypertonic saline for termination of pregnancy.[128] Other causes include diabetes insipidus, acute renal failure, nonketotic hyperosmolar coma, renal tubular damage, dialysis in chronic uremia, dehydration secondary to elevated ambient temperatures, ingestion of sea water, aldosteronism, corticosteroid therapy, and excessive intravenous administration of sodium bicarbonate to newborn infants or adults following cardiac arrest.[11] Hypernatremia has been described in intracranial lesions including hypothalamic tumors (such as craniopharyngioma and pinealoma), Hand-Christian-Schüller disease, and nonspecific inflammation of the neurohypophysis.[53, 213, 295, 341] All of these conditions appear to result in loss of the normal response to thirst due to osmoreceptor damage in the anterior hypothalamus. Some cases appear to tolerate the condition well and develop chronic or "essential" hypernatremia without symptoms.

The abrupt elevation of plasma osmolality in hypernatremia establishes an osmotic gradient between blood and brain, and there is a rapid movement of water from the brain and a rapid shrinking in brain volume. This produces tearing of intracerebral veins and intracerebral hemorrhage in some cases. Other cases show multiple petechial hemorrhages in the cortex and white matter with thrombosis of capillaries, veins, and dural sinuses. Dehydration may lead to permanent brain damage.[142]

Clinical Features

In the initial stages, there is increasing somnolence leading to stupor and coma, with muscle rigidity, meningism, opisthotonus, and decerebrate rigidity. Transient chorea, myoclonus or seizures may occur during the stage of dehydration or rehydration and may be due to a concomitant hypocalcemia or hypomagnesemia.[319] About one third of the patients die, one third survive with neurologic abnormalities, and one third recover. The sequelae include transient choreoathetosis,[213] mono- or hemiparesis, seizures, and mental retardation.[234]

Treatment

Hypernatremia should be treated by slow rehydration, using plasma expanders to correct the hypovolemia. The use of intravenous dextrose and water may dilute the extracellular fluid and lead to secondary intracellular edema.

Treatment with intravenous isotonic solutions composed of equal parts of 5.5 per cent glucose and 0.9 per cent sodium chloride combined with peritoneal dialysis with a slightly hypertonic dialysate (347 mosmol per liter), which produces slower correction of the hypertonicity, has been recommended.[181] Administration of cortisone acetate may be followed by return of thirst in some cases of chronic hypernatremia, suggesting that cortisone may be necessary for normal functioning of the osmoreceptors in the hypothalamus.[341]

Neurologic Complications of Hypokalemia

The main causes of hypokalemia are given in Table 5–2. Familial periodic paralysis is discussed elsewhere (p. 745).

Hypokalemia produces an alteration in the resting cell potential owing to loss of intracellular potassium into the extracellular compartment. There is hyperpolarization of the cell membrane and a change in the cell response to stimuli. The change is particularly marked in muscle but also affects other cells, including neurons.

Clinical Features

Patients with hypokalemia complain of muscle weakness and easy fatigue. These are usually of minor degree in the majority of conditions given in Table 5–2. The condition presents with generalized weakness and lethargy followed by clouding of consciousness, confusion, or delirium, which may progress to semicoma or coma. Respiratory weakness may be evident in severe cases. Severe hypokalemia with paralysis may occur in hypo-

TABLE 5–2

Hypokalemia

1. *Deficient intake of potassium*
   a. Excessive water ingestion
   b. Intestinal obstruction
   c. Parenteral fluid therapy

2. *Intestinal loss of potassium*
   a. Vomiting
   b. Diarrhea

3. *Renal loss of potassium*
   a. Chronic renal disease
   b. Congenital renal defects
   c. Secondary aldosteronism following severe hypertension

4. *Following dialysis for chronic renal insufficiency*

5. *Endocrine abnormalities*
   a. Primary aldosteronism
   b. Cushing's disease
   c. Hyperthyroidism
   d. Primary and secondary aldosteronism

6. *Pharmacologic causes*
   a. Excessive use of diuretics, corticosteroids, and licorice

7. *Metabolic alkalosis*

8. *Treatment of diabetic acidosis without potassium replacement*

9. *Familial periodic paralysis of hypokalemic type* (see Chap. 12)

chloremic acidosis complicating renal disease and in the hypochloremic alkalosis secondary to severe vomiting. Acute quadriplegia has been reported in diabetic ketoacidosis with hypokalemia.[214, 256]

Potassium depletion has a profound effect on impulse formation and conduction in the heart. There is enhanced ectopic activity in pacemaker cells with depression of conduction velocity at the AV node. Arrhythmias with occasional development of life-threatening ventricular tachycardia are not uncommon when the potassium levels fall below 3.2 mEq/liter.[72]

Diagnostic Procedures

1. Serum potassium levels are below 3.5 mEq/liter.
2. The electrocardiogram shows depression of the S-T segment, prolonged Q-T interval, and inverted T waves. There may be the appearance of U waves and fusion of T and U waves.

Primary Aldosteronism

This condition is due to an adrenocortical adenoma and also may cause profound hypokalemia. Symptoms include muscular weakness, easy fatigue, and intermittent paralysis in some cases, often provoked by the administration of thiazides. There may be frontal headaches, paresthesias of the extremities, polydipsia, polyuria, and tetany. Mild hypertension is a usual but not invariable finding. Chvostek and Trousseau signs are present in some cases. Urinalysis usually reveals proteinuria, with normal sodium and excess potassium concentration. Serum sodium levels are elevated, with decreased sodium concentration in sweat and saliva. Serum potassium is markedly reduced, and serum angiotensin and renin levels are very low or absent. There is metabolic alkalosis and increased plasma volume. The electrocardiogram shows the hypokalemic changes already described.

Diagnostic aspects of primary aldosteronism are as follows:

1. The serum potassium is low and sodium is high.
2. Final diagnosis depends on the demonstration of excess urinary aldosterone (normal, 3 to 30 μg in 24 hours).[28]
3. If urinary aldosterone determinations are not available, the patient should be placed on a high-sodium diet and urinary potassium clearance should be determined before and after the administration of spironolactone. The high urinary clearance of potassium before spironolactone is followed by a profound fall in urinary potassium clearance and a rise in serum potassium levels after administration of this drug.[41]

Secondary Aldosteronism

This condition rarely produces the severe hypokalemia of primary aldosteronism. Secondary aldosteronism is due to renal arteriolar stenosis and is associated with an increase in renin and angiotensin production leading to excess aldosterone production by the normal adrenals. There are severe hypertension, normal serum sodium levels, and slight depression in serum potassium levels.

Diagnosis depends on the demonstration of elevated plasma renin and angiotensin levels and impaired renal function.

Treatment

In the majority of patients, hypokalemia is one facet of a complex metabolic abnormality, such as metabolic alkalosis or diabetic acidosis, and responds to appropriate treatment. Primary aldosteronism can be cured by surgical removal of the adrenal adenoma unless irreversible hypertension and adrenal damage have occurred. In order to restore potassium levels to normal, it is safer to give potassium by mouth rather than by intravenous administration, which may result in sinus bradycardia or even cardiac arrest in systole if plasma levels are increased too rapidly. The suggested oral daily dose of potassium is 2 to 6 gm/day (28 to 80 mEq of potassium). Intravenous dosage should not exceed 50 to 100 mEq, given no faster than at a rate of 20 mEq per hour. Serum potassium levels should be checked frequently.

Neurologic Complications of Hypermagnesemia and Hypomagnesemia

The magnesium ion is essential for the activation of many enzymatic systems and is mainly intracellular in distribution.[106] It is also important in synaptic transmission and membrane excitability. Highest concentrations occur in bone, liver, brain, and muscle. Normal serum magnesium levels vary from 1.6 to 2.1 mEq/liter.

Since magnesium is present in most foodstuffs, depletion does not occur with a normal diet. However, hypomagnesemia may be encountered in patients with inadequate diet and excess gastrointestinal loss, particularly in vomiting associated with intestinal obstruction. Low serum magnesium levels can occur in diabetic acidosis, steatorrhea, long-term diuretic therapy, and hyperaldosteronism. The risk of hypomagnesemia is increased by prolonged use of intravenous fluids without magnesium added, malabsorption syndromes, pancreatitis, porphyria, malignant osteolytic disease, and extensive bowel resection. Hypomagnesemia is also associated with impaired release and probably lack of end-organ response to parathormone. Thus, it is not uncommon to find severe hypomagnesemia associated with hypocalcemia.[362] A transient hypomagnesemia is common in the alcohol withdrawal phase, following a period of chronic intoxication. It probably contributes to the seizures and other symptoms that characterize alcoholic withdrawal. Hypomagnesemia decreases intracellular myocardial potassium and sensitizes the myocardium to the effects of digoxin. Low serum magnesium levels increase the risk of digoxin intoxication.[316]

Hypermagnesemia may occur in renal failure due to administration of magnesium salts, usually antacids.

Clinical Features

Symptoms of hypomagnesemia include mental confusion, irritability, agitation, muscle twitching, hallucinations, coma, and myoclonic jerks with marked tachycardia. There may be associated tremors, generalized hyperreflexia, athetoid and choreiform movements, and seizures in some cases. Chvostek and Trousseau signs may be present. There is a prompt response to magnesium replacement.

The magnesium ion is concerned with the release of acetylcholine at the motor end plate, and high concentrations produce motor paralysis. Hypermagnesemia may result in lethargy leading to coma, respiratory failure, and death. Respiratory death has been reported in infants with elevated serum magnesium levels due to administration of magnesium salts to their mothers in the treatment of preeclampsia.

Diagnostic Procedures

In hypomagnesemia, the serum magnesium levels are below 1.6 mEq/liter, and low magnesium levels are found in the CSF.[54] In hypermagnese-

mia, the serum levels are in excess of 2.1 mEq/liter.

Treatment

Hypomagnesemia should be treated by intravenous infusion of magnesium sulfate. The solution is prepared by dissolving 20 ml of 10 per cent magnesium sulfate in 250 to 500 ml of 5 per cent dextrose and 0.2 N saline and should be infused slowly over a two- to four-hour period to prevent depression of the cardiovascular or nervous systems. Particular care should be taken in giving parenteral magnesium to patients with renal disease since hypermagnesemia may result.

Hypermagnesemia is treated by intravenous administration of fluids plus 10 per cent calcium gluconate solution. In severe cases renal dialysis may be necessary.

Cerebral Anoxia and Anoxic Encephalopathy

Common causes of cerebral anoxia are given in Table 5–3. The terms "anoxic," "stagnant," "anemic," and "histotoxic" have been retained because they are well-established in the literature, but there is considerable overlap between these major groups in many cases. The role of anoxia neonatorum in cerebral palsy is discussed in Chapter 2.

Etiology and Pathology

Brain metabolism is almost entirely dependent on oxygen and glucose. The demand is high, and anoxic or hypoxic changes will occur if either or both are lacking. When the cerebral venous P_{O2} falls below 25 mm Hg, the brain progressively shifts to anaerobic glucose metabolism. Anaerobic metabolism in the brain is less efficient than oxidative, and if oxygen consumption is reduced by more than about 30 per cent, neurologic impairment follows despite anaerobic glycolysis. There is, however, wide variation in the damage to the central nervous system caused by hypoxia depending on its duration, the body temperature, blood pressure (perfusion pressure), the cerebral metabolic rate for oxygen, and different susceptibilities of various parts of the nervous system to the effects of hypoxia.

In general, the gray matter of the brain has a higher metabolic rate than the white matter, and hypoxia initially damages the cerebral neurons.[199] The frontal cortex has a high metabolic rate,

TABLE 5–3

Classification of Causes of Anoxic Encephalopathy

1. *Anoxic anoxia*
   a. Obstruction to airway—strangulation, foreign bodies, laryngeal spasm, drowning
   b. Impairment of respiratory muscles—poliomyelitis, high spinal cord lesions, postinfectious polyneuritis, myasthenia gravis
   c. Depression of brainstem respiratory center—encephalitis, tumors, granulomas, porphyria, barbiturate poisoning, cerebral hemorrhage, and trauma
   d. Impaired gaseous exchange in lungs—severe pneumonia, chlorine poisoning, emphysema
   e. Anesthesia—nitrous oxide, ether
   f. High altitude (flying or mountain climbing)

2. *Stagnant anoxia*
   a. Cardiac arrest
   b. Some forms of strangulation

3. *Anemic anoxia*
   a. Carbon monoxide poisoning
   b. Blood loss

4. *Histotoxic anoxia*
   a. Cyanide poisoning

whereas the metabolic rates of the occipital, parietal, and temporal cortex, the basal ganglia, and the cerebellum are lower. The brainstem has a lower metabolic requirement, with the longest survival time in the medulla. Hence, during progressive anoxia, the first clinical sign is impaired judgment, followed later by perceptual and visual difficulties and unconsciousness. Decortication appears next and decerebration follows. Thereafter, there is progressive paralysis of cranial nerve function followed by a failure of respiration.

In fatal cases of anoxic encephalopathy, the changes in the brain depend on the duration of survival after the hypoxic episode.[30] There are three possibilities, each producing a characteristic pathologic picture:

1. Death occurs during or immediately after the anoxic episode.
2. There is a period of coma, followed by the development of signs indicating diffuse damage to the central nervous system. Death occurs after a period varying from a few days to several months.
3. Rarely, the period of coma is followed by an interval of two or three weeks during which time the patient appears to have recovered partially or even completely. This is followed by the development of progressive neurologic deficit and death or severe neurologic residual.[266]

When death occurs during or immediately after the anoxic episode, the brain shows acute congestion with diffuse dilatation of all blood vessels.

There are scattered petechial hemorrhages and occasional large hemorrhages throughout the central nervous system. In cases caused by carbon monoxide poisoning, the brain is pink owing to the presence of carboxyhemoglobin in the blood.

When death occurs about 48 hours after the anoxic episode, the brain is edematous, with capillary and venous dilatation and petechial hemorrhages. There is early necrosis of the globus pallidus, and occasionally similar necrotic changes are found in the reticular zone of the substantia nigra. Survival for longer periods intensifies the necrosis in the globus pallidus and also results in extensive necrosis in the cortical gray matter, which may be focal or laminar in type. The neurons are necrotic or show irreversible changes, and there is both astroglial and microglial proliferation. Similar degenerative changes can be seen in the neurons in the brainstem and in the Purkinje cells of the cerebellum.

The pathologic findings in patients who have recovered from anoxic coma and exhibit a period of apparent recovery followed by delayed neurologic deterioration are quite different from the changes found predominantly in gray matter as described above. Delayed postanoxic encephalopathy is predominantly a disorder of the white matter rather than gray matter[84] and is characterized by widespread demyelination throughout the cerebral hemispheres. Neuronal loss is often minimal or absent in the cortical gray matter, brainstem, and cerebellum, and the basal ganglia may be normal or show small areas of necrosis. The pathogenesis of this type of leukoencephalopathy is unclear. The deeper cerebral white matter has a poor blood supply with few anastomoses compared to the cortical matter. This suggests that the white matter may be particularly vulnerable to anoxic-ischemic damage.[125] Most cases of delayed anoxic leukoencephalopathy appear to have suffered prolonged anoxic hypotension and acidosis, which suggests that these factors may be important in the development of white matter damage. The delay in the development of symptoms may be due to anoxic-ischemic damage to oligodendroglial cells, which are responsible for the formation and metabolic integrity of myelin. Failure to replace myelin and the gradual removal of myelin by microglia would occur over a period of several weeks.

A totally different type of delayed hypoxic damage to the brain has been reported after apparent recovery from strangulation. These cases show marked cavitation of the caudate nucleus, putamen, and globus pallidus with sparing of white matter.[89] This type of delayed reaction may be due to the combined effects of anoxia, lactic acidosis, and severe venous stasis.

Clinical Features

Patients who survive the initial period following the anoxic episode may show various degrees of recovery depending on the severity and duration of the anoxic episode. They may (1) recover completely, (2) show varying degrees of neurologic deficit, which may improve or remain as a permanent deficit, or (3) pass through a period of apparent recovery followed by the development of neurologic signs after an interval of two or three weeks. Such cases may show progressive deterioration and death or eventually stabilize with variable neurologic deficits.

Some patients exhibit intellectual deterioration which begins immediately after the anoxic episode. There may be generalized rigidity with mild parkinsonian-like tremor. The more severely affected remain semicomatose and restless, with involuntary movements, myoclonic jerks, or decerebrate rigidity. Recovery may continue over a period of many months, but many patients show permanent deficits, particularly in the intellectual areas. Recovery usually begins with return of brainstem and cerebellar function, basal ganglia function next, followed by return of visual and perceptual function, and of insight and judgment last. Some patients develop severe myoclonus

(posthypoxic intention myoclonus) in which violent myoclonic jerks occur during voluntary motor activity. This is believed to be due to a deficiency of cerebral serotonin metabolism, and cerebrospinal fluid 5-hydroxyindolacetic acid (5-HIAA) levels are low in the cerebrospinal fluid.[129a]

The clinical picture of delayed postanoxic encephalopathy is somewhat different. There is a history of severe anoxia, exposure to carbon monoxide, cardiac arrest, severe respiratory depression from drugs, or respiratory arrest due to anaphylactic shock or anesthesia. The initial coma is followed by recovery in most cases, but some patients show a chronic state of altered consciousness varying from stupor to akinetic mutism. Patients who show apparent recovery are well for a period varying from 48 hours to several weeks, when they become withdrawn and irritable, or apathetic and confused. Motor activity is slowed, and there may be generalized rigidity with parkinsonian features. Since the anoxic episode is remote by this time, a diagnosis of depression or other psychiatric illness may be entertained in some cases. The course may be one of steady deterioration, and death or a second period of recovery, which may or may not be complete, may ensue.

Diagnostic Procedures

1. When the patient is admitted in coma, carboxyhemoglobin and serum barbiturate levels should be obtained to exclude carbon monoxide and barbiturate poisoning.
2. Hemoglobin levels should be obtained at frequent intervals since it is important to correct any anemia, which may compound the effect of anoxia.
3. Arterial P_{O_2}, P_{CO_2}, and pH values should be obtained every day together with serum electrolytes.
4. Roentgenograms of the chest should be taken to rule out pulmonary causes for the anoxic attack or pulmonary complications that might be an additional factor in producing anoxia.
5. The electroencephalogram is extremely useful in assessing the cerebral damage and progress. In severe cases there is absence of electrical activity, which indicates an extremely grave prognosis. The persistence of an isoelectric recording after a period of 24 hours, if barbiturate intoxication is excluded, probably indicates irreversible brain damage. Rarely, recovery has been reported in cases with iso-

electric EEGs associated with barbiturate intoxication. Less severely affected patients show diffuse delta activity over both hemispheres. As improvement occurs, this is replaced by diffuse theta activity and the eventual appearance of sporadic alpha activity. The alpha activity increases in amount as recovery proceeds until a normal record is obtained, usually some weeks or months following the anoxic episode.[159]

6. An electrocardiogram and serial serum enzyme studies (LDH, SGOT) should be obtained in patients who are believed to have had cardiac arrest due to myocardial infarction.

7. Computed tomography with contrast enhancement may show increased densities in the region of the basal ganglia and dentate nucleus several days after cabon monoxide poisoning.[244a]

Treatment

As soon as a patient is admitted after an alleged anoxic episode, he should be examined to make sure that the airways are clear and given pure oxygen to breathe by mask or nasal catheter. Fluid and electrolyte balance should be maintained during prolonged coma. Records of intake and output and daily electrolyte estimations should be maintained during this period. Good nursing care with frequent changes of posture will prevent decubiti and pulmonary atelectasis. Attention should also be given to the prevention of pulmonary and urinary tract infections.

If there is any obstruction to the respiratory passages, it should be removed by laryngoscopy or bronchoscopy. Endotracheal intubation may be necessary. A P_{O_2} level below 50 mm Hg or a P_{CO_2} level above 50 mm Hg is an indication for intermittent positive pressure respiration using a mechanical respirator. Impaired respiratory exchange due to chronic emphysema may also require the use of a mechanical respirator. Any concomitant bronchitis and pneumonia require prompt antibiotic therapy and the use of bronchodilator drugs. If the anoxic episode follows cardiac arrest, the patient should have an electrocardiographic monitor and pacemaker attached to the chest.

The anoxia or hypoxia of carbon monoxide poisoning is due to the presence of circulating carboxyhemoglobin. The carbon monoxide is firmly bound to hemoglobin, unlike the loose binding of oxygen in oxyhemoglobin, so that oxygen can no longer combine with the carboxyhemoglobin. This means that the hemoglobin is not available for oxygen transport. Such patients should be given pure oxygen by mask and treated in a hyperbaric chamber, if this is available. Another method of treatment includes exchange transfusion to remove the carboxyhemoglobin and restore circulating oxyhemoglobin. Patients with posthypoxic infection myoclonus show considerable reduction in myoclonic activity following oral replacement therapy with L-5-hydroxytryptophan, 5 to 15 mg/kg body weight per day, and carbidopa, 100 mg/day. Clonazepam is also reported to be effective in the treatment of posthypoxic intention myoclonus.[128a]

Irreversible Coma and Determination of Brain Death

Accurate definition of irreversible coma (coma dépassé or brain death) has assumed major importance now that reliable methods are available to support cardiac and respiratory function by artificial means.

It is now possible to maintain cardiac and respiratory function in an individual suffering from irreversible coma for several weeks or even months, imposing a major burden on the patient's family and hospital facilities. In addition, the development of organ transplant programs (particularly renal transplantation) has led to a considerable demand for healthy donor organs. These should be obtained as soon as possible after declaration of irreversible coma or "brain death" in the donor, since prolonged resuscitation is associated with deterioration in the condition of potential donor sites such as the kidney and cornea of the eye.

Since the neurologist is usually called in consultation in such cases, and because international standards have not yet been established for the definition of irreversible coma, the following guidelines may prove helpful:

Criteria for Establishing Brain Death[2, 8, 10, 86, 184, 230, 293, 315, 354]

1. Hypothermia should not be present.
2. There should be no history of drug ingestion or measurable sedative drug level (particularly of barbiturate and glutethimide) present in the blood.[269]

3. Spontaneous respiratory movements should be absent. The patient is given 5 per cent CO_2 in oxygen through the mechanical respirator, which should be disconnected when the Pa_{CO_2} reaches 40 to 45 mm Hg. The respirator remains disconnected for three minutes while the patient is observed for signs of spontaneous respiration. Hypoxia can be prevented during this period by delivering oxygen at 6 liters/minute through a catheter in the trachea.

4. All spontaneous movements should be absent both at rest and following stimulation by pain, sound, or light.

5. The brainstem reflexes should be absent, resulting in:
   a. Dilated and fixed pupils
   b. Absent corneal reflexes
   c. Absent ciliospinal reflex
   d. Absence of reflex eye movements on head turning
   e. Absent gag, swallowing, and coughing reflexes
   f. Absent vestibulo-ocular reflexes. There is absence of eye movement during or after the slow injection of 20 ml of ice-cold water into each external auditory meatus in turn. Clear access to the tympanic membrane must be established by inspection.
   g. Absent tonic neck reflexes

6. Metabolic and endocrine disturbances that can cause coma must be excluded. There should be no profound abnormality in serum electrolytes, acid-base balance, or blood glucose levels.

7. The limbs should be flaccid with no spontaneous movement, although spinal reflexes such as the tendon jerks may be elicited in some cases.

8. The blood pressure may be low, and it may not be possible to maintain blood pressure without the use of drugs.

9. The temperature shows a tendency to fall below 98°F if the body is uncovered.

10. Electroencephalographic signs. There is absence of electrical activity, usually termed "electrocerebral silence," when there is no discernible electrical activity greater than 2 μv in amplitude. In order for this important electroencephalographic diagnosis to be made, certain technical requirements are essential. These include:
    a. Recording by a competent technician
    b. Use of ear reference electrodes and a minimum of ten scalp electrodes
    c. One channel should be used for an electrocardiogram so that electrocardiogram artefact can be readily identified in the EEG record
    d. A second channel should be used for a noncephalic lead (e.g., dorsum of the hand) to pick up other artefacts that may be recorded in an intensive care unit
    e. Interelectrode resistance should be under 10,000 ohms but over 100 ohms
    f. Interelectrode distance of at least 10 cm
    g. The EEG should be recorded at standard gains (50 μv/5 mm) for ten minutes and at twice standard gains for a similar period of time
    h. The EEG machine should be run at its slowest speed for a short period of time
    i. A brief recording at maximum gains should also be obtained
    j. Tests for electrical reactivity to intense stimuli such as pain, loud noise, and strong lights should be performed

When the above criteria have been met, the patient is reexamined in 24 hours and a second EEG is taken. If the results are unchanged, the criteria for irreversible coma have been reasonably established.

Additional Procedures That Are Useful in Establishing Brain Death

1. The early and late components of the orbicularis oculi reflex are absent in irreversible coma.[224]

2. There is absence of bolus tracing from the head in the presence of bolus recording from the femoral artery after the injection of technetium 99 m pertechnetate in irreversible coma.[183] Two negative bolus studies one hour apart indicate a condition incompatible with cerebral survival.[257]

3. Intravenous isotope angiography using a mobile gamma camera at the bedside will demonstrate absence of cerebral blood flow in irreversible coma.[132]

4. Auditory-evoked potentials using far-field recording techniques show total absence of response or the presence of just the initial component (wave 1) which has a prolonged latency.[321]

Further Suggestions for Evaluating Patients and Establishing Criteria of Brain Death

1. The team evaluating patients who are considered to be suffering from brain death should consist of two physicians, one of whom is a neurologist or neurosurgeon. Neither physician should be a member of the transplantation team.
2. The two evaluating physicians should examine the patient with attention to the above-suggested criteria to establish brain death, and they should record their findings with the time and date of examination in the progress notes of the patient's chart.
3. The physicians should repeat their evaluation after 24 hours and again record their findings in the chart.
4. If the patient meets the criteria at each examination, death may be declared. The time of death is recorded and signed by the evaluating physicians. The respirator may then be discontinued.

Discussion with Relatives

The relatives should be informed of the possibility of brain death when the patient is first examined, using the criteria outlined here. The subject of permission for donation of organs should the patient be declared dead may be discussed at that time. If this is acceptable to the relatives, they may be introduced to the leader of the transplant team who may explain the technical procedure and answer any questions. The relatives should be informed as soon as brain death has been established and be told that the patient has been pronounced dead. The respirator may then be discontinued or the body removed, with the respirator still functioning, to the operating room for purposes of organ donation.

Encephalopathy in Chronic Pulmonary Failure

Encephalopathy may occur in patients during treatment for chronic pulmonary insufficiency. This condition is due to the combined effects of hypoxia, cerebral alkalosis, and hypotension[96] and may be potentiated by the administration of aminophylline.

Patients who are in chronic pulmonary failure develop myoclonus due to cortical neuronal hypoxia,[220] multifocal and occasional generalized seizures, and appear to be semicomatose or in a coma. Treatment should be directed toward correction of metabolic abnormalities; aminophylline should be discontinued, and seizures should be controlled with anticonvulsants. The alkalosis can be reversed by deliberate hypoventilation or the use of acetazolamide, 500 mg intravenously.

Pulmonary Encephalopathy and Carbon Dioxide Narcosis

In chronic pulmonary disease and in extreme obesity,[227] pulmonary function may be sufficiently impaired so that the lungs fail to remove carbon dioxide and the arterial carbon dioxide levels rise steadily. This causes headache and cerebral congestion, resulting in papilledema. As the P_{CO_2} rises to 60 and 80 mm Hg, the patient lapses into lethargy, drowsiness, stupor, and coma. The brainstem respiratory center becomes refractory to CO_2, and the respiratory center is now driven by the rise and fall of the P_{O_2}.

Clinical Features

These patients have either chronic long-standing lung disease such as bronchiectasis or partial respiratory paralysis or obesity which impairs cardiopulmonary function. They are lethargic, confused, apathetic, and disoriented, and progress to stupor and coma. Myoclonic jerks of the extremities are seen. Papilledema is present. The tendon jerks are depressed and symmetric. The plantar reflexes may be extensor.[127]

Diagnostic Procedures

1. The EEG shows high-voltage delta activity.
2. The CSF pressure is increased but the fluid is clear and the chemical analysis is normal.
3. The P_{CO_2} is elevated above 50 mm Hg and the P_{O_2} is reduced.

Treatment

Assisted respiration with a mechanical respiratory with oxygen mixtures of 30 to 40 per cent should result in rapid improvement. The blood pH, P_{CO_2}, and P_{O_2} should be checked daily.

Pure oxygen breathing, without assisted respiration, is highly dangerous and may prove fatal since the respiratory center is refractory to changes in P_{CO_2} and only responds to hypoxia.

Bronchoscopy with aspiration of secretions, tracheostomy, and the use of antibiotics are necessary in cases of pulmonary encephalopathy. In cases due to obesity, weight reduction usually results in restoration of adequate ventilation.

Cheyne-Stokes Respiration

In bilateral cerebral disease, cerebral anoxia, cerebral ischemia, or toxic and metabolic conditions causing depression of the respiratory center (such as morphine or barbiturate poisoning), the respirations may become periodic. Periods of apnea, which may last for half a minute or more, are followed by a crescendo and decrescendo of hyperventilation. During the apneic phase the patient may be comatose or unresponsive, but in the hyperventilation phase he may become communicative. The pupils may constrict and dilate alternately, and there may be a hiccough or an involuntary myoclonic jerk with each onset of respiration. The EEG may show periodic slowing during apnea. Studies of arterial and cerebral blood gases show that cerebral venous P_{CO_2} moves in a direction opposite to that of arterial blood P_{CO_2}; i.e., the cerebral venous P_{CO_2} rises during the phase of hyperventilation and falls during the apneic phase. Cerebral venous oxygen levels are not necessarily at their lowest during the apneic, stuporous phase with EEG slowing. The pattern of blood gases indicates that Cheyne-Stokes respiration is caused by a depression of the brainstem which is periodically driven by a rising P_{CO_2}, and this is followed by posthyperventilation apnea. The fluctuations in cerebral function also seem to be mediated by depression of the reticular formation of the brainstem with periodic stimulation by the rising P_{CO_2} and improved responsiveness.[135]

Neurologic Disorders Due to Endocrine Abnormalities

Neurologic Complications of Diabetes Mellitus

The frequent association of diabetes mellitus and cerebral atherosclerosis is discussed in Chapter 9. There are a number of other important neurologic complications of diabetes.

Diabetic Neuropathy

A symmetric peripheral neuropathy and, more rarely, a single or multiple mononeuropathy may occur.

Etiology and Pathology. The etiology is not entirely clear. Diabetic peripheral neuropathy is probably a syndrome caused by a chronic metabolic disturbance affecting the cell body and/or the axon or the Schwann cell. A disturbance of sorbitol metabolism has been described in diabetes mellitus with excess production of sorbitol under conditions of hyperglycemia and insulin deficiency.[187] The excess sorbitol damages the Schwann cell resulting in peripheral demyelination and secondary axonal degeneration. Alternatively, the effect of insulin deficiency and hyperglycemia is believed to be a defect in myoinositol in the peripheral nerve with axon loss.[369] There is also a possibility that diabetic peripheral neuropathy is an axonal disorder.[42] There may be a "dying back" of axons secondary to an impairment of axonal transport of proteins synthesized in the neuron.

The pathologic picture is patchy loss of neurons in the anterior horns, sensory root ganglia, and sympathetic ganglia associated with the loss of large axons and to a lesser extent small unmyelinated fibers in peripheral nerves and nerve roots. There is evidence of damage to Schwann cells with some "onion bulb" formation around surviving axons. The capillary basement membrane is thickened, and the capillary changes are typically those of diabetic microangiopathy.[350]

Clinical Features. The neuropathy may occur at any time in patients with diabetes mellitus and is not related to the severity of the disturbance in carbohydrate metabolism. It is commonly quite severe in mild untreated chronic diabetes, although the most advanced neuropathy occurs following long periods of inadequate treatment. When it appears during treatment, it seems to follow a period of poor control. Statistics from diabetic clinics indicate that about half the diabetic population eventually develop some neurologic complications. Some clinicians believe that some degree of neuropathy will eventually occur in all diabetics at some time. Certainly, the majority of elderly diabetic patients have decreased vibration sense and ankle jerks. There are unpredictable remissions and relapses in diabetic neuropathy, and sometimes spontaneous improvement occurs despite poor clinical control.

Peripheral Neuropathy

There is evidence that some degree of peripheral neuropathy develops in all diabetics with progressive motor unit loss[43] and slowing of motor nerve conduction velocities, which decline progressively with increased duration of disease.[215]

Symptoms are frequently mild, and distal neuropathy may be an incidental finding in a patient with diabetes mellitus who has no complaints. Other patients develop pain, numbness, paresthesias, and distal burning in the limbs, which tend to be worse at night. The course is chronic, but distal muscle weakness and wasting may occur. There is a glove-and-stocking type of hypalgesia to pinprick, reduced or absent vibration sense peripherally, and loss of ankle jerks. In the more chronic cases, there may be generalized areflexia.

Diabetic Mononeuropathy

This is a less common neurologic complication of diabetes than the symmetric peripheral neuropathy. It usually involves a single nerve or nerve root at one time. Occasionally a polymononeuropathy occurs with an asymmetric involvement of two or more nerves. It is possible that some cases are due to infarction of the nerve tissue as the vasa nervorum become occluded.[272, 273] Many cases appear to be due to peripheral nerve entrapment. The most common site is the sciatic nerve and its lumbosacral roots, but other sites include the roots, trunks, or nerves of the brachial plexus and individual peripheral nerves, such as the lateral cutaneous nerve of the thigh, and the peroneal, median, and ulnar nerves. The major symptom is pain in the distribution of the affected nerve and motor weakness. Diabetic mononeuropathy may be responsible for sudden ocular palsies in children and adults,[139] unilateral or bilateral facial palsy,[148] meralgia paresthetica (Chap. 11), and the carpal tunnel syndrome (Chap. 11). Patients with lumbosacral root involvement may develop pain and weakness similar to that produced by a herniated disk. It should be noted, however, that sudden onset of pain in the lower limbs in a diabetic can be due to infarction of muscle.[17]

Diabetic mononeuropathy usually resolves completely or improves remarkably within a six- to eight-week period.

Diabetic Autonomic Neuropathy

The demyelination and axonal loss of diabetic neuropathy can extend to the autonomic nervous system. There may be loss of sensory impulses from the bladder, producing incomplete emptying and a hypotonic "tabetic" type of bladder paralysis, with painless overdistention predisposing to repeated infections of the bladder and urinary tract.[44] Impotence, with loss of penile erection, is a common complaint in the diabetic male. Loss of vasomotor activity in the lower limbs in association with the peripheral neuropathy can lead to severe postural hypotension and the development of painless and indolent ulcers of the feet.

Diminished gastrointestinal tone can result in gastroparesis diabeticorum characterized by a large atonic stomach with slow and erratic emptying of ingested material into the small bowel. This is accompanied by nausea, vomiting, postprandial distress, weight loss, and debility. Small-bowel autonomic dysfunction produces nocturnal diarrhea and malabsorption.[194] An established diabetic autonomic neuropathy with postural hypotension and an impaired cardiovascular response to the Valsalva maneuver should be regarded as a major complication of diabetic neuropathy and carries a high mortality.[95]

Diabetic Pseudotabes

This is a combination of severe myeloradiculoneuropathy and autonomic involvement. There is a marked sensory loss in the lower limbs with the development of ulcers on the feet. The ankle, knee, and hip joints may show the typical painless and degenerative changes of Charcot joints (Fig. 5–1). Severe changes in the sensory root ganglia lead to degeneration of the posterior columns of the spinal cord with the development of locomotor ataxia. The bladder develops a painless distention with overflow. Involvement of the autonomic

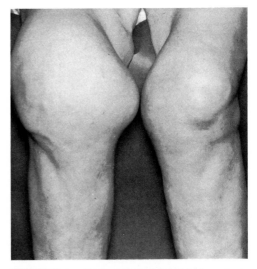

FIGURE 5–1. Charcot joint of the right knee in a patient with advanced peripheral neuropathy of diabetes with "pseudotabes diabetica."

connections to the pupil produces an irregular miotic pupil, which fails to react to light[79] (Argyll Robertson pupil, Chap. 1).

Subacute Proximal Diabetic Neuropathy (Diabetic Amyotrophy)

A condition of symmetric proximal muscle weakness occurs in some diabetics and has been called diabetic myelopathy or diabetic amyotrophy. The condition is a subacute diabetic neuropathy in which there is evidence for a generalized diabetic peripheral neuropathy.[368]

Other Complications of Diabetes Mellitus

Children and less frequently adults with diabetes mellitus frequently show wide fluctuations in blood glucose levels and occasional hypoglycemic reactions with confusion and coma. These reactions predispose to seizures, and all patients with seizures should have glucose tolerance tests to exclude diabetes and hypoglycemia. Many diabetics have decreased resistance to infection, and this includes infections of the central nervous system. Unusual infections, such as mucormycosis, may produce a subacute meningoencephalitis in diabetics. It should also be borne in mind that diabetic acidosis is a common cause of stupor or coma and should be considered in the differential diagnosis of patients with coma of unknown cause. Diabetic coma occurs in severe cases, usually following infection or stress, including surinadequate therapy. The onset is insidious, and the patient passes through confusion and stupor to coma. The face is flushed and dry, and there are marked dehydration, vomiting, hyperpnea (Kussmaul breathing), a smell of acetone on the breath, and hyporeflexia.

Diagnostic Procedures

1. The diagnosis of diabetes mellitus is established by fasting and two-hour blood glucose determinations, urinary glucose levels, and the five-hour glucose tolerance test in mild cases. In diabetic acidosis, ketoacids are present in the urine and plasma, and the pH of both is low.
2. Motor and sensory nerve conduction velocities are slowed in most diabetics.
3. Patients with diabetic autonomic neuropathy and diabetic pseudotabes should have a urologic evaluation of bladder function.

Treatment

1. In all of the complications of diabetes mellitus, the carbohydrate metabolism should be well-controlled by diet, weight control, and the use of oral hypoglycemic agents or insulin as indicated.
2. Painful diabetic peripheral neuropathy is reported to respond to combined therapy with fluphenazine hydrochloride, 1 mg every eight hours, and amitriptyline, 75 mg at night.[77]
3. Diabetic mononeuropathies are often entrapment neuropathies and respond to infiltration of the nerve at the site of entrapment with 1 to 2 ml of 2 per cent xylocaine and 40 mg of methylprednisolone.
4. The atonic bladder of diabetic autonomic neuropathy is often infected, and the patient needs appropriate antibiotic therapy. A parasympathetic drug such as bethanechol chloride, 10 to 25 mg every four to six hours, is effective in stimulating bladder contraction and emptying in some cases.
5. Conscientious care of the feet is essential in severe diabetic peripheral neuropathy to prevent the development of ulceration. This is a frequent complication of diabetic pseudotabes and may be associated with neuroarthropathy of ankle, tarsal, or tarsometatarsal joints. The latter complication requires treatment directed at preventing weight bearing on the affected joints for three to six months.

Neurologic Complications of Hypoglycemia

Hypoglycemia is an important disorder of metabolism that manifests itself by neurologic signs. Since glucose and oxygen are almost the exclusive metabolic substrates of the brain, the symptoms of glucose lack are similar and the pathology is almost identical to that described under cerebral anoxia. There are glucose stores in the brain, however, which delay the onset of symptoms for 30 to 45 minutes when the blood glucose falls rapidly. In cerebral anoxia, since there are no stores of oxygen, the onset of symptoms is more rapid.

The most frequent causes of hypoglycemia are listed in Table 5–4. Hypoglycemia is an important cause of seizures, mental confusion, and coma in the adult, and of mental retardation and seizures in infancy. It occasionally complicates alcoholic intoxication in chronic alcoholics.[167]

TABLE 5–4

Causes of Hypoglycemia

1. *Deficient supply of carbohydrate*—Starvation, esophageal obstruction, anorexia nervosa

2. *Malabsorption*—Sprue, chronic diarrhea

3. *Excessive utilization*—Hyperthyroidism, fever, certain neoplasms including hepatoma and fibrosarcoma

4. *Excessive secretion of insulin*—Hyperplasia of beta cells
   Neoplasia of beta cells (insulinoma)

5. *Inappropriate secretion of insulin*—Idiopathic postprandial hypoglycemia
   Alimentary (postgastrectomy hypoglycemia)
   Leucine sensitivity

6. *Hepatic*—Acute necrosis, cirrhosis, hepatitis, glycogen storage disease

7. *Endocrine*—Hypopituitarism, hypoadrenalism, hypothyroidism

8. *Drugs or toxic agents*—Biguanides, guanides, sulfonylurea, alloxan, certain amino acids, hydrazine, pyribenzamine, alcohol, salicylates, propoxyphene, factitious administration of insulin

9. *Diabetes mellitus*—Prediabetic states, "brittle" diabetes, overtreated diabetes

10. *Infantile hypoglycemias*—See Chapter 2

Pathology

The cerebral cortex shows areas of focal or laminar necrosis, which are irregular in distribution. Ammon's horn, in the hippocampus, is usually severely involved, while the visual cortex is frequently spared. There are various degrees of degeneration of neurons, many of which are irreversibly damaged and surrounded by microglia and proliferating astrocytes. The white matter is usually spared. The subcortical gray matter is also susceptible to hypoglycemia, and changes in the caudate nucleus and putamen vary from total necrosis to loss of smaller neurons. There may also be some loss of Purkinje cells in the cerebellum.

Clinical Features

The symptoms, signs, and residual cerebral damage due to hypoglycemia, like cerebral hypoxia, depend on the rapidity of onset, duration, and severity of the hypoglycemia.

Minor degrees of hypoglycemia may be responsible for repeated attacks of sweating, pallor, confusion, syncope, and seizures in adults as well as children. For this reason, it is wise for all patients with seizures to have a glucose tolerance test.

Mild hypoglycemic episodes produce attacks of hunger, weakness, irritability, sweating, tachycardia, tremor, and anxiety. The majority of these symptoms are due to sympathetic overactivity.

Repeated attacks of hypoglycemia can produce chronic cerebellar ataxia and tremor without other symptoms.

A severe attack of hypoglycemia produces the initial symptoms of hunger, weakness, and anxiety, as described above, followed by abnormal behavior, sweating, emotional instability, personality change, confusion, psychosis, and loss of consciousness. Once coma has developed, unless glucose is administered, irreversible changes can be expected and there may be loss of reflex activity, irregular respirations, and death. Other cases recover consciousness with different degrees of damage to the nervous system, similar to anoxic encephalopathy. Damage includes loss of insight and judgment, perceptual disorders, and decerebrate and decorticate states. In older patients, with poor areas of perfusion in the brain, a clinical picture resembling stroke may result with hemiparesis, hemianopia, cerebellar ataxia, or a parkinsonian-like picture.[228] Repeated and severe attacks of hypoglycemia may result in progressive dementia and, rarely, signs of myeloneuropathy with generalized muscle wasting, fasciculations, and peripheral sensory loss.

Diagnostic Procedures

1. Estimations of blood glucose should be obtained in patients with the warning symptoms of hypoglycemia listed above. This is particularly true in diabetics who receive insulin or oral hypoglycemic agents and who feel excessively hungry or develop personality changes.

2. In questionable cases, attacks of hypoglycemia may be provoked by fasting for 12, 24, or even 36 hours if necessary.

3. Plasma insulin assay should be carried out if facilities for the measurement are available. The demonstration of Whipple's triad (the association of symptoms of hypoglycemia with low serum glucose levels and relief of symptoms after administration of glucose) suggests the presence of an insulinoma.[308]

4. Testing for leucine sensitivity (Chap. 2) should be considered in adults as well as children. A test dose of 1-leucine, 150 mg/kg of body weight, will be followed by hypoglycemia within 30 to 40 minutes in leucine-sensitive patients. Positive results have occasionally been obtained in patients with insulinomas.

5. Tests of liver function and tests for malabsorption should be performed in all obscure cases of hypoglycemia.

6. The electroencephalogram is diffusely abnormal in severe hypoglycemia with symmetric theta and delta activity over both hemispheres. The slowing is rapidly accentuated by hyperventilation.

7. A tolbutamide sensitivity test may be performed alone or in association with serum insulin determinations in suspected cases of insulinoma. The patient should be given a high-carbohydrate (150 to 300 gm) diet daily for three days prior to the test. A fasting blood glucose is drawn on the morning of the test, and 1 gm of tolbutamide in 20 ml of sterile water is injected intravenously at a constant rate over a three-minute period. Blood specimens are then withdrawn at 20, 30, 45, 60, 90, 120, 150, and 180 minutes. The procedure is then terminated by giving a meal containing carbohydrate. If severe hypoglycemic symptoms develop during the test, it should be terminated immediately by the intravenous injection of 50 ml of 50 per cent glucose solution.

If serum insulin determinations are made, specimens should be drawn at 10, 20, and 30 minutes after the injection of tolbutamide.

Healthy subjects show a decrease in blood glucose levels of 38 to 79 per cent of the fasting level following the injection of the tolbutamide, with a return to normal or near-normal levels between 90 and 120 minutes. Patients with insulinoma tend to have a more prolonged fall in blood glucose values, and the hypoglycemia is maintained throughout the 180 minutes of testing with values below 40 to 64 per cent of normal. The serum insulin levels are abnormally high and rise to a peak within 30 minutes of injecting the tolbutamide in patients with an insulinoma. The test can be terminated after 30 minutes when insulin assay is available.

Treatment

The treatment of hypoglycemia is dependent on the cause. Postprandial and alimentary hypoglycemia are best treated with frequent feedings and a diabetic type of diet.[258] Small doses of anticholinergic drugs such as probanthine, 7.5 mg 30 minutes before each meal, will delay gastric emptying and help to prevent hypoglycemia. Insulinoma and hyperplasia of the beta cells may be cured or alleviated by surgical removal of the tumor or partial resection of the pancreas. Hypoglycemias complicating various endocrinopathies respond to endocrine treatment by appropriate substitution therapy.

Neurologic Complications of Hyperglycemia

Patients with diabetes mellitus may develop acute cerebral complications due to (1) diabetic ketoacidotic coma or (2) hyperglycemic hyperosmolar coma resulting from (a) hyperosmolality due to hyperglycemia, hypernatremia, or both, (b) lactic acidosis, or (c) cerebral edema.

Diabetic Ketoacidotic Coma

This is the most common cerebral complication of diabetes and is usually seen in juvenile diabetes with low plasma levels of insulin resulting in catabolism of adipose tissue. There is a subsequent increase of free fatty acid levels in the blood, and their metabolism by the liver with excessive production of acetone, acetoacetate, and beta-hydroxybutyrate results in acidosis. The low arterial pH produces hyperventilation with Kussmaul breathing, which reduces arterial P_{CO2} and plasma bicarbonate concentrations. The osmotic diuresis due to the hyperglycemia results in dehydration and depletion of sodium and potassium, which themselves may cause impaired cerebral and cardiac function. Diabetic coma may be due to the acidosis, dehydration, and/or ionic depletion.

Treatment of diabetic coma requires administration of frequent small doses of insulin[58] to restore carbohydrate utilization and replacement of depleted water and electrolytes. Serum sodium, potassium, and bicarbonate levels should be frequently measured during replacement therapy.

Hyperglycemic Hyperosmolar Coma

This form of coma can occur in diabetes and results from hyperosmolality of the extracellular fluids as a result of severe hyperglycemia (plasma glucose levels in excess of 600 mg/100 ml) or severe hypernatremia.[144, 162] In severe hyperglycemia, serum sodium levels may be normal and ketosis may not be present. The primary disorder is extracellular hyperosmolality with dehydration of cells.

Hyperglycemic hyperosmolar coma is primarily a syndrome of the aged, infirm, or alcoholic patient who has mild to moderate diabetes mellitus. However, the condition has been described in children and in nondiabetics who have severe burns, acromegaly, or thyrotoxicosis, or where there has been prolonged use of such drugs as diuretics, diazoxide, steroids, propranolol, and diphenylhydantoin. The hyperglycemic hyperosmolar state has also been reported following dialysis with hypertonic glucose solutions and during the treatment of cerebral edema with glycerol.[305] The syndrome is often precipitated by infection, cerebral infarction, acute pancreatitis, limited water intake, or heat stroke. The state of consciousness varies from alert to deep coma. Other clinical signs include a coarse flapping of the arms, hallucinosis, focal and generalized seizures, and paralysis. Thrombosis of the mesenteric and cerebral vessels may result. The mortality rate is high, around 50 per cent. Therapy consists of correction of hypovolemia and dehydration, correction of electrolyte imbalance, reduction of serum glucose levels and hyperosmolality, and simultaneous management of the precipitating illness.[133]

Neurologic Complications of Hyperthyroidism

Excessive production of thyroid hormone which results in the clinical picture of hyperthyroidism may occur at any age, although the condition is rare in children. Females are involved more frequently than males in a ratio of about 8:1. The condition is most commonly due to excessive stimulation by the thyrotropic hormone secreted by the anterior pituitary. This produces diffuse overactivity of the thyroid gland and the clinical picture of Graves' disease. Hyperthyroidism due to toxic nodular goiter is probably autonomous and independent of pituitary influences. In either case, there is an increase in the production of thyroid hormone and an increase in metabolic activity.

Clinical Features

Thyrotoxicosis is characterized by increasing nervousness, irritability, emotional instability, and hyperkinesis.[201] The appetite is good, but there is progressive weight loss, diarrhea, sweating, palpitation, and intolerance to heat. Examination reveals excess pigmentation, a warm, moist skin, a fine tremor of the fingers and tongue, and brisk deep-tendon reflexes. There is unilateral or bilateral exophthalmos associated with lid lag, frequent blinking, and poor convergence. The thyroid may contain nodules or show diffuse enlargement and a bruit on auscultation. Cardiovascular signs include tachycardia at rest or atrial fibrillation and a wide pulse pressure. Cardiac signs are particularly marked in patients with toxic nodular goiter, and atrial fibrillation may be the only sign of thyrotoxicosis in older patients.

Neurologic manifestations of hyperthyroidism include a symmetric peripheral neuropathy with equal involvement of proximal and distal muscles and a relatively minor impairment of sensation.[98] There may be progressive weakness of the extraocular muscles resulting in ophthalmoplegia and involvement of bulbar muscles producing weakness in chewing, swallowing, and talking. A reversible corticospinal tract disease resembling motor neuron disease with weakness, spasticity, hyperreflexia, extensor plantar responses, and normal sensory function has been described.[117] Repeated attacks of cerebellar ataxia during infection and fever have also been recorded in chronic hyperthyroidism.[1] Optic neuritis is a rare complication of thyrotoxicosis.

Thyroid Crisis

Some patients with Graves' disease may develop thyroid crisis following infection, trauma, an emotional upset, or surgery on the thyroid gland. There is a period of extreme agitation, frequently accompanied by delirium, mania, hyperpyrexia, tachycardia, vomiting, diarrhea, dehydration, and seizures in some cases. The condition culminates in exhaustion and may be complicated by hypotension and adrenal insufficiency unless promptly treated. Thyroid crises are occasionally mistaken for acute manic psychoses.

Thyroid myopathy and the relationship between thyrotoxicosis, myasthenia gravis, and hypokalemic periodic paralysis are discussed elsewhere (Chap. 12).

Diagnostic Procedures

1. The protein-bound iodine (PBI), ^{131}I-L-tri-iodothyronine (T_3), and the thyroxine-iodine (T_4 iodine) levels in serum are consistently elevated in thyrotoxicosis. Radioactive iodine uptake is increased.
2. The EEG shows nonspecific changes including an increase in low-voltage alpha activity and the appearance of diffuse theta and low-voltage fast activity in the central regions. Paroxysmal spike wave activity is not infrequent.
3. Computed tomography of the orbit is abnormal in patients with exophthalmos and hyperthyroidism. The CT scan shows swelling of the extraocular muscles[39a] and will differentiate patients with thyrotoxicosis from those with pseudotumor of the orbit or orbital tumors.[248]

Treatment

Thyroid crisis requires emergency treatment with intravenous fluids, hydrocortisone, and propranolol. Propranolol relieves tremor, high-output failure, bulbar dysfunction, and many of the neuromuscular features of thyrotoxicosis.[362a] Any electrolyte imbalance should be corrected by the intravenous route and the patient sedated by the use of adequate doses of barbiturates. Hyperpyrexia requires the use of ice packs or a refrigerated mattress. If the patient develops cardiovascular shock, intravenous hydrocortisone should be increased and pressor agents will be required. Patients with thyrotoxicosis are sensitive to pressor agents, and the intravenous infusion requires monitoring of blood pressure levels. The thyroid-blocking agents propylthiouracil or methimazole (Tapazole) should be given during the crisis. They will not have an immediate effect since it takes some days for them to reduce thyroid activity.

Neurologic Complications of Hypothyroidism

The infantile form of hypothyroidism (cretinism) has already been described in Chapter 2. The adult form of the disease (myxedema) is easily recognized in its fully developed form. However, milder forms of hypothyroidism are quite frequent in adults and result in a number of symptoms such as lassitude, slowness of mentation,

and headache, which are frequently not recognized to be due to lack of thyroid hormone.

Etiology and Pathology

The main causes of hypothyroidism in the adult are listed in Table 5–5. Deficiencies in hormone production may result from a familial defect in certain enzymes that participate in thyroid hormone synthesis. The causes of thyroid atrophy are not clear. The condition is more common in females and usually occurs after the age of 40. The development of thyroid deficiency after thyroidectomy is often an insidious condition or may be the result of the patient discontinuing thyroid medication some months or years after surgery.

A number of patients develop hypothyroidism following thyrotoxicosis, apparently resulting from exhaustion of a chronically overstimulated gland. Hypothyroidism may be seen following treatment for thyrotoxicosis with either radioactive iodine or the thyroid suppressive drugs. Other drugs that are toxic to the thyroid gland include para-aminosalicylic acid, iodides, iodopyrine, lithium carbonate, methimazole, perchlorates, phenylbutazone, resorcinol, sulfonamides, sulfonylureas, and thiocyanates which may have been prescribed for various reasons.[311] However, most of these drugs have a weak and inconsistent effect on the thyroid gland.

Chronic thyroiditis (of both the Hashimoto and Riedel types) is frequently associated with hypothyroidism.

Hypothyroidism may also result from panhypopituitarism as a result of tumors and disease of the pituitary gland. Occasionally, pituitary function will be normal except for a specific defi-

---

TABLE 5–5

Causes of Hypothyroidism

Deficient thyroid function
1. Deficiencies in hormone production
2. Thyroid atrophy
3. Postthyroidectomy
4. "Burnt-out" thyrotoxicosis
5. Overtreatment of thyrotoxicosis by thyroid suppressive drugs or radioactive iodine
6. Chronic thyroiditis (Hashimoto-Riedel)
7. Effect of drugs (thiouracil, iodides, thiocyanates)
8. Panhypopituitarism
9. Deficient TSH production

Dietary deficiency
1. Iodine-deficient diet

ciency of thyroid-stimulating hormone. Finally, an endemic form of chronic hypothyroidism has been reported in certain areas of the world where the diet is deficient in iodine.

The pathology of the thyroid gland varies according to the conditions causing the hypothyroidism. The gland is usually small and atrophic in thyroid atrophy, often almost totally absent following thyroidectomy, and enlarged in chronic thyroiditis and in iodine-deficient states.

Certain abnormalities of the nervous system have been reported to occur in severe hypothyroidism. These include cerebellar degeneration with loss of Purkinje cells in the cerebellar cortex. The maximum loss of Purkinje cells is found in the vermis. In the atrophic areas of the cerebellum and also in the spinal cord unusual round and granular structures (neural myxedema bodies) are found that resemble amyloid bodies. Wallerian degeneration occurs in the peripheral nerves, and hypothyroid myopathy may also be present. The latter condition is described in detail in Chapter 12.

Clinical Features

The clinical picture of well-established hypothyroidism includes mental dullness and marked motor retardation. The hearing is poor, and the patient complains of a dull headache. There is a characteristic hoarseness of the voice. Vague complaints include neuralgic types of pain and weakness of the muscles. The patient frequently complains of intolerance to cold. Other associated features of myxedema are often striking. They include frontal baldness in women, a dry scaling skin, and puffiness around the eyes and cheeks. There are often supraclavicular deposits of fat. The hair is dry and brittle, and the lateral third of the eyebrows is missing. There is bradycardia, bradykinesis, and a subnormal temperature. In many cases the neurologic examination is negative except for slowness in the response of the tendon reflexes (Chap. 5). Sometimes these reflexes are termed "hung-up" or pseudomyotonic. A certain number of patients display striking neurologic abnormalities:

Myxedema and Dementia. Occasionally, psychomotor retardation and mental dullness are so startling in myxedema that the patient appears to be demented and confused. There may be disorientation, delusions, and illusions. Some cases show marked change in personality with psychotic and paranoid features.

Coma. Patients with severe myxedema may develop coma and hypothermia. This is often precipitated by an infection and requires immediate treatment. The coma may follow a seizure.

Cerebellar Degeneration. This is an unusual complication of hypothyroidism. It presents as a truncal ataxia and ataxia involving the lower limbs with relative sparing of the upper limbs.[163, 270] There is usually no nystagmus. The diagnosis is confirmed by complete recovery within six weeks of instituting replacement therapy with thyroid hormone preparations.

Myopathy. Although muscular weakness is a feature of myxedema, a number of patients with hypothyroidism develop a more specific myopathy. This condition is discussed in more detail in Chapter 12.

Peripheral Neuropathy. A certain number of patients with myxedema show symmetric peripheral sensory loss with depression or loss of the tendon jerks involving all four limbs due to peripheral nerve degeneration.[102] The condition is associated with a marked loss of large myelinated nerve fibers and is believed to be due to a metabolic disorder of the Schwann cell related to hypothyroidism.[311]

Carpal Tunnel Syndrome. Symptoms of carpal tunnel syndrome (Chap. 11) are commonly the presenting complaints in patients with hypothyroidism.

Increased Frequency of Atherosclerosis. The incidence of atherosclerotic heart disease and cerebrovascular disease is increased in patients with hypothyroidism. Routine measurements of protein-bound iodine and radioactive iodine uptake in a series of patients with established cerebrovascular disease have shown chemical evidence of hypothyroidism in as many as 30 per cent of cases in one large series (Chap. 9).

Diagnostic Procedures

The diagnosis of hypothyroidism is established by measuring the blood levels of protein-bound iodine, by the serum thyroxine-iodine levels (T_4 iodine test), by measuring the radioactive iodine uptake of the thyroid gland, or by the ^{131}I-L-triodothyronine test (T$_3$ test). The protein-bound iodine determination is low (normal values, 4 to 8 mg/100 ml of blood), both the T$_4$ iodine test and T$_3$ test are decreased, and there is marked reduction of the uptake of radioactive iodine by the thyroid gland. The serum cholesterol is elevated in hypothyroidism.

Lumbar Puncture. Many patients with hypothyroidism, particularly when myxedema is present, show elevation of CSF protein, which may be as high as 100 mg/ml.

Electroencephalogram. The electroencephalogram in myxedema shows reduction in amplitude or loss of alpha activity, with diffuse, low-voltage slowing in the theta range. The EEG improves progressively with thyroid hormone substitution therapy.

Treatment

Hypothyroidism and myxedema should be treated with desiccated thyroid or the more refined hormonal preparations, such as sodium 1-thyroxine (0.1 mg of sodium 1-thyroxine is equivalent to 60 mg of desiccated thyroid). Initial treatment should be started with 0.03 gm desiccated thyroid, which can be increased in steps of 0.03 gm every two or three weeks until optimum results are obtained. Rapid increase of medication may lead to the development of angina pectoris and myocardial infarction in patients with myxedema because of the generalized increase in the metabolic rate of all organs, including the brain, as a result of substitution therapy. The effectiveness of treatment should be assessed by both clinical examination and serial determinations of protein-bound iodine or serum thyroxine-iodine levels (T$_4$) and serum cholesterol.

All the neurologic complications of hypothyroidism including dementia, coma, cerebellar degeneration, neuropathy, and carpal tunnel syndrome respond well to replacement therapy within six to eight weeks.

Neurologic Complications of Hyperparathyroidism

Primary hyperparathyroidism owing to tumor or hyperplasia of the parathyroid glands is the main cause of hypercalcemia. Other common causes of hypercalcemia include hypervitaminosis D, malignancy with or without metastases, thia-

zide and chlorthalidone therapy, multiple myeloma, sarcoidosis, and the milk-alkali syndrome.[271]

Primary hyperparathyroidism is due to autonomous hyperfunction of one or more of the parathyroid glands with increase in production of parathyroid hormone leading to hypercalcemia, decalcification of bone, and nephrolithiasis.[59, 283]

Etiology and Pathology

About 90 per cent of cases are due to an adenoma is one or more of the parathyroid glands, while the remaining cases result from hyperplasia. This latter group contains some cases of familial hyperparathyroidism. Hyperplasia may also occur in secondary hyperparathyroidism, which follows retention of phosphorus in chronic renal disease. Serum calcium levels are rarely elevated in secondary hyperparathyroidism.

The effect of the increase in circulating parathyroid hormone is to promote bone resorption over new bone formation and to increase calcium absorption from the distal renal tubules.

Clinical Features

Systemic changes due to hypercalcemia include osteitis fibrosa cystica with numerous cysts of bone, fractures, and skeletal deformities. However, diffuse demineralization of bone is encountered more frequently. Many patients complain of joint stiffness and arthralgia due to the deposition of calcium in the articular surfaces and synovial membranes of joints with calcification of joint capsules and muscle tendons. The development of renal calculi and repeated attacks of renal colic may be the only symptoms of hypercalcemia for many years. Nephrocalcinosis, renal failure, polyuria, and uremia may occur in advanced cases. There is a high incidence of peptic ulceration of the duodenum and stomach in hyperparathyroidism, while acute cases may present with nausea, vomiting, anorexia, abdominal colic, and constipation. The incidence of hypertension is increased in hyperparathyroidism, and 70 per cent of patients are hypertensive.[33]

Neurologic symptoms vary but are of considerable interest. The more chronic cases complain of intermittent headache for many years. Other patients complain of weakness, easy fatigue, headache, and anxiety. A proximal myopathy with a gradually increasing proximal muscle weakness has been reported in some cases.[284] The more fulminating cases with marked elevation of serum calcium levels to as high as 16 or 17 mg per cent develop rigidity, tremor, agitation, disorientation, psychotic behavior with hallucinations, and paranoid delusions. There is extreme muscle weakness with hypotonia and loss of tendon reflexes. Tachycardia is a prominent feature. These cases present as an emergency, as coma and death rapidly follow if the tumor is not removed.

Diagnostic Procedures

1. Serum calcium levels are elevated above 11 mg per cent. There is less consistent depression of serum phosphorus levels below the normal level of 3 mg per cent.
2. Levels of serum immunoreactive parathyroid hormone are elevated in primary hyperparathyroidism. The levels are depressed in other conditions causing hypercalcemia such as hypervitaminosis D, sarcoidosis, and the milk-alkali syndrome.
3. Early roentgenographic changes are seen in the hands with fraying of the distal phalangeal tufts, subperiosteal resorption at the margins of the phalanges, cysts in the carpal bones, and chondrocalcinosis of the triangular fibrocartilage of the wrist. Later changes include generalized demineralization of the skeleton, the presence of multiple cysts in bone, loss of the lamina dura around the teeth sockets, the presence of giant cysts (epules) in the mandible, and metastatic calcification of the kidneys and tendons. The combination of chondrocalcinosis and cysts in bone in any situation should raise the possibility of primary hyperparathyroidism.[325]
4. Patients with chronic hyperparathyroidism may have a normochromic normocytic anemia.
5. Slit lamp examination may reveal calcium deposition in the cornea. Smaller deposits in the conjunctiva lead to inflammation and lacrimation.
6. The electrocardiogram shows shortening of the Q-T interval.

Treatment

Surgical removal of a parathyroid adenoma or removal of sufficient parathyroid tissue in patients with hyperplasia effects complete cure.[173]

Some patients, particularly those with renal failure, must be treated medically before and after surgery. Postoperative tetany is effectively controlled with 50,000 to 100,000 units of vitamin D daily. Magnesium levels are usually low and should be corrected. Acute hypercalcemia often presents as a medical emergency with anorexia, nausea, vomiting, pyrexia, dehydration, mental confusion, psychosis, and eventually coma. The most important initial step is rehydration with parenteral fluids since urinary calcium excretion is enhanced by saline infusion. If hypercalcemia persists, 50-mg doses of ethacrynic acid can be given intravenously, and the resulting fluid lost by diuresis should be replaced and the electrolyte balance maintained. Corticosteroids also lower the serum calcium and can be given in large doses, such as 250 to 500 mg of cortisone every eight hours. Oral or parenteral administration of phosphate (Na_2PO_4 or Na_2HPO_4) is also helpful in lowering the serum calcium of patients with severe renal impairment. Mithramycin, a cytotoxic antibiotic, also has a hypocalcemic effect.

Neurologic Complications of Hypoparathyroidism

Hypoparathyroidism results in a deficiency of parathyroid hormone manifested by low serum calcium and high serum phosphorus levels.[88, 282, 324] It appears within 24 hours after surgical removal of the glands during thyroidectomy. There is a rare congenital hypoparathyroidism of unknown etiology. Hypoparathyroidism rarely occurs in Hashimoto's autoimmune thyroiditis.

The essential features of hypoparathyroidism are the presence of hypocalcemia and normal or elevated serum inorganic phosphorus in patients with destroyed or hypofunctioning parathyroid glands. This excludes other causes of hypocalcemia including gastrointestinal malabsorption, jejunoileal bypass as a treatment of morbid obesity,[50] hypocalcemia with hypermagnesemia after therapeutic use of magnesium sulfate,[94] and renal insufficiency. Two other conditions are of interest, namely, pseudohypoparathyroidism in which there is a failure of peripheral response to parathormone (Chapter 2) and hypohyperparathyroidism in which there is a defective endogenous parathyroid hormone.[64]

Etiology

There are two main causes of hypoparathyroidism: (1) postoperative, following thyroidectomy, and (2) idiopathic, which may be due to an autoimmune mechanism. Antibodies to parathyroid tissue (and occasionally to thyroid and adrenal tissue) have been demonstrated in some cases of idiopathic hypoparathyroidism.

Clinical Features

Hypocalcemia causes hyperexcitability of the peripheral and central nervous system with tetany and convulsions. Chvostek, Trousseau, and Erb signs are present with carpopedal spasm. These signs are enhanced by hyperventilation or alkalosis. Spasm of the larynx and diaphragm may cause death, and spasm may be evident in the urinary bladder, iris, bronchioles, cilia, and gastrointestinal tract. Cardiac dysrhythmias may occur.

Seizures may be of the generalized, focal, motor, sensory, absence, or akinetic type. All signs are rapidly reversible by the intravenous administration of calcium. Paresthesias of the face, fingers, and toes may occur, and muscle cramps are not uncommon. Headache due to increased intracranial pressure and seizures are both more common in the idiopathic group. Examination shows positive Chvostek and Trousseau signs, and many patients have a dry, rough skin and poor dentition. The ocular signs of hypoparathyroidism include cataracts, blepharospasms, keratoconjunctivitis, and loss of eyelashes.[322] Papilledema associated with increased intracranial pressure occurs in about 20 per cent of cases of hypoparathyroidism. Optic neuritis is rare.[15] There seems to be an increased incidence of hypertension in hypoparathyroidism, but the reason for this is not clear. Calcification of the basal ganglia with neuronal degenerative changes may lead to symptoms of Parkinson's disease. Dementia may be the sole neurologic symptom of hypocalcemia in idiopathic hypoparathyroidism.[316a]

Diagnostic Procedures

1. The serum calcium levels are depressed and the serum inorganic phosphorus levels are normal or increased.
2. Urinary calcium excretion is decreased.
3. Roentgenographic changes include calcification of the basal ganglia[203] and choroid plexus and occasional calcification of the meninges[238] (Fig. 5–2). There may be separation of the sutures due to increased intracranial pressure in children with idiopathic hypoparathyroidism. The bones have a normal appearance in about 50 per cent of cases. In the others, there may be demineralization with coarse trabeculae. This may be severe enough to produce collapse of vertebral bodies. Calcification of bursae, par-

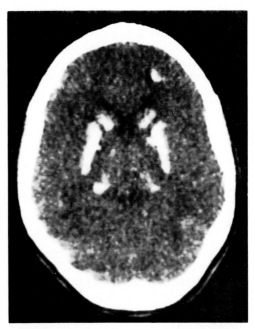

FIGURE 5–2. Computed tomography in hypoparathyroidism. There is symmetric calcification of the caudate nucleus and putamen.

ticularly around the shoulder, is not uncommon.
4. Computed tomography will demonstrate calcification of the basal ganglia before the calcification is visible on skull roentgenograms (Fig 5–2).
5. The electrocardiogram shows prolonged Q-T intervals due to hypocalcemia.
6. The electroencephalogram may show epileptic discharges in patients with seizures.

Treatment

Hypocalcemia may present as a medical emergency requiring the immediate intravenous administration of 20 to 30 ml of 10 per cent calcium gluconate over a 15-minute interval.

Vitamin D_2, 8,000 IU/kg/day, is given orally until the serum calcium concentration reaches 9.0 mg/100 ml. Supportive therapy with intravenous calcium gluconate is given for three days. When the serum calcium level reaches 9.0 mg/100 ml, the dose of vitamin D_2 is reduced to a maintenance level of 2,000 IU/kg/day.

Tetany as a Neurologic Symptom

The neuromuscular hyperexcitability of tetany may result from hypocalcemia or alkalosis or a

TABLE 5–6

Causes of Tetany

1. *Decreased calcium intake*
   a. Malnutrition

2. *Hypovitaminosis D*
   a. Rickets
   b. Osteomalacia

3. *Malabsorption of calcium*
   a. Nontropical sprue
   b. Ileocolic fistula
   c. Jejunoileal bypass for morbid obesity

4. *Loss of calcium*
   a. Vomiting
   b. Therapeutic use of magnesium sulfate

5. *Endocrine causes*
   a. Hypoparathyroidism
   b. Hyperaldosteronism

6. *Renal causes*
   a. Congenital renal lesions
   b. Chronic renal disease, hyperphosphatemia, and hypocalcemia

7. *Alkalosis*
   a. Hyperventilation
   b. Metabolic

combination of these two conditions. Tetany is commonly seen following prolonged hyperventilation, and this may occur in anxious people (hyperventilation syndrome). A lowering of calcium ion concentration increases the irritability of the presynaptic membrane at the myoneural junction and of muscle fibers. Spontaneous discharges or tetany may occur or may be easily provoked by stimulation. Sensory nerve endings are similarly affected. Table 5–6 lists common causes of tetany. Motor symptoms include carpopedal spasm, laryngeal stridor, muscle cramps, and seizures. The sensory manifestations are usually paresthesias of the lips, tongue, and extremities.

Neurologic Disorders Due to Disturbances of Hypothalamic-Hypophyseal Relationships

Of all the neurologic disorders due to endocrine disturbances, those due to lesions in the region of the hypothalamus and pituitary gland are among the most dramatic. The anatomic and functional relationships of the hypothalamus and hypophysis are summarized diagrammatically in Figures 5–3 and 5–4. The neurologic disorders will be briefly listed and discussed.

Diabetes Insipidus

Lesions of the hypothalamus and posterior pituitary may give rise to diabetes insipidus, characterized by excessive thirst and excessive urinary output of low specific gravity. This results from insufficient secretion of antidiuretic hormone, and the lesion is in the region of the supraoptic nucleus, the supraopticohypophyseal tract, or the posterior pituitary. This may follow trauma, primary and metastatic tumors, neurosurgical procedures, and infections and inflammatory conditions (particularly sarcoidosis.)

Treatment

The administration of *l*-desamino-8-*d*-arginine-vasopressin (DDAUP) by intranasal spray produces 8 to 20 hours of antidiuresis and is extremely effective in controlling diabetes insipidus.[285] Carbamazepine, 400 mg daily, is also effective in some cases of diabetes insipidus.[27]

Syndrome of Diabetes Insipidus, Diabetes Mellitus, Optic Atrophy, and Deafness in Childhood (DIDMOAD)

This syndrome is inherited as an autosomal recessive trait and consists of the development of polyuria in juvenile diabetes, despite satisfactory diabetic control, followed by the gradual development of optic atrophy and high-frequency neurosensory hearing loss.[141] The early diagnosis by adequate monitoring of juvenile diabetics is important, since the optic atrophy and hearing loss are progressive and the diabetes insipidus will respond to treatment.[265]

Inappropriate Secretion of Antidiuretic Hormone

Inappropriate secretion of antidiuretic hormone (ADH) causes an encephalopathy due to hyponatremia. The condition is caused by a derangement of hypothalamic control of secretion of ADH, with an imbalance of facilitating and inhibiting influences acting on the supraoptic and paraventricular nuclei of the hypothalamus, resulting in excessive secretion of ADH. Rarely, excessive secretion of ADH may result from extracerebral neoplasms. The result of excessive ADH secretion is water retention, hyponatremia, and renal salt loss. It is possible that excessive ADH secretion results from a disturbance of osmoreceptor sensitivity in the hypothalamus or from abnormalities in secretion of renin, angioten-

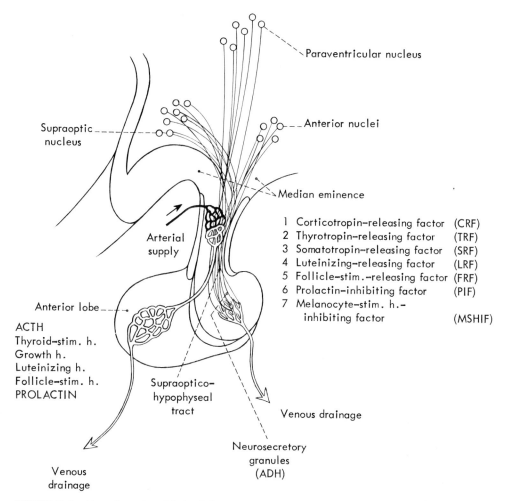

1 Corticotropin–releasing factor (CRF)
2 Thyrotropin–releasing factor (TRF)
3 Somatotropin–releasing factor (SRF)
4 Luteinizing–releasing factor (LRF)
5 Follicle-stim.–releasing factor (FRF)
6 Prolactin–inhibiting factor (PIF)
7 Melanocyte-stim. h.–
   inhibiting factor (MSHIF)

FIGURE 5–3. Hypophyseal-portal circulation.

sin, or aldosterone, all of which seem to regulate hypothalamic control of ADH secretion.

Inappropriate secretion of ADH has been reported as a complication of hydrocephalus, brain trauma, encephalitis, meningitis, gliomas and metastatic tumors involving the hypothalamus, acute intermittent porphyria, remote effects of neoplasm (particularly bronchogenic carcinoma), subarachnoid hemorrhage, postinfectious polyneuritis, metastatic infiltration of the vagus nerves, and after intracranial surgery.

Clinical Features

Neurologic signs regularly occur when the serum sodium levels decrease below 110 mEq/liter. The first complaint is muscular weakness with decreased reflexes. This is followed by signs of bulbar palsy, stupor, convulsions, and extensor plantar responses. When the serum sodium level decreases below 90 to 105 mEq/liter, coma ensues.[19]

The metabolic findings include hyponatremia with hypo-osmolality of the serum and extracellular fluid, continued renal loss of sodium, normal blood pressure, signs of overhydration, urine osmolality greater than that of the plasma (which is reduced), normal renal function, and normal adrenal function.

The diagnosis and treatment of inappropriate secretion of ADH are discussed on page 492 (Chap. 8).

Neurogenic Fever and Poikilothermia

Injury to the hypothalamus may interfere with temperature control due to abnormal vasomotor activity, piloerection, and shivering response. The

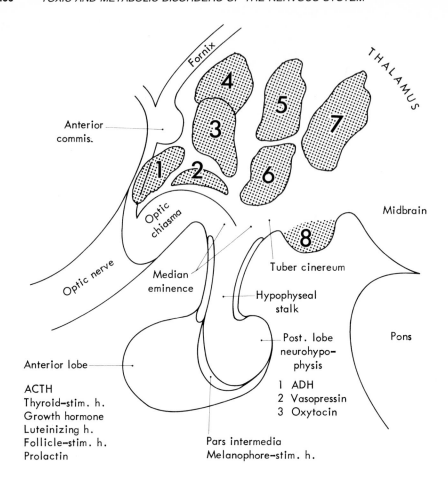

HYPOTHALAMIC NUCLEI:

1 PREOPTIC
2 SUPRAOPTIC
3 ANTERIOR
4 PARAVENTRICULAR
5 DORSOMEDIAL
6 VENTROMEDIAL
7 POSTERIOR
8 MAMMILLARY BODY

FUNCTIONS:

1 TEMPERATURE REGULATION
  Thermoreceptors
    a. preoptic nuclei
    b. anterior nucleus
2 WATER BALANCE and OSMOLALITY
  Supraoptic nucleus
3 GLUCOSE HOMEOSTASIS
  Ventromedial – satiety
  Dorsomedial – hunger

FIGURE 5–4. Hypothalamic nuclei and hypophysis.

lesions producing this change include hemorrhage, tumors, and infections of this area. Cerebral neurogenic fever is characterized by body temperatures of 104° to 108°F., with a cool skin due to vasoconstriction. The high fever itself may lead to degeneration of Purkinje cells of the cerebellum. Autonomic diencephalic epilepsy has been postulated to be due to seizure discharges in the hypothalamus and results in increases of blood pressure, heart rate, and body temperature accompanied by piloerection and tonic postures of the limbs and joints (Chap. 6). Poikilothermia, which is the inability to regulate temperature, with the body temperature following that of the environment, can also occur following injury to the hypothalamus.

Treatment

The primary hypothalamic lesion should be treated. Elevated temperatures above 104°F should be controlled with ice packs and acetylsalicyclic acid. Autonomic diencephalic seizures should be treated with anticonvulsive drugs (Chap. 6).

Hypothalamic Obesity and Cachexia

Lesions of the hypothalamus may result in obesity or cachexia. "Pituitary cachexia" is probably due to hypothalamic damage. The lesions are usually tumors, or the changes may follow infections such as encephalitis.

Treatment is directed at removal or amelioration of the primary lesion and dietary control or supplementation.

Frolich's Syndrome or Adiposogenital Dystrophy

Children with hypothalamic lesions in the region of the tuber cinereum often show a characteristic picture of flabby obesity and failure of genital development.

Treatment

Removal of the primary lesion when possible should be followed by hormonal replacement therapy and dietary control.

Thyrotoxic Ophthalmoplegia

Excessive secretion of thyrotropic hormone may lead to thyrotoxicosis and exophthalmos with ophthalmoplegia (Chap. 12).

Pituitary Gigantism and Acromegaly

Eosinophilic adenomas of the anterior lobe of the pituitary cause gigantism in children and adolescents prior to closure of the epiphyses, and acromegaly in adults. Some cases with normal pituitary fossae are due to microadenomatous change or hyperplasia of the growth-hormone-producing cells in the anterior pituitary. There have also been several reports of hypothalamic tumors with increased serum levels of growth hormone. Acromegaly is characterized by personality changes, muscular weakness, bony overgrowth with enlarged fingers, hands, and feet, enlarge-

ment of the frontal bones, and prognathism. Most patients develop a mild or moderate degree of diabetes mellitus. Some patients complain of symptoms of the carpal tunnel syndrome (Chap. 11) and may show evidence of a proximal myopathy.[261]

Diagnostic Procedures

1. The skull roentgenogram may show enlargement of the pituitary fossa.
2. Computed tomography may show a suprasellar or intrasellar mass.
3. Serum levels of growth hormone are elevated.
4. The glucose tolerance test shows a diabetic curve.
5. Electromyography and nerve conduction velocity studies are indicative of a proximal myopathy or a carpal tunnel syndrome in some cases.

Treatment

Treatment is by irradiation of the pituitary or surgical removal. In pituitary tumors with increasing visual field defects, surgical removal is advisable in order to preserve vision (Chap. 10).

Cushing's Syndrome

Tumors of the beta cells of the anterior lobe of the pituitary may rarely lead to adrenal hyperplasia and Cushing's syndrome with personality changes, obesity, purple striae of the skin, hypertension, hypernatremia, diabetes mellitus, hypokalemia, demineralization of bone, amenorrhea, moon facies, acne, and increase of body hair. Occasionally some features of the syndrome are seen in chromophobe adenomas.

Diagnostic Procedures

1. The blood count shows a polycythemia with lymphopenia and eosinopenia.
2. The skull roentgenograms show enlargement of the sella turcica in cases due to chromophobe adenomas.
3. The spinal fluid may be under increased pressure with increased protein content.
4. The visual fields may show characteristic changes such as a bitemporal hemianopsia.
5. ACTH and plasma steroid levels are increased.
6. Computed tomography may reveal a suprasellar mass lesion.

Treatment

Treatment is by irradiation of the pituitary or surgical removal. In pituitary tumors with visual field defects, surgical removal is advisable to preserve vision (Chap. 10).

Panhypopituitarism

This may result from destructive tumors of the hypothalamus and lesions of the pituitary gland, such as chromophobe adenoma or craniopharyngioma,[370] leukemic infiltration, or sarcoidosis following head injury, and is much more common in diabetes mellitus.[204] Panhypopituitarism also occurs as a result of infarction of the pituitary gland during pregnancy (pituitary apoplexy, Sheehan syndrome). There are weakness, dryness of the skin, premature aging, weight loss, signs of hypothyroidism, hypoadrenalism (Addison's disease), and loss of secondary sex characteristics, including loss of axillary and pubic hair with impotence in the male and amenorrhea in the female. Patients are sensitive to cold and are subject to hypotension and hypoglycemic episodes.

Diagnostic Procedures

1. There may be bitemporal hemianopia and optic atrophy.
2. The plasma and urinary 17-ketosteroids and 17-hydroxysteroids and the urinary FSH levels are all low. Protein-bound iodine levels and radioactive iodine uptake levels are in the hypothyroid range.
3. There may be ballooning of the sella turcica or suprasellar calcification by roentgenographic examination.
4. Computed tomography may show the presence of pituitary, parapituitary, or hypothalamic tumors.

Treatment

Tumors may be treated by surgical removal or irradiation. Surgical exploration is advised in cases with involvement of the visual fields. Replacement hormone therapy is necessary in most cases.

Pituitary Apoplexy

This may be due to infarction of the pituitary gland during pregnancy particularly in patients with diabetes mellitus (see above) or due to infarction of a pituitary tumor.[40]

There is a sudden onset of headache, photophobia, and neck stiffness lasting several days. Signs of pituitary insufficiency develop two or three months later. The cerebrospinal fluid shows a pleocytosis with 20 to 100 monocytes or polymorphonuclear leukocytes during the acute phase of the illness. The patient may become comatose with shock due to addisonian crisis.

Treatment

This includes intravenous therapy with hypertonic saline and cortisone to correct the addisonian crisis.

Neurologic Complications of the Hemoglobinopathies and Blood Dyscrasias

The hemoglobinopathies are genetically determined conditions in which the red cells contain an abnormal hemoglobin. Sickle cell disease and sickle cell hemoglobin C disease are both associated with similar neurologic complications.

Sickle Cell Anemia

Etiology

Sickle cell trait is a heterozygous condition in which red cells contain a mixture of hemoglobin S and normal hemoglobin A. Sickle cell disease is the homozygous state in which the red cells contain only hemoglobin S, which causes the erythrocyte to be fragile and form a gel under conditions of low oxygen tension. The composition of hemoglobin S reduces the life-span of the red cell resulting in both hemolytic anemia and crises in the homozygous condition and anemia as the sole manifestation in the heterozygous condition.

Hemoglobin S results from a single amino acid replacement of valine for glutamic acid in the beta polypeptide chain of hemoglobin. The abnormality is associated with a change in the hemoglobin molecule, which converts the normally fluid content of the erythrocyte into a solid gel when the cells are exposed to low concentrations of oxygen. This results in the development of rigid sickle cells, which may block the microcirculation of any organ due to a "logjamming" of cells, resulting in infarction. This is the generally accepted explanation for the painful crisis of sickle cell disease.[101, 241, 267]

Clinical Features

Patients with sickle cell disease are usually short and underweight with dorsal kyphosis, lumbar lordosis, and chronic ulceration of the legs.

There is a moderately severe anemia (about 8 gm/100 ml) with erythroid hyperplasia of the bone marrow. Cardiomegaly, hepatomegaly, and splenomegaly usually occur. There is a marked increase in the circulating blood volume with increased cardiac output and cerebral blood flow.

The sickle cell crisis occurs when the regional or arterial oxygen saturation decreases and often results in partial infarction of several organs. The crisis may present with acute abdominal pain, pleuritic pain, bone pain, and hematuria. Infarction of long bones is common and may be complicated by osteomyelitis.

The frequency as well as the severity of the neurologic complications of homozygous sickle cell disease have been underestimated in the past, and neurologic abnormalities occur in about 25 per cent of patients with this condition. The symptoms include hemiparesis, seizures, meningeal irritation, and subarachnoid hemorrhage, all of which may progress to coma. Repeated optic nerve involvement may be followed by optic atrophy and blindness. Sudden deafness has been reported during sickle cell crises and is due to bilateral cochlear and auditory nerve involvement.[250] Other cranial nerve palsies and spinal nerve radiculopathies may occur. Sudden paraplegia with loss of sphincter control is a major complication secondary to infarction of the spinal cord.[140] Pituitary infarction and hypopituitarism, vitreous hemorrhages, and a high risk of pneumococcal pneumonia are additional hazards in this disease. Repeated episodes of cerebral infarction may lead to dementia and retardation.

Diagnostic Procedures

1. The in vitro slide test with reduced oxygen tension produces typical sickling of red cells.
2. Roentgenograms of the skull usually show thickening of the diploe with fine radial striations. The long bones may show irregular areas of sclerosis.
3. Hemoglobin electrophoresis will reveal the presence of the abnormal hemoglobin (S hemoglobin).
4. Arteriography has been safely performed in patients with sickle cell anemia after reduction of the hemoglobin S concentration to less than 20 per cent by exchange transfusion or repeated transfusion of packed red cells. This may reveal multiple stenosis or occlusions involving the terminal portions of the internal carotid arteries, the circle of Willis, and the

proximal portions of its major branches.[323]
5. Serial electroencephalography is useful in the assessment of cerebral involvement during sickle cell crisis. The procedure should be performed without hyperventilation, which may induce cerebral vasoconstriction from hypocapnea and increase the risk of cerebral infarction.[7]

Treatment

1. Pain is severe and should be adequately controlled during the crisis. This may require narcotics such as meperidine and morphine.
2. Oxygen therapy, particularly hyperbaric oxygenation, reduces sickle cell formation and improves the microcirculation in ischemic organs.

Sickle Cell Trait

There are a number of reports indicating that sickle cell trait is not invariably a benign condition. Sickle cell trait has been associated with an increased risk of cerebral infarction, chorioretinal infarction, central retinal artery occlusion, and retinal detachment. There is an increased incidence of complicated migraine[251] and transient monocular blindness[103] in individuals with sickle cell trait.

Sickle Cell Hemoglobin C Disease

The prevalence of stroke has been reported to be higher in this rare hemoglobinopathy than in those with normal hemoglobin.

Neurologic Complications of Polycythemia

Both polycythemia vera and secondary polycythemia may be associated with neurologic complications. Polycythemia vera may be defined as a condition with persistent elevation in erythrocyte count, hemoglobin content, and circulating blood volume. Secondary polycythemia occurs as a physiologic adaptive mechanism in those living at high altitudes and as a complication of a number of abnormalities, including congenital heart disease, chronic pulmonary disease, chronic renal disease, renal carcinoma, and hemangioblastoma of the cerebellum (Chap. 10). Because of the increased viscosity of the blood in polycythemia, cerebral blood flow is greatly reduced, the transit time is greatly prolonged, and consequently the liability to cerebral thrombosis is increased.

Patients with polycythemia vera frequently complain of headache, vertigo, blurring of vision, somnolence, and lethargy without evidence of abnormalities on neurologic examination. For reasons already mentioned, there is increased liability to transient ischemic episodes (Chap. 9) and stroke due to cerebral thrombosis in polycythemia vera and also in secondary polycythemia. Many patients develop hypertension, which increases the risk of intracerebral hemorrhage. Spontaneous subarachnoid hemorrhage is rare but has been described.

Papilledema and headache can also occur in polycythemia vera owing to increased intracranial pressure, suggesting the possibility of brain tumor. There is an association between hemangioblastoma of the cerebellum and polycythemia, and this diagnosis should be considered in tumors of the posterior fossa associated with polycythemia. This is one of the causes of cerebellar hemorrhage.

Diagnostic Procedures

1. The complete blood count shows elevation of the erythrocyte count and repeated hemoglobins in excess of 16 gm.
2. In primary polycythemia, the circulatory blood volume is increased, as are the white count and thrombocyte count. The liver and spleen may be enlarged.
3. Intravenous pyelograms, chest films, and skull roentgenograms may reveal the cause of secondary polycythemia.

Treatment

Venesection should be used cautiously if the platelet count is increased because of the danger of causing cerebral thrombosis. In secondary polycythemia, cautious venesection with removal of small aliquots of blood may be used. The volume removed should be replaced with low-molecular-weight dextran. Levodopa has been reported to produce marked improvement in polycythemia in some cases.[151] A therapeutic trial of levodopa is worthwhile prior to the use of more hazardous forms of therapy. Melphalan, the phenylalanine derivative of nitrogen mustard (Alkeran), or busulfan (Myleran) may be used to suppress erythropoiesis.

Neurologic Complications of Leukemia

Neoplastic proliferation of white blood cells or their precursors may be followed by diffuse infiltration of many organs including the nervous system.[158, 263] The nervous system is affected in about 25 per cent of cases of leukemia of both acute and chronic types.[364]

The major complications of leukemia may be listed as follows:

1. The Virchow-Robin spaces of the brain and, less frequently, the spinal cord may be infiltrated by leukemic cells in acute leukemia. Tumor formation and sagittal sinus thrombosis may occur[16a] and result in personality changes, hallucinations, mental deterioration, dysphasia, paraparesis, and the development of a voracious appetite with weight gain. Cerebral atrophy may occur, particularly in cases treated with intrathecal methotrexate alone or in combination with radiation therapy.[70a] Brainstem infiltrates may produce respiratory disturbances, including hyperpnea and Cheyne-Stokes respirations.
2. Intracerebral hemorrhage is not infrequent in acute leukemia.[111] It occurs predominantly in the white matter. It appears that leukemic cells block the penetrating vessels in the brain and infiltrate the vessel wall to form a leukemic nodule from which there is hemorrhage into the white matter. The associated depression of the platelet count with hemorrhagic diathesis is a contributing factor. Subarachnoid hemorrhage and hemorrhage into the spinal cord are uncommon.
3. Meningeal infiltration by leukemic cells is probably the most common neurologic complication of leukemia in children.[147] This produces increased intracranial pressure with headache, vomiting, papilledema, and separation of the sutures. The cerebrospinal fluid is under increased pressure with an increased white cell count, elevated protein content, and depressed glucose content in 50 per cent of patients. The meningeal involvement is usually a complication of acute or subacute leukemia. It can occur at any time during the illness and, paradoxically, can occur when the disease seems to be under chemotherapeutic remission. Infiltration around the base of the brain and brainstem results in progressive cranial nerve involvement, usually beginning with oculomotor paralysis and complaints of diplopia.
4. An autopsy finding of an unsuspected subdural hematoma is not uncommon in acute leukemia. A subdural hematoma should be suspected in patients with known meningeal leukemia who

become lethargic and show focal neurologic abnormalities.[20] It can be readily demonstrated by CT scan.

5. Epidural compression by leukemic deposits usually arises in the spinal canal and results in progressive paraparesis with sensory level and loss of sphincter control. More diffuse infiltration of the epidural space with involvement of the nerve roots may produce widespread peripheral or cranial neuropathy.

6. The peripheral nerves may be infiltrated at any point by leukemic cells. These have been described in the proximal nerve roots, posterior root ganglia, and peripheral nerves. A clinical picture resembling postinfectious polyneuropathy (Guillain-Barré syndrome) may be due to widespread nerve root involvement by leukemia[145] or to demyelination of nerve roots due to the remote "toxic" effects of neoplasia. It should be borne in mind that peripheral neuropathies may arise as a complication of the chemotherapy in the treatment of leukemia.[232]

7. Other remote effects of a neoplastic process without direct cellular infiltration may occur in leukemia and include progressive multifocal leukoencephalopathy and polymyositis.[195]

8. Leukemic patients are susceptible to infections of the nervous system, particularly when under treatment with cytotoxic agents. As a result, the incidence of herpes zoster neuritis, encephalitis, acute and subacute meningitis, and brain abscess is increased during the course of the disease.

9. The toxic effects of chemotherapy can produce a number of changes in the nervous system. Intrathecal methotrexate administration has resulted in arachnoiditis with transient or permanent paraplegia.[116] Children receiving long-term chemotherapy for acute leukemia may develop a leukoencephalopathy with axonal degeneration, patchy demyelination, mural thickening of the microvasculature, and reactive astrocytosis.[85] This condition presents with seizures, progressive dementia, spasticity, and ataxia.[263]

Neurologic Complications of Hodgkin's Disease

Approximately 10 per cent of patients with Hodgkin's disease show evidence of neurologic complications due to direct involvement of the nervous system or to its remote effects.

Etiology and Pathology

Hodgkin's disease is a neoplastic condition of lymphoid tissue which originates in lymphatic or reticuloendothelial tissues.[120, 205] The cells exhibit local invasiveness and the ability to spread to other parts of the body. Any organ may be involved. The condition is more common in males, with the highest incidence between 20 and 40 years of age.

Four types of Hodgkin's disease have been recognized according to cell content and mean survival time.

1. Those with lymphocytic predominance comprise 10 per cent of cases, and this is the most benign form of the disease.

2. Those with so-called "nodular sclerosis" of lymph nodes comprise 45 per cent, and these lesions occur predominantly in the mediastinum and cervical lymph nodes.

3. Those with mixed cellularity comprise 35 per cent. The pleomorphism and the presence of Reed-Sternberg cells indicate more active disease with higher malignancy.

4. Those with lymphocytic depletion comprise 10 per cent of cases including cases previously termed "Hodgkin's sarcoma."

Neurologic involvement, particularly direct invasion of nervous tissue, predominantly occurs in those categories with mixed cellularity and lymphocytic depletion.[318]

Clinical Features

General symptoms of Hodgkin's disease, including fever, weight loss, weakness, and anemia, are usually present for some time before the occurrence of neurologic complications.

The neurologic manifestations include the following:

Direct Invasion of the Brain or Spinal Cord. This is very rare and may present as a solitary lesion of Hodgkin's sarcoma.[114, 177, 178] There appears to be a tendency toward invasion of the hypothalamus and optic chiasm, with the production of diabetes insipidus (see p. 258) and visual field defects or invasion of the temporal lobes and focal epileptic activity.

Noninvasive Encephalopathy and Dementia. An encephalopathy with axonal swelling and a moderate degree of gliosis has been described as a nonmetastatic complication of Hodgkin's disease. The condition presents as a progressive dementia and is believed to represent an unknown response to Hodgkin's disease rather than a reaction to chemotherapy or radiation therapy.[280]

Involvement of the Meninges and Base of Skull. Invasion of the floor of the skull by extension from the cervical area, nasopharynx, or oropharynx results in cranial nerve compression or infiltration. Hypopituitarism is possible, owing to invasion of the pituitary fossa. A diffuse involvement of the leptomeninges has been described, and subarachnoid hemorrhage is a possible complication.

Compressive Lesions. Hodgkin's disease is one of the most common causes of epidural compression of the spinal cord. Epidural involvement is rare intracranially, but subdural involvement with a subdural effusion may occur.[222]

Peripheral Nerve Involvement. Local invasion of peripheral nerves is common, including infiltration of the brachial plexus, cervical sympathetics (Horner's syndrome), and vagus, phrenic, and recurrent laryngeal nerves in the mediastinum or the lumbosacral plexus. A condition resembling postinfectious polyneuropathy (Guillain-Barré syndrome) may occur in Hodgkin's disease, possibly as a "toxic" manifestation or owing to direct involvement of multiple nerve roots by tumor cells. A mild peripheral neuropathy of the "carcinomatous" neuropathy type has also been described. Herpes zoster is not uncommon in Hodgkin's disease and results from the lowered resistance to infection associated with this disease owing to reduction of gamma globulins.

Remote Effects of Malignancy. At least three of the remote nonmetastatic effects of malignancy, namely progressive multifocal leukoencephalopathy (Chap. 3), cerebellar degeneration with demonstrable antibodies to cerebellar Purkinje cells,[337] and a subacute motor neuropathy with prominent degeneration of anterior horn cells,[301a] have been recorded in Hodgkin's disease.

Predisposition to Infection. The increased incidence of herpes zoster has already been mentioned. There is also an increased risk of cerebral abscess, cryptococcosis, and meningitis due to bacteria or fungi in Hodgkin's disease. The associated lowered resistance to infection may be enhanced by chemotherapy.

Treatment

Compression or direct invasion of nerve tissue usually shows a good response to irradiation or chemotherapy, including cytotoxic agents, and/or surgical decompression. The paraplegia of epidural cord compression should be decompressed surgically and also may be treated, in addition, with a combination of irradiation and chemotherapy, which gives superior results compared to one type of therapy alone.

Neurologic Complications of Multiple Myeloma

This disorder is a malignant neoplasm arising from plasma cells of the bone marrow and showing protean manifestations. The disorder may present as a single tumor (plasmacytoma) or as disseminated neoplasia, possibly arising from metastatic cells or from multiple sites in response to some unknown stimulus. A significant proportion of myeloma cells exhibit aneuploidy, with chromosome counts ranging from 43 to 92, and it is possible that the presence of abnormal chromosomes confers the ability to produce the abnormal globulins usually present in this disease.[63, 240]

Pathology

The neurologic complications of multiple myeloma may result from several factors, all of which may cause disorders of the nervous system.

1. The plasma cell tumors produce osteolytic lesions in bone.
2. There may be direct invasion of the brain or spinal cord.
3. Extradural deposits produce compression of the brain, cranial nerves, and spinal cord.
4. Macroglobulinemia or macrocryoglobulinemia may occur.
5. Amyloidosis has been reported in 10 to 15 per cent of patients.
6. There is an interference with coagulation mechanisms with the possibility of hemorrhage in the nervous system.
7. The immunoglobulin mechanisms are abnormal, producing increased risk of infection of the nervous system.

8. Hypercalcemia and hyperuricemia are not unusual in multiple myeloma.
9. Many of the nonmetastatic effects of cancer have been described in this disease, including neuropathy and progressive multifocal leukoencephalopathy.[81]

Clinical Features

Osteolytic lesions of bone may lead to collapse of vertebral bodies and compression of nerve roots with severe segmental pain. Compression of the cord and spastic paraplegia are usually due to extradural proliferation of plasma cells. This type of compression of the brain is less common, but a plasmacytoma involving the body of the sphenoid or the apex of the petrous temporal bone with extradural extension may produce cranial nerve palsies.[5, 326] Focal cerebral symptoms including seizures may occur if there is extension of the extradural masses into the brain. Occasionally, a large solitary plasma cell tumor develops in the brain with all the features of a primary brain tumor.

The most common of the neurologic complications of multiple myeloma is probably a sensorimotor peripheral neuropathy. Amyloidosis may cause a bilateral carpal tunnel syndrome due to compression of the median nerve beneath the flexor retinaculum. In addition, a rapidly progressive polyneuropathy somewhat similar to the postinfectious polyneuropathy of the Guillain-Barré syndrome can occur. A more chronic form of neuropathy, similar to that seen in Waldenstrom's macroglobulinemia, occurs in some cases.

Interference with coagulation mechanisms increases the risk of intracerebral and subarachnoid hemorrhage, although these are not common complications. The abnormality in immunoglobulins may permit infections such as herpes zoster, meningitis, or encephalitis to develop owing to lowering of defense mechanisms.

Hypercalcemia, with elevation of serum calcium levels as high as 16 or 18 mg/100 ml, can occur and is probably due to hyperproteinemia, increased bone destruction, and decreased renal function. The mental changes, weakness, and apathy associated with hypercalcemia are not unusual in multiple myeloma. This disease may also be associated with the remote effects of malignancy in common with other neoplasms, so that progressive multifocal leukoencephalopathy, myelopathy, and peripheral neuropathy are possible complications.

Diagnostic Procedures

1. The blood picture is usually that of a normocytic anemia with the presence of plasma cells in the blood smear in some cases.
2. Examination of a bone marrow biopsy shows the characteristic "myeloma" cells in 80 per cent of cases.
3. At least 75 per cent of patients have an abnormality in serum proteins by electrophoresis. This is usually in the gamma fraction, but it occasionally appears in the alpha or beta fractions. Both macroglobulinemia and cryoglobulinemia may be present.
4. About 50 per cent of patients have Bence Jones protein in the urine.
5. Roentgenograms of bone may reveal osteolytic lesions. These are clearly defined areas, frequently multiple, and sometimes associated with compression fractures of vertebral bodies. Patients with an obscure sensorimotor neuropathy and a raised CSF protein level should have a full skeletal survey to detect a possible solitary plasmacytoma.[277a]

Treatment

Spinal cord compression by vertebral collapse or extradural compression should be relieved immediately by laminectomy and decompression of the cord.

Intermittent combination therapy, using cyclophosphamide, steroids, urethane, and chlorambucil, is effective in this disease,[291] while radiation therapy is useful if directed toward specific lesions causing painful symptoms. The neuropathy often improves with treatment of the myeloma.

Neurologic Complications of Macroglobulinemia

An increase in serum gamma globulin in the macroglobulin range may occur as an apparent primary disease or secondary to multiple myeloma, leukemia, lymphosarcoma, and primary amyloidosis.[134] Some 25 per cent of patients with macroglobulinemia develop neurologic symptoms (Bing-Neel syndrome).

Etiology and Pathology

Many of the neurologic symptoms are related to increased serum viscosity due to the presence of abnormal macroglobulins, which results in aggregation of the cellular elements of the blood in small blood vessels. The macroglobulins are probably produced by abnormal activity of lymphocytes and plasma cells in such conditions as myeloma and leukemia. The primary form of macroglobulinemia is associated with widespread proliferation of lymphocytes and plasma cells and may, in fact, represent a more diffuse form of any one of these conditions.

The brain and spinal cord show infiltration of the meninges and Virchow-Robin spaces, with plasma cells and lymphocytes in many patients with scattered areas of hemorrhage or ischemic infarction. Changes in the peripheral nerves consist of modification of the myelin sheath which contains IgM deposits.[173a]

Clinical Features

Cerebral symptoms can be related to decreased cerebral blood flow due to increased viscosity which produces hypoxic changes in the blood vessels and the brain. Headache and mental dullness may occur with frankly psychotic behavior in some cases. Others develop typical transient ischemic attacks of cerebrovascular insufficiency or more permanent deficits, including dysphasia, hemiparesis, cerebellar ataxia, and cranial nerve palsies. Subarachnoid hemorrhage has occasionally been reported and is a manifestation of the defect in blood coagulation that occurs in macroglobulinemia. Tinnitus and gradual decrease in auditory acuity are probably due to hemorrhage into the cochlea.

Visual deterioration is quite common in patients with macroglobulinemia due to papilledema or retinal or vitreous hemorrhages.

Spinal cord compression by extradural masses of plasma cells or softening due to vascular occlusion may result in a progressive spastic paraparesis. A syndrome similar to the progressive muscular atrophy type of amyotrophic lateral sclerosis (see p. 209) may occur.[259]

Peripheral neuropathy is usually of sensory type with distal sensory loss and ataxia. However, distal muscle weakness and wasting can occur.[74, 202]

Diagnostic Procedures

1. Serum protein electrophoresis shows the presence of an abnormal macroglobulin.
2. Serum viscosity levels are markedly elevated.
3. The cerebrospinal fluid contains macroglobulins, and the total protein content is usually increased.

4. Slit lamp examination can be used to demonstrate sludging in the conjunctival vessels.

Treatment

Symptoms may be alleviated by plasmapheresis.[304] This procedure consists of the removal of venous blood, separation of red cells and plasma, and infusion of the red cells into the patient. This will produce a decrease in serum viscosity. A viscosity threshold may be estimated in each patient and is defined as the viscosity level at which symptoms recur. The serum viscosity is then maintained below that level by plasmapheresis weekly or biweekly.

In the occasional patient with neurologic symptoms and low serum viscosity levels, a whole-blood viscosity threshold should be determined and treatment should be governed by this level.[207]

Neurologic Complications of Cryoglobulinemia

In this condition, the gamma globulins are precipitated by a fall in body temperature, resulting in increased viscosity and sludging or thrombosis in smaller vessels. There are two types of cryoglobulins: (1) single-component cryoglobulins, which are made up of monoclonal immunoglobulins and occur in myeloma, Waldenström's macroglobulinemia, and benign monoclonal gammopathy; and (2) mixed cryoglobulins, which occur in rheumatoid arthritis, systemic lupus erythematosus, lymphomas, several chronic infections, and "essential cryoglobulinemia."

Clinical Features

Systemic signs of cryoglobulinemia include Raynaud's phenomenon, purpura, hemoptysis, loss of appetite, abdominal colic, hematemesis, and diarrhea. Renal involvement produces albuminuria, hypertension, and uremia. A mixed motor and sensory peripheral neuropathy occurs in about 20 per cent of cases.[68]

Treatment

The treatment of cryoglobulinemia depends on identification of the type of cryoglobulin. Chronic infection must be excluded in mixed cryoglobulinemia. Antimetabolite drugs may be used in cases of myeloma or lymphoma. Plasmapheresis is also effective. Essential cryoglobulinemia responds to melphalan (L-phenylalanine mustard) and corticosteroid therapy.[284]

Nonmetastatic Effects of Carcinoma on the Nervous System

Interest in the nonmetastatic effects of neoplasm is relatively recent,[39] but a number of clinical syndromes have been recognized, and it is possible to attempt classification of these abnormalities (Table 5–7).

Etiology and Pathology

The etiology is uncertain, and it is possible that multiple factors are involved.

The presence of a tumor may lead to the production of autoimmune antibodies to a number of tissues including nervous tissue.[366] If these antibodies can penetrate the blood-brain barrier or attach themselves to peripheral nerve or muscle, pathologic change may arise in the affected tissues, which would be compatible with changes seen in a number of the abnormalities to be described here. The theory of antibody formation has received some support from the description of antibrain antibodies in "carcinomatous neuromyopathy" and antibodies against neurons in sensory carcinomatous neuropathy.[367]

It is also possible that some of the conditions described in this section are due to chronic viral infection. This is supported by the description of intraneuronal inclusion bodies in some cases of progressive multifocal leukoencephalopathy. Infection by a neurotropic virus could conceivably occur following reduction in body defenses secondary to the development of neoplasia.

Finally, some of the abnormalities occurring in association with malignancy may be the result of concomitant endocrine or metabolic disturbances. Some tumors are known to produce endocrine-like substances that may have the effect of the true hormone. In addition, nonendocrine disturbances of cation metabolism of unknown etiology have occasionally been described.

Although each condition is described as a distinct entity in this section, it should be realized that it is typical to find a number of conditions arising in one patient.[372] The term "carcinomatous neuromyopathy" has been used to cover disorders affecting the central and peripheral nervous system and muscle in a single patient.[236] It seems worthy of retention unless a clear-cut clinical condition exists.[70]

Nonmetastatic Involvement of the Brain

Dementia

Dementia may occur as a remote manifestation of neoplasia alone or in association with other degenerative conditions, including cerebellar degeneration and encephalomyelopathy.

Pathology. Some patients may show patchy loss of neurons, microglial proliferation, and perivascular cuffing in the basal ganglia and brainstem, but the changes are not consistent.

Clinical Features. There is a moderately rapid progressive dementia, with loss of judgment, insight, retention, and recent memory. Occasionally, agitation, depression, or anxiety may occur with intermittent confusion and disorientation.

Progressive Multifocal Leukoencephalopathy

This is a rare complication of neoplasm and occurs mainly in association with Hodgkin's disease, leukemia, and neoplastic conditions of the reticuloendothelial system. It is fully described elsewhere (Chap. 2).

Encephalomyelopathy

This is usually associated with the oat cell type of bronchial carcinoma and may occasionally occur with carcinoma of the breast or uterus.[150]

TABLE 5–7

Nonmetastatic Effects of Carcinoma on the Nervous System

1. *Involvement of the brain*
   a. Dementia
   b. Progressive multifocal leukoencephalopathy
   c. Encephalomyelopathy
   d. Subacute cerebellar degeneration

2. *Spinal cord syndromes*
   a. Posterolateral column degeneration
   b. Necrotizing myelopathy
   c. Carcinomatous amyotrophic lateral sclerosis

3. *Peripheral nerve involvement*
   a. Sensory neuropathy

4. *Myopathic features*
   a. Carcinomatous myopathy
   b. Carcinomatous polymyositis
   c. Myasthenic syndrome

5. *Endocrine and metabolic disturbances*
   a. Hypoglycemia
   b. Hypercalcemia
   c. Cushing-like syndrome
   d. Hyponatremia and water intoxication

Pathology. There is perivascular cuffing, with lymphocytes, some neuronal loss, and microglial proliferation in the hippocampal formation, amygdala, cingulate gyrus, and orbital cortex (limbic encephalitis). Similar changes occur throughout the brainstem, with a variable loss of neurons of the motor nuclei. There is some loss of anterior horn cells and demyelination of the posterior columns in the spinal cord, which may be secondary to loss of ganglion cells in the posterior root ganglia and wallerian degeneration of the posterior nerve roots. The peripheral nerves are also affected by some degree of demyelination.

Clinical Features. There is progressive dementia, with intellectual impairment, fluctuating levels of awareness, and alternating periods of consciousness and somnolence. Bulbar involvement results in external ophthalmoplegia, nystagmus, vertigo, ataxia, dysarthria, and dysphagia.

Damage to anterior horn cells produces proximal muscle wasting and fasciculations in some cases. The peripheral nerve and posterior column involvement produces sensory loss to touch and pinprick at the periphery of the limbs, with more extensive loss or impairment of vibration and joint position sense.

Subacute Cerebellar Degeneration

This may appear at any time during tumor growth and is occasionally the initial symptom of an undetected neoplasm.[218a] The association between ovarian and bronchial carcinoma with cerebeller degeneration is particularly high. Other tumors, including carcinoma of the breast, are also associated with this condition.

Pathology. There is a diffuse loss of Purkinje cells in all parts of the cerebellum. The molecular layer is thinner, with microglial proliferation, and there is some loss of cells in the granular layer. The dentate nucleus may be normal or show moderate loss of neurons.

The degenerative process may affect areas outside the cerebellum, particularly the spinal cord. Demyelination of the long tracts is selective and tends to be marked in the spinocerebellar tracts and dorsal columns with slight involvement of the corticospinal pathways. Changes in the brainstem include demyelination of the superior cerebellar peduncles and degeneration of bulbar motor nuclei. Anterior horn cells may show similar degenerative changes in some cases.

Clinical Features. The condition presents as a rapidly progressive ataxia, beginning with a difficulty in walking due to early involvement of the lower limbs. This is followed by truncal ataxia and loss of coordination in the upper limbs. Bulbar involvement produces ptosis, ophthalmoplegias, and nystagmus, with bilateral facial weakness and a progressive dysarthria. Sudden deafness has been reported occasionally. Other associated symptoms include progressive dementia, numbness, and paresthesias of the extremities and signs of posterior column dysfunction. There may be proximal weakness in all four limbs. The reflexes have been described as decreased, normal, or increased with equal frequency. The plantar responses may be flexor or extensor.

Diagnostic Procedures. The cerebrospinal fluid protein content is occasionally elevated as high as 120 mg per cent.

Nonmetastatic Spinal Cord Syndromes
Posterolateral Column Degeneration

This occasionally occurs as an isolated form of spinal cord disease in association with carcinoma. Symptoms consist of weakness involving the lower limbs with increased deep tendon reflexes and extensor plantar responses. The dorsal column involvement results in distal sensory loss to touch with more prominent loss of vibration and position sense. The condition usually occurs in association with peripheral neuropathy or anterior horn cell degeneration.

Necrotizing Myelopathy

This is an infrequent but acute complication of a malignant tumor, usually a bronchial carcinoma.[211]

Pathology. There is a fairly symmetric and often patchy necrosis of myelin and axis cylinders in the spinal cord with a mild microglial reaction. The anterior horn cells are swollen, with central chromatolysis.

Clinical Features. The illness begins suddenly in patients who are known to have a visceral malignancy and who have often received radiation or chemotherapy. However, there may be a delay of many months following treatment, which does not seem to be related to the myelopathy. There is some pain in the back and weakness in both lower limbs initially, followed by ascending numbness and paresthesias and loss of sphincter control. The deep tendon reflexes are increased with bilateral extensor plantar responses. The weakness and sensory deficit show rapid progression, with ascending sensory levels on the trunk. Eventually, the upper limbs are involved, and death occurs with involvement of muscles of respiration.

Carcinomatous Amyotrophic Lateral Sclerosis

This has been described in association with a variety of neoplasms including bronchial carcinoma; carcinoma of the breast, colon, thymus, and prostate; seminoma of the testes; leukemia; astrocytoma; and basal cell carcinoma of skin.

Pathology. The changes show some difference from those described in classic amyotrophic lateral sclerosis. There is loss of anterior horn cells and motor fibers in the anterior nerve roots, with denervation atrophy of muscle. However, neuronal loss in the posterior root ganglia with wallerian degeneration in the posterior nerve roots is not uncommon. This latter finding is not seen in amyotrophic lateral sclerosis.

Clinical Features. The signs and symptoms are similar to those of classic amyotrophic lateral sclerosis (Chap. 4). The patients tend to be somewhat older on the average than patients with amyotrophic lateral sclerosis, and the carcinomatous type may run a somewhat milder course.[38]

Nonmetastatic Peripheral Nerve Involvement

Sensory Neuropathy

A predominantly sensory neuropathy may occur in patients with malignancy, most commonly bronchial carcinoma.[69, 78] The condition is not confined to this type of neoplasm, however, and has been described as a complication of other malignant tumors. The neuropathy may occur alone or present as the dominant feature, with evidence of involvement of other parts of the neuraxis.

Pathology. There are inflammation and degeneration of the posterior root ganglia with secondary wallerian degeneration of fibers in the posterior columns and peripheral nerves.[155]

Clinical Features. Symptoms present as numbness and paresthesias in hands and feet, and the course is that if a subacute progressive sensory loss involving all four limbs. All sensory modalities are involved, and there may be marked ataxia and postural lapses in the upper limbs (pseudoathetosis). The condition tends to become arrested after some three months and remains unchanged thereafter.[268]

Diagnostic Procedures. An elevation in cerebrospinal fluid protein content is not unusual. Significant levels of antibrain antibodies have been detected in the sera of some patients.

Motor Neuropathy

A more acute symmetric, predominantly motor peripheral neuropathy may also occur as a nonmetastatic complication of neoplasia. The peripheral nerves show severe demyelination with some axonal loss.[118] A rarer form with wallerian degeneration and microvasculitis of the vasa nervorum has been reported.[170a] The symptoms begin insidiously with fatigue followed by progressive proximal or distal muscular weakness.[18a]

Myopathic Features

Carcinomatous Myopathy

About 16 per cent of patients with carcinoma of the lung, breast, stomach, or ovary develop a progressive proximal muscle weakness. The condition also occurs as a rare complication in other forms of malignancy.

Pathology. There is some variation in the changes seen on muscle biopsy. Typical findings of polymyositis (Chap. 12) are found in a few cases, while others show atrophy of type II muscle fibers without inflammation or have a normal appearance. It is possible that the findings reflect the intensity of the disease process rather than differing pathologic conditions. Serum enzyme levels, serum creatinine phosphokinase (CPK), aldolase, and serum glutamic oxalacetic transaminase (SGOT) may be elevated.

Clinical Features. Acute cases, which usually occur in men over the age of 50 years, present with a rash, followed by muscular weakness and atrophy. The usual picture consists of a progressive proximal weakness and wasting of muscle, and it may be difficult to decide whether the condition is a myopathy or due to neurogenic atrophy. The signs of peripheral neuropathy and spinal cord involvement are often present (carcinomatous neuromyopathy). The EMG shows evidence of disturbed function of the motor units.[312] Some cases have myasthenic features (see Myasthenic Syndrome, Chap. 12).

Endocrine and Metabolic Disturbances Due to Neoplasia That Affect the Nervous System

The secretion of insulin-like material by tumors may produce symptoms of hypoglycemia and lead to encephalopathy in severe cases with recurrent attacks. Hypercalcemia is not unusual in malignancy with bone metastases, but may also occur in the absence of metastases owing to the secretion of a parathyroid hormone-like material. Elevated serum calcium levels may lead to muscular weakness, headache, anxiety, and, in severe cases, psychotic episodes.

The production of a corticotrophin-like material may lead to adrenocortical hyperplasia, hypokalemia, and muscular weakness. This may further progress to a state resembling Cushing's syndrome, with proximal muscle weakness and wasting.

Hyponatremia and symptoms of water intoxication have been reported in association with malignant tumors. The reason for inappropriate secretion of antidiuretic hormone in these cases is not known.

Neurologic Effects of Alcohol

Almost all the neurologic complications of alcohol are due to concomitant nutritional deficiencies rather than any direct neurotoxic effect of alcohol itself.[344] The chronic alcoholic neglects his diet to such an extent that classic deficiency diseases such as Wernicke's encephalopathy or beriberi may develop. Apart from acute intoxication and delirium tremens, all the conditions listed in Table 5–8 that may occur in alcoholics are probably of nutritional origin or intimately related to nutritional factors.

Acute Intoxication and Coma

The symptoms of acute alcoholic intoxication are well known, and the condition is usually regarded as reversible. However, imbibing large quantities of alcohol over a short period of time

TABLE 5–8

Neurologic Effects of Alcohol

1. Acute intoxication and coma
2. Delirium tremens
3. Marchiafava-Bignami disease (see Chap. 3)
4. Wernicke's encephalopathy and Korsakow's psychosis
5. Alcoholic seizures and accentuation of epilepsy in epileptics
6. Dementia
7. Central pontine myelinolysis (see Chap. 3)
8. Cerebellar degeneration
9. Myelopathy
10. Peripheral neuropathy
11. Alcoholic myopathy (see Chap. 12)

may lead to coma and death unless treated promptly.

Etiology and Pathology

Alcohol is absorbed directly from the stomach and upper intestine and, consequently, enters the bloodstream rapidly after ingestion. It is then metabolized via acetaldehyde and acetic acid to carbon dioxide and water. The cerebral effect of alcohol seems to be due to a direct inhibitory effect on excitable membranes with reduction in neuron excitability.[14, 174] Since death is rare in acute intoxication, the description of pathologic changes is scanty. The changes that have been described are probably those of cerebral congestion and edema due to asphyxiation and respiratory depression.

Clinical Features

The effect of acute alcoholic intoxication is to produce progressive paralysis of cerebral function beginning at the highest levels. There is, at first, some loss of inhibition with a feeling of relaxation and freedom of conversation. This is followed by progressive loss of judgment with the inability to sustain or to follow critical argument. Further intake produces changes that depend on the personality, varying from excitement to depression or paranoid behavior. There are impairment of retention and memory, irrational behavior, and dysarthria. Coordination is affected, resulting in ataxia of gait and upper limbs. The conjunctivae are often injected, the face is flushed, the pupils are dilated, and the respiratory rate is increased, frequently with the odor of ethanol in the expired air from the lungs. Additional ingestion of alcohol leads to disorientation and stupor followed by coma. The EEG is helpful in differentiating coma due to other causes, such as brain tumor and trauma,[332] from coma due to acute intoxication.

Death may occur from three possible causes: (1) the effect of alcohol in lethal amounts, (2) aspiration of stomach contents due to vomiting during semicoma, and (3) hypoglycemia, which may occur in certain susceptible individuals.

Treatment

The majority of patients with acute intoxication who reach the stage of disorientation and stupor usually fall into a deep sleep and literally "sleep it off." Some hours later, they awaken, dehydrated and tremulous, with headache, nausea, anorexia, fatigue, and the generalized muscle weakness termed "the hangover." This usually lasts 24 hours, then resolves after a further night of sleep. During "the hangover" period, light nourishment, adequate fluid intake, and aspirin for headache may render existence tolerable. A diagnosis of alcoholic intoxication, alone, should never be assumed in any patient who presents in coma smelling of alcohol or even after a known alcoholic bout. A full neurologic examination must be performed and blood drawn for blood glucose and barbiturate levels. The patient should be observed with recording of vital signs every 15 minutes. This should be a routine procedure in any case of acute coma until the patient regains consciousness. Catheterization and emptying of a distended bladder may allay restlessness. The airway must be cleared by suction, if necessary, and the patient turned on his side to drain secretions from the oropharynx. Intravenous fluids, consisting of 5 per cent dextrose in 0.2 N saline, will help to prevent dehydration and may partially alleviate the aftereffects.

Gastric lavage is useful in acute alcoholic coma that is known to have occurred immediately before the patient is examined. Alcohol is rapidly absorbed, and the procedure is of little value at a later stage.

Delirium Tremens

"DT's," or "delirium tremens," is one of the most dramatic complications of alcoholism. It presents as an acute psychosis occurring in chronic alcoholics in the withdrawal stages following a severe bout of drinking or occasionally precipitated by infection, trauma, or malnutrition.[247, 345]

Etiology and Pathology

Delirium tremens is probably related to the sudden withdrawal of the sedative effects of alcohol on nerve cells with a marked release of autonomic activity and neuronal irritability. The chronic alcoholic has a depressed respiratory sensitivity to carbon dioxide. Withdrawal of alcohol is associated with a rebound hypersensitivity to CO_2 with an increase in depth of respiration, hyperventilation, and the development of respiratory alkalosis. There appears to be a direct relationship between the degree of respiratory alkalosis and the severity of clinical manifestations of delirium tremens.[23] However, other factors including dehydration and electrolyte imbalance are important once the syndrome has developed.

Clinical Features

The condition is usually heralded by a change in personality. The patient becomes withdrawn, morose, restless, and irritable. There is an aversion to food, and sleep is disturbed, with terrifying dreams and the development of fleeting fragmentary illusions and hallucinations when awake. This is followed by an increase in hallucinations, which may be visual, and usually take the form of animals or insects, or auditory and rarely olfactory or tactile. The patient is extremely restless and vocalizes freely, crying out at one moment, then muttering unintelligibly, or replying to an apparent conversation with an hallucinatory colleague. Consciousness is clouded, the patient is disoriented, and the speech is often incoherent. Seizures may also occur in some cases but always precede the delirium. On examination, the temperature is elevated, the skin dry, and dehydration may be quite marked. There are hyperpnea and tachycardia, and life-threatening ventricular tachycardia has been observed secondary to hypokalemia and hypomagnesemia.[105] There is a coarse tremor involving the tongue, lips, face, and limbs, which is particularly marked in the extended fingers. The deep tendon reflexes are hyperactive, and the muscles may be tender on palpation.

Treatment

Therapy should be directed toward combating infection, restoring fluid and electrolyte balance, and sedating the patient.

1. The patient should be forbidden alcohol. The practice of giving alcohol as prophylaxis in incipient delirium tremens is unnecessary since there are now a number of effective drugs available to treat delirium tremens.
2. Infections such as pneumonia should be treated with adequate dosage of antibiotics parenterally.
3. Most patients have a severe water loss often in the range of 5,000 to 6,000 ml/day. Strict attention must be given to fluid replacement by infusing 5 per cent dextrose in 0.2 N saline intravenously with 20 mEq of potassium in every 100 ml or modifications of this solution based on serum electrolyte determinations.
4. Frequent determinations of serum electrolytes should be made to detect electrolyte imbalance, which must be corrected.
5. Hypomagnesemia can be corrected by the administration of up to 8 gm/day of magnesium sulfate intramuscularly.
6. Vital signs, i.e., pulse, temperature, blood pressure, and intake and output, should be monitored regularly.
7. Sedation requires the use of adequate doses of chlorpromazine (up to 1.0 gm daily in divided doses intramuscularly) or chlordiazepoxide (Librium) (80 mg every six hours intramuscularly). Sodium pentobarbital, 200 mg every six hours, or paraldehyde, 10 to 12 ml every three hours orally or rectally, is very effective in severe cases of delirium tremens.
8. Supplementary thiamine hydrochloride, 200 mg daily, may be given intravenously or intramuscularly, and a multivitamin preparation containing the vitamin B group should be added to the intravenous fluids.
9. As the patient improves, intravenous fluids can be discontinued and a high-protein, high-carbohydrate diet with oral vitamin supplements substituted, unless there is evidence of incipient hepatic failure requiring curtailment of protein intake.

Wernicke-Korsakow Encephalopathy

The association of Korsakow's psychosis with Wernicke's encephalopathy is so common that the two conditions may be regarded as part of one syndrome. Wernicke's encephalopathy is a nutritional disorder due to acute thiamine deficiency that is most commonly seen in alcoholics, but not exclusively so. It has been described in starvation, malnutrition, intravenous hyperalimentation without concomitant vitamin therapy,[188] hyperemesis gravidarum, and pernicious vomiting due to high gastrointestinal obstruction.

Etiology and Pathology

The syndrome is due to thiamine deficiency (vitamin B_1), although a lack of other vitamins of the B complex may contribute to the pathologic changes. The pathogenesis is unclear. Some patients apparently have a genetically determined predisposition to this syndrome and show an abnormality in transketolase activity that would be unimportant if the diet was adequate.[31] The lack of thiamine and hence cocarboxylase, with impairment of glucose and pyruvate metabolism and accumulation of pyruvic acid, undoubtedly interferes with nerve cell metabolism, which is so heavily dependent on carbohydrate as a source of energy.

The lesions of Wernicke's encephalopathy are confined to the zones around the aqueduct, the third and fourth ventricles, and the mammilary bodies (Fig. 5–5). The histopathologic changes consist of degeneration of parenchymal elements in these zones, myelinated fibers being more vulnerable than nerve cells. Capillaries and astrocytes proliferate in the affected zones. Petechial hemorrhages occur in only a small proportion of cases. Most cases also show a loss of Purkinje cells, most prominent in the anterosuperior vermis. Thalamic changes, which are most marked in the medial dorsal, pulvinar, and anteroventral nuclei, tend to be more prominent in patients with Korsakow's psychosis.

Clinical Features

The essential features of Wernicke's encephalopathy are the triad of ophthalmoplegia, ataxia, and dementia. The onset is often abrupt, with appearance of all three abnormalities. Occasionally, the ophthalmoplegia and ataxia precede the mental symptoms for a period of several days. The eye signs are characterized by horizontal and vertical nystagmus followed by bilateral lateral rectus weakness, internal strabismus, and diplopia. Ptosis is rare, and the pupil is generally spared.[351] The condition may progress to a complete external ophthalmoplegia. The ataxia is cerebellar in type, involving the trunk and lower limbs, but with little change in the upper limbs. The gait is wide-based, and the disability varies but may be so severe that walking is impossible.

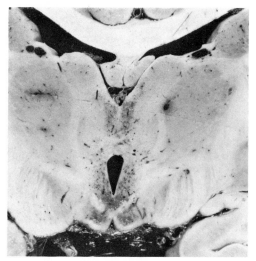 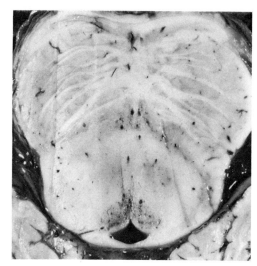

A B

FIGURE 5–5. Typical changes on cut section of the brain in a fatal case of Wernicke's encephalopathy due to alcoholism and malnutrition.

A. Coronal section at the level of the mammillary bodies and third ventricle, showing marked pericapillary diapedesis and atrophy of the mammillary bodies and hypothalamic nuclei.

B. Section through the pons, showing the same changes in the periaqueductal gray matter, which were also present in the upper cranial nerve nuclei.

Hypothermia may result from hypothalamic involvement. Sudden death is not unusual.[147a]

Mental symptoms present, with drowsiness and a tendency to sleep. When aroused, the patient shows paucity of conversation and is disoriented. This develops into the marked lack of retention and recent memory with confabulation characteristically associated with Korsakow's psychosis.

The essential clinical features of Korsakow's psychosis are a confabulatory dementia with marked loss of recent memory with a relatively intact remote memory.[4a] Korsakow's psychosis almost always results from alcoholism, although cases have been demonstrated following trauma and malnutrition. The condition often follows recovery from Wernicke's encephalopathy. The loss of recent memory is often so severe that the patient cannot recall three objects such as an apple, an orange, and an umbrella 15 to 30 seconds after the examiner has requested that they be remembered. Confabulation can be regarded as an attempt by the patient without recent memory to function by reference to his remote memory only.[108] He mistakenly identifies the hospital as a place he has known in the past and identifies new acquaintances based on his memory of individuals whom he has known previously. For example, the physician may ask the patient, "Have you seen me before?" "Oh yes, doctor, down at the Silver Dollar Bar." "What was I wearing?" "A green tie, a blue shirt, and a suit." "Was I wearing an orange plaid suit?" "Yes, doctor, indeed you were!" These answers are typical of confabulation.

Diagnostic Procedures

1. The blood pyruvate levels are usually elevated in established cases.
2. There is a reduction in transketolase activity of erythrocytes, which first appears in incipient cases of thiamine deficiency. This test is the most sensitive index of thiamine deficiency at this time.

Treatment

The ocular and ataxic signs of Wernicke's encephalopathy respond promptly to adequate diet and parenteral vitamin B_1 (thiamine hydrochloride, 100 mg b.i.d., intramuscularly). Other vitamins of the B complex should also be given orally.

Failure to respond may be due to thiamine refractoriness secondary to hypomagnesemia, which should be corrected as soon as possible.[334] The mental symptoms do respond in early cases but less well in long-standing symptoms, particularly when there are marked signs of Korsakow's psychosis, and many patients of this type are left with permanent defects in retention and recent memory.

Alcoholic Seizures and Accentuation of Epilepsy in Alcoholics

There is no doubt that seizures occur as a complication of chronic alcoholism, and the condition is usually termed "rum fits."[346] A number of possibilities concerning the relationship between alcohol and seizures deserve consideration.[126] In a large group of alcoholic patients with seizures reported in the literature, one large group comprising 90 per cent of the cases and two smaller groups were delineated. In the large group, the seizures ("rum fits") began in adult life and were generalized seizures that occurred as single or bursts of attacks during withdrawal of alcohol after chronic intoxication. The EEG was normal except in immediate relation to the seizures. About 50 per cent showed sensitivity to photic stimulation during the withdrawal interval. Of the two small groups, one consisted of patients with idiopathic epilepsy who became alcoholic after the onset of seizures. The other group consisted of patients with a history of head injury associated with alcoholism. This group was distinguished by focal seizures and localized EEG abnormalities. In this group, seizures occurred whether the patients were drinking or not but were more severe when drinking. The EEG findings supported the view that alcoholic seizures are engendered by alcohol itself and negate the idea that alcohol precipitates seizures in patients who are "constitutionally predisposed" to them. The most important factor in the genesis of alcoholic seizures and delirium tremens is the withdrawal of alcohol after chronic abuse.[346, 349]

Alcoholic Dementia

There is no doubt that some chronic alcoholics develop a slowly progressive dementia that is quite distinct from the dementia of the Wernicke-Korsakow syndrome. In some cases, alcoholic dementia may be due to increased use of alcohol during the early stages of Alzheimer's presenile dementia occasioned by the failing judgment, poor insight, decreased social restraint, and depression seen in the early stages of Alzheimer's disease. Other causes of alcoholic dementia include repeated head trauma, chronic seizures, and the development of an undetected chronic subdural hematoma. The chronic alcoholic may also suffer from insidious hepatic encephalopathy, which can present as a progressive dementia with few signs of the more overt forms of hepatic encephalopathy.

However, when all of the above causes have been considered, there remains a group of patients who have abused the use of alcohol for many years and who show signs of a chronic dementia.

Diagnostic Procedures

1. Computed tomography of the brain shows diffuse cerebral cortical atrophy in most cases with relatively less enlargement of the lateral ventricles.[109]
2. The electroencephalogram shows more slowing of the background activity than would be expected for age and the presence of transient theta and delta activity in the temporal leads bilaterally.[246]

Treatment

1. Withdrawal from alcohol and total abstinence produce improvement in mentation and reversal of the EEG abnormalities.
2. Lithium therapy is reported to reduce drinking and improve functioning in chronic alcoholics with depression but is not effective in the nondepressed chronic alcoholic.[226]

Central Pontine Myelinolysis

This condition has been described as a complication of chronic alcoholism and has also occurred in association with certain neoplastic conditions and poor nutrition. The majority of cases have been reported in alcoholics (p. 272). Central pontine myelinoysis can be diagnosed clinically, and patients may recover if treated in an intensive care unit with nasogastric feeding and immediate antibiotic therapy for intercurrent infection.[361]

Alcoholic Cerebellar Degeneration

This type of cerebellar degeneration is quite unique and is apparently a nutritional form of cerebellar degeneration since it has been described occasionally in nonalcoholic nutritional disorders.[348]

Pathology

The appearance of the cerebellum is characteristic with marked atrophy of the superior aspect of the vermis and the anterior lobe of the cerebellum. These areas show loss of Purkinje cells and loss of neurons in both granular and molecular layers of the cortex. Advanced cases also show neuronal loss in the dentate nucleus and inferior olives.[9]

Clinical Features

The disorder may be classified into acute transient cerebellar ataxias in alcoholics with a good prognosis and the more common subacute and chronic forms, which have a bad prognosis. The clinical picture in alcoholic cerebellar degeneration is unique. There is an ataxia more or less limited to the lower limbs and trunk, which develops over a period of several weeks or months. This produces a severe ataxia of gait, which contrasts with the paucity of cerebellar signs in the upper limbs and the absence of nystagmus and dysarthria in most cases.[252] Standing with the feet together and the eyes closed (Romberg test) may produce a rhythmic extension and flexion of the feet, and standing with flexed knees produces a rhythmic bobbing of the body.[313] The condition may progress to the extent that the patient cannot walk even with canes and is confined to a wheelchair.

Treatment

In the acute forms the immediate prognosis is good, if the condition is treated early. This should be carried out in the hospital away from any source of alcohol. There is usually a gradual improvement after a few weeks of a wholesome diet with vitamin B supplements. Full recovery can be expected in the majority of acute cases. Unfortunately, the relapse rate is high if the patient begins to take alcohol again, and after two or three episodes of cerebellar ataxia with recovery, the condition enters the subacute and chronic stages. If drinking is continued, the patient becomes permanently ataxic and severely disabled.

Alcoholic Myelopathy

A spastic paraparesis may rarely occur in the alcoholic, presumably due to nutritional deficiencies, since it is frequently combined with Wernicke's encephalopathy, optic neuritis, and beriberi.

Clinical Features

There is a spastic weakness of the lower limbs, with ankle clonus, increased deep tendon reflexes, and extensor plantar responses. Some loss of vibration and position sense in the feet and ankles suggests that there is posterior column as well as corticospinal tract involvement.

Treatment

Withdrawal from the source of alcohol and a nutritious diet with vitamin supplements may arrest the process, but permanent damage will result if treatment is not instituted early.

Alcoholic Peripheral Neuropathy

The majority of cases of peripheral neuropathy in alcoholics appear after many years of excessive drinking and are often mild or insidious in onset.

Etiology and Pathology

There has been disagreement concerning the etiology of peripheral neuropathy in alcoholism. The peripheral nerve lesions have been attributed to nutritional deficiency or to the toxic effects of alcohol on the peripheral nerve.[24] Given the poor dietary habits of the alcoholic, it is reasonable to suggest that both factors are involved in the development of peripheral neuropathy. The pathologic changes consist of a wallerian degeneration of peripheral nerves with loss of myelin and axis cylinders. Advanced cases may show involvement of anterior and posterior nerve roots with neuronal loss in the posterior root ganglia.

Clinical Features

Many chronic alcoholics have a mild subclinical peripheral neuropathy with some loss of muscle bulk in the distal lower limbs, tenderness on squeezing the calf muscles, depressed deep tendon reflexes, and a mild degree of hypalgesia to pinprick over the feet and lower legs. In more advanced cases, there are complaints of weakness in all four limbs, and pain, which may be quite severe with a lancinating quality or a sensation of burning, involving the hands and feet. Sometimes the dysesthesia of the feet is so intense that the patient is unable to tolerate the contact of clothing or bedclothes that touch the feet and legs. In advanced patients, examination reveals bilateral foot and wrist drop, and varying degrees of peripheral weakness occur in other patients. There are muscle wasting, tenderness, loss of deep tendon reflexes, and peripheral sensory loss to all modalities.

Treatment

The response to adequate diet, thiamine intravenously in doses of 100 mg twice daily, other vitamin B supplements, and abstinence from alcohol is good, but recovery is usually slow.

Alcoholic Myopathy

The acute and chronic forms of alcoholic myopathy are discussed elsewhere (Chap. 12).

Fetal Alcohol Syndrome

Alcohol appears to have a teratogenic effect on the developing fetus, and the chronic use of alcohol affects fetal development during early embryogenesis. The affected infants exhibit growth retardation and diminished intellectual performance and have a typical appearance with short palpebral tissues, micrognathia, low nasal bridge, long convex upper lip (fishmouth), and epicanthic folds. Infants born to chronic alcoholic mothers may show signs of acute withdrawal symptoms in the neonatal period characterized by irritability, increased muscle tone, tremors, and tonic seizures often accompanied by abdominal distention and vomiting.

Treatment

Chlorpromazine (2 mg/kg/day) or phenobarbital (5 mg/kg/day) is effective in reducing symptoms and improving the clinical condition of the affected infants.[264]

Disulfiram Encephalopathy

A large number of chronic alcoholics are maintained on disulfiram to deter alcohol abuse. This drug inhibits aldehyde dehydrogenase for desired effect but also inhibits dopamine metabolism resulting in increased dopamine and decreased norepinephrine levels in the brain.

Clinical Features

Disulfiram encephalopathy presents with impaired concentration, poor memory, anxiety, depression, and insomnia several days to several months after the initiation of therapy. The condition may progress to disorientation, paranoid delusions, and hallucinations with dysarthria, ataxia, and corticospinal tract involvement.[156]

Treatment

The encephalopathy resolves after withdrawal of disulfiram.

Neurologic Manifestations Due to the Vitamin Deficiencies

This is an important subject in the practice of neurology, since neurologic signs and symptoms due to vitamin deficiencies are common and they may pose as other neurologic disorders or complicate them.[343]

Vitamin A

Deficiency of vitamin A is rare except in children with malabsorption syndromes. The earliest symptom is night blindness, which is difficult to detect in infants and young children. This is followed by keratinization of epithelium, including the conjunctiva and cornea (xerophthalmia), and absence of tearing due to blockage of the lacrimal ducts. Hydrocephalus, mental retardation, and cranial nerve palsies have also been described in some cases.

Excessive vitamin A intake has also been reported to cause raised intracranial pressure, papilledema, and bulging of the fontanel (see Benign Intracranial Hypertension).

Vitamin B_1 (Thiamine)

Vitamin B_1 deficiency is the major cause of Wernicke's encephalopathy and is the major factor leading to the development of beriberi, peripheral neuropathy, and retrobulbar neuritis. Beriberi is endemic among people who use milled rice as a major food or may occur under conditions of malnutrition or starvaton. A high obstruction in the gastrointestinal tract, particularly carcinoma of the stomach or esophagus with little or no passage of food into the intestine, may also lead to vitamin B_1 deficiency.

Wernicke's encephalopathy occurs predominantly in the chronic alcoholic in the United States, but the peripheral neuropathy in alcoholics is probably due to the toxic effects of alcohol on the nerve rather than beriberi.

Beriberi neuropathy is an axon degeneration occurring in individuals who take hard exercise or indulge in manual labor while subsiding on a high-carbohydrate, low-thiamine diet. The clinical picture is one of cardiac enlargement, peripheral edema, and peripheral neuropathy.[330] There is dramatic improvement after a single administration of thiamine.

Niacin or Nicotinic Acid

Nicotinic acid deficiency is one of the major factors responsible for the development of pellagra. The disease was endemic in the southern United States in the early part of the century but has now practically disappeared. Sporadic cases may occur in infants who are given a restricted diet over a period of months. Adults with pellagra are usually impoverished chronic alcoholics with chronic pancreatitis.

Etiology and Pathology

Pellagra should be regarded as a disease with severe protein malnutrition and a deficiency of other vitamins as well as niacin. The protein lack causes a fall in serum tryptophan, which is the source of endogenous synthesis of niacin. Deficiencies of thiamine, riboflavin, and pyridoxine probably contribute to the signs and symptoms of pellagra, and these vitamins also act as cofactors in the synthesis of niacin. The adult pellagrin may compound multiple-vitamin deficiency because of alcohol abuse. The chronic diarrhea that is often due to chronic pancreatitis causes electrolyte imbalance including hypomagnesemia.[320]

The essential lesion in pellagra consists of central chromatolysis affecting neurons at many levels. The nerve cells in the cerebral cortex, particularly the large pyramidal cells in the motor cortex, are swollen with eccentric nuclei and loss of Nissl substance. Similar changes are seen in other parts of the cerebral cortex, basal ganglia, and most of the nuclei of the brainstem. The anterior horn cells are involved in some, but not all, cases. There is little glial reaction, and axonal damage is inconsistent.

Degenerative changes have been described in the posterior and lateral columns of the spinal cord, with loss of myelin and axis cylinders. Similar wallerian degeneration occurs in the nerve roots and peripheral nerves. Occasionally, there is some loss of myelin in the optic nerves.

Clinical Features

The triad of diarrhea, dermatitis, and dementia has historically described pellagra, but the symptoms are in fact more complex. The disease presents with gastrointestinal and cutaneous symptoms. There are anorexia, weight loss, and chronic diarrhea, sometimes alternating with constipation. The cutaneous lesions begin as sharply defined erythema in those areas exposed to sunlight, such as the dorsum of the hands, wrists, elbows, feet, legs, nose, cheeks, and neck. This is followed by desquamation and, finally, a brownish area of pigmentation. Glossitis, stomatitis, and gingivitis are often present. Infection is a common complication in pellagra because of the lowered defense mechanisms due to protein deficiency. Initial signs of involvement of the nervous system consist of headache, insomnia, and irritability.

Children with this disease are listless and dull and have little interest in their surroundings. Adults may present with symptoms of anxiety or depression. This is followed by an acute psychosis, with hallucinations, disorientation, and delirium in some cases. Patients show a progressive dementia unless treated early. Seizures are not uncommon. Involvement of the spinal cord produces a spastic paraparesis or ataxia. The deep tendon reflexes vary in response, but there may be bilateral extensor plantar responses. Distal weakness, atrophy, and sensory loss occur in patients with peripheral neuropathy.[35] Visual symptoms are usually mild, but associated retrobulbar or optic neuritis may lead to complaints of blurring of vision.

Diagnostic Procedures

1. Anemia, hypokalemia, hypomagnesemia, and hypocalcemia are usually present. Hypoalbuminuria occurs in profound malnutrition.
2. The electroencephalogram shows progressive development of diffuse slowing with the appearance of symmetric theta and delta activity as clinical signs of dementia appear.

Treatment

Patients with pellagra require a protein intake of about 1 gm/kg/day with restricted fat and adequate carbohydrate. Niacinamide, 200 mg daily, is preferable and avoids the gastrointestinal and vasodilator effects of niacin. Thiamine, riboflavin, and pyridoxine should be administered at the same time. Infections require prompt treatment with antibiotics.

Pantothenic Acid

It is possible that lack of pantothenic acid may contribute to the pathologic changes of Wernicke's encephalopathy, beriberi, and pellagra, although experimentally the first two conditions have been produced by thiamine deficiency alone. A particularly unpleasant symptom is paresthesias in the lower limbs, the burning feet syndrome, which has been attributed to pantothenic acid deficiency and has been said to respond promptly to administration of this vitamin.

Vitamin B₆ (Pyridoxine)

The dermatitis, peripheral neuropathy, and perhaps the cerebral cortical changes of pellagra may be due, in part, to vitamin B_6 deficiency. Pyridoxine deficiency may cause seizures in the neonate or infant.

Etiology

Pyridoxine is incorporated into a number of coenzymes that are concerned with the metabolism of both tryptophan and glutamic acid. In pyridoxine deficiency, there is a block in the conversion of tryptophan to nicotinic acid, with excess production of xanthurenic acid. Another block occurs in the conversion of glutamic acid to gamma amino butyric acid, which interferes with mitochondrial activity in neurons.

Clinical Features

Seizures associated with both pyridoxine deficiency and pyridoxine dependency have been described.[112] In pyridoxine deficiency, the infant develops generalized seizures between the ages of one and four months. A family history for seizures is negative, and there is a good response to anticonvulsants or pyridoxine. The interictal EEG is normal, and there is an excess of xanthurenic acid in the urine on administration of tryptophan. Children with pyridoxine deficiency usually develop normally.

Pyridoxine dependency appears to be due to an endogenous metabolic block, as yet undetermined. Seizures begin in the neonatal period and are generalized, with so-called "infantile spasms." There is a family history of unexplained neonatal deaths or repeated stillbirths in some cases, and the condition may be genetically determined. The response to anticonvulsants is poor, but large doses of pyridoxine (14 mg/kg of body weight per day) orally produce a cessation of seizures. The electroencephalogram shows continuous irregular high-voltage spike wave discharges with shifting foci (hypsarrhythmia) in untreated cases.

Tryptophan loading does not produce an excess of xanthurenic acid in the urine in pyridoxine dependency, and these children show mental retardation unless treated early. An adult form of pyridoxine dependency with anemia and peripheral neuropathy has also been described that responds well to parenteral followed by oral pyridoxine therapy.[22]

Vitamin B₁₂ (Cyanocobalamin)

The syndrome resulting from deficiency of vitamin B_{12} is unique in that it is rarely due to lack of the vitamin in the diet.[335] Vitamin B_{12} is absorbed only in the presence of an intrinsic factor produced in the gastric mucosa. Atrophy of the gastric mucosa is followed after several months by the development of pernicious anemia and, in some cases, by subacute combined degeneration of the spinal cord. Other causes of pernicious anemia include gastric resection for carcinoma of the stomach, subtotal gastrectomy for peptic ulcer, gastrocolic fistula, and malabsorption syndromes.

Etiology and Pathology

The relationship of vitamin B_{12} deficiency to pernicious anemia and subacute combined degeneration of the cord is not clear. There is little relationship between the degree of anemia and the onset of the neurologic deficit. The place of vitamin B_{12} in cellular metabolism has not been determined nor has its role in myelin formation.

The lesions of subacute combined degeneration can be seen as pale areas with the naked eye in sections stained for myelin. The earliest changes consist of a patchy loss of myelin and axis cylinders in the posterior columns which is maximal in the thoracic area and later spreads to involve the lateral columns. The degenerative process appears to affect myelin earlier and perhaps to a greater extent than axis cylinders. The primary lesions are followed by secondary wallerian degeneration up and down the cord. There is an appropriate glial reaction and the damaged areas have a vacuolated appearance. The gray matter is spared.[4]

Advanced cases show patchy areas of demyelination and axon degeneration in the centrum semiovale and internal capsule of the cerebral hemisphere. Some cases show severe demyelination and axon loss involving the papulomacular bundle in the optic nerve. There may be loss of myelin and axons in the intramedullary portion and the most proximal segments of the cranial nerves. The peripheral nerves have been reported to show a mild segmental demyelination.

Clinical Features

The symptoms of subacute combined degeneration usually occur in the presence of anemia. This may be mild in some cases, and occasionally, the neurologic syndrome will antedate the development of pernicious anemia.

The first symptom is usually paresthesias of the extremities. These are persistent and often distressing to the patient and are followed by numbness and distal weakness in the limbs. The gait becomes ataxic, and there are variable degrees of spasticity in the lower limbs depending on the predominance of lateral column involvement. About 50 per cent of cases show hyperactivity of the deep tendon reflexes and bilateral extensor plantar responses. In untreated cases, the ataxia and sensory loss in the lower limbs increase until the patient is unable to walk. The patient then becomes confined to bed and usually dies from a urinary tract infection.

The majority of patients exhibit mental changes, which are probably due, in part, to the associated anemia and cerebral anoxia and in rare instances to demyelination of the hemispheres.[110] The mental changes consist of forgetfulness, dullness, moroseness, suspiciousness, and irritability, initially, with the development of frank dementia in advanced cases. Progressive visual deterioration first presenting as a cecocentral scotoma and progressing to optic atrophy occurs in some cases of subacute combined degeneration and has occasionally been reported as the first manifestation of pernicious anemia.[196]

Diagnostic Procedures

1. The complete blood count in pernicious anemia usually shows a low hemoglobin and a low red cell count. Since this is a macrocytic normochromic anemia, the mean corpuscular volume (MCV) and mean corpuscular hemoglobin (MCH) are increased, while the mean corpuscular hemoglobin concentration (MCHC) is normal. The reticulocyte count is low, and occasional nucleated red cells of the megaloblastic type may be found in the peripheral blood. There is usually some degree of leukopenia and a slight to moderate thrombocytopenia.
2. The bone marrow shows the changes of megaloblastic erythropoiesis.

3. There is a histamine-fast achlorhydria. The deficiency in intrinsic factor is reflected in an abnormal Schilling test. This test measures the urinary excretion of radioactive vitamin B_{12} following oral administration, and low values are obtained in pernicious anemia.
4. Serum vitamin B_{12} levels are decreased, while plasma iron and serum bilirubin levels may be elevated.
5. Atrophy of the gastric mucosa can be seen on gastroscopy.
6. Nerve conduction velocities are decreased in all cases with active subacute combined degeneration.
7. Visual evoked potentials are significantly delayed at an early stage in the absence of visual impairment.[335a]

Treatment

Pernicious anemia shows an immediate and dramatic response to parenteral vitamin B_{12}. The neurologic abnormalities usually show rapid improvement except in the most advanced cases, but the process is always arrested by adequate therapy. The recommended dosage is 100 μg of vitamin B_{12} intramuscularly daily for the first week followed by three times weekly until the blood picture is normal. The maintenance dose of 100 μg monthly must be continued for the rest of the patient's life.

Heavy Metals and Industrial Toxins

Neurologic Complications of Lead Poisoning

The increasing release of lead into the environment is reflected in rising blood levels of lead in children and adults throughout the world.[200] More than 15 per cent of preschool children in urban areas in the United States have blood lead concentrations that exceed 40 mg/100 ml, which is the currently accepted upper limit of safety.[60]

Etiology and Pathology

The most common cause of lead poisoning in children is still the ingestion of lead paint. Since lead paint is no longer available for interior decorating, children living in older houses and, consequently, in the lower socioeconomic groups are more likely to be exposed. In recent years, there has been an increase in lead poisoning following the inhalation of fumes from burning car batteries used as fuel. Other causes have included chewing lead toy soldiers and drinking contaminated water.[137] Lead poisoning is an industrial hazard for demolition workers who cut lead-painted steel with acetylene torches, for workers exposed to lead dust or lead fumes from molten lead, and for those who use sprays containing lead. Non-industrial causes of lead poisoning include gasoline sniffing and drinking lead-contaminated "moonshine" whiskey.

All parts of the nervous system are vulnerable to the effects of lead. There is increasing deposition of lead in the central nervous system with increasing blood levels of lead. However, lead is retained in the brain when blood levels fall so that intermittent exposure produces an incremental rise in the concentration of lead in the brain. The child's brain shows an increased susceptibility to the toxic effects of lead, and acute exposure may produce lead encephalopathy which occurs almost exclusively in children. The main pathologic findings in acute encephalopathy consist of interstitial edema and hemorrhage, more prominent in the cerebellum but also affecting other regions of the brain. It is believed that lead damages the capillary endothelium in the brain, producing increased capillary permeability and edema.[129]

Chronic exposure to lead in both children and adults produces neuronal damage at all levels in the central nervous system, including the anterior horn cells in the spinal cord.

The peripheral neuropathy of lead poisoning consists of an initial segmental demyelination with later damage to axons and cells in the spinal cord.

Clinical Features

Children with lead encephalopathy usually have a past history of pica, abdominal colic, vomiting, and constipation. The development of cerebral edema produces drowsiness and ataxia or may be heralded by focal or generalized seizures. There may be postictal coma, with papilledema or focal paralysis at this stage. Repeated seizures or status epilepticus is not uncommon. Many children who survive the acute phase continue to have seizures. Other complications include varying degrees of mental retardation, and some cases have optic atrophy. Death may occur from brain edema and herniation.

Chronic exposure to lead produces anemia, recurrent abdominal colic, and constipation at all ages. When exposure is insufficient to produce acute encephalopathy in children, the more chronic effects of lead include mental retardation, behavior problems, learning disabilities, and hyperactivity.[21, 76] There is a possible association between chronic exposure to lead and the development of astrocytomas in children.[302]

Adults exposed to toxic levels of lead develop a chronic encephalopathy with signs of a personality change, dementia, spasticity, and rigidity. A condition resembling amyotrophic lateral sclerosis has been described in lead industry workers.

The peripheral neuropathy of lead poisoning occurs after many months of exposure and may be seen in children or adults.[99] This condition frequently presents with weakness of the hands and wrist drop.

Diagnostic Procedures

1. There are varying degrees of anemia, with the presence of basophilic stippling in the red cells.
2. Lead concentrations of above 150 μg/liter of urine per 24-hour collection and 0.07 mg per cent of blood are considered indicative of lead intoxication in adults.
3. Coproporphyrinogen III is elevated in the urine.
4. Roentgenographic examination of the long bones may reveal a dense "lead line" at the metaphysis. Similar changes occur in the iliac crests and tips of the scapula. The increased intracranial pressure of lead encephalopathy may lead to separation of the cranial sutures.
5. In lead encephalopathy the electroencephalogram shows diffuse slowing in proportion to the degree of cerebral edema and mental obtundity. Focal or generalized epileptic discharges may also occur.
6. Motor nerve conduction velocities are decreased in lead neuropathy. This test is useful in screening lead-exposed workers for early signs of lead intoxication, since a significant decrease in motor nerve conduction velocities occurs in subclinical lead exposure.

Treatment

The child with plumbism should be removed immediately from the source of infection. Laxatives and enemas are useful in eliminating ingested lead in the gastrointestinal tract. Lead encephalopathy requires immediate treatment in order to control seizures (see Treatment of Status Epilepticus in Children, Chap. 6). The cerebral edema may be reduced by restricting fluids and giving intravenous urea solution or mannitol.[176] Steroid therapy may be of value. If there is no improvement within six hours, bitemporal cranial decompression should be performed.

Lead in the soft tissues may be mobilized, using the chelating agent calcium disodium edetate (EDTA). The initial dose of 25 mg/kg of body weight twice daily is gradually increased to 75 mg/kg over a period of five days. A second course may be given after a rest period of three weeks. Additional five-day courses of calcium EDTA may be given if the blood level of lead is greater than 0.10 mg per cent.

Neurologic Complications of Arsenic Poisoning

Ingestion of arsenic may occur from a number of sources including medicinal preparations, paints and plasters, fruit and vegetables contaminated by arsenical sprays, and accidental ingestion of arsenical rodenticides or insecticides. Arsenic may also be used in attempted suicide or homicide and occasionally contaminates illicitly distilled alcohols.[164]

Etiology and Pathology

The metal interferes with the tricarboxylic acid cycle by blocking the pyruvate oxidase and alpha glutarate oxidase systems. Damage to the nervous system is usually confined to the peripheral nerves, which show demyelination and loss of axis cylinders.[51]

Clinical Features

In acute cases the patient experiences a burning pain in the esophagus and stomach after ingestion of arsenic, followed by vomiting and diarrhea. Death may occur from myocardial poisoning or renal failure. Survivors develop conjunctivitis, epistaxis, erythematous and exfoliative rashes, transverse white depressions on the fingernails, transient jaundice, anemia, and increased capillary permeability. Symptoms of neuropathy appear at any time between 1 and 14 days after ingestion of arsenic. The earliest symptoms consist of numbness and paresthesias, usually appearing in the lower before the upper extremities. There is generalized muscle pain and cramps, and tenderness on palpation of muscles may be present. Some patients experience an intense unpleasant burning sensation involving the feet. Examination shows a symmetric, peripheral sensory loss involving all four extremities with some degree of wrist and foot drop. The ankle jerks are absent and other tendon jerks are absent or depressed. Recovery is slow, over a period of many months, and is frequently incomplete.

A rare encephalopathy has been described after ingestion of arsenic, with clouding of consciousness, delirium, cerebellar ataxia, and signs suggesting Wernicke's encephalopathy. Seizures may occur, and there may be a residual dementia with Korsakoff's psychosis. Subacute combined degeneration of the spinal cord has been described as a rare complication of arsenic poisoning.[330a]

The chronic ingestion of sublethal amounts of arsenic results in a generalized pigmentation of the skin, more marked on exposed surfaces, and an exfoliative dermatitis. These patients also develop peripheral neuropathy with marked wasting of the distal muscles of all four limbs.[221] A myelopathy has been reported following administration of neoarsphenamine.

Diagnostic Procedures

1. The cerebrospinal fluid protein may be elevated but the glucose content is normal.
2. The blood count may show an eosinophilia as high as 40 per cent.
3. Nerve conduction velocities are prolonged, and frequently the end point cannot be recorded.
4. The arsenic level in the blood exceeds 7 nanograms/100 ml, and the body hair and fingernail levels exceed 1 nanogram/gramine. The arsenic level in the urine exceeds 0.1 mg in 24 hours.
5. The arsenic level in the liver exceeds 0.1 mg/100 gm.
6. Sural nerve biopsy shows demyelination with characteristic ovoid bodies.

Treatment

1. The source of arsenic poisoning must be removed.
2. Acute cases should be treated with gastric lavage using 1 per cent sodium thiosulfate in warm water or milk.
3. D-Penicillamine administered orally in doses of 25 mg/kg four times a day is effective in the treatment of acute arsenic intoxication.[260]
4. The use of intravenous fluids and maintenance of electrolyte balance may be lifesaving during the acute phase of intoxication.
5. Acute arsenic intoxication associated with transient renal failure should be treated by

hemodialysis[122] followed by D-penicillamine when renal function improves.

Neurologic Effects of Manganese Intoxication

Chronic manganism or manganese poisoning is not rare, and the psychiatrist or the neurologist may be the first physician consulted. It has long been known in the manganese mines of Chile, but also occurs in ore-crushing mills and steel-making plants where manganese ore is used for hardening the steel. It is a preventable condition if adequate precautions are taken for removing the manganese dust from the environment and preventing its inhalation and ingestion.[292]

Etiology and Pathology

Workers in the manganese industries are exposed to the metal primarily by inhalation of the dust. Signs of nervous system involvement may be delayed for 2 to 25 years after exposure. Manganese is absorbed from the lungs, enters the bloodstream, and is concentrated in the liver and excreted into the upper intestine.[352] Healthy workers appear to have a more rapid turnover of manganese than those who suffer poisoning.[225] Manganese absorption seems to be enhanced by heavy smoking.[294] In patients with manganism, the metal is present in high levels in body tissues such as the scalp and chest hair and exerts a chronic deleterious effect on the catecholamine metabolism of the brain. There is neuronal loss in the basal ganglia, cerebellum, and substantia nigra.[67]

Clinical Features

The initial symptoms suggest a psychiatric disorder, with nervousness, irritability, and a tendency to compulsive acts, which makes the victim a potential hazard to his fellow workers. There is emotional instability, and anger is easily provoked. There are spells of crying and occasional hallucinations, impaired judgment, poor concentration, and memory impairment.[18] This is followed by the development of generalized muscular weakness and rigidity with an expressionless masklike face, a stooped flexed posture, and a shuffling gait. There is generalized headache, and the speech becomes slurred and unintelligible in some cases. Less frequent symptoms include sialorrhea, a Parkinson-like tremor, dystonic posturing of the trunk and limbs, sexual impotence, and muscle cramps.

Diagnostic Procedures

1. Blood-serum manganese levels are elevated to about 0.075 ppm (normal, 0.015 ppm or less).
2. A 24-hour urine collection is made after 1 gm of the chelating agent, edetic acid, is given intravenously. Normally there is no manganese in the urine. In cases of manganism, after administration of edetic acid, urinary manganese levels usually increase to 0.035 to 0.052.[292]
3. Manganese levels are increased in hair, urine, feces, and brain.

Treatment

Levodopa in doses of 6 to 12 gm/day relieves or improves the rigidity, bradykinesis, dystonia, and tremor (Fig. 5–6).[66] The dosage is slowly increased to avoid nausea and vomiting (see Treatment of Parkinson's Disease). Higher doses of levodopa are tolerated in manganism than in Parkinson's disease.

Neurologic Complications of Mercury Poisoning

Poisoning by metallic mercury, which was once an industrial hazard, is now rare, but may occur in dental office personnel who inhale mercury vapor in the preparation of dental amalgam.[160] There is a greater risk of poisoning from exposure to organic mercury compounds, which are widely used as fungicides, weed killers, and seed disinfectants. Poisoning may occur from handling the compounds, by the ingestion of pretreated cereal seeds intended for planting, or by consuming meat from animals that have been fed with contaminated grain.

Pathology

Organic mercury compounds produce a toxic encephalopathy, with marked loss of neurons in the granular layer of the cerebellum and patchy loss of neurons in the cerebral cortex, which is most marked along the borders of the calcarine fissure. Degenerative changes may also occur in the peripheral nerves, posterior nerve roots, and posterior columns of the spinal cord.

Clinical Features

The acute cases of organic mercury poisoning present with confusion, drowsiness, and stupor alterating with periods of excitement and restlessness. There may be progressive deterioration to coma and death. In subacute cases, there are

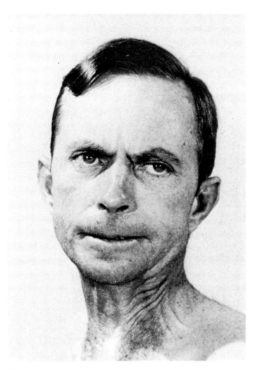
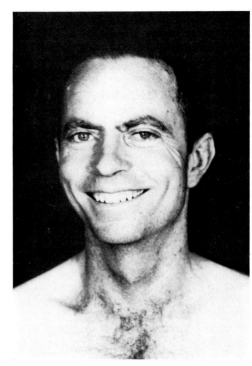

A   **B**

FIGURE 5–6. Chronic manganese poisoning. *A.* Dystonia and masklike facies in a patient exposed to manganese. *B.* Return of normal facial expression following treatment with levodopa.

numbness of the extremities, dysarthria, ataxia, and visual deterioration. The ataxia and dysarthria are of the cerebellar type, while the visual symptoms appear to be due to constriction of the visual fields due to involvement of the visual cortex. Seizures and choreoathetosis are occasional occurrences. Severe and permanent sensory loss has been described due to a combination of peripheral neuropathy and cortical neuronal loss in the postcentral gyrus.[328]

Diagnostic Procedures

Mercury may be detected by spectrophotometric methods in the urine and body or scalp hair in suspected cases.

Treatment

Metallic mercury poisoning responds to penicillamine therapy, but there is no specific treatment for organic mercury poisoning, and recovery of function can only be helped by long-term physical therapy and speech therapy.

Much can be done in the prevention of poisoning, however, by abandoning the manufacture of the more toxic methyl and ethyl mercury compounds and employing adequate safety precautions in factories. The hazards of handling mercury fungicides as a spray or in treated seeds should be stressed to farmers and market gardeners. Protective clothing must be worn in spraying crops in fields and greenhouses to prevent contact with the skin or inhalation of dust.

Neurologic Complications of Bismuth Salts

A toxic encephalopathy following therapeutic administration of insoluble bismuth salts has been described.[47, 327] The salts, either bismuth subgallate or bismuth subnitrate, are used in the treatment of constipation.

Etiology and Pathology

The insoluble bismuth salts are probably converted to soluble substances by the action of intestinal flora. Bismuth is then absorbed into the systemic circulation and crosses the blood-brain barrier into the brain. High levels of bismuth have been found in the brain in cases of fatal bismuth encephalopathy.

Clinical Features

There is a prodromal phase of several weeks when the patient appears to be anxious, depressed, irritable, and even paranoid with insomnia and in some cases visual hallucinations. This phase is followed by the abrupt onset of mental confusion, myoclonus, and ataxia. Conscious patients may be euphoric and show evidence of memory failure and perceptual difficulties. Seizures have been observed in about 50 percent of cases.

Diagnostic Procedures

1. The electroencephalogram shows loss of alpha activity, which is replaced by symmetric 4–5HZ activity occurring symmetrically over both hemispheres. Most patients show low-voltage beta activity in the anterior leads. There are no spikes or paroxysmal discharges corresponding to the myoclonic jerks.
2. Blood levels of bismuth are elevated.

Treatment

Most patients recover from the encephalopathy 3 to 12 weeks after bismuth administration is stopped.

Neurologic Complications of Carbon Tetrachloride Poisoning

The solvent carbon tetrachloride is commonly used in fire extinguishers and may be toxic if the fumes are inhaled after use in an enclosed space. Because of its solvent properties, it has also been used for the cleaning of clothes, usually by removal of fluid from a fire extinguisher, with serious or fatal results. Toxicity is enhanced when it is used in conjunction with alcohol.

Pathology

There are usually severe changes in the liver in fatal cases, with diffuse cellular necrosis and fatty infiltration, particularly in the central part of the lobule. The kidneys may show diffuse tubular necrosis. Toxic effects may also be severe in the brain, with necrosis of blood vessels and extravasation of red blood cells. This change is more

marked in the pons and cerebellum, which may show patchy areas of hemorrhage. In addition, there is diffuse patchy perivasular edema involving the cerebrum as well as the brainstem and cerebellum.[206]

Clinical Features

There are early symptoms of headache, vertigo, and blurring of vision, which may develop into visual loss or complete blindness. Lethargy and coma occur in some cases with a fairly rapid deterioration to a fatal outcome in seven to ten days. Those who recover or patients who do not have severe symptoms, initially, may develop intellectual impairment, optic atrophy, cerebellar ataxia, parkinsonism, or peripheral neuropathy.[210]

Treatment

Since the principal change in the central nervous system consists of perivascular edema, treatment with steroids might possibly help in cases with cerebral symptoms. There is, however, no definite indication that this type of therapy influences the course of the disease.

Neurologic Complications of Methyl Bromide

Methyl bromide is widely used in industry as a refrigerant, in fire extinguishers, as a fumigant, and as an insecticide. It is colorless and practically odorless and may produce toxic effects if inhaled.

Clinical Features

Severe cases develop acute ataxia, apathy, nausea, vomiting, headache, diplopia, vertigo, and dysarthria, and may die from pulmonary edema or renal failure. Survivors may pass into a stage of convulsions, delirium, or acute mania. The condition may resemble Reye's syndrome in children.[310] Cases with acute but less severe exposure are apathetic and ataxic, with marked nystagmus and vertigo. Recovery usually takes several months.

Chronic exposure to methyl bromide fumes results in a peripheral neuropathy, mainly affecting the lower limbs, with weakness, numbness, paresthesias, and ataxia of gait.

Treatment

There is no specific treatment. Recovery from the neuropathy takes several months after removal from the source of the methyl bromide.

Neurologic Complications of Organophosphorus Insecticide Poisoning

Organophosphorus compounds are used extensively throughout the world in industry and as agricultural insecticides. One of these compounds, triorthocresylphosphate, has occasionally contaminated cooking oils or fats, and major outbreaks of poisoning have been reported in Morocco and India due to ingestion of adulterated cooking oils.[317] Another organophosphorus, parathion, has probably been responsible for more cases of accidental poisoning and death than any other organophosphorus compound. Organophosphorus compounds act by inhibiting the enzyme cholinesterase.

Clinical Features

Symptoms of poisoning are nausea, vomiting, diarrhea, abdominal pain, tightness of the chest, muscular fasciculations, muscular weakness, and paralysis. Paralysis of the respiratory muscles may result. Ataxia, slurred speech, convulsions, and coma with loss of reflexes also occur. Death results from vasomotor collapse and respiratory paralysis. Symptoms of peripheral neuropathy appear within a few days and may be quite severe resembling acute postinfectious polyneuropathy (Guillain-Barré syndrome).[308] Chronic peripheral neuropathy and corticospinal tract damage[232a] may persist for months or permanently after poisoning.[371]

Diagnostic Procedures

The cholinesterase activity of the erythrocytes is reduced to less than 25 per cent of normal.

Treatment

General Measures. CUTANEOUS CONTAMINATION. The patient should shower or should be washed immediately and all clothing should be discarded. The hair must be thoroughly washed, and the fingernails cleaned.
INGESTION. The insecticide must be removed by emesis or lavage immediately.

Specific Measures. Specific measures include the following:

1. Atropine is specific and highly effective. It should be given in doses of 2 to 4 mg intravenously every ten minutes until full atropinization occurs. This is indicated by dilated pupils, dry flushed skin, and a rising pulse rate. The dose of atropine is then adjusted to maintain full atropinization for 24 hours.
2. Neuromuscular paralysis may be reversed by pralidoxime, a cholinesterase reactivator. In moderate or severe intoxications 1 gm should be injected intravenously. The injection must not be administered in less than two minutes. If there is failure of the drug to reverse the paralysis or if there is a recurrence within 20 minutes, the dosage may be repeated.
3. Endotracheal intubation may be required to ensure an adequate airway.
4. A mechanical respirator should be used for respiratory failure.

Neurologic Complications of Thallium

Although the use of thallium sulfate as a depilatory agent has been abandoned, accidental ingestion of thallium-containing pesticides may still occur, particularly in children. In addition, thallium poisoning is occasionally encountered in adults due to chronic inhalation of thallium-containing dusts generated in some industrial processes.[278]

Etiology and Pathology

Thallium acts by inhibition of intracellular enzymatic systems. In acute cases, there is swelling of the brain and chromatolysis in the neurons of the cortex, basal ganglia, and brainstem. Chronic cases may show neuronal loss in the brain, but changes are more marked in the anterior horn cells of the spinal cord. There is also marked loss of neurons in the posterior root ganglia and wallerian degeneration of peripheral nerves.

Clinical Features

Ingestion of large doses produces an acute gastroenteritis with hemorrhages, abdominal colic, and diarrhea. Acute neurologic symptoms appear in two to five days and consist of disorientation, delirium, hallucinations, and seizures with death from respiratory paralysis in less than a week. Smaller doses produce encephalopathy, with obtundity, disorientation, and confusion associated with choreoathetosis, myoclonus, and occasional seizures. Blurring of vision or visual loss may occur owing to optic neuritis. Paresthesias occur at an early stage in the lower limbs, and there is a marked ataxia. Cardiac signs, including tachycardia, hypertension, and angina-like pain, are seen during the second week following ingestion of thallium. Alopecia occurs at ten days. The patient may recover completely, recover with some intellectual impairment, or develop signs of chronic peripheral neuropathy.

More chronic exposure to thallium in industry usually leads to peripheral neuropathy without evidence of cerebral damage. There are paresthesias in the lower limbs and weakness and atrophy of the calf muscles with quite severe muscle cramps and ataxia.

Diagnostic Procedures

Thallium sulfate may be detected in the urine in patients who have ingested thallium or who have been exposed in industry to thallium-containing dusts.

Treatment

In the acute phase, ingested thallium sulfate should be removed by immediate gastric lavage and oral activated charcoal. Urinary excretion may be increased by abundant intake of fluids and potassium chloride, 3 to 5 gm daily, for ten days.

Symptomatic treatment requires adequate sedation, including morphine for severe pain and anticonvulsant drugs when indicated.

The use of chelating agents such as dimercaprol (BAL) or calcium disodium edetate (EDTA) has not been effective in removing thallium sulfate from the tissues.

Neurologic Complications of Hydroxyquinolines (Clioquinol)

Clioquinol-containing drugs have been in wide clinical use for more than 30 years for the treatment of intestinal disorders, particularly amebiasis and acrodermatitis enteropathica.[73] Signs of damage to the optic nerve have been reported,[26] and polyneuritic symptoms have been observed in association with long-term administration of hydroxyquinolines. Nevertheless, other long-term studies carried out in a large number of patients have failed to provide evidence of specific neurotoxic properties of clioquinol.[121]

A remarkable neurologic syndrome was recognized in Japan in the 1950s and was given the name "subacute myelo-optic neuropathy" (SMON). This disorder, affecting the spinal cord, peripheral nerves, and optic nerves, is believed to be due to the ingestion of clioquinol for the treatment of gastrointestinal disturbances.[57] The use of hydroxyquinolines has now been banned by the Japanese authorities, and the number of reported cases has decreased.[182] SMON has rarely been reported from countries other than Japan, but reports of cases from India[353] carry the implication that clioquinol is the etiologic agent. Clioquinol is still available in most countries, and fears have been expressed that the continued use of the drug may lead to a second outbreak of SMON in any part of the world.[146]

Pathology

Optic nerves and dorsal columns, corticospinal tracts of the spinal cord, and dorsal roots may show demyelination.

Clinical Features

The neurologic syndrome is characterized by paresthesias and blurred vision usually preceded by abdominal pain. The dysesthesias ascend from legs to arms. There is impairment of sensation of the lower limbs with or without pyramidal signs.[244] Involvement of the upper limbs occurs late in the disease. There is bilateral impairment of vision with cecocentral scotoma in up to 20 per cent and optic atrophy in 2 to 3 percent.[182]

Diagnostic Procedures

Diagnostic facts include the following:

1. CSF and blood are normal.
2. Related findings: a history of ingestion of hydroxyquinolines during the phase of gastrointestinal disturbance has been reported in 85 per cent of the patients.[182]

Differential Diagnosis

Multiple sclerosis and vitamin B deficiency syndromes should be excluded.

Treatment

Treatment is symptomatic, supportive, and rehabilitative.

Neurologic Complications of Toluene

Toluene is an organic solvent which is extensively used in industry and which has a natural affinity for the lipids of the nervous system. Toluene "sniffing" by glue sniffers produces euphoria and perceptual disorders and has been popular among solvent sniffers because of the ready availability of glue and contact cements in hobby shops and hardware stores.

Etiology and Pathology

The neuropathologic changes induced by toluene are unknown, but hydrocephalus and cerebral atrophy have been demonstrated by computed tomography.[36]

Clinical Features

Chronic exposure to or chronic abuse of toluene produces cerebellar ataxia and corticospinal tract involvement with spasticity and hyperreflexia. Chronic inhalation of toluene by addicts results in personality change with flat affect, indifference, and dementia. The peripheral neuropathy reported in glue sniffers is probably due to the presence of n-hexane in the inhalant rather than a toxic effect of toluene.[185]

Treatment

Patients accidentally exposed to toluene will recover once the contact is removed. Chronic toluene abusers may suffer permanent brain damage.

Neurologic Complications Due to Liver Failure

Hepatic Encephalopathy

Three types of hepatic encephalopathy have been recognized depending on the severity of hepatic failure.[298] Acute hepatic coma occurs in fulminant hepatic failure, most often secondary to viral or toxic hepatitis, where coma is a grave and usually irreversible prognostic sign. Reversible hepatic encephalopathy occurs in cirrhotic patients and often has a recognizable precipitating cause. There is usually a good response to treatment. The hepatocerebral degeneration syndrome is a complication of long-standing liver disease with a spontaneous or surgical portosystemic shunt. The course is one of slow progression, and the response to treatment is poor.

Etiology and Pathology

The main causes of hepatic coma and reversible hepatic encephalopathy are given in Table 5–9. There are two common factors in all cases of liver failure: (1) failure to detoxify metabolites, which have a profound effect on many cerebral metabolic processes, and (2) shunting of portal venous blood carrying neurotoxic substances ab-

TABLE 5–9

Hepatic Encephalopathy

Acute hepatic failure
1. Viral hepatitis
2. Homologous serum jaundice
3. Drugs and toxins, including halothane anesthesia
4. Acute failure following portacaval shunt

Chronic liver failure
1. Laennec's cirrhosis
2. Postnecrotic cirrhosis
3. Schistosomiasis
4. Terminal failure following portacaval shunt

sorbed directly from the gastrointestinal tract into the systemic circulation.

When hepatic coma occurs, the loss of liver function has crippled the internal environmental control, and the plasma contains degradation products released from necrotic liver cells, some of which may be toxic. Other abnormal substances are absorbed from the bowel, and since the liver is unable to detoxify these substances, they enter the systemic circulation unchanged.[180] The final result is an acute and profound disturbance of neuronal metabolism with loss of function and the clinical state of coma.

Reversible hepatic encephalopathy and the hepatocerebral degeneration syndrome are the result of the metabolic disorder of the central nervous system that complicates advanced hepatic cirrhosis. Both of the encephalopathic syndromes are believed to be caused by ammonia or other substances such as methionine, short-chain fatty acids, and biogenic amines that escape degradation in the liver, accumulate in systemic circulation, and cross the blood-brain barrier. One important factor in reversible hepatic encephalopathy is the direct entry of portal blood into the systemic circulation through intrahepatic anastomoses or portosystemic surgical shunts.[161] However, other factors must also be involved in the chronic hepatic encephalopathies. These include deficiencies in carbohydrate metabolism, particularly in the tricarboxylic acid cycle, which have a profound effect on cerebral metabolism. This is compounded by hypoglycemia in some cases. Elevated serum bilirubin levels are usually present and reach high levels in acute hepatic failure. Hypokalemia and hyponatremia are not unusual, particularly after repeated paracentesis to remove ascitic fluid. The hyperventilation that often accompanies hepatic encephalopathy results in respiratory alkalosis, but any respiratory obstruction will rapidly produce cerebral hypoxia and a sudden metabolic acidosis, both of which are poorly tolerated in hepatic failure.

Pathology

The brain grossly does not show any change of note in acute hepatic coma. Chronic cases show some neuronal loss with diffuse gliosis involving the cerebral cortex, basal ganglia, brainstem, and cerebellum. Enlarged and irregular nuclei of astrocytes (Alzheimer type II cells) are a distinctive feature. There is also proliferation of astrocytes, which have edema and swelling of the cytoplasm.

Clinical Features

Acute hepatic coma carries a high mortality. The patient with acute hepatic failure and jaundice develops confusion followed by delirium, stupor, and coma. There are dysconjugate eye movements, hypertonia, clonus, and hyperreflexia in the early stages followed by decerebration, areflexia, coma, and respiratory arrest. Seizures often precede decerebration and probably indicate cerebral edema. The manifestations of reversible hepatic encephalopathy include periodic waxing and waning of consciousness and confusion, which may be mistaken for a psychiatric illness. A carefree and euphoric attitude with constructional dyspraxia is not uncommon. The latter may be tested, using the same tests daily as an assessment of improvement or deterioration. However, marked intellectual impairment can be demonstrated even when the patient is alert and apparently neurologically intact.[279] At other times the same patients develop drowsiness, slurred speech, a curious alternating flexion and extension of the hands at the wrists (liver flap, flapping tremor, asterixis), myoclonic jerks, seizures, ocular bobbing,[274] choreoathetosis, extrapyramidal rigidity, or spastic paraparesis. The hepatocerebral degeneration syndrome presents as a progressive dementia with rigidity, asterixis, spastic paraparesis,[237] and increased reflexes. This may show little change for many months, but eventually will terminate in hepatic coma.

Diagnostic Procedures

1. Uremia may also follow massive gastrointestinal bleeding and may confuse the diagnosis.
2. Other blood abnormalities include elevated ammonia levels, hypokalemia, hyponatremia, elevated serum bilirubin, alkalosis, or metabolic acidosis. Hypoglycemia is occasionally present.
3. The electroencephalogram shows progressive slowing with the development of hepatic encephalopathy and the appearance of diffuse delta activity during coma. Bilateral, synchronous, high-voltage triphasic waves sometimes appear anteriorly and symmetrically on the two sides (Fig. 5-7).

Treatment

Acute Hepatic Failure

1. The precoma state should be treated by correcting electrolytic imbalance and maintaining fluid balance with intravenous fluids containing adequate amounts of glucose.
2. Absorption of ammonia and other toxins from the bowel can be reduced by a daily enema and the use of oral antibiotics that are not absorbed from the bowel. These include neomycin, 4 to 8 gm daily, and streptomycin, 0.5 to 1 gm twice daily. The absorption of ammonia can also be reduced by giving the synthetic disaccharide lactulose orally or by retention enema.[186]
3. If the prothrombin time ratio (test time in seconds divided by control time in seconds) exceed 2, one unit of fresh frozen plasma every 12 hours will reduce the risk of bleeding.
4. Anemia should be corrected by infusion of packed cells.
5. Seizures can be controlled by low doses of intravenous diazepam.
6. Cerebral edema may be reduced by intravenous dexamethasone.
7. Any infection should receive immediate and vigorous treatment.
8. If impairment of consciousness occurs, treatment with levodopa (3 to 5 mg daily) or bromocriptine[233] may rapidly reverse stupor, improve the EEG, and restore normal awareness presumably by replenishing depleted dopamine in the basal ganglia.[254] Other methods of treatment to be considered in progressive hepatic failure with coma are exchange transfusions,[25, 119, 172] cross-circulation,[297, 360] peritoneal dialysis, or hemodialysis.[297, 360]

Chronic Hepatic Failure. Ammonia production in the intestine can be decreased by a low-protein diet and the administration of a daily dose of 4 to 8 gm of neomycin orally to reduce ammo-

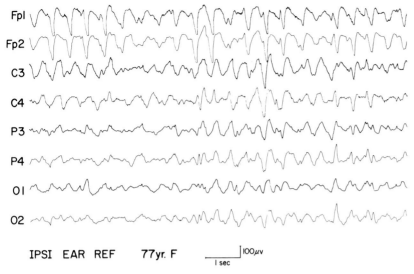

Fpl
Fp2
C3
C4
P3
P4
Ol
O2

IPSI EAR REF   77yr. F   ⌐100μv
                          I sec

FIGURE 5–7. Electroencephalogram in hepatic coma showing typical high-voltage triphasic waves anteriorly and symmetrically on the two sides.

nia-producing bacteria. Since gastrointestinal hemorrhage from esophageal varices is the most important cause of hepatic coma, it should be treated promptly with a Sengstaken-Blakemore tube. Blood ammonia levels may then be reduced by the methods described above and liver transplantation may be considered.

Neurologic Manifestations of Renal Failure (Uremia)

The neurologic complications of uremia consist of a number of conditions which are either related to the complex metabolic dysfunctions of uremia or which arise as a complication of dialysis (Table 5-10).

Uremic Encephalopathy

Both acute and chronic forms of uremic encephalopathy have been recognized and appear to be related to the rate of development of renal failure.

Etiology and Pathology

A variety of neuropathic changes have been described in the brain, most of which are nonspecific and not necessarily related to uremia. Areas of cortical necrosis and neuronal degeneration are probably related to terminal hypoxia, and focal demyelination may be related to lacunar infarc-

TABLE 5–10

Neurologic Aspects of Uremia

1. *Uremic encephalopathy*
2. *Uremic neuropathy*
   a. Restless leg syndrome
   b. Burning feet
   c. Sensorimotor peripheral neuropathy

3. *Uremic myopathy*
   a. Muscle cramps
   b. Myopathy
   c. Myositis
   d. Hyperparathyroidism
   e. Neuromuscular transmission defect

4. *Complications of dialysis*
   a. Dialysis encephalopathy
   b. Dialysis dementia
   c. Chronic meningeal infection
   d. Subdural hematoma
   e. Wernicke's encephalopathy
   f. Central pontine myelinolysis
   g. Reticulum cell sarcoma

tion from coexisting hypertensive cerebrovascular disease. Cerebral edema is not a failure of uremia[12] but does occur in the acute encephalopathy associated with dialysis. Uremic encephalopathy is probably a metabolic encephalopathy resulting from chronic acidosis in which there are numerous secondary metabolic changes affecting neuronal function.

Clinical Features

The earliest signs of uremic encephalopathy consist of increased fatigue, decreased alertness, and inability to concentrate. As the condition progresses, the patient appears to be apathetic, then obtunded and stuporous. Examination at this stage reveals disorientation, perceptual errors, and defective memory; some patients may develop hallucinations and delirium. Myoclonic jerks, diffuse muscle twitching, and muscle cramps may precede frank seizure, which may be partial or generalized in type. The muscle tone is increased, and there are asterixis and tremors of the upper limbs. The deep tendon reflexes are increased, and release phenomena such as sucking, rooting, and grasp reflexes are usually present. Further progression of the encephalopathy leads to decortication, hemiparesis, decerebration, and coma.[276]

Diagnostic Procedures

The electroencephalogram shows progressive slowing with increasing severity of uremia. Symmetric bursts of slower theta or delta activity are seen in some cases, and focal spike activity occurs in patients with partial seizures.[331]

Treatment

1. Status epilepticus should be treated with intravenous diazepam, 10 to 20 mg, or diphenylhydantoin given at 50 mg/minute to a total of 1,000 mg.
2. Seizures in chronic uremic encephalopathy can be controlled by oral anticonvulsants, but it should be noted that serum diphenylhydantoin levels are depressed in uremia and a patient may be receiving an adequate dose of the drug with low serum levels.

Uremic Neuropathy

At least 50 per cent of patients with uremia develop symptoms of neuropathy.

Etiology and Pathology

The cause of uremic peripheral neuropathy remains unknown, but the improvement documented after adequate hemodialysis suggests that the neuropathy is the result of a retained metabolite.[193, 281] The histopathologic changes consist of a decrease in myelinated nerve fibers with areas of demyelination and remyelination, indicating a concomitant degenerative and reparative process.[92]

Clinical Features

One of the earliest features of uremic peripheral neuropathy is the restless leg syndrome. The patient complains of creeping, crawling, pruritic sensations within the lower limbs, worse at night and relieved by movement of the limbs. Another distressing symptom, burning feet, is also a manifestation of early uremic neuropathy.[179] The earlier symptoms are followed by the development of a distal symmetric sensorimotor neuropathy affecting the lower limbs with little evidence of upper limb involvement.

Diagnostic Procedures

Slowing of motor and sensory nerve conduction velocities can be recorded in uremic patients before clinical signs of peripheral neuropathy. This is a labile abnormality and often improves after dialysis.

Treatment

1. Cholestyramine, 5 mg two to four times a day, is reported to reduce the symptoms of the restless leg syndrome.[314]
2. Ultraviolet phototherapy will reduce pruritus after two or three weeks of therapy.[124]

Uremic Myopathy

Muscle cramps are an early symptom in uremia, but whether they indicate the presence of a uremic myopathy or early peripheral neuropathy is unknown. Proximal muscle weakness is quite common in uremic patients, but evidence of myositis by muscle biopsy is more likely to indicate an underlying vasculitis rather than a uremic myopathy. Other causes of proximal muscle weakness in uremia include the hyperparathyroidism of the chronic uremic state.[130] A defect in neuromuscular transmission has been reported in uremia in which patients show a curare-like response to antibiotics such as kanamycin, streptomycin, neomycin, gentamicin, polymyxin B, and sodium colistimethate. The weakness shows a partial response to anticholinesterase drugs.[339]

Complications of Dialysis

A number of neurologic abnormalities have been described after hemodialysis or peritoneal dialysis. Dialysis encephalopathy, or the dysequilibrium syndrome is probably due to cerebral edema and presents with headache, nausea, vomiting, muscle cramps, irritability, agitation, delirium, and seizures. Symptoms usually appear toward the end of a dialysis period or within 24 hours after dialysis.

A progressive and fatal dialysis dementia has been described in several patients undergoing chronic hemodialysis. The cause is obscure. Affected patients develop progressive dysarthria and dementia with choreoathetosis, asterixis, and seizures. There is some remission of symptoms following dialysis in the early stages of this condition, but dialysis dementia eventually becomes progressive and unresponsive to therapy.

A number of neurologic complications have been reported in uremic patients receiving chronic hemodialysis and should be considered when the physician is faced with a puzzling problem. Chronic meningitis or encephalitis due to the mycoses, toxoplasmosis, or cytomegalovirus may occur in patients who have had renal transplantation and are immunosuppressed. There is also an increased risk of subdural hematoma in chronic uremia. Wernicke's encephalopathy and central pontine myelinolysis are rare complications in uremic patients on restrictive diets.[97] The development of persistent progressive neurologic symptoms in a uremic patient may indicate the presence of a reticulum cell sarcoma. This tumor occurs with higher-than-expected frequency in immunosuppressed patients.[262]

Progressive Dialysis Encephalopathy

The development of successful extracorporeal dialysis has led to considerable improvement in the prognosis of chronic renal failure. The success of dialysis has been tempered somewhat by complications in some cases including the development of anemia, hemosiderosis, pulmonary embolism, osteomalacia, pericarditis, cardiomegaly, accelerated atherosclerosis, subdural hematoma, peripheral neuropathy, and psychologic disturbances. Some patients have developed an acute encephalopathy immediately after dialysis with confusion, disorientation, and convulsions followed by coma and death. Acute dialysis encephalopathy is probably due to cerebral edema and differs from subacute progressive dialysis encephalopathy, which has a characteristic clinical picture with distinctive although not characteristic electroencephalographic abnormalities.

Etiology and Pathology

The cause is unknown. It is assumed that progressive dialysis encephalopathy is a metabolic abnormality, and elevated levels of trace metals such as tin, rubidium, aluminum,[6] copper, zinc, lead, and cadmium may be present in some cases. Alternatively, it has been suggested that there may be a chronic deficiency of dopamine or asparagine in the brain. There is a similarity between the encephalopathy of hypophosphatemia and progressive dialysis encephalopathy suggesting that the latter condition may be related to high aluminum absorption and hypophosphatemia.[37] It has also been suggested that progressive dialysis encephalopathy is the result of chronic accumulation of sedatives such as the phenothiazines or diazepam because of poor excretion in chronic renal failure.[329]

The pathologic changes are nonspecific and are either normal[52] or mildly abnormal and consistent with a toxic encephalopathy[45] but are quite distinct from uremic encephalopathy.

Clinical Features

Progressive dialysis encephalopathy begins between 14 months and seven years after the start of dialysis treatments. Early symptoms consist of intermittent dysarthria or dysphasia, which may progress to severe dysphasia in some cases. There is a progressive dementia associated with disturbances in behavior, including agitation, delirium, paranoia, and hallucinations. Focal neurologic deficits such as hemiparesis may develop in some cases. Seizures and myoclonus are not uncommon. The condition is progressive, and death occurs 3 to 15 months after onset.

Diagnostic Procedures

The electroencephalogram shows normal or moderate slowing of background activity with intermittent appearance of bisynchronous delta activity and occasional epileptic activity in the frontocentral areas. This type of change is seen in a number of metabolic abnormalities.

Treatment

There is no known treatment for progressive dialysis encephalopathy. Chronic use of sedatives should be discontinued in all cases.

Pancreatic Encephalopathy

Acute encephalopathy has been reported to occur occasionally during the course of acute pancreatitis.

Etiology and Pathology

It is unlikely that pancreatic encephalopathy is a distinct clinical entity. The encephalopathy is probably due to one of the following conditions which are known to occur in acute pancreatitis:[170]

1. Hypoxic encephalopathy secondary to pulmonary fat embolism.
2. Fat embolism of the brain.
3. Disseminated intravascular coagulation.
4. Hyperglycemic-hyperosmolality syndrome.

Clinical Features

The illness begins with symptoms typical of acute pancreatitis including the sudden onset of abdominal pain, nausea, constipation, and a rigid abdomen. The diagnosis of acute pancreatitis is established by elevated serum amylase levels. In the following interval of approximately one to five days, the patient develops mental confusion, disorientation, and hallucinations and may progress to seizures, stupor, decerebrate rigidity, coma, and death in some cases. Focal signs such as dysphasia may occur.[309]

Diagnostic Procedures

1. The serum amylase level is elevated.
2. The cerebrospinal fluid may show a mild lymphocytic pleocytosis with slight elevation of protein.
3. The EEG shows diffuse slowing compatible with an encephalopathy. Focal delta activity may be noted particularly in patients with focal neurologic deficits.
4. Appropriate studies should be made to confirm or exclude disseminated intravascular coagulation (p. 402) and the hyperglycemic hyperosmolar syndrome (p. 252).

Treatment

1. Fluid and electrolyte balance should be maintained by use of intravenous fluid therapy. Daily records of fluid intake and output should be maintained together with frequent determination of the serum electrolytes.
2. Adequate ventilation and supplementary oxygen are indicated in suspected cases of hypoxic encephalopathy. Arterial blood gases should be determined at regular intervals. Patients who are stuporous or comatose with depressed respiration will require endotracheal intubation and assisted respiration with a mechanical respirator.
3. Disseminated intravascular coagulation or the hyperglycemic hyperosmolality syndrome should be treated promptly if present.

Neurologic Complications of the Porphyrias

There are two main types of porphyria: the erythropoietic type, which is without neurologic manifestations, and the hepatic type, which is associated with neurologic abnormalities (Table 5–11). The porphyrins are formed during the biosynthesis of heme (Fig. 5–8).

The initial step is the conversion of succinate or alpha ketoglutarate, both of which are derived from the tricarboxylic acid cycle into succinyl CoA.[46, 300] The condensation of succinyl with glycine in the presence of pyridoxine-phosphate-biotin and aminolevulinic acid synthetase produces delta aminolevulinic acid (ALA). Two molecules of ALA are condensed in the presence of ALA dehydrogenase to form the porphyrin precursor porphobilinogen. The metabolic pathway proceeds from porphobilinogen through uroporphyrinogen 111, coproporphyrinogen 111, protoporphyrinogen 111, to protoporphyrin 111. The latter unites with iron to form heme. The formation of uroporphyrinogen 1 and coproporphyrinogen 1 occurs as a by-product of porphobilinogen metabolism, and the amounts formed are very small under physiologic conditions. The porphyrins of the type 1 series do not have any physiologic action.

Acute Intermittent Porphyria

Acute intermittent porphyria is inherited as an autosomal dominant trait, but many latent cases occur and the history of inheritance may not be obtained. The condition is associated with an excess in production of delta aminolevulinic acid (ALA) and the porphyrin precursor porphobilinogen and may be due to an excess production of the enzyme delta aminolevulinic acid synthetase in the level due to a faulty feedback mechanism.

During an acute attack of porphyria there is a marked increase in the plasma levels of ALA, and brain levels of ALA attain values about half as great as plasma levels.[223] The increased concentrations of ALA in the brain mimic the effects of gamma aminobutyric acid (GABA) by binding at GABA receptor sites. Thus the neurologic symptoms of acute intermittent porphyria are

TABLE 5–11

Classification of the Porphyrias

Type	"Defect in Porphyria" Metabolism	Neurologic Manifestations
A. *Erythropoietic type*		
1. Erythropoietic porphyria	In developing red cells	Nil
2. Erythropoietic protoporphyria	In developing red cells	Nil
B. *Hepatic type*		
1. Acute intermittent porphyria	Liver	Yes

probably due to facilitation by ALA of synaptic transmission at GABA receptor sites.[239]

Pathology

The brain shows diffuse neuronal loss in the cortex and focal areas of infarction. The latter finding probably represents the effects of vascular spasm secondary to hypertension.

Clinical Features

Abdominal Symptoms. Attacks usually begin with abdominal colic, which may be followed by abdominal distention, nausea, vomiting, constipation, or diarrhea. An attack may last from several days to weeks, with considerable weight loss and emaciation.

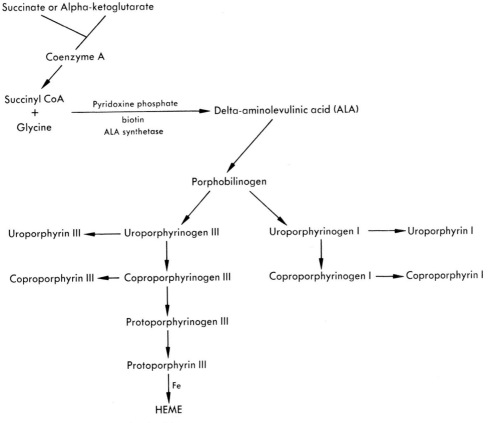

FIGURE 5–8. The biosynthesis of heme.

Hypertension. Hypertension and tachycardia are not infrequent during acute episodes.

Neurologic Manifestations. These are protean and include the following.

1. Mental changes may occur, with periods of excitement or mania, agitation, tremor, delirium, and hallucinations. Occasionally paranoid ideas or depression may occur.
2. Peripheral neuropathy may vary in intensity from a mild degree of peripheral motor weakness to a rapidly progressive involvement of all peripheral nerves with flaccid quadiparesis and respiratory failure. Electromyographic studies have suggested that this rapid type of porphyric polyneuropathy may be due to a failure of acetylcholine release at the neuromuscular junction; a condition resembling botulism.[369a] Sensory loss is usually less extensive than the motor involvement and if present is confined to the periphery of the limbs.
3. Brainstem or cranial nerve involvement is manifested by ophthalmoplegia, facial diplegia, dysarthria, and dysphagia. Involvement of the respiratory center will produce either hypo- or hyperventilation.[16] When hypoventilation occurs, it may compound the difficulties of a patient already in respiratory failure from peripheral neuropathy.
4. Seizures are not uncommon.
5. Transient amaurosis and permanent visual loss have been described due to spasm of the retinal vessels. Blindness of cerebral origin has been described from bilateral infarction of the occipital lobes.[191]

Latent forms of the disease may be precipitated into overt attacks following ingestion of barbiturates, sulfonamides, or griseofulvin, or following exposure to industrial solvents. Barbiturates probably potentiate the action of ALA at GABA receptor sites.

Diagnostic Procedures

1. Some patients excrete a brown-red urine (port wine urine) during an attack of acute intermittent porphyria. In the majority of cases, the "port wine urine" appearance occurs only after the urine has stood for some time. In all cases of suspected porphyria the urine should be placed in sunlight and observed for the development of the deep brownish-red color.
2. The diagnosis of acute intermittent porphyria requires the demonstration of excess porphobilinogen in the urine. The Watson-Schwartz or Hoesh tests, both of which use Ehrlich's aldehyde reagent, are sensitive screening tests for porphobilinogen. Quantitative determination of porphobilinogen levels should be carried out if the screening test is positive.[192]

Treatment

1. Patients with porphyria should avoid known agents that precipitate attacks, such as barbiturates, alcohol, sulfonamides, estrogen, chloroquine, griseofulvin, and alpha-methyldopa.[13] Attacks may increase during pregnancy and may be precipitated by infection.
2. The mental changes, particularly manic episodes, delirium, and excitement, may be controlled with adequate amounts of parenteral phenothiazines. Abdominal pain may require meperidine. Carbamazepine has been recommended for control of seizures.[208]
3. Fluid and electrolyte balance should be maintained by the intravenous route in all seriously ill patients.
4. A mechanical respirator will be required in patients with respiratory difficulties due to peripheral neuropathy or to involvement of the respiratory center. Respiratory failure may occur with alarming speed and has been associated with a high mortality (80 per cent) prior to the widespread use of respirators.
5. In severe cases hemodialysis may be considered.

Wilson's Disease (Hepatolenticular Degeneration)

Although Wilson was not the first to report this condition, his paper entitled "Progressive Lenticular Degeneration" led to its wide recognition, and the eponym Wilson's disease seems to be generally accepted. The condition is essentially a neuronal degeneration, possibly due to the toxic effects of copper in the cerebral parenchyma, with particular involvement of the basal ganglia and associated with cirrhosis of the liver.[356, 359]

Etiology and Pathology

Wilson's disease is inherited as an autosomal recessive trait and is associated with a disturbance in copper metabolism.

Normal Copper Metabolism. Copper is normally absorbed in small amounts from the intestinal tract and is transported to various parts of the body bound loosely to serum albumin. The majority of the copper in the copper/albumin complex is converted to ceruloplasmin by binding it to alpha 2 globulin. Copper forms specific copper protein complexes in a number of organs including the liver (hepatocuprein), brain (cerebrocuprein), and red cells (erythrocuprein). Copper is excreted in small amounts in sweat, bile, and urine.

Copper Metabolism in Wilson's Disease. There is an increased absorption of copper from the intestinal tract. The copper bound to albumin is not converted to ceruloplasmin at the normal rate and is deposited in the tissues. This results in an elevation of serum copper levels, decreased ceruloplasmin levels, and increased excretion of copper in the urine.[357]

The deposition of copper in the liver cells is increased, and it is possible that the development of cirrhosis of the liver and cerebral damage is due to the interference of specific enzyme systems by the tissue copper.[347] This would explain the peculiar sensitivity of neurons in the basal ganglia. The deposition of copper in the kidneys produces damage to the proximal renal tubules and impairment of the renal reabsorptive mechanisms. This results in aminoaciduria in some chronic cases of Wilson's disease with occasional glycosuria, an alkaline urine due to excess excretion of bicarbonate, and low serum uric acid and phosphate levels due to excess loss in the urine. The deposition of excess copper in Descemet's membrane in the cornea results in the development of the characteristic Kayser-Fleischer ring of Wilson's disease.

The brain, in Wilson's disease, may appear grossly normal or there may be some evidence of cortical atrophy. On coronal section, there may be atrophy of the globus pallidus and putamen with less severe involvement of the caudate nucleus. These areas may show staining and appear darker than usual, and cavitation occurs in some cases. Similar changes may occur in the dentate nuclei of the cerebellum. There also may be some staining of the internal capsule and central white matter. Microscopic examination shows a diffuse neuronal degeneration throughout the cortical gray matter with secondary gliosis. There may be almost complete neuronal loss in the basal ganglia with the presence of large hypertrophied astrocytes.

Clinical Features

Wilson's disease occurs equally in both sexes and has been identified in all races. The age of onset varies from 5 to 40 years, and there is often a familial similarity in the age of onset, clinical features, and biochemical findings. The earlier the onset, the worse the prognosis.

Clinical Types

1. The dystonic form is characterized by generalized rigidity, bradykinesis, dysarthria, and masklike facies. The gait is of the festinant type, resembling parkinsonism with a forward stoop and absence of arm swinging. Tremor is mild or absent. This form occurs in patients with onset after the age of 20 years.
2. The choreoathetotic form occurs in children and is more rapidly progressive. It is dominated by dystonic movements. There is marked facial grimacing and a characteristic open-mouthed appearance. Choreoathetotic movements of the upper limbs are prominent and may be interrupted by a proximal flapping tremor. Similar dystonic movements interfere with the gait, which has a curious dancing quality.
3. An acute hepatic form has been described with liver failure, acute intravascular hemolysis, marked hypercupremia, and cupriuria occurring as the first manifestation of Wilson's disease.[287, 288]
4. The disease may present as a fulminating hepatitis in children.[3]
5. A chronic active hepatitis without neurologic symptoms has been described in adults.[171]

All forms show the presence of Kayser-Fleischer rings in the cornea (Fig. 5–9). These rings are usually brownish-red or brownish-green (khaki or olive) and occur at the limbus, beginning as crescents in the superior and inferior aspects and gradually extending to join and form a complete ring.

All cases, if untreated, eventually show progressive dementia, with impaired judgment, failing memory, and emotional lability, epileptic seizures, progressive muscular weakness, and some degree of cirrhosis of the liver.

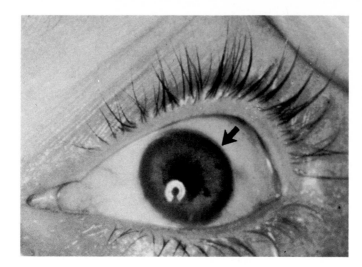

FIGURE 5–9. The appearance of Kayser-Fleischer rings of Wilson's disease. The rings are brownish-green ("olive drab" or khaki) and are located at the sclerocorneal junction. With treatment, the rings lose their brown color, which is caused by copper deposition.

Death usually occurs four or five years following the onset of symptoms, but patients with the later onset run a more chronic course and may survive for ten years or more. The prognosis has improved with penicillamine therapy.

Diagnostic Procedures

1. Serum ceruloplasmin levels are reduced below 20 mg/dl.
2. Serum copper levels are usually but not invariably elevated in Wilson's disease (above 80 to 150 mg/dl), and urinary copper excretion is increased (more than 10 to 30 mg/24 hours)
3. The presence of Kayser-Fleischer rings may be confirmed by slit lamp examination. Corneal copper content may be measured by x-ray–excitation spectometry, which provides a fast and reliable method for the early diagnosis of Wilson's disease.[24a] Sunflower cataracts occur in about 20 per cent of cases.[365]
4. Chronic cases show aminoaciduria, glycosuria, and alkaline urine due to excess bicarbonate excretion and low serum phosphate and uric acid levels.
5. Cirrhosis of the liver is usually mild in Wilson's disease, but there may be some increase in the bromsulfalein retention test. Hepatic copper concentrations are elevated (above 18 to 45 mg/gm dry weight) in symptomatic and asymptomatic Wilson's disease and can be measured after liver biopsy.
6. If there is doubt about the diagnosis of Wilson's disease, either a radioactive copper kinetic study using 64 Cu or 67 Cu or a liver biopsy with measurement of hepatic copper concentration can be done.[107]

Treatment

The treatment of Wilson's disease should be directed toward inhibiting absorption of copper from the intestinal tract and promoting excretion of tissue copper in the urine. The dietary copper should be restricted to 1 mg/day. Potassium sulfide, 40 mg given with meals, will "bind" dietary copper and prevent absorption. The best of the chelating agents for copper is penicillamine, which has replaced BAL in the treatment of Wilson's disease.[358] It has the advantage of oral administration and appears to be more effective than BAL with fewer side effects. Penicillamine is given in doses of from 1 to 4 gm/day in divided doses on an empty stomach. Vitamin B$_6$, pyridoxine, should be given during the period of penicillamine therapy to minimize the risk of optic neuritis. Side effects including optic neuritis are infrequent. There have been reports of acute sensitivity to the drug with fever, morbilliform rashes, leukopenia, thrombocytopenia, lymphadenopathy, and systemic lupus erythematosus. These reactions may be controlled by oral corticosteroids and penicillamine; therapy may then be reinstituted beginning with smaller doses. Other reactions, including anorexia, nausea, vomiting, and nephrosis, are infrequent. Administration of penicillamine can be continued during pregnancy.[333]

Nonclinically affected siblings should be treated with penicillamine if there are low ceruloplasmin levels and elevated hepatic copper content is found by liver biopsy.

Neurologic Complications of Amyloidosis

A classification of amyloidosis is given in Table 5–12.

The hereditary forms are discussed under the familial neuropathies. The nonhereditary forms of amyloidosis are of three types. Nonhereditary amyloidosis may occur in association with a chronic infection such as chronic tuberculosis, syphilis, or chronic septic infections of bones and joints. It has also been described in chronic pulmonary diseases such as empyema, bronchiectasis, and lung abscess and in association with rheumatoid arthritis, Hodgkin's disease, ulcerative colitis, and chronic pyelonephritis.

The second of the nonhereditary forms of amyloidosis is found in association with multiple myeloma or other major plasma cell dyscrasias, including Waldenström's macroglobulinemia and H-chain disease. The remaining cases of nonhereditary amyloidosis have often been called primary amyloidosis in the past, but they all probably have some plasma cell dyscrasia and immunoglobulin abnormality.

The clinical and pathologic lesions in amyloidosis depend on the site of deposition of amyloid. In some cases, it is deposited in the reticulum, in which case amyloid is found in the intima of blood vessels. It involves the liver, spleen, tongue, gastrointestinal tract, and kidneys, usually without involvement of peripheral nerves.[64] In other cases, there is deposition of amyloid in collagenous tissue, producing lesions in the adventitia of blood vessels. This pattern of amyloidosis is usually associated with peripheral neuropathy and amyloid deposition in the peripheral nerves.

Pathology

Amyloidosis of the brain and spinal cord has not been described although deposits may occasionally occur in the choroid plexus, pia mater, and adventitia of blood vessels within the central nervous system. In cases with peripheral neuropathy, amyloid may be found in both the posterior roots and sympathetic ganglia as well as in the epineurium and in the blood vessels of the peripheral nerves.

This results in axonal degeneration probably due to a toxic metabolic process affecting neuronal integrity.[336] Alternatively, the peripheral neuropathy may represent a compression neuropathy due to amyloid deposits within nerves.[82]

Clinical Features

Systemic involvement produces the following conditions: generalized weakness and weight loss; diplopia and ptosis due to external ophthalmoplegia; blurring of vision and progressive loss of visual acuity due to hemorrhagic retinitis and vitreous opacities; dysphagia, hoarseness, dysarthria, and respiratory distress due to involvement of the tongue (macroglossia), larynx, pharynx, esophagus, and trachea. Myocardial involvement produces cardiomegaly and chronic heart failure. Dermatologic signs are common and include pruritus, purpura, ecchymoses, scleroderma-like lesions, papules, nodules, and polypoid-like masses. Abdominal colic, constipation, diarrhea, bloody stools, or melena can result from gastrointestinal involvement. Generalized lymphadenopathy occurs in some cases.

The earliest symptoms of neurologic involvement consist of aching or burning pain often accompanied by lancinating pains in the lower extremities. This is followed by the development of distal numbness or hyperesthesia, which shows a symmetric progression proximally in the lower extremities. Involvement of the upper extremities and trunk occurs later. Distal muscle weakness is also a later phenomenon and is more pronounced in the lower extremities. Autonomic nervous system dysfunction is prominent with impotence in the male, postural syncope, orthostatic hypotension, and gastrointestinal disturbances with intermittent constipation and diarrhea. Loss of bladder sensation may occur with bladder distention and incomplete emptying of the bladder.

Diagnostic Procedures

1. Roentgenography of the chest may show hilar lymph node enlargement or cardiomegaly.
2. Liver function tests are usually abnormal.
3. Electrocardiographic changes are common.

TABLE 5–12

Classification of Amyloidosis

A. *Hereditary amyloidosis*
B. *Nonhereditary amyloidosis*
  1. Amyloidosis in chronic infection
  2. Amyloidosis with major plasma cell dyscrasias (multiple myeloma, Waldenström macroglobulinemia, H-chain disease)
  3. Amyloidosis with minor plasma cell dyscrasias

4. Lumbar puncture may reveal elevated protein levels due to nerve root involvement.
5. Serum and urine protein electrophoresis and immunoelectrophoresis will show the presence of a monoclonal immunoglobulin abnormality.[245]
6. Electromyography shows typical changes of denervation. Motor nerve conduction velocities are abnormal.
7. Tissue biopsy will ultimately confirm the diagnosis.[32] Rectal biopsy is the most successful method of tissue biopsy in amyloidosis. There is a higher percentage of positive results when compared with biopsy of other sites, and rectal biopsy has the advantage of being a relatively painless procedure. Renal or muscle biopsy is recommended in cases where amyloidosis is suspected, with a negative rectal biopsy. Sural nerve biopsy should be used in cases with primarily neurologic complaints.

Treatment

Associated diseases should be eradicated in the hope that this will delay or arrest the progress of the amyloidosis.

Long-term, high-single-dose, alternate-day corticosteroid therapy has been suggested on the basis that amyloidosis is an anomalous immune disorder.

Neuropathy of Adult Celiac Disease

A degenerative disease, bearing some resemblance to subacute combined degeneration of the spinal cord, has been described in adult celiac disease and may also occur in other forms of intestinal malabsorption. The condition is chronically progressive and does not respond to the usual treatment with vitamin B_{12}.[65]

Etiology and Pathology

The etiology is not clear, but the disease may represent the cumulative effect of multiple vitamin B complex deficiencies, including vitamins B_1, B_2, B_6, pyridoxine, pantothenic acid, and folic acid. There is diffuse loss of neurons in the cortical gray matter, basal ganglia, hypothalamus, cerebellum, brainstem, and anterior horns of the spinal cord. The posterior and lateral columns show demyelination, and there is a peripheral neuropathy with degeneration of muscle fibers on a neurogenic basis.

Clinical Features

The symptoms of malabsorption, including chronic diarrhea and weight loss, usually begin in childhood or adolescence and are present for many years. The neurologic symptoms usually begin later with ataxia and numbness of hands and feet with progressive deterioration and gradual impairment of memory. Examination reveals cerebellar ataxia, muscle weakness and wasting, decreased deep tendon reflexes, and peripheral sensory loss with impaired position and vibration sense in the lower limbs.

Diagnostic Procedures

1. Intestinal malabsorption can be demonstrated by the *d*-xylose absorption test and by analysis of the stool for fat, which usually exceeds 6 gm in 24 hours.
2. Serum folate levels are usually low.

Treatment

Injection of vitamin B_{12}, gluten-free diets, and corticosteroids have all been ineffective. Cases appear to be arrested or improve slowly when given high doses of parenteral vitamin B complex.

Neurologic Complications of Whipple's Disease

Whipple's disease is a rare disorder that is believed to be caused by a bacterial infection occurring on a background of defective immunologic mechanisms.[55]

Etiology and Pathology

There is considerable evidence pointing to an infection by bacteria in Whipple's disease: The pathologic changes are unique with deposits of periodic-acid-Schiff (PAS-positive) staining material in the intestinal and mesenteric lymphatic systems. The material may be intracellular, lying in foamy macrophages, or extracellular.

Examination of macrophages by electron microscopy shows that they contain bacilli in an intact form and in various stages of degradation that are responsible for the strongly PAS-positive staining.[290] Similar changes have been described in the central nervous system.

Clinical Features

Whipple's disease is characterized by intestinal malabsorption with chronic diarrhea, steatorrhea, weight loss, and multiple arthritis. Encephalopathy produces dementia, supranuclear paralysis of gaze, and seizures progressing to akinetic mutism and death. Bilateral uveitis occurs in some cases.[104] A myelopathy, with demyelination of the posterolateral column of the spinal cord and patchy demyelination of the peripheral nerves, has also been described.

Diagnostic Procedures

1. The cerebrospinal fluid shows a monocytic pleocytosis in most cases with normal glucose and protein content.
2. The diagnosis is established by intestinal biopsy; however, brain biopsy will be necessary when systemic manifestations are absent.

Treatment

A number of antibiotics have been reported to be effective in Whipple's disease. A regimen of 1.2 million units of procaine penicillin G and 1 gm of streptomycin daily for 14 days followed by 1 gm of tetracycline daily for 12 months has been used in the treatment of the systemic form of the disease.[209]

Tropical (Jamaican) Neuropathy

A syndrome of myeloneuropathy has been described in widely separated tropical countries, particularly Jamaica and the West Indian Islands.[231]

Etiology and Pathology

The condition is probably syndromic and may be the result of neurosyphilis complicated by chronic vitamin deficiencies or by the action of toxins ingested in locally grown foodstuffs, many of which contain cyanide. Clinically, it is closely related to neurolathyrism, a cause of myeloneuropathy due to ingestion of the Lathyrus bean in India.

The pathologic changes are mainly confined to the spinal cord, which shows a chronic meningomyelitis. There are thickening of the pia arachnoid and marked shrinkage of the posterior columns, which are pale owing to loss of myelin. The inflammatory process appears to be maximal around the pia vessels, and there is a perivascular inflammatory response around the pentrating vessels of the cord. The vessels show thickening and hyaline degeneration, and the exudate is chiefly lymphocytic, with some macrophages and a few plasma cells. There is marked loss of myelin and axis cylinders in the posterior columns and posterior nerve roots with degenerative changes in the anterior horn cells.

Clinical Features

Two distinct types of disturbance have been recognized: (1) an ataxic group in which there is optic atrophy, nerve deafness, marked ataxia due to posterior column involvement, mild spasticity, and distal wasting of the muscles in the lower limbs, particularly affecting the peroneal group; and (2) a spastic group, which presents with progressive spastic paraparesis associated with ataxia of the posterior column type in about 50 per cent of cases. Nerve deafness, optic atrophy, and bladder involvement may occur in later stages.

The course tends to be chronic with apparent arrest of symptoms after several years in both groups.

Diagnostic Procedures

1. There is a positive serologic test for syphilis in about 30 per cent of the ataxic group and 60 per cent of the spastic group.
2. The spinal fluid is abnormal in the majority of cases in the spastic group with lymphocytic pleocytosis and an elevated protein content. The postive type of colloidal gland reaction may be present in some of these cases, but the serologic test for syphilis is usually negative.

Treatment

The use of adequate doses of penicillin in serologic positive cases does not seem to alter the course of the disease. Adequate diet, vitamin supplements, and intense physical therapy produce improvement in early cases.

Metabolic Abnormalities Involving the Skull

Fibrous Dysplasia of the Skull

The replacement of bone by fibrous tissue in this disease may be limited to one bone or present as a generalized process. Involvement of the skull occurs in 50 per cent of cases of fibrous dysplasia, with one or both frontal or sphenoid bones affected. There is progressive asymmetry of the skull, with visual loss due to compression of the optic nerve in the optic foramen. Optic atrophy will occur unless the compression is relieved by surgery. Stenosis of the external canal and middle ear may lead to progressive hearing loss and deafness in some cases. Precocious puberty and an increased incidence of seizures have also been recorded.

Osteopetrosis

The formation of dense, compact, but abnormally brittle bone is inherited as an autosomal recessive trait in children and as an autosomal dominant trait in the more benign form seen in adults. When the skull is involved, there may be narrowing of the optic foramina with optic atrophy and blindness. The disorder may be complicated by hydrocephalus, mental retardation, subdural hematoma, and anemia in children.[296] The adult form runs a more benign course.[169]

Benign Intracranial Hypertension

The term "pseudotumor cerebri" is widely used for this condition, particularly by neurosurgeons, although "benign intracranial hypertension" is nosologically more accurate since it describes the essential features. The condition is usually a benign elevation of cerebrospinal fluid pressure without evidence of infection, any intracranial mass, or hydrocephalus.[130] The majority of cases show spontaneous resolution, and major decompressive procedures are rarely needed.

Etiology and Pathology

The main causes are listed in Table 5–13. The condition is a syndrome, not a disease, and appears to be a nonspecific change in the blood vessels or blood-brain barrier caused by a number of unrelated disorders. There is, however, some evidence of endocrine imbalance and coagulation disorder in many of the causative conditions.[91] Since the disorder is benign, autopsy reports are rare, but the brain is edematous with diminution of ventricular size.

Some cases show an increase in cerebral blood volume,[216] and it is possible that there are varying degrees of increased cerebral blood volume and increased tissue water content of the brain in the syndrome of benign intracranial hypertension.[274a]

Clinical Features

Benign intracranial hypertension occurs in infants, children, and adults. In infancy, the presenting signs are irritability, lack of appetite, and

TABLE 5–13

Benign Intracranial Hypertension

1. *Vitamin A excess*
2. *Vitamin A deficiency* in infants
3. *Tetracycline therapy* in infants
4. *Hypoparathyroidism*
5. *Following withdrawal of corticosteroids*
6. *Addison's disease*
7. *Occurrence at the menarche*—water retention in response to ovarian hormones
8. *Obesity in adolescent females*—possible imbalance in adrenocortical, other hormonal, and estrogen imbalance
9. *Pregnancy*—early in pregnancy, when there may be falling adrenal corticosteroid levels, *thrombophlebitis and cryofibrinogenemia* with sudden change in hormonal levels
10. *Menstrual irregularity*—presumably associated with abnormalities in endocrine activity—often a protracted condition
11. *Carbon dioxide retention* (pulmonary encephalopathy, hypoventilation syndrome of extreme obesity)
12. *Dural sinus thrombosis associated with thrombophlebitis and cryofibrinogenemia*

vomiting. The only physical abnormality is a bulging fontanel. There have been reports of intracranial hypertension and mental retardation in infants receiving diets deficient in vitamin A.

Older children usually complain of headache and "dizziness" with occasional nausea and vomiting. They may be lethargic or irritable, and there is papilledema on funduscopic examination. The neurologic examination is normal in all other aspects.

The symptoms usually begin with headache in the adult followed by "dizziness," which is usually a feeling of lightheadedness or unsteadiness and occasional nausea and vomiting. Lethargy and some loss of visual acuity (usually described as blurring of vision) occur at a later stage. Examination reveals papilledema without any neurologic abnormalities. The visual fields may be constricted, with enlargement of the blind spot in more protracted cases.

The diagnosis of benign intracranial hypertension is usually indicated by the history. Possibly there has been excessive vitamin A intake[255] for the treatment of acne, or vitamin A has been deficient in the diet of infants, or there has been recent tetracycline or nitrofurantoin[243] therapy, all of which are known causes of benign intracranial hypertension. The physician should inquire about recent corticosteroid therapy and consider this diagnosis at the menarche or in the obese adolescent female. When the condition occurs in older female patients, there is usually a history of prolonged menstrual irregularity.

Diagnostic Procedures

1. Despite the clinical impression of benign intracranial hypertension, the diagnosis of a possible brain tumor has to be excluded in all patients, unless there is rapid resolution of symptoms.
2. The skull roentgenogram shows separation of the sutures in infants and children with thinning of the dorsum sellae in chronic cases.
3. The electroencephalogram is often abnormal, particularly in children, the abnormalities ranging from bilateral synchronous frontal slow wave activity to bursts of 3-Hz generalized spike and wave activity.[34]
4. Computed tomography shows a normal scan with normal appearance of the ventricular system,[80, 157] although excessively small ventricles have been reported.[143] If the CT scan is normal in a patient with clinical findings compatible with the diagnosis of benign intracranial hypertension, no further neuroradiologic tests are indicated unless there is further deterioration in the patient's neurologic condition.[363]
5. The cerebrospinal fluid is under increased pressure without any increase in cells or protein elevation. All chemical tests are normal.

Treatment

When the cause is known, e.g., the infant is receiving tetracycline, the condition will resolve rapidly when the use of the drug is discontinued. If the condition follows corticosteroid therapy, there is usually some response on restoring the medication, and most cases will resolve over a period of weeks with gradual withdrawal. The obese adolescent girl requires a reducing diet, which is effective in most cases. Older women with menstrual irregularities may respond to hormonal regulation.

The course of benign intracranial pressure is usually self-limiting with spontaneous remission or improvement following repeated lumbar puncture. More protracted cases show a good response

to corticosteroid therapy[336] (methylprednisolone, 64 mg daily). The effect of therapy should be monitored by measuring cerebrospinal fluid pressure by lumbar puncture.

Surgical procedures such as lumbar-peritoneal shunts or subtemporal decompression are rarely necessary.

Neurologic Complications Due to the Use of Oral Contraceptives

Oral contraceptives have been used extensively since the early 1960s, and the results of long-term prospective studies involving large numbers of women are now becoming available.[235, 342] In essence, these studies indicate that the risk of circulatory disease increases with the duration of oral contraceptive use and that this risk is concentrated in older women who are cigarette smokers.[277] The circulatory diseases identified in the group of women include subarachnoid hemorrhage, malignant hypertension, cardiomyopathy, and mesenteric artery thrombosis. Oral contraceptives are anovulary agents which consist of an estrogen or varying mixtures of estrogens and progesterones. This means that women taking these agents may possibly be subjected to some of the physiologic changes associated with pregnancy, such as salt and water retention and an increased tendency to thromboembolic phenomena.

Some women suffering from migraine have reported increased symptoms when using oral contraceptive agents, but this does not seem to be supported by prospective studies and there have been reports of improvement in migraine in some cases by the use of oral contraceptives.

There have been a series of cases studied of acute stroke occurring in young women taking oral contraceptives with implications that these agents were solely responsible for the thromboembolic episode.[61, 307] Some retrospective studies have shown an increase in the incidence of stroke in young women using oral contraceptives.[62] Others have failed to do so.[165] There are no prospective studies showing a significant association between oral contraceptives and stroke due to thromboembolism at this time.[90, 113] However, the physician should prudently avoid prescribing oral contraceptive agents to women with a history of thromboembolism, diabetes, migraine, or hypertension[212] who may be prone to cardiovascular disease.

Neurologic Complications of the Phenothiazine and Antipsychotic Drugs

The use of phenothiazine, butyrophenones, and thioxanthenes has greatly improved the medical care of the mentally ill, the agitated states, and chronic anxiety, as well as the treatment of nausea and vomiting. However, side effects are seen occasionally in patients under treatment with these drugs. Nonneurologic side effects include drowsiness, miosis, dryness of the mouth, nasal congestion, constipation, and mild fever. Jaundice and agranulocytosis have been rarely reported as serious complications. Other rare effects, such as skin pigmentation, urticaria, photosensitivity, exfoliative dermatitis, hypotension, lactation and breast engorgement, and lens opacities, have also been reported. The neurologic side effects are not uncommon and will be discussed in detail.[217]

Etiology and Pathology

Since the neurologic side effects can be categorized as "extrapyramidal," it is probable that all the drugs in this group act at a cellular level in the basal ganglia and substantia nigra by interfering with the neurotransmitter balance, particularly the catecholamines, and by depleting dopamine. Pathologic and biochemical evidence is, however, incomplete at this time.

Clinical Features

There are three types of neurologic disorders resulting from administration of the phenothiazines, butyrophenones, and thioxanthenes, and all are characterized by abnormal movements. In certain individuals who are predisposed, a single dose may produce neurologic complications.

Acute Dystonia. This type of disorder usually occurs shortly after injection or oral administration of a phenothiazine. The patient experiences intermittent pulling of the face, tongue, or neck, which is followed by a prolonged dystonic posturing of the affected parts. The head and eyes may be tonically deviated upward or to one side, and speech may be difficult or impossible. The back, arm, and leg muscles may be affected resulting in bizarre movements of the pelvis and difficulty with gait. The tongue may be protruded or the neck maintained in an abnormal posture. Opisthotonos may occur in some cases. Acute dystonia is often mistaken for tetanus and may be of sufficient severity to cause dislocation of the jaw.

Tardive Dyskinesia. There is a tendency for this type of side effect to occur after weeks or months of phenothiazine, butyrophenone, or thioxanthene therapy. The principal features of tardive dyskinesia are:

1. Involuntary movements of the mouth, tongue, and lips associated with choreoathetoid movements of the trunk and extremities.
2. Late occurrence of these movements in the course of neuroleptic treatment. The movements may appear after reduction in dosage or discontinuation of therapy.
3. The movements persist for months or years.
4. Antiparkinsonian agents are ineffective in reducing the dyskinetic movements and may aggravate the condition.

Parkinsonism. This is probably the most common form of akinesia occurring in patients taking phenothiazine drugs. The symptoms vary from a mild bradykinesia to a marked generalized rigidity with lack of facial expression, flexed posture, loss of associated movements, and a festinant gait. Tremor is less frequent but may occur in some cases.

Treatment

The acute dystonia responds to withdrawal of the phenothiazine and intravenous injections of diazepam (Valium), 5 to 10 mg, diphenhydramine hydrochloride (Benadryl), 25 to 50 mg, or procyclidine. The response is prompt and in many cases dramatic. A single treatment with withdrawal of phenothiazine may be all that is required in the majority of cases, although some few patients show a return of symptoms, requiring further injections.

Tardive dyskinesia is persistent but is not necessarily irreversible if all antipsychotic drugs are withdrawn, particularly in young patients. The development of symptoms of tardive dyskinesia may be delayed and the symptoms diminished by frequent administration during the day rather than using a single daily dose.[166] Oral choline, 150 to 200 mg/kg/day, will decrease involuntary movements in some patients with tardive dyskinesia.[138] but may induce depression. Haloperidol may produce improvement in some cases of tardive dyskinesia induced by phenothiazines. A combination of tricyclic antidepressant and lithium is reported to give good results in patients with tardive dyskinesia but can only be used if the patient has been withdrawn from antipsychotic medication.[291a]

Phenothiazine-induced parkinsonism does not respond to levodopa but can be controlled by the anticholinergic drugs, particularly procyclidine.[229]

Neurologic Complications of Quinidine

Quinidine is used extensively for the control of cardiac arrhythmias, and many elderly patients with neurologic problems receive the drug for concomitant heart disease. Quinidine has been associated with a progressive dementia with symptoms resembling Alzheimer's disease. There is a rapid recovery when quinidine is discontinued.[123] There is also an interaction between quinidine and anticonvulsant drugs with low plasma levels and rapid excretion of quinidine in patients receiving barbiturates or diphenylhydantoin.[75]

Neurologic Complications of Barbiturate Poisoning

Barbiturates are still the most common agents among all the solids and liquids causing death by poisoning,[168] and barbiturate intoxication should always be considered in the differential diagnosis of coma of undetermined etiology. Accidental ingestion also occurs, particularly in children.[218]

Etiology and Pathology

Barbiturates in large doses depress cerebral blood flow and metabolism and interfere with cerebral synaptic action and probably alter neuronal membrane excitability. At autopsy, the brain shows changes secondary to cardiopulmonary collapse such as congestion and edema.

Clinical Features

The diagnosis may be difficult because other drugs such as bromide, chlordiazepoxide, meprobamate, and phenothiazines may have been ingested also. In suicide attempts, alcohol may also be ingested, and the odor on the breath may lead to a mistaken diagnosis of acute alcoholism.

Moderate barbiturate intoxication resembles al-coholic intoxication except that nystagmus is evident and there is vertical gaze palsy.[99] The voice is thick and dysarthric, insight is impaired, or there is ataxia; and other signs of cerebellar incoordination are evident.

In severe intoxication, the patient is comatose and the tendon jerks are markedly depressed or absent. There may be bilateral extensor plantar responses. The pupils show hippus or, later in deep coma, may be dilated and fail to respond to light. Respiration is depressed and respiratory arrest may occur. Hypoxia and respiratory acidosis are common. The blood pressure falls owing to depression of the vasomotor center and the patient develops shock. Renal failure may result. Respiratory complications such as atelectasis, pneumonia, and pulmonary edema are common and are the leading cause of morbidity and mortality.

Diagnostic Procedures

1. Barbiturate levels in the blood and urine are elevated and can be measured accurately by ultraviolet spectrophotometric analysis as an emergency screening procedure.[303] Barbiturate levels of 10 mg per cent for long-acting barbiturates and 3 mg per cent for short-acting barbiturates are said to be "potentially lethal," but these figures are unreliable, and treatment should be based on the clinical state of the patient rather than serum barbiturate levels.

2. The EEG in profound coma shows slow waves or may become flat[29] with the potential still present for recovery. The EEG may appear strikingly normal in light coma (Fig. 5–10).

Treatment

General Measures. The patient should be treated in an intensive care unit.[286] Gastric lavage and aspiration of any recently ingested drug should be performed. This is effective if performed within four hours of drug ingestion. Oxygen should be given by nasal catheter and a patient airway preserved by frequent suctioning of secretions. A low-pressure cuffed endotracheal tube should be inserted if there is a tendency for the accumulation of secretions. The blood P_{CO_2}, P_{O_2}, and pH should be monitored. Roentgenograms of the chest should be taken daily since pneumonia is a frequent complication in barbiturate intoxication. Bronchoscopy is advised for the aspiration of tracheobronchial obstruction if there is

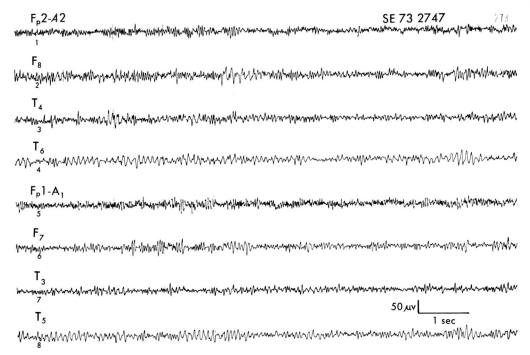

FIGURE 5–10. Electroencephalogram made from a patient in coma following ingestion of an overdose of barbiturates. There is diffuse fast activity in all leads, which is characteristic of this condition. F_p, frontopolar; F, frontal; T, temporal. Even numbers, right hemisphere. Odd numbers, left hemisphere.

evidence of atelectasis. Mechanical respiration should be instituted as soon as the blood gas analysis indicates inadequate respiration.

Shock requires prompt treatment with intramuscular metaraminol (Aramine), intravenous infusions of low-molecular-weight dextran, or whole blood if necessary. Should renal failure occur, hemodialysis is required.

Removal of Barbiturate. Hemodialysis is the most effective way of removing the barbiturate. Other methods include peritoneal dialysis and forced alkaline mannitol diuresis. The majority of patients can, however, be managed successfully without using these methods, and they are recommended only for the deeply comatose patient. Any of these procedures carries the risk of inducing electrolyte imbalance.

The use of analeptic agents is no longer recommended.

Treatment of Hypothermia. A number of patients who take potentially lethal doses of barbiturates remain outdoors in cold weather and develop hypothermia and coma. The hypothermia should be treated by gentle rewarming. This can be accomplished by peritoneal dialysis with warm fluid, which serves the double purpose of removal of barbiturate and slow elevation of body temperature.

Neurologic Complications of Antibiotics

Many antibiotics can cause severe neurotoxic reactions. These reactions include vestibular and auditory ototoxicity, optic neuritis, neuropathy, neuromuscular blockade, and increased intracranial pressure.

Streptomycin and gentamicin can produce dysfunction of the vestibular division of the eighth cranial nerve, and streptomycin, neomycin, kanamycin, and vancomycin can produce dysfunction of the auditory division of the eighth cranial nerve with irreversible deafness in some cases. An acute psychosis with visual hallucinations has been reported in patients receiving gentamicin therapy.[48]

Streptomycin and chloramphenicol have also been reported to cause impairment of vision due to optic neuritis. Chloramphenicol, streptomycin, neomycin, kanamycin, polymyxin B, colistin, amphotericin B, and nitrofurantoin may cause peripheral neuropathy in susceptible individuals.

Neomycin, streptomycin, kanamycin, polymyxin B, and colistin may produce muscular weakness in susceptible individuals due to neuromuscular blockade.

As described earlier in this chapter, tetracycline may cause benign intracranial hypertension.[249] Massive intravenous injections of penicillin compounds may cause seizures and cerebral toxicity. This is extremely common when penicillin is injected directly into the spinal fluid or directly into the brain. Amphotericin B can cause tremor, incontinence, mental cloudiness, weakness of the respiratory muscles, and flaccid paralysis of the limbs.[340]

Neurologic Complications of Griseofulvin

Griseofulvin is a widely used fungistatic for the chronic treatment of a number of epidermophytoses (particularly so-called "athlete's foot"). Prolonged usage may cause a peripheral neuropathy with paresthesias of the hands and feet and occasionally signs of involvement of the spinal cord. Withdrawal of the drug usually is associated with prompt recovery.

Neurologic Complications of Vincristine

Vincristine sulfate is widely used as an oncolytic agent in the treatment of leukemias and lymphomas. The toxic side effects of vincristine are mainly neurologic and include seizures, mental changes, myalgias with muscle atrophy, and peripheral neuropathy. The latter is a mixed motor and sensory neuropathy which is symmetric and usually appears after about two months of treatment.[149] The motor nerve conduction velocities are normal or slightly prolonged. The peripheral neuropathy is reversible after stopping vincristine. A mononeuropathy has also been reported during vincristine therapy.[198]

Neurologic Complications of Poisoning by Anticholinergic Drugs

Atropine, scopolamine, belladonna, tricyclic antidepressants, and phenothiazines have anticholinergic properties and all may produce symptoms of poisoning. Accidental ingestion of tricyclic antidepressants or phenothiazines by young children is not uncommon, and deliberate overdosage may occur in depressed patients. Toxic effects are also seen in parkinsonian patients treated with anticholinergic drugs.

Pathogenesis

Atropine-like substances stimulate the medulla and cerebral cortex. The rate and depth of respiration are increased. Cerebral excitation leads to confusion and excitement. Eventually, large enough doses produce cerebral depression.

Clinical Features

Clinical signs appear within 30 to 45 minutes of ingestion. The mouth becomes dry, the vision is blurred, and there is photophobia. The skin is hot, dry, and flushed. A rash may appear over the face and upper trunk. The body temperature rises to alarming heights. The pulse is weak and rapid. The patient is agitated, anxious, restless, and confused and may be "picking invisible objects from the air." Visual hallucinations may occur. Gait is ataxic and speech is thick. Memory and articulation are impaired. Mania and delirium may occur.

Diagnostic Procedures

A slow intravenous injection of 2 mg physostigmine will improve consciousness as well as life-threatening cardiac arrhythmias. If there is no response, a second injection should be given after 20 minutes.[48] Physostigmine crosses the blood-brain barrier and effectively reverses the neurologic effects of anticholinergic drugs.

Treatment

1. Gastric lavage should remove any unabsorbed alkaloid.
2. Once the patient shows response to the diagnostic dose of physostigmine, additional injection of 1 to 4 mg may be given every 30 to 60 minutes as necessary.[249]
3. Oxygen should be administered.
4. The temperature should be maintained at or

below 102°F with ice packs or nursing on a refrigerated blanket.

Neurologic Effects of Bromide Intoxication

Acute bromide intoxication is rare because the drug is irritating to the gastrointestinal tract, but the drug is slowly excreted by the kidney.

Bromide levels may gradually increase in the cerebrospinal fluid and central nervous system if the drug is ingested daily. There is an equally slow fall in concentration after discontinuation of the drug with a half-life of about 12 days.[190]

Clinical Features

Mental disturbance is the most common feature, consisting of impaired thought and memory, drowsiness, irritability, and emotional disturbances. Delirium, delusions, hallucinations, lethargy, and coma follow the ingestion of large doses. There are tremors, dysarthria, incoordination, cerebellar signs, decreased tendon jerks, and extensor plantar responses. Rarely, papilledema and/or symptoms resembling neuropathy may be present.[175] A skin rash is common, beginning on the face and hair roots, and spreading over the entire body. Signs of permanent neurologic damage with dysarthria and cerebellar ataxia have been reported after withdrawal of bromides.

Diagnostic Procedures

1. The EEG shows diffuse high-voltage slow waves.
2. Blood bromide levels above 18 mEq/liter are almost invariably associated with toxic signs.

Treatment

1. Intravenous administration of normal saline (at least 6 gm daily) increases the excretion of bromide.
2. Oral thiazides increase bromide excretion.
3. Hemodialysis may be used in comatose patients.

Neurologic Complications of Methyl Alcohol Poisoning

Poisoning by methyl alcohol results usually from ingestion by alcoholics who are under the impression that it is ethyl alcohol. It is obtained as a heating agent ("canned heat") or as cleaning or rubbing alcohol. It is rapidly absorbed from the stomach and causes depression of the central nervous system similar to that of ethyl alcohol. In addition, it causes severe metabolic acidosis due to the production of formic acid and has a tragic but specific toxicity for the optic nerves. It is postulated that formic acid diffuses into the optic nerve head from the adjacent choroid or cerebrospinal fluid, producing damage and swelling of the oligodendroglial cells. This in turn causes axonal compression, axoplasmic flow stasis, axonal swelling, and papilledema.[149]

Clinical Features

Eight to thirty-six hours after ingestion of methyl alcohol the patient complains of headache, vertigo, vomiting, abdominal pain, restlessness, and blurring of vision. The optic disks appear congested and swollen. The visual symptoms may progress to blindness, with optic atrophy and loss of the pupillary light reaction. Restlessness and delirium may be marked, and the severe acidosis results in Kussmaul breathing. Coma may suddenly develop.

Diagnostic Procedures

1. The blood pH is low and the plasma bicarbonate is low.
2. Methanol and formic acid are present in the blood and urine.
3. The cerebrospinal fluid pressure is often elevated owing to cerebral edema. The spinal fluid is normal is appearance and content.

Treatment

Correction of the acidosis is the most important aspect of treatment. The intravenous use of alkalizing agents, such as bicarbonate, is recommended. Water and electrolyte balance should be maintained. Ethanol slows down the oxidation of methanol and may be administered if alkali therapy is not available.

The patient usually recovers from the acute intoxication, but the damage to the optic nerve is irreversible and many have a severe reduction in visual acuity or permanent blindness.

Neurologic Complications of Gold Therapy

Chrysotherapy is still used in the treatment of rheumatoid arthritis and may be responsible for a number of neurologic complications. A reversible gold encephalopathy with disorientation and impaired memory has been described.[219] Other toxic effects include seizures, cranial nerve palsies, transverse myelitis, and a symmetric peripheral neuropathy.[355]

Treatment

Corticosteroids have been advised on the assumption that the neurologic complications are due to immunologic hypersensitivity. D-Penicillamine will increase the excretion of gold.

Cited References

1. Aberg, H. E.; Herbai, G. L.; and Westerberg, C.-E. Recurrent and reversible cerebellar ataxia with concomitant episodes of hyperthyroidism. *Acta Med. Scand.,* **199:**331–34, 1976.
2. A definition of irreversible coma. Report of the Ad Hoc Committee of the Harvard Medical School to Examine the Definition of Brain Death. *J.A.M.A.,* **205:**337–40, 1968.
3. Adler, R.; Mahnovski, V.; et al. Fulminating hepatitis—a presentation of Wilson's disease. *Am. J. Dis. Child.,* **131:**870–72, 1977.
4. Agamanolis, D. P.; Chester, E. M.; et al. Neuropathology of experimental vitamin B_{12} deficiency in monkeys. *Neurology* (Minneap.), **26:**905–14, 1976.
4a. Albert, M. S.; Butters, N.; and Levin, J. Temporal gradients in the retrograde amnesia of patients with alcoholic Korsakoff's disease. *Arch. Neurol.,* **36:**211–16, 1979.
5. Alexander, M. P.; Goodkin, D. E.; and Poser, C. M. Solitary plasmacytoma producing cranial neuropathy. *Arch. Neurol.,* **32:**777–78, 1975.
6. Alfrey, A. C.; LeGendre, R.; and Kaehny, W. D. Dialysis encephalopathy syndrome: possible aluminum intoxication. *N. Engl. J. Med.,* **294:**184–88, 1976.
7. Allen, J. P.; Imbus, C. E.; et al. Neurologic impairment induced by hyperventilation in children with sickle cell anemia. *Pediatrics,* **58:**124–26, 1976.
8. Allen, N. Life or death of the brain after cardiac arrest. Guest editorial. *Neurology* (Minneap.), **27:**805–806, 1977.
9. Allsop, J., and Turner, B. Cerebellar degeneration associated with chronic alcoholism. *J. Neurol. Sci.,* **3:**238–58, 1966.
10. An appraisal of the criteria of cerebral death—a summary statement (Final report: Collaborative study of cerebral survival HEW NIH NINDS Contract 1-MS-1-2316 Bethesda M.D. April 1974). *J.A.M.A.,* **237:**982–86, 1977.
11. Arieff, A. I., and Guisado, R. Effects on the central nervous system of hypernatremic and hyponatremic states. *Kidney Int.,* **10:**104–16, 1976.
12. Arieff, A. I.; Giusado, R.; and Massry, S. G. Uremic encephalopathy: studies on biochemical alterations in the brain. *Kidney Int.,* suppl. **2:**194–99, 1975.
13. Asbury, A. K.; Victor, M.; and Adams, R. D.

Uremic polyneuropathy. *Arch. Neurol.,* **8:**413–28, 1963.
14. Ashby, P.; Carlen, P. L.; et al. Ethanol and spinal presynaptic inhibition in man. *Ann. Neurol.,* **1:**478–80, 1977.
15. Bajandas, F. J., and Smith, J. D. Optic neuritis in hypoparathyroidism. *Neurology* (Minneap.), **26:**451–54, 1976.
16. Baker, N. H., and Messert, B. Acute intermittent porphyria with central neurogenic hyperventilation. *Neurology* (Minneap.), **17:**559–66, 1967.
16a. Ballard, J. O.; Towtighe, J.; et al. Neurologic complications of acute myelomonoblastic leukemia of four years duration. *Neurology* (Minneap.), **28:**174–78, 1978.
17. Banker, B. Q., and Cheski, C. S. Infarction of thigh muscle in diabetic patient. *Neurology* (Minneap.), **23:**667–77, 1973.
18. Banta, R. G., and Markesbery, W. R. Elevated manganese levels associated with dementia and extrapyramidal signs. *Neurology* (Minneap.), **27:**213–16, 1977.
18a. Barron, S. A., and Heffner, R. R., Jr. Weakness in malignancy: evidence for a remote effect of tumor on distal axons. *Ann. Neurol.,* **4:**268–74, 1978.
19. Bartter, F. C., and Schwartz, W. B. The syndrome of inappropriate secretion of antidiuretic hormone. *Am. J. Med.,* **42:**790–806. 1967.
20. Bean, C., and Ladisch, S. Chorea associated with a subdural hematoma in a child with leukemia. *J. Pediatr.,* **90:**255–56, 1977.
21. Beattie, A. D., Moore, M. R.; et al. Role of chronic low-level lead exposure in the aetiology of mental retardation. *Lancet,* **1:**589–92, 1975.
22. Beaupre, E. M., and Growney, P. M. Pyridoxine-responsive anemia with neuropathy. *Ann. Intern. Med.,* **59:**724–30, 1963.
23. Behnke, R. H. Recognition and management of alcohol withdrawal syndrome. *Hosp. Pract.,* **11:**79–84, 1976.
24. Behse, F., and Buchthal, F. Alcoholic neuropathy: Clinical electrophysiological and biopsy findings. *Ann. Neurol.,* **2:**95–110, 1977.
24a. Beltern, M.; Chajek, T.; et al. Non-invasive quantitation of corneal copper in hepatolenticular degeneration (Wilson's disease). *Lancet,* **1:**341–92, 1976.
25. Berger, R. L.; Stanton, J. R.; Liversage, R. M., Jr.; Goldrick, D. M.; Graham, J. H.; and Stohlmann, F., Jr. Blood exchange in the treatment of hepatic coma. *J.A.M.A.* **202:**267–74, 1967.
26. Berggren, L., and Hansson, O. Absorption of intestinal antiseptics derived from 8-hydroxyquinolines. *Clin. Pharmacol. Ther.,* **9:**67–70, 1968.
27. Bickler, R. N. Treatment of diabetes insipidus with carbamazepine. *Lancet,* **2:**749, 1976.
28. Birchall, R., and Batson, H. M., Jr. Primary aldosteronism; unusual manifestations and a practical approach to diagnosis. *Med. Clin. North Am.,* **51:**861–70, 1967.
29. Bird, T. D., and Plum, F. Recovery from barbiturate overdose coma with a prolonged isoelectric encephalogram. *Neurology* (Minneap.), **18:**436–60, 1968.

30. Blackwood, W.; McMenemey, W. H.; Meyer, A.; Norman, R. M.; and Russel, D. S. Anoxic poisons and the problems of anoxia and selective vulnerability In *Greenfield's Neuropathology.* Williams & Wilkins, Baltimore, 1963, pp. 237–61.

31. Blass, J. P., and Gibson, G. E. Abnormality of a thiamine requiring enzyme in patients with Wernicke-Korsakoff syndrome. *N. Engl. J. Med.,* **297:**1367–70, 1977.

32. Blum, A., and Sohar, E. The diagnosis of amyloidosis; ancillary procedures. *Lancet,* **1:**721–24, 1962.

33. Blum, M.; Kirsten, M.; and Worth, M. H. Reversible hypertension caused by the hypercalcemia of hyperparathyroidism, vitamin D toxicity and calcium infusion. *J.A.M.A.,* **237:**262–63, 1977.

34. Bodensteiner, J., and Matsuo, F. EEG in benign intracranial hypertension. *Dis. Nerv. System,* **38:**1007–10, 1977.

35. Bomb, B. S.; Bedi, H. K.; and Bhatnagar, L. K. Post-ischemic paresthesiae in pellagrins. *J. Neurol. Neurosurg. Psychiat.,* **40:**265–67, 1977.

36. Boor, J. W., and Hurtig, H. I. Persistent cerebellar ataxia after exposure to toluene. *Ann. Neurol.,* **2:**440–42, 1977.

37. Boxer, M.; Ellman, L.; et al. Anemia in primary hyperparathyroidism. *Arch. Intern. Med.,* **137:**588–90, 1977.

38. Brain, W. R.; Croft, P. B.; and Wilkinson, M. Motor neurone disease as a manifestation of neoplasm (with a note on the course of classical motor neurone disease). *Brain,* **88:**479–500, 1965.

39. Brain, W. R., and Norris, F. (eds.). *The Remote Effects of Cancer on the Nervous System.* Grune & Straton, New York, 1965.

39a. Brismar, J.; Davis, K. R.; et al. Unilateral endocrine exophthalmos. Diagnostic problems in association with computed tomography. *Neuroradiology,* **12:**21–24, 1976.

40. Brooks, M. R.; Baylis, P. H.; and Heath, D. A. Diabetes insipidus and panhypopituitrism after pituitary infarction in a case of acromegaly. *Br. Med. J.,* **2:**369, 1977.

41. Brown, J. J.; Chinn, R. H.; Davies, D. L.; Dusterdieck, G.; Fraser, R.; Lever, A. F.; Robertson, J. I. S.; Tree, M.; and Wiseman, A. Plasma electrolytes, renin and aldosterone in the diagnosis of primary hyperaldosteronism. *Lancet,* **2:**55–59, 1968.

42. Brown, M. J.; Martin, J. R.; and Asbury, A. K. Painful diabetic neuropathy: Morphometric study. *Arch. Neurol.,* **33:**164–71, 1976.

43. Brown, W. F., and Feasby, T. E. Estimates of functional motor axon loss in diabetes. *J. Neurol. Sci.,* **23:**275–93, 1974.

44. Buck, A. C.; Reed, P. I.; et al. Bladder dysfunction and neuropathy in diabetics. *Diabetologia,* **12:**251–58, 1976.

45. Burks, J. S.; Alfrey, A. C.; et al. A fatal encephalopathy in chronic hemodialysis patients. *Lancet,* **1:**764–68, 1976.

46. Burnham, B. F., and Lascelles, J. Control of porphyrin biosynthesis through a negative-feedback mechanism. *Biochem. J.,* **87:**462–69, 1977.

47. Burns, R.; Thomas, W.; and Barron, V. J. Reversible encephalopathy possibly associated with bismuth subgallate ingestion. *Br. Med. J.,* **1:**220–23, 1974.

48. Byrd, G. I. Acute organic brain syndrome associated with gentamicin therapy. *J.A.M.A.,* **238:**53–54, 1977.

49. Caccia, M. R.; Comotti, B.; et al. Vincristine polyneuropathy in man. A clinical and electrophysiological study. *J. Neurol.,* **216:**21–26, 1977.

50. Campbell, J. M.; Hunt, T. K.; et al. Jejunoileal bypass as a treatment of morbid obesity. *Arch. Intern. Med.,* **137:**602–10, 1977.

51. Chhuttani, P. N.; Chawla, L. S.; and Sharma, T. D. Arsenical neuropathy. *Neurology* (Minneap.), **17:**269–74, 1967.

52. Chokroverty, S.; Bruetman, M. E.; et al. Progressive dialytic encephalopathy. *J. Neurol. Neurosurg. Psychiat.,* **39:**411–19, 1976.

53. Christie, S. B., and Ross, E. J. Ectopic pinealoma with adipsia and hypernatremia. *Br. Med. J.,* **2:**669–70, 1968.

54. Chutkow, J. G., and Meyers, S. Chemical changes in the cerebrospinal fluid and brain in magnesium deficiency. *Neurology* (Minneap.), **18:**963–74, 1968.

55. Clancy, R. L.; Romkins, W. A. F.; et al. Isolation and characterization of an aetiological agent in Whipple's disease. *Br. Med. J.,* **3:**568–70, 1975.

56. Clift, G. V.; Schletter, F. E.; Moses, A. M.; and Streetan, D. H. P. Syndrome of inappropriate vasopressin secretion; studies on the mechanism of the hyponatremia in a patient. *Arch. Intern. Med.,* **118:**453–60, 1967.

57. Clioquinol and neurological disease (Editorial). *Br. Med. J.,* **2:**291–92, 1971.

58. Clumeck, N.; DeTroyer, A.; et al. Treatment of diabetic coma with small intravenous insulin doses. *Br. Med. J.,* **2:**394–96, 1976.

59. Clunie, G. J. A.; Gunn, A.; and Robson, J. S. Hyperparathyroid crisis, *Br. J. Surg.,* **54:**538–41, 1967.

60. Cohen, C. J.; Bowers, G. N.; and Lewpow, M. L. Epidemiology of lead poisoning. A comparison between urban and rural children. *J.A.M.A.,* **226:** 1430–33, 1973.

61. Cole, M. Strokes in young women using oral contraceptives. *Arch. Intern. Med.,* **120:**551–55, 1967.

62. Collaborative Group for the Study of Stroke in Young Women. Oral contraception and increased risk of cerebral ischemia or thrombosis. *N. Engl. J. Med.,* **288:**871–78, 1973.

63. Coltman, C. A., Jr. Multiple myeloma without a paraprotein; report of a case with observations on chromosomal composition. *Arch. Intern. Med.,* **120:**687–96, 1967.

64. Connors, M. H.; Ircas, J. J.; and Golabi, M. Hypo-hyperparathyroidism: Evidence for a defective parathyroid hormone. *Pediatrics,* **60:**343–48, 1977.

65. Cooke, W. T., and Smith, W. T. Neurological disorders associated with adult coeliac disease. *Brain,* **89:**683–722, 1966.

66. Cotzias, G. C. Metabolic modification of some

neurologic disorders. *J.A.M.A.,* **210:**1255–62, 1969.

67. Cotzias, G. C.; Hoviuchi, K.; Fuenzalida, S.; and Mena, I. Chronic manganese poisoning: clearance of tissue manganese concentrations with persistence of the neurological picture. *Neurology* (Minneap.), **18:**376–82, 1968.

68. Cream, J. J.; Hern, J. E. C.; et al. Mixed or immune complex cryoglobulinaemia and neuropathy. *J. Neurol. Neurosurg. Psychiat.,* **37:**82–87, 1974.

69. Croft, P. B.; Henson, R. A.; Urich, H.; and Wilkinson, P. C. Sensory neuropathy with bronchial carcinoma; a study of four cases showing serological abnormalities. *Brain,* **88:**501–14,1965.

70. Croft, P. B., and Wilkinson, M. Incidence of carcinomatous neuromyopathy in patients with various types of carcinoma. *Brain,* **88:**427–34, 1965.

70a. Crosby, C. J.; Rorke, L. B.; et al. Central nervous system lesions in childhood leukemia. *Neurology* (Minneap.), **28:**678–85, 1978.

71. Crumpacker, R. W., and Kriel, R. L. Voluntary water intoxication in normal infants. *Neurology,* **23:**1251–55, 1973.

72. Curry, P.; Fitchett, D.; et al. Ventricular arrhythmias and hypokalemia. *Lancet,* **2:**231–33, 1976.

73. Danbolt, N., and Closs, K. Akrodermatitis enteropathica. *Acta Derm. Venereol.* (Stockh.), **23:**127–69, 1942.

74. Darnley, J. D. Polyneuropathy in Waldenstrom's macroglogulinemia. *Neurology* (Minneap.), **12:**617–23, 1962.

75. Data, J. L.; Wilkinson, G. R.; and Nies, A. S. Interaction of quinidine with anticonvulsant drugs. *N. Engl. J. Med.,* **294:**699–702, 1976.

76. David, O.; Clark, J.; and Voeller, K. Lead and hyperactivity. *Lancet,* **2:**900–903, 1972.

77. Davis, J. L.; Lewis, S. B.; et al. Peripheral diabetic neuropathy treated with amitryptyline and fluphenagine. *J.A.M.A.,* **238:**2291–92, 1977.

78. Dayan, A. D.; Croft, P. B.; and Wilkinson, M. Association of carcinomatous neuromyopathy with different histological types of carcinoma of the lung. *Brain,* **88:**435–48, 1965.

79. DeJong, R. N. CNS manifestations of diabetes mellitus. *Postgrad. Med.,* **61:**101–107, 1977.

80. Delaney, P., and Schellinger, D. Computerized tomography and benign intracranial hypertension. *J.A.M.A.,* **236:**951–52, 1976.

81. DelDuca, V., Jr., and Morningstar, W. A. Multiple myeloma associated with progressive multifocal leukoencephalopathy. *J.A.M.A.,* **199:**671–73, 1967.

82. DeNavasguez, S., and Treble, H. A. A case of generalized amyloid disease with involvement of nerves. *Brain,* **61:**116–28, 1974.

83. De Troyer, A., and Demanet, J. C. Clinical biological and pathogenic features of the syndrome of inappropriate secretion of antidiuretic hormone. *J. Med.,* **45:**521–31, 1976.

84. Devereaux, M. W., and Partnow, M. J. Delayed hypoxic encephalopathy without cognitive dysfunction. *Arch. Neurol.,* **32:**704–705, 1975.

85. Devivo, D. C.; Malas, D.; et al. Leukoen-

cephalopathy in childhood leukemia. *Neurology* (Minneap.), **27:**609–13, 1977.

86. Diagnosis of brain death. Statement issued by the honorary secretary of the Conference of Medical Royal Colleges and Their Faculties in the United Kingdom on 11 October 1976. *Br. Med. J.,* **2:**1187–88, 1976.

87. Dialysis dementia. *Br. Med. J.,* **2:**1213–14, 1976.

88. Dimich, A.; Bedrossian, P. B.; and Wallach, S. Hypoparathyroidism; clinical observations in 34 patients. *Arch Intern. Med.,* **120:**449–58, 1967.

89. Dooling, E. C., and Richardson, E. P. Delayed encephalopathy after strangling. *Arch. Neurol.* **33:**196–99, 1976.

90. Drill, V. A. Oral contraceptives and thromboembolic disease. I. Prospective and retrospective studies. *J.A.M.A.,* **219:**583–96, 1972.

91. Dunsker, S. B.; Torres-Reyes, E.; and Peden, J. C., Jr. Pseudotumor cerebri associated with idiopathic cryofibrinogenemia. *Arch. Neurol.,* **23:**120–27, 1970.

92. Dyek, P. J.; Johnson, W. J.; et al. Detection and evaluation of uremic peripheral neuropathy in patients on hemodialysis. *Kidney Int.,* suppl. **2:**201–205, 1975.

93. Edis, R. H., and Mastraglia, F. L. Vertical gaze palsy in barbiturate intoxication. *Br. Med. J.,* **1:**144, 1977.

94. Eisenbud, E., and LoBue, C. C. Hypocalcemia after therapeutic use of magnesium sulphate. *Arch. Intern. Med.,* **136:**688–91, 1976.

95. Ewing, D. J.; Campbell, I. W.; and Clarke, B. F. Mortality in diabetic autonomic neuropathy. *Lancet,* **1:**601–603, 1976.

96. Faden, A. Encephalopathy following treatment of chronic pulmonary failure. *Neurology* (Minneap.), **26:**337–39, 1976.

97. Favis, A. A. Wernicke's encephalopathy in uremia. *Neurology* (Minneap.), **22:**293–97, 1972:

98. Feibel, J. H., and Campa, J. F. Thyrotoxic neuropathy (Basedow's paraplegia). *J. Neurol. Neurosurg. Psychiat.,* **39:**491–97, 1976.

99. Feldman, R. G.; Hayes, M. K.; et al. Lead neuropathy in adults and children. *Arch. Neurol.,* **34:**481–88, 1977.

100. Fichman, M. P.; Vorheer, M.; et al. Diuretic-induced hyponatremia. *Ann. Intern. Med.,* **75:**853–63, 1971.

101. Finch, C. A. Pathophysiologic aspects of sickle cell anemia. *Am. J. Med.,* **53:**1–6, 1972.

102. Fincham, R. W., and Cape, C. A. Neuropathy in myxedema. *Arch. Neurol.,* **19:**464–66, 1968.

103. Finelli, P. F. Sickle cell trait and transient monocular blindness. *Am. J. Ophthalmol.,* **81:**850–51, 1976.

104. Finelli, P. F.; McEntee, W. J.; et al. Whipple's disease with predominantly neuroophthalmologic manifestations. *Ann. Neurol.,* **1:**247–52, 1977.

105. Fisher, J., and Abrahms, J. Life-threatening ventricular tachyarrhythmias in delirium tremens. *Arch. Intern. Med.,* **137:**1238–41, 1977.

106. Fishman, R. A. Neurological aspects of magnesium metabolism. *Arch. Neurol.,* **12:**562–69, 1965.

107. Fitzgerald, M. A.; Gross, J. B.; et al. Wilson's disease (hepatolenticular degeneration) of late

adult onset. Report of case. *Mayo Clin. Proc.,* **50:**438–42, 1975.

108. Follender, A. B. Neurologic problems prevalent in alcoholics. *Postgrad. Med.,* **61:**166–71, 1977.

109. Fox, J. M.; Ramsey, R. G., et al. Cerebral ventricular enlargement: Chronic alcoholics examined by computerized tomography. *J.A.M.A.,* **236:**365–68, 1976.

110. Fraser, T. N. Cerebral manifestation of Addisonism in pernicious anemia. *Lancet,* **2:**458–59, 1960.

111. Freireich, E. J.; Thomas, L. B.; Frei, E.; Fritz, R. D.; and Forkner, C. E. A distinctive type of intracerebral hemorrhage associated with "blastic crisis" in patients with leukemia. *Cancer,* **13:**146–54, 1960.

112. French, J. H.; Grueter, B. B.; Druckman, R., and O'Brien, D. Pyridoxine and infantile myoclonic seizures. *Neurology* (Minneap.), **15:**101–13, 1965.

113. Fuertes De La Haba, A.; Curet, J. O.; Pelegrina, I.; and Bangdiavala, I. Thrombophlebitis among oral and non-oral contraceptive users. *Obstet. Gynecol.,* **38:**259–63, 1971.

114. Gaelen, L. H., and Levitan, S. Solitary intracranial metastasis by Hodgkin's disease. *Arch. Intern. Med.,* **120:**740–45, 1967.

115. Gafni, J.; Merker, H.-J.; Shibolet, S.; Sohar, E.; and Heller, H. On the origin of amyloid; study of an amyloid tumor in multiple myeloma. *Ann. Intern. Med.,* **65:**1031–44, 1966.

116. Gagliano, R. G., and Costanzi, J. J. Paraplegia following intrathecal methotrexate. Report of a case and review of the literature. *Cancer,* **37:**1663–68, 1976.

117. Garcia, C. A., and Fleming, R. H. Reversible corticospinal tract disease due to hyperthyroidism. *Arch. Neurol.,* **34:**647–48, 1977.

118. Garofalo, M.; Danon, M. J.; et al. Peripheral neuropathy associated with primary malignant lymphoma of the brain. *Arch. Neurol.,* **35:**50–52, 1978.

119. Gelfand, M. L.; Sussman, L.; Caimol, B. C.; Florita, C.; and Joson, F. Successful treatment of hepatic coma by exchange transfusions. *J.A.M.A.,* **201:**630–33, 1967.

120. Geller, W., and Lacher, M. J. Hodgkin's disease. *Med. Clin. North Am.,* **50:**819–32, 1966.

121. Gholz, L. M., and Arons, W. L. Prophylaxis and therapy of amebiasis and shigellosis with iodochlorhydroxyquin. *Am. J. Trop. Med. Hyg.,* **13:**396–401, 1964.

122. Gilberson, A.; Vaziri, D.; et al. Hemodialysis of acute arsenic intoxication with transient renal failure. *Arch. Intern. Med.,* **136:**1303–1304, 1976.

123. Gilbert, G. J. Quinidine dementia. *J.A.M.A.,* **237:**2093–94, 1977.

124. Gilchrest, B. A.; Rowe, J. W.; et al. Relief of uremic pruritus with ultraviolet phototherapy. *N. Engl. J. Med.,* **297:**136–38, 1977.

125. Ginsberg, M. D.; Henley-White, E. T.; and Richardson, E. P. Hypoxic-ischemic leukoencephalopathy in man. *Arch. Neurol.,* **33:**5–14, 1976.

126. Giove, G., and Gastaut, H. Epilepsie alcoolique et déclenchement alcoolique des crises chez les épileptiques. (Une approche clinique et électro-éncephalographique). *Rev. Neurol.* (Paris), **113:**347–57, 1965.

127. Glaser, G. H. Metabolic encephalopathy in hepatic, adrenal and pulmonary disorders. *Postgrad. Med.,* **27:**611–19, 1960.

128. Goldman, J. A., and Eckerling, B. Intracranial dural sinus thrombosis following intrauterine instillation of hypertonic saline. *Am. J. Obstet. Gynecol.,* **112:**1132–33, 1972.

128a. Goldberg, M. A., and Dorman, J. D. Intention myoclonus: Successful treatment with clonazepam. *Neurology* (Minneap.), **26:**24–26, 1976.

129. Goldstein, G. W.; Asbury, A. I.; and Diamond, I. Pathogenesis of lead encephalopathy. Uptake of lead and reaction of brain capillaries. *Arch. Neurol.,* **31:**382–89, 1974.

129a. Growdon, J. H.; Young, R. R.; and Shahani, B. T. L-5-Hydroxytryptophan in treatment of several different syndromes in which myoclonus is prominent. *Neurology* (Minneap.), **26:**1135–40, 1976.

130. Goodhue, W. W.; David, J. N.; and Porro, R. S. Ischemic myopathy in uremic hyperparathyroidism. *J.A.M.A.,* **222:**911–12, 1972.

131. Goodman, J. M.; Bischel, M. D.; et al. Barbiturate intoxication morbidity and mortality. *West. J. Med.,* **124:**179–86, 1976.

132. Goodman, J. M., and Heck, L. L. Confirmation of brain death at bedside by isotope angiography. *J.A.M.A.,* **238:**966–68, 1977.

133. Gordon, E. E., and Kabadi, U. M. The hyperglycemic hyperosmolar syndrome. *Am. J. Med.,* **271:**252–68, 1976.

134. Gotham, J. E.; Wein, H.; and Meyer, J. S. Clinical studies of neuropathy due to macroglobulinemia (Waldenstrom's syndrome). *Can. Med. Assoc. J.,* **89:**806–9, 1963.

135. Gotoh, F.; Meyer, J. S.; and Takagi, Y. Cerebral venous and arterial blood gases during Cheyne-Stokes respiration. *Am. J. Med.,* **47:**534–45, 1969.

136. Greer, M. Benign intracranial hypertension (pseudotumor cerebri). *Pediatr. Clin. North Am.,* **14:**819–30, 1967.

137. Griggs, R. C.; Sunshine, J.; Newill, V. A.; Newton, B. W.; Buchanan, S.; and Rasch, C. A. Environmental factors in childhood lead poisoning. *J.A.M.A.,* **187:**703–707, 1964.

138. Growdon, J. H.; Hirsch, M. J.; et al. Oral choline administration to patients with tardive dyskinesia. *N. Engl. J. Med.,* **297:**524–27, 1977.

139. Grunt, J. A.; Destro, R. L.; et al. Ocular palsies in children with diabetes mellitus. *Diabetes,* **25:**459–62, 1976.

140. Guillozet, N. Sickle cell SS genotype and paralysis in children. *J. Pediatr.,* **89:**605–607, 1976.

141. Gunn, T.; Bartolussi, R.; et al. Juvenile diabetes mellitus optic atrophy sensory nerve deafness and diabetes insipidus—a syndrome. *J. Pediatr.,* **89:**565–70, 1976.

142. Habel, A. H., and Simpson, H. Osmolar relation between cerebrospinal fluid and serum in hyperosmolar hypernatremic dehydration. *Arch. Dis. Child.,* **51:**660–66, 1976.

143. Hahn, F. J. Y., and Schapiro, R. L. The excessively small ventricle on computed axial tomography of the brain. *Neuroradiology,* **12:**137–39, 1976.

144. Halmos, P. B.; Nelson, J. K.; and Lowry, R. C. Hyperosmolar nonketoacidotic coma in diabetics. *Lancet,* **1:**675–79, 1966.

145. Hansen, M. M.; Baadsgaard, B.; and Vistebaek, A. Diffuse lymphosarcomatous infiltration in the central nervous system. *Scand. J. Haematol.,* **16:**70–74, 1976.

146. Hansson, O. Toxicity of oxyquinolines. *Lancet,* **1:**1152, 1977.

147. Hardisty, R. M., and Norman, P. M. Meningeal leukaemia. *Arch. Dis. Child.,* **42:**441–47, 1967.

147a. Wernicke's encephalopathy: A more common disease than realized: A neuropathological study of 51 cases. *J. Neurol. Neurosurg. Psychiatry,* **4–2:**226–31, 1979.

148. Hattori, T., and Schlangenhauft, R. E. Bilateral facial palsy: Occurrence in diabetes mellitus. *N. Y. State J. Med.,* **77:**1492–94, 1977.

149. Hayreh, M. S.; Hayreh, S. S.; et al. Methyl alcohol poisoning. III. Ocular toxicity. *Arch. Ophthalmol.,* **95:**1851–58, 1977.

150. Henson, R. A.; Hoffman, H. L.; and Urich, H. Encephalomyelitis with carcinoma. *Brain,* **88:**449–64, 1965.

151. Herishanu, Y., and Rosenberg, P. Effect of L-dopa on polycythemia. *J. Am. Geriatr. Soc.,* **25:**218–19, 1977.

152. Hess, R.; Koella, W. P.; Krinke, G.; Petermann, H.; Thomann, P.; and Zák, F. Absence of neurotoxicity following prolonged administration of iodochloro-8-hydroxyquinoline to beagle dogs. *Arzneim. Forsch.,* **23:**1566–71, 1973.

153. Hilden, T., and Svendsen, T. L. Electrolyte disturbances in beer drinkers. *Lancet,* **2:**245–46, 1975.

154. Hogan, G. R.; Dodge, P. R.; Gill, S. R.; Master, S.; and Sotos, J. F. Pathogenesis of seizures occurring during restoration of plasma tonicity to normal in animals previously chronically hypernatremic. *Pediatrics,* **43:**54–64, 1969.

155. Horwich, M. S.; Cho, L.; et al. Subacute sensory neuropathy: A remote effect of carcinoma. *Ann. Neurol.,* **2:**7–19, 1977.

156. Hotson, J. R., and Langston, J. W. Disulfiram-induced encephalopathy. *Arch. Neurol.,* **33:**141–42, 1976.

157. Huckman, M. S.; Fox, J. S.; et al. Computed tomography in the diagnosis of pseudotumor cerebri. *Radiology,* **119:**593–97, 1976.

158. Hyman, C. B.; Bogle, J. M.; Brubaker, C. A.; Williams, K.; and Hammond, D. Central nervous system involvement by leukemia in children. I. Relationship to systemic leukemia and description of clinical and laboratory manifestations. *Blood,* **25:**1–12, 1965.

159. International Colloquium on Anoxia and the EEG, Marseille, 1959. In Meyer, J. S., and Gastaut, H. (eds.). *Cerebral Anoxia and the Electroencephalogram.* Thomas, Springfield, Ill., 1961.

160. Iyer, K.; Goodgold, J.; et al. Mercury poisoning in a dentist. *Arch. Neurol.,* **33:**788–90, 1976.

161. Jacobson, S., and Bell, B. Recognition and management of acute and chronic hepatic encephalopathy. *Med. Clin. North Am.,* **57:**1567–77, 1973.

162. Jefferson, A., and Clark, J. Treatment of benign intracranial hypertension by dehydrating agents with particular reference to the measurement of the blind spot as a means of recording improvement. *J. Neurol. Neurosurg. Psychiat.,* **39:**627–39, 1976.

163. Jellinek, E. H., and Kelly, R. E. Cerebellar syndrome in myxedema. *Lancet,* **2:**225–27, 1960.

164. Jenkins, R. B. Inorganic arsenic and the nervous system. *Brain,* **89:**479–98, 1966.

165. Jennett, W. B., and Cross, J. N. Influence of pregnancy and oral contraception on the incidence of strokes in women of childbearing age. *Lancet,* **1:**1019–23, 1967.

166. Jeske, D. V.; Olgiati, S. G.; and Ghali, A. Y. Masking of tardive dyskinesia with four-time-a-day administration of chlorpromazine. *Dis. Nerv. System,* **38:**755–58, 1977.

167. Joffe, B. I.; Shires, R.; et al. Plasma insulin C-peptide and glucagon levels in acute phase of ethanol-induced hypoglycemia. *Br. Med. J.,* **2:**678, 1977.

168. Johns, M. W. Self-poisoning with barbiturates in England and Wales during 1959–74. *Br. Med. J.,* **1:**1128–30, 1977.

169. Johnson, C. C., Jr.; Lary, N.; Lord, T.; Vellcos, F.; Merritt, A. D.; and Deiss, W. P., Jr. Osteopetrosis. *Medicine,* **47:**149–67, 1968.

170. Johnson, D. A., and Tong, N. T. Pancreatic encephalopathy. *South. Med. J.,* **70:**165–67, 1977.

170a. Johnson, P. C.; Rolak, L. A.; et al. Paraneoplastic vasculitis of nerve. A remote effect of cancer. *Ann. Neurol.,* **5:**437–44, 1979.

171. Johnson, R. C.; DeFord, J. W.; and Gebhart, R. J. Chronic active hepatitis and cirrhosis in Wilson's disease. *South. Med. J.,* **70:**753–54, 1977.

172. Jones, E. A.; Clain, D.; Clink, H. M.; MacGillivray, M.; and Sherlock, S. Hepatic coma due to acute hepatic necrosis treated by exchange blood-transfusion. *Lancet,* **2:**169–72, 1967.

173. Judd, D. R.; Heimburger, I.; and Johnston, C., Jr. Parathyroid adenoma. *Ann. Surg.,* **164:**1077–84, 1966.

173a. Julien, J.; Vital, C.; et al. Polyneuropathy in Waldenstrom's macroglobulinemia. Deposits of M components on myelin sheaths. *Arch. Neurol.,* **35:**423–25, 1978.

174. Kalant, H. Direct effect of ethanol on the nervous system. *Fed. Proc.,* **34:**1930–41, 1975.

175. Kantarjian, A. D., and Shaheen, A. S. Methyl bromide poisoning with nervous system manifestations resembling polyneuropathy. *Neurology* (Minneap.), **13:**1054–58, 1963.

176. Katz, R. A. Intravenous urea in the therapy of increased intracranial pressure with lead encephalopathy. *N. Engl. J. Med.,* **262:**870–72, 1960.

177. Kaufman, G. Hodgkin's disease involving the

central nervous system. *Arch. Neurol.,* **13:**555–58, 1965.

178. Keidan, S. E. Paraplegia in childhood malignant disease. *Acta Paediat. Scand. Suppl.,* **172:**110–18, 1967.

179. Kersh, E. S.; Kronfield, S. J.; et al. Automatic neuropathy in uremia. *N. Engl. J. Med.,* **290:**650–53, 1974.

180. Knell, A. J. Acute liver failure. *Practitioner,* **218:**230–37, 1977.

181. Kolendorf, K., and Moller, B. B. Peritoneal dialysis in hypernatremia: Ketoacidotic diabetic coma. *Acta Med. Scand.,* **200:**75–77, 1976.

182. Kono, R. Subacute myelo-optic-neuropathy, a new neurological disease prevailing in Japan. *Jap. J. Med. Sci. Biol.,* **24:**195–216, 1971.

183. Korein, J.; Braunsteen, P.; et al. Brain death. 1. Angiographic correlation with the radioisotopic bolus technique for evaluation of cortical deficit of cerebral blood flow. *Ann. Neurol.,* **2:**195–205, 1977.

184. Korein, J., and Maccario, M. On the diagnosis of cerebral death: A prospective study on 55 patients to define irreversible coma. *Clin. EEG,* **2:**178–99, 1971.

185. Korobkin, R.; Asbury, A. K.; et al. Glue-sniffing neuropathy. *Arch. Neurol.,* **32:**158–62, 1975.

186. Kosmar, M. E. Lactulose (cephulae) in portosystemic encephalopathy. *J.A.M.A.,* **236:**2444–45, 1976.

187. Kozak, G. P.; Yoo, J.; and Ganz, K. Diabetic neuropathies. *Am. Physician,* **15:**122–22, 1977.

188. Kramer, J., and Goodwin, J. A. Wernicke's encephalopathy. Complication of intravenous hyperalimentation. *J.A.M.A.,* **14:**2176–77, 1977.

189. Krebs, R., and Flynn, M. Treatment of hepatic coma with exchange transfusion and peritoneal dialysis. *J.A.M.A.,* **199:**430–32, 1967.

190. Kunze, U. Chronic bromide intoxication with a severe neurological deficit. *J. Neurol.,* **213:**149–52, 1976.

191. Lai, C.-W.; Hung, T.-P.; and Lin, W. S. J. Blindness of cerebral origin in acute intermittent porphyria. *Arch. Neurol.,* **34:**310–12, 1977.

192. Lamon, J. M.; Frykholm, B. C.; and Tschudy, D. P. Screening tests in acute porphyria. *Arch. Neurol.,* **34:**709–12, 1977.

193. Lang, A. H., and Forsström, J. Transient changes of sensory nerve function in uraemia. *Acta Med. Scand.,* **202:**495–500, 1977.

194. Lawrence, A. M., and Abraira, C. Diabetic neuropathy: a review of clinical manifestations. *Ann. Clin. Lab. Sci.,* **6:**78–83, 1976.

195. Layzer, R. B.; Shearn, M. A.; and Satya-Murti, S. Eosinophilic polymyositis. *Ann. Neurol.,* **1:**65–71, 1977.

196. Lerman, S., and Feldman, A. L. Centrocecal scotomata as the presenting sign of pernicious anemia. *Arch. Ophthalmol.,* **65:**427–32, 1969.

197. Leventhal, J. M., and Reid, D. E. Oxytocin-induced water intoxication with grand mal convulsions. *Am. J. Obstet. Gynecol.,* **102:**310–11, 1968.

198. Levitt, L., and Prager, D. Mononeuropathy due to vincristine toxicity. *Neurology* (Minneap.), **25:**894–95, 1975.

199. Levy, D. E.; Brierley, J. B.; et al. Brief hypoxia-ischemia initially damages cerebral neurons. *Arch. Neurol.,* **32:**450–56, 1975.

200. Lin-Fu, J. S. Vulnerability of children to lead exposure and toxicity. *N. Engl. J. Med.,* **289:**1229–33, 1973.

201. Logothetis, J. Neurologic and muscular manifestations of hyperthyroidism. *Arch. Neurol.,* **5:**533–44, 1961.

202. Logothetis, J.; Silverstein, P.; and Coe, J. Neurologic aspects of Waldenstrom's macroglobulinemia. *Arch. Neurol.,* **3:**564–73, 1960.

203. Löwenthal, A., and Bruyn, G. W. Calcification of the striopallidodentate system. In Vinken, P. J., and Bruyn, G. W. (eds.). *Handbook of Clinical Neurology.* North-Holland Publishing Company, Amsterdam, 1968, Vol. 6, pp. 703–25.

204. Lufkin, E. G.; Reagan, T. J.; et al. Acute cerebral dysfunction in diabetic ketoacidosis: Survival followed by panhypopituitrism. *Metabolism,* **26:**363–69, 1977.

205. Lukes, R. J.; Butler, J. J.; and Hicks, E. B. Natural history of Hodgkin's disease as related to its pathologic picture. *Cancer,* **19:**317–44, 1966.

206. Luse, S. A., and Wood, W. G. The brain in fatal carbon tetrachloride poisoning. *Arch. Neurol.,* **17:**304–12, 1967.

207. Mackenzie, M. R., and Lee, T. K. Blood viscosity in Waldenström macroglobulinemia. *Fed. Proc.,* **49:**507–10, 1977.

208. Magnussen, C. R. Grand mal seizures and acute intermittent porphyria: The problem of differential diagnoses and treatment. *Neurology* (Minneap.), **25:**1121–25, 1975.

209. Maizel, H.; Ruffin, J. M.; and Dobbins, W. O. Whipple's disease: A review of 19 patients from one hospital and a review of the literature since 1950. *Medicine,* **49:**175–205, 1970.

210. Malamed, E., and Lavy, S. Parkinsonism associated with chronic inhalation of carbon tetrachloride. *Lancet,* **1:**1015, 1977.

211. Mancall, E. L., and Rosales, R. K. Necrotizing myelopathy associated with visceral carcinoma. *Brain,* **87:**639–56, 1964.

212. Mann, J. I.; Vessey, M. P.; Thorogood, M.; and Doll, R. Myocardial infarction in young women with special reference to oral contraceptive practice. *Br. Med. J.,* **2:**241, 1975.

213. Mann, T. P. Transient choreo-athetosis following hypernatremia. *Dev. Med. Child Neurol.,* **11:**637–40, 1969.

214. Manzano, F., and Kozak, G. P. Acute quadriplegia in diabetic hyperosmotic coma with hypokalemia. *J.A.M.A.,* **207:**2278–81, 1969.

215. Marcus, J.; Ehrlich, R.; et al. Nerve conduction in childhood diabetes. *Can. Med. Assoc. J.,* **108:**1116–19, 1973.

216. Mathews, N. T.; Meyer, J. S.; and Ott, E. O. Increased cerebral blood volume in benign intracranial hypertension. *Neurology* (Minneap.), **25:**646–49, 1975.

217. Matholone, M. B. R. Ocular effects of phenothiazine derivatives and reversibility. *Dis. Nerv. Syst.,* **29:**29–35, 1968.

218. Matthew, H., and Lawson, A. A. H. Acute barbi-

turate poisoning; review of two years experience. *Q. J. Med.,* **35:**539–52, 1966.

218a. Mayne, N. The short-term prognosis in diabetic neuropathy. *Diabetes,* **17:**270–73, 1968.

219. McAuley, D. L. F.; Lecky, B. R. F.; and Earl, C. J. Gold encephalopathy. *J. Neurol. Neurosurg. Psychiat.,* **40:**1021–22, 1977.

220. McCutchen, C. B.; Vignaendra, V.; and Chatrian, G. E. Electrographic and clinical effects of intra-carotid sodium amobarbital on bilateral myoclonic status epilepticus. *Neurology* (Minneap.), **27:**252–56, 1977.

221. McCutchen, J. J., and Utterback, R. A. Chronic arsenic poisoning resembling muscular dystrophy. *South. Med. J.,* **59:**1139–45, 1966.

222. McDonald, J. V., and Burton, R. Subdural effusion in Hodgkin's disease. *Arch. Neurol.,* **15:**649–52, 1966.

223. McGillion, F. B.; Thompson, G. G.; et al. The passage of δ aminolevulinic acid across the blood brain barrier of the rat: effect of ethanol. *Biochem. Pharmacol.,* **23:**472–74, 1974.

224. Mehta, A. J., and Seshia, S. S. Orbicularis oculi reflex in brain death. *J. Neurol. Neurosurg. Psychiat.,* **39:**784–87, 1976.

225. Mena, I.; Marin, R.; Fuenzalida, S.; and Cotzias, G. C. Chronic manganese poisoning; clinical picture and manganese turnover. *Neurology* (Minneap.), **17:**128–36, 1967.

226. Merry, J.; Reynolds, C. M.; et al. Prophylactic treatment of alcoholism by lithium carbonate. *Lancet,* **2:**481–82, 1976.

227. Meyer, J. S.; Gotham, J.; Tazaki, Y.; and Gotoh, F. Cardiorespiratory syndrome of extreme obesity with papilledema. Report of a fatal case with EEG, metabolic and necropsy studies. *Neurology* (Minneap.), **11:**950–58, 1961.

228. Meyer, J. S., and Portnoy, H. Localized cerebral hypoglycemia simulating stroke. A clinical and experimental study. *Neurology* (Minneap.), **8:**601–14, 1958.

229. Mindhom, R. M.-S.; Lamb, P.; and Bradley, R. A comparison of piribedil procyclidine and placebo in the control of phonothiazine-induced parkinsonism. *Br. J. Psychiat.,* **130:**581–85, 1977.

230. Mohandas, A., and Chou, S. N. Brain death. A clinical and pathological study. *J. Neurosurg.,* **35:**211–18, 1971.

231. Montgomery, R. D.; Cruikshank, E. R.; Robertson, W. B.; and McMenemey, W. H. Clinical and pathological observations on Jamaican neuropathy; report of 206 cases. *Brain,* **87:**425–62, 1964.

232. Moress, G. R.; D'Agostino, A. N.; and Jarcho, L. W. Neuropathy in lymphoblastic leukemia treated with vincristine. *Arch. Neurol.,* **16:**377–84, 1967.

232a. Morgan, J. P., and Penovich, P. Jamaica ginger paralysis. Forty-seven year follow-up. *Arch. Neurol.,* **35:**530–32, 1978.

233. Morgan, M. Y.; Jakobovitz, A.; et al. Successful use of bromocriptine in the treatment of a patient with chronic portosystemic encephalopathy. *N. Engl. J. Med.,* **296:**793–94, 1977.

234. Morris-Jones, P. H.; Houston, I. B.; and Evans, R. C. Prognosis of the neurological complications of acute hypernatraemia. *Lancet,* **2:**1385–89, 1967.

235. Mortality among oral-contraceptive users. Royal College of General Practitioners Oral Contraception Study. *Lancet,* **2:**727–31, 1977.

236. Morton, D. L.; Itaboshi, H. H.; and Grimes, O. F. Nonmetastatic neurologic complications of bronchogenic carcinoma: the carcinomatous neuromyopathies. *J. Thorac. Cardiovasc. Surg.,* **51:**14–29, 1966.

237. Mousseau, R., and Reynolds, T. Hepatic paraplegia. *Am. J. Gastroenterol.,* **66:**343–48, 1976.

238. Mueater, M. D., and Whisnant, J. R. Basal ganglia calcification hypoparathyroidism and extrapyramidal motor manifestations. *Neurology* (Minneap.), **18:**1075–83, 1968.

239. Muller, W. E., and Snyder, S. H. δ aminolevulinic acid: Influences on synaptic GABA receptor binding may explain CNS symptoms of porphyria. *Ann. Neurol.,* **2:**340–42, 1977.

240. Multiple myeloma; clinicopathologic conference. *Am. J. Med.,* **43:**912–21, 1967.

241. Murayama, M. Molecular mechanism of red cell "sickling." *Science,* **153:**145–49, 1966.

242. Murphy, J. J. Inappropriate secretion of antidiuretic hormone in urologic patients. *J. Urol.,* **97:**755–57, 1967.

243. Mushet, G. R. Pseudotumor and nitrofurantoin therapy. *Arch. Neurol.,* **34:**239, 1977.

244. Nakae, K.; Yamamoto, S-I.; and Igata, A. Subacute myelo-optico-neuropathy. (S.M.O.N. in Japan). *Lancet,* **2:**510–12, 1971.

244a. Nardizzi, L. R. Computerized tomographic correlate of carbon monoxide poisoning. *Arch. Neurol.,* **36:**38–39, 1979.

245. Neundorfer, B.; Meyer, J. G.; and Volk, B. Amyloid neuropathy due to monoclonal gammopathy. A case report. *J. Neurol.,* **216:**207–15, 1977.

246. Newman, S. E. The EEG manifestations of chronic ethanol abuse: Relation to cerebral atrophy. *Ann. Neurol.,* **3:**299–304, 1978.

247. Nielsen, J. Delirium tremens in Copenhagen. *Acta Psychiat. Scand.,* **41:**Suppl. 187:1–92, 1965.

248. Nikoskelainen, E.; Enzmann, D. R.; et al. Computerized tomography of the orbits. A report of 196 patients. *Acta Ophthalmol.,* **55:**885–900, 1977.

249. Ohlrich, G. D., and Ohlrich, J. G. Papilledema in an adolescent due to tetracycline. *Med. J. Aust.,* **1:**334–35, 1977.

250. Orchik, D. J., and Dunn, J. W. Sickle cell anemia and sudden deafness. *Arch. Otolaryngol.,* **103:**369–70, 1977.

251. Osuntokun, O., and Osuntokun, G. O. Complicated migraine and hemoglobin AS in Nigeria. *Br. Med. J.,* **2:**621, 1972.

252. Packard, R. C. The neurologic complications of alcoholism. *Am. Fam. Physician,* **14:**111–15, 1976.

253. Pampiglione, G. The effect of metabolic disorders on brain activity. *J. Roy. Coll. Physicians Lond.,* **7:**347–64, 1973.

254. Parkes, J. D.; Sharpstone, P.; and Williams, R.

Levodopa in hepatic coma. *Lancet,* **2:**1341–43, 1970.

255. Pasquariello, P. S.; Schut, L.; and Borns, P. Benign increased intracranial hypertension due to chronic vitamin A overdosage in a 26 month old child. *Clin. Pediatr.,* **16:**379–82, 1977.

256. Patel, A. N. Hypokalemic quadriparesis as a presenting manifestation of diabetic ketoacidosis. *Indian J. Med. Sci.,* **22:**633–35, 1968.

257. Pearson, J.; Korein, J.; et al. Brain death. II. Neuropathological correlation with the radioisotopic bolus technique for evaluation of cortical deficits of cerebral blood flow. *Ann. Neurol.,* **2:**206–210, 1977.

258. Permutt, M. A. Postprandial hypoglycemia. *Diabetes,* **25:**719–33, 1976.

258a. Perrura, E.; Garratt, A.; et al. Water intoxication in epileptic patients receiving carbamazepine. *J. Neurol. Neurosurg. Psychiatry,* **41:**713–18, 1978.

259. Peters, H. A.; and Chatanoft, D. V. Spinal muscular atrophy secondary to macroglobulinemia. Reversal of symptoms with chlorambucil therapy. *Neurology* (Minneap.), **18:**101–108, 1968.

260. Peterson, R. G., and Rumack, B. H. D-Penicillamine therapy of acute arsenic poisoning. *J. Pediatr.,* **91:**661–66, 1977.

261. Pickett, J. B. E.; Layzer, R. B.; et al. Neuromuscular complications of acromegaly. *Neurology* (Minneap.), **25:**638–45, 1975.

262. Pierce, J. C.; Madge, G. E.; et al. Lymphoma, a complication of renal allotransplantation in man. *J.A.M.A.,* **219:**1593–97, 1972.

263. Pierce, M. I. Neurologic complications in acute leukemia in children. *Pediat. Clin. North Am.,* **9:**425–42, 1962.

264. Pierog, S.; Chandavasu, O.; and Wexler, I. Withdrawal symptoms in infants with the fetal alcohol syndrome. *J. Pediatr.,* **90:**630–33, 1977.

265. Pilley, S. F. J., and Thompson, H. S. Familial syndrome of diabetes insipidus, diabetes mellitus, optic atrophy and deafness (Didmoad) in childhood. *Br. J. Ophthalmol.,* **60:**294–98, 1976.

266. Plum, F.; Posner, J. B.; and Hain, R. F. Delayed neurological deterioration after anoxia. *Arch. Intern. Med.,* **110:**18–25, 1962.

267. Portnoy, B. A., and Herron, J. C. Neurological manifestations in sickle cell disease. *Ann. Intern. Med.,* **76:**643–52, 1972.

268. Powles, R. L., and Malpas, J. S. Guillain-Barre syndrome associated with chronic lymphatic leukemia. *Br. Med. J.,* **3:**286–87, 1967.

269. Powner, D. Drug associated isoelectric EEGs—a hazard in brain-death certification. Commentary. *J.A.M.A.,* **236:**1123, 1976.

270. Price, T. R., and Netsky, M. D. Myxedema and ataxia, cerebellar alterations. Neural myxedema bodies. *Neurology* (Minneap.), **16:**957–62, 1966.

271. Purnell, D. C.; Scholz, D. A.; and Smith, L. H. Diagnosis of primary hyperparathyroidism. *Surg. Clin. North Am.,* **57:**543–56, 1977.

272. Raff, M. C., and Asbury, A. K. Ischemic mononeuropathy and mononeuropathy multiplex in diabetes mellitus. *N. Engl. J. Med.,* **279:**17–22, 1968.

273. Raff, M. C.; Sangaland, V.; and Asbury, A. K. Ischemic mononeuropathy multiplex associated with diabetes mellitus. *Arch. Neurol.,* **18:**487–99, 1968.

274. Rai, G. S.; Buxton-Thomas, M.; and Scanlon, M. Ocular bobbing in hepatic encephalopathy. *Br. J. Clin. Pract.,* **30:**202–205, 1976.

274a. Raichle, M. E.; Grubb, R. L.; et al. Cerebral hemodynamics and metabolism in pseudotumor cerebri. Ann. Neurol., **4:**104–11, 1978.

275. Raskind, M. Psychosis polydypsia and water intoxication. Report of a fatal case. *Arch. Gen. Psychiat.,* **30:**112–14, 1974.

276. Rashin, N. H., and Fishman, R. A. Neurologic disorders in renal failure. *N. Engl. J. Med.,* **294:**143–48, 294–10, 1976.

277. Recommendations from the findings by the RCGP oral contraceptive study on the mortality risks of oral contraceptive users. *Br. Med. J.,* **2:**947, 1977.

277a. Read, D., and Warlow, C. Peripheral neuropathy and solitary plasmocytoma. *J. Neurol. Neurosurg. Psychiatry,* **41:**177–84, 1978.

278. Reed, D.; Crawley, J.; Faro, S. N.; Pieper, S. J.; and Kurland, L. T. Thallotoxicosis. *J.A.M.A.,* **183:**516–22, 1963.

279. Rehnström, S.; Simart, G.; et al. Chronic hepatic encephalopathy. A psychometrical study. *Scand. J. Gastroenterol.,* **12:**305–11, 1977.

280. Reyes, M. G.; Chokroverty, S.; and Masden, J. Thalamic neuroaxonal dystrophy and dementia in Hodgkin's disease. *Neurology* (Minneap.), **26:**251–53, 1976.

281. Rezner, R. H.; Salway, J. G.; and Thomas, P. K. Plasma-myxinositol concentrations in uraemic neuropathy. *Lancet,* **1:**675–76, 1977.

282. Richter, P. L., and Chutorian, A. M. Familial hypoparathyroidism: Case reports and review of the literature. *Neurology* (Minneap.), **18:**75–80, 1968.

283. Riddick, F. A. Primary hyperparathyroidism. *Med. Clin. North Am.,* **51:**871–81, 1967.

284. Ristow, S. C.; Griner, P. F.; et al. Reversal of systemic manifestations of cryoglobulinemia. Treatment with melphalan and prednisone. *Arch. Intern. Med.,* **136:**467–70, 1976.

285. Robinson, A. G. DDAUP in the treatment of central diabetes insipidus. *N. Engl. J. Med.,* **294:**507–11, 1976.

286. Robinson, R. R.; Hayes, C. P., Jr.; and Gunnells, J. C., Jr. Treatment of acute barbiturate intoxication. *Mod. Treatm.,* **4:**679–96, 1967.

287. Robitaille, G. A., and Piscatelli, R. L. Hemolytic anemia in Wilson's disease. A report of three cases with transient increase in hemoglobin A. *J.A.M.A.,* **237:**2402–2403, 1977.

288. Roche-Sicot, J., and Benhaman, J.-P. Acute intravascular hemolysis and acute liver failure as a first manifestation of Wilson's disease. *Ann. Intern. Med.,* **86:**301–303, 1977.

289. Rollinson, R. D., and Gilligan, B. S. Primary hyperparathyroidism presenting as a proximal myopathy. *Aust. N. Z. J. Med.,* **7:**420–21, 1977.

290. Romanul, F. C. A.; Radvany, J.; and Rosales,

R. K. Whipple's disease confined to the brain: A case studied clinically and pathologically. *J. Neurol. Neurosurg. Psychiat.,* **40:**901–909, 1977.

291. Rosen, B. J. Multiple myeloma. A clinical review. *Med. Clin. North Am.,* **59:**375–86, 1975.

291a. Rosenbaum, A. H. Pharmacotherapy for tardive dyskinesia. *Psychiatr. Ann.,* **9:**51–61, 1979.

292. Rosenstock, H. A.; Simons, D. G.; and Meyer, J. S. Chronic manganism. Neurologic and laboratory studies during treatment with Levodopa. *J.A.M.A.,* **217:**1354–61, 1971.

293. Samuel, V. N. Brain Death. *Dis. Nerv. Syst.,* **38:**691–93, 1977.

294. Saric, M.; Markicevic, A.; and Hrustic, O. Occupational exposure to manganese. *Br. J. Indust. Med.,* **34:**114–118, 1977.

295. Sarto, T.; Yoshida, S.; Nakao, K.; and Takanoshi, R. Chronic hypernatremia associated with inflammation of the neurohypophysis. *J. Clin. Endocrinol.,* **31:**391–96, 1970.

296. Sassin, J. F., and Rosenberg, R. N. Neurological complications of fibrous dysplasia of the skull. *Arch. Neurol.,* **18:**363–69, 1968.

297. Saunders, S. J.; Terblanche, J.; Bosman, S. C. W.; Harrison, G. G.; Watts, R.; Hickman, R.; Biebuyck, J.; Dent, D.; Pearce, S.; and Barrard, C. N. Acute hepatic coma treated by cross circulation with a baboon and by repeated exchange transfusions. *Lancet,* **2:**585–88, 1968.

298. Schenker, S.; Breen, K. J.; and Hoyumpa, A. M., Jr. Hepatic encephalopathy: Current status. *Gastroenterology,* **66:**12–151, 1974.

299. Schmid, K.; Krinke, G.; Früh, F.; and Keberle, H. Studies of the distribution and excretion of clioquinol in the animal. *Arzneim. Forsch.,* **23:**1560–66, 1973.

300. Schmidt, W. R., and Jarcho, L. W. Persistent dyskinesias following phenothiazine therapy; report of five cases and a review of the literature. *Arch. Neurol.,* **14:**369–77, 1966.

301. Schoeller, J.-P. Mise au point sur les neuropathies survenues cours de traitements par le clioquinol. *Therapie,* **28:**401–404, 1973.

301a. Schold, S. C.; Cho, E.-S.; et al. Subacute motor neuropathy: A remote effect of lymphoma. *Ann. Neurol.,* **5:**271–87, 1979.

302. Schreier, H. A.; Sherry, N.; and Shaughnessy, E. Lead poisoning and brain tumors in children. A report of two cases. *Ann. Neurol.,* **1:**599–600, 1977.

303. Schumann, G. B.; Lauenstein, K.; et al. Ultraviolet spectrometric analysis of barbiturates. Current assessment as an emergency screening procedure. *Am. J. Clin. Pathol.,* **66:**823–30, 1976.

304. Schwab, P. J., and Fahey, J. L. Treatment of Waldenstrom's macroglobulinemia by plasmopheresis. *N. Engl. J. Med.,* **263:**574–79, 1960.

305. Sears, E. S. Nonketotic hyperosmolar hyperglycemia during glycerol therapy for cerebral edema. *Neurology* (Minneap.), **26:**89–94, 1976.

306. Selby, G. Subacute myelo-optic neuropathy in Australia. *Lancet,* **1:**123–25, 1972.

307. Seigel, D., and Corfman, P. Epidemiological problems associated with studies of the safety of oral contraceptives. *J.A.M.A.,* **203:**950–54, 1968.

308. Service, F. J.; Dale, A. J. D.; et al. Insulinoma. Clinical and diagnostic features of 60 consecutive cases. *Mayo Clin. Proc.,* **51:**417–29, 1976.

309. Sharf, B., and Bental, E. Pancreatic encephalopathy. *J. Neurol. Neurosurg. Psychiat.,* **34:**357–61, 1971.

310. Shield, L. K.; Coleman, T. L.; and Markesbery, W. R. Methyl bromide intoxication: Neurologic features including simulation of Reye syndrome. *Neurology* (Minneap.), **27:**959–62, 1977.

311. Shirabe, T.; Tawara, S.; et al. Myxoedatous polyneuropathy: A light and electron microscopic study of the peripheral nerve and muscle. *J. Neurol. Neurosurg. Psychiat.,* **38:**241–47, 1975.

312. Shy, G. M., and Silverstein, I. Study of the effects upon the motor unit by remote malignancy. *Brain,* **88:**515–28, 1965.

313. Silfverskiöld, B. P. Cortical cerebellar degeneration associated with a specific disorder of standing and locomotion. *Acta Neurol. Scand.,* **5:**257–72, 1977.

314. Silverberg, D. S.; Iaina, A.; et al. Cholestyramine in uraemic pruritus. *Br. J. Med.,* **1:**752–53, 1977.

315. Silverman, D.; Saunders, M. G.; Schwab, R. S.; and Masland, R. L. Cerebral death and the electroencephalogram. Report of the ad hoc committee of the American Electroencephalographic Society on EEG Criteria for determination of cerebral death. *J.A.M.A.,* **209:**1505–10, 1969.

316. Singh, R. B.; Duke, K. P.; and Srwastav, P. K. Hypomagnesemia in relation to digoxin intoxication in children. *Am. Heart J.,* **92:**144–47, 1976.

316a. Slyter, H. Idiopathic hypoparathyroidism presenting as dementia. *Neurology* (Minneap.), **29:**393–94, 1979.

317. Smith, H. V., and Spalding, J. M. Outbreak of paralysis in Morocco due to orthocresyl phosphate poisoning. *Lancet,* **2:**1019–21, 1959.

318. Sohn, D.; Valensi, Q.; and Miller, S. P. Neurologic manifestations of Hodgkin's disease. *Arch. Neurol.,* **17:**429–36, 1967.

319. Sparacio, R. R.; Anziska, B.; and Schutta, H. S. Hypernatremia and chorea. A report of two cases. *Neurology* (Minneap.), **26:**46–50, 1976.

320. Spivak, J. L., and Jackson, D. L. Pellagra: An analysis of 18 patients and a review of the literature. *Johns Hopkins Med. J.,* **140:**295–309, 1977.

321. Starr, A. Auditory brain-stem responses in brain death. *Brain,* **99:**543–54, 1976.

322. Stieglitz, L. N.; Kind, H. P.; et al. Keratitis with hypoparathyroidism. *Am. J. Ophthalmol.,* **84:**467–72, 1977.

323. Stockman, J. A.; Nigro, M. A.; Mishkin, M. M.; and Oski, F. A. Occlusion of intracrainal major vessels in sickle-cell anemia. *N. Engl. J. Med.,* **287:**846–49, 1972.

324. Sugar, O. Cerebral neurological complaints of hypoparathyroidism. *Arch. Neurol. Psychiat.,* **70:**86–107, 1953.

325. Sundaram, M., and Scholz, C. Primary hyperparathyroidism presenting with acute paraplegia. *Am. J. Roentgenol.,* **128:**674–76, 1977.

326. Sundaresan, N.; Noronha, A.; et al. Oculomotor palsy as initial manifestation of myeloma. *J.A.M.A.,* **238:**2052–53, 1977.

327. Supino-Viterbo, V.; Sicard, C.; et al. Toxic encephalopathy due to ingestion of bismuth salts: Clinical and EEG studies of 45 patients. *J. Neurol. Neurosurg. Psychiat.,* **40:**748–52, 1977.

328. Synder, R. D., and Seelinger, D. F. Methylmercury poisoning—clinical follow-up and sensory nerve conduction studies. *J. Neurol. Neurosurg. Psychiat.,* **39:**701–704, 1976.

329. Taclob, L., and Needle, M. Drug-induced encephalopathy in patients on maintenance dialysis. *Lancet,* **2:**704–705, 1976.

330. Takabashi, K., and Nakamura, H. Axonal degeneration in beriberi neuropathy. *Arch. Neurol.,* **33:**836–41, 1975.

330a. Tay, C. H., and Seah, C. S. Arsenic poisoning from anti-asthmatic herbal preparations. *Med. J. Aust.,* **2:**424–28, 1975.

331. Teschan, P. E. Electroencephalographic and other neurophysiological abnormalities in uremia. *Kidney Int.,* Suppl **2:**210–16, 1975.

332. Thompson, G. N. Electroencephalogram in acute pathological alcoholic intoxication. *Bull. Los Angeles Neurol. Soc.,* **28:**217–24, 1963.

333. Toaff, R.; Toaff, M. E.; et al. Hepatolenticular degeneration (Wilson's disease) and pregnancy. A review and report of a case. *Obstet. Gynecol. Surv.,* **32:**497–507, 1977.

334. Traviesa, D. C. Magnesium deficiency: A possible cause of thiamine refractoriness in Wernicke-Korsakoff encephalopathy. *J. Neurol. Neurosurg. Psychiat.,* **37:**959–62, 1974.

335. Traviesa, D. C.; Schwatzman, R. J.; et al. Familial benign intracranial hypertension. *J. Neurol. Neurosurg. Psychiat.,* **39:**420–23, 1976.

335a. Troncoso, J.; Marcall, E. L.; and Schatz, N. J. Visual evoked responses in pernicious anemia. *Arch. Neurol.,* **36:**168–69, 1979.

336. Trotter, J. D.; Engel, W. K.; and Ignaczak, T. F. Amyloidosis with plasma cell dyscrasia. An overlooked cause of adult onset sensorimotor neuropathy. *Arch. Neurol.,* **34:**209–14, 1977.

337. Trotter, J. L.; Hendin, B. A.; and Osterland, C. K. Cerebellar degeneration with Hodgkin's disease. An immunological study. *Arch. Neurol.,* **33:**660–61, 1976.

338. Tsubaki, T.; Toyokura, Y.; and Tsukagoshi, H. Subacute myelo-optico-neuropathy following abdominal symptoms, a clinical and pathological study. *Jap. J. Med.,* **4:**181–84, 1965.

339. Tyler, H. R. Neurological aspects of uremia: An overview. *Kidney Int.,* suppl **2:**188–93, 1975.

340. VanOmmen, R. A. Adverse effects of antimicrobial agents on major organ systems. *Clevel. Clin. Q.,* **37:**59–71, 1970.

341. Vejjajiva, A., and Sitprija, V. Chronic sustained hypernatremia and hypovolemia in hypothalamic tumor. *Neurology* (Minneap.), **19:**161–66, 1969.

342. Vessey, M. P.; McPherson, K.; and Johnson, B. Mortality among women participating in the Oxford/Family Planning Association Contraceptive Study. *Lancet,* **2:**731–33, 1977.

343. Victor, M. Effects of nutritional deficiency on the nervous system; comparison with the effects of carcinoma. In Brain, W. R., and Norris, F. H., Jr. (eds.). *Remote Effects of Cancer on the Nervous System.* Grune & Stratton, New York, 1965, pp. 134–61.

344. Victor, M., and Adams, R. D. On the etiology of the alcoholic neurologic diseases; with special reference to the role of nutrition. *Am. J. Clin. Nutr.,* **9:**379–97, 1961.

345. Victor, M. Treatment of alcoholic intoxication and the withdrawal syndrome. *Psychosom. Med.,* **28:**636–50, 1966.

346. Victor, M. The pathophysiology of alcoholic epilepsy. *Proc. Res. Nerv. Ment. Dis.,* **46:**431–54, 1968.

347. Victor, M.; Adams, R. D.; and Cole, M. The acquired (non-Wilsonian) type of chronic hepatocerebral degeneration. *Medicine,* **44:**345–96, 1965.

348. Victor, M.; Adams, R. D.; and Mancall, E. L. Restricted form of cerebellar cortical degeneration occurring in alcoholic patients. *Arch. Neurol.,* **1:**579–688, 1959.

349. Victor, M., and Brausch, C. The role of abstinence in the genesis of alcoholic epilepsy. *Epilepsia,* 1–20, 1967.

350. Vital, C.; Vallat, J. M.; et al. Peripheral neuropathies of diabetes mellitus: Ultrastructural study of biopsies from 12 cases. *J. Neurol. Sci.,* **18:**381–98, 1973.

351. Vogel, R. M., and Lee, R. V. Bilateral ptosis in Wernicke's disease. *Neurology* (Minneap.), **17:**85–86, 1967.

352. Wacker, W. E. C., and Parisi, A. F. Magnesium metabolism. *N. Engl. J. Med.,* **278:**658–63, 712–17, 772–76, 1968.

353. Wadia, N. H. Some observations on SMON from Bombay. *J. Neurol. Neurosurg. Psychiat.,* **40:**268–75, 1977.

354. Walker, A. E., and Molinari, G. E. Criteria of cerebral death. *Trans. Am. Neurol. Assoc.,* **100:**29–35, 1975.

355. Walsh, C. J. Gold neuropathy. *Neurology* (Minneap.), **20:**455–58, 1970.

356. Walshe, J. M. Wilson's disease; the presenting symptoms. *Arch. Dis. Child.,* **37:**253–56, 1962.

357. Walshe, J. M. Filterable and nonfilterable serum copper. I. Action of penicillamine. *Clin. Sci.,* **25:**405–11, 1963.

358. Walshe, J. M. Penicillamine. *Practitioner,* **191:**789–95, 1963.

359. Walshe, J. M., and Cummings, J. N. (eds.). *Wilson's Disease: Some Current Concepts.* Blackwell, Oxford, 1961.

360. Watts, J. Mck.; Douglas, M. C.; Dudley, H. A. F.; Gurr, F. W.; and Owen, J. A. Heterologous liver perfusion in acute hepatic failure. *Br. Med. J.,* **2:**341–45, 1967.

361. Weiderholt, W. C.; Kobayashi, R. M; et al. Central pontine myelinolysis: A clinical reappraisal. *Arch. Neurol.,* **34:**220–23, 1977.

362. Weigmann, T., and Kaye, M. Hypomagnesemic hypocalcemia. Early serum calcium and late

paralhormone increase with magnesium therapy. *Arch. Intern. Med.,* **137:**953–55, 1977.

362a. Weinstein, R.; Schwartzman, R.; and Levey, G. S. Proprananol reversal of bulbar dysfunction and proximal myopathy in hyperthyroidism. *Ann. Intern. Med.,* **82:**540, 1975.

363. Weisberg, L., and Nue, C. N. Computed tomographic evaluation of increased pressure without localizing signs. *Radiology,* **122:**133–36, 1977.

364. Wells, C. E., and Silver, R. T. Neurologic manifestations of the acute leukemias; clinical study. *Ann. Intern. Med.,* **46:**439–49, 1957.

365. Wiebers, D. O.; Hollenhorst, R. W.; and Goldstein, N. P. The ophthalmologic manifestations of Wilson's disease. *Mayo Clin. Proc.,* **52:**409–16, 1977.

366. Wilkinson, P. C. Serological findings in carcinomatous neuromyopathy. *Lancet,* **1:**1301–3, 1964.

367. Wilkinson, P. C., and Zeromski, J. Immunofluorescent detection of antibodies against neurones in sensory carcinomatous neuropathy. *Brain,* **88:**529–38, 1965.

368. Williams, I. R., and Mayer, R. F. Subacute proximal diabetic neuropathy. *Neurology* (Minneap.), **26:**108–16, 1976.

369. Winegrad, A. I., and Greene, D. A. Diabetic polyneuropathy: Importance of insulin deficiency hyperglycemia and alteration in myoinositol metabolism in its pathogenesis. *N. Engl. J. Med.,* **295:**1416–21, 1976.

369a. Wolchnic-Dygas, D.; Niewiadomski, M.; and Kostrzewska, E. Porphyric polyneuropathy and its pathogenesis in the light of electrophysiological investigations. *J. Neurol. Sci.,* **35:**243–56, 1978.

370. Wright, F. W., and Hamilton, W. S. A large craniopharyngioma with panhypopituitrism. *Br. J. Clin. Pract.,* **30:**224–27, 1976.

371. Zavon, M. R. Treatment of organophosphorus and chlorinated hydrocarbon insecticide intoxication. *Mod. Treatm.,* **4:**625–32, 1967.

372. Zangemeister, W. H.; Schwendemann, G.; and Colmant, H. J. Carcinomatous encephalomyelopathy in conjunction with encephalomyeloradiculitis. *J. Neurol.,* **218:**63–71, 1978.

6 HEADACHE, MIGRAINE, EPILEPSY, AND SYNCOPE

Headache: General Considerations

Headache is one of the most common of physical complaints and is listed almost invariably as an accompanying symptom in most of the diseases discussed in any textbook of medicine. Headache can be mild and of short duration or it can be severe enough to be totally incapacitating. The majority of headaches are not serious and respond rapidly to mild analgesics; others are prolonged, have serious implications, and may require narcotics.

The term "headache" has been defined as the occurrence of pain or discomfort over the upper part of the head from the orbits to the suboccipital area. This definition is, however, too restricted since the source of the pain may originate in the face, teeth, or neck and spread into the area defined above. Consequently, a discussion of headache should consider a number of painful conditions which arise primarily in the face and neck as well as those arising from disorders of the upper part of the head.

In neurologic practice, three types of headache are most commonly encountered. These are migraine, cluster, and tension headaches. These conditions and their treatment will be considered after a brief review of the mechanisms of pain in the head. Thereafter, special types of headache will be discussed.

Mechanisms of Pain in the Head

Careful observations have been recorded during intracranial operations, carried out under local anesthesia, on conscious patients. Traction and electrical stimulation revealed that only certain intracranial structures are sensitive to pain. Structures sensitive to pain included the venous sinuses and cortical veins which drain into them; the arteries at the base of the brain which form the circle of Willis and proximal portions of the major vessels arising from them; the dura lining the floor of the anterior and posterior fossae; and the cranial nerves (mainly the fifth, ninth, and tenth which carry pain fibers from these intracranial structures). In contrast, the bones of the cranium, most of the pia, arachnoid, and remaining portions of dura, the parenchyma of the brain, the ependymal lining of the ventricles, and the choroid plexus were insensitive.

When structures sensitive to pain above the tentorium cerebelli were stimulated, the pain was referred to the frontotemporal or anterior parietal regions of the head. Such pain was transmitted via the trigeminal nerve. Pain arising from structures in the posterior fossa was referred to the occipital, suboccipital, and upper cervical areas and was transmitted via the ninth and tenth cranial nerves and the upper three cervical nerves.

Virtually all the structures of the scalp and face were sensitive to pain. These included the skin and arteries of the scalp and face; the muscles of the scalp, face, and neck; the orbital contents; the mucous membrane of the nasal and paranasal spaces; the external and middle ears; and the teeth. Pain arising from any of these structures is usually well-localized but often spreads to cover a wide area of the head.

Pain in the head has been shown to be induced in a number of ways. These include:

1. Traction on the circle of Willis and its major branches.
2. Dilatation of intracranial and extracranial blood vessels.
3. Induced spasm of intracranial and extracranial blood vessels.
4. Inflammation involving blood vessels (arteritis).
5. Inflammation of intracranial and extracranial structures including the leptomeninges.
6. Sustained contraction of the muscles in the scalp and neck such as occurs in tension states.
7. Changes in the intracranial pressures and intracavitary pressures within the nasal or paranasal cavities, orbits, ears, and teeth.
8. Direct pressure on nerves containing pain fibers.

In addition to the strictly mechanical factors described above, headache is commonly caused by emotional disturbances including anxiety and depression. The cause of these psychogenic headaches appears to be sustained muscular contraction of the muscles of the head and neck and possibly dilatation of the cephalic vessels.

Vascular Headaches of the Migraine Type

In migraine there is periodic instability of cranial arteries with episodes of vasoconstriction followed by vasodilatation. The aura of classic migraine occurs during vasoconstriction, and the pain arises during dilatation of the arteries supplying the brain and scalp.[15] Variations in the clinical manifestations of certain types of migraine depend on the site of the blood vessels involved and the duration of the vascular distention.

Etiology and Pathology

Many factors may contribute to the development of migraine, and it may be that migraine is not a single pathogenetic entity.

Migraine is often familial, and a positive family history is obtained in at least 60 per cent of cases. The tendency to suffer from migraine has been described as an autosomal dominant and as an autosomal recessive trait with a penetrance of approximately 70 per cent in the latter. Nevertheless, some studies indicate that hereditary factors are much less important in migraine than is usually supposed.[230]

There is a high incidence of migraine in intelligent people, in the higher socioeconomic group, and in professional occupations. However, the impression of a higher incidence may be spurious due to the tendency of individuals in these groups to seek medical advice. It has been said that the migraine sufferer is a hard-driving, ambitious, and compulsive individual, but there is obviously a wide variation in the types of personality encountered in patients with migraine. Nevertheless, there is some evidence that migraine victims are more neurotic, less extroverted, and more hostile with inadequate emotional expression.[172]

In women there is frequently a relationship between attacks of migraine and their menstrual periods.[231] Many women experience migraine at the onset of each menstrual period or complain that their attacks are more severe at that time. There may be an exacerbation in women during the menopause. Some women report that they are free of attacks during pregnancy. In others, their headaches are exacerbated during the early months of pregnancy.[25] The relationship to menstruation and pregnancy has long suggested that migraine was triggered by changes in endocrine balance[14, 202] and perhaps an associated disturbance in salt and water metabolism. It is known that the attacks always occur as estrogen levels fall[203] and may be delayed or abolished if levels are artificially maintained at a high level of administration of estrogens. This view is supported by some reports of exacerbation or relief of headache in young women who take oral contraceptive pills.[120, 184b]

The relationship of allergy to migraine is not clear. There is no association between migraine and known hypersensitivity states such as allergic asthma or hay fever.[140] However, complement is activated during a migraine attack, suggesting the possibility of an antibody-antigen reaction.[129]

Many patients develop migraine during or after stressful situations,[66, 85] particularly those causing frustration and tension. This stress is often well tolerated by others; is nonspecific; and includes fatigue, exposure to bright light, mild hypoglycemia,[162] meteorologic changes, exposure to high altitudes, the use of various drugs (including vasodilators and reserpine), and repeated mild trauma to the head (as in soccer players).[136]

Some migraine sufferers develop headache during a period of hunger in which they do not develop hypoglycemia.[162] This suggests that there may be involvement of more complex metabolic factors in these cases. Many patients relate the onset of migraine headaches to ingestion of certain foods, particularly chocolate, cheese, citrus fruits, smoked fish, and alcohol.[41] A number of these foods have a high tyramine content. It has been postulated that patients with dietary migraine may have a deficiency of tyramine-o-sulphatase, and excess tyramine could act by releasing catecholamines that in turn initiate the vasoconstrictive stage of migraine.[65, 198]

Patients who suffer from migraine show hyperaggregability of platelets when free from headache.[37] Platelet aggregation increases during the prodromal stage of migraine. This may be due to an increase in epinephrine, thrombin, or arachidonic acid in the circulation in response to anxiety, stress, starvation, smoking, ingestion of foods containing tyramine, phenylethylamine, or ingestion of alcohol. Increased platelet aggregation in the prodromal stage is followed by a decrease in platelet aggregation during the headache.[40] These changes parallel the increase

in plasma serotonin levels reported during the prodromal stage of migraine and the decrease in serotonin levels that occurs during the headache.[4] Platelets contain virtually all of the serotonin present in the blood and release serotonin during aggregation. This suggests that changes in plasma serotonin levels during migraine are secondary to changes in platelet aggregation.[44]

Platelet aggregation is enhanced by adenosine diphosphate (ADP), epinephrine, and arachidonic acid, and aggregated platelets release ADP, serotonin, histamine, epinephrine, norepinephrine, and arachidonic acid. Thus, the initial platelet aggregation releases substances that produce a second phase of platelet aggregation. The released catecholamine may precipitate vasoconstriction while arachidonic acid is transformed into several types of prostaglandins including prostaglandin F_2 alpha which also cause cerebral vasoconstriction,[164] cerebral ischemia, and reduction in cerebral blood flow. Prostaglandins also have the property of causing nausea and vomiting, which are frequent symptoms in migraine.[94] Flufenamic acid, an inhibitor of prostaglandin synthesis, relieves migraine[221] possibly by inhibition of the vasoactivity of prostaglandins.

The cerebral vasodilatation and increased blood flow that occur during the headache phase of migraine are possibly due to depletion of serotonin and catecholamine from platelets or may represent a reactive vasodilatation from the cerebral ischemia and lactacidosis of the prodromal phase. Serotonin may be released into the extracellular space around the dilated blood vessels which produces an increase in sensitivity of cranial pain receptors. The migraine headache could be the result of the action of bradykinin or other tissue kinins on the sensitized pain receptors.

There is an interesting association between migraine and REM sleep. Migraine that awakens patients from sleep occurs immediately after a period of REM sleep when there is a sudden fall in plasma serotonin levels.[45] There is a demonstrable increase in plasma noradrenaline levels during sleep in migraine patients for about three hours before they awaken with headache.[96] The causes of the biochemical changes and their relation to REM sleep and headache are unclear.

The role of gamma amino butyric acid in migraine is also intriguing in that the concentration of GABA in the cerebrospinal fluid is increased during migraine attacks.[113] GABA is an inhibitory neurotransmitter, and it is possible that local

GABA release may depress neuronal function during the ischemic phase of the migraine attack, producing the reversible neurologic deficits of the aura.[168]

It has long been claimed that there is a relationship between migraine and seizures.[11, 97, 190] The family histories of patients with migraine are said to show a higher incidence of seizures compared to the general population. Data of this type were collected before the precision of neurologic diagnosis available today. It is possible that some epileptic subjects whose seizures were manifested by recurrent headaches were incorrectly classified as having migraine, and some migrainous subjects whose attacks were predominantly those of photopsia and hemiparesthesias, with little headache, were incorrectly classified as having seizure disorders. The great majority of patients suffering from migraine have normal electroencephalograms when they are free of attacks, although focal slowing on the side of the headache is frequent during an attack. It is unusual for subjects with migraine to be afforded relief by the use of anticonvulsant drugs, although a trial is justifiable in rare patients with migraine-like symptoms who have abnormal EEGs when free of attacks. Certain patients with intermittent headache, who show spike and slow-wave or other paroxysmal disorders in the EEG and who respond to anticonvulsant drugs, should be regarded as cases of seizures with headache as a manifestation of seizure activity.

Clinical Features

It is difficult to assess the true incidence of such a common disorder as migraine since many patients do not seek medical advice or treatment. The majority of epidemiologic studies have been carried out among highly selected groups; however, it is probable that migraine occurs in about 5 to 10 per cent of the population.

Attacks of migraine sometimes begin in childhood, although the first attack may be experienced as late as the thirties. In general, the first symptoms are usually noted in late adolescence and the twenties. The frequency of attacks varies a great deal from case to case, but they occur less than once per week in 60 per cent of patients. Rarely, patients may complain of migraine headaches three or four times per week but this is unusual. Daily headaches are usually not due to migraine but may be cluster headaches or caused by anxiety, states of tension, or some related condition.

Prodromal Symptoms. A number of patients with migraine experience prodromata for several hours preceding the attack. There may be generalized fluid retention at the beginning of the attack with a feeling of tightness of the skin, inability to remove rings, and a measurable gain in weight. Some patients experience a feeling of restlessness and creativity; others describe a sensation of mounting tension.

Classic Migraine. The classic aura of migraine consists of the complaint that for 20 to 40 minutes preceding the headache the patient develops visual symptoms, usually referred to as photopsia, which impair vision in part of the visual field. In children the aura may be the outstanding feature, while in older patients the visual symptoms may occur without the subsequent development of headache. Visual symptoms include scintillating scotomata or "seeing stars." The visual scotomata may have different shapes and configurations and are often bordered by moving streaks of light. They are sometimes described as jagged in outline or resembling the battlements of a medieval castle. The latter type is termed "fortification spectra." The scotomata are homonymous, and the majority of patients develop a temporary homonymous hemianopia, which begins as a central scotoma and gradually spreads out toward the periphery of the homonymous visual field. Almost all complain of photophobia, sometimes with an aversion to a particular color or black and white (chromophobia).

The prodromal symptoms of photopsia develop to a maximum just before the headache begins and then recede. They are confined to or are maximal in the homonymous visual field opposite the headache. Additional symptoms may include hemiparesthesias, mild hemiparesis, dysphasia, and monocular photopsia.

The headache begins as a dull ache in the supra-orbital, retro-orbital, or frontotemporal area on one side. Occasionally, it develops in the parietal or occipital region, but this is unusual. It is unilateral, and as the pain increases in intensity, it takes on a pulsating or throbbing character, rises to a crescendo, and then persists as an intense, constant pain. At this stage, the headache often spreads from the original site to involve the whole of the hemicranium and extends down into the upper cervical area. The patient is pale, nauseated (and usually vomits), prostrated by pain, and complains of marked photophobia. The pupils are dilated and the patient prefers to lie in a darkened room. Rarely, some patients develop flushing of the face, constricted pupils, and diffuse perspiration. In some cases there is marked diuresis toward the end of an attack.

The headache usually lasts all day but is terminated by sleep. There is a feeling of relief on awakening and being free of the headache.

Occasionally the headache, nausea, and vomiting will last for two or three days accompanied by increasing weakness, prostration, and distress. This may leave the patient with a feeling of fatigue and listlessness for several days after the headache abates.

Common Migraine. Many patients experience periodic vascular headaches that do not have the stereotyped characteristics of classic migraine. The prodromal symptoms are sometimes absent or consist of a brief period of photopsia or blurred vision, and the headache is occasionally bilateral from the onset. The same degree of prostration, nausea, vomiting, and retching accompanies the headache in most cases, and the condition is similar to classic migraine in every way except for the lack of the prominent prodromal phase.

Migraine in Children. It has been estimated that migraine affects 5 per cent of children aged 11 years, the onset of the attacks occurring in most children between the ages of six and ten years.[178] Children with migraine often have an antecedent history of periodic or cyclic vomiting, episodic vertigo, or transient neurologic deficits such as hemiparesis, ptosis, diplopia, or ataxia, all without headache.[50] Many children experience bilateral headaches at the onset of migraine with later development of unilateral pain, usually located in the forehead and temple. Some children develop the typical symptoms of classic migraine, which often occurs in the late afternoon after school or seems to be precipitated by fatigue or stress. It is not uncommon to see children in whom the headaches are less troublesome than the accompanying vomiting and prostration. On the whole, vomiting seems to be more prominent in children who have an increased tendency to suffer from motion sickness. A migraine variant called subintrant migraine has been described in childhood.[59] There are successive attacks of unilateral headache which are similar to cluster headaches in the adult but without the autonomic concomitants. The attacks occur daily for about seven days, resolve, and then recur two or three times a year.

Childhood migraine usually responds to phenobarbital, 15 to 30 mg three times a day. Ergotamine preparations and prophylactic medications such as methysergide maleate or clonidine are rarely needed.

Hemiplegic Migraine. An occasional migraine patient may experience symptoms of numbness and/or weakness preceding the onset of headaches. The symptoms often begin in the hand or lower limb and spread progressively until the whole of one side of the body is involved. Some patients develop dysphasia or aphasia depending on whether the right or left side is involved. The headache begins 20 to 60 minutes after the onset of symptoms, may be ipsilateral or contralateral, and lasts from several hours to two or three days. The weakness and/or numbness may last for several days and usually resolves. Permanent deficits have occurred in rare cases. Hemiplegic migraine is occasionally preceded by the visual symptoms of classic migraine. Impairment of consciousness has been reported in some cases.

Two types of hemiplegic migraine are recognized.[88]

1. Familial hemiplegic migraine in which the symptoms are similar in all affected family members who never have migraine of any other type.
2. Hemiplegic migraine, which may be familial or nonfamilial, in which the affected patients have occasional attacks of classic or common migraine without hemiplegic symptoms.

Hemiplegic migraine sufferers may have motor weakness alone, sensory symptoms alone, or a combination of motor and sensory symptoms. Symptoms are usually unilateral but bilateral deficits may occur in some cases.

The association of familial hemiplegic migraine, retinitis pigmentosa, and sensorineural deafness has been reported.[242] However, repeated attacks of familial hemiplegic migraine may lead to retinal degeneration due presumably to ischemic infarction of the retina.[74]

The onset of hemiparesis or hemisensory deficit is believed to be due to vasoconstriction, and the persistence of symptoms for several days is probably due to cerebral edema which can be seen by CT scan. Treatment by prophylaxis (i.e., propranolol, imipramine, methysergide) rather than vasoconstrictive agents is recommended.[76]

Basilar Migraine. This unusual form of migraine presents with vertigo, ataxia, dysarthria, bilateral visual symptoms, and motor weakness, often of hemiparetic type. There may be impairment of consciousness with stupor or restless behavior in which the patient is incoherent and dysphasic (see Migrainous Psychosis). The headache is usually bilateral and occipital,[235] and the symptoms of neurologic deficit can persist for several hours in the presence of headache. Spasm of the basilar artery has been demonstrated by angiography in basilar migraine, and the electroencephalogram may show a typical photoconvulsive response during an attack.[211a]

Ophthalmoplegic Migraine. This rare migraine variant consists of the combination of migraine headache and ipsilateral ophthalmoplegia. The ophthalmoplegia is due to paresis of the third nerve, and the fourth and sixth nerves and ophthalmic division of the fifth nerve are rarely involved. Ophthalmoplegic migraine is believed to be the result of vasodilatation of the intracavernous carotid artery of sufficient degree to compress the third nerve in the lateral wall of the cavernous sinus.

Patients with ophthalmoplegic migraine usually have a history of migraine headaches without oculomotor involvement, often from childhood, before the development of ophthalmoplegia. The typical attack begins with the development of a unilateral migrainous headache, followed by nausea and vomiting. The attack is more severe and protracted than the majority of migraine headaches experienced by the patient, lasting one or two days and occasionally longer. Finally, as the pain begins to decrease in intensity, the patient develops an ipsilateral ptosis and diplopia. The oculomotor paresis lasts several days and slowly improves. However, paresis may be present for as long as two weeks in chronic recurrent cases.

Ophthalmoplegic migraine is strictly unilateral with the pain and the paresis always on the same side. Very few cases have been described in which the attacks shift from side to side. This migraine variant usually occurs without an aura, but the headache precedes the oculomotor defect by hours or even days in some cases. The paresis occurs as the pain abates and therefore outlasts the pain. Remission is usually complete between attacks although some chronic cases develop a partial permanent oculomotor deficit.

Migrainous Psychosis. Most migraine sufferers experience some mild depression, mental slowing, and personality change during an attack of migraine. These symptoms are usually overshadowed by the severity of the headache, nausea, and vomiting. However, migraine may be accompanied by or present with prominent mental symptoms including confusion, abnormal behavior, anxiety, fear, hallucinations, restlessness, or stupor.[122] These symptoms occur without headache in some cases and mimic an acute encephalopathy. Symptoms of marked mental aberration are occasionally seen in families with hemiplegic migraine, and it is possible that these attacks are produced by vasoconstriction in the vertebral basilar system resulting in ischemia of the brainstem and diencephalic structures.

Complicated Migraine. Migraine is usually regarded as a benign condition that resolves completely after each attack without evidence of damage to the central nervous system. This statement is undoubtedly true in the majority of cases, but there have been descriptions of permanent neurologic deficits which cannot be ascribed to an associated disorder such as a vascular malformation. The demonstration of focal cortical atrophy by CT scan indicates that ischemic atrophy can occur in severe recurrent cases of migraine. Clinical reports include permanent visual field defects and visual deterioration due to ischemic retinopathy, indicating damage to both occipital lobes and the retina. Hemiparesis and hemisensory loss may be permanent but rare complications of hemiplegic migraine and fatal cerebral infarction have been reported.[144] Respiratory arrest is a possible complication in basilar migraine.[150]

Migraine Equivalents. Symptoms of almost any type of migraine may occur without the accompanying headache. The most common migraine equivalent is the scintillating scotoma,[177] which occasionally occurs as an isolated symptom in individuals who have never had migraine headaches. Similar symptoms are not unusual in migraine sufferers who are surprised and relieved when the expected headache fails to develop. The symptoms of any of the more complex forms of migraine may also occur without headache and frequently lead to erroneous diagnosis and needless investigative procedures, unless the diagnosis is established by an adequate history.

Diagnostic Procedures

The blood count, urinalysis, and roentgenograms of the skull are all normal in patients with migraine. Between attacks of migraine the EEG is usually normal. Transient EEG slowing is recorded during an attack of migraine and usually consists of alpha asymmetry with the appearance of localized and rhythmic theta or delta activity in the posterior head region on the side of the headache (Fig. 6–1).

A CT scan may show evidence of focal cerebral edema if the scan is taken within several days following a migraine attack.[135] Ventricular enlargement and focal cortical atrophy have been reported by CT scan in patients who have had severe migraine for many years.[23, 98]

Many patients experience fluid retention and weight gain prior to an attack, and daily weight

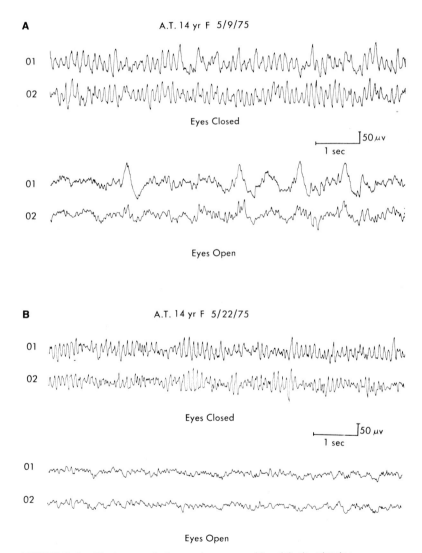

FIGURE 6–1. Electroencephalogram in a case of hemiplegic migraine. *A* taken during the acute phase shows a focus of high-voltage slow activity in the posterior portion of the left hemisphere. *B* shows recovery with a normal pattern two weeks later.

records are of some use in predicting attacks and attempting prophylactic therapy.

In cases with focal neurologic signs such as "ophthalmoplegic migraine," it is important to exclude aneurysms of the terminal portion of the internal carotid, posterior communicating, or terminal basilar arteries. A cerebral arteriovenous malformation may also mimic migraine. An intracranial bruit can be heard in two thirds of these cases.[163] An iodine-enhanced CT scan and/or arteriography is recommended in patients with focal neurologic signs.

Treatment

Since the pain of migraine is due to vasodilatation of the cephalic circulation, any agent or mechanism that produces vasoconstriction is likely to lessen the intensity of the headache. It has long been known that measures such as pressure on the scalp over the superficial temporal arteries and compression of the common carotid and external carotid arteries afford temporary relief during an attack. Application of an icebag to the painful area is also helpful. Inhalation of 100 per cent oxygen and drugs such as caffeine, ephedrine, epinephrine, and amphetamine afford temporary relief since they all have some vasoconstrictive action on either the extra- or intracranial vessels.

If the attack cannot be aborted by early treatment, the patient should be removed from any aggravating stimuli and rest quietly in bed in a darkened room. Attacks often terminate during sleep, and the patient awakes pain-free several hours later.

Use of Ergotamine Preparations in Migraine. Both ergot and ergotamine preparations such as ergotamine tartrate have been used effectively for many years in the symptomatic control of migraine. Ergotamine is generally more satisfactory than other ergot preparations and is used almost exclusively at the present time. The treatment of migraine should begin with oral preparations of ergotamine, usually combined with caffeine. The patient with classic migraine should be instructed to take the tablets at the onset of premonitory symptoms while those with atypical migraine should take them as soon as the headache begins.[237]

The most widely used preparation for treatment of migraine consists of a combination of ergotamine tartrate, 1 mg, and caffeine, 100 mg (Cafergot). Two tablets are taken orally and repeated in 30 minutes if the headache does not abate. Another two tablets may be taken 30 minutes later if necessary. However, if no relief is obtained after 6 mg, no further ergotamine should be administered, although analgesics may be taken and at this time are usually effective. Doses in excess of 6 mg/24 hours may lead to ergot poisoning (ergotism). In cases in which the oral preparations are ineffective, usually because of nausea and vomiting, ergotamine can be given sublingually since it is absorbed rapidly. The sublingual tablets consist of ergotamine tartrate, 2 mg. These are placed beneath the tongue at the onset of the warning symptoms or at the onset of headache. If the initial dose is ineffective, the medication can be repeated at 30-minute intervals for two further doses. A number of patients with nausea and vomiting find that rectal suppositories of ergotamine and caffeine (Cafergot suppositories) are effective if administered at the beginning of an attack. These suppositories contain 2 mg of ergotamine tartrate. The second suppository may be given after one hour if the headache is still present.

The great majority of patients with migraine respond to either oral or rectal preparations of ergotamine.[134a] However, in severe attacks, the physician may elect to administer the drug by the intramuscular route. It is usually given intramuscularly in doses of 0.25 to 0.5 mg. If this is the only method of administration that affords relief, the patient may be taught to administer the drug by intramuscular injection to himself. Following the administration of ergotamine preparations in any form, the patient should be instructed to rest in bed until the headache has subsided.

TOXIC EFFECTS. The majority of patients tolerate the dosage of ergotamine tartrate outlined above well, but side effects occasionally occur. However, they are rarely of sufficient magnitude to necessitate abandoning the use of the drug. The most common complaint is that the drug produces lightheadedness and drowsiness. Some patients experience paresthesias in the extremities and muscle stiffness, particularly in the thigh muscles owing to vasoconstriction of the peripheral vessels.

Ergotamine preparations can also cause gastric irritation, nausea, and vomiting, although these may be hard to distinguish from the nausea and vomiting caused by the migraine itself. Rare complications include thrombophlebitis, angina pectoris, and peripheral neuropathy.[89a] There have been a few reports of ergotism with ischemia of the extremities following habitual and excessive use of ergotamine tartrate.[239]

Since ergotamine preparations act as vasoconstrictors and stimulate uterine contraction, they should be used with caution in hypertensive subjects and are contraindicated during pregnancy and in patients with peripheral vascular disease and angina pectoris.

Use of Analgesics in Migraine. If the migraine headache develops despite ergotamine or if ergotamine is administered too late in the course of the attack, the patient may require analgesics to control pain. Acetylsalicylic acid can be given orally before the stage of nausea and vomiting in some cases, although acetylsalicylic acid is poorly absorbed during a migraine attack and may increase gastric irritation. Propoxyphene hydrochloride (Darvon), 65 mg or 100 mg, or codeine, 30 to 60 mg, is required during severe attacks of migraine. When it is impossible to administer oral preparations because of vomiting, intramuscular codeine in doses of 30 to 60 mg may be necessary to control pain. Narcotics such as meperidine hydrochloride (Demerol) or morphine should be avoided if possible because of the dangers of drug addiction.

The headache frequently resolves after a period of sleep, and an oral or intramuscular injection of 250 to 500 mg of amobarbital sodium (Amytal sodium) may help to induce sleep.

Treatment of Migraine Status. Rarely, patients develop a migraine with continuous headache which lasts several days accompanied by severe prostration and intermittent vomiting. Such patients should be treated in the hospital. The fluid and electrolyte imbalance induced by vomiting should be corrected with intravenous saline, glucose, and potassium if necessary. The vomiting can usually be controlled with intramuscular injection of chlorpromazine in doses of 25 to 50 mg every six hours.

Ergotamine preparations are ineffective when the headache is well-established and prolonged, and they should be discontinued. The headache usually abates after the induction of sleep. The patient should take one capsule of 250 mg amobarbital sodium. If this fails to induce sleep, a further capsule of 250 mg amobarbital sodium

should be taken after one and a half hours. The migraine status will usually resolve during a prolonged period of sleep.

Prophylactic Therapy of Migraine. The use of formal psychotherapy in an attempt to reduce the incidence of migraine attacks is rarely necessary, and the sympathetic physician can usually help the patient ventilate any repressed hostility and frustrations without difficulty. Patients with obvious disturbances in behavior and who exhibit obsessive and compulsive personality traits that appear to trigger attacks will benefit by counseling.[28, 147] This can usually be carried out effectively by the internist or neurologist rather than a psychiatrist.

METHYSERGIDE MALEATE (SANSERT). The role of 5-hydroxytryptamine (serotonin) in the complex vascular changes that accompany a migraine attack is widely accepted, although the exact action of serotonin is not established. There is no doubt that serotonin antagonists are effective in the prophylaxis of migraine and methysergide maleate will prevent migraine if taken regularly every day. The action of methysergide maleate is not fully understood. The drug does not induce vasoconstriction, although it renders the cephalic arteries more susceptible to the action of vasoconstricting drugs such as norepinephrine. The drug is indicated only in severe cases of migraine since potentially dangerous side effects have been reported as rare complications.

The dosage of methysergide should be gradually increased to avoid side effects. A starting dose of a single tablet (2 mg) daily should be followed by an additional tablet every four days to a total of three or four tablets daily. This minimizes side effects such as drowsiness, ataxia, and nausea, which sometimes occur during the institution of methysergide therapy.

The patient should be required to keep a record of the intensity and frequency of headaches, which usually decrease or cease in the majority of cases after several weeks of methysergide therapy. If the patient remains free from attacks for six months, attempts may be made to withdraw the drug by progressively reducing the dose. The drug should not be used continuously for longer than a year without some planned interval of withdrawal for one to two months.

Apart from drowsiness, nausea, and ataxia, other side effects have been noted. These include vomiting, abdominal pain, diarrhea, and mild changes in personality with euphoria, lightheadedness, and hallucinations. Papuloerythematous skin rashes and hair loss have been reported, and some patients report edema and gain in weight.

Retroperitoneal fibrosis with obstruction of the ureters and hydronephrosis has been reported in a few cases treated without interruption for prolonged periods.[81, 110] Retroperitoneal fibrosis may also compress arteries and result in the Leriche syndrome and intermittent claudication.[109] There have been even rarer reports of pleuropulmonary and cardiac fibrosis with dysphagia, chest pain, pleural effusion, angina pectoris, and the development of cardiac murmurs.

In view of these potentially dangerous side effects, patients on this form of therapy should be under regular supervision with periodic estimations of the erythrocyte sedimentation rate and blood urea nitrogen. If the drug should be used on a long-time basis, an intravenous pyelogram is advised every year to detect any evidence of ureteral obstruction and hydronephrosis.

The development of any symptoms suggestive of retroperitoneal, pulmonary, or cardiac fibrosis should prompt immediate cessation of methysergide therapy. Inflammatory and fibrotic manifestations as well as loss of hair usually regress when the drug is stopped, and surgery is usually not required. There is some indication that steroid therapy (methylprednisolone, 80 mg once every 48 hours) may hasten the resolution of the inflammatory process.

Use of Phenobarbital in Migraine. Migraine is common in children and can result in loss of schooling if attacks are frequent. Many children respond to phenobarbital taken regularly in doses of 15 to 30 mg three times daily, depending on the age of the child. Simple psychotherapy by the physician and involving both the parents as well as the child is often helpful. The parents and the child are often overly fastidious and ambitious.

Use of Propranolol in Migraine. The beta sympathetic blocking agent propranolol is an effective drug in the prophylactic treatment of migraine.[232] The drug should be given in doses of 10 mg four times a day, gradually increasing the dosage to 40 mg four times a day if necessary. Propranolol seems to be a safe and effective drug but should not be given to patients with bradycardia, congestive heart failure, asthma, or hypoglycemia.

Use of Amitryptyline in Migraine. Amitryptyline, a tricyclic antidepressant, is an effective prophylactic agent in the treatment of common migraine.[79] It appears to be less effective in classic migraine and in patients who have migraine headaches of long duration. A dose of 25 to 50 mg at night is recommended. Side effects, including drowsiness, disturbed sleep, disturbing dreams, dry mouth, and excessive perspiration, are occasionally troublesome.

Use of Clonidine in Migraine. The hypotensive agent clonidine is an effective prophylactic in some cases of adult and childhood migraine.[195] The initial dose should be 25 μg daily, with a gradual increase to 25 μg three times a day. Side effects include fatigue, nausea, and disturbed sleep and usually resolve within a week or two after beginning treatment.

Use of Other Drugs in Migraine. A combination of ergotamine, belladonna, and phenobarbital (Bellergal) is effective as a prophylactic in some cases of migraine if given on a regular basis. The usual dosage is four to six tablets daily with reduction to a maintenance dose when control of the headache is obtained. Cyproheptadine is an effective antagonistic of histamine and serotonin and may be used prophylactically in doses of 4 mg qid. The most prominent side effect is drowsiness.

A combination of isometheptene, acetaminophen, and dichloralphenazone (Midrin) is a useful alternative to ergotamine in the treatment of migraine. The capsules should be taken at the beginning of a headache followed by one capsule after an hour if needed. The isometheptene combination produces less nausea than ergotamine preparations and is equally effective if given at the beginning of a migraine attack.[47]

Cluster Headaches

A certain type of recurrent headache with distinctive clinical features has been described under a number of titles, including cluster headaches, periodic migrainous neuralgia (Harris), histaminic cephalgia (Horton), sphenopalatine ganglion neuralgia, and Sluder's syndrome. The clinical picture is quite distinct, yet the diagnosis is often delayed, and the victims of this particularly distressing condition are not given the benefit of treatment which may well control the attacks of pain.[114]

Although there are some similarities between cluster headaches and migraine, there are obvious differences in the two conditions. Both are associated with vasodilatation. However, the distribution of vascular involvement is different. Migraine often presents with bilateral dilatation of the large extracranial vessels, but the scalp and facial capillaries are constricted. In cluster headaches the scalp and facial capillaries show unilateral dilatation on the side of the headache, and there is increased blood flow through the external carotid system. At the same time, there is marked intraocular vasodilatation with increased intraocular pressure,[95] while intraocular pressure does not change in migraine. The occasional occurrence of Horner's syndrome in cluster headaches suggests that the sympathetic innervation may be paralyzed due to dilatation of the internal carotid artery. Increased cerebral blood flow recorded in cluster headaches is consistent with this hypothesis.[155]

There may also be biochemical differences in migraine and cluster headaches. Plasma serotonin levels are reported to fall and plasma histamine levels are unchanged in migraine, while serotonin levels are unchanged and histamine levels are increased in cluster headaches.[3] Significantly low plasma testosterone levels have been reported in males during cluster headaches when compared to males during remission of cluster headaches or to a control population.[112]

Both alcohol and nitroglycerine can precipitate attacks of cluster headaches, and the relief of angina pectoris reported during cluster headache suggests that a vasodilatory agent may be circulating during an attack.[52] An unusual association of peptic ulcer and cluster headache has also been reported. This association and the demonstrable increase in gastric acidity during attacks led to the hypothesis that patients with cluster headaches suffered from hypersensitivity to histamine.

Histamine desensitization has been recommended but has generally been ineffective in cluster headaches. Nevertheless, evidence points to a sudden local discharge of histamine at the onset of cluster headaches, and the condition may be a hypersensitivity reaction involving the cranial arteries.[33]

Clinical Features

Cluster headaches occur mainly in men aged 20 to 50 years. A headache may be precipitated by ingestion of alcohol or vasodilatory drugs or may occur spontaneously.[118] Attacks may occur once or several times a day, often wake the patient at night, and last from 30 to 120 minutes. An episode of cluster headaches lasts from 4 to 12 weeks. When remission occurs, the patient is free from this type of headache for months or years. The pain occurs without warning, is sudden in onset, excruciating in intensity, and is localized to one orbit and frontotemporal region. An attack is associated with photophobia, lacrimation, unilateral nasal congestion, and occasionally Horner's syndrome. A chronic form of cluster headaches has been described where attacks occur without remission and can incapacitate the patient. A variant known as "lower-half headache" has also been described in which the episodic pain is confined to the cheek and lower jaw and is often accompanied by Horner's syndrome and peptic ulceration.

Treatment

1. Patients should avoid known precipitating factors such as alcohol.
2. Ergotamine, 0.5 mg, can be given by intramuscular injection one hour before an expected attack or by suppository (1 or 2 mg) every 8 or 12 hours prophylactically. Treatment should be withheld for one day every ten days to determine if the episode of cluster headaches has ended.
3. A course of methysergide should be given to those who fail to respond to ergotamine preparations. It is better to begin with 1 tablet (2 mg) at night and in the morning and increase by one tablet every three days to a total of two tablets four times a day if necessary.
4. Oral prednisone or methylprednisolone may produce dramatic relief from cluster headaches in some cases.[104] Methylprednisolone, 64 mg daily, may relieve symptoms, but recurrence often occurs when the dose is reduced.[37a]
5. Cyproheptadine (Periactin) has powerful antihistaminic and antiserotonin properties. It is reported to be effective in doses of 4 mg qid.
6. Propranolol, 10 to 40 mg qid, is effective in some cases, and the low incidence of side effects adds to the usefulness of this drug.
7. Chronic cluster headaches that fail to respond

to other measures may be treated with lithium carbonate beginning with 300 mg a day and gradually increasing the dose to produce a serum level of 1 to 2 mEq/liter.[113, 135a]

Painful Ophthalmoplegia

The causes of painful ophthalmoplegia are listed in Table 6–1. The majority of these conditions are discussed elsewhere.

Painful ophthalmoplegia (Tolosa-Hunt) is a rare but distinct clinical entity. It is believed to be due to a nonspecific chronic inflammatory lesion usually involving the carotid artery and the contiguous walls of the cavernous sinus[99] but occasionally spreading into the orbit, the clivus, or the middle cranial fossa.[184a] The Tolosa-Hunt syndrome presents with a steady, boring pain behind the eye on the involved side which usually precedes the ophthalmoplegia by several days but occasionally follows the development of ophthalmoplegia. Third-nerve paralysis is often accompanied by paralysis of the fourth, sixth, and ophthalmic division of the fifth cranial nerves. Sympathetic paralysis with Horner's syndrome and optic nerve involvement are present in some cases. The condition persists for several days and occasionally weeks. Further attacks may occur after months or even years of remission. There is a good response to corticosteroid therapy.[212a]

Tension Headaches

The majority of headaches are due to states of anxiety, tension, and depression. They are extremely common, and probably most of the population have suffered from tension headache at some time. It has been shown that the headache results from sustained contraction of skeletal muscles in the scalp, face, neck, and shoulders. This has been verified by electromyography. The frown or furrowed brow of depression is literally more than skin deep and is accompanied by prolonged contraction of the cephalic musculature resulting in muscular pain referred to the head.

There are three possible causes of sustained contraction of the muscles of the head and neck: it may be the direct result of anxiety or depression with associated tension; it may occur as a secondary phenomenon when there is headache from other causes or pain elsewhere in the body; and it may occur when there is faulty posture of the head, neck, and shoulder girdles. This last feature may be prominent in the depressed patient.

The patient with tension headaches usually complains of generalized headache with a tight and strained feeling in the head as though it were constricted by a band. The pain is described as a constant ache, in contrast to the throbbing quality of headache due to vascular causes. It is common for patients to describe the pain with descriptive embellishments including such terms as "viselike," "crushing," "unbearable," and "bursting." When the pain occurs in the occipital area, it is often associated with pain in the cervical area which radiates down into the shoulders. The headaches often last for days, and patients may claim that they are "never" free from headache. The vivid description of pain is often at variance with the calm and absorbed appearance of the patient who may claim to be suffering from headache at the time of the interview.

Treatment

Patients with tension headaches need attention and reassurance. The physician should express concern and sympathy and listen with patience and attention to the account of suffering. He should not casually dismiss the complaint as being "just a tension headache." Every patient with complaint of severe headache should receive a general physical and neurologic examination. This is the first step in reassurance and treatment.

The mechanism of the headache should be explained in simple terms and any emotional problems discussed with the patient. The patient should be encouraged to ventilate his fears and frustrations and should be asked about any repressed feelings of hostility. In tense and anxious patients a mild tranquilizer such as a phenothia-

TABLE 6–1

Conditions That Can Produce Painful Ophthalmoplegia

1. Carotid cavernous sinus fistula
2. Periostitis of the orbital fissure
3. Syphilitic meningitis with oculomotor palsy
4. Ethmoidal sinusitis and orbital cellulitis
5. Cavernous sinus thrombosis
6. Orbital neoplasms
7. Aneurysm of the internal carotid artery
8. Temporal arteritis
9. Polyarteritis nodosa
10. Dilated arteriosclerotic carotid artery with pressure on oculomotor nerve
11. Ophthalmoplegic migraine
12. Painful ophthalmoplegia (Tolosa-Hunt syndrome)

zine derivative may be helpful. Psychic energizers such as imipramine hydrochloride (Tofranil) are useful when the headaches are due to depression. The patient should also be offered adequate sedation to ensure sound sleep at night. If there is difficulty in getting to sleep, one of the short-acting barbiturates, amobarbital sodium, 150 mg, or sodium secobarbital, 100 mg (Seconal), is usually effective. Those who are unable to stay asleep require a longer-acting barbiturate such as pentobarbital (Nembutal), 100 mg. If these measures fail and a serious emotional disturbance is apparent, the patient should be referred to a psychiatrist for consultation and treatment.

Headache in Cerebrovascular Disease

Headache is frequently one of the initial symptoms of hypertensive encephalopathy, hypertensive intracerebral hemorrhage, and subarachnoid hemorrhage due to rupture of an intracranial vascular malformation. Control of hypertension relieves the headache of hypertensive encephalopathy. Patients with hypertensive intracerebral and subarachnoid hemorrhage, if they are able to communicate, complain bitterly of headache, and the restlessness of patients with these conditions is usually due to pain in the head. The headache is described as generalized and "bursting" in type, but is usually maximal in the occipital area and radiates down the neck. The neck is stiff and, unlike migraine headache, the stiffness persists for many days. Such patients require adequate doses of narcotics at regular intervals (e.g., meperidine hydrochloride [Demerol], 100 mg every four hours) to control the headache and neck pain and to allay restlessness.

Headaches are unusual in patients with congenital saccular and arteriosclerotic aneurysms prior to rupture and subarachnoid bleeding. However, unilateral headache may occur episodically for several weeks prior to the rupture of a berry aneurysm. This "sentinel headache" is due to leakage of blood through a small tear in the wall of the aneurysm.[9] Unilateral headache may also result from an enlarged aneurysm arising at the terminal bifurcation of the internal carotid artery which exerts pressure on parasellar structures. On the other hand, unilateral headache is not unusual in cases of arteriovenous malformation and may be located over the site of the abnormality. The pain, which resembles migraine in about one third of the cases,[227] presumably results from excessive dilatation of extracranial and intracra-nial vessels supplying the malformation and possibly traction on the meningeal nerve endings.

In general, headache is not a common symptom of cerebral infarction due to thromboembolism although it is highly characteristic of intracranial hemorrhage of all types. However, headache regularly precedes cerebral infarction as a symptom of cerebrovascular insufficiency. Patients with carotid insufficiency usually complain of headache on the affected side, while those with vertebral basilar insufficiency complain of suboccipital headache. The headache is episodic and occurs during or immediately after the transient ischemic attack.[141]

Patients with multi-infarct or arteriosclerotic dementia frequently complain of episodic headache probably due to cerebrovascular insufficiency. This may be of some help in the differential diagnosis of dementia since headache is unusual in dementia due to neuronal degeneration. Arteriosclerotic dementia is the most likely diagnosis if headache is accompanied by, or follows, episodic confusion, dysphasia, hemiparesis, or ataxia and if there are signs of emotional lability and pseudobulbar palsy.

Cerebral arteritis, particularly temporal arteritis, can cause severe and incapacitating headache. It should be differentiated from the pain of temporomandibular arthritis. The unilateral headache and tender temporal artery of temporal arteritis have been described elsewhere. Headache in polyarteritis nodosa is probably caused by disease affecting the branches of the trigeminal and cervical nerves supplying the scalp. Headache is also common in systemic lupus erythematosus with cerebral involvement, but in this condition cerebral infarction and brain swelling may be the cause.

Elevated Blood Pressure as a Cause of Headache

Headaches are no more frequent in mild and moderate hypertension than in normotensive persons. However, in patients with severe hypertension (e. g., a blood pressure over 200/110) occipital and frontal headaches, which are aggravated by bending or straining, are the rule. Hypertensive headaches are also worse on awakening in the morning, probably because of the carbon dioxide retention and increased cerebral blood flow that occur during sleep with resulting increases in intracranial pressure.

Headache is a prominent feature of malignant

hypertension with hypertensive encephalopathy, where it is often associated with a marked increase in intracranial pressure. Other signs, including dysphasia, confusion, seizures, and papilledema, are usually present.

Attacks of intense pulsatile headache, often of short duration and accompanied by anxiety, perspiration, pallor, tachycardia, nausea, and vomiting, are characteristic of pheochromocytoma. The blood pressure is elevated during these attacks.

Headache Due to Anemia and Polycythemia

In patients with severe anemia there may be complaints of headache due to increased cerebral blood flow resulting from the decreased cerebral vascular resistance. These patients may have a bruit over their head and papilledema. The patient with polycythemia also complains of headache in addition to fatigue, visual disturbances, generalized pruritus, and abdominal pain. The cause of the headache in polycythemia is not clear, but it may result from cerebral ischemia, which commonly occurs in this condition.

Headache in Meningeal Inflammation

The inflammation of acute or subacute meningitis produces edema of the meninges and irritation of the nerve endings supplying them as well as those supplying the blood vessels at the base of the brain. Inflammatory involvement of the nerve roots emerging from the cervical cord produces reflex muscle spasm, which produces stiffness and pain in the neck and suboccipital area.

Consequently, the headache in meningitis is usually generalized, although often worse in the occipital area, and subsides as the inflammatory process resolves. It is increased by activity and by flexing of the neck and is reduced by lying immobile in bed.

Headache Due to Changes in Intracranial Pressure

Lumbar Puncture Headache

There is considerable variation in the incidence of headache following lumbar puncture from one service to another. A lot depends on the technical skill of those performing the procedure, the type of patients examined, whether the procedure is carried out on hospitalized inpatients or ambulatory outpatients, whether a period of bed rest is ordered following the procedure, and the closeness of the patient-doctor relationship.

Postlumbar puncture headache does not occur for some hours or even days after the procedure and is usually rare. When it does occur, it may be the result of slow leakage of cerebrospinal fluid at the site of puncture and is probably more common if multiple punctures have been made. As a result there is gradual reduction of the volume and pressure of the cerebrospinal fluid, resulting in traction on the cerebral arteries and venous sinuses at the base of the brain. If scrupulous aseptic technique is not used, an inflammatory reaction in the subarachnoid space may follow the procedure and this will cause headache. Patients with anxiety are more prone to complaints of headache and require reassurance.

The pain varies from mild discomfort to severe pain in the head with prostration lasting from a few hours to several days. Usually, it lasts a few hours and disappears after a night's sleep. The pain is usually described as a dull frontal and occipital headache. The condition is characterized by severe worsening on sitting up, improvement when lying flat, and moderate exacerbation by lateral motion of the head.

As already indicated, scrupulous attention to technique will reduce the incidence of postlumbar puncture headache. With strict asepsis a 19-gauge spinal needle should be examined prior to use to see that the point is sharp. The bevel should be turned so that it is parallel to the fibers of the posterior longitudinal ligament. Multiple punctures must be avoided. The occurrence of headache is greatly reduced by requiring the patient to lie in the prone position for at least six hours after the performance of the procedure. If headache does occur, the patient should remain in bed, oral fluids should be encouraged, and adequate analgesics should be given to control the pain. In severe cases, the patient should lie prone with the foot of the bed elevated. Intravenous saline and inhalation of 5 per cent CO_2 in oxygen are helpful. Unusual cases with prostration may possibly require a short course of fludrocortisone acetate (Florinef), 0.1 mg four times a day.

Headache Following Pneumoencephalography

The introduction of computed tomography has been followed by a remarkable decrease in the use of pneumoencephalography in neurologic practice. Nevertheless, pneumoencephalography is still needed in the diagnosis of some difficult problems. The mechanism of headache is basically the same as a postlumbar puncture headache with low pressure resulting from leakage of cerebrospinal fluid and the introduction of air, which acts as a foreign substance. If the cerebrospinal fluid continues to leak, the brain is no longer supported efficiently by the cerebrospinal fluid and becomes easily displaced within the cranial cavity; this produces traction on the arteries at the base of the brain and the meninges. Because of the presence of a foreign substance there is usually some inflammatory reaction. The headache usually resolves after 48 hours of rest in bed, adequate fluid intake, and the use of analgesics. If it is unusually severe with prostration, fludrocortisone acetate, 0.1 mg taken orally four times a day, may be prescribed.

Headache in Patients with Increased Intracranial Pressure

Headache that occurs in patients with increased intracranial pressure is probably due to displacement and traction of the meninges and blood vessels rather than the pressure itself. Patients with brain tumor complain of headaches whether or not they have increased intracranial pressure. Patients with benign intracranial hypertension complain of generalized headache despite the fact that there is no displacement of brain structure. It is probable that the headache in such cases is caused by the associated edema of the brain, which stretches the nerve endings of the meninges and cerebral blood vessels.

Headaches and Brain Tumor

The headache of brain tumor may be due to displacement of the arteries at the base of the brain, the cortical veins, the venous sinuses, and the cranial nerves, and their intracranial branches. As already discussed, increased intracranial pressure by itself is probably not an important cause of headache. The site of headache in a large brain tumor with massive increased intracranial pressure is of limited value in localization since traction on pain-sensitive structures may be caused by displaced or herniated brain and the remote effects of hydrocephalus.

Headache is usually of more value in localizing tumor if papilledema is absent, since it has been reported to occur over or near the site of tumor in about two thirds of cases. Unilateral headache without papilledema is almost invariably on the same side as the tumor. Headache is commonly the first symptom in posterior fossa tumors and begins in the occipital area. In tumors of the cerebellopontine angle, headache develops months or years after the onset of unilateral deafness and then is localized over the mastoid area. Headache is often absent in supratentorial tumors but is the first symptom in about one third of cases and is usually frontal or temporal in location.

Headache due to brain tumor is usually intermittent and described as a dull ache. Later, as the tumor becomes larger, headache may be continuous. The pain is aggravated by assuming an erect posture, by stooping over, and by coughing, straining, or sneezing and tends to be worse in the morning.

Posttraumatic Headache

The occurrence of headache following minor head injury is common and has been discussed in detail elsewhere. In brief, headaches that develop after head injury are usually due to contraction of the cervical muscles and are similar to tension headaches.

Injury to the anterior neck may be followed by a unique type of dysautonomic headache due to damage to sympathetic pathways in the neck. Patients experience episodic, unilateral, frontotemporal headache associated with ipsilateral mydriasis and facial hyperhidrosis, followed by ptosis and miosis. The condition responds to oral propranolol.[223]

Headaches Due to Toxic and Metabolic Causes

There are numerous systemic causes of headache due to toxic or metabolic abnormalities, which usually have one or more of three causative factors in common:

1. Excessive cephalic circulation.
2. Altered intracranial dynamics due to either cerebral edema or dehydration.
3. Other factors including electrolyte imbalance and alterations in cellular metabolism of the brain.

A number of the more important systemic conditions that commonly cause headache will now be considered.

Infectious Diseases

Almost all infectious diseases with fever are associated with headache. Fever causes an increase of cerebral blood flow and metabolism. The elaboration of toxins may also be responsible for the dilatation of intracranial blood vessels. The severity of headache varies with the severity of the infectious agent.

A mild generalized discomfort in the head is regularly associated with the common cold and upper respiratory tract infections. Severe headache is characteristic of typhoid fever, malaria, and typhus. Patients with severe headache in the course of an infectious illness should be observed for abnormal neurologic signs indicating direct involvement of the meninges or brain by the infectious process. In the majority of infectious diseases, the headache subsides with the reduction of fever and the use of antibiotics. If it is troublesome, antipyretic and analgesic drugs usually relieve the pain. If fever is severe, alcohol sponging or a hypothermic blanket and the use of acetylsalicylic acid and codeine may be necessary. Dehydration should be avoided, and adequate fluid and electrolyte balance should be maintained by the use of intravenous saline and glucose.

Hangover Headache

The generalized throbbing headache that occurs the morning after heavy ingestion of alcohol and commonly called a "hangover" is also due to vascular dilatation. This may be due to alcohol itself, which is a vasodilator of the cephalic vessels, or to the circulation of small quantities of aromatic compounds that are imbibed with the alcoholic drink. The severity of hangover headache varies not only according to the amount ingested but also according to how much of these aromatic compounds were ingested. Hangover headache is often minimal or absent in the chronic alcoholic. The severe hangover that sometimes prostrates the occasional drinker should be treated with rest, forced fluids by mouth, and analgesics such as acetylsalicylic acid and codeine.

Hypoglycemia

Headache is usually a prominent feature at the onset of hypoglycemia. There are many causes of hypoglycemia (p. 250), and severe episodes present with a variety of dramatic symptoms that overshadow the headache. However, most hypoglycemic patients develop headache, which usually occurs three or four hours after a meal. Cerebral blood flow is decreased during hypoglycemia so that the headache may be due to dilatation of the scalp vessels. The majority of cases with mild postprandial hypoglycemia are relieved of symptoms by a high-protein, low-carbohydrate diet.

Hypercapnia

Certain pulmonary disorders are associated with the retention of carbon dioxide and increased levels of P_{CO_2} in the arterial blood. Cerebral blood flow becomes greatly increased, and the patient complains of headache. This may occur in chronic emphysema, bronchiectasis, and pulmonary infection. It has also been described in patients with the hypoventilation syndrome of extreme obesity (pickwickian syndrome). In all these conditions, the headache is relieved by improvement in pulmonary function and by the use of such measures as antibiotics, mechanical respirators, and weight reduction (the latter in the pickwickian syndrome).

Headache in Anoxia

Reduction of the arterial oxygen tension also causes increased cerebral blood flow and headache. This is a striking complaint in carbon monoxide poisoning. Treatment should be directed toward correction or removal of the cause of the anoxic state.

Headache in Heat Exhaustion

The mechanism of headache in heat exhaustion and heat stroke is probably due, in part, to the increased cerebral blood flow accompanying hyperpyrexia and possibly also results from cerebral dehydration, lowered cerebrospinal fluid pressure, and traction on the pain-sensitive structures within the cranium. The condition usually responds to replacement of fluids and correction of any electrolyte imbalance.

Headaches During the Menopause

Headache is a common complaint of women during the menopause and may be related to the hormonal imbalance, although a more likely explanation is that the headaches result from anxiety and depression. In the latter case they may be considered a form of tension headache and should be treated accordingly.

Headache and Sexual Activity

The development of headache during intercourse is often regarded as an ominous sign, and subarachnoid hemorrhage due to rupture of a berry aneurysm has been recorded after coitus.[161] There is a benign paroxysmal headache which can occur suddenly during sexual intercourse appearing a minute or so before, during, or shortly after orgasm. The headache may be occipital, generalized, or restricted to one frontal area. The majority of cases are probably due to muscle contraction in the neck, jaw, and scalp.[117]

Headaches and Diseases of the Eye

"Eyestrain" is generally thought to be a common cause of headache. Actually, this is a rather uncommon cause of headache in adults, although errors of refraction may be a more common cause of headache in children.

Certain diseases of the eye commonly cause headache, but with few exceptions the cause is apparent on examination. In superficial inflammation of the eye, such as conjunctivitis, dacryocystitis, meibomitis, hordeolum, keratitis, and episcleritis, there is usually local pain in the eye and headache is either absent or mild. Inflammation of the orbital tissues with orbital cellulitis results in severe pain in the orbit radiating into the frontal area. There is often proptosis, with exacerbation of orbital pain on attempting to move the eye. Some conditions affecting the structures within the eye, such as uveitis, iritis, and endo- or panophthalmitis, are associated with severe frontal headache. In neurologic practice optic neuritis is probably the most frequent of the ocular conditions associated with pain in the eye and frontal headache. The causes of optic neuritis have been discussed elsewhere (p. 156), but symptoms of sudden visual loss associated with pain on movement of the eye are characteristic of this condition.

Errors of refraction may cause headache in children. This usually occurs when the child begins school and is found in those suffering from astigmatism and hypermetropia. The child is usually free from headache on awakening, but develops frontal headache at school, particularly following close work such as reading. Similar complaints may occur in children with imbalance of the extraocular muscles, since these children usually suffer from hypermetropia. The myopic child does not usually complain of headaches.

Chronic glaucoma is an important and serious cause of chronic frontal headache, which can be established by tonometry by an opthalmologist. In an acute attack of glaucoma, the diagnosis is more obvious than in chronic glaucoma. The patient complains of severe pain in the eye, the pupils are often asymmetric, and the affected cornea is steamy with circumcorneal injection. There may be a nasal defect in the visual field, and the optic cup is deeper than normal.

Headaches Due to Disease of the Nose, Paranasal Sinuses, and Throat

The mucous membranes of the turbinates and ostia of the nasal sinuses are sensitive to inflammatory processes and pressure caused by tumors and empyemas. The pain that results is referred to the frontal or frontotemporal regions as a headache. The mucous membranes within the sinuses themselves appear to be less sensitive.

A deviated nasal septum may rarely cause chronic frontal or temporal headaches by displacement and pressure on the turbinates. The location of the headache depends on the site of the septal deviation.

The location of pain due to acute sinusitis depends on the site of involvement, but acute sinusitis is usually associated with severe headache. Maxillary sinusitis usually produces pain that begins in the face and may radiate to the forehead and sometimes to the teeth of the upper jaw. Frontal, ethmoidal, and sphenoidal sinusitis are all associated with frontal headache, although the pain may radiate into the orbit and occasionally into the frontotemporal area.

The patient with acute sinusitis is usually febrile, with conjunctival injection, nasal congestion or discharge, and tenderness over the affected sinus. In acute maxillary sinusitis there may be freedom from pain in the morning, but it begins in the early afternoon and increases toward evening. Acute frontal sinusitis almost invariably causes severe frontal headache. This usually radiates into the medial aspect of the orbit of the affected side. The headache is usually present on awakening, continues all day, and improves in the evening. Acute sphenoid and ethmoid sinusitis are occasionally a cause of pain behind the eye, sometimes associated with swelling due to orbital cellulitis in the case of ethmoid sinusitis. Cavernous sinus thrombosis may result, with paralysis of the cranial nerves that pass through the sinus and proptosis.

Chronic sinusitis does not usually cause headache, but the development of a mucocele in the maxillary or frontal sinus may be associated with considerable pain if the cyst increases in size to occupy the whole of the sinsus.

"Vacuum headache," or headache due to relatively negative pressure within the nasal passages and eustachian tube, often occurs when there is a sudden increase in atmospheric pressure that is not transmitted to the paranasal sinuses or the middle ear, usually because of nasal congestion. This frequently occurs in modern commercial aircraft during a rapid descent since they are usually pressurized to an equivalent atmospheric pressure of 8,000 ft. The onset is sudden, with severe pain over the affected sinus or ear, with headache that is relieved by the use of a nasal decongestant.

Headache is usually a late manifestation of malignant tumors involving the paranasal sinuses. A carcinoma in the maxillary sinus usually causes pain over the maxilla and upper teeth with epistaxis, followed by the development of unilateral headache as the condition progresses. Expanding tumors of the ethmoid sinus may cause pain over the bridge of the nose, while carcinoma of the frontal sinus produces unilateral frontal headache. Carcinoma of the nasopharynx may cause unilateral headache associated with nasal obstruction, epistaxis, unilateral deafness, and pain in the throat, which is also referred to the ear on the same side. As the tumor expands, there is involvement of the maxillary and mandibular divisions of the fifth cranial nerve and pain over the maxilla and mandible. The nasopharynx should always be examined in cases with persistent unilateral headache, particularly if the pain is referred to the ear.

Headache Due to Arthritis and Disease of the Cervical Spine

Injury or disease of the cervical spine is commonly associated with headache. There are four possible causes of headache arising from disease of the cervical spine:

1. Prolonged muscular contraction of the strap muscles of the neck.
2. Injury to cervical nerve roots with spasm of the neck muscles.
3. Disease of the joints, intervertebral disks, or vertebral bodies with compression of nerve roots.
4. Vascular insufficiency in the territory of the vertebral-basilar arterial system.

Any of these factors may occur alone or in combination as a result of injury or disease of the cervical spine. The headache is usually described as a diffuse pain in the occipital area, which occasionally radiates forward bitemporally and may reach the frontal areas. The headache of vascular insufficiency is also occipital in distribution and is believed to be due to a vasodilatation of collateral channels in the neck and base of the skull.

Headache is a common complaint in chronic degenerative changes of the cervical spine including osteoarthritis, cervical spondylosis, and degeneration of the cervical disks. All these conditions produce abnormalities in posture of the cervical spine, resulting in prolonged contraction of the muscles of the neck and irritation of the cervical nerve roots. Severe headaches can also result from temporomandibular arthritis and malocclusion of the teeth of the upper and lower jaws.

Epilepsy

There have been numerous attempts to define epilepsy, which vary depending on the scientific knowledge available at the time. In physiologic terms, epilepsy can be regarded as a periodic and excessive discharge of electrical activity from cerebral neurons which may result in loss of consciousness, involuntary movements, abnormal sensory phenomena, increased autonomic activity, and a variety of psychic disturbances.

The seizure, whether subjective or objective, should be considered to indicate a disturbance of neuronal function. The disturbance may arise from many different causes since epilepsy is a symptom and not a disease. The use of terms such as "cryptogenic" or "idiopathic" seizures in certain cases is really an admission that their cause is unknown. This group is gradually being reduced as our knowledge of intracellular physiology and chemistry is increased. Fortunately, despite lack of knowledge of the cause of seizures in some cases, advances in symptomatic treatment are progressing steadily. Over 85 per cent of individuals suffering from epilepsy can have their seizures controlled or reduced to an acceptable minimum with anticonvulsant medication.

Epilepsy still remains an important public health problem. In view of the effectiveness of presently available anticonvulsive medication, the physician who cares for epileptic patients assumes considerable responsibility and should establish effective control as soon as possible. Whenever feasible, the least toxic medications should be used.

Epidemiology

Epidemiologic studies concerned with epilepsy have usually been restricted to highly selected populations, and it is difficult to give an accurate estimation of the incidence or prevalence in the general population. The problem is made more difficult since patients with seizures are unfortunately discriminated against and conceal the fact that they suffer from the disorder. The prevalence probably lies between four and seven per 1,000, which would mean that there are between 800,000 and 1.4 million epileptics in the United States.

Estimates of incidence also show considerable variation owing to differences in the definition of the term "epilepsy." The figure probably lies between 0.3 and 0.7 per thousand persons per year. The incidence of febrile convulsion is about 5.0 per thousand per year.[115, 125]

Epilepsy occurs in all races, and there seems to be little or no variation in geographic distribution. It is more common in males than females.[123] Although seizures can occur at any age, there are marked differences in the frequency with which seizures begin in relation to age. Thirty per cent of epileptics experience their first seizure before the age of four years. This increases to 50 per cent by the age of ten years and 75 per cent by the age of 20 years. Only 15 per cent of patients experience their first seizure after the age of 25 years, and less than 2 per cent begin having seizures after the age of 50 years. There is a higher incidence of epilepsy in the first child born in a family, presumably due to the higher incidence of difficult labor and fetal anoxia occurring among primiparae compared to multiparae.

Etiology and Pathology

Epileptic seizures are symptomatic of numerous conditions. Despite the rather extensive list in Table 6–2, the etiology is unknown in about 50 per cent of children and in a smaller percentage of adults. In a large series of cases of seizures of unknown cause, the brain has been shown to be macroscopically and microscopically normal, so that a biochemical or metabolic cause or causes may be reasonably assumed.

These conditions, many of which have been discussed in detail in other sections of the book, will now be considered in relation to epilepsy as a symptom.

Hereditary and Familial Conditions Causing Seizures

A number of the hereditary degenerative diseases, including the lipidoses and aminoacidurias, are regularly accompanied by epileptic seizures. Most of them are known to be associated with a metabolic defect that interferes with or alters intracellular metabolism. This is also believed to be the case in children with chromosomal abnormalities in which seizures may be one of the signs and symptoms, e.g., trisomy D syndrome.

There is a familial incidence of certain types of seizures including absence or petit mal and psychomotor epilepsy, indicating that genetic factors are important in this condition.[18] Furthermore, epidemiologic studies of electroencephalograms in parents and siblings of children with these types of seizures disclose an even higher incidence of EEG abnormalities. The abnormalities of the EEGs of relatives include epileptic discharges, even though there are no overt epileptic seizures.[181]

Developmental Defects Causing Seizures

Patients with developmental defects such as tuberous sclerosis and Sturge-Weber disease suffer from epileptic seizures. The incidence of seizures is also high in acquired developmental defects due to infection in utero by viruses such as rubella or cytomegalovirus. There is both clinical and pathologic evidence that other unidentified viruses cause cerebral maldevelopment and seizures. Furthermore, maternal infection with toxoplasmosis or irradiation of the uterus during gestation with injury to the developing embryo has been shown to impair cerebral embryogenesis with the production of epileptic seizures as a symptom. Certain drugs are suspected of having similar effects if taken during the first months of pregnancy.

Birth Trauma as a Cause of Seizures

During parturition there may be cerebral anoxia or contusion, and more rarely cerebral thrombosis or embolism.[171] These conditions may lead to what is loosely termed "cerebral palsy" and are often associated with seizures. Excessive moulding of the head during parturition may lead to herniation of the medial aspect of the temporal lobe over the free edge of the tentorium in the infant. This may compress the posterior cerebral artery. Such herniation may spontaneously reduce, but the ischemic area undergoes

TABLE 6–2

Classification of Seizures According to Known Causes

1. *Hereditary and familial conditions*
   These include genetic factors and chromosomal abnormalities (also see p. 87).

2. *Development defects*
   This group includes defects caused by tuberous sclerosis, Sturge-Weber disease, cerebral embryogenetic defects due to intrauterine rubella, cytomegalovirus, other viruses, toxoplasmosis, toxic effects of drugs, and irradiation (also see p. 512).

3. *Birth trauma*
   The causes include perinatal anoxia, cerebral contusion, and cerebral thrombosis and embolism.

4. *Anoxia in infancy and childhood*

5. *Acute cerebral anoxia*

6. *Trauma to the head*
   This includes open and closed injuries to the head in childhood and adult life (also see Chap. 8).

7. *Infections of the brain*
   Examples of this include viral encephalitides, bacterial and fungal infections of the brain and meninges, neurosyphilis, brain abscess, and cerebral cysticercosis (also see p. 440).

8. *Neoplasia of the nervous system*
   This group includes primary and metastatic brain tumors (also see Chap. 10).

9. *Nutritional and metabolic disorders*
   This includes conditions such as alcoholism, pyridoxine deficiency and dependency, aminoacidurias, hypoglycemia, hypocalcemia, hypomagnesemia, uremia, and water intoxication.

10. *Toxic conditions*
    There are a large group of toxic agents and drugs which cause seizures including lead encephalopathy, ACTH and the corticosteroids, atropine, chloroquine, diphenhydramine, camphor, caffeine, insulin, penicillin, lidocaine, and procaine.

11. *Vascular disease*
    Certain forms of cerebrovascular disease such as arteriovenous malformations of the brain, cerebral arteriosclerosis, and lupus erythematosus may give rise to seizures (also see Chap. 9).

12. *Degenerative conditions*
    Seizures may occur in many of these conditions, such as Alzheimer's disease, Pick's disease, Jakob-Creutzfeld disease, and Huntington's disease.

---

gliosis (incisural sclerosis) and may give rise to temporal lobe seizures in later life.

Anoxia in Infancy and Childhood as a Cause of Seizures

An alternative theory concerning the development of mesial sclerosis postulates that it is the result of an anoxic episode in infancy or childhood. At that time the neuronal population of the hippocampus and amygdala are particularly vulnerable to anoxic damage, and neuronal loss may be followed by gliosis in this area.[57, 58, 214] An epileptic attack during infancy is one possible cause of anoxia, and in this sense the notion that epilepsy begets epilepsy would be appropriate.

Acute Cerebral Anoxia as a Cause of Seizures

Improved methods of resuscitation following cardiac arrest and other conditions producing acute cerebral anoxia have resulted in much greater survival in recent years. Many of these patients have permanent and widespread neuronal damage with diffuse abnormal electrical discharges usually resulting in bilateral and synchronous myoclonus epilepsy.[55]

Trauma of the Head as a Cause of Seizures

Seizures occurring in the first week after head injury are unlikely to be followed by further episodes in the majority of cases.[107] However, patients who have the first seizure two to seven weeks after head injury have a 20 per cent chance of another seizure.[233] The development of seizures is unusual in closed head injuries, but the incidence increases when the injury has resulted in penetration of the dura and increases further with increasing degrees of brain damage.[29] Early seizures are usually of the focal motor type, while seizures that occur later are often of the psychomotor type. The psychomotor seizure pattern is never seen in the first week after head injury.

Infections of the Brain as a Cause of Seizures

In addition to prenatal infections of the brain already discussed, postnatal infections of the brain may also be a cause of epileptic seizures. The viral encephalitides,[1a] particularly in children, are a common cause of epilepsy, and less commonly, seizures may result from the meningoencephalitides due to bacterial, fungal, and yeast infections. A blocking of inhibitory transmitter receptor sites by antibodies produced in response to antigens released during tissue destruction or infection could explain the focal character of some seizures.[56] Prior to the advent of antibiotics, neurosyphilis and brain abscess were common causes of seizures. Cysticercosis of the brain is a frequent cause of epilepsy in countries where these is a high incidence of *Taenia solium* infestation.[6] Hydatid cyst of the brain is highly epileptogenic and must be considered in the differential diagnosis when epilepsy of recent onset occurs in countries with a high rate of hydatinosis.[185]

Tumors of the Brain and Seizures

Primary and metastatic tumors of the brain may cause seizures at any age, but in particular, the late onset of focal seizures should be considered to be due to brain tumor until proven otherwise. Slowly growing tumors and those involving the cerebral cortex are more likely to produce seizures.[7] The subject is discussed further in the chapter dealing with tumors of the brain (see Chap. 10).

Nutritional and Metabolic Disorders as a Cause of Seizures

The causative relationship between pyridoxine deficiency and pyridoxine-dependent epilepsy in some children with this disorder has been demonstrated. Pyridoxine-dependent seizures are associated with increased glutamic acid and reduced GABA concentrations in the brain.[128a] Other hereditary metabolic defects such as the aminoacidurias and certain of the hypoglycemic conditions of infancy and childhood may also be associated with seizures.[55] There are many causes of hypoglycemia in children, and determination of the fasting blood sugar levels is an important part of the evaluation of all children with seizures. Other disturbances of electrolytes, including hypocalcemia,[109a, 139a] hypomagnesemia,[26, 92] uremic alkalosis, and water intoxication, are also associated with seizures and should be considered in the diagnostic evaluation.

Toxic Conditions Affecting the Nervous System and Causing Seizures

Poisoning by heavy metals such as lead is frequently associated with epileptic seizures in children. Patients with alcohol-related seizures, form a large subgroup with seizure disorders in general city hospitals[51] (see Chap. 5). Certain drugs, including ACTH and corticosteroids, atropine, chloroquine,[215] diphenhydramine (Benadryl), tricyclic antidepressants,[39] camphor, caffeine, insulin, penicillin,[16, 169] lidocaine, and procaine, are occasionally associated with the development of seizures in susceptible individuals. Certain sedative drugs, such as barbiturates, may cause seizures if they are suddenly withdrawn after prolonged use. The intra-amniotic injection of prostaglandin F_{2a} has resulted in seizures, which is a further indication of the active role of prostaglandins in nervous system metabolism.[133]

Vascular Diseases and Seizures

In general, seizures are not a common symptom of cerebral infarction. However, they may result from cerebral embolism, small ischemic infarcts due to diabetic vascular disease, and the inflammatory arteritides such as meningovascular syphilis, periarteritis nodosa, and lupus erythematosus. They may herald the onset of a cerebral hemorrhage, and seizures are frequently seen in arteriovenous malformation of the brain as well as cortical thrombophlebitis and phlebothrombosis. The overall incidence of seizures arising from acute strokes of all kinds is about 15 per cent, but chronic recurrent seizures develop in less than 5 per cent.

The assumption that the majority of elderly patients with a first seizure are suffering from cerebrovascular disease is erroneous. It is only possible to identify a cause for the seizures in 50 per cent of cases, and only 30 per cent of the total group have cerebrovascular disease.[187]

Degenerative Diseases and Seizures

The neuronal degenerations, including Alzheimer's disease, Pick's disease, Jakob-Creutzfeldt disease and Huntington's chorea, and the demyelinating diseases, including multiple sclerosis, may give rise to seizures, but these are not characteristic of the clinical manifestations of these conditions since they are present in only about 10 to 20 per cent of patients.

Pathogenesis

An epileptic seizure may be considered an uncontrolled discharge of a neuronal population within the central nervous system. The discharge has been recorded in cortical and subcortical regions in both animals and man.[229] The discharge may involve a limited number of the neuronal population, in which case it will manifest as a focal discharge and remain localized, or it may spread to involve other levels of the brain and brainstem.[19] In generalized or "grand mal" seizures, the entire or a large part of the neuronal population of the brain participates in the epileptic discharge.

In absence or petit mal seizures, which are characterized by brief staring spells with loss of awareness, the discharge is presumed to originate from the cell population within the upper brainstem (reticular formation). These discharges are then propagated bilaterally through cortical inhibitory pathways, and loss of awareness or "absence" represents paroxysmal activity in cortical inhibitory systems.[67]

The discharge in focal motor seizures is confined to the neuronal population within the motor areas of the brain. In focal sensory seizures, the discharge involves the neuronal population of the sensory neurons, particularly those in the parietal lobe.

Psychomotor seizures or seizures arising in the temporal lobe involve primarily the neuronal population of one temporal lobe, although commissural transmission to both temporal lobes and the limbic system is likely to follow. A discharge which is localized to a specific group of neurons may spread to involve the entire or a large part of the neuronal population of the central nervous system (as a generalized seizure). The discharge may spread with extreme rapidity so that the delay in the development of abnormal discharges between one site and another is in the order of milliseconds and can only be measured by the use of depth electrodes and computer analysis.[225]

The development of the primary epileptic discharge results from instability or irritability of a certain neuronal population, which transmits its electrical discharges more or less in unison, producing the clinical seizure. This may be due to disorders of the metabolism within the neuron or of the ionic homeostasis of its membrane or to factors outside the neuron that alter neuronal and synaptic excitability.

The role of neurotransmitters in the genesis, spread of, or inhibition of seizure activity is not clear. There is some evidence that increased concentrations of acetylcholine and glutamate will increase neuronal excitability and initiate seizure activity. Norepinephrine and gamma aminobutyric acid inhibit neuronal activity, and reduction of brain concentrations of these two transmitters or blocking of receptor sites might lead to an increase in neuronal excitability and seizure activity.[139] The nonphysiologic discharge of the abnormal neurons is transmitted to other neurons, which are forced to discharge periodically and synchronously. This results in synchronous neuronal discharges of extremely high amplitude which can be recorded on an EEG and appear as spikes or high-voltage spike and slow wave discharges.

As the seizure develops, the amplitude of the discharge increases as more neurons are recruited and begin to discharge synchronously with their neighbors. At the end of the discharge, in the exhaustion phase, the frequency of the synchronous discharges decreases, there is progressive lengthening of the refractory period, and finally, the synchronous discharges cease altogether. The termination of the seizure discharge is probably due to a number of factors, including exhaustion of energy reserves, changes in intracellular and extracellular electrolyte concentrations, anoxia, the accumulation of toxic metabolites, and possibly inhibitory discharges.[143]

Clinical Symptoms That May Precede the Seizure and the Aura

Many patients experience symptoms that are present for some time or immediately precede an epileptic seizure. Such prodromal symptoms are recognized by the patient as the warning symptoms of a seizure. Two types of prodromal symptoms can be recognized: *premonitory symptoms,* which persist for a period of hours, or, in some cases, days, prior to the seizure; and *the aura,* which occurs seconds or minutes before the seizure. Premonitory symptoms are often affective in nature and manifest themselves as changes in mood, depression, irritability, sullenness, apprehension, and mental dullness which persists for a number of hours or even as long as several days prior to the convulsive episode. The patient complains of difficulty in thinking and organizing his thoughts or briefly describes himself as "stupid" during this period. Usually, these prodromal symptoms are described as unpleasant, but rarely patients describe feelings of physical and mental well-being with hypomanic features.

Changes in autonomic function may also precede a seizure. These changes include alterations in heart rate, appetite, constipation, borborygmi, dyspepsia, urinary frequency, and the desire to defecate. Keen observers may note pupillary dilation and an unusual complexion due to pallor or flushing of the skin prior to a seizure. The aura immediately preceding the seizure is an integral part of the seizure and is of considerable importance in diagnosis. The aura frequently indicates the location of the localized neuronal population giving rise to the seizure. Since the aura is the result of a local discharge of a neuronal population, there are an almost infinite number of symptoms that can occur, depending on the site and local spread of the abnormal discharge. The aura may be relatively simple, such as the clonic jerking of a thumb, indicating neuronal activity in the opposite motor cortex; or more complex, such as an olfactory hallucination followed by an impairment of awareness, indicating a neuronal discharge in the uncinate gyrus which spreads into the temporal lobe. The seizure begins as a focal discharge, and this type of seizure activity should be regarded as a partial seizure. The rapid spread of the epileptic discharge from this point through the brain results in a generalized seizure, which may follow the local discharge within a few seconds. These seizures are now termed "secondary generalized seizures," and their incidence is probably higher than earlier published figures have indicated. Many generalized seizures are still incorrectly diagnosed as "grand mal" despite the fact that they are preceded by an aura of focal epileptic activity. It is important to recognize these seizures as secondary generalized seizures, since this diagnosis dictates the course of further investigation and treatment in such cases.

Clinical Classification of Different Types of Epileptic Seizures

Epileptic seizures (the epilepsies) are classified according to their clinical manifestations in Table 6–3. These manifestations will now be discussed in detail.

Generalized Convulsive Seizures
Tonic-Clonic (Grand Mal) Seizures

Tonic-clonic ("grand mal") seizures occur in two forms:

1. The seizure occurs suddenly without prodromal symptoms.
2. The seizure is preceded by prodromal symptoms (an aura) indicating focal onset when the term "secondarily generalized seizures" should be used.

The two conditions are not necessarily different, since the onset of the seizure may be focal, but the spread of electrical activity is so rapid that there is no appreciation of prodromal symptoms by the patient or an observer. The seizure is the clinical manifestation of a generalized discharge which affects most, if not all of, the neuronal population of the central nervous system including the autonomic division. There are generalized tonic contractions of all voluntary muscles, and the patient falls to the floor, if he happens to be standing, "as stiff as a board."

Loss of consciousness occurs concurrently with the tonic seizure. All muscles contract, including the respiratory muscles, resulting in expulsion of air from the lungs and prolonged apnea and cyanosis. If the tonic contraction of muscle occurs with partial closure of the vocal cords, this produces the characteristic "epileptic cry." The cry is an involuntary phenomenon and sounds like a high-pitched wheeze or the plaintive, choking, high-pitched sob of a child.

The tonic contraction of the muscles involves the limbs and the trunk, and to the trained neurologic observer, it may resemble decerebrate rigidty. However, there may be slight abduction of the arms as well as flexion of the elbows and adduction of the thumbs into the palms. The lower limbs are always extended and the feet plantar-flexed. As long as the tonic phase persists, the patient remains deeply cyanotic with marked venous congestion. There is marked sympathetic discharge with release of epinephrine,[216] resulting in tachycardia, elevation of blood pressure, mydriasis, and increased intravascular pressure. This stage usually lasts about 20 to 60 seconds and is one of rapid tetanic discharge of neurons which results in tonic contraction of muscle.

As the rate of neuronal discharge slows, the clonic phase begins. Initially there is brief relaxation at first, but the clonic contractions begin and

TABLE 6–3

Clinical Classification of the Epilepsies

I. *Generalized seizures*
  A. Generalized convulsive seizures
    1. Tonic-clonic seizures (grand mal)
    2. Infantile spasm
    3. Myoclonic seizures and akinetic (astatic) seizures
    4. Clonic seizures
    5. Tonic seizures
    6. Generalized convulsive seizures with focal onset (secondary generalized seizures)
  B. Generalized nonconvulsive seizures
    1. Typical absence (petit mal)
    2. Atypical absence (atypical petit mal, petit mal variant)
    3. Continuing absence (petit mal status)

II. *Unilateral seizures*

III. *Partial seizures* (focal seizures; seizures beginning locally)
  A. With motor symptoms
    1. Partial without spread
    2. Partial with spread (jacksonian seizures)
    3. Adversive seizures
    4. Epilepsia partialis continua
    5. Partial tonic seizures
    6. Partial seizures with a loss of speech
  B. With sensory symptoms
    1. Somatosensory seizures
  C. With complex symptomatology (temporal lobe or psychomotor seizures)
    1. With disturbance of thinking
      Amnesia, forced thinking, *déjà vu*
    2. With disturbance of language
    3. With complex motor behavior
    4. With antisocial behavior
    5. With affective disturbances
    6. With subjective visceral or sensory symptoms
      a. Auditory
      b. Olfactory
      c. Visual
      d. Vertiginous
      e. Gustatory
      f. Alimentary
      g. Cardiovascular
  D. Partial seizures secondarily generalized

IV. *Reflex seizures*
  A. Photic, visual, and pattern-induced epilepsy
  B. Musicogenic seizures
  C. Reading epilepsy
  D. Arithmetical epilepsy
  E. Seizures induced by movement
    1. Paroxysmal choreoathetosis

V. *Miscellaneous forms of seizures*
  A. Running epilepsy
  B. Laughing epilepsy
  C. Diencephalic autonomic epilepsy
  D. Cephalgic seizures and headache
  E. "Cerebellar fits"
  F. Hysterical seizures

VI. *Status epilepticus*

become more powerful as time passes. All voluntary muscles are involved in clonic movement, including the respiratory muscles and the jaw. This produces rapid and stertorous respiration with characteristic frothing of saliva in the mouth. If an airway is not maintained, smothering and fatal asphyxia may result.

The clonic contraction of the jaw usually produces biting of the tongue, sometimes with laceration and bleeding. Intermittent contractions of the bladder and its sphincters result in involuntary emptying of the bladder, if it is full. Lacerations of the forehead and scalp and fractures of the teeth and bones may result if the patient falls on a hard surface. Burns and scalding may occur if he falls near hot objects or boiling water. The clonic phase usually lasts about 40 seconds but may be prolonged. The patient then lies in deep coma with trismus and tonic contraction of the axial muscles followed by generalized flaccidity, moderately dilated pupils that react sluggishly to light, absent corneal reflexes, absence of response to painful stimuli, and bilateral extensor plantar responses. The stage of coma usually lasts about one minute, following which the patient begins to respond to painful stimuli.

After a generalized seizure the patient lapses into deep sleep, which lasts for two or three hours. If aroused during this period, most patients complain of severe headache and appear confused. They are often obtunded, disoriented, and unaware of the seizure. Headache occurs in about 80 per cent of patients and persists after the seizure for the rest of the day and abates after sleep, but may remain as a dull ache for a day or two. The period of confusion varies; some patients are apparently mentally normal within a few minutes, but the mental dullness can last up to seven to ten days in others. Following a seizure, there is usually a feeling of extreme fatigue with pain in the muscles that persists for 24 to 48 hours. There may be amnesia for events immediately prior to the seizure and for the period of confusion after the seizure. Mentation may be slowed and the patient may feel dull-witted for several days. If a generalized seizure follows a localized discharge of neurons, those neurons may show postictal exhaustion, which is manifested, for example, by paralysis or sensory loss in the area innervated by them.

As mentioned earlier, patients suffering from generalized seizures frequently suffer traumatic injuries during the attack. These include laceration of the tongue; broken teeth, or loss of teeth; fracture of bones, particularly compression fractures of the vertebrae due to sustained muscular contraction; head injury; and bruises and lacerations of various parts of the body. If a seizure occurs while the patient is driving an automobile, death or severe injury may result to himself and others. If a seizure occurs while he is swimming, drowning may result. If it occurs while he is working or climbing at a height, a fatal fall may result. Unexpected and sudden death is a rare phenomenon in young epileptics, but when it occurs it may be due to acute involvement of cardiac and respiratory centers in the brainstem.[89]

The Electroencephalogram. The electroencephalogram taken during a tonic-clonic seizure usually shows artefact due to the generalized tonic and clonic muscle activity. Records that are free from muscle artefact show generalized 8- to 14-cps rhythmic spike activity, which decreases in frequency and increases in amplitude as the tonic phase proceeds. In the clonic phase, the spike activity is interrupted by periods of electrical silence. Each group of spikes corresponds to a clonic muscular contraction, and the periods of electrical silence tend to become more prolonged just before the seizure ceases.

When the spikes cease, the clinical seizure ceases, and there is a short period of electrical silence followed by generalized delta activity. Thereafter, the EEG frequency gradually increases with the appearance of theta activity and the return to a normal resting record over a period of hours. Occasionally, slowing may persist for several days after a seizure. The interictal EEG in patients with generalized seizures may be normal with symmetric alpha activity, or it may show paroxysmal bursts of polyspike and slow waves or bursts of spike and wave or sharp and slow wave activity, which is usually symmetric and diffuse.

Tonic Type of Generalized Seizures

Tonic seizures may be defined as seizures manifested by sustained and uninterrupted muscular contraction throughout the attack. They probably occur almost as frequently as mixed tonic and clonic seizures in children. However, purely tonic seizures are rare in infants, adolescents, and adults.

The seizure begins with immediate loss of consciousness, and the patient falls to the ground in a tonic posture identical to that already described in the tonic phase of mixed tonic and clonic seizures. The tonic contraction seldom lasts longer than five or ten seconds and is associated with mydriasis, tachycardia, and hypertension. After the tonic phase, the patient immediately passes into a stage of flaccid coma without an intervening clonic phase. The stage of recovery is the same as that described for mixed tonic and clonic seizures.

The Electroencephalogram. In tonic seizures the electroencephalogram shows low-voltage symmetric 10- to 14-cps spike activity at the beginning of the seizure, which decreases in frequency and increases in amplitude during the seizure. There is a period of generalized delta activity immediately after the seizure, with gradual increase in frequency until normal activity returns.

Infantile Spasms (Salaam Seizures, Massive Myoclonic Spasms)

This characteristic form of epilepsy occurs in infants as a result of perinatal infection, developmental abnormalities, trauma, or degenerative disorders of the brain. It carries a serious prognosis, since almost all these children become severely retarded. The seizures usually begin in the first four to six months of life, but the onset has been reported as late as one year of age.

The terms "infantile spasm" and "salaam" seizures are descriptive of the clinical manifestations of the seizure. These consist of sudden brief flexion movements of the neck and trunk with adduction and flexion of the limbs so that the hands tend to meet the bowed head in a "salaam" or double-handed salute. The movements are lightning-like and usually brief and sometimes consist of extensor thrusts of the arms. The attacks are accompanied by pallor and less commonly cyanosis with sweating, rapid breathing, and pupillary dilatation. They may be preceded by a period of hyperventilation. The child may cry during or immediately following the episode. The eyes have a fixed stare and may be conjugately deviated to one side. The frequency of attacks varies from case to case, but they are usually frequent with as many as 50 to 100 occurring in a single day. They tend to be more frequent during drowsiness and on awakening.

After five years of age generalized seizures, focal seizures, and psychomotor seizures replace the infantile spasms in about half the cases, and the EEG patterns change from hypsarrhythmia (see description below) to an abnormal spike pattern. In the remaining cases the seizures cease. More than 90 per cent of children who have had an EEG pattern of hypsarrhythmia show severe mental retardation.

The Electroencephalogram (Hypsarrhythmia). The name "hypsarrhythmia" is derived from the characteristic electroencephalographic picture of mountainous slow waves in the delta range. The record shows synchronous and asynchronous high-voltage delta activity, with single or multiple spikes occurring in all leads in apparently asynchronous and random fashion. This activity is present when the child is awake or asleep, sometimes during the ictus, and also when he is free of apparent clinical seizures. Ictal episodes are usually accompanied by low-voltage activity (decremental response) lasting up to 15 seconds and followed by gradual resumption of the hypsarrhythmic pattern.

Myoclonic Seizures and Akinetic (Astatic) Seizures

Myoclonic jerks are brief unexpected muscular contractions, usually bilateral, often asymmetric, and occasionally unilateral. This type of seizure activity may be the only sign of epilepsy, or myoclonic seizures may occur in patients who suffer from other forms of epilepsy, particularly those with tonic-clonic seizures. They usually occur on awakening or during the first hour after getting up in the morning. There may be one or two of these myoclonic jerks during this period, and they are occasionally of sufficient intensity to throw the patient to the ground. The maximal involvement is usually in the upper limbs and occurs when the patient is performing a task such as brushing the hair or drinking coffee. Objects held in the hand such as a hairbrush or coffee cup may be flung with considerable force by a sudden

involuntary movement of the shoulder and arm.

Akinetic seizures or drop attacks are seen in children who have a sudden loss of muscle tone often with a precipitous drop to the ground. Akinetic seizures are sometimes associated with myoclonic jerks in the same individual. Occasionally the akinetic seizure is very brief, and the individual only "bobs" the head or stumbles.

Both myoclonic seizures and akinetic seizures are sensitive to sound, and attacks may be precipitated by a sudden noise, which need not be loud.

The Electroencephalogram. The record may show symmetric or asymmetric generalized slow spike and wave discharges or complex polyspike wave discharges. Attacks sometimes occur without correlated EEG discharges.

Clonic Type of Generalized Seizures

This type of generalized seizure occurs in young children and infants and is the type of seizure that is characteristic of febrile convulsions (p. 373). The clonic movements vary in rate from 3 to 12 per second and appear as repetitive generalized jerks of the whole body. These attacks may occasionally last for as long as an hour. The child is unconscious throughout the seizure and passes into a deep sleep after the clonic movements cease. Discharge within the autonomic nervous system must be slight in this type of seizure because mydriasis, sweating, and urinary incontinence are seldom noted.

The Electroencephalogram. The EEG shows 10-cps, bifrontal, spike discharges during the ictus. The interictal record is normal in children with febrile convulsions. Occasional paroxysmal spike-wave or polyspike and wave discharges are seen in the interictal record of epileptic children with this type of seizure.

Generalized Convulsive Seizures with Focal Onset (Secondary Generalized Seizures)

Any seizure discharge beginning in a localized population of neurons with focal clinical manifestations may spread to involve the entire central nervous system and thus produce a generalized seizure. The focal episode is often brief and may be described by the patient as the warning or "aura" of an impending generalized seizure. In some cases this "aura" is so brief that it is not mentioned by the patient or noticed by those who observe the seizure and is only elicited by direct questioning. In seizures with a brief aura, localized spike activity may only appear in the electroencephalogram for a few seconds prior to generalized epileptic discharge. In some patients who describe an aura, it is not possible to record the localized discharge using standard scalp electrodes, and the seizure appears as a diffuse burst of spike activity without preceding focal abnormality. The use of nasopharyngeal, tympanic, and sphenoidal electrodes in such cases may show a deep subcortical focus in the medial temporal regions. There is increasing evidence that secondary generalized seizures may originate in the prefrontal cortex with secondary involvement and dissemination of electrical activity through the mesial thalamus.[78, 153] It is probable that secondary generalized seizures are more common than can be established by presently available EEG recording techniques.

The Electroencephalogram. In the majority of cases, the EEG shows focal spike and slow wave activity, which becomes generalized at the onset of the generalized seizure (Fig. 6–2). The interictal record frequently shows focal paroxysmal activity.

Generalized Seizures of Nonconvulsive Type

Typical Absence or Petit Mal

The diagnosis of typical absence or petit mal seizures is based on both clinical and electroencephalographic findings. It may be defined as loss of consciousness (initially of brief duration with staring or rhythmic blinking of the eyes) and associated symmetric 3-cps spike and slow wave activity in the EEG. Minor seizures with brief lapses of consciousness are frequently misdiagnosed on clinical grounds as "petit mal" in children with brief spells unassociated with convulsive movements. Many such patients are later found to have focal seizures of psychomotor epilepsy. The diagnosis of typical absence or petit mal should be reserved for those cases having both the clinical and EEG findings indicative of this condition.

Typical absence occurs almost exclusively in childhood after the age of three years, and there is a positive family history in about 40 per cent of cases. It is characterized by brief episodes of loss of consciousness lasting 5 to 15 seconds during which time the patient's activities are suspended and the child stares with a vacant expression. There may be 3-cps blinking of the eyelids or myoclonic jerks, and very occasionally turning of the head, swallowing, or movement of an arm.[165] The frequency of the attacks shows considerable variation from a single episode every two or three months to several hundred per day. The neurologic examination is normal, except that the seizures may often be induced by hyperventilation during the examination. When the seizures are frequent, mentation becomes seriously impaired (due to frequent lapses of consciousness), and these children may present as misdiag-

C.C. 7/5/77

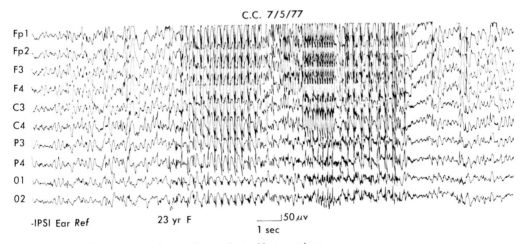

-IPSI Ear Ref   23 yr F   50 μv
                                        1 sec

FIGURE 6–2. Electroencephalogram in a patient with secondary generalized seizures. Ictal discharges consist of irregular 2½- to 6-Hz spike-and-wave discharges bilaterally. Interictal pattern showed multiple foci of spike discharges.

nosed cases of mental retardation or with learning problems in school.

The majority of patients cease to have absence attacks in adolescence, but some do continue into adult life at a much reduced rate. In about one third of patients the seizure pattern changes and the patient develops generalized seizures in adolescence that may continue into adult life. The most favorable prognosis is seen in those who have an early onset of absence with a positive family history, normal intelligence, and normal neurologic examination.[38]

The Electroencephalogram. Each clinical seizure is accompanied by highly characteristic diffuse 3-cps symmetric spike and wave (spike and dome) discharges in the EEG (Fig. 6–3).

Atypical Absence or Petit Mal Variant

This condition, variously called atypical absence or petit mal variant, must also be diagnosed on the basis of the combined clinical and electroencephalographic abnormality. The pathogenesis may resemble that of typical absence with paroxysmal discharges arising in brainstem inhibitory systems which project bilaterally to both hemispheres. In addition, this activity may be initiated by focal epileptic discharges in other areas of the brain, such as the mesial aspect of the temporal lobe, which discharge down into a damaged brainstem inhibitory system.[207]

The clinical picture of the seizure is variable but characterized by a brief period of unresponsiveness (absence), sometimes associated with a brief tonic seizure. The condition often occurs in children with cerebral damage; so there may be additional features such as mental retardation or abnormalities on neurologic examination.

The Electroencephalogram. The electroencephalogram is characterized by sharp and slow wave discharges which are usually rhythmic but either faster or slower than the 3-cps activity of petit mal. In addition, they may show some asymmetry and lack of bifrontal onset. The majority show a focal onset in one frontal lobe with diffuse spread probably by firing with thalamic and brainstem neurons which have diffuse cortical projections. This is sometimes called "secondary bilateral synchrony" and contrasts with the EEG features seen in typical absence.

Continuing Absence or Petit Mal Status

Unlike brief typical absence seizures, the condition of continuing absence (petit mal status) tends to occur in young adults rather than in children. It is characterized by long periods, varying from hours to several days, of clouding of consciousness

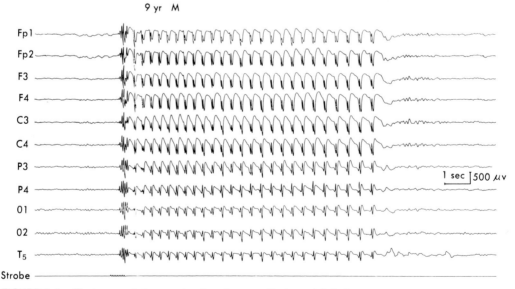

FIGURE 6–3. Electroencephalogram showing absence attack precipitated by photic stimulation. There are rhythmic 2½- to 3-Hz generalized spike-and-wave discharges. The interictal pattern was normal for age.

during which the electroencephalogram shows continuous, more or less symmetric, and diffuse 3-cps spike and wave activity as described under either atypical absence or petit mal. The patient is not unconscious but is obtunded and the reaction time is slowed. For example, when such a patient is questioned and requested to perform tasks, the response is slow and the response time is lengthy compared to the patient's normal reactions.[82] If a series of simple tests of mentation or motor performance is attempted, many will be omitted or incorrectly performed.

Although the treatment of epilepsy will be discussed in detail later, the treatment of petit mal status receives special consideration.

Continuing absence can be terminated by the injection of diazepam intravenously. The drug is usually given at the rate of 1 mg every 30 seconds, and it is helpful if the electroencephalogram is recorded during the injection. The injection can be terminated when there is clinical improvement and disappearance of the 3-cps spike wave activity and the appearance of normal background activity. Further episodes can be prevented by the use of oral diazepam or ethosuximide (Zarontin).

Unilateral Seizures

Unilateral seizures commonly occur in children and are much less frequent in adults, but when they occur, brain tumor should be suspected. The most common type of unilateral seizures in children is clonic and is often incorrectly referred to as a "jacksonian seizure." The jacksonian type of march is rare in children, but is not uncommon in focal seizures of adults.

The unilateral clonic seizure may be accompanied by impairment or loss of consciousness and clonic movements involving one side of the body. The head and eyes are deviated toward the side showing the clonic movements. The frequency and amplitude of the clonic movements vary, and the seizure may last from several minutes to several hours. During prolonged seizures, there may be waxing and waning of the clonic activity, which may give rise to the erroneous impression that the jerking is restricted to part of a limb or to one side of the face. Careful observation will show that the whole side is affected. It is this waxing and waning that gives rise to the faulty impression of a jacksonian march. In such cases, the epileptic activity remains unchanged in the electroencephalogram during the periods of waxing and waning of hemiclonic activity. The seizure is regularly followed by a postictal paralysis (Todd's paralysis) involving the affected side and lasting for an hour or so after clonic movements have ceased.

Many children have hemiclonic seizures, which may alternate from time to time to involve either side of the body. The seizure may even alternate from one side to the other during the same episode or both sides may simultaneously be briefly involved.

The Electroencephalogram. The EEG usually shows bilateral spike and wave discharges during a hemiclonic seizure with higher voltage activity arising from the hemisphere on the side opposite to the clonic movements. There is marked slowing over this hemisphere after the seizure, particularly during the period of postictal paralysis. The interictal record usually shows bilateral synchronous paroxysmal activity.

Partial Seizures (Focal Seizures)

Partial Motor Seizures

Classification. There are six types of partial motor seizures, which will be discussed separately. These are:

1. Partial motor seizures without spread.
2. Partial motor seizures with spread (jacksonian epilepsy).
3. Adversive seizures.
4. Epilepsia partialis continua with motor manifestations.
5. Partial tonic seizures.
6. Partial seizures with loss of speech.

PARTIAL MOTOR SEIZURES WITHOUT SPREAD. This type consists of brief seizures of clonic movements of one or more muscles on one side of the body. The thumb, thumb and index finger, hand, face, or foot is commonly involved. The movement is maximal at the onset and terminates in a few seconds to a few minutes.

PARTIAL MOTOR SEIZURES WITH SPREAD (Jacksonian Epilepsy). In this type of seizure, there is rhythmic clonic jerking of part of the body followed by an orderly spread of activity to involve adjacent muscles. This type of "jacksonian march" often begins in the thumb with spread to the fingers, wrist, forearm, upper arm, and then upper face with clonic movements of the eyelids on the same side. The spread of activity may occasionally involve the whole of one side of the body, then suddenly spread to the opposite side and develop into a generalized tonic and clonic seizure of the secondary generalized type.

ADVERSIVE SEIZURES. This type of motor seizure results in turning of the head or body owing to synergistic contraction of muscles during a seizure discharge. In its simplest form, there may be conjugate deviation of the eyes to one side. In more complex forms, the eye movement may be accompanied by head turning in the same direction. This may be followed by turning of the body as though the patient were turning to look at an object of interest. The turning movement is often accompanied by abduction and elevation of the arm. Occasionally, the turning may continue until the patient has completed several rotations (gyratory epilepsy).

EPILEPSIA PARTIALIS CONTINUA. Some patients with partial motor seizures may experience clonic movements, at intervals of one or two seconds, of a part of the body which persists for many hours without ceasing. These may periodically develop into more complex partial motor seizures (Fig. 6–2).

PARTIAL TONIC SEIZURES. These seizures present with tonic spasm of muscle groups producing abnormal postures of the affected limb. When this occurs in the thumb or fingers, it resembles a dystonic posturing of the hand. Partial tonic seizures may be induced by repeated voluntary movement of the hand on the affected side.[68]

All types of partial motor seizure may be followed by a postictal paralysis of the muscles involved by the seizure activity (Todd's paralysis). This may result in a paralyzed limb with slow recovery of strength over a period of several hours.

PARTIAL SEIZURES WITH LOSS OF SPEECH. A partial seizure discharge may cause simple vocal arrest, that is loss of speech without difficulty in recalling symbols of language. Other patients experience transient aphasia with difficulty in comprehension and motor performance of language.

The Electroencephalogram in Partial Seizures. There are focal contralateral epileptic discharges during the seizure (Fig. 6–4). Brief discharges may be seen in some cases in the interictal period.

Partial Somatosensory Seizures

These sensory seizures are comparable to partial motor seizures in that they are localized, may spread in orderly fashion, and may persist for long periods of time (epilepsia partialis continua of the sensory type).

Somatosensory seizures are characterized by an abnormal sensation which usually involves part of or occasionally the whole of one side of the body. These sensations are usually reported as aberrations of primary sensation, such as numbness, tingling, loss of feeling, formication, electrical sensations, or paresthesias in the affected area.

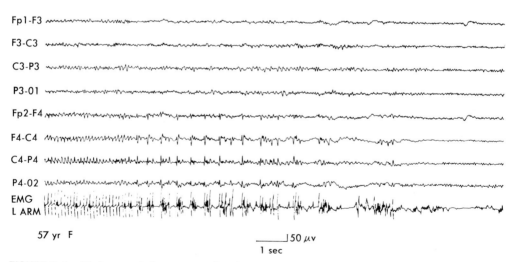

FIGURE 6–4. Electroencephalogram recording the termination of a partial motor seizure involving the left upper extremity. The EEG showed rhythmic sharp discharges over the right central region. The interictal recording was normal.

When the abnormality involves proprioceptive sensation, there is a feeling of abnormal posture or position of the limb, or occasionally it feels absent. Other sensations are described as an "electric shock" or feeling of warmth or cold in the affected parts.

Sensory seizures usually involve the thumb, hand, or face (particularly in the region of the lips and involving half the tongue). In most cases, the abnormal sensation is confined to one area throughout the seizure,[136b] while in others, there is an orderly march of symptoms as, for example, from the thumb to the fingers, hand, angle of the mouth, cheek, and half the tongue.

Some patients report that the seizures may be triggered by certain stimuli such as a sudden shock or an unexpected blow to the affected limb. Others claim that they are able to stop the march of somatosensory seizures by painful stimuli to the affected part such as tying a tight ligature around the limb.

A patient with partial somatosensory seizures should have complete diagnostic studies as a brain tumor suspect because of the high rate of focal pathologic changes.[124] Computed tomography is particularly useful as an early screening procedure and is likely to reveal abnormalities in more than one third of the patients.[17]

The Electroencephalogram. This may show focal paroxysmal abnormality in the parietal region on the side opposite the involved extremities, but the record is often normal in the interictal period. When a record is obtained during a seizure, focal high-voltage spike activity usually appears in the parietal area.

Partial Seizures with Complex Symptomatology (Psychomotor Seizures)

The terms "psychomotor seizures" and "seizures arising in the temporal lobe" have been applied with some looseness to all partial seizures that are believed to originate within the temporal lobe. This may be true in the majority of conditions that will be described under the title of "Psychomotor Seizures," but it is also likely that many of these seizures have their origin in the orbital area of the frontal lobe and the insula. Both these structures have rich projections to the temporal lobe.

Classification. Psychomotor seizures are categorized according to the initial symptoms. During this initial phase, the seizure may present with one symptom such as an unusual smell (gustatory hallucination). The seizure may terminate or develop into a more complex seizure pattern involving a wide variety of disorders of perception[64] due to the spread of epileptic activity within the temporal lobe. In other cases, the seizure that follows the initial temporal lobe manifestation is a secondary generalized seizure, usually of a generalized tonic and clonic type.

SEIZURES WITH DISTURBANCE OF THINKING. A frequent manifestation of psychomotor seizures is the "dreamy state" in which there is clouding of consciousness with associated illusional or hallucinatory experiences resembling a dream. These may be described in many ways but certain experiences are so frequently described by patients that they have become in some ways synonymous with psychomotor seizures. There may be an intense feeling of reliving events that have occurred in the past, often in childhood, or a strange feeling of familiarity when in strange surroundings. Both conditions are described as *déjà vu* (already seen) phenomena.[35] The opposite illusion in which the patient is unable to recognize familiar surroundings *(jamais vu)* does not occur as commonly as the *déjà vu* phenomenon.

Visual illusions in which objects appear smaller (micropsia) or larger (macropsia) or in which objects change shape or position (metamorphosis) are often described. Similarly, illusions involving hearing in which sounds become fainter (microacusia) or louder (macroacusia) can occur. Feelings of incongruity in which the patient has a sensation of being detached from what is going on around him or that he is observing himself and the scene from outside of his body may also be described. Other patients experience feelings of unreality and feel that the activity going on around them is not really happening.

Complex hallucinations with recall of scenes from the past, often including great detail, such as hearing the voices of persons present in the hallucination who are no longer alive, can be an unusual manifestation of psychomotor seizures. This type of seizure pattern involves controlled activity of memory patterns and is too complex to be regarded as a visual or auditory hallucination alone. A somewhat similar situation involves the experience of sudden compulsive thoughts, usually of an unpleasant nature, or of compulsive ideas that force themselves into the patient's mind to the exclusion of all others.

Occasionally the patient is able to alter the thought by an extreme effort of will but it is promptly changed to another repetitive thought or idea sometimes of an even more bizarre nature.

SEIZURES WITH DISTURBANCE OF LANGUAGE. Two types of language disturbance are encountered in psychomotor epilepsy.[194] There may be dysphasia when the epileptic form lies in the dominant hemisphere, or there may be speech automatisms with utterance of identifiable words during an attack for which the patient is subsequently amnesic. The latter automatism does not show correlation with dominant hemisphere involvement.

SEIZURES WITH COMPLEX MOTOR BEHAVIOR. Innumerable patterns of behavior have been described in psychomotor epilepsy since attacks differ in each patient and sometimes the pattern of behavior differs from seizure to seizure in the same patient.

A common example is the patient who experiences automatisms with amnesia. At the beginning of the attack, the patient is motionless and stares for about ten seconds. This is followed by a brief period of stereotyped automations such as rapid chewing, blinking, or swallowing.[54] The patient then enters a third stage in which he answers questions incorrectly or ignores the questioner and may repeat phrases or mumble incoherently as though sleepwalking. Some patients perform repetitive actions such as stroking the face or arm; others engage in more complex activity such as undressing or wandering around a room or office rearranging furniture or papers. If an attempt is made to restrain the patient, force is met by force, and many patients exhibit an unexpected degree of strength under such circumstances. This is an unconscious reaction on the part of the patient to resist attempted interference with previously programmed and automatic behavior and is the major reason for the belief that patients with psychomotor seizures are dangerous.

Some patients enter what has been termed a "fugue state"[77] and may walk or travel for hours or occasionally days before they regain consciousness. During the period of the seizure, the behavior is normal to the extent that some patients can use quite complex transportation systems such as trains or airlines without appearing to behave abnormally. Other patients have driven cars for many hours in a similar fugue state, obeying traffic lights and road signs. There is amnesia for the event, yet the patient responds to his environment.[61] Some forms of running epilepsy (p. 356) are due to psychomotor seizures and are closely related to the group of so-called "fugue states."

SEIZURES WITH ANTISOCIAL BEHAVIOR. Some patients with psychomotor epilepsy exhibit antisocial behavior. Automatisms simulating exhibitionism have been reported.[91] There may be moodiness, irritability, and outbursts of anger on slight provocation which occur periodically.[167] These patients are usually young men of lower-than-average intelligence who have a history of behavioral disturbance in school.[179] It may be that anger is a reactive phenomenon in many cases due to the stress of the social pressure imposed by the disease, or it may reflect more diffuse brain damage in some psychomotor epileptics.[213]

The question of inflicting harm on others during an epileptic seizure has been debated. It is most unusual for an epileptic subject to harm others during an attack[20] unless an attempt is made to restrain him or to prevent his carrying out some form of automatism. Epileptic violence is not premeditated, is unprovoked and senseless, and the patient usually has no recollection of the episode.[48]

SEIZURES WITH AFFECTIVE DISTURBANCES. The most common affective disturbance described in psychomotor seizures is a feeling of fear. This occurs in about 80 per cent of patients with psychomotor seizures and may remain as an isolated phenomenon or precede other manifestations such as hallucinations or forced thinking. Sometimes the patient has amnesia for the events that occur during the seizure and can remember only the intense feeling of fear.

Sensations of pleasure or well-being are much rarer than an aura of fear. Short periods of compulsive laughter may occur and are described as "laughing epilepsy," but the laugh is not a natural or amusing one and sounds entirely artificial. Epileptic laughter may occur with other symptoms such as *déjà vu* phenomena or automatisms and the patient is unaware afterward of the period of laughter. In some cases, however, the patient recalls the laughter with embarrassment and may try to explain it away in a rather unconvincing manner. Uncontrolled episodes of crying occurring without provocation and unassociated with feelings of sadness or depression have also been reported in psychomotor epilepsy.

SEIZURES WITH AUDITORY SYMP-
TOMS. Auditory symptoms that occur during
seizures consist of elementary noises. The patient
may describe a continuous and shrill whistle or
a deep-toned roar. The sound may be intermittent
and occasionally rhythmic. The most complex
sound of this type of seizure is hallucinatory pealing of bells. The sounds are usually appreciated
in both ears. The seizure discharge originates in
the posterior aspect of the superior temporal gyrus or in the supratemporal region in the lateral
fissure.

SEIZURES WITH OLFACTORY SYMP-
TOMS. An intense hallucination of smell is a
common complaint in patients with epilepsy. This
type of sensation can occur as an isolated phenomenon but is often followed by other forms of psychomotor epilepsy or by a generalized seizure.
The smell is usually described as powerful and
is unpleasant in about 80 per cent of cases. Patients describe a hallucination of "burnt blood"
or "bad eggs." Occasionally the sensation is pleasant and may be described as "the smell of flowers"
or, more specifically, as the smell of "geraniums"
or "jasmine." The symptoms are often associated
with masticatory movements such as licking and
smacking of the lips and a clouding of consciousness or "dreamy state."

The epileptic focus lies in the uncus of the hippocampal formation, and the term "uncinate fits"
has been used by some neurologists to describe
olfactory seizures.

SEIZURES WITH VISUAL SYMP-
TOMS. Visual sensations may be elementary
in form, but complex visual hallucinations also
occur. The patient may experience floating balls
of light or stars, wheels, or disks, which are multi-
colored and frequently increase in size. In other
cases, there may be scintillating scotomata. These
phenomena occur in the visual field opposite to
the seizure discharge and, occasionally, in both
visual fields at the same time. This type of seizure
is frequently due to discharges arising in the occipital region (areas 18 and 19 of Brodmann) as
well as from posterior temporal foci.

More complex hallucinations of familiar scenes
and of human figures or animals, sometimes of
bizarre appearance, are occasionally described.
These are most frequently associated with EEG
discharges arising from posterior temporal foci.
As an example, one particular patient could recall
scenes from a television cartoon she watched in
childhood. The epileptic focus, in this case, lay
in the posterior part of the temporal lobe adjoining the visual association areas.

SEIZURES WITH VERTIGINOUS
SYMPTOMS. One of the most common symptoms of psychomotor seizures is a sense of spinning, usually around a vertical axis. Other symptoms that are encountered are suggestive of a
labyrinthine disturbance and include a sense of
vertical or lateral movement or a feeling of falling.
The symptoms are frequently associated with epigastric sensations, sensory disturbances, dreamy
states, and loss of consciousness. Crude visual
and auditory hallucinations are not uncommonly
associated with vertiginous seizures. This suggests
that the epileptic discharge arises in the posterior
part of the temporal lobe near the angular gyrus,
which is known to be the cortical area receiving
vestibular connections from the brainstem.[196]

SEIZURES WITH GUSTATORY SYMP-
TOMS. It is often difficult to distinguish between gustatory and olfactory seizures since both
are associated with masticatory movements and
"dreamy states." The patient usually describes a
bitter taste, although occasional hallucinations of
a pleasant taste have been reported.

The epileptic discharge originates in the oper-
culum of the insula, just above the lateral fissure.

SEIZURES WITH ABDOMINAL AND
ALIMENTARY SENSATIONS. This is a
relatively common form of psychomotor epilepsy
in which the patient experiences epigastric sensations, often described as "butterflies in the stomach." This may be accompanied by the desire
to defecate. It is usually followed by other manifestations of psychomotor epilepsy or by a generalized seizure. In children it may be associated
with recurrent abdominal pain and may be referred to as "abdominal epilepsy." The condition
should be considered in children who have paroxysmal pain of relatively short duration, some disturbance of awareness or responsiveness, an electroencephalographic abnormality, and a favorable
response to anticonvulsants.[46]

The epileptic focus lies in the posterior part
of the insula.

SEIZURES WITH CARDIOVASCULAR
SYMPTOMS. Patients with psychomotor epilepsy have described a sensation of precordial discomfort, fluttering in the left chest or mediastinum, and tachycardia as isolated symptoms or
as part of the seizure pattern.

SEIZURES SIMULATING SCHIZO-
PHRENIA. Occasionally, patients with psy-

chomotor seizures are misdiagnosed as schizophrenic. This occurs when the seizure activity presents with an acute episode of withdrawal and hallucinations followed by agitated behavior and decreased organization of thought processes. However, episodes tend to be stereotyped, and there is an obvious impairment of consciousness and amnesia for the event.[1] Patients with psychomotor seizures simulating schizophrenia are emotionally labile and show rapid swings of mood in the interictal phase unlike the true schizophrenic patient.[180]

Diagnosis. The diagnosis of psychomotor seizures can usually be made on clinical history alone. This requires a careful reconstruction of episodes by the patient and observers which may be time-consuming. The neurologic examination is usually normal, but many patients with psychomotor seizures show facial asymmetry due to slight unilateral weakness, particularly when smiling.[173]

The Electroencephalogram. Many patients who have seizures of psychomotor epilepsy show the presence of rapid paroxysmal discharges or spike activity over one or both temporal areas during the attack (Fig. 6–5). This is not universal, however, and there may be little or no abnormality in some records. This is to be expected when it is recognized that much of the electrical activity of the temporal lobe is not recorded by the standard scalp electrodes. Consequently, abnormal electric discharges emanating from the inferior or medial surface of the temporal lobe usually do not appear in the electroencephalogram made with routine scalp leads. The use of nasopharyngeal, tympanic, or sphenoidal electrodes increases the chances of recording epileptic activity from the inferior or medial surface of the temporal lobe.[43] However, these electrodes cause some discomfort, and their placement is time-consuming and requires skill.

The interictal record may also show focal spike activity or short runs of focal theta activity. Many are normal. Epileptic activity can be activated by drowsiness and light sleep in the majority of cases, and a sleep EEG should be obtained in cases of suspected psychomotor epilepsy. Activation by a single intravenous dose of methohexital not greater than 1 to 5 mg/kg of body weight appears to be safe and superior to other activation techniques in enhancing temporal lobe epileptic activity.[149] More information on epileptic activity occurring in the depth of the temporal lobe may be obtained in selected cases by depth electrography.[119] This has clinical application in patients with chronic seizure disorders who may benefit from surgical treatment.

The Reflex Epilepsies

Certain seizures may be precipitated by sensory stimuli and therefore have been classified as reflex

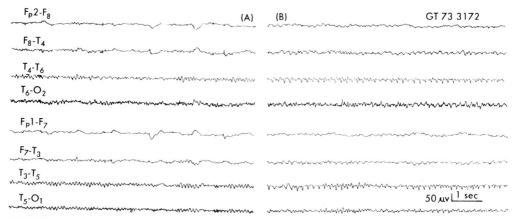

FIGURE 6–5. Electroencephalogram in a case of psychomotor epilepsy. The resting recording *(A)* shows occasional sharp waves in T_6-O_2. During a psychomotor seizure the activity is superseded by rhythmic sharp wave activity occurring over both temporal lobes *(T_4, T_6, T_3, and T_5)*. Electrode positions: F_p, frontopolar; *F*, frontal; *T*, temporal; *O*, occipital. Even numbers, right hemisphere. Odd numbers, left hemisphere.

epilepsies. The resulting seizure pattern is usually of the generalized or psychomotor type.

Seizures Provoked by Photic or Visual Stimuli (Photogenic Epilepsy)

A certain number of patients with epilepsy may have seizures induced by visual stimuli such as flashing or flickering lights.[87] Such individuals report that seizures may be provoked when driving a car and being subjected to the flicker of sunlight passing through the branches of trees, or when passing telephone poles when in a train. Others are sensitive to the flicker induced by passing streetlights at regular intervals when driving at night or to the flickering lights of television sets or psychedelic discotheques. Quite a number of reports have now accumulated of epilepsy induced by watching television.[13] The adequate stimulus appears to be the flickering of badly adjusted sets.

Photogenic epilepsy is most prevalent in children between the ages of 6 and 14 years. Photosensitivity may be readily demonstrated while recording the electroencephalogram by the use of a stroboscopic light. Photogenic epilepsy responds well to anticonvulsant medication (see p. 361). Adjuvant treatment includes conditioning methods using stroboscopic stimulation and the use of tinted glasses or contact lenses that filter out the portion of the light spectrum to which the patient responds.

Musicogenic Epilepsy

This is a rare form of epilepsy in which seizures are induced by listening to certain musical themes or tones. The adequate stimulus may be highly specific and has been reported to occur regularly when the patient is listening to certain passages of music or to the pealing of church bells or even in response to music made only by certain specific musical instruments. The electroencephalogram shows epileptic activity when the patient listens to recordings containing the adequate musical stimulus.

Reading Epilepsy

The precipitation of epilepsy by reading is rare, but both generalized and focal psychomotor seizures have occasionally been described as a result of this unusual stimulus.[121] The patient experiences involuntary movements of the jaw while reading, which usually cease when the reading is stopped. Occasionally, the jaw movements may be followed by a period of automatic behavior with loss of consciousness or a generalized tonic and clonic seizure. The type of reading material has little effect on the production of involuntary jaw movements, and in some patients seizures may follow the reading of a foreign language that the patient does not understand or the chewing of gum.[21] This suggests that there are two forms of this condition: a primary reading epilepsy and epilepsy induced by articulatory and other jaw movements.

The Electroencephalogram. The EEG is usually normal in the resting and alert state, with the appearance of generalized bilaterally synchronous 3- to 6-cps spike wave activity during reading. This activity begins in brief bursts, which become more frequent as reading continues and stop when reading ceases. Patients learn to avoid seizures by ceasing to read when the involuntary jaw movements begin.

Arithmetical Epilepsy

An extremely rare form of epilepsy has been described in which minor seizures are provoked by attempts to calculate. The seizures are brief, with a lapse of consciousness and the unconscious performance of automatic movements lasting up to 15 seconds. They can be initiated by presenting the patient with a simple arithmetic problem.[103] The patient may suffer from generalized seizures that are independent of the stimulus.

The Electroencephalogram. The resting record may show short bursts of slow waves and irregular spike wave activity. Recordings taken during attempted calculation show a bilateral synchronous 3-cps spike wave pattern, which begins immediately after the presentation of an arithmetic problem.

Paroxysmal Choreoathetosis (Kinesigenic Seizures)

There are some reasons for classifying this condition either as a movement disorder or as a reflex form of epilepsy, although its nature is not entirely accepted. It has been included in this section on epilepsy for practical reasons since the attacks are abolished by diphenylhydantoin (Dilantin) in most cases, and in one case the condition seemed to be epileptic in nature. It is unfortunate, although understandable, that the condition is often misdiagnosed as conversion hysteria rather than an unusual form of epilepsy.

Etiology and Pathology. Paroxysmal choreoathetosis is inherited as an autosomal dominant trait with low penetrance, but there is no evidence that has been demonstrated as yet of a metabolic abnormality in patients suffering from this condition.

The condition is benign and autopsy reports are meager, but in the few reported cases the brain appeared to be normal.

Clinical Features. Symptoms usually begin in childhood around the age of seven years with sudden, brief, and intermittent paroxysmal choreoathetoid movements of the extremities and face. The episodes usually occur several times a day. When they occur, the child or adolescent exhibits bizarre doubling up or choreoathetoid movements of the hands and feet so that walking during the attack appears bizarre or impossible. Some attacks are so severe that the patient is hurled to the floor, where the movements continue for a few seconds.[205] There is no loss of consciousness, tonic or clonic movements do not occur, and there is no incontinence. Attacks last up to 30 seconds, and the patient seems and feels perfectly normal as soon as the movements cease. The choreoathetoid movements are sometimes preceded by a sensory "aura," such as paresthesias or shocklike sensations in the limbs, since patients occasionally experience the sensory phenomenon, without the development of the motor component. Others believe they are able to abort an attack by concentrating or making some repetitive motor movement such as crossing the legs or gripping an object tightly when the sensory symptoms occur.

Nearly all patients report that the attacks occur immediately after a period of immobility followed by a brisk movement.[111] Hyperventilation may induce attacks in some cases. In others, episodes occur spontaneously without specific precipitants.[176] The patients are of normal intelligence with a normal neurologic examination and have no associated signs of anxiety or reason for emotional disorder. They suffer considerable embarrassment from these attacks and as a result may become withdrawn and depressed.

Diagnostic Procedures. All investigations, including roentgenograms of the skull, examination of the cerebrospinal fluid, serum calcium and phosphorus determination, and computed tomography, are within normal limits. The electroencephalogram is normal at rest, but occasional higher-voltage paroxysmal theta activity has been reported during hyperventilation. There is no definite epileptic activity in the EEG at rest during hyperventilation or in attempted recordings during an attack of paroxysmal choreoathetosis.[166] The condition is completely prevented or the attacks are sharply reduced by the anticonvulsant drug diphenylhydantoin (Dilantin). This lends support to the view that the disorder is epileptic in nature.

Other Reflex Epilepsies

Seizures induced by the voices of certain radio announcers (voice-induced epilepsy) have been reported.[62] Another unusual form of reflex epilepsy is the induction of seizure activity in a case of psychomotor epilepsy by irrigation of the external auditory canal with warm or cold water.[27]

Miscellaneous Types of Epilepsy

Running Epilepsy (Cursive Epilepsy)

Compulsive running has occasionally been reported as a type of seizure. The condition is rare, and four distinct types have been described. In each case the patient suffers from seizures but displays some sort of running movements as a manifestation of it.[208]

1. As part of the onset of seizure, the patient runs for as long as 30 minutes while in a state of disturbed consciousness. If questioned during the spell, he is confused and disoriented. He is able to avoid objects during the period of running and has complete amnesia for the episode when he recovers consciousness. The electroencephalogram shows temporal lobe spike activity. This type of running epilepsy falls into the category of a psychomotor seizure in which the automatism of running occurs at the onset of the fugue state.[31]

2. Compulsive running may occur in the period of confusion after a seizure. Under these circumstances, the running is part of the postictal state.

3. During a seizure, some patients make short running movements, usually for only a few steps before falling down and having a generalized convulsion. They are unable to recall the stage of running.

4. Another type has been described in which the entire attack consists of the compulsion to run. There is no loss of consciousness, and the desire can be suppressed by a marked effort of will. The electroencephalogram shows paroxysmal activity, including spike activity arising from the frontal lobes.

Laughing Epilepsy (Gelastic Epilepsy)

The occurrence of laughter during a seizure is rare and has been described as an isolated phenomenon[42, 49] or occasionally associated with running epilepsy. Patients usually show clouding of consciousness with sudden inappropriate laughter and amnesia for the event in the postictal period.[130, 184] There is no characteristic pattern of electroencephalographic change in this condition, but the record usually shows focal activity over one or both hemispheres. This suggests that epileptic foci in different sites may cause laughing epilepsy if they discharge through limbic pathways associated with production of laughter.

Diencephalic Autonomic Epilepsy

An unusual and rare form of epilepsy has been described in adolescents and young adults. The epileptic discharge is believed to arise in the hypothalamus and anterior thalamus since many of such cases had tumors or cysts in this area, hence the term "diencephalic autonomic epilepsy" (Penfield). The clinical picture is stereotyped in each patient, although there are individual differences in each case. The patient may or may not be conscious throughout the episode, and the diencephalic autonomic discharge may be followed by other types of seizure, particularly psychomotor epilepsy or tonic seizures. In a typical attack, the patient develops a feeling of fear or detachment followed by a sensation of fullness in the abdomen, nausea, difficulty in breathing, and a feeling of suffocation. This is followed by tachycardia, elevation of blood pressure, flushing, lacrimation, salivation, perspiration, piloerection, and, occasionally, vomiting and hypothermia.[63] The episode lasts from 30 seconds to several minutes and terminates or progresses into a more generalized seizure.

Except for those cases associated with obvious signs of brain tumor, the condition may be incorrectly diagnosed as anxiety neurosis. Correct diagnosis depends on a careful history, the onset, whether in adolescence or early adult life, the presence of other manifestations of epilepsy, abnormalities in the EEG, and amelioration by anticonvulsant medication.

The Electroencephalogram. The EEG is usually normal between attacks, but the patient develops bilateral symmetric medium- or high-voltage 4- to 6-cps theta activity during the episode of diencephalic autonomic epilepsy. This tends to confirm the view that the seizure discharge arises within deep central structures, such as the hypothalamus, and from here the discharges are propagated symmetrically into both hemispheres.

Cephalgic Seizures and Headache

While headache is almost an invariable complaint in the postictal period following a generalized tonic-clonic seizure, it is possible that paroxysmal headaches may be a major if not the only manifestation of an epileptic seizure. The diagnosis should be considered in children with paroxysmal headaches resembling migraine headaches, who have paroxysmal sharp waves and spike discharges in the electroencephalogram. This is particularly true if there is a history of head injury.

While the differential diagnosis may be difficult, some patients cease to have headaches when treated with anticonvulsant medication but do not respond to caffeine, ergotamine, or methysergide (Sansert). Occasionally, children with paroxysmal headaches have epileptic seizures that are so brief they are not noticed by parents or teachers. The fleeting alteration in consciousness sometimes lasts no longer than a few seconds and consists of staring. The seizures can be observed and recognized by the neurologist, however, and confirmed during recording of the EEG.

"Cerebellar Fits"

This condition is not epileptic but is mentioned here because a lot of experts in the past have considered it a form of epilepsy. The term "cerebellar fits" continues to be used to describe patients who are usually in coma owing to a space-occupying lesion in the intracranial cavity, such as a brain tumor with uncal herniation. During the so-called "cerebellar fit," the patient shows intermittent attacks of decerebration or decerebrate rigidity with tonic extension of all four limbs and extension of the neck. The attacks are precipitated by painful stimulation, which produces rapid and brief extensor spasms of the axial muscles and all four limbs. They are simply attacks of intermittent decerebrate rigidity due to brainstem damage, since apart from their intermittency, they resemble that condition in all other respects. The condition, like decerebrate rigidity, carries a grave prognosis, with evidence of brainstem damage at necropsy.

The EEG does not show spike activity during the "cerebellar fit," and the intravenous injection of anticonvulsant drugs is also without effect.

Hysterical Seizures (Hysteroepilepsy)

Although the name "hysteria" is derived from ancient medical theories of uterine displacement as its cause and hysteria is more common in the female sex, the condition of hysterical seizure is seen in both sexes. The attacks are usually precipitated at a time and in a situation in which the disability will provide some secondary gain. The somatic conversion reaction indicates some deepseated emotional problem, usually at an unconscious level, which requires expert psychotherapy by a psychiatrist.

It is the neurologist's responsibility to diagnose the condition, to reassure the patient and family, and to provide psychiatric referral if it is needed. Hysterical seizures are bizarre and almost always occur in a dramatic and well-timed setting for the observer. The onset is often gradual with complaints of dizziness, palpitation, and nonspecific feelings of being unwell. There is a gradual collapse, usually onto a bed or chair without harm to the patient, and this is followed by motor movements in which the patient thrashes the limbs around and throws the body into wildly contorted postures. There is no incontinence, tongue biting, or loss of consciousness.[126]

The patient may even respond when questioned during the height of this activity. Recovery may be sudden, with the patient suddenly opening his eyes and asking, "What happened?" or "Where am I?" and there is no evidence of postictal coma, stupor, or confusion. In other cases, the patient lies in a flaccid state following the period of motor activity; but the neurologic examination is normal, and attempts to open the eyelids to examine the pupils result in tight closure of the eyelids by the patient. The neurologic examination is normal in the interictal period, and the EEG does not show abnormalities either during or after the seizure.

A more difficult situation occurs when a patient with bonafide epilepsy develops hysterical seizures in addition. The diagnosis depends on careful observation of all types of seizures by the physician.

Fortunately, this complex situation is not frequent, but when it does occur, the patient is usually admitted to a hospital because of seizures that fail to respond to anticonvulsant medication. The seizures usually continue following admission, which permits observation of the complete epidose by a trained observer and performance of a neurologic examination during or immediately following the seizure.

Status Epilepticus

The occurrence of generalized epileptic seizures, one after another, without recovery of consciousness between attacks, is defined as status epilepticus and is a medical emergency. The seizures are usually of the generalized tonic and clonic type, although seizures of continuing absence (p. 348) can occur, which do not present the same problem in emergency treatment. When partial motor or partial sensory seizures present with continuous seizure activity, the condition is termed "epilepsia partialis continua" (p. 350), and such continuing seizures do not carry the grave prognosis of status epilepticus. The sudden onset of status epilepticus in an otherwise healthy adult is highly suggestive of a brain tumor involving the frontal lobe.[156, 157]

The treatment of status epilepticus is discussed on page 367.

Seizures in Infants and Children

Seizures in the very young pose particular problems in diagnosis and treatment. The problem can be considered by age.[72a]

1. Birth to three months. Neonatal seizures are usually due to birth injury, hypoxia, or hypoglycemia. Attacks beginning after the first few weeks of life suggest pyridoxine deficiency or dependency, or hypocalcemia in bottle-fed babies.
2. Three months to nine months. Attacks beginning in this period are more likely to be due to meningitis or encephalitis. Infantile spasms usually appear after three months of age.
3. Nine months to three years. The onset of seizures in this period may also be related to meningitis or encephalitis. However, the common seizure type in this age group is the febrile convulsion, which must be differentiated from epilepsy induced by fever (p. 374). The "adult" forms of epilepsy also begin to develop in children between two and three years of age.

Diagnostic Evaluation

About 90 percent of epileptic patients have histories of epilepsy beginning in childhood. The extent of the investigation of children with epilepsy depends to a great degree on the clinical experience of the attending physician, but the following evaluation has proved helpful.

All children should be interviewed together with the parents. The history concerned with the pregnancy and the perinatal period is important and may disclose possible perinatal causes of cerebral injury. Inquiry should be made concerning the history of the delivery together with the length of labor, manner of presentation of the fetal head, use of instruments, and anesthesia. It is important to know whether the child cried immediately after birth or whether resuscitation was required. Episodes of cyanosis in the first few days of life indicate cerebral anoxic damage of cerebral embolism.

The developmental history up to the time of the first seizure should be documented in detail. A careful description of the seizure should be recorded since this often permits the diagnosis of the type of seizure disorder.

The past history and family history should be established. For example, a past history of encephalitis or meningitis is a likely cause of seizures. A positive family history of epilepsy usually limits the number of investigational procedures that will be necessary if the neurologic examination is within normal limits.

The social history should be obtained in some detail, including any possible exposure to chemicals or toxins (such as lead) that might cause seizures. A complete neurologic examination is performed and decisions are then made regarding treatment and further investigative procedures.

If the neurologic examination is normal and the family history is positive for epilepsy, the child requires only roentgenograms of the skull, EEG, and fasting blood sugar determination to exclude one of the familial hypoglycemias and serum calcium and phosphorus levels to exclude hypocalcemia.

The mentally retarded child with epilepsy requires a more extensive evaluation (see Mental Retardation, p. 63).

Diagnostic Considerations in the Child with One Convulsion

The child with the one convulsion should have a complete history and physical examination. This should be followed by roentgenograms of the skull and an electroencephalogram. If the seizure was a febrile convulsion (p. 373), further investigations are not necessary and the parents can be reassured. Other cases should have a blood count, estimation of serum calcium and phosphorus levels, a five-hour glucose tolerance test, and a CT scan.[70]

Diagnostic Considerations When the Onset of Epilepsy Is in Adolescence and Early Adult Life

The program of investigation in such cases will again be modified by the history and neurologic examination. When the family history is positive for epilepsy and the neurologic examination is negative, investigation can be terminated after skull roentgenogram, fasting blood sugar, serum calcium and phosphorus, electroencephalogram, and CT scan, unless any of these procedures indicate a neoplasm or structural abnormality, in which case arteriography may be indicated.

Diagnostic Considerations When the Onset of Epilepsy Is After 50 Years of Age

Patients who are over 50 should be assumed to have a brain tumor until proven otherwise. When the neurologic examination is normal, the investigation should include skull roentgenogram, fasting blood glucose, serum calcium and phosphorus, electroencephalogram, and a CT scan. Patients with an abnormal neurologic examination or CT scan will usually require arteriography. The patient who has had generalized seizures but whose neurologic examination, CT scan, cerebrospinal fluid, and EEG are normal has a good prognosis.[101, 222] However, he should be examined at repeated intervals of several weeks as an outpatient to exclude tumor, and further investigations may be deferred at this time.[206] The electroencephalogram should be repeated after six weeks and then at intervals of three months for at least one year, and the CT scan should be repeated at intervals of six months. Any indication of localized cerebral abnormality is an indication for arteriography. It should be remembered that patients with late onset of epilepsy who are suspected on clinical grounds of having a brain tumor (the "brain tumor suspect") may have a normal battery of tests, including CT scan and arteriogram. However, months or years later these patients may develop overt signs of brain tumor. Any patient with a reported generalized seizure and a normal neurologic examination who has a cardiac irregularity should be monitored for cardiac arrhythmias. Sudden loss of consciousness of cardiac origin can mimic a generalized seizure.[188]

Medical Treatment

General Principles

The majority of seizures will be adequately controlled by the use of anticonvulsive drugs alone. It is, therefore, essential that the physician concerned with the care of neurologic disorders know which drugs are effective in controlling the different types of the epilepsies and what toxic effects may result from the use of these different drugs.

Certain principles are helpful in instructing resident physicians in the control of seizure disorders with anticonvulsive drugs. These are as follows:

1. The physician should be familiar with the use of at least a small number of effective anticonvulsant drugs.

There are many anticonvulsant drugs available and the number is steadily increasing. New drugs for the treatment of epilepsy are often prematurely and enthusiastically reported, and they have often been introduced for general use before sufficient clinical experience has been gained in neurologic clinics concerned with the investigation and treatment of epilepsy. Most neurologists, even those whose major concern is with the treatment of epilepsy, tend to become highly experienced in the use of five or six drugs, since they find that they can control the majority of seizures with them. This group of "favorite" drugs tends to differ somewhat from one neurologist to another. New drugs should be used with caution and held under a certain healthy suspicion until their worth and lack of toxicity have been verified.

2. Anticonvulsant drugs with minimum toxicity should be used whenever possible.

Many anticonvulsant drugs are effective in controlling certain types of epilepsy but are potentially toxic. Trimethadione (Tridione) in the management of absence (petit mal) and phenacemide (Phenurone) in the treatment of psychomotor seizures are two examples. With the wide choice of anticonvulsant drugs available at the present time, drugs of low toxicity should be used first in all types of epilepsy and the toxic drugs instituted only if all other medications fail.

3. There is no "standard dose" of any anticonvulsant drug.

The tolerance of different patients for different drugs differs enormously, and if *slowly* increased, certain anticonvulsant drugs, such as phenobarbital, primidone, and clonazepam can be given in some individuals in large doses. One drug should be instituted at a time and the dose slowly increased until seizures are controlled or toxic signs persist before abandoning the drug and attempting the use of another. Great disservice to the patient may result from skipping rapidly from one drug to another without careful and fair trial. This may lead to erroneous conclusions that the drugs with minimum toxicity are ineffective or, even worse, that no drug is effective.

4. At the beginning of treatment the use of one anticonvulsant drug alone is advised.

In general, treatment should begin with one drug, which should be increased to the limits of tolerance. If no effective decrease in seizures results, another drug should be substituted, but if partial or near-complete control results, another drug may reasonably be added in combination with the first.

The practice of beginning treatment with more than one drug is common. It is, however, undesirable since this practice increases the chances of toxic effects and adds an additional problem of drug interaction.[174]

5. Withdrawal of one anticonvulsant drug because of substitution of another must be a gradual process.

The sudden withdrawal of an anticonvulsant can precipitate either a marked increase in the frequency of seizures or status epilepticus. This will be avoided if introduction and withdrawal of anticonvulsive drugs are carried out gradually.

6. The patient should be observed for signs of toxicity when anticonvulsant drugs are initiated or the dosage is increased.

In children, the parents should be instructed to observe the child for any unusual signs such as drowsiness, staggering, skin rash, or sore throat and to call the physician if they occur. Both adults and children need examination at regular and frequent intervals by the physician during this period.

7. When an anticonvulsant drug is used that may depress hematopoiesis, the patient requires periodic blood counts.

Parents should be instructed to inform the physician immediately if the child develops signs such as sore throat, purpura, bruising, epistaxis, fever, and rectal, renal, or vaginal bleeding. A blood count should be obtained before treatment and at monthly intervals when using trimethadione (Tridione), paramethadione (Paradione), mephenytoin (Mesantoin), phenacemide (Phenurone), and carbamazepine (Tegretol). This can be increased to three-month intervals after one year.

8. Patients must agree that they will take the medication regularly, as prescribed, and for a protracted period of time.

The parent or patient should be carefully instructed that once medication is used, it must be taken regularly. Control of seizures is not an indication to stop or reduce the medication, and the dose of medication should not be changed unless a responsible physician is consulted.

Useful Anticonvulsant Drugs

Diphenylhydantoin (Dilantin [U.S.], Epanutin [U.K.]). The introduction of diphenylhydantoin as an anticonvulsant in 1938 began an era of more effective anticonvulsant medication. Diphenylhydantoin is one of the most powerful anticonvulsants available and has a relatively low rate of side effects. It is particularly effective in the control of generalized seizures and has some usefulness in the treatment of psychomotor epilepsy. It is not effective in absence (petit mal) and may even increase the frequency of this type of seizure.

The dosage of diphenylhydantoin varies with each patient. Some patients have a low tolerance to the drug, which is caused by congenital enzymatic deficiency, liver disease, or metabolic interference by other drugs. Other patients show refractoriness, which is due to excessive metabolism, deficient absorption, or unreliable intake.[116] To be therapeutically effective, sufficient diphenylhydantoin must be given to maintain adequate blood levels. These can be measured in many laboratories, and the therapeutic level is now accepted as 10 to 20 μg/ml with better seizure control at 20 μg/ml. Nystagmus usually appears at the 17-μg/ml level, but frank toxicity is unusual below 30 μg/ml.[84]

Diphenylhydantoin is supplied in 100-mg capsules (these are white with a red band around them), also as a long-acting preparation (Dilantin, Delayed Action, or DA) in 100-mg capsules, in 50-mg tablets (Dilantin Infatabs), and as a suspension containing 100 mg/4 ml (teaspoonful). The average adult dose varies between 300 and 500 mg daily. The drug should be given in divided doses at 12-hour intervals, with frequent monitoring of blood levels during the early weeks of therapy in an attempt to establish a therapeutic blood level and optimum control of seizures.[73] Constancy of plasma diphenylhydantoin levels through a 24-hour period can be obtained most satisfactorily by oral administration every 12 hours,[217] and more frequent administration is unnecessary.[214a]

Infants and young children can be treated with the suspension of diphenylhydantoin if they refuse to take the tablet, which is rare. The bottle should be shaken thoroughly before each dose since the suspended drug tends to gravitate to the bottom of the bottle. The 50-mg tablets (Dilantin Infatabs) should be substituted as soon as the child is willing to swallow tablets since the dosage is more accurately regulated with tablets or capsules.

TOXIC EFFECTS. Symptoms of mild overdosage include ataxia, lightheadedness, tremors, nystagmus, titubation, diplopia, blurred vision, ptosis, ocular pain, and dysarthria.[127, 160] The drug may reduce the rate of heart action, probably by reducing conduction time in the bundle of His. Such signs resolve quickly with reduction in dosage, and it is not usually necessary to discontinue diphenylhydantoin if the patient develops signs of toxicity.

Diphenylhydantoin occasionally causes skin rashes, particularly in children. These are usually erythematous or morbilliform rashes, but urticaria or purpura may also be seen. Exfoliative dermatitis and erythema multiforme bullosum are serious, but rare, complications which respond to intravenous steroid therapy. Diphenylhydantoin should be discontinued immediately after the appearance of any skin reaction but may be prescribed once again after the rash has faded.

Gastrointestinal symptoms may be encountered due to diphenylhydantoin therapy. These include gastric discomfort, nausea, and vomiting. These have been minimized in many cases by giving the drug at mealtimes.

Disturbances in connective tissue growth occur during diphenylhydantoin therapy, and hypertrophy of the gums is a common side effect. It is occasionally of sufficient severity to warrant withdrawal of the drug or require excision of hyperplastic tissue by an oral surgeon. Other connective tissue changes include enlargement of the lips and nose and generalized thickening of the subcutaneous tissues of the face, producing coarsening of the features in patients receiving prolonged high doses of diphenylhydantoin. There is also a suggestion that diphenylhydantoin produces Dupuytren's contracture in some patients.

Hirsutism of the face, arms, and trunk, pigmentation of the face, and acne are distressing side effects in some patients and are apparently unrelated to drug dose or drug levels.

There have been a few reports of leukopenia during diphenylhydantoin therapy, but agranulocytosis is rare. Megaloblastic anemia has also been reported[80] and responds to a combination of folic acid and vitamin B_{12} therapy. Folic acid should not be given alone since it lowers serum vitamin B_{12} levels.[100] The same combination of drugs is said to prevent mental deterioration in epileptic children receiving diphenylhydantoin[151] but has no effect on frequency of seizures.[170]

Unusual complications of diphenylhydantoin therapy include chronic encephalopathy with dementia, which resolves on withdrawal of the drug, cerebellar atrophy,[93] and peripheral neuropathy.[131] Liver enzyme induction may have important implications including an increased demand for folic acid as a coenzyme leading to folic acid deficiency.[137]

Hemorrhage due to a coagulation defect has been reported in infants born to mothers taking phenobarbital and diphenylhydantoin. Epileptic mothers should be given small doses of vitamin K before delivery and the neonate should be given 1 mg of vitamin K at birth.[200]

The effect of chronic diphenylhydantoin therapy on the endocrine system includes a reduced capacity for the reflex release of ACTH, interference with release of antidiuretic hormone,[60] and impaired insulin response to glucose producing transient hyperglycemia.[90]

Hypocalcemia, elevated alkaline phosphatase, rickets, and osteomalacia have been reported in chronic diphenylhydantoin administration in about 30 per cent of patients. The condition can be reversed with small doses of hydroxycholecalciferol (10 to 45 μg/day) by mouth.

Lymphocytic counts are often low, and lymphadenopathy, which has been mistaken for malignant lymphoma, may be associated with hydantoin drugs; it resolves spontaneously after therapy is stopped.[2] Diphenylhydantoin inhibits the action of bishydroxycoumarin, and withdrawal of the anticonvulsant may lead to serious hemorrhage.[148]

Carbamazepine (Tegretol). It is now widely accepted that carbamazepine is an excellent primary anticonvulsant drug.[183] Carbamazepine is effective in generalized convulsive seizures and partial seizures of all types and may be used alone or in combination with diphenylhydantoin or other anticonvulsants. Carbamazepine is a rapidly acting drug with a short half-life and must be given at least three times a day. The initial dose of one 200-mg tablet at night can be increased over several days to 800 to 1,200 mg in divided doses three times a day. The therapeutic serum level of carbamazepine is between 7 and 12 mg/ml. Carbamazepine has the effect of depressing serum diphenylhydantoin levels, and the dose of diphenylhydantoin may need to be adjusted if the two drugs are used together.

Side effects of carbamazepine include nausea, gastric distress, anorexia, constipation and diarrhea, skin rashes, vertigo, and ataxia, but there is less mental dullness compared to diphenylhydantoin or primidone.[182] Aplastic anemia has been reported as a rare complication of carbamazepine therapy. Therefore, a complete blood count and platelet count should be obtained before treatment and at each month for one year, then at three-monthly periods thereafter. Other side effects which are unusual include abnormalities in liver function tests, peripheral neuropathy, urinary retention, cardiac arrhythmias, hypertension, edema, syncope, and lymphadenopathy.

Phenobarbital. Prior to 1938, when diphenylhydantoin (Dilantin) was introduced, phenobarbital and the bromides were the only drugs available for the treatment of epilepsy. Phenobarbital still remains one of the most effective drugs for this purpose, since it has a low incidence of toxic effects in therapeutic dosage. Another advantage is the low cost of the drug. This is an important consideration in the treatment of epilepsy since relatively large amounts of the drug must be taken regularly for many years or even a lifetime.

Phenobarbital selectively and reversibly depresses excitatory postsynaptic potentials.[10] The drug may be effective in all types of epilepsy in doses of 30 to 60 mg three or four times a day. The therapeutic blood level of phenobarbital is 10 to 20 μg/ml. Plasma levels are representative of concentration in the brain.[193]

Phenobarbital has largely been displaced to a secondary role in seizure control with the introduction of newer drugs such as carbamazepine. However, phenobarbital is still widely used, particularly in combination with diphenylhydantoin, but there may be marked depression of serum levels of diphenylhydantoin after adding phenobarbital, and regular estimations of serum drug levels are recommended.

TOXIC EFFECTS. Signs of toxicity are unusual with phenobarbital. Some patients experience drowsiness, but this generally disappears after a few weeks of treatment. Erythematous rashes have been reported but are rare. The drug sometimes produces excitement in children and, paradoxically, may increase hyperactive behavior in the retarded child.

Mephobarbital (Mebaral). This is an effective drug in the treatment of generalized seizures and psychomotor seizures. However, it is a barbiturate that is almost identical in chemical formula to phenobarbital and does not appear to have any advantages over it. It is claimed that mephobarbital (Mebaral) causes less drowsiness than phenobarbital, but the claim is not supported by clinical experience. The drug is more expensive than phenobarbital.

Metharbital (Gemonil). Like mephobarbital, there is little evidence that metharbital has any advantage over phenobarbital (to which it is closely related in chemical structure) in the treatment of epilepsy.

Primidone (Mysoline). This drug is widely used, particularly in the treatment of psychomotor and focal epilepsy, where it seems to have equal effectiveness with carbamazepine in seizure control. There is biochemical evidence that the metabolic pathway of primidone is the same as that of phenobarbital, and measurement of blood levels after injection of the drug suggests that, metabolically, it has the same effect as phenobarbital. The equivalent dose is phenobarbital, 25 mg, or primidone, 100 mg. Despite this biochemical evidence of similarity of the action to phenobarbital, the chemical structure of primidone is different and the tolerance to toxic effects after its ingestion is different from that of phenobarbital.

Primidone induces drowsiness and ataxia if initially administered in full dosage; so therapy should begin with a single 125-mg dose. The dose is increased by 125 mg every three or four days to full dosage, which is usually 250 mg four times daily in the adult. Effective therapeutic levels of primidone seem to be between 5 and 10 mg/ml.

The toxic effects of primidone are similar to those of phenobarbital, but primidone does seem to produce excessive drowsiness, depression, and loss of libido in some patients. The prominent mental dullness seen in some children taking primidone may interfere with their performance in school. In addition, megaloblastic anemia has been reported as a complication of the drug. This responds to folic acid, 15 mg daily, and it is not necessary to discontinue primidone.

Sodium Valproate (Depakene). Sodium valproate has been available in Europe for about ten years now but has only recently been released for therapeutic use in the United States. Sodium valproate is a new chemical form of anticonvulsant that is believed to act by increasing concentrations of gamma aminobutyric acid in the central nervous system.

Clinical experience indicates that sodium valproate is effective in the treatment of generalized tonic-clonic seizures, absence seizures, and partial seizures with complex symptomatology. It should be used as an adjuvant to other anticonvulsants in treatment of these seizure types when the control of seizure activity is poor.

Sodium valproate is supplied in 250-mg capsules. Treatment should begin with 15 mg/kg/day, increasing to 30 gm/kg/day by increments every three to five days. Side effects include gastrointestinal upsets with occasional vomiting, abnormal hepatic function tests,[237a] somnolence, hair loss, and, rarely, thrombocytopenia.[106] Sodium valproate has a relatively short half life of 8.7 hours and should be administered in divided daily doses. It causes a decline in serum diphenylhydantoin concentrations and an increase in free diphenylhydantoin when the two drugs are used for seizure control.[136a]

Clonazepam. Clonazepam, a benzodiazepine derivative, is an effective drug in the treatment of most forms of epilepsy.[145] However, because of an unpredictable occurrence of tolerance in about one third of patients treated with clonazepam, the drug should be used as a "second-line" agent in patients who fail to achieve complete control with other medications. Clonazepam is useful in absence, atypical absence, myoclonus epilepsy, infantile spasms, and akinetic seizures, and in partial seizures with complex symptomatology (psychomotor seizures). There may be increased seizure activity if clonazepam is used in the treatment of generalized tonic-clonic seizures.

The usual dose in adults is 0.5 mg three times a day, increasing by 0.5 mg increments every three days to a total of 5 to 6 mg. Children between three and six years should receive up to 3 mg daily, and children under three years of age 1 to 2 mg daily. The most common side effects are drowsiness and ataxia, which can be minimized by using small starting doses and small increments when increasing dosage.[22] Other side effects are irritability, dysarthria, and behavior disturbance in children. Skin rashes are rare.

Mephenytoin (Mesantoin). This hydantoin derivative is effective in the control of generalized seizures as well as psychomotor and focal epilepsy. Mephenytoin has less tendency to produce mental dullness and ataxia than diphenylhydantoin, and mephenytoin does not produce gingival hyperplasia. However, mephenytoin can produce aplastic anemia, and its use should be restricted to cases with poor seizure control when it can be used to supplement or substitute for diphenylhydantoin.

Mephenytoin is supplied in tablets of 100 mg. Treatment is started with one half of one tablet daily, increasing by one tablet per week until the seizures are controlled. Children require one to four tablets and adults up to eight tablets daily. The therapeutic range of serum levels is the same as that of diphenylhydantoin.

Side effects of mephenytoin include drowsiness, ataxia, dysarthria, and skin rashes. Agranulocytosis has been reported, and, therefore, complete blood count and platelet count should be obtained before beginning treatment and every two weeks while the dose is being adjusted. Patients on long-term treatment with mephenytoin should have a complete blood count and platelet count every month for the first year, then every three months for the duration of treatment.

Ethosuximide (Zarontin). This is one of the group of succinimide drugs and it has proved to be more effective than other members of the group. Ethosuximide is the most effective drug available for the treatment of typical absence and atypical absence.[189] Since it is less toxic than trimethadione (Tridione), it has largely superceded trimethadione in the treatment of absence. Ethosuximide is supplied in 250-mg capsules, and the average dose is 250 mg three or four times daily. The capsules are rather large and small children find it difficult to swallow them. The liquid ethosuximide can be removed from the capsule and the unpleasant taste disguised with cola syrup.

Toxic effects of ethosuximide therapy are unusual but nausea, drowsiness, and skin rashes may occur. Most complications abate if the dosage is reduced and it is rarely necessary to discontinue the drug.

Trimethadione   (Tridione). Trimethadione used to be the most effective drug in the treatment of absence. However, with the occurrence of serious side effects and the availability of less toxic preparations that are equally effective, it is rarely used now.

The drug is supplied in capsules of 300 mg, tablets of 50 mg, or in a solution in which each fluidounce contains 1.2 gm. The child with absence should be started on 150 mg twice daily and the dose increased to 300 mg three times daily if this is necessary to obtain control of seizures.

Toxic effects of trimethadione therapy are quite common and include hiccough, nausea, vomiting, and skin rashes. Changes in visual perception described as yellow vision may be a complaint. Leukopenia and anemia occur in about 5 per cent of cases and agranulocytosis has been reported. Complete white blood counts must be performed on all patients before treatment with trimethadione and repeated at monthly intervals during therapy.

Paramethadione (Paradione). This drug is closely related to trimethadione and is also effective in the treatment of absence. Paramethadione is supplied in capsules of 150-mg and 300-mg strength. The treatment and dosage are the same as for trimethadione. Toxic effects are similar, although paramethadione is said to be less toxic than trimethadione.

Phenacemide (Phenurone). This is an example of an effective anticonvulsant in the treatment of psychomotor seizures whose usefulness is limited because of serious side effects. Phenacemide is also said to be effective in generalized as well as psychomotor seizures. It is supplied in 500-mg tablets, which are purple-colored and unusually large. The usual starting dose in the adult is 500 mg three times daily, increasing slowly to as much as 1,000 mg three times daily.

The drug produces headache, insomnia, and

personality changes, with irritability and destructive behavior in some cases. Other serious effects include hepatitis and aplastic anemia. Carbamazepine and primidone are more effective and much safer in the treatment of psychomotor seizures.

Diazepam (Valium). Diazepam, which was originally used as a tranquilizer, is an excellent anticonvulsant for intravenous use but is ineffective orally. The use of diazepam is now restricted to the treatment of status epilepticus (see Table 6–4).

Treatment of Specific Types of Epilepsy

Tonic and Clonic (Generalized) Seizures. The majority of patients can be controlled with diphenylhydantoin.[175] Serum levels should be monitored to assure maintenance of therapeutic levels. If other drugs are required, carbamazepine, sodium valproate, mephytoin, or phenobarbital may be added or substituted in that order of preference.

Infantile Spasms (Hypsarrhythmia). There have been encouraging reports on the use of ACTH and corticosteroids in the treatment of salaam seizures or infantile spasms. However, the initial enthusiasm has been replaced by more cautious assessment of results as it has become apparent that most of the children who survive following steroid therapy are mentally retarded. Although the seizures may be ameliorated by steroid therapy, they are seldom abolished and anticonvulsant medication is necessary.

Infantile spasms are due to widespread epileptic activity in a severely damaged brain. Cerebral damage results from developmental abnormalities or degenerative processes, and those who survive are usually severely retarded. Children who develop infantile spasms and hypsarrhythmia resulting from viral encephalitis during infancy sometimes have a better outlook if they survive. It is probable that this is the group that benefits most from ACTH or steroids, and they fare better than the group with developmental deficits or degenerative conditions.

The response of infantile spasms to anticonvulsant drugs such as diphenylhydantoin, carbamazepine, and barbiturates is unpredictable. The multifocal seizure discharges that arise in the damaged brain are very difficult to control and combinations of anticonvulsants are often used. The best results are obtained when therapy is

TABLE 6–4

Treatment of Specific Types of Epilepsy

Seizure Type	First Choice	Second Choice	Other Drugs
Generalized tonic-clonic seizures	Diphenylhydantoin	Carbamazepine	Phenobarbital, primidone, sodium valproate
Generalized tonic seizures	As above	As above	As above
Generalized clonic seizures	As above	As above	As above
Myoclonus epilepsy	As above	As above	As above
Secondary generalized seizures	As above	As above	Clonazepam
Infantile spasm	ACTH	Carbamazepine	Clonazepam, diphenylhydantoin, phenobarbital
Absence	Ethosuximide	Sodium valproate	Clonazepam
Atypical absence Akinetic seizures	Ethosuximide	Clonazepam	
Continuing absence	IV diazepam		
Partial seizure with complex symptomatology	Diphenylhydantoin	Carbamazepine	Primidone, sodium valproate, clonazepam

monitored, with frequent determinations of serum anticonvulsant levels.

Secondary Generalized Seizures.   Treat as for generalized epilepsy.

Clonic Seizures.   Treat as for generalized epilepsy.

Typical Absence and Atypical Absence. Children with typical absence (petit mal) or atypical absence (petit mal variant) may respond to phenobarbital, and the drug may be tried before resorting to the more expensive preparations. When phenobarbital is ineffective, ethosuximide should be substituted. This will control the great majority of seizures of this type and it is rarely necessary to use trimethadione.

Continuing Absence (Petit Mal Status).   The attack can be terminated by the intravenous injection of diazepam (Valium) at the rate of 1 mg every 15 to 30 seconds. The electroencephalogram is monitored during this period, and the disappearance of the 3-cps spike wave activity will indicate control of the seizure. Treatment is continued with ethosuximide to prevent recurrence of absence attacks.

Partial Seizure with Complex Symptomatology (Psychomotor Seizures.)   This is the most difficult common form of seizure to treat. Therapy can be begun with diphenylhydantoin, and later carbamazepine or primidone may be added or substituted. Plasma levels of these drugs should be monitored and therapeutic levels maintained.

Sodium valproate is useful in some refractory cases of psychomotor seizures, probably as an adjuvant to other anticonvulsant drugs. Ethosuximide (Zarontin) is another alternative drug and is occasionally helpful, in combination with other anticonvulsants, in controlling psychomotor seizures.

Despite the impression that psychomotor seizures are the most difficult to control, 40 per cent of patients become seizure-free on anticonvulsant medication and a further 33 per cent have a marked reduction in seizure activity.[108]

Status Epilepticus.   The treatment of status epilepticus in adults and children is outlined in Table 6–5.

Status epilepticus is a medical emergency, and the patient should be under the supervision of a physician or treated in an intensive care unit until the condition is controlled. This is necessary because status epilepticus is often fatal if untreated. Treatment includes maintenance of an airway, restoration of fluid and electrolyte balance by the use of intravenous fluids, and control of infection by the use of antibiotics. An oral pharyngeal tube or endotracheal tube should be inserted to maintain an adequate airway and to prevent tongue biting and damage to the teeth. Excess secretions should be removed by suction to prevent aspiration and atelectasis. In untreated cases, death occurs from asphyxiation, aspiration, pneumonitis, and exhaustion.

Surgical Treatment

The surgical excision of focal lesions causing epilepsy, such as arteriovenous malformations, porencephalic cysts, abscesses, granulomas, and tumors, is usually performed for other reasons rather than the control of epilepsy. However, there is an increase in the surgical treatment of focal epileptogenic foci that are the cause of intractable seizures. This treatment has been facilitated by the use of CT scanning, electrocorticography, and the recording from depth microelectrodes,[228] which help to localize active epileptogenic foci.

The majority of cases treated by surgical excision are suffering from psychomotor seizures. These patients should fulfill the following criteria before surgery is considered.[211]

1. Failure to respond to adequate drug treatment, which includes monitoring of serum anticonvulsant levels.
2. Evidence of a predominantly or wholly unilateral temporal lobe epileptic focus shown by electroencephalography.
3. If there is bilateral epileptic activity, it should be at least four times more frequent on the side where surgery is contemplated.
4. The patient should have a chronic seizure disorder with reasonable certainty that all potentially epileptic foci have been identified.
5. The patient must have an IQ of at least 60.

The extent of the surgical excision can be determined by EEG electrodes recording from and in the temporal lobe at the time of surgery. Under ideal circumstances the excision of tissue will be completed when all spike discharges have disap-

TABLE 6–5

Treatment of Status Epilepticus

Establishment of an adequate airway, oxygen inhalation (8 liters/min), and an intravenous infusion of 500 ml of 5 per cent dextrose in 0.2 N saline are administered. The vital signs should be recorded at 15-minute intervals on a chart and notes of progress should be recorded in the hospital chart. A hypothermic blanket or ice-water and alcohol sponging should be used to prevent hyperthermia. The patient is best treated in the intensive care unit. The following program is suggested.

Adults

1. Seizure activity should be controlled in most cases by the intravenous injection of diazepam given at a rate not faster than 1 mg every 30 seconds, until 10 to 20 mg is administered. The injection should be stopped if respiratory depression results.[12] If the seizures continue, an additional 100 mg of diazepam may be infused slowly in 500 ml of 5 per cent dextrose and 0.2 N saline over a 12-hour period.[8,152,159,186]

2. Draw blood for glucose, calcium, and electrolyte determinations. If there is any suspicion of hypoglycemia, give 25 ml of 50 per cent dextrose IV.

3. If seizure activity still persists, which is unlikely, 500 mg of sodium amobarbital (Sodium Amytal) may be given intravenously at the rate of 50 mg every 30 seconds. This rate should not be exceeded, and careful observation for respiratory depression or hypotension should be made.

4. Seizures can be controlled almost invariably if diazepam or sodium amobarbital is given intravenously. When seizures cease, sodium phenobarbital, 120 mg intramuscularly, can be given every four hours until oral diphenylhydantoin and phenobarbital can be *initiated.*

5. As an alternative to phenobarbital, diphenylhydantoin can be given in doses of 1,000 mg intravenously at the rate of 100 mg per minute. This should be supplemented by 500 mg orally or intravenously every day as a maintenance dose.[226] Plasma diphenylhydantoin levels should be obtained daily.

6. In refractory cases, sodium valproate, 200 to 800 mg every 6 hours, administered rectally in 200-mg lipid-based suppositories, can be given.[218a]

Should hypotension or respiratory depression occur at any stage in the above program of treatment, anticonvulsant drugs should be temporarily discontinued. Reduction in frequency of seizures is acceptable as an alternative to drug intoxication, which itself is potentially fatal.

Children

1. The first drug of choice is diazepam, 5 to 10 mg, diluted to 1 mg/ml, by slow intravenous injection.[24] This may be repeated after ten minutes if necessary.[197] Respiratory arrest is a rare complication and must be treated immediately by artificial respiration.

2. If seizures persist, give phenobarbital by intramuscular injection of 3 mg/lb of body weight.

3. If seizures continue, give paraldehyde, 0.15 ml/lb of body weight. Dissolve each milliliter of paraldehyde in 10 ml of 5 per cent dextrose and 0.2 N saline. This can be infused as a slow intravenous drip.

4. A record should be kept of the exact time and duration of each attack, including the length of the apneic periods and the exact time and dose of phenobarbital, paraldehyde, and diazepam.

5. The rate and depth of respirations, the pupillary size, and the corneal and tendon reflexes should be examined before further injections of phenobarbital to test for barbiturate intoxication. The drug may be repeated every 60 minutes if there are no signs of toxicity.

6. In children, the following anticonvulsants should be avoided: the intravenous administration of sodium amobarbital or diphenylhydantoin and the inhalation of ether or vinyl ether.

---

peared. There are, of course, limitations to the extent of the surgical excision particularly in the dominant hemisphere. The results of surgical treatment are good in carefully selected cases. About 40 per cent of patients are entirely free from seizures, while another 20 per cent have a marked reduction in the number of seizures and 15 per cent a reduction to less than one half the preoperative number of seizures. Patients also show improvement in mental status and personality, particularly a decrease in aggressive behavior.[224]

Children with uncontrolled intractable seizures due to multiple epileptic foci in one severely dam-aged hemisphere may benefit from disconnection of the cerebral hemispheres.[238]

This operation requires division of the corpus callosum from rostrum to splenium, and section of the anterior commissure, fornix, and hippocampal commissure. Disconnection is preferable to the alternative operation of hemispherectomy.

Disorders Related to Epilepsy

Narcolepsy and Cataplexy

Narcolepsy may be defined as a condition where there are abnormal and irresistible attacks of the desire to sleep. These occur after adequate sleep at night and in inappropriate places and under inappropriate circumstances. The condition tends to be familial and is often associated with recurrent attacks of loss of tone (cataplexy) and paralysis of voluntary movements of muscles during emotional states such as laughing (lachschlag) or anger. Attacks of paralysis during the stage between sleep and arousal (sleep paralysis) may accompany the condition, and vivid visual or auditory sensations may occur at the onset of sleep (hypnogenic or hypnagogic hallucinations).[243]

Clinical Features

The patient with narcolepsy experiences an intense desire to sleep, which is overwhelming and results in a brief period of sleep no matter where he happens to be at that time. The attacks usually last for a few minutes and are often associated with weird dreams. The patient then awakens refreshed. These episodes usually occur many times daily, usually when the patient is carrying out sedentary tasks or attending conferences, and, as may be imagined, this becomes a threat to the patient's continued employment. Some patients experience long periods of freedom from attacks lasting several months.

Attacks of cataplexy often begin after the development of narcolepsy and consist of sudden attacks of loss of muscle tone and paralysis, which are precipitated by an emotional situation. This usually takes the form of amusement, but a sudden fright, sudden elation, sudden bodily contact, tickling, or occasionally sudden anger may precipitate attacks in susceptible individuals.

After the stimulus, the affected individual loses all voluntary muscle tone and sinks to the floor, where he or she lies completely paralyzed for a short period of time, usually for a matter of seconds. Recovery then follows and there is no evidence of weakness or neurologic abnormality after the attack.

Patients with both narcolepsy and cataplexy occasionally experience two associated conditions that are of special interest, hypnogogic or hypnogenic hallucinations and sleep paralysis. Hypnogogic hallucinations are usually described as visual in type and frightening. Auditory hallucinations may occasionally occur but are rare and occur just as the patient is falling asleep. Sleep paralysis occurs when the patient is going to sleep or if the patient is aroused suddenly or on awakening in the morning. The patient is fully conscious but is totally unable to move or perform any voluntary movements for periods varying from a few seconds to two or three minutes.

Diagnostic Procedures

The diagnosis depends entirely on the history because the neurologic examination, electroencephalogram, cerebrospinal fluid, and roentgenograms of the skull are all within normal limits. When serial night sleep recordings are made, the EEG shows rapid eye movements (REM) as the patient falls asleep and increased REM activity throughout natural sleep. This consists of rapid eye movements, decreased muscle tone, and an asynchronous EEG. The REM activity is not always present in sleep attacks during the day, and its absence does not negate the diagnosis of narcolepsy.[158]

Treatment

Both methylphenidate (Ritalin) and dextroamphetamine sulfate (Dexedrine) are effective in the treatment of narcolepsy. If dextroamphetamine sulfate is prescribed, it should be given in doses of 5 mg three times daily and the dose should gradually be increased until the attacks are controlled. Methylphenidate is the drug of choice and the dosage is usually started at 10 mg two or three times daily and gradually increased if necessary. Some patients require large doses of either drug, e.g., methylphenidate, 60 mg daily, before the attacks of narcolepsy cease. The attacks of sleep paralysis and hypnagogic hallucinations also improve with the above treatment. Cataplexy, which is a less troublesome complaint, may improve under treatment but is often persistent and refractory to therapy.

Imipramine (75 mg to 100 mg daily) may relieve cataplexy and can be combined with methylphenidate. Clomipramine hydrochloride, in doses of 25 to 75 mg/day, is also effective in stopping cataplexy, sleep paralysis, and hypnagogic hallucinations.[192]

Sleep Apnea

Individuals who awaken frequently during the night often sleep excessively during the day and may be erroneously diagnosed as narcoleptic. One of the causes of interruption of nocturnal sleep is sleep apnea in which the individual suffers sudden obstruction to the upper respiratory tract. There is posterior displacement of the genioglossus muscle due to retrognathia, and the tongue lies unusually close to the pharyngeal wall.[102] Further relaxation of the jaw produces apposition of the tongue and pharyngeal wall during sleep and airway obstruction. Sleep apnea leads to pulmonary and systemic hypertension, hypercapnea and hypoxemia, and the development of cardiac arrhythmias.[34] Sleep apnea may be one of the causes of the sudden infant death syndrome.

Adults with sleep apnea are often obese, snore loudly, or have a "birdlike" face due to retrognathia. They complain of interrupted sleep at night and have a tendency to sleep during the day when inactive. However, unlike narcolepsy, the patient with sleep apnea is not bothered by sleep when active.

Treatment consists of weight reduction and tracheotomy.

Myoclonus

Myoclonus may be defined as a neuromuscular disorder originating in the cerebral nervous system in which there are irregular, asynergic, and jactitious contractions of muscle, producing nonrepetitive, brief, involuntary movements, which can occur in any part of the body. The contractions may be provoked or enhanced by various stimuli, including auditory or photic stimulation and changes in posture. Myoclonus tends to increase during drowsiness and emotional disturbance. This interesting phenomenon is a symptom, not a disease entity, and occurs as part of the clinical picture in many disorders[69] (Table 6–6).

Myoclonus Without Seizures or Neurologic Abnormalities

Paramyoclonus Multiplex (Hereditary Essential Myoclonus)

The presence of myoclonus does not necessarily denote a progressive and degenerative condition. It occurs in paramyoclonus multiplex, which is a benign condition. The symptoms usually begin during the first or second decade of life and consist of myoclonus principally involving the face, neck, and proximal muscles of the limbs. The jerking is absent during sleep but is aggravated by emotional stimuli or movement. The condition affects both sexes and is inherited as an autosomal dominant trait. It runs a benign course and is compatible with a normal life-span.[134] There are no other neurologic abnormalities, and in particular, there is no evidence of dementia, ataxia, or epilepsy.

TABLE 6–6

Classification of Myoclonus

A. *Myoclonus without seizures or neurologic abnormalities*
  1. Paramyoclonus multiplex (hereditary essential myoclonus)

B. *Myoclonus with seizures*
  1. Myoclonic seizures and akinetic (astatic) seizures
  2. Myoclonic jerks in patients with other types of seizure disorder

C. *Myoclonus and nonprogressive neurologic disorders*
  1. Viral encephalitides
  2. Hypoxic or anoxic encephalopathy
  3. Toxins—methylbromide, mercury, strychnine, penicillin, contrast media (angiography)
  4. Metabolic—uremia, hepatic insufficiency
  5. Cerebrovascular disease—infarction

D. *Myoclonus and degenerative diseases*
  1. Familial myoclonus and ataxia
  2. Unverricht-Lundberg disease
  3. Lafora disease
  4. Dysynergia cerebellaris myoclonica
  5. Ganglioside storage diseases
  6. Leukodystrophies
  7. Aminoacidurias
  8. Neuronal degenerations of infancy
  9. Slow virus diseases of the nervous system
    a. Jakob-Creutzfeldt disease
    b. Subacute sclerosing panencephalitis
  10. Adult dementias
    a. Alzheimer's disease
    b. Pick's disease
  11. Hepatolenticular degeneration
  12. Tuberous sclerosis
  13. Multiple sclerosis
  14. Amyotrophic lateral sclerosis
  15. Tumors of the brainstem
  16. Nonmetastatic degenerative disease

E. *Myoclonus and disease of the spinal cord*
  1. Tetanus
  2. Syringomyelia
  3. Spinal cord tumors
  4. Traumatic paraplegia
  5. Multiple sclerosis

The cerebrospinal fluid and electroencephalogram are normal.

Familial Myoclonus and Ataxia

Patients suffering from this condition may have been included in the syndrome of dyssynergia cerebellaris progressiva or myoclonica described by Ramsay Hunt. A great deal of confusion has resulted from the use of this eponymic term since Hunt described several other disease entities which have been named after him (see p. 682). Familial myoclonus with ataxia and in some families associated deafness is an uncommon condition that is inherited as an autosomal dominant trait with incomplete penetrance.[75] The affected patients usually develop symptoms during childhood. The condition is usually benign, although some of the cases described by Hunt showed deterioration with age. The symptoms consist of myoclonic jerks affecting the neck and proximal muscles of the limbs, nystagmus, intention tremor, and ataxia of gait of a cerebellar type. These are not necessarily symmetric, and there may be a preponderance of both myoclonus and cerebellar signs on one side of the body. The muscle tone, strength, and the deep tendon reflexes are normal and the plantar responses are flexor. The sensory examination is within normal limits. The cerebrospinal fluid and electroencephalogram are also normal.

A similar condition of familial myoclonus, ataxia, and deafness has also been described.[138] The symptoms are essentially the same as those of familial myoclonus and ataxia with the addition of a progressive loss of hearing, which begins in early adult life.

Myoclonus with Seizures

Myoclonic seizures and myoclonic jerks occurring as sudden isolated symptoms in patients with generalized tonic clonic or occasionally psychomotor seizures have been discussed elsewhere (p. 351).

Myoclonus and Nonprogressive Neurologic Disorders

Myoclonus is an occasional symptom in viral encephalitides occurring during the acute phase of the infection or as a sign of chronic neuronal damage. Myoclonus was reported to be common in patients with encephalitis lethargica and is likely to occur after any severe viral encephalitis, particularly herpes simplex encephalitis. Children with predominantly brainstem encephalitis occasionally develop myoclonus and opsoclonus, an irregular jerking of the eyes in any direction.

The severe brain damage of hypoxic encephalopathy due to cardiac or respiratory arrest is frequently accompanied by myoclonus.

A number of toxic substances, including methylbromide, mercury, strychnine, and penicillin, can cause acute myoclonus. A sudden myo-clonic jerk may accompany the injection of io-dinized contrast material during angiography. Metabolic encephalopathies such as uremia and hepatic encephalopathy are also associated with myoclonus. The condition is rare in cerebrovascular disease but may occur following brainstem or deep hemisphere infarction.

Myoclonus and Degenerative Diseases of the Central Nervous System

Myoclonus occurs in many degenerative diseases. Many authorities regard Unverricht-Lundberg disease and Lafora disease as one disease, but there is evidence that they are separate clinical entities.

Lafora Disease

The disorder is a progressive dementia of adolescents associated with myoclonus and generalized seizures.

Etiology and Pathology. The disease is inherited as an autosomal recessive trait and is due to an inborn error of metabolism.[105] The material in the Lafora bodies shows histochemical properties resembling amylopectin,[241] while ultrastructural studies have shown a protein core surrounded by polyglucosan.[210]

The brain is normal in appearance without evidence of atrophy. Intracellular and extracellular Lafora bodies are found in all parts of the central nervous system, particularly in the gray matter. The neurons of the substantia nigra, dentate nucleus, thalamus, and globus pallidus are usually heavily peppered with these bodies, and it is probable that extracellular Lafora bodies originated within cells that degenerated. The inclusions are not confined to neurons and occur to a lesser extent in astrocytes, oligodendrocytes, axons, and white matter. They range in size from 3 to 40, stain dark purple with hematoxylin, brown with iodine, and red with Best's carmine, and they are PAS-positive. Neurons containing the bodies show considerable structural abnormality with displacement of the nucleus and Nissl substance.

Lafora bodies are also present in the retina, heart, liver, peripheral nerves, and striated muscle.

Chemical analysis of Lafora bodies has shown them to be 90 per cent of glucose, which is contained in a structural form related to glycogen and resembling the plant starch amylopectin.

Clinical Features. The symptoms begin in late childhood or adolescence and consist of progressive dementia, usually presenting as deterioration of scholastic achievement and the development of generalized seizures. Within a year, it is apparent that the dementia and seizure disorder are getting progressively worse. Examination reveals dysarthria, irregular myoclonic jerks, which may be precipitated by various types of stimuli, hypotonia, intention tremor, and truncal ataxia. The deep tendon reflexes have been reported to be hyperactive in some cases. The condition progresses over a period of about ten years and terminates in a condition of severe dementia, blindness, and seizures. The myoclonic jerks and seizures are a characteristic of the entire course of the disease. Terminally, on examination there is flaccid quadriparesis, generalized muscle wasting, and extensor plantar responses.

Diagnostic Procedures. Diagnostic procedures include the following:

1. The electroencephalogram shows a normal background activity with episodic generalized high-voltage spike and wave discharges in the early stages of the illness. Gradually, the alpha becomes replaced by slowing of background activity and the appearance of generalized theta and delta activity with bursts of symmetric but atypical spike and wave activity. The spike and wave discharges may be induced by stimulation with flashes of light, loud sounds, tactile stimulation, and other stimuli in some cases.
2. The diagnosis can be established during life by liver or brain biopsy. Muscle biopsy is not a reliable means of diagnosis in the early stages of the disease.

Treatment. The seizures and myoclonus can usually be controlled or effectively reduced by anticonvulsant medication.

Unverricht-Lundberg Disease

This disease is inherited as an autosomal recessive trait and is characterized by generalized myoclonus, seizures, and dementia. The seizures begin in childhood or early adolescence and myoclonus appears several months later. There is a slowly progressive dementia with the development of dystonia and rigidity in the terminal stages of the disease. Unverricht-Lundberg disease is a slowly progressive condition and death occurs 10 to 60 years after the onset.

Myoclonus and Disease of the Spinal Cord

The acute myoclonus of tetanus is due to the effects of tetanus endotoxin on the anterior horn cells. Chronic irritation of anterior horn cells occasionally occurs in syringomyelia and spinal cord tumors with focal myoclonus. Sudden myoclonic jerks are not uncommon in patients with traumatic paraplegia or paraplegia in multiple sclerosis and are presumed to be the result of removal of inhibiting influences on the anterior horn cells.

Treatment of Myoclonus

There is evidence that there is depletion of brain serotonin (5-hydroxytryptamine) levels in degenerative diseases with myoclonus and that repletion of serotonin may lead to clinical improvement.[219] The patient is pretreated with 100 to 300 mg/day of alpha-methyldopa hydrazine (Carbidopa) for two days, and the treatment with carbidopa is maintained during treatment with L-5-hydroxytryptophan, the precursor of serotonin. Carbidopa reduces the peripheral effects of serotonin and enhances the passage of L-5-hydroxytryptophan into the brain. L-5-hydroxytryptophan is given in capsules with meals beginning with 1 mg/kg of body weight per day and increasing slowly until side effects appear or until the myoclonus is controlled.[83] Side effects include nausea, vomiting, anorexia, increased seizure activity, and toxic psychosis. The response to L-5-hydroxytryptophan appears to be good when the myoclonus is associated with anoxic encephalopathy or head trauma. The response is equivocal or poor in patients with degenerative diseases of the brain.

The anticonvulsant clonazepam and monoaminoxidase inhibitors are also reported to reduce myoclonus by increasing serotonin concentrations in the brain.[30]

Palatal Myoclonus or Palatal Nystagmus

This condition, called palatal myoclonus or nystagmus, may be defined as a rhythmic, side-to-side or rarely up-and-down movement of the uvula or pharynx, which occurs at different rates but usually at a rate of 60 to 180 per minute. There may be complaints of clicks in the ears with each movement. Palatal nystagmus is probably the better term, since the movements are rhythmic and not irregular jerks, as connoted by the term "myoclonus." Furthermore, as can be seen from the previous discussion of myoclonus, this term has become one of the most confused in neurology. Palatal nystagmus is a sign and not a disease and is caused by numerous diseases.

Pathophysiology

The lesion involves the olivary-cerebello-midbrain relay system, which probably provides tonic inhibition on the rostral midbrain reticular formation.[86] Causes of the lesion include hemorrhage, thrombosis, embolism, tumor, and abscess. It is presumed that such semiautomatic actions as yawning, changes in respiration, chewing, and swallowing are integrated at this level in the brainstem and that loss of inhibition releases a rhythmic tremor of the pharynx.

Clinical Features

Palatal myoclonus is basically rhythmic but the movements under certain circumstances may become temporarily irregular. The pharyngeal muscles can be seen to contract rhythmically, and the intensity and the rhythm of contraction can be altered by such reflex acts as swallowing and speech. The palatal movements persist during sleep and are about the same or twice as frequent as the pulse rate. The contractions are usually confined to the soft palate and pharynx, but in some cases, there may be synchronous movements of the muscles of facial expression. Contractions of the cervical muscles, particularly the sternocleidomastoid, may produce titubation of the head. Synchronous movements have also been reported in the larynx, esophagus, diaphragm, tongue, upper limbs, and eyes ("ocular bobbing") in some cases.[240] Treatment should be directed at the cause of the lesion in the olivodentatorubral projection system.

Exaggerated Startle Reaction

A number of conditions have been described in which an unexpected stimulus is followed by an exaggerated startle reaction.[71] The condition is uncommon, but its recognition is important since it can be mistaken for epilepsy. An exaggerated startle reaction is an excessive psychologic response to an unexpected stimulus arising from hyperexcitability of brain reticular formation, which is presumed to be responsible for the normal startle reaction. Apart from delirium tremens, barbiturate withdrawal, and excessive ingestion of analeptic drugs, the following naturally

occurring conditions are also related to an excessive startle reaction.

The Jumping Frenchmen of Maine

This condition was first described among certain families of French Canadian extraction. It is a familial condition in which an exaggerated startle reaction begins in childhood and persists throughout life. An unexpected sound, command, or visual stimulus induces a single violent jump, which may literally lift the patient from the ground. This may be accompanied by an involuntary exclamation or a reiteration of the command with automatic and involuntary execution of the order even though harmful or foolish.[204] The neurologic examination and EEG are both normal.

Similar conditions have been described in Siberia (Myrrachit) and Malaya (Latah), although the latter may be a form of essential hyperexplexia.

Hereditary Hyperexplexia

This is inherited as an autosomal dominant trait. The first symptoms are hypertonus and hypokinesia, which last for three or four months.[209] These symptoms are followed by the development of an exaggerated startle reaction, which is often severe enough that the patient falls to the ground. The reaction is increased by emotional tension, nervousness, and fatigue. Violent generalized jerks may occur as the patient falls asleep. There are no seizures and no loss of consciousness. General physical examination reveals the presence of inguinal, umbilical, or epigastric hernias in a large percentage of cases. The neurologic examination is normal except for exaggeration of the cerebral bulbar reflexes, such as the snout, glabellar, palmar-mental, and head retraction reflex. The EEG is normal or shows nonspecific slowing at rest. There is no evidence of epileptic activity in the EEG during the startle response. Nocturnal startle responses may be suppressed by phenobarbital or chlordiazepoxide (Librium).

Exaggerated Startle Reactions in Cerebral Palsy

These are rare but have been observed on occasion.

Essential Hyperexplexia

Essential hyperexplexia is also rare and occurs in patients who appear to have disturbed emotional and psychologic states. The exaggerated startle response occurs without any alteration in consciousness. The patients experience violent nocturnal jumps when asleep, triggered by switching on the light, a noise, or any type of somatic stimuli. The general physical and neurologic examinations are normal. The EEG is normal at rest but shows generalized desynchronization with loss of alpha rhythm during the startle response, but there is no epileptic activity.[72]

There may be some difficulty in the differential diagnosis between an exaggerated startle reaction and myoclonic seizures. In myoclonic seizures the myoclonus occurs without stimulation. Myoclonic seizures may occur as a single phenomenon or may be associated with other types of seizure activity. The electroencephalogram is abnormal.

Tic Convulsif (Gilles de la Tourette Syndrome)

This condition is difficult to classify since there is no general agreement as to its cause. It used to be considered a purely psychiatric disorder, but there is sound evidence that a neurologic disorder underlies the syndrome.[212] There is also some evidence that Gilles de la Tourette syndrome[53] is a genetically determined biochemical disorder of purine metabolism,[220] or alternatively may represent an imbalance between the central transmitters dopamine and serotonin.[195a]

1. Subtle neurologic abnormalities occur in 50 per cent of cases.
2. Left-handedness or an ambidextrous state occurs in more than 30 per cent.
3. Affected families contain an excessive number of individuals with chronic motor tics.[76b]
4. EEG abnormalities occur in from 25 to 75 per cent.[132]
5. The condition often responds to haloperidol, a compound that blocks dopa receptors, suggesting that there may be a dopamine excess in this condition.[199]

The first symptom is the appearance of a simple tic which usually involves the eyes, head, or face but can involve almost any part of the body. The onset occurs between ages 2 and 13 years and may follow exposure to central nervous system stimulants, particularly methylphenidate.[76a] The development of tics may be accompanied by various noises, but vocalization usually occurs later when the movements are accompanied by grunting, barking, screaming, yelling, sniffing, or hissing. These sounds gradually give way to coprolalia over a period of years in about 60 per cent of cases. In coprolalia, words or phrases are repetitive and usually obscene, antisocial, and scatologic in nature. Eventually, the words or phrases may be compulsively yelled in a loud voice that is hard to dampen.

Treatment

1. There is a good response to haloperidol, 2 to 4 mg daily, in most cases.[142, 191]
2. A combination of L-5-hydroxytryptophan and carbidopa may also be effective in this disease (see p. 244).

Febrile Convulsions

There has been considerable controversy concerning the relationship between febrile convulsions and epilepsy. Much of the current diversity of opinion is the result of a failure of definition, with some investigators classifying all seizures of infancy and childhood occurring during a febrile episode as "febrile convulsions." However, it is possible to recognize a distinct condition when convulsions occur during a fever in which the prognosis is excellent. This condition can be differentiated from epilepsy induced by fever, which may be associated with the seizures in later life.

Etiology and Pathology

It is possible that there is a genetic predisposition to febrile convulsions, and a positive family history may be obtained in parents and siblings.[64]

The febrile convulsion is a pathologic response of the immature brain to a sudden elevation in temperature. Fever increases cerebral blood flow and metabolism and induces changes in water and electrolyte content of the cerebral tissue, which are associated with a reduction of the seizure threshold because of alterations of the membrane potential and neuronal excitability. It has been shown, both in experimental animals and in infants, that two factors are of major importance in the development of febrile convulsions: the age of the subject and the rapidity of temperature elevation.[146] It is relatively simple to induce febrile convulsions in young rats or kittens by subjecting them to a rapid rise in body temperature, but not in adult animals. After the febrile seizure in these young animals, the brain appears normal grossly and microscopically.

Clinical Features

Certain differences between febrile convulsions and epileptic seizures due to other causes but induced by fever are outlined in Table 6–7.

The febrile convulsion is a generalized tonic-clonic or clonic seizure, of relatively short dura-

TABLE 6–7

Differences Between Febrile Convulsions and Epilepsy

Febrile Convulsions	Epilepsy Induced by Fever
1. Generalized tonic-clonic or clonic seizure	1. May be generalized or focal in type
2. Single episodes of short duration; recovery within 15 minutes	2. Multiple seizures are not uncommon; recovery often slow; status epilepticus may occur
3. Convulsion occurs early in the febrile episode within 10 hours of onset	3. May occur at any time during febrile episode
4. Always associated with fever often due to an upper respiratory infection	4. Attacks may occur at times when it is doubtful if child is febrile and there are no signs of infection.
5. No family history of epilepsy	5. Family history of epilepsy is commonly present
6. Convulsions first noticed between 6 months and 3 years of age; they usually cease at 4 and do not occur after 6 years	6. Begin at any time during infancy and childhood and continue beyond the age of 6 years
7. Neurologic examination normal	7. Neurologic examination may be abnormal
8. Electroencephalogram is normal between attacks	8. Electroencephalogram is usually abnormal with epileptic or paroxysmal activity in interictal period

tion, which occurs within ten hours of the onset of fever. The cause of the fever is often a mild infection, such as in the upper respiratory tract. Febrile convulsions will be noticed by the parents between the ages of six months and three years. They usually cease by age four and do not occur after age six. There is no history of epilepsy in the family, and both the neurologic examination and the electroencephalogram are normal.

Treatment

Febrile convulsions often cause a good deal of anxiety in the parents, and they should be reassured that febrile convulsions are common and do not lead to epilepsy with the liability to repeated seizures throughout life. There is no evidence of a decrease in intellegence or academic performance in children who have had febrile convulsions.[53a]

Anticonvulsant drugs have little or no effect in preventing febrile convulsions, and treatment is better directed toward preventing fever. The use of aspirin at the beginning of a fever and the application of an icebag or towels soaked in ice water may prevent a sudden rise in temperature and the febrile convulsion.

Fainting and Syncope

The correct diagnosis of a syncopal episode is dependent upon an accurate and detailed history in the great majority of cases. When the physician is faced with the problem of syncope, the patient should be asked to give a detailed account, in chronologic order, of all events leading up to the loss of consciousness. This is followed by an account of events experienced by the patient after the return of consciousness, up to the time that he believes he had returned to a normal state. This subjective impression should be augmented by a step-by-step account of what happened to the patient before, during, and immediately after loss of consciousness as observed by those who witnessed the patient during the syncopal episode.

The history may be entirely dependent on observations of another, and this is usually the mother in the case of syncopal episodes occurring in infants and children. However, quite young children may give much valuable information about their attacks, and the pediatric patient should always be given the opportunity to describe symptoms in cases of syncope. Nevertheless, the information supplied by the mother is often critical in the differential diagnosis of syncope in a child, and an effort should be made to obtain the maximum amount of information in an orderly fashion, avoiding personal interpretations of events by the mother or her desire to relay gratuitous diagnoses offered by the best-intentioned relatives or friends who have not seen any of the syncopal episodes.

The following scheme is suggested when interviewing a patient or relative to obtain the maximum information in the case of fainting or syncope:

Questions to the Patient

1. What were you doing before the attack?
2. What was the first thing you noticed that seemed to be abnormal?
3. What happened after that until you lost consciousness?
4. What was the first thing you remembered after return of consciousness?
5. Were you confused?
6. Did you have a headache?
7. Had you lost control of your bladder?
8. Had you bitten your tongue?
9. Were you tired and did you go to sleep?
10. Did your muscles ache?

Questions to the Observer

1. All of the questions given to the patient.
2. In addition, between questions 3 and 4 above, obtain a detailed account of the ictus.
   a. How did it start?
   b. Did the head turn? Were there any movements of the mouth?
   c. Were there any clonic movements?
   d. Was there a tonic phase?
   e. What was the appearance of the face? Pale? Cyanosed? Flushed?

Syncope, whatever its cause, is associated with a sudden decrease in blood pressure to zero or to extremely low levels in which the cerebral autoregulatory mechanisms are no longer effective, resulting in a sudden arrest or decrease in cerebral blood flow. The factors regulating cerebral blood flow have been discussed in detail elsewhere (see p. 543). Cerebral blood flow is well maintained in the healthy young adult until the systolic blood pressure falls below 50 mm Hg in the erect posture. If it falls much below this level, there is lightheadedness, fainting, and loss of consciousness, with collapse to the ground. After the collapse, as soon as the head is at the level of the heart, consciousness is usually regained.

Hypotensive Syncope Due to Lowered Peripheral Vascular Resistance

Fainting (Psychogenic or Vasovagal Syncope)

The typical vasovagal syncopal attack occurs on the background of an emotional or painful stimulus in most cases. This results in vagal over-activity, producing peripheral vasodilatation and slowing of the heart with fall in blood pressure. The patient experiences a period of lightheadedness, tinnitus, and unsteadiness followed by loss of consciousness and collapse to the ground. At this stage, the muscles are relaxed but control of the sphincters is maintained. There is marked pallor during the faint, sometimes accompanied by a slight degree of cyanosis of the lips, and occasionally there are one or two clonic jerks of the extremities during the phase of unconsciousness, so that a diagnosis of a convulsive disorder may be entertained. In view of this, the history is all-important in differential diagnosis since the physical examination is unlikely to reveal any abnormality.

Orthostatic Hypotension

This condition results in impairment of consciousness on suddenly assuming the erect position, particularly after lying down for some time.

Etiology. The causes are numerous, but include:

1. Venous pooling in the lower extremities following prolonged standing, particularly in members of the armed forces or in those with severe varicose veins.
2. Poor muscle and vascular tone occurring in individuals who have had a prolonged period of confinement in bed.
3. Impairment of sympathetic vasomotor reflex activity: syringomyelia; diabetic neuropathy; tabes dorsalis; postinfectious polyneuropathy; subacute combined degeneration; familial dysautonomia; surgical sympathectomy; some cases of Parkinson's disease; Shy Drager syndrome.
4. Drugs: use of hypotensive agents; phenothiazines; certain tranquilizers; levodopa.
5. Corticosteroid deficiency: Addison's disease; deficiency of ACTH in hypopituitarism and in elderly patients with cerebrovascular disease.
6. Chronic orthostatic hypotension. Chronic orthostatic hypotension is an unusual condition in which the blood pressure falls rapidly as soon as the patient assumes an upright position. There is no sympathetic response and absence of tachycardia, pallor, and sweating. Symptoms of cerebral ischemia may occur with dysarthria and disorientation. Loss of con-

sciousness may occur very quickly with equally rapid recovery when the patient is recumbent.

Treatment. When the prodromata occur or if the patient faints, he should be kept in the horizontal position with the head at the level of the heart. Contributing factors, such as pituitary insufficiency, Addison's disease, diabetes, and peripheral neuropathy, should be treated, and the use of peripheral vasodilatory drugs, if prescribed, should be discontinued. Symptomatic treatment of orthostatic hypotension can be achieved with an elasticized leotard for the lower extremities, oral metaraminol (Aramine), and, in severe cases, fludrocortisone acetate, 0.1 to 0.3 mg daily.

Patients with orthostatic hypotension should, of course, avoid sudden changes in posture. They should sit on the edge of the bed and dangle their toes for 30 seconds or so on getting up in the morning, and then stand by the side of the bed for 30 seconds to see if they are "lightheaded" before attempting to walk.

Hypotension Secondary to Decreased Venous Return to the Heart

Valsalva Maneuver

Among adolescents, a forced Valsalva maneuver is sometimes performed by school-boys as a trick or "a dare." The victim is asked to take a deep inspiration and to hold the breath while he is clasped tightly around the chest, which is then compressed by a colleague. The intrathoracic pressure rises steeply, exceeding the venous pressure, and the venous return to the heart abruptly ceases with decreased cardiac output, hypotension, and syncope.

Breath-Holding Spells

This benign condition is encountered more by the general practitioner or pediatrician but is occasionally referred to the neurologist when the attacks terminate in convulsions or prolonged unconsciousness. It may be defined as a condition peculiar to childhood in which the breath is held for prolonged periods of time, with the appearance of cyanosis of pallor and often terminating in loss of consciousness. The condition carries a good prognosis in the vast majority of cases.

Etiology. Breath-holding spells occur in a small percentage of children, and there is usually a family history of the disorder in affected chil-

dren. Characteristically, there is some factor that provokes each attack, such as a sudden fright, an emotional upset, or frustration. The condition is often mistaken for epilepsy by the anxious parent who should be assured that the condition is not epileptic and that the prognosis is good. The loss of consciousness is due to cerebral anoxia, which may result from a number of factors, including anoxic anoxia from respiratory arrest and cardiac inhibition or reduced cerebral blood flow occasioned by self-induced Valsalva maneuver.

Two types of breath-holding spells have been described.[128]

CYANOTIC FORM. The probable series of pathogenic events is as follows: Violent crying with hyperventilation, which produces hypocapnia. This is followed by apnea, which results in hypoxemia, cerebral vasoconstriction, and reduced cerebral blood flow. The child turns cyanotic and now performs a self-induced Valsalva maneuver. This increased intrathoracic pressure impairs venous return and reduces cardiac output. The cerebral vasoconstriction induced by the hypocapnia prevents compensatory cerebral vasodilation, and cerebral anoxia results, with loss of consciousness.

PALLID FORM. The stimulus, which may be quite trivial, produces violent crying and sobbing, and then the breath is held, which results in vagal hyperactivity with cardiac arrest. The circulatory failure results in loss of consciousness.

Clinical Features. Breath-holding spells usually develop before 18 months of age and may be seen as early as the first few weeks of life. There is said to be a high incidence of behavior problems but not a high incidence of mental retardation associated with the condition. The frequency of attacks varies from a single episode to several attacks each day. The condition usually ceases by the age of five years, but attacks have persisted up to ten years of age in some cases. These children also have frequent spells of "fainting" and "syncope" in adolescence and early adult life.

The cyanotic form usually follows an unpleasant stimulus, such as a painful experience, physical injury, punishment, or frustration. The attack begins with a vigorous crying, sobbing, and hyperventilation, which is suddenly climaxed by a period of apnea, which leads to cyanosis and loss of consciousness in a flaccid state. There may be a few jerking movements of the limbs or occasionally a period of opisthotonus or generalized convulsive jerks. The period of unconsciousness is usually brief but may persist for as long as two minutes. Unlike epilepsy, incontinence and tongue biting are rare in breath-holding spells and recovery is not associated with a period of postical confusion. After the attack the child usually complains of fatigue. The pallid form also follows an apparently trivial but frustrating stimulus. The child has a brief period of crying and becomes apneic, usually after a single deep gasp. Marked pallor, loss of consciousness, opisthotonus, and convulsive movements are seen in some cases. Again, recovery occurs after a brief interval without postictal confusion, although fatigue may be a complaint.

Diagnostic Procedures. These include the following:

1. Between attacks of breath-holding spells, the electroencephalogram is within normal limits. During an attack the EEG record is typical of acute hypoxia with hypersynchrony of the background activity followed by high-voltage, theta, and later diffuse delta rhythms. Clonic jerking may occur during the period of delta activity, while the stage of opisthotonus is usually associated with a flat electroencephalogram.
2. The ocular compression test is one in which the examiner applies sudden pressure to the eyes during electroencephalographic and electrocardiographic recording. This often initiates a breath-holding spell in susceptible children. The breath-holding spell is associated with a period of asystole of more than two seconds' duration in children with the pallid type of attack. The EEG changes are typically those of acute hypoxia in either the cyanotic or pallid form of attack. The EEG shows no paroxysmal sharp wave or spike activity during breath-holding spells.

Treatment. Many children with breath-holding spells are regarded as epileptic, "borderline epileptic," or "possibly epileptic" and are given anticonvulsant medication, which is unnecessary.

The parents should be reassured and a brief explanation should be given of the mechanism of the attacks. They should be told to avoid, as much as is possible, frustrating situations for the child. In cases of the pallid type, where the car-dioinhibitory reflex is marked, treatment with small doses of atropine may be effective.

Tussive Syncope

Episodes of syncope may occur after paroxysms of coughing in adults, particularly in those individuals suffering from cerebrovascular disease, chronic bronchitis, and emphysema. The repeated coughing results in an increase of intrathoracic pressure including venous return to the heart and decreasing cardiac output as described under the Valsalva maneuver.

Sneeze Syncope

Repeated sneezing may occasionally produce syncope due to a Valsalva-like mechanism. However, syncope can be precipitated by coughing or sneezing in patients who have an Arnold-Chiari malformation with herniated cerebellar tonsils or basilar invagination. The mechanism is obscure but must involve sudden pressure changes affecting the lower brainstem.[36]

Micturition Syncope

Loss of consciousness following micturition sometimes occurs in older individuals, particularly a man with prostatic hypertrophy. The mechanism seems to be at least threefold. The individual usually gets out of bed at night to empty the bladder. This may induce some fall in blood pressure. There is straining to empty the bladder, which results in the patient performing a Valsalva maneuver and increasing the intrathoracic pressure.[155a] The impairment of venous return to the heart is further implemented by pooling of blood in the abdominal area following emptying of the distended bladder, which produces a decrease in volume of abdominal contents. The combination of these events is followed by syncope in susceptible individuals.

Hypotension Due to Decreased Cardiac Output

Carotid Sinus Sensitivity

Although a number of healthy adolescents and young adults have carotid sinus sensitivity, the condition is most often seen in patients with arteriosclerotic plaques involving the bifurcation of the internal carotid artery. The carotid sinus is part of the baroreceptor system, which regulates blood pressure by altering heart rate and vasomotor tone. Slight stimulation in the area of the carotid sinus produces an exaggerated baroreceptor reflex, with bradycardia, hypotension, and syncope. Temporary asystole may result (the cardioinhibitory reflex). In other cases, hypotension occurs without alteration of the heart rate (vasodepressor reflex).

The history is usually that of loss of consciousness following compression of the carotid sinus while shaving or turning the head. This may be preceded by a short period of lightheadedness and ataxia.

The diagnosis is established by recording the electrocardiogram with the patient comfortably seated and the examiner lightly massaging the carotid sinus. In the majority of cases, massage produces asystole and the patient complains of "dizziness."[32]

In the vasodepressor type of carotid sinus sensitivity, the symptoms occur without bradycardia, and the hypotension is best demonstrated by recording the blood pressure during carotid sinus stimulation. If the carotid artery is occluded rather than massaged, the test becomes one of patency of the other carotid and vertebral vessels.

Treatment. Patients with carotid sinus sensitivity should be treated by insertion of a permanent demand pacemaker.

Cardiogenic Syncope

Syncope of cardiac origin may occur in three ways: (1) sudden increase in heart rate, (2) sudden decrease in heart rate, and (3) obstruction to flow of blood from the heart.[154]

A sudden increase in heart rate with a feeling of lightheadedness or actual syncope occurs in supraventricular tachycardia or ventricular tachycardia. Sudden slowing of heart rate and syncope occurs in heart block, tachycardia, bradycardia syndrome, and carotid sinus sensitivity. A myxoma of the heart may produce sudden obstruction to the flow of blood from the heart and sudden syncope. A similar attack may occur in patients with aortic stenosis, pericarditis with effusion, and severe myocardial fibrosis.

The diagnosis can usually be established by history, clinical examination of the heart, and electrocardiography. Echocardiography and cardiac catheterization may be required in difficult cases of suspected cardiac lesions such as a left atrial myxoma.

Deglutition Syncope

The unusual and rare condition of syncope provoked by swallowing occurs in patients who have coexistent esophageal and heart disease.[236] The esophageal disorder may be a diverticula stricture spasm or carcinoma that produces increased sensitivity of receptors in the esophageal wall and an enhanced vasovagal reflex. The inhibitory reflex activity acting on a diseased conduction system produces sinus bradycardia, sinus arrest, or heart block with failure of cardiac output and syncope. Deglutition has also been reported to produce tachyarrhythmias, followed by bradycardia and syncope. Deglutition syncope is treated by insertion of a pacemaker.

Primary Cerebral Causes of Syncope

Epileptic Seizures

A number of nonconvulsive seizures may be confused with fainting or syncope in children and adults. The diagnosis may only be established by a careful and detailed historic account of the event by both the patient and those who have observed the attacks as outlined above, and by the use of serial electroencephalograms.

Cerebrovascular Insufficiency

Syncopal attacks can occur due to transient ischemic episodes associated with cerebrovascular insufficiency. These are encountered in both carotid and vertebral-basilar insufficiency and are discussed in detail in Chapter 9.

It should be noted that transient ischemic attacks and carotid sinus sensitivity may coexist in the same patient, particularly when there is evidence of carotid artery stenosis.[218]

Conversion Reaction (Hysteria)

Syncopal episodes may occur in emotionally disturbed patients as a manifestation of a conversion reaction. The physician may be alerted to this possibility from the incompatible history obtained in these cases, and of course, many patients may well have a normal electroencephalogram. The occurrence of conversion reactions in patients who already have an established form of seizure disorder may present great difficulties to the clinician who has to treat such cases. There is often a marked secondary gain, and the response to therapeutic measures is frequently poor. A combination of neurologic and psychiatric treatment may be necessary.

Hematologic Causes of Syncope

Hypoglycemia

Although hypoglycemia may be associated with a feeling of lightheadedness and fainting and the patient may experience tachycardia and sweating due to sympathetic overactivity, sudden loss of consciousness is unusual unless the hypoglycemia precipitates an epileptic seizure. Hypoglycemia usually produces a prolonged period of mental confusion before loss of consciousness, which occurs at very low blood glucose levels. This is particularly likely to occur in individuals who are receiving a long-acting insulin preparation for the treatment of diabetes mellitus.

Anemia

Patients with anemia from any cause may be subject to syncopal episodes, presumably because the oxygen supply to the brain is marginal. The small changes in blood pressure associated with changes in posture are sufficient to produce a slight reduction in cerebral blood flow and loss of consciousness in susceptible patients.

Hyperventilation

The sudden onset of hyperventilation followed by syncope is usually a manifestation of anxiety neurosis or psychoneurosis from other causes and is one form of a conversion reaction producing syncope. Treatment has already been discussed above.

Cited References

1. Adebimpe, V. R. Complex partial seizures simulating schizophrenia. *J.A.M.A.*, **237:**1339–41, 1977.
1a. Aguilar, M., and Rasmussen, T. Role of encephalitis in pathogenesis of epilepsy. *Arch. Neurol.*, **2:**666–76, 1960.
2. Anthony, J. J. Malignant lymphoma associated with hydantoin drugs. *Arch. Neurol.*, **22:**450–54, 1970.
3. Anthony, M., and Lance, J. W. Histamine and serotonin in cluster headaches. *Arch. Neurol.*, **25:**225–31, 1971.
4. Anthony, M., and Lance, J. W. Current concepts in the pathogenesis and interval treatment of migraine. *Drugs*, **3:**153–58, 1972.
5. Aring, C. D. The migrainous scintillating scotoma. *J.A.M.A.*, **220:**519–22, 1972.
6. Arseni, C., and Cristescu, A. Epilepsy due to cysticercosis. *Epilepsia*, **13:**253–58, 1972.
7. Arseni, C., and Petrovici, I. N. Epilepsy in temporal lobe tumors. *Eur. Neurol.*, **5:**201–14, 1971.
8. Bailey, D. W., and Fenichel, G. M. The treatment of prolonged seizure activity with intravenous diazepam, *Pediatr. Pharmacol. Therap.*, **73:**923–27, 1968.
9. Ball, M. J. Pathogenesis of the "sentinel headache" preceding berry aneurysm rupture. *Can. Med. Assoc. J.*, **112:**78–79, 1975.
10. Barker, J. L., and Gainer, H. Pentobarbital: Selective depression of excitatory postsynaptic potentials. *Science*, **182:**720–22, 1973.
11. Basser, L. S. Relation of migraine and epilepsy. *Brain*, **92:**285–300, 1969.
12. Bell, D. S. Dangers of treatment of status epilepticus with diazepam. *Br. Med. J.*, **1:**159–61, 1969.
13. Binnie, C. D., Darby, C. E., and Hindley, A. T. Electroencephalographic changes in epileptics while viewing television. *Br. Med. J.*, **4:**378–79, 1973.
14. Blau, J. N. Migraine research. *Br. Med. J.*, **2:**751–54, 1971.
15. Blau, J. N., and Davis, E. Small blood vessels in migraine. *Lancet*, **2:**740–42, 1970.
16. Bloomer, H. A., Barton, L. J., and Maddock, R. K., Jr. Penicillin-induced encephalopathy in uremic patients. *J.A.M.A.*, **200:**131–33, 1967.
17. Bogdanoff, B. M.; Stafford, C. R.; et al. Computerized transaxial tomography in the evaluation of patients with focal epilepsy. *Neurology* (Minneap.), **25:**1013–17, 1975.
18. Bray, P. F., and Wiser, W. C. The relation of focal to diffuse epileptiform EEG discharges in genetic epilepsy. *Arch. Neurol.*, **13:**223–37, 1965.
19. Brazier, M. A. B. Spread of seizure discharges in epilepsy: Anatomical and electrophysiological considerations. *Exp. Neurol.*, **36:**263–72, 1972.
20. Brewer, C. Homicide during a psychomotor seizure. The importance of air-encephalography in establishing insanity under the McNaughten Rules. *Med. J. Aust.*, **1:**857–59, 1971.
21. Brooks, J. E., and Jerauch, P. M. Primary reading epilepsy: A misnomer. *Arch. Neurol.*, **25:**97–104, 1971.
22. Browne, T. R. Clonazepam. A review of a new anticonvulsant drug. *Arch. Neurol.*, **33:**326–32, 1976.
23. Cala, L. A., and Mastaglia, F. L. Computerized axial tomography findings in patients with migrainous headache. *Br. Med. J.*, **1:**49–50, 1976.
24. Calderon-Gonzales, R., and Mireles-Gonzales, A. Management of prolonged motor seizure activity in children. *J.A.M.A.*, **204:**544–46, 1968.
25. Callaghan, N. The migraine syndrome in pregnancy. *Neurology* (Minneap.), **18:**197–201, 1968.
26. Canelas, H. M.; De Assis, L. M.; and De Jorge, F. Disorders of magnesium metabolism in epilepsy. *J. Neurol. Neurosurg. Psychiat.*, **28:**378–81, 1965.
27. Cantor, F. K. Vestibular-temporal lobe connections demonstrated by induced seizures. *Neurology* (Minneap.), **21:**507–16, 1971.
28. Carroll, J. D. Migraine-general management. *Br. Med. J.*, **2:**756–57, 1971.
29. Caveness, W. F. Epilepsy, a product of trauma of our time. *Epilepsia*, **17:**207–15, 1976.
30. Chadwick, D.; Harris, R.; et al. Manipulation

of brain serotonin in the treatment of myoclonus. *Lancet,* **2:**434–35, 1975.

31. Chen Rong-Chi, and Forster, F. M. Cursive epilepsy and gelastic epilepsy. *Neurology* (Minneap.), **23:**1019–29, 1973.

32. Chughtai, A. L.; Yans, J.; and Kwata, M. Carotid sinus syncope. Report of two cases. *J.A.M.A.,* **237:**2320–21, 1977.

33. Cluster headache. *Br. Med. J.,* **4:**25–26, 1975.

34. Coccagna, G.; Donato, G.; et al. Hypersomnia with periodic apneas in acquired micrognathia. *Arch. Neurol.,* **33:**769–76, 1976.

35. Cole, M., and Zangwell, O. L. Déjà vu in temporal lobe epilepsy. *J. Neurol. Neurosurg. Psychiat.,* **26:**37–38, 1963.

36. Corbett, J. J.; Butler, A. B.; and Kaufman, B. Sneeze syncope, basilar invagination and Arnold Chiari type I malformation. *J. Neurol. Neurosurg. Psychiat.,* **39:**381–84, 1976.

37. Couch, J. R., and Hassanein, R. S. Platelet aggregability in migraine and relation of aggregability to clinical aspects of migraine. *Neurology* (Minneap.), **27:**843–48, 1977.

37a. Couch, J. R., and Ziegler, D. K. Prednisone therapy for cluster headache. *Headache,* **18:**219–21, 1978.

38. Currier, R. D.; Kooi, K. A.; and Saidman, L. J. Prognosis of "pure" petit mal. A follow up study. *Neurology* (Minneap.), **13:**959–67, 1963.

39. Dallos, V., and Heathfield, K. Iatrogenic epilepsy due to antidepressant drugs. *Br. Med. J.,* **4:**80–82,1969.

40. Dalessio, D. J. Migraine platelets and headache prophylaxis. *J.A.M.A.,* **239:**52–53, 1978.

41. Dalton, K. Food intake prior to a migraine attack. Study of 2313 spontaneous attacks. *Headache,* **15:**188–93, 1975.

42. Daly, D. D., and Mulder, D. W. Gelastic epilepsy. *Neurology* (Minneap.), **7:**189–92, 1957.

43. De Jesus, P. V., Jr., and Masland, W. S. Role of nasopharyngeal electrodes in clinical electroencephalography. *Neurology* (Minneap.), **20:**869–78, 1970.

44. Deshmukh, S. V., and Meyer, J. S. Cyclic changes in platelet dynamics and the pathogenesis and prophylaxis of migraine. *Headache,* **17:**101–108, 1977.

45. Dexter, J. D., and Riley, T. L. Studies in nocturnal migraine. *Headache,* **15:**51–62, 1975.

46. Douglas, E. F., and White, P. T. Abdominal epilepsy—a reappraisal. *J. Pediatr.,* **78:**59–67, 1971.

47. Dramond, S. Treatment of migraine with isometheptene, acetaminophen and dichloralphenazone combination: A double blind crossover trial. *Headache,* **15:**282–87, 1976.

48. Dreifuss, F. E. The differential diagnosis of partial seizures with complex symptomatology. In Penry, J. K., and Daly, D. D. (eds.). *Advances in Neurology,* Vol. 11. Raven Press, New York, 1975, Chap. 9.

49. Druckman, R., and Chao, D. Laughter in epilepsy. *Neurology* (Minneap.), **7:**26–36, 1957.

50. Dyken, P. R. Headaches in children. *Am. Fam. Pract.,* **11:**105–11, 1975.

51. Earnest, M. P., and Yarnell, P. R. Seizure admissions to a city hospital: The role of alcohol. *Epilepsia,* **17:**387–93, 1976.

52. Ekbom, K. Patterns of cluster headache with a note on the relations to angina pectoris and peptic ulcer. *Acta Neurol. Scand.,* **46:**225–37, 1970.

53. Eldridge, R.; Sweet, R.; et al. Gilles de la Tourette syndrome: Clinical, genetic, psychologic, and biochemical aspects in 21 selected families. *Neurology* (Minneap.), **27:**115–24, 1977.

53a. Ellenberg, J. H., and Nelson, K. B. Febrile seizures and later intellectual performance. *Arch. Neurol.,* **35:**17–21, 1978.

54. Escueta, A. V.; Kunze, U.; et al. Lapse of consciousness and automatisms in temporal lobe epilepsy: A videotape analysis. *Neurology* (Minneap.), **27:**144–54, 1977.

55. Etheridge, J. E., and Millichap, J. G. Hypoglycemia and seizures in childhood. *Neurology* (Minneap.), **14:**397–404, 1964.

56. Ettinger, G., and Lowrie, M. B. An immunological factor in epilepsy. *Lancet,* **1:**1386, 1976.

57. Falconer, M. A. Significance of surgery for temporal lobe epilepsy in childhood and adolescence. *J. Neurol. Neurosurg. Psychiat.,* **33:**233–51, 1970.

58. Falconer, M. A. Temporal lobe epilepsy in children and its surgical treatment. *Med. J. Aust.,* **1:**1117–21, 1972.

59. Fenichel, G. M. Migraine in childhood. *Clin. Pediatr.,* **7:**192–94, 1968.

60. Fichman, M. P.; Klennman, C. R.; and Bethune, J. E. Inhibition of antidiuretic hormone secretion by Diphenylhydantoin. *Arch. Neurol.,* **22:**45–53, 1970.

61. Forster, F. M., and Liske, E. Role of environmental clues in temporal lobe epilepsy. *Neurology* (Minneap.), **13:**301–305, 1963.

62. Forster, F. M.; Hansotia, P.; Cleeland, C. S.; and Ludwig, A. Case of voice-induced epilepsy treated by conditioning. *Neurology* (Minneap.), **19:**325–31, 1969.

63. Fox, R. H., et al. Spontaneous periodic hypothermia: Diencephalic epilepsy. *Br. Med. J.,* **2:**693–95, 1973.

64. Frantzen, E.; Lennox-Buchthal, M.; Nygaard, A.; and Stone, J. Genetic study of febril convulsions. *Neurology* (Minneap.), **20:**909–17, 1970.

65. Friedman, A. P. Metabolic abnormalities in migraine. *Ann. Intern. Med.,* **75:**801–802, 1971.

66. Friedman, A. P. Migraine headaches. *J.A.M.A.,* **222:**1399–1402, 1972.

67. Fromm, G. H., and Kohli, C. M. The role of inhibitory pathways in petit mal epilepsy. *Neurology* (Minneap.), **22:**1012–20, 1972.

68. Gabor, A. J. Focal seizures induced by movement without sensory feedback mechanisms. *Electroenceph. Clin. Neurophysiol.,* **36:**403–408, 1974.

69. Gastaut, H. Les Myoclonies. Séméiologie des myoclonies et nosologie analytique des syndromes myoclonique. *Rev. Neur. Paris,* **119:**1–30, 1968.

70. Gastaut, H., and Gastaut, J. L. Computerized transverse axial tomography in epilepsy. *Epilepsia,* **17:**235–36, 1976.

71. Gastaut, H., and Tassinari, C. A. Triggering mechanisms in epilepsy. The electroclinical point of view. *Epilepsia,* **7:**85–138, 1966.

72. Gastaut, H., and Villeneuve, A. A startle disease of hyperexplexia: pathological surprise reaction. *J. Neurol. Sci.,* **5:**523–42, 1967.

72a. Gibberd, F. B. Diseases of the central nervous system. Epilepsy. *Br. Med. J.,* **2:**270–72, 1975.

73. Gibberd, F. B.; Dunne, J. F.; Handley, A. J.; and Hazelman, B. L. Supervision of epileptic patients taking phenytoin. *Br. Med. J.,* **1:**147–49, 1970.

74. Gilbert, G. J.; Rappaport, A.; and Trump, R. Retinal degeneration in hemiplegic migraine. *Headache,* **14:**77–80, 1974.

75. Gilbert, G. J.; McEntee, W. J., III; and Glaser, G. H. Familial myoclonus and ataxia. *Neurology* (Minneap.), **13:**365–72, 1963.

76. Glista, G. G.; Mellinger, J. F.; and Rooke, E. D. Familial hemiplegic migraine. *Mayo Clin. Proc.,* **50:**307–11, 1975.

76a. Golden, G. S. The effect of central nervous system stimulants on Tourette syndrome. *Ann. Neurol.,* **2:**69–70, 1977.

76b. Golden, G. S. Tics and Tourette's. A continuum of symptoms. *Ann. Neurol.,* **4:**145–48, 1978.

77. Goldensohn, E. S., and Gold, A. P. Prolonged behavioural disturbances as ictal phenomena. *Neurology* (Minneap.), **10:**1–9, 1960.

78. Goldring, S. The role of prefrontal cortex in grand mal convulsion. *Arch. Neurol.,* **26:**109–19, 1972.

79. Gomersall, J. D., and Stuart, A. Amitryptyline in migraine prophylaxis. Changes in pattern of attacks during a controlled clinical trial. *J. Neurol. Neurosurg. Psychiat.,* **36:**684–90, 1973.

80. Gordon, N. Folic acid deficiency from anticonvulsant therapy. *Dev. Med. Child Neurol.,* **10:**497–504, 1968.

81. Graham, J. R.; Suby, H. I.; Le Compte, P. R.; and Sadowsky, N. L. Fibrotic disorders associated with methysergide therapy for headache. *N. Engl. J. Med.,* **274:**359–68, 1966.

82. Grisell, J. L.; Levin, S. M.; Cohen, B. D.; and Rodin, E. A. Effect of subclinical seizure activity on overt behaviour. *Neurology* (Minneap.), **14:**133–35, 1964.

83. Growdan, J. H.; Young, R. R.; and Shahari, B. T. L-5-Hydroxytryptophan in treatment of several different syndromes in which myoclonus is prominent. *Neurology* (Minneap.), **26:**1135–40, 1976.

84. Haerer, A. F., and Grace, J. B. Studies of anticonvulsant levels in epileptics. I. Serum diphenylhydantoin concentrations in group medically indigent outpatients. *Acta Neurol. Scand.,* **45:**18–31, 1969.

85. Henryk-Gutt, R., and Rees, W. L. Psychological aspects of migraine. *J. Psychosom. Res.,* **17:**141–53, 1973.

86. Herrmann, C., and Brown, J. W. Palatal myoclonus: A reappraisal. *J. Neurol. Sci.,* **5:**473–92, 1967.

87. Hess, R. F.; Harding, G. F. A.; and Drasdo, N. Seizures induced by flickering light. *Am. J. Optom. Physiol. Optics,* **51:**517–29, 1974.

88. Heyck, H. Varieties of hemiplegic migraine. *Headache,* **12:**135–42, 1973.

89. Hirsch, C. S., and Martin, D. C. Unexpected death in young epileptics. *Neurology* (Minneap.), **21:**682–90, 1971.

89a. Hokkanen, E.; Waltimo, O.; and Kallanrante, M. T. Toxic effects of ergotamine used for migraine. *Headache,* **18:**95–98, 1978.

90. Holcomb, R.; Lynn, R.; Harvey, B. Jr.; Sweetman, B. J.; and Gerber, N. Intoxication with 5.5-diphenylhydantoin (Dilantin). *J. Pediatr.,* **80:**627–32, 1972.

91. Hooshmand, H., and Brawley, B. W. Temporal lobe seizures and exhibitionism. *Neurology* (Minneap.), **19:**1119–24, 1969.

92. Hopkins, I. J. Seizures in the first weeks of life. *Med. J. Aust.,* **2:**647–51, 1972.

93. Horne, P. D. Long term anticonvulsant therapy and cerebellar atrophy. *J. Irish Med. Assoc.,* **66:**147–52, 1973.

94. Horrobin, D. F. Hypothesis: Prostaglandins and migraine. *Headache,* **17:**113–17, 1977.

95. Horven, I., and Sjaastad, O. Cluster headache syndrome and migraine. *Acta Ophthalmol.,* **55:**35–51, 1976.

96. Hsu, L. K.; Crisp, A. H.; et al. Early morning migraine. *Lancet,* **1:**447–51, 1977.

97. Hughes, J. R. EEG in headache. *Headache,* **11:**162–70, 1972.

98. Hungerford, G. D.; duBoulay, G. H.; and Zilkha, K. J. computerized axial tomography in patients with severe migraine. A preliminary report. *J. Neurol. Neurosurg. Psychiat.,* **39:**990–94, 1976.

99. Hunt, E. S.; Meagher, J. N.; et al. Painful ophthalmoplegia. Its relation to indolent inflammation of the cavernous sinus. *Neurology* (Minneap.), **11:**56–62, 1961.

100. Hunter, R.; Barnes, J.; and Mathews, D. M. Effect of folic acid supplement on serum vitamin B_{12} levels in patients on anticonvulsants. *Lancet,* **2:**666–67, 1969.

101. Hyllested, K., and Pakkenberg, M. Prognosis in epilepsy of late onset. *Neurology* (Minneap.), **13:**641–44, 1963.

102. Imes, N. K.; Orr, W. C.; et al. Retrognathia and sleep apnea. *J.A.M.A.,* **237:**1596–97, 1977.

103. Ingvar, D. H., and Nyman, G. E. Epilepsia arithmetices. A new psychologic trigger mechanism in a case of epilepsy. *Neurology* (Minneap.), **12:**282–87, 1962.

104. Jammes, J. L. The treatment of cluster headaches with prednisone. *Dis. Nerv. Syst.,* **3:**75–76, 1900.

105. Janeway, R., et al. Progressive myoclonus epilepsy with Lafora inclusion bodies I. Clinical genetic histopathologic and biochemical aspects. *Arch. Neurol.,* **16:**565–82, 1967.

106. Jeavons, P., and Clark, E. Sodium valproate in treatment of epilepsy. *Br. Med. J.,* **2:**584–86, 1974.

107. Jennett, W. B. Early traumatic epilepsy: Definition and identity. *Lancet.* **1:**1023–25, 1969.

108. Kattan, K. R., Calvarial thickening after Dilantin medication. *Am. J. Roentgenol.,* **110:**102–105, 1970.

109. Katz, J., and Vogel, R. M. Abdominal angina as a complication of methysergide maleate therapy. *J.A.M.A.,* **199:**160–61, 1967.

109a. Keen, J. H. Significance of hypocalcemia in neonatal convulsions. *Arch. Dis. Child.,* **44:**356–61, 1961.

110. Kerbel, N. C. Retroperitoneal fibrosis secondary to methysergide bimaleate. *Can. Med. Assoc. J.,* **96:**1420–22, 1967.

111. Keretesz, A. Paroxysmal kinesigenic choreoathetosis: An entity within the paroxysmal choreotosis syndrome; description of 10 cases including one autopsied. *Neurology* (Minneap.), **17:**680–90, 1967.

112. Kudrow, L. Plasma testosterone levels in cluster headaches. Preliminary results. *Headache,* **16:**28–31, 1976.

113. Kudrow, L. Lithium prophylaxis for chronic cluster headache. *Headache,* **17:**15–18, 1977.

114. Kunkel, R. S. Cluster headache. *Ohio State M.J.,* **73:**131–38, 1977.

115. Kurland, L. T. The incidence and prevalence of convulsive disorders in a small urban community. *Epilepsia,* **1:**143–61, 1960.

116. Kutt, H., and McDowell, F. Management of epilepsy with diphenylhydantoin sodium. Dosage regulation for problem patients. *J.A.M.A.,* **203:**969–72, 1968.

117. Lance, J. W. Headaches related to sexual activity. *J. Neurol. Neurosurg. Psychiat.,* **39:**1226–30, 1976.

118. Lance, J. W., and Anthony, M. Migrainous neuralgia or cluster headache. *J. Neurol. Sci.,* **13:**401–14, 1971.

119. Larsen, L. E., and Cornee, J. An analytic case study of periparaxysmal events in an implanted temporal lobe epileptic. *Brain Res.,* **38:**93–108, 1972.

120. Larsson-Cohn, U., and Lundberg, P. O. Headache and treatment with oral contraceptives. *Acta Neurol. Scand.,* **46:**267–78, 1970.

121. Lasater, G. M. Reading epilepsy. *Arch. Neurol.,* **6:**492–95, 1962.

122. Lee, C. H., and Lance, J. W. Migraine stupor. *Headache,* **17:**32–38, 1977.

123. Leibowitz, U., and Alter, M. Epilepsy in Jerusalem Israel. *Epilepsia,* **9:**87–105, 1968.

124. Lende, R. A., and Popp, A. J. Sensory jacksonian seizures. *J. Neurol. Neurosurg. Psychiat.,* **44:**706–11, 1976.

125. Lessell, S., Torres, J. M., and Kurland, L. T. Seizure disorders in a Guamanian village. *Arch. Neurol.,* **7:**37–44, 1962.

126. Liske, E., and Forster, F. M. Pseudoseizures: A problem in the diagnosis and management of epileptic patients. *Neurology* (Minneap.), **14:**41–49, 1964.

127. Logen, W. J., and Freeman, J. M. Pseudodegenerative disease due to diphenylhydantoin intoxication. *Arch. Neurol.,* **21:**631–37, 1969.

128. Lombroso, C. T., and Lerman, P. Breath holding spells (cyanotic and pallid infantile syncope). *Pediatrics,* **39:**563–81, 1967.

128a. Lott, I. T.; Coulombe, T.; et al. Vitamin B_6-dependent seizures: pathology and chemical findings in brain. *Neurology* (Minneap.), **28:**47–54, 1978.

129. Lord, G. D. A.; Duckworth, J. W.; and Charlesworth, J. A. Complement activation in migraine. *Lancet,* **1:**781–82, 1977.

130. Lorseau, P.; Cohadan, F.; and Cohadan, S. Gelastic epilepsy: A review and report of five cases. *Epilepsia* (Amst.), **12:**313, 1971.

131. Lovelace, R. E., and Horwitz, S. J. Peripheral neuropathy in long-term diphenylhydantoin therapy. *Arch. Neurol.,* **18:**69–77, 1968.

132. Lucas, A. R. Gilles de la Tourette's disease: An overview. *N.Y. State J. Med.,* **70:**2197–2200, 1970.

133. Lyneham, R. C., et al. Convulsions and electroencephalogram abnormalities after intraamniotic prostaglandin F_{2a} *Lancet,* **2:**1003–1005, 1973.

134. Mahloudji, M., and Pikielny, R. T. Hereditary essential myoclonus. *Brain,* **90:**669–74, 1967.

134a. Mann, P.; Sutherland, J. M.; and Eadie, M. J. A critical review of the treatment of migrainous neuralgia. *Proc. Aust. Assoc. Neurol.,* **7:**49–53, 1970.

135. Mathew, N. T.; Meyer, J. S.; et al. Abnormal CT scans in migraine. *Headache,* **17:**272–79, 1977.

135a. Mathew, N. T. Clinical subtypes of cluster headache and response to lithium therapy. *Headache,* **18:**26–30, 1978.

136. Mathews, W. B., Footballers migraine. *Br. Med. J.,* **2:**326–27, 1972.

136a. Mattson, R. H.; Cramer, J. A.; et al. Valproic acid in epilepsy: clinical and pharmacological effects. *Ann. Neurol.,* **3:**20–25, 1978.

136b. Mauguiere, F., and Courgon, J. Somatosensory epilepsy. A review of 127 cases. *Brain,* **101:**307–32, 1978.

137. Maxwell, J. D.; Hunter, J.; et al. Folate deficiency after anticonvulsant drugs; an effect of hepatic enzyme induction. *Br. Med. J.,* **1:**297–99, 1972.

138. May, D. L., and White, H. H. Familial myoclonus cerebellar ataxia and deafness. *Arch. Neurol.,* **19:**331–38, 1968.

139. Maynert, E. W.; Marezynski, T. J.; and Browning, R. A. The role of neurotransmitters in the epilepsies. In Friedlander, Walter J. (ed.). *Advances in Neurology,* Vol. 13. Raven Press, New York, 1975, pp. 79–147.

139a. McInerny, T. K., and Schubert, W. K. Prognosis of neonatal seizures. *Am. J. Dis. Child.,* **117:**261–64, 1969.

140. Medina, J. L., and Diamond, S. Migraine and atopy. *Headache,* **15:**271–73, 1976.

141. Medina, J. L.; Diamond, S.; and Rubino, F. A. Headaches in patients with transient ischemic attacks. *Headache,* **15:**194–97, 1975.

142. Messiha, F. S.; Knapp, W.; Vanecko, S.; O'Brien, V.; and Carson, S. A. Haloperidol therapy in Tourette's syndrome: Neurophysiological, biochemical and behavioral correlates. *Life Sciences* Part **10:**449–557, 1971.

143. Meyer, J. S.; Kanda, T.; Shinohara, Y.; and Fukuuchi, Y. Changes in cerebrospinal fluid sodium and potassium concentrations during seizure activity. *Neurology* (Minneap.), **20:**1179–84, 1970.

144. Migrainous cerebral infarction. *Br. Med. J.,* **1:**532–33, 1977.

145. Mikkelsen, B.; Birket-Smith, E.; et al. Clonazepam in the treatment of epilepsy. A controlled clinical trial in simple absences, bilateral massive epileptic myoclonus and atonic seizures. *Arch. Neurol.,* **33:**322–25, 1976.

146. Millichap, J. G.; Madsen, J. A., and Aledort, L. M. Studies in febrile seizures, V. Clinical and electroencephalographic study in unselected patients. *Neurology* (Minneap.), **10:**643–53, 1960.

147. Mitchell, K. R. A psychological approach to the treatment of migraine. *Br. J. Psychiat.,* **19:**533–34, 1971.

148. Mølholm, J., et al. Effect of diphenylhydantoin on the metabolism of dicoumarol in man. *Acta Med. Scand.,* **189:**15–19, 1971.

149. Musella, L.; Wilder, B. J.; and Schmidt, R. P. Electroencephalographic activation with intravenous methohexital in psychomotor epilepsy. *Neurology* (Minneap.), **21:**594–602, 1971.

150. Neligan, P.; Harriman, D. G.; and Pearce, J. Respiratory arrest in familial hemiplegic migraine: a clinical and neuropathological study. *Br. Med. J.,* **2:**732–34, 1977.

151. Neubauer, C. Mental deterioration in epilepsy due to folate deficiency. *Br. Med. J.,* **2:**759–61, 1970.

152. Nicol, C. F., Tutton, J. C., and Smith, B. H. Parenteral diazepam in status epilepticus. *Neurology* (Minneap.), **19:**332–43, 1969.

153. Niedermeyer, E.; Laws, E. R.; and Walker, A. E. Depth EEG findings in epileptics with generalized spike-wave complexes. *Arch. Neurol.,* **21:**51–58, 1969.

154. Noble, R. J. The patient with syncope. *J.A.M.A.,* **237:**1372–76, 1977.

155. Norris, J. W.; Hachinski, V. C.; and Cooper, P. W. Cerebral blood flow changes in cluster headaches. *Acta Neurol. Scand.,* **54:**371–74, 1976.

155a. O'Connor, P. J. Syncope. *Practioner,* **216:**276–80, 1976.

156. Oxbury, J. M., and Whitty, C. W. M. Causes and consequences of status epilepticus in adults. A study of 86 cases. *Brain,* **94:**733–44, 1971.

157. Oxbury, J. M., and Whitty, W. M. Syndrome of isolated epileptic status. *J. Neurol. Neurosurg. Psychiat.,* **34:**182–84, 1971.

158. Parkes, J. D.; Fenton, G.; et al. Narcolepsy and cataplexy. Clinical features, treatment and cerebrospinal fluid findings. *Q. J. Med.,* **43:**525–36, 1974.

159. Parsonage, M. J., and Norris, J. W. Use of Diazepam in treatment of severe convulsive status epilepticus. *Br. Med. J.,* **3:**85–88, 1967.

160. Patel, H., and Crichton, J. U. Neurologic hazards of diphenylhydantoin in childhood. *J. Pediatr.,* **73:**676–84, 1968.

161. Paulson, G. W., and Klawans, H. L. Benign orgasmic cephalgia. *Headache,* **13:**181–87, 1974.

162. Pearce, J. Insulin-induced hypoglycemia in migraine. *J. Neurol. Neurosurg. Psychiat.,* **34:**154–56, 1971.

163. Pearce, J. M. S., and Foster, J. B. An investigation of complicated migraine. *Neurology* (Minneap.), **15:**333–40, 1965.

164. Penrick, M.; White, R. P.; Crockarell, J. T.; et al. Role of prostaglanden $F_2\alpha$ in the genesis of experimental vasospasm. *J. Neurosurg.,* **37:**398–406, 1972.

165. Penry, J. K., and Dreifuss, F. E. Automatisms associated with absence or petit mal epilepsy. *Arch. Neurol.,* **21:**142–49, 1969.

166. Perez-Borja, C.; Tassinari, A. C.; and Swanson, A. G. Paroxysmal choreoathetosis and seizures induced by movement (reflex epilepsy). *Epilepsia,* **8:**260–70, 1967.

167. Peters, U. H. Pseudopsychopathic emotion syndrome of temporal lobe epileptic. Investigation into problem of behavioural change in psychomotor epilepsy. *Nervenarzt,* **40:**75–82, 1969.

168. Pollask, M. A., and French, J. M. Hypothesis: Glutamic acid in migraine. Headache, **15:** 114–17, 1975.

169. Raichle, M. E.; Kutt, H.; Louis, S.; and McDowell, F. Neurotoxicity of intravenous administered penicillin G. *Arch. Neurol.,* **25:**232–39, 1971.

170. Ralston, A. J.; Snaith, R. P.; and Hinley, J. B. Effect of folic acid and fit frequency and behaviour in epileptics on anticonvulsants. *Lancet,* **1:**867–68, 1970.

171. Rasmussen, T., and Gossman, H. Epilepsy due to gross destructive brain lesions: results of surgical therapy. *Neurology* (Minneap.), **13:**659–69, 1963.

172. Rees, W. L. Personality and psychodynamic mechanisms in migraine. *Psychother. Psychosom.,* **23:**111–22, 1974.

173. Remillard, G. M.; Andermann, F.; et al. Facial asymmetry in patients with temporal lobe epilepsy. *Neurology,* 27:109–14, 1977.

174. Reynolds, E. H. Chronic antiepileptic toxicity: A review. *Epilepsia,* **16:**319–52, 1975.

175. Reynolds, E. H.; Chadwick, D.; and Galbraith, A. W. One drug (phenytoin) in the treatment of epilepsy. *Lancet,* **1:**923–26, 1976.

176. Richards, R. N., and Barnett, H. J. M. Paroxysmal dystonic choreoathetosis: A family study and review of the literature. *Neurology* (Minneap.), **18:**461–69, 1968.

177. Riffenburgh, R. S. Migraine equivalent: The scintillating scotoma. *Ann. Ophthalmol.,* **3:**787–88, 1971.

178. Rigg, C. A. Migraine in children and adolescents. *Acta Paediatr. Scand., suppl.,* **256:**62–64, 1975.

178a. Roberts, S. A.; Cohen, M. D.; and Forfar, J. O. Antenatal factors associated with neonatal hypoglycemic convulsions. *Lancet,* **2:**809–14, 1973.

179. Rodin, E. A. Psychomotor epilepsy and aggressive behavior. *Arch. Gen. Psychiat.,* **28:**210–13, 1973.

180. Rodin, E. A. Psychosocial management of patients with complex partial seizures. In Penry, J. K., and Daly, D. D. (eds.). *Advances in Neurology,* Vol. 11. Raven Press, New York, 1975, Chap. 22.

181. Rodin, E. A., and Gonzales, S. Hereditary components in epileptic patients, EEG family studies. *J.A.M.A.,* **198:**221–25, 1966.

182. Rodin, E. A.; Rim, C. S.; et al. A comparison of the effectiveness of primidone versus carbamazepine in epileptic outpatients. *J. Nerv. Ment. Dis.,* **163:**41–46, 1976.

183. Rodin, E. A.; Rim, C. S.; and Rennick, P. M. The effects of carbamazepine on patients with psychomotor epilepsy: Results of a double-blind study. *Epilepsia,* **15:**547–61, 1974.

184. Roger, J.; Lob, H.; Waltregay, A.; et al. Attacks of epileptic laughter in five cases. *Electroencephalogr. Clin. Neurophysiol.,* **22:**279, 1967.

184a. Rosenbaum, D. H.; Davis, M. J.; and Song, I. S. The syndrome of painful ophthalmoplegia. A case with intraorbital mass and hypervascularity. *Arch. Neurol.,* **36:**41–43, 1979.

184b. Ryan, R. E., Sr. A controlled study of the effect of oral contraceptives on migraine. *Headache,* **17:**250–52, 1978.

185. Saus, A. B.; Gaudin, E. S.; et al. Hydatid cyst of the brain as an epileptogenic factor. *Acta Neurol. Lat. Am.,* **19:**78–88, 1973.

186. Sawyer, G. T.; Webster, D. D.; and Schut, L. J. Treatment of uncontrolled seizure activity with diazepam. *J.A.M.A.,* **203:**913–18, 1968.

187. Schold, C.; Yarnell, P. R.; and Earnest, M. P. Origin of seizures in elderly patients. *J.A.M.A.,* **238:**1177–78, 1977.

188. Schott, G. D.; McLeod, A. A.; and Jewitt, D. E. Cardiac arrhythmias that masquerade as epilepsy. *Br. Med. J.,* **1:**1454–57, 1977.

189. Schwartz, J. F. Recent advances in treating epileptic children. *Postgrad. Med.,* **44:**107–111, 1968.

190. Scott, D. F.; Moffett, A.; and Swash, M. Observations on the relation of migraine and epilepsy. An electroencephalographic psychological and clinical study using oral tyramine. *Epilepsia* (Amst.), **13:**365–75, 1972.

191. Shapiro, A. K., and Shapiro, E. Treatment of Gilles de la Tourette's syndrome with haloperidol. *Br. J. Psychiat.,* **114:**345–50, 1968.

192. Shapiro, W. R. Treatment of cataplexy with clomipramine. *Arch. Neurol.,* **32:**653–56, 1975.

193. Sherwin, A. L.; Eisen, A. A.; and Sokolowski, C. D. Anticonvulsant drugs in human epileptogenic brain. *Arch. Neurol.,* **29:**73–77, 1973.

194. Sicuteri, F. M. D. Headache as a possible expression of deficiency of brain 5-hydroxytryptamine (central denervation supersensitivity). *Headache,* **12:**69–72, 1972.

195. Silanpaa, M. Clonidine prophylaxis of childhood migraine and other vascular headaches. A double blind study of 57 children. *Headache,* **17:**28–31, 1977.

195a. Singer, H. S.; Pepple, J. M.; et al. Gilles de la Tourette syndrome: Further studies and thoughts. *Ann. Neurol.,* **4:**21–25, 1978.

196. Smith, B. H. Vestibular disturbances in epilepsy. *Neurology* (Minneap.), **10:**465–69, 1960.

197. Smith, B. T., and Masotti, R. E. Intravenous diazepam in the treatment of prolonged seizure activity in neonates and infants. *Dev. Med. Child Neurol.,* **13:**630–34, 1971.

198. Smith, I.; Kellow, A. H.; and Hannington, E. A clinical and biochemical correlation between tyramine and migraine headache. *Headache,* **10:**43–52, 1970.

199. Snyder, S. H.; Taylor, K. M.; Coyle, J. T.; and Meyerhoff, J. L. The role of brain dopamine in behavior regulation and the activity of psychotropic drugs. *Am. J. Psychiat.,* **127:**199–207, 1970.

200. Solomon, G. E.; Hilgartner, M. W.; and Kutt, H. Coagulation defects caused by diphenylhydantoin. *Neurology* (Minneap.), **22:**1165–71, 1972.

201. Somerville, B. W. The influence of hormonal changes upon migraine in women. *Proc. Aust. Assoc. Neurol.,* **8:**47–53, 1971.

202. Somerville, B. W. The role of progesterone in menstrual migraine. *Neurology* (Minneap.), **21:**853–59, 1971.

203. Somerville, B. W. The role of estradiol withdrawal in the etiology of menstrual migraine. *Neurology* (Minneap.), **22:**355–65, 1972.

204. Stevens, H. "Jumping Frenchmen of Main," myriachit. *Arch. Neurol.,* **12:**311–14, 1965.

205. Stevens, H. Paroxysmal choreo-athetosis. A form of reflex epilepsy. *Arch. Neurol.,* **14:**415–20, 1966.

206. Stevens, H., and Ammerman, B. J. Late onset epilepsy. *Med. Ann. D.C.,* **41:**236–39, 1972.

207. Stevens, J. R. Focal abnormality in petit mal: Intracranial recordings and pathologic findings. *Neurology* (Minneap.), **20:**1069–76, 1970.

208. Strauss, H. Paroxysmal compulsive running and the concept of epilepsia cursiva. *Neurology* (Minneap.), **10:**341–44, 1960.

209. Suhren, O.; Bruyn, G. W.; and Tuynman, J. A. Hyperexplexia. A hereditary startle syndrome. *J. Neurol. Sci.,* **3:**577–605, 1966.

210. Sulibhavi, D. G., and Schneck, L. Myoclonus epilepsy in progressive disease. In Charlton, M. H. (ed.). *Myoclonic Seizures.* Roche Monograph Series Exerpta Medica, Amsterdam, 1975, pp. 60–76.

211. Surgery for epilepsy. *Br. Med. J.,* **1:**924, 1976.

211a. Swanson, J. W., and Vick, N. A. Basilar artery migraine. 12 patients with an attack recorded electroencephalographically. *Neurology* (Minneap.), **28:**782–86, 1978.

212. Sweet, R. D.; Solomon, G. E.; Wayne, H.; Shapiro, E.; and Shapiro, A. K. Neurological features of Gilles de la Tourette's syndrome. *J. Neurol. Neurosurg. Psychiat.,* **36:**1–9, 1973.

212a. Takeoka, T.; Gotoh, F.; et al. Tolosa-Hunt syndrome. Arteriographic evidence of improvement in carotid narrowing. *Arch. Neurol.,* **35:**219–23, 1978.

213. Taylor, D. C. Aggression and epilepsy. *J. Psychosom. Res.,* **13:**229–36, 1969.

214. Taylor, D. C., and Ounsted, C. Biological mechanisms influencing the outcome of seizures in response to fever. *Epilepsia,* **12:**33–45, 1971.

214a. Terrance, C., and Alberts, M. Phenytoin dosage in ambulant epileptic patients. *J. Neurol. Neurosurg. Psychiatry,* **41:**463–65, 1978.

215. Torrey, E. F. Chloroquine seizures. *J.A.M.A.,* **204:**115–18, 1968.

216. Toyada, M., and Meyer, J. S. Effects of cerebral ischemic seizures and anoxia on arterial concen-

trations of catecholamines. *Cardiovasc. Res. Cent. Bull.,* **8:**59–73, 1969.

217. Triedman, H. M.; Fishman, R. A.; and Yahr, M. D. Determination of plasma and cerebrospinal fluid of Dilantin in the human. *Trans. Am. Neurol. Assoc.,* **85:**166–70, 1960.

218. Uesu, C. T.; Eisenman, J. I.; and Stemmer, E. A. The problem of dizziness and syncope in old age: Transient ischemic attacks versus hypersensitive carotid sinus reflex. *J. Am. Geriatr. Soc.,* **24:**126–35, 1976.

218a. Vajda, F. J. E.; Mihaly, G. W.; et al. Rectal administration of sodium valproate in status epilepticus. *Neurology* (Minneap.), **28:**897–99, 1978.

219. Van Woert, M. M.; Rosenbaum, D.; et al. Longterm therapy of myoclonus and other neurologic disorders with L-5-hydroxytryptophan and carbidopa. *N. Engl. J. Med.,* **296:**70–75, 1977.

220. Van Woert, M. H.; Yip, L. C.; and Bales, M. E. Purine phosphororibosyltransferase in Gilles de la Tourette syndrome. *N. Engl. J. Med.,* **296:**210–12, 1977.

221. Vardi, Y.; Rabay, J. M.; et al. Migraine attacks. Alleviation by an inhibitor of prostaglandin synthesis and action. *Neurology* (Minneap.), **26:**447–50, 1976.

222. Vercelletto, P., and Delobel, R. Etiology and prognosis of epilepsy after age 60 years. *Sem. Hôp. Paris,* **60:**3133–37, 1970.

223. Vijayan, N. A new post-traumatic headache syndrome: Clinical and therapeutic observations. *Headache,* **17:**19–22, 1977.

224. Walker, A. E. Critique and perspectives. In Purpura, D. P.; Penry, J. K.; and Walker, R. D. (eds.). *Advances in Neurology,* Vol. 8. Raven Press, New York, 1975, pp. 333–49.

225. Walker, D. O. Spectral analysis of electroencephalograms, Mathematical determination of neurophysiological relationships from records of limited duration. *Exp. Neurol.,* **8:**155–81, 1963.

226. Wallis, W.; Kutt, H.; and McDowell, F. Intravenous diphenylhydantoin in treatment of acute repetitive seizures. *Neurology* (Minneap.), **18:**513–25, 1968.

227. Waltimo, O.; Hokkanen, E.; and Pirskanen, R. Intracranial arteriovenous malformations and headache. *Headache,* **15:**133–35, 1975.

228. Ward, A. A., Jr. Theoretical basis for surgical therapy in epilepsy. In Purpura, D. P.; Penry, J. K.; and Walter, R. D. (eds.). *Advances in Neurology,* Vol. 8. Raven Press, New York, 1975, pp. 23–35.

229. Ward, A. A.; Jr., and Schmidt, R. P. Some properties of single epileptic neurons. *Arch. Neurol.,* **5:**308–13, 1961.

230. Waters, W. E. Migraine: Intelligence, social class and familial prevalence. *Br. Med. J.,* **2:**77–81, 1971.

231. Waters, W. E., and O'Connor, P. J. Epidemiology of headache and migraine in women. *J. Neurol. Neurosurg. Psychiat.,* **34:**148–53, 1971.

232. Weber, R. B., and Reinmuth, O. M. The treatment of migraine with proprananol. *Neurology* (Minneap.), **22:**366–69, 1972.

233. Weiss, G. H.; and Caveness, W. F. Prognostic factors in the persistence of posttraumatic epilepsy. *J. Neurosurg.,* **37:**164–69, 1972.

234. Welch, K. M. A.; Chabi, E.; et al. Cerebrospinal fluid gamma aminobutyric acid levels in migraine. *Br. Med. J.,* **4:**516–17, 1975.

235. Whitty, C. W. M. Migraine variants. *Br. Med. J.,* **1:**38–40, 1971.

236. Wik, B., and Hillestad, L. Deglutition syncope. *Br. Med. J.,* **2:**747, 1975.

237. Wilkinson, M. Migraine—Treatment of acute attack. *Br. Med. J.,* **2:**754–55, 1971.

237a. Willmore, L. J.; Wilder, B. J.; et al. Effect of valproic acid on hepatic function. *Neurology* (Minneap.), **28:**961–64, 1978.

238. Wilson, D. H.; Culver, C.; et al. Disconnection of the cerebral hemispheres. An alternative to hemispherectomy for the control of intractable seizures. *Neurology* (Minneap.), **25:**1149–53, 1975.

239. Yao, S. T., Goodwin, D. P.; and Kenyon, J. R. Case of ergot poisoning. *Br. Med. J.,* **3:**86–87, 1970.

240. Yap, C.-B.; Mayo, C.; and Barron, K. Ocular bobbing in palatal myoclonus. *Arch. Neurol.,* **18:**304–10, 1968.

241. Yokoi, S.; Austin, J.; Witmer, F.; and Sakai, M. Studies in myoclonus epilepsy (Lafora body form), 1) Isolation and preliminary characterization of Lafora bodies in two cases. *Arch. Neurol.,* **19:**15–33, 1968.

242. Young, G. F.; Leon-Barth, C. A.; and Green, J. Familial hemiplegic migraine, retinal degeneration, deafness and nystagmus. *Arch. Neurol.,* **23:**201–209, 1920.

243. Zarcone, V. Narcolepsy. *N. Engl. J. Med.,* **288:**1156–66, 1973.

7 INFECTIONS OF THE CENTRAL NERVOUS SYSTEM

Anatomic Considerations

Mechanisms to counter infection within the central nervous system are perhaps less effective and not as well developed as elsewhere in the body. Hence, organisms of relatively mild pathogenicity may cause severe infections such as meningitis or brain abscess. Although antibody production within the nervous system does occur, it is not a particularly active process. Furthermore, the passage of antibodies and inflammatory cells into the central nervous system is hindered by the blood-brain barrier. The situation is complicated further because cerebrospinal fluid provides an almost ideal culture medium for infectious agents. Under normal circumstances, the central nervous system is well protected by the surrounding tissues (including skin, mucous membrane, muscle, bone, meninges, and the blood-brain barrier) which prevent the entry of bacteria, viruses, and toxic substances into the central nervous system.

The Blood-Brain Barrier

The so-called "blood-brain barrier" is more of a physiologic concept than a well-defined anatomic structure. The term was first introduced when it was demonstrated that, under normal circumstances, injected vital dyes, e.g., trypan blue, failed to leave the circulation and stain the gray and white matter of the central nervous system. The blood-brain barrier, however, is not complete since trypan blue will regularly stain certain areas such as the pituitary gland, infundibulum, tuber cinereum, supraoptic area, pineal gland, area postrema, and choroid plexus. These areas also tend to concentrate radioactive materials following intravenous injection. Why the blood-brain barrier is incomplete at these sites is unknown. They do not appear to act as sites of reduced "resistance" during systemic infections.

The demonstration that endothelial cells of cerebral capillaries possess tight junctions between the plasmalemma of adjacent cells provides an anatomic basis for a blood-brain barrier. Since the endothelial cells form what is essentially a continuous membranous barrier between the blood and the brain parenchyma, the two-way flux of substances across the blood-brain barrier is probably both diffusion- and carrier-mediated. At least eight independent carrier systems have been identified, and each system mediates the transport of an essential substrate into the brain.[243]

The difference in ion content between the blood plasma and brain extracellular fluid (i.e., CSF) suggests that the blood-brain barrier acts as a two-way pump. The activities of a transport system and a pump require ATPase-dependent energy consumption, and the high concentration of mitochondria in the capillary endothelia suggests that the blood-brain barrier is a high-energy-consuming structure.[237]

Routes of Infection

The central nervous system may be infected by a number of routes, not all of which entail passing across the blood-brain barrier. These are:

1. Blood-borne infections
   a. Arterial
   b. Arterial with passage through the choroid plexus into the cerebrospinal fluid
   c. Venous with retrograde infection of the central nervous system
2. Direct infection
   a. Traumatic due to penetrating wounds
   b. Nontraumatic with passage of infection by direct extension from nearby structures
3. Retrograde passage along nerve trunks
4. Direct infection of the cerebrospinal fluid. This is rare, although it may result from trauma or poor technique during lumbar puncture.

Once infection has gained access to the cerebrospinal fluid, it flourishes and frequently invades the central nervous system since the cerebrospinal fluid-brain barrier is a less effective defense mechanism compared to the blood-brain barrier.

Abscess, Empyema, and Effusion

Infection may extend from a focus immediately adjacent to or within the skull (e.g., from sinusitis or mastoiditis) and produce the following:

1. Epidural abscess
2. Subdural empyema
3. Leptomeningitis
4. Cerebral or brain abscess

Cranial Epidural Abscess

The dura mater is firmly attached to the inner table of the cranial cavity so that cranial epidural abscesses are usually small. A cranial epidural abscess usually arises from extension into the epidural space from acute or chronic sinusitis, acute or chronic mastoiditis, or osteomyelitis of the skull.[99] The infection may progress through the dura to produce a subdural empyema, leptomeningitis, or brain abscess. Occasionally the abscess is iatrogenic and represents postoperative sepsis following craniotomy and the use of foreign material such as a graft, dural substitutes, or a tantalum button.[105]

Clinical Features

A small epidural abscess should be suspected when pain and fever persist after surgical drainage of infected mastoid air cells or chronic sinusitis.

Occasionally, a cranial epidural abscess may reach a sufficient size and cause headache, contralateral focal motor seizures, hemiparesis, drowsiness, stupor, and papilledema.

A cranial epidural abscess situated at the tip of the petrous temporal bone and usually associated with apical petrositis characteristically produces paralysis and irritation of the overlying fifth and sixth cranial nerves. The signs are almost pathognomonic and are termed Gradenigo's syndrome. Irritation of the fifth cranial nerve produces pain over the face, particularly in the retroorbital area. Involvement of the sixth cranial nerve produces paralysis of the lateral rectus muscle on the same side, with internal strabismus, diplopia, and inability to abduct the eye.

Diagnostic Procedures

1. Roentgenograms of the skull usually show clouding of the mastoid air cells or paranasal sinuses which indicate the initial focus of infection or reveal changes compatible with osteomyelitis of the skull.
2. Computed tomography shows a crescent-

shaped area of reduced density between the inner table of the skull and the brain.[200] There is contrast enhancement of the displaced dura which forms a thin rim on the inner aspect of the abscess cavity.

3. Lumbar puncture reveals clear cerebrospinal fluid or several hundred cells. When cell numbers are elevated, they are usually polymorphonuclear leukocytes and are indicative of an adjacent but sterile inflammatory reaction. The protein content of the cerebrospinal fluid may be increased but the glucose and chloride levels are usually normal.

4. Any discharge (e.g., from the middle ear or sinuses) should be cultured and tests for sensitivity to various antibiotics should be performed to aid in selection of the appropriate antibiotic therapy.

Treatment

The abscess should be drained surgically with removal of infected bone or foreign body. The source of the infection may also need surgical treatment, particularly in the case of chronic sinus infection or chronic mastoiditis. Appropriate antibiotics should be given in adequate dosage until the symptoms have subsided, the wound is healing, and the spinal fluid is free of cells. This usually requires a course of three to four weeks of vigorous therapy. The resolution of the abscess can be monitored by serial CT scans.

Cranial Subdural Empyema

This is not a common condition and is less frequently encountered since the advent of antibiotics. The term "subdural empyema" is correct since empyema denotes the presence of pus within a preformed cell-lined cavity.

Like epidural abscess, subdural empyema is usually secondary to infection of the paranasal sinuses or middle ear[60] but may also occur following penetrating wounds of the skull, osteomyelitis of the skull, infection of a subdural hematoma, and as a complication of a leptomeningitis or brain abscess. The subdural space may be infected by direct spread of infection from the middle ear or nasal sinus, but the most common route appears to be spread of infection via thrombophlebitis of the emissary veins traversing the subdural space.[141] This accounts for the development of an abscess some distance away from the original focus of infection.

The most common sites of subdural empyema are over the dorsolateral aspects of the hemispheres, over the frontal lobes, or medially in the subdural space of the falx cerebri. It rarely occurs over the inferior surface of the brain owing, presumably, to the close application of this surface to the floor of the cranial vault. The infection tends to spread through the subdural space, and an empyema beginning over the frontal lobe may extend as far back as the parietal lobe. Loculation is common with the formation of granulation tissue which binds together the surfaces of the dura and arachnoid. The most common infecting organisms are the β-hemolytic group A species of *Streptococcus* or *Staphylococcus aureus*. A tuberculous infection of the subdural space may result in the development of scattered miliary tubercles throughout the space or a tuberculoma en plaque. Syphilis may produce a granulomatous pachymeningitis.

Clinical Features

The clinical features are those of the initial infection, such as otitis media or sinusitis, with fever, leukocytosis, and a meningeal reaction with a positive Kernig's sign in most cases.

There is usually rapid progression with the appearance of focal neurologic signs such as fixed deviation of the eyes to the side opposite the lesion, focal seizures, hemiparesis, aphasia, and visual field defects.[33] In the case of empyema of the falx, the initial symptoms may include weakness and sensory changes in both lower limbs. There are often signs of increased intracranial pressure, with headache, vomiting, papilledema, and drowsiness. There may be rapid deterioration with unilateral dilatation of a pupil, Cheyne-Stokes respirations, decerebrate rigidity, and signs of progressive brainstem dysfunction. The mortality is approximately 40 per cent, and the persistent high fatality rate is due to late or delayed surgery in many cases.[324]

Diagnostic Procedures

1. Roentgenograms of the skull may show signs of otitis media, sinusitis, osteomyelitis, and displacement of the pineal gland.

2. Computed tomography shows an elliptic area of decreased density adjacent to the inner table of the skull. There may be displacement of the ipsilateral ventricle and midline structures.[169] Contrast enhancement produces a thin, dense crescent adjacent to the cortex in some cases.[173] The parasagittal empyema pre-

sents as a lucent area that separates the hemispheres. The demonstration of a subdural empyema by CT scanning is sufficient to permit surgery without arteriography in most cases. Postoperative CT scanning should be used to verify complete evacuation of the subdural empyema.

3. Lumbar puncture may be hazardous in subdural empyema and may be followed by acute brainstem compression. The lumbar puncture should not be performed if a diagnosis of subdural empyema is considered, and a CT scan should be obtained in such cases whenever there are signs of acute neurologic deficits. The CT scan will establish the presence of a subdural mass and the lumbar puncture will not be required.

4. The electroencephalogram shows unilateral slowing, frequently with voltage suppression recorded from head regions overlying the area of the empyema.

5. Arteriography will be required if CT scanning is not available. The arteriogram shows displacement of the cerebral vessels away from the skull by the subdural mass.

Differential Diagnosis

An extradural abscess seldom shows such well-marked focal features, and the cerebrospinal fluid is normal. Cortical thrombophlebitis is often indistinguishable clinically from subdural empyema, and angiography should be performed in disputed cases. A superficially located abscess of the brain may present greater difficulty in differential diagnosis but usually has a more protracted course with absence of rigidity.

Treatment

Adequate surgical drainage of both the subdural empyema and the focus of infection should be carried out and appropriate antibiotics should be given in adequate doses. Anticonvulsant drugs are usually necessary to control focal seizures.

Subdural Effusion

This condition occasionally occurs as a complication of meningitis in infants, particularly *Haemophilus influenzae,* type B. There is a transudate into the subdural space comparable to the sterile postpneumonia pleural effusions which complicate pneumococcal pneumonia. The fluid is usually clear or xanthochromic but may be bloody.

The condition should be suspected in an infant who had meningitis that appeared to respond to treatment with reduction of fever and improvement of the signs of meningitis but the child remained ill. Signs of increased intracranial pressure develop with bulging of the fontanel, separation of the sutures, seizures, and vomiting. The diagnosis is established by skull transillumination, aspiration of the fluid by means of a needle carefully inserted into the subdural space through the skin overlying the lateral angle of the anterior fontanel, or computed tomography.

Treatment

The fluid should be removed by serial subdural punctures via the lateral aspects of the fontanels. If the fluid cannot be removed by this means, craniotomy may be necessary.

Brain Abscess

Etiology

The incidence of abscess of the brain decreased following the introduction of antibiotic therapy, but there is evidence of stabilization or even some increase in the incidence of this condition in recent years.[100, 185, 342] There seems little doubt that there has been a continued reduction of brain abscess as a complication of middle ear infection. There is, however, more frequent isolation of anaerobic bacteria in cases of brain abscess, reflecting a change in the types of organisms responsible for this condition.[122, 194, 196, 267]

Direct Extension. Infection may spread from otitis media and mastoiditis or from frontal, ethmoidal, sphenoidal, or maxillary sinusitis.[108]

Cortical Thrombophlebitis. Infection from the middle ear or from the paranasal sinuses may extend into the cortical venous system and the dural sinuses. This commonly results in cortical thrombophlebitis and brain abscess. Similarly, but less frequently, the focus of infection giving rise to the brain abscess may be osteomyelitis of the skull, cellulitis, erysipelas of the face, or an abscess around an infected tooth.[224]

Penetrating Wounds of the Skull. Brain abscesses are encountered following gunshot wounds, particularly those which drive foreign material and soil into the brain. They were more common in World War I than in World War II, owing to improved emergency care, dressing of wounds, early surgery, and the use of sulfonamides. The incidence was further reduced in the Korean and Vietnam conflicts owing to the availability of wide-spectrum antibiotics and rapid evacuation of casualties to hospital facilities by air.

Septic Emboli. THORACOGENIC. Brain abscess may complicate chronic plumonary infections such as bronchiectasis, empyema, or abscess of the lung due to passage of septic material into the pulmonary veins and hence to the systemic circulation.

FROM THE HEART. Septic emboli arise directly from the heart in acute and subacute bacterial endocarditis. These are usually small and lodge in the peripherally located cerebral vessels and within their vasa vasorum. These may cause mycotic aneurysms, which usually respond to antibiotics. Emboli from *Candida endocarditis* tend to be larger, often resulting in a frank necrotic process of the brain. Brain abscess is also a frequent complication of congenital heart disease, with right-to-left shunt allowing emboli to bypass the lungs and enter the aorta and the cerebral arterial circulation.[185, 194, 196]

Unknown Etiology. Most published series show a considerable number of cases of unknown etiology. The surgeon may occasionally encounter an abscess when operating for what is believed to be a solid brain tumor.[185]

Location. The most common sites of brain abscess are the frontal and the parietal lobes.[108, 185, 196] They are also found in the temporal lobe as a complication of otitis media, and in the cerebellum and brainstem as a complication of mastoiditis.

Types of Organisms Causing Brain Abscess

Various types of bacteria, fungi, yeasts, and other organisms have been isolated from abscesses within the brain. The most common organisms found are streptococci (including anaerobic streptococci and enterococci),[69] *Staphylococcus aureus,* pneumococci and meningococci, organisms of the *Bacteroides* group, typhoid bacillus, *Escherichia coli, Proteus,* and *Bacillus pyocyaneus.*

Mixed infections usually occur in abscesses of the temporal lobe secondary to infection of the middle ear.[70] Yeasts are unusual causes of brain abscess, but blastomycosis, actinomycosis, nocar-

diosis, coccidioidomycosis, cryptococcosis, and *Candida albicans* organisms have all been isolated. The protozoal and metazoal infections are rare causes of brain abscess. These include amebiasis, paragonimiasis, and schistosomiasis. Later in this chapter, many of these infections will be considered separately.

Possibly because of the widespread use of antibiotics in the last 20 years, there has been a change in the incidence of bacterial types isolated from brain abscess, with an increased isolation of anaerobic streptococci and bacteroides. Prompt inoculation of pus and prompt incubation are mandatory in order to obtain cultures of anaerobic bacteria. Antibiotic inhibitors must be added to culture media if antibiotics have been used.

Pathology

Brain abscesses arising from blood-borne infection, whether arterial or venous, begin at the junction of gray and white matter. Multiple brain abscesses may occur, particularly when they result from septic emboli arising from the lung owing to bronchiectasis or lung abscess. The infection tends to spread into the white matter rather than the gray matter, probably because white matter has a relatively poor blood supply and a less rapid inflammatory response. Hence, brain abscesses tend to be found deep within the hemisphere rather than immediately below the surface.

The initial reaction within the brain is one of edema and congestion. This is followed by central necrosis and liquefaction with the formation of pus. There is marked edema around the abscess with proliferation of the fibroblasts that surround the blood vessels. The astroglia also proliferate and join with the fibroblasts to form a fibroglial capsule. There is always the danger, however, that the abscess will rupture into the ventricle or subarachnoid space and produce a fulminating and purulent meningitis.

Clinical Features

Brain abscess occurs at all ages, with a marked increase in incidence in the first ten years of life and between 20 and 50 years of age.[267] Childhood cases are predominantly associated with congenital heart disease.

There are four distinct clinical types of brain abscess.[344]

Type 1. Abscess Presenting as an Acute Expanding Focal Mass. A brain abscess often presents as a rapidly expanding intracranial mass lesion with a neurologic progression extending over a period of several hours to several weeks. The clinical signs are well-developed, permitting localization of the lesion to the cerebral hemisphere, cerebellum, or brainstem. The clinician tends to think in terms of a high-grade astrocytoma, metastatic tumor, or intracerebral hematoma unless the patient is known to have had an antecedent infection or shows signs of infection such as otitis media, sinusitis, pneumonia, bronchiectasis, or bacterial endocarditis.

Type 2. Abscess Presenting with Focal Neurologic Deficits Only. A chronic brain abscess may present with well-defined focal neurologic deficits with slowly progressive features. There is little or no evidence of raised intracranial pressure. The clinician tends to think in terms of a meningioma, low-grade astrocytoma, or subdural hematoma.

Type 3. Abscess with Signs of Rapidly Increasing Intracranial Pressure. There may be few localizing neurologic signs and a rapid increase in intracranial pressure when there are multiple abscesses or when the abscess is located in the prefrontal area or in the posterior part of the occipital lobe. Signs of increasing intracranial pressure with headache, vomiting, obtundation, mental dullness, personality change, and severe papilledema are prominent. Early diagnosis often depends on recognition of a focus of infection elsewhere.

Type 4. Abscess with Diffuse Brain Destruction. Multiple and often bilateral signs of neurologic impairment and progressive deterioration over a period of several days can occur in patients with multiple brain abscesses. The neurologic deficits are not due to increased intracranial pressure, and papilledema is mild or absent. The course of the disease is similar to that of a patient with multiple cerebral emboli.

Diagnostic Procedures

1. The white blood count is above 10,000/cu mm, with a polymorphonuclear leukocytosis in about 50 per cent of cases. The sedimentation rate is usually elevated, suggesting the presence of an abscess when an intracranial space-occupying lesion is suspected.[185]
2. Roentgenograms of the skull may reveal evidence of mastoiditis, sinusitis, or displacement of the pineal gland.

3. Computed tomography has significantly improved the diagnosis of brain abscess and should contribute to a reduction in mortality.[229] The plain CT scan shows low attenuation (decreased density) in the area of the abscess cavity and the surrounding edema. There is a shift of the midline and ventricular structures because of mass effect. Contrast enhancement produces a scan with a well-defined annular rim which may be irregular or regular in outline, representing peripherally displaced or newly formed blood vessels[231] (Fig. 7–1). The CT scan may show the presence of gas in the abscess cavity in some cases. Computed tomography will also demonstrate multiple abscess cavities more accurately than any other study.[175] Serial CT scans should be obtained in all cases treated with antibiotics for the pre-abscess stage of "cerebritis" and after surgical treatment of an abscess to demonstrate resolution of the disease.[256a]
4. The electroencephalogram is useful in the more chronic types of cerebral abscess. The EEG shows marked focal slowing around the site of the abscess. Occasionally there are spikes as well as high-voltage delta activity with phase reversal indicating the site of the abscess when the bipolar recording is used. A normal EEG is strong evidence against the presence of brain abscess.
5. Cerebral arteriograms with serial exposure are

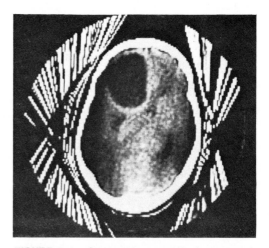

FIGURE 7–1. Computed tomography in a case of brain abscess showing a circumscribed area of decreased density in the left frontal area surrounded by a rim of contrast-enhanced tissue. There is a marked distortion of the ventricular system.

recommended in suspected cases of brain abscess when CT scanning is not available or when the neurosurgeon feels that additional information on the relationship of the blood vessels and the abscess is necessary. The radiologic picture is often highly suggestive of brain abscess. In addition to the displacement of blood vessels, owing to the mass effect of the abscess, there is a striking vascular blush with a translucent center in about 50 per cent of cases due to the crowding of numerous blood vessels surrounding the abscess and the proliferation of vessels in the capsule of the abscess.[232]

6. Lumbar puncture can be extremely hazardous in the presence of a brain abscess and increased intracranial pressure.[317, 324] Uncal or cerebellar tonsillar herniation may occur within minutes or hours of lumbar puncture, and the procedure is not recommended in suspected cases of brain abscess. It is unusual for brain abscess to present as "meningitis," and the lumbar puncture does not yield critical information in cases of brain abscess. If there are clinical signs of meningitis with lateralizing neurologic signs, computed tomography should be performed before lumbar puncture. However, lumbar puncture is occasionally performed as part of a diagnostic evaluation in more obscure cases of brain abscess. The opening pressure is usually increased. There are usually several hundred cells per cubic millimeter in the cerebrospinal fluid, which are predominantly polymorphonuclear in type. The culture will be sterile unless the abscess has ruptured into the subarachnoid or ventricular space. Glucose levels in the CSF are usually normal, but there tends to be an increase in the protein content.

Treatment

A brain abscess usually requires drainage. In most cases the neurosurgeon elects to make a wide craniotomy followed by extensive drainage of the abscess. However, repeated aspiration may be necessary for abscesses deeply situated in the cerebral hemispheres. The primary focus of infection should also be treated adequately and surgical drainage employed if necessary.[280]

Appropriate antibiotics should be used in adequate doses. This may produce resolution without surgical intervention in some early cases of cerebritis that have not yet undergone central necrosis and abscess formation. The patient should be given 20 million units of aqueous penicillin G daily in all cases of frontal lobe abscess and the same dose of aqueous penicillin G plus metronidazole, 400 to 600 mg every eight hours, for all other types of brain abscess[153, 317] due to the probable presence of anaerobic *Bacteroides* in these cases. Antibiotic therapy can be modified once the results of culture of the abscess material are available. Vigorous antibacterial therapy should be continued for three to four weeks. Focal epilepsy should be controlled with anticonvulsant drugs. Supportive care should include adequate fluid intake, replacement of the serum electrolytes so that they are controlled within the normal range, and good nursing care.

Prognosis

The mortality is known to correlate with the level of consciousness of the patient when the diagnosis of brain abscess is made. The comatose patient has an extremely poor prognosis.[172] Rupture of a brain abscess into the ventricular system is particularly lethal, and survivors may require a ventriculoatrial shunt for hydrocephalus. Multiple abscesses, particularly those associated with remote infection and septicemia, have a high mortality. However, the increasing use of CT scanning and improved methods of bacterial culture leading to the earlier use of appropriate antibiotics in brain abscess should reduce the mortality.

Thrombosis of the Dural Sinuses

Thrombosis or thrombophlebitis of the dural sinuses is usually a complication of infection of the middle ear, sinuses, nasopharynx, scalp, or face. Cavernous sinus thrombosis may be an unusual complication of infection by a species of the yeast mucormycosis in the diabetic patient. Cortical phlebothrombosis may also occur in noninfectious conditions such as during the hypercoagulable state that occurs following childbirth.

Anatomic Considerations

The dural or cerebral venous blood sinuses receive the venous drainage of the brain via the cerebral veins. The dural veins are endothelial tubes, lying within a strong, rigid layer of dura.

The Superior Longitudinal (Sagittal) Sinus. This begins at the foramen caecum, where it may communicate with the veins of the nasal mucosa and pass backward in the upper border of the falx cerebri. It grooves the vault of the skull to the torcular Herophili at the internal occipital protuberance. At the torcular Herophili about two thirds usually drains to the right and becomes continuous with the right lateral or transverse sinus. Small tributaries of the superior longitudinal sinus may include the nasal veins from the nasal mucous membrane, the middle meningeal veins, and the diploic veins, but the great preponderance of flow comes from the cerebral veins draining the hemispheres. The latter enter the sagittal sinus at an angle and empty blood against the current of flow in the sinus. The majority of venous flow from the right hemisphere drains into the right lateral and transverse sinuses, while blood from the left hemisphere drains into the left transverse sinus.

The sagittal sinus communicates with the middle cerebral vein through the great anastomotic vein of Trolard and indirectly with the lateral sinus via the inferior anastomotic vein of Labbé.

The Transverse Sinuses. These begin at the internal occipital protuberance on the right as a continuation of the superior sagittal sinus and on the left as a continuation of the straight sinus. The transverse sinuses pass laterally in the edge of the tentorium cerebelli, groove the occipital bone to the posteroinferior angle of the parietal bone, and then become continuous with the sigmoid sinuses.

The Sigmoid Sinuses. These pass downward and medially to the jugular foramen and groove the mastoid portion of the temporal bone. Both sinuses empty into the internal jugular veins.

The tributaries of the transverse sinuses include the ipsilateral cerebellar veins from the cerebellar hemispheres. A few tributary veins from the mastoid process of the temporal bone, and the veins from the base of the skull via the condylar foramina drain into the sigmoid sinuses, but less than 10 per cent of the venous drainage is of extracerebral origin.

The Cavernous Sinus. The cavernous sinus arises from the ophthalmic vein behind the superior orbital fissure and passes along the floor of the middle cranial fossa and grooves lateral aspect of the sphenoid bone. It ends at the level of the dorsum sellae by dividing into the superior and inferior petrosal sinuses.

The medial wall of the sinus is closely related to the pituitary gland and the infundibulum. The lateral wall contains the third, fourth, sixth, and ophthalmic division of the fifth cranial nerves. The internal carotid artery enters the sinus inferiorly and posteriorly and passes anteriorly for a short distance before leaving by bending sharply upward and penetrating the roof of the sinus opposite the anterior clinoid process.

The two cavernous sinuses communicate with each other through the intercavernous sinuses, which pass anteriorly and posteriorly to the dorsum sellae. The ophthalmic veins are tributaries that drain into the cavernous sinus anteriorly. These veins receive blood from the anterior facial vein and the pterygoid plexus of veins and form an important means for spread of infection from these structures to the cavernous sinus. The superior and inferior petrosal sinuses form a communication posteriorly between the cavernous sinus and the transverse sinus and jugular vein, respectively.

Pathogenesis

Thrombosis of a dural sinus without involvement of the cortical veins is relatively rare, and the signs and symptoms associated with thrombosis of any dural sinus are frequently those of the associated cortical thrombophlebitis.

Dural sinus thrombosis and cortical thrombophlebitis and phlebothrombosis may be seen in association with the following conditions:

1. Primary Thrombosis of the Dural Sinuses and Cortical Veins. This includes:

a. Heart disease associated with heart failure due to congenital lesions, rheumatic heart disease, hypertension, and arteriosclerotic heart disease.

b. Cachexia in terminal malignancy or severe dehydration in chronically debilitated patients.

c. Marasmatic infants.

d. Dehydration due to gastrointestinal infections such as dysentery or typhoid fever.

e. Postoperative hypercoagulable state following abdominal, thoracic, or thyroid surgery.

f. Hypernatremia, owing to intrauterine instillation of hypertonic saline in therapeutic abortion.[114]

g. Posttraumatic states following closed head injury.

h. After cerebral arterial thrombosis or hemorrhage.

i. Post partum.

j. In blood dyscrasias, particularly leukemia.

k. Following fever therapy in the past or hyperpyrexia.

2. Secondary (Septic) Thrombosis of Dural Sinuses and Cortical Veins. This is seen:

a. Following infections of scalp, skull, middle ear, mastoid air cells, paranasal sinuses, or face.

b. Following a generalized septicemia.

Superior Longitudinal (Sagittal) Sinus Thrombosis: General Considerations

Thrombosis of the superior longitudinal sinus may be an incidental finding at autopsy. It may, however, be associated with thrombosis of the cortical veins in the postpartum period or following the spread of a nearby infectious process.

Postpartum Thrombosis of the Superior Longitudinal Sinus

This condition is a rare complication of pregnancy and usually occurs several hours to several weeks after delivery. The etiology is unknown, but certain factors such as increased blood volume, hypercoagulability, increased serum fibrinogen levels, and sudden decrease in blood pressure may contribute to thrombosis during the puerperium.[115, 199, 252]

Pathology

In puerperal cases, the cortical veins and the superior longitudinal sinus contain thrombus, which seems to arise from a plug of gray thrombus lying at the junction of the cortical veins with the superior longitudinal sinus.

The brain shows numerous small hemorrhages at the junction of the cortical venules and the obstructed cortical veins. There may be severe cerebral edema and hemorrhages or nonhemorrhagic cerebral infarction in areas of cortical venous thrombosis.

Clinical Features

Symptoms may occur in a period varying from a few hours to several weeks after delivery. There is severe headache often followed by one or more generalized seizures or by partial seizures and hemiparesis. Status epilepticus and coma occur in some cases. In others, involvement of the dominant hemisphere produces aphasia with contralateral hemiplegia. A fluctuating hypertension develops in response to any rise in intracranial pressure. Noncomatose patients may exhibit confusion and psychotic symptoms.

When the condition has been present for a few days, papilledema with fullness of the temporal veins, and edema of the scalp may be found on the side of the cortical venous thrombosis. Computed tomography appearances are compatible with diffuse cerebral edema.

Nonpuerperal Thrombosis of the Superior Longitudinal Sinus

Superior longitudinal sinus thrombosis has also been described following trauma, dehydration and cachexia, congestive heart failure,[311] polycythemia vera, hemolytic anemia, thrombocytopenia, sickle cell disease, cryofibrinogenemia, diffuse intravascular coagulation, paroxysmal nocturnal hemoglobinuria, ulcerative colitis, diabetes mellitus, and cerebral arterial occlusion.

A number of cases of idiopathic thrombosis of the superior longitudinal sinus have been described, and the condition is known to occur in some cases of benign intracranial hypertension (pseudotumor cerebri). There are several case reports of superior longitudinal sinus thrombosis in young women using oral contraceptives.[110]

Secondary (Septic) Thrombosis of the Superior Longitudinal Sinus

Superior longitudinal sinus thrombosis may occur during infections of the middle ear or mastoid air cells. An initial thrombosis of the lateral sinus may spread through the torcular Herophili to the superior longitudinal sinus. Extension may also occur via the anastomotic veins of the cortex from the transverse sinus to the superior longitudinal sinus.

Pathology

Infection of the middle ear or paranasal sinus may be complicated by extradural, subdural, intracerebral, or cerebellar abscess. The transverse sinus, superior longitudinal sinus, and cortical veins contain a red thrombus, and there are scattered areas of hemorrhagic or nonhemorrhagic infarction of the brain, particularly in the cortex and subjacent white matter in the parasagittal region, bilaterally.

Clinical Features

The clinical signs include those due to the initial infection such as otitis media and sinusitis, plus seizures, hemiparesis, paraparesis, perceptual disorders, hemianopia, and dysphasia.

Diagnostic Procedures

1. Roentgenogram of the skull may show clouding of the nasal sinuses or mastoid air cells.
2. Lumbar puncture usually reveals a clear cerebrospinal fluid under increased pressure. There is a small or moderate number of red cells, but occasionally the fluid will be bloody in cases where there has been marked cortical venous hemorrhage.
3. Electroencephalography shows focal slowing over the affected hemisphere but this may be obscured by generalized slowing in a semicomatose or comatose patient.
4. Angiography with serial exposures will demonstrate absence of filling of the superior longitudinal sinus in the venous phase.
5. Computed tomography shows severe cerebral edema and areas of infarction in the superior cortical regions of the hemispheres.
6. Dynamic radionuclide scanning is a rapid noninvasive procedure that will demonstrate dural sinus thrombosis using an 80-lens optical camera.[18]

Treatment

1. In secondary (septic) cases the appropriate antibiotic therapy should be given to control infection and surgical drainage should be instituted when necessary.
2. In all cases:
   a. Status epilepticus requires immediate control by emergency use of anticonvulsant drugs.
   b. Occasional generalized or focal seizures can be controlled by adequate oral drugs.
   c. Intracranial pressure should be reduced by repeated lumbar puncture or by the use of agents that control cerebral edema such as dexamethasone or mannitol. Subtemporal decompression should be reserved for acute cases with life-threatening increase in intracranial pressure or for those who might suffer irreversible neurologic deficits from a chronic increase in intracranial pressure.
   d. The fluid and electrolyte balance should be maintained by daily measurement of fluid intake and output and measurement of the serum electrolytes.
   e. Anticoagulant therapy is not recommended because of the danger of cerebral hemorrhage.

Transverse Sinus Thrombosis

Since the transverse sinus lies in close relationship to the middle ear, thrombosis may result from acute otitis media, mastoiditis, or chronic middle ear infections associated with cholesteatoma. It is possible that infections of the neck may result in thrombosis of the jugular vein, with retrograde extension of the thrombus to cause transverse sinus thrombosis.

Pathology

Thrombosis of the transverse sinus usually has little effect unless it spreads to involve the superior longitudinal sinus and the cortical veins. The effects of this type of thrombosis have been described under Superior Longitudinal Thrombosis.

Clinical Features

Transverse sinus thrombosis is frequently asymptomatic. It may produce symptoms of headache and raised intracranial pressure without focal features. This usually occurs in children, tends to resolve spontaneously, and is similar to benign intracranial hypertension (p. 302). The term "otitic hydrocephalus" has also been used for this condition.

An extension of the thrombosis into the jugular vein is followed by tenderness and swelling on that side of the neck and paralysis of the ninth, tenth, and eleventh cranial nerves. Paralysis of the twelfth nerve occurs less commonly and is due to thrombosis of the anterior condylar vein. Spread to the inferior petrosal sinus may produce sixth-nerve (lateral rectus) paralysis. Extension of the thrombosis into the superior longitudinal sinus and to the cortical veins will produce symptoms similar to those described under the heading Superior Longitudinal Sinus Thrombosis.

Diagnostic procedures and treatment have been outlined under Superior Longitudinal Sinus Thrombosis (p. 395).

Cavernous Sinus Thrombosis

Thrombosis of the cavernous sinus may be due to:

1. Secondary (septic) thrombosis
   a. Acute
   b. Chronic
2. Primary thrombosis, which is rare and is usually associated with trauma, tumor growth at the base of the skull, or polycythemia vera[211]

Acute Cavernous Sinus Thrombosis

This condition is usually secondary (septic) in type. Most commonly, it is caused by infections that originate on the face and spread through the angular vein into the sinus. It may also occur following infection of the sphenoidal, ethmoidal, and frontal sinuses or by spread of infection from the transverse sinus or jugular vein through the petrosal sinuses to the cavernous sinus. Unilateral thrombosis of one sinus commonly spreads to the other within a few days via the intercavernous sinuses.

Clinical Features

The clinical picture is highly characteristic. It includes signs of a generalized septic infection with fever, rigors, headache, nausea, and vomiting. There are also neurologic signs of involvement of the third, fourth, sixth, and ophthalmic divisions of the fifth cranial nerves in their passage through the cavernous sinus.

Obstruction of the ophthalmic veins produces edema of the orbit and eyelids, with ptosis, chemosis, and edema of the periorbital structures, forehead, and face (Fig. 7–2). The obstruction of venous return from the eye produces marked venous engorgement, hemorrhage, edema of the retina, and papilledema, with reduction or loss of vision. Obstruction of the pterygoid plexus produces edema of the pharynx.

Involvement of the third, fourth, and sixth nerves results in complete internal and external

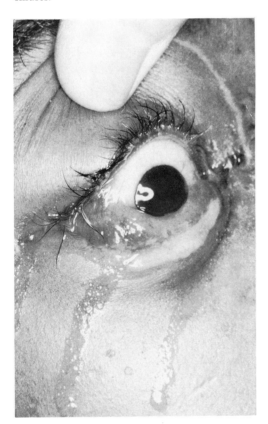
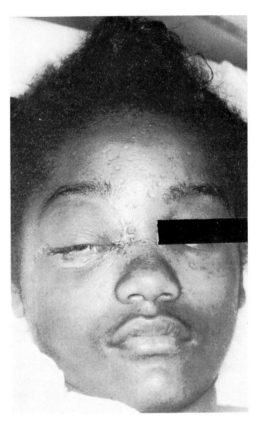

A　　　　　　　　　　　　　　**B**

FIGURE 7–2. A case of unilateral cavernous sinus thrombosis due to an infected penetrating wound in the region of the ethmoid sinus. *A.* Edema and congestion of the orbit with ptosis and extraocular paralysis. *B.* Facial appearance.

ophthalmoplegia, and involvement of the carotid sympathetic plexus contributes to the ptosis. Involvement of the ophthalmic division of the fifth nerve produces pain in the eye which radiates over the supraorbital zone to the forehead and scalp. Initially there is excess lacrimation, but later this may become reduced and anesthesia of the cornea may occur. Spread of the thrombosis through the intercavernous sinuses results in bilateral cavernous sinus thrombosis and the appearance of identical signs on the opposite side.

Differential Diagnosis

Orbital cellulitis may produce many of the symptoms of cavernous sinus thrombosis and may be a precursor of the latter condition. Exophthalmic ophthalmoplegia is not so rapid in onset and the patient does not exhibit the toxic and febrile features of cavernous sinus thrombosis. Orbital and retro-orbital tumors are more chronic, with the gradual development of signs and symptoms. Carotid-cavernous fistula produces similar signs, is acute in onset, and usually follows head injury. Both spontaneous and posttraumatic carotid-cavernous fistulas present with pulsating exophthalmos and loud murmurs over the eye and forehead, which may be modified by compression of the ipsilateral carotid artery.

Diagnostic Procedures

1. Roentgenograms of the skull usually reveal infection of the paranasal sinuses or of the orbit.
2. Lumbar puncture usually reveals clear cerebrospinal fluid with normal or slightly increased pressure. In a number of cases acute meningitis may complicate cavernous sinus thrombosis, and the CSF will then be cloudy with increased pressure, a polymorphonuclear pleocytosis, increased protein, and decreased glucose content. The infecting organism can be obtained by culture.
3. Serial angiography, using a submental view, may reveal absence of filling of the cavernous sinus.
4. Injection of contrast material into the frontal vein will show filling of the veins of the apex of the orbit but no filling of the cavernous and inferior petrosal sinuses.[195] Orbital and skull base phlebography is the only method that will demonstrate or exclude cavernous sinus thrombosis with any degree of certainty.[38]

Treatment

Infection should be controlled as soon as possible with appropriate and adequate antibiotic therapy. If penicillins are used while awaiting a report of culture and sensitivity, penicillin G and methicillin should be administered by vein (e.g., approximately 42 million units of penicillin G and 8 gm of methicillin). Amphotericin B (25 to 35 mg per day by vein) should be used immediately in cavernous sinus thrombosis accompanying acute diabetic acidosis.

Surgical drainage of infected paranasal sinuses, orbits, and cellulitis of the face will be necessary in some cases. The use of intravenous thrombolytic enzymes such as activated human plasmin is believed by some to benefit cases of cavernous sinus thrombosis.

Cavernous sinus thrombosis was almost invariably fatal in the preantibiotic era. The course and prognosis have changed dramatically, since the introduction of penicillin. Although the condition should always be regarded as a grave complication of an infectious process, the prognosis is good with adequate antibiotic therapy.

Chronic Cavernous Sinus Thrombosis

Chronic thrombosis of the cavernous sinus is a much rarer condition than the acute fulminating disease. The infection begins as a slowly progressive thrombophlebitis of one of the efferent channels that drains the cavernous sinus with chronic extension and slow obliteration of the cavernous sinus. The focus of infection may be in the mouth, nasopharynx, paranasal sinuses, or middle ear.

Clinical Features

Chronic cavernous sinus thrombosis presents with recurrent fever and signs of infection followed by the development of retro-orbital pain. Signs of oculomotor and trigeminal nerve involvement appear after several weeks of discomfort, and there is little or no evidence of the periorbital edema that is so characteristic of the acute form of the disease.[300] Diagnostic procedures and treatment have been described under Acute Cavernous Sinus Thrombosis (p. 397).

Meningitis

The term "meningitis" is synonymous with leptomeningitis and denotes an infection of the cerebrospinal fluid with inflammation involving the pia-arachnoid, subarachnoid space, and, to a lesser extent, the superficial tissues of the brain and spinal cord. The meningeal infections are divided into two main groups for purposes of description and discussion:

1. Acute bacterial meningitis
2. Subacute and chronic meningitis

Both groups have shown a remarkable reduction in mortality and morbidity since the introduction of antibiotics. Nevertheless, meningitis remains a serious illness and a medical emergency requiring early diagnosis and prompt treatment. There is evidence that antibiotics have reduced the frequency of meningeal infection by certain organisms and have increased the isolation of what were formerly rare forms. An increase in *Staphylococcus aureus* and gram-negative organisms as common causes of meningitis has recently been reported from some centers. Should this trend continue, the mortality may increase again and add to the problems of selection of appropriate antibiotic treatment.

Acute Bacterial Meningitis

A wide variety of organisms produce acute purulent meningitis once they enter the cerebrospinal fluid. The prevention of infection depends on the blood-brain and blood-CSF barriers, but once the organism crosses the barrier and enters the subarachnoid space, it flourishes in an ideal culture medium that has little or no capacity for antibody formation. Immunoglobulins in serum have scant access to the cerebrospinal fluid. Furthermore, the circulation of the CSF aids in the rapid dissemination of the infecting organisms throughout the subarachnoid space.

There are considerable differences in the type of meningeal infection according to age. The incidence of the commonly isolated bacteria according to age is shown in Table 7–1. Infections by gram-negative enterobacilli, particularly *Escherichia coli,* are commonest in the neonatal period up to 30 days of age. In infants 31 to 60 days of age the majority of cases of acute purulent meningitis are caused by β-hemolytic streptococci, followed by *Haemophilus influenzae* and *Neisseria meningitidis,* and there is a marked reduction in meningeal infection due to gram-negative enterobacilli. From two months to four years of age the major pathogen is *H. influenzae* followed by *N. meningitidis* and *Streptococcus pneumoniae.* However, infection by *H. influenzae* decreases abruptly after three years of age, and meningitis in older children and adults is caused predominantly by *S. pneumoniae* and *N. meningitidis.*

When *H. influenzae* meningitis occurs after ten years of age, it is nearly always associated with an immunoglobulin deficiency, a dural defect, or direct spread of infection from a nearby focus.[190] There has been an increase in the past 20 years of cases of acute purulent meningitis where attempted culture of the organisms has been unsuccessful, presumably owing to the adminstration of antibiotics to the patient before admission to hospital. As mentioned previously, a number of centers have reported a decrease in the number of cases of meningitis caused by *Streptococcus pyogenes* and an increase in the number due to *Staphylococcus aureus* and gram-negative bacilli.

TABLE 7–1

Incidence of Acute Purulent Meningitis (Columns in Descending Order of Frequency)

Neonatal Period (up to 30 Days)	Infants (31 to 60 Days)	Children (2 mo to 4 yr)	Older Children and Adults
Gram-negative enterobacilli	β-hemolytic streptococci	*Haemophilus influenzae*	*Streptococcus pneumoniae*
β-hemolytic streptococci	*Haemophilus influenzae*	*Neisseria meningitidis*	*Neisseria meningitidis*
Listeria monocytogenes	*Neisseria meningitidis*	*Streptococcus pneumoniae*	*Staphylococcus aureus*
Staphylococcus aureus	Gram-negative enterobacilli		*Haemophilus influenzae*
Streptococcus pneumoniae			

Most of these cases occurred in hospital as complications of serious neoplastic or congenital diseases. The change in the epidemiology of such hospitalized cases of meningitis, with reduction of hemolytic streptococci as a cause, is almost certainly due to the widespread use of antibiotics with emergence of resistant strains of *Staphylococcus aureas* within the hospital environment.

Pathogenesis and Pathology

Infection may reach the leptomeninges and subarachnoid space by the following routes:

1. Direct implantation after open head wounds
2. Direct extension from an infectious process involving the middle ear, paranasal sinuses, scalp, or face
3. Via the bloodstream during septicemia or bacteremia
4. By extension from cortical thrombophlebitis
5. By extension from extradural, subdural, or brain abscesses
6. Via the cribriform plate in chronic or recurrent cerebrospinal fluid rhinorrhea

Once infection reaches the leptomeninges, it is rapidly disseminated throughout the ventricular system and the subarachnoid space. In bloodborne infections it is possible that the organisms reach the meninges through the choroid plexus and are disseminated by the circulating cerebrospinal fluid.

The initial reaction to infection is an acute inflammatory response. The meninges develop a cloudy or milky appearance, owing to the production of an inflammatory exudate from the congested vessels. The exudate accumulates in the cisterns around the base of the brain, but in some cases becomes particularly thick over the superior aspects of the convexities of the hemispheres where the circulating cerebrospinal fluid is absorbed by the arachnoid villi, which are relatively impermeable to the inflammatory cells. The exudate is also seen covering the choroid plexus and lining the walls of the ventricular system. There is a gradual obstruction to the circulation of the cerebrospinal fluid, both internally and externally, with progressive ventricular dilatation in cases of several weeks' duration. Cortical venous thrombosis is not uncommon, and dural sinus thrombosis may be a terminal feature.

The cellular content of the exudate is almost entirely polymorphonuclear in the early stages of infection, with a gradual increase in lymphocytes and the appearance of larger mononuclear cells after several days. The appearance of mononuclear cells is accelerated and the amount of fibrin may be increased by antibiotic therapy. The infecting organisms are seen within the inflammatory cells and occasionally lying free in the subarachnoid space.

The superficial layers of the brain and spinal cord show perivascular cuffing by inflammatory cells, and there may be inflammation and thrombosis of both arteries and veins with surrounding edema and degeneration of neurons. This is always present to some degree and is no doubt responsible for some of the symptoms seen in this disease. Consequently, acute purulent meningitis should also be regarded as a superficial encephalitis.

Clinical Features

In the neonate acute purulent meningitis may present as a severe febrile illness with few localizing signs. There is frequently a history of premature or traumatic delivery, premature rupture of the membranes, cesarean section, or maternal infection prior to delivery. The onset is sudden, with high fever, dyspnea, poor feeding, jaundice, drowsiness, and a poor Moro response. This may be followed by convulsions and coma, the development of opisthotonus with apneic spells, and the detection of a bulging fontanel and cranial nerve palsies.

Infants and younger children show a somewhat different clinical picture with poor feeding, irritability, and confusion at the onset, followed by lethargy, convulsions, and coma. Older children may complain of headache and pain in the neck. Examination shows fever, skin petechiae, a high-pitched cry, and a bulging fontanel. The Kernig and Brudzinski signs are positive, and there are cranial nerve palsies and generalized hyperreflexia. Lumbar puncture will confirm the diagnosis and should be performed in all cases of suspected meningitis.[164]

Meningitis in older children and adults can be classified into three clinical groups:

Group 1. A rapid onset with fever, headache, and stiffness of the neck followed by drowsiness, confusion, and loss of consciousness.

Group 2. A slowly progressive illness characterized by fever, headache, and nuchal rigidity developing over a period of one to seven days with signs of associated upper respiratory tract infection and drowsiness but no loss of consciousness.

Group 3.   A sudden onset with fever and headache followed by acute shock with hypotension and tachycardia due to an overwhelming septicemia.

In groups 1 and 2, examination usually reveals neck stiffness with positive Kernig and Brudzinski signs, unless the patient is deeply comatose. A petechial rash is to be expected in meningococcal meningitis and can occur in both pneumococcal and *Haemophilus* infections. Cranial nerve involvement occurs in the subarachnoid space resulting in inequality of the pupils, paresis, or paralysis of eye movement and strabismus. Other focal signs, such as hemiparesis, deviation of the head and eyes, inequality of reflexes, and extensor plantar responses, are present in some cases. These lateralizing signs may indicate a complicating cortical thrombophlebitis.

Associated Diseases

Examination of the ears to exclude otitis media should be a routine procedure in any febrile illness, particularly in a suspected case of meningitis. Other associated diseases or abnormalities such as pneumonia, diabetes mellitus, head trauma, brain abscess, furunculosis, cellulitis, or decubitus ulcers should be suspected. Meningitis may also be a complication of certain debilitating illnesses such as Hodgkin's disease and leukemia. Patients whose symptoms fall under group 2 have a high incidence of pharyngitis.

Diagnostic Procedures

1. The cerebrospinal fluid is usually under increased pressure, particularly if there is some obstruction to its circulation by fibrin deposits in the aqueduct of Sylvius or in the foramina of the fourth ventricle or by pus in the subarachnoid space. It may vary in appearance from turbid to purulent according to its cellular content. In the early stages, the cell count may vary from 500 to 35,000 white cells per cubic millimeter, of which over 95 per cent are polymorphonuclear leukocytes. As the disease progresses, there is a gradual increase in lymphocytes and large mononuclear cells. These mononuclear cells are particularly prominent in the early stages in patients receiving antibiotics. All specimens should be centri-

fuged and the smear stained by Gram's method, which may reveal intracellular or extracellular organisms provided the patient has not received antibiotics. Pneumococcal meningitis is characterized by myriads of extracellular diplococci, while in meningococcal meningitis, meningococci are sparse extracellularly. The ratio of leukocytes to bacteria is high with meningococci, while the reverse is true for pneumococci. Culture of the CSF should be obtained using blood agar, blood chocolate agar, and thioglycolate broth media incubated in 10 per cent carbon dioxide. If penicillin has already been given, penicillinase should always be added to the culture medium.

Chemical analysis of the cerebrospinal fluid in acute purulent meningitis shows reduction of the glucose content below 45 mg/100 ml, with occasional values as low as zero. The chloride level is usually decreased below 700 mg/100 ml and the protein content elevated above 70 mg and occasionally as high as 500 mg/100 ml. While changes in protein and chloride levels may be seen in a number of conditions, the lowering of cerebrospinal fluid glucose levels is highly suggestive of bacterial meningitis even in the absence of confirmation by stained smear and by cultures. Low glucose levels are, however, a feature of meningeal carcinomatosis, but this condition is usually subacute with a white cell count of less than 100 per cubic millimeter.[220]

The increase in protein in the spinal fluid is the result of injury to the pia-arachnoid by the inflammatory process and subsequent passive diffusion of albumin from serum. Glucose, on the other hand, is actively transported across the blood-brain barrier. Transport decreases with the buildup of inflammatory exudate. Glucose utilization by leukocytes during phagocytosis is also increased.

2. Roentgenograms of the skull and chest sometimes reveal unsuspected infection of the paranasal sinuses and middle ear or pneumonia with a lung abscess. There may be a recent fracture of the skull in cases of posttraumatic meningitis or separation of the sutures in children with subdural effusions.

3. Blood culture should be obtained along with a culture from the throat and from the ear or any other sites that may be draining infected material. The culture of the primary focus should produce an organism that corresponds

to that obtained from the cerebrospinal fluid. Should the latter be sterile, culture of the primary focus may be the only means of identifying the organism responsible for the meningitis.

4. The cerebrospinal fluid can be tested for the presence of antigens to *H. influenzae, S. pneumoniae,* or *N. meningitidis,* using counterimmunoelectrophoresis. This is a rapid, reliable, and inexpensive screening test for the identification of the causative organism in bacterial meningitis.[129, 223]

5. A subdural effusion is a possible complication in any infant or young child with meningitis who fails to improve after 72 hours of antibiotic therapy. These children usually show continuing lethargy, nuchal rigidity, opisthotonus, deepening coma, and frequent seizures. There is an increase in diameter of the head with bulging fontanels. The diagnosis is confirmed by performing subdural taps through the lateral angles of the fontanels or by computed tomography in older children. There should be no hesitation in obtaining a CT scan in any child who appears to respond poorly to treatment or in those who show persistent focal signs despite improvement in the cerebrospinal fluid.

6. The electroencephalogram usually shows diffuse slowing over both hemispheres, but there may be a decrease in voltage over a subdural effusion or focal delta activity in the case of an associated cerebral abscess.

Treatment

General Measures. These are as follows:

1. Complete bed rest should be ordered as well as appropriate isolation when the risk of transmission is high. The patient should be turned in bed every two hours to avoid bedsores and to drain dependent areas of the lung. An endotracheal tube may be necessary in stuporous or comatose patients with depressed respiratory function. If assisted respiration is used, arterial blood gases are monitored daily and the P_{O_2} is kept above 50 mm Hg and the P_{CO_2} between 35 and 40 mm Hg.

2. The fluid intake should be adequate. A central venous catheter should be inserted and dehydration corrected, with the central venous pressure maintained within normal range (2.5 to 4.5 cm of water in children; 7.5 to 15 cm of water in adults). The average adult requires 3,000 ml of fluid in 24 hours; children, proportionately less.

3. Accurate charts of intake and output should be kept to calculate daily fluid requirements.

4. Daily serum electrolyte levels are necessary to maintain electrolyte balance. There is usually little disturbance in electrolyte levels with the use of 5 per cent dextrose in 0.2 N saline with 20 mEq of potassium chloride added to each 1,000 ml of intravenous fluid. Hyponatremia may occur owing to inappropriate secretion of antidiuretic hormone, which is not uncommon in children with meningitis. The diagnosis is made by demonstrating a low serum sodium with elevated urine sodium, depressed serum osmolality, elevated urine osmolality, and a normal or low blood urea nitrogen. Treatment requires restriction of fluids.

5. Stuporous or comatose patients will require a urinary catheter with a three-way or tidal drainage.

6. Overwhelming septicemia and shock are rare complications of meningococcus and *Haemophilus influenzae* infections. It had been assumed for many years that such cases suffered acute adrenal failure, but adrenal hemorrhages have not been found in all cases coming to autopsy, and adrenal insufficiency is no longer considered a likely cause.

   Treatment of shock consists of administration of fluids to elevate the central venous pressure to normal range (see above). If hypotension persists, isoproterenol (5 mg in 1,000 ml of 5 per cent dextrose in 0.2 N saline at 1 ml/minute) should be used. There is little evidence to support the view that patients benefit from steroid therapy. Some studies indicate that cases treated with steroids have a higher mortality rate. Steroids are therefore not recommended for the treatment of shock.

7. Seizures are not infrequent and require intravenous diazepam (Valium), 10 mg in 10 ml of water injected at the rate of 1 ml every 30 seconds (see Treatment of Status Epilepticus, p. 367). This can be supplemented by intramuscular injection of phenobarbital, 3 mg/pound of body weight in children.

8. Disseminated intravascular coagulation with the presence of thrombin in the systemic circulation can occur in any form of meningitis but is usually a complication of meningococ-

cal meningitis.[56] Signs include the presence of petechiae in the skin, bleeding from one or more sites, acrocyanosis, signs of peripheral venous or arterial thrombosis, and hypotension. The diagnosis is established if the prothrombin time is prolonged; fibrinogen levels are depressed and the platelet count is abnormally low. Other tests, including prolonged thrombin time, decreased euglobulin clot lysis time, and the presence of fibrinogen degradation products, are available in some laboratories. Treatment consists of:

a. Adequate therapy of the acute meningitis.

b. Inhibition of the effects of thrombin with heparin. This is given in doses of 100 USP units/kg of body weight every four hours intravenously. The clotting time should be maintained two to three times that of the normal control.

c. In a severe case, consumed clotting factors can be replaced with fresh frozen plasma.

9. Hyperthermia with rectal temperatures exceeding 106°F is an occasional complication in infants and children. Most cases respond to tepid sponging and nursing on a refrigerated blanket.

10. Cerebral edema, leading to brainstem compression and death, is always a potential complication in acute purulent meningitis. this is the one situation that may benefit from the use of corticosteroids, beginning with dexamethasone, 12 mg intravenously, followed by 4 mg intramuscularly every four hours for three days. Hyperosmotic agents such as mannitol, 2 gm/kg administered intravenously in a 20 per cent solution or glycerol, 2 gm/kg by nasogastric tube as a 50 per cent solution, or 1.24 gm/kg as a 10 per cent solution given intravenously, will also decrease acute cerebral edema.

11. Thrombophlebitis in the lower limbs is likely to occur in comatose or semicomatose adults. The risk of this complication and subsequent pulmonary embolism can be reduced by the use of elastic stockings and the movement of all limbs through full range of passive movement several times twice a day.

Antibiotic Therapy. There are frequent changes in the recommended antibiotic treatment of acute purulent meningitis because of the steady development of new drugs as well as the development of drug-resistant strains of certain organisms. The sulfonamide drugs, which were frequently prescribed during the period 1940–1960, are now seldom used, but penicillin G remains the antibiotic of choice in many infections. Once a diagnosis is made by culture, treatment should be started as outlined in Table 7–2. In cases of unknown etiology in infants and children, penicillin or ampicillin is recommended with gentamicin (see Neonatal Meningitis, p. 407). Meningitis due to mixed infections should be treated with adequate doses of antibiotics, as determined by culture and sensitivity tests, in order to eradicate all organisms. Intrathecal therapy is no longer recommended in acute purulent meningitis since it does not have any advantages over other forms of parenteral therapy. Exceptions include gram-negative meningitis, caused by *Pseudomonas* and neonatal meningitis.

The majority of cases of acute purulent meningitis can be treated with penicillin G (pneumococcus, meningococcus, *Streptococcus,* penicillinase-negative staphylococci) or the semisynthetic penicillin known as ampicillin (all of the preceding plus *Haemophilus influenzae*), as outlined in Table 7–2. Ampicillin has the advantages of being a broad-spectrum antibiotic with fewer side effects than chloramphenicol or the tetracycline group of drugs. The disadvantage of recommending either penicillin G or ampicillin is that since both drugs belong to the penicillin group, both are likely to produce drug reactions if there is a sensitivity to penicillin. Several alternatives have been suggested to meet such a situation and also to provide antibiotic therapy in the few cases of acute purulent meningitis that are resistant to both penicillin G and to ampicillin. Gentamicin sulfate is currently recommended as the drug of choice in *E. coli* and *Pseudomonas* meningitis.

The toxic reactions that may be encountered during antibiotic therapy are listed in Table 7–3. Reactions other than hypersensitivity to the penicillin group of drugs are infrequent and less potentially dangerous than those encountered when using chloramphenicol. Any reaction other than a minor skin irritation is an indication for a change in antibiotic, provided an adequate alternative is available as indicated by culture and sensitivity testing.

Complications Arising During Treatment of Acute Purulent Meningitis. These are as follows:

1. Subdural effusions should be suspected in any infant or child who fails to improve after 72

TABLE 7–2

Treatment of Acute Purulent Meningitis

	Antibiotic	Duration of Therapy (Weeks)
Streptococcus pneumoniae		
Adults 1 million units every 1–2 hours IM or IV by bolus or 2 million units every 1–2 hours by constant IV drip	Penicillin G	3–4
Children 1 million units IM or IV immediately, then 500,000 units IM or IV by bolus every 1–2 hours	Penicillin G	2
Neisseria meningitidis		
Adults 1 million units every 1–2 hours IM or IV by bolus or 2 million units every 1–2 hours by constant IV drip	Penicillin G	3
Children 1 million units IM or IV immediately, then 500,000 units IM or IV by bolus every 1–2 hours	Penicillin G	2
Group A streptococci		
Adults 1 million units every 1–2 hours IM or IV by bolus or 2 million units every 1–2 hours by constant IV drip	Penicillin G	3
Children 1 million units IM or IV immediately, then 500,000 units IM or IV by bolus every 1–2 hours	Penicillin G	2
*Staphylococcus aureus**		
Adults 1 million units every 1–2 hours IM or IV by bolus or 2 million units every 1–2 hours by constant IV drip	Penicillin G	4
Children 1 million units IM or IV immediately, then 500,000 units IM or IV by bolus every 1–2 hours	Penicillin G	3
Adults 1 gm IV by bolus immediately, then 1 gm IM every 3 hours	Ampicillin	3
Children 100–200 mg/kg/day in divided doses every 3 hours	Ampicillin	3
Adults 2.0 gm IV every 4 hours if organism is penicillin-resistant; 10 mg in 1 ml 0.85% saline IT daily for 7 days, then every other day for 10 days	Methicillin	4
Children 100 mg/kg/day IV in divided doses every 4 hours if organism is penicillin-resistant; 5 mg in 1 ml 0.85% saline daily for 7 days, then every other day for 10 days	Methicillin	3
Haemophilus influenzae		
Adults 1 gm IV by bolus immediately, then 1 gm IM every 3 hours	Ampicillin	3
Children 100–200 mg/kg/day in divided doses every 3 hours	Ampicillin	2
Children† 75 mg/kg/day in divided doses every 6 hours	Chloramphenicol (alternate therapy)	2

TABLE 7-2 (Continued)

	Antibiotic	Duration of Therapy (Weeks)
Escherichia coli, Pseudomonas		
Adults		
3–4 mg/kg/day IM in divided doses every 8 hours; 5 mg in 1 ml 0.85% NaCl IT daily for 7 days, then every other day for 10 days	Gentamicin	4
Children		
5.0 mg/kg/day IM in divided doses every 8 hours; 2 mg in 1 ml 0.85% NaCl daily for 7 days, then every other day for 10 days	Gentamicin	3
Adults		
1 gm IV by bolus immediately, then 1 gm IM every 3 hours	Ampicillin (alternate therapy)	4
Children		
100–200 mg/kg/day in divided doses every 3 hours	Ampicillin (alternate therapy)	3
Children		
50 mg/kg/day in divided doses every 6 hours	Chloramphenicol (alternate therapy)	3
Unknown etiology‡		
See above recommendations for dosage and duration		

* Penicillin G and methicillin should be used initially. After sensitivity testing one of these agents may be omitted. Intrathecal (IT) methicillin is necessary.

† Ampicillin is preferred to chloramphenicol. Chloramphenicol should not be used for a period exceeding two weeks. When chloramphenicol is used, platelet counts should be done every three days.

‡ Penicillin G and gentamicin are recommended for adults and children.

hours on appropriate antibiotic therapy. Diagnostic subdural taps may be performed in infants and children under 18 months of age if the anterior fontanel is still patent. If fluid is obtained, daily taps should be performed with removal of 20 to 30 ml of fluid until the effusion resolves. Surgical drainage of chronic subdural effusions should be performed after the failure of repeated daily subdural taps.[39]

2. Ventriculitis should be considered in all cases of neonatal meningitis who show persistent positive culture of organisms from the cerebrospinal fluid after 48 hours of treatment. Ventriculitis should be considered in children without subdural effusion who are deteriorating despite antibiotic therapy.[266] The diagnosis can be confirmed by ventricular puncture with the recovery of purulent fluid. Treatment consists of the insertion of a Salmon Rickman or Ommaya type of ventriculostomy reservoir and the daily instillation of the appropriate antibiotic through the reservoir.

3. Foci of infection that have produced the meningeal infection may require surgical drainage. This includes intracranial and intracerebral abscesses and extracranial foci such as otitis media, mastoiditis, and paranasal sinusitis.

4. Hydrocephalus, which occurs as a complication of meningitis, should be treated by surgical shunting of cerebrospinal fluid from the lateral ventricles to the internal jugular vein by the use of a ventriculoatrial catheter and low-pressure valve.

Prognosis

Early diagnosis and prompt treatment, including the use of appropriate antibiotics, are undoubtedly major factors in the determination of prognosis in acute meningitis. The prognosis is poorer and the mortality higher in infants and in patients of all ages with pneumococcal meningitis[74] and in those who are semicomatose or comatose at the time of admission to the hospital.[56]

Escherichia coli Meningitis

Acute purulent meningitis due to *E. coli* is usually seen in infants.[210] The predilection for the infant may be due to impaired antibody formation in the first few months of life or to increased

TABLE 7–3

Complications of Antibiotic Therapy

Penicillin
Ampicillin
Methicillin
	Fever
	Skin rash
	Angioedema
	Serum sickness
	Anaphylaxis
		(Leukopenia has been reported with ampicillin,
		  hematuria with methicillin at dosages of
		  greater than 10 gm a day)

Chloramphenicol	Vomiting Glossitis Skin rash Bone marrow depression	
Gentamicin	Vertigo Tinnitus Hearing loss (involvement of vestibular and auditory divisions of eighth nerve) Convulsions Renal toxicity	
Tetracyclines	Skin rash Gastrointestinal irritation Thrombophlebitis (IV) Discoloration of teeth Fatal hepatorenal syndrome	
Amphotericin B	Headache Fever and chills Vomiting Hepatic and renal toxicity	
Polymyxin B	Flushing of face Dizziness Paresthesias, convulsions, respiratory arrest Renal toxicity	

permeability of the gastrointestinal mucosa and meninges to *E. coli.* Many infants with *E. coli* meningitis have a history of prematurity, a difficult labor, or congenital defects such as meningomyelocele or congenital dermal sinus. A few cases of traumatic *E. coli* meningitis have been reported in adults, and these usually followed penetrating head and spine wounds.[271] A number of cases have occurred following craniotomy and neurosurgical procedures.

Treatment

The drug of first choice is gentamicin, 4 mg/kg every 24 hours in eight hourly doses IM for four weeks supplemented by 4 mg/day for seven to ten days given intrathecally. Ventriculitis should be suspected if the spinal fluid culture remains positive after two days, and treatment should be changed to intraventricular gentamicin, 4 mg/day, rather than using the intrathecal route.[49]

Meningitis Due to Gram-Negative Bacilli Other Than *E. Coli*

Gram-negative rods other than *E. coli* are occasionally encountered in cases of meningitis. Infection is usually seen in infants but may occur at any age following penetrating wounds of the head or spine and in the presence of craniocerebral fistulas, following craniotomy, following radiotherapy, or in patients suffering from a chronic debilitating disease such as leukemia. The organisms in this group include *Pseudomonas, Enterobacter alcaligenes, Proteus, Salmonella,* and paracolon bacilli. *Pseudomonas* infections may begin as an otitis externa in adult diabetes and spread through the bone to involve the meninges.[276] In each case the symptoms are those of an acute purulent meningitis. The cerebrospinal fluid shows an increased pressure. It may have a greenish tinge and a green fluorescence under ultraviolet light in *Pseudomonas* meningitis.

Treatment

The antibiotic of choice is gentamicin.[102] The second choice is ampicillin. Intrathecal administration may be required because of poor passage of drug into the subarachnoid space, even in the presence of inflammation (see Table 7–2). Intraventricular gentamicin, 4 mg/day, should be used to treat ventriculitis if the spinal fluid culture remains positive after two days of intrathecal therapy.

Neonatal Meningitis

Cases of purulent meningitis in the neonatal period in which there is a failure to culture organisms are not infrequent. This is probably due to the widespread use of antibiotics in infancy prior to admission to the hospital. Such cases should be treated under the assumption that either *E. coli* or β-hemolytic streptococci are present and should be given gentamicin, 8 mg/kg every 24 hours IM in eight-hourly doses, and intravenous ampicillin, 200 to 400 mg/kg every 24 hours IV in six-hourly doses. Lumbar punctures are performed daily to monitor spinal fluid changes and for intrathecal instillation of gentamicin, 4 mg daily (low-birth-weight infants 2 mg daily) for seven days.[343] If the cerebrospinal fluid shows a persistent positive culture after two days of therapy, the administration of gentamicin is changed from the intrathecal to the intraventricular route. Intrathecal or intraventricular gentamicin is continued until the spinal fluid shows a negative growth for three days and there are no demonstrable organisms on gram stain. If a gram-positive organism is identified by culture during the first 24 to 48 hours of therapy, the gentamicin therapy can be stopped and treatment continued with ampicillin or intrathecal methicillin for a staphylococcal infection.

Bacterium anitratum Meningitis (Also Described as Belonging to the Genus *Herellea*)

Bacterium anitratum has been described as a cause of urethritis in man and may occasionally contaminate open wounds. Other closely related organisms include *Mima polymorpha, Herellea vaginicola,* and *Colliodes anoxydana.*[236] They have been isolated in patients with pneumonia, septicemia, bacterial endocarditis, and conjunctivitis and are a rare cause of cerebral abscess and meningitis. These organisms are gram-negative diplobacilli frequently mistaken for *N. meningitidis.* The similarity may be carried further since *B. anitratum* meningitis may resemble the acute purulent meningitis due to *N. meningitidis* with a rapid and fulminating course, and associated petechial skin rashes.[330]

Treatment

The drug of choice is ampicillin. The drug of second choice is chlortetracycline. The adult dose of chlortetracycline is 500 mg every six hours orally or 500 mg every 12 hours when given intravenously. For children the dose is 25 mg/kg of body weight every six hours by mouth or 25 mg/kg of body weight every 12 hours if given intravenously.

Streptococcal Meningitis

There has been a reduction in the incidence of meningitis due to streptococci. The incidence began to decrease with the introduction of the sulfonamide drugs and has been further decreased following the use of penicillin. The majority of cases of streptococcal meningitis are secondary to otitis media and mastoiditis and occur in the neonatal period. Streptococcal meningitis is rare in adults.

Acute purulent meningitis due to *Streptococcus faecalis* may occur following penetrating head wounds, neurosurgical procedures, or due to the presence of a craniocerebral fistula. These organisms show resistance to penicillin G.

The symptoms of streptococcal meningitis are usually those of an acute purulent meningitis. The cerebrospinal fluid shows increased pressure with a pleocytosis of polymorphonuclear leukocytes and the presence of gram-positive cocci occurring in pairs or short chains.

Treatment

The drug of first choice is penicillin G. The drug of second choice is ampicillin. In meningitis due to *Streptococcus faecalis* ampicillin may be the first choice.

Staphylococcal Meningitis

Staphylococcal meningitis is predominantly an infection of infancy, but it may occur at any age and is usually a sequel to a staphylococcal infection elsewhere in the body which results in staphylococcal septicemia or bacteremia. It also occurs following penetrating wounds of the head and spine, as a complication of craniocerebral fistulas, and following neurosurgical procedures. Infections by *Staphylococcus aureus* produce a fulminating purulent meningitis. *Staphylococcus albus* infections are more insidious and are usually associated with shunting procedures to relieve hydrocephalus.[316]

The symptoms of *Staphylococcal aureus* meningitis are those of an acute purulent meningitis with gram-positive cocci in the smear. Culture and sensitivity testing is imperative since many of the organisms are resistant to penicillin G.

Treatment

Penicillin G and either methicillin or ampicillin should be used together initially. One of these drugs should be omitted after results of sensitivity are available. In Europe, methicillin-resistant strains have become clinically important. Tests of sensitivity then determine therapy.

Treatment should be continued for at least three to four weeks after the temperature has been reduced to normal levels to minimize the risk of relapse. Abscesses and foci of infection elsewhere in the body should be treated by surgical drainage.

Pneumococcal Meningitis

This type of acute purulent meningitis is predominantly a disease of adults but it may occur at any age. It is the most common cause of recurrent meningitis in all ages, and there is a frequent history of head trauma or cerebrospinal fluid rhinorrhea in patients with recurrent pneumococcal meningitis.[59] It is most commonly seen as a complication of a debilitating disease such as chronic alcoholism in adults.[253] Other predisposing factors include splenectomy, sickle cell disease, and conditions producing an altered immune response. The risk of pneumococcal meningitis in individuals with sickle cell disease is approximately five hundred times greater than in the general population.

Pneumococcal meningitis may be a complication of otitis media, mastoiditis, or paranasal sinusitis. The symptoms are those of an acute purulent meningitis, and gram-positive diplococci are usually abundant in the stained smear of the CSF.

Treatment

The drug of choice is penicillin G, usually given in a dosage of 12 to 20 million units/day for adults.

To prevent recurrence, treatment should be continued for at least three to four weeks. Surgical drainage of a focus of infection such as a mastoiditis or a paranasal sinusitis may be necessary.

Prognosis

The mortality in pneumococcal meningitis varies from 17 per cent to more than 60 per cent in some centers.[336] This is due to differences in the patient population. The disease is particularly deadly in the chronic alcoholic with pneumonia. The following signs also indicate a poor prognosis:[12, 142, 331]

1. Coma on admission
2. Age above 60 years
3. Pneumonia
4. Convulsions
5. Absence of nuchal rigidity
6. Pneumonic septicemia
7. Elevated cerebrospinal fluid protein
8. A positive smear from the cerebrospinal fluid

In the majority of cases death is probably due to acute hydrocephalus resulting from the inflammatory exudate.

Haemophilus influenzae Meningitis

Meningitis due to *Haemophilus influenzae* type B is predominantly an infection of children under four years of age, with few cases reported in adults. The organism is frequently found in the upper respiratory tract and passes to the meninges during an upper respiratory tract infection. The history of such an infection is quite common prior to the onset of meningitis in children. Symptoms of meningitis are usually abrupt in onset and may be fulminating with death within 24 hours. In the majority of cases, however, the symptomatology is that of an acute purulent meningitis. Infection in adults tends to be milder than in children and is frequently associated with some condition that impairs resistance to infection, such as cerebrospinal fluid rhinorrhea, otorrhea, hypogammaglobulinemia, diabetes mellitus, and alcoholism.

Although antibiotic therapy has reduced the mortality of *H. influenzae* meningitis from 100 per cent in the preantibiotic era to less than 10 per cent, there is still a high incidence of permanent neurologic damage in surviving children. In most cases these deficits are minor, but severe neurologic damage can be expected in about 10 per cent of survivors.[92]

Diagnostic Procedures

1. The cerebrospinal fluid shows a polymorphonuclear pleocytosis with intra- and extracellular gram-negative organisms in the stained smear.
2. Persistent coma may be the result of acute hydrocephalus. This can be confirmed by computed tomography with the demonstration of generalized symmetric ventricular dilatation.

Treatment

1. The drug of first choice is ampicillin[19, 128] and that of second choice is chloramphenicol or tetracycline, 50 mg/kg/day intravenously in divided doses.[227] If ampicillin-resistant strains of *H. influenzae* are known to be present in the geographic area, it is advisable to begin therapy with intravenous ampicillin and chloramphenicol. Sensitivity tests should be performed on the cultured organisms. Treatment with chloramphenicol must be continued if the organisms are resistant to ampicillin. In the rare event that the *H. influenzae* is resistant to ampicillin and chloramphenicol or when chloramphenicol induces bone marrow depression, treatment should be changed to a combination of streptomycin, 30 mg/kg/day, and sulfadiazine, 150 mg/kg/day, or tetracycline.[17]
2. Subdural effusion is a particularly common complication of *Haemophilus* meningitis in infants and young children. Subdural taps should be performed in any child who fails to show prompt improvement after 48 hours of antibiotic therapy.
3. Acute hydrocephalus requires a ventriculoatrial or ventriculoperitoneal shunt procedure.
4. Ventriculitis should also be considered in children who fail to respond to treatment. This requires a ventriculostomy reservoir and the daily instillation of antibiotic into the ventricles.[266]

Meningococcal Meningitis

Epidemics of meningococcal meningitis have been recognized for more than 150 years and tend to occur in persons living in confined and overcrowded conditions.[345] Outbreaks in military camps have usually been among recruits who were crowded together, permitting easy transmission of nasopharyngeal droplet infection. There is usually a marked increase in upper respiratory tract infections and a rise in the nasopharyngeal carrier rate of *Neisseria meningitidis* to about 90 per cent or more immediately preceding the epidemic of meningitis. The organism becomes rapidly disseminated among such a susceptible group, and an increase in virulence may culminate in an outbreak of meningitis.

In addition to the epidemic form, sporadic cases occur at any age, usually in the winter months when there is increased spread of *N. meningitidis* due to infections of the upper respiratory tract.

The responsible organism, *N. meningitidis,* is a gram-negative diplococcus that can be classified into four serologically distinct groups on the basis of agglutination reactions induced by their capsular polysaccharides. Nearly all epidemics have been caused by organisms belonging to group A. Occasionally group B or C has been responsible. Group D infections are rare.

Clinical Features

The majority of infections are in the form of an acute nasopharyngitis. Septicemia may produce a mild systemic illness with arthralgia and a macular or maculopapular rash resembling rubella. More chronic forms of meningococcemia with low-grade fever and mild systemic symptoms may persist for many weeks.

Acute purulent meningitis usually presents with rapid onset, high fever, vomiting, neck stiffness, and symptoms of encephalitis leading to coma. There is a maculopapular or petechial rash involving skin and mucous membranes. The onset may be more gradual in some cases which run a less fulminating course. These patients have a much better prognosis.

Occasionally, an overwhelming septicemia may occur with abrupt onset and rapid progression to coma, shock, and death within 24 hours. These patients frequently show confluent hemorrhages and necrotic skin lesions of disseminated intravascular coagulation.[27]

Diagnostic Procedures

1. Blood culture should be obtained in all cases before antibiotic therapy.
2. The cerebrospinal fluid is occasionally clear and without cells if lumbar puncture is performed at a very early stage in the illness. However, *N. meningitidis* can be cultured from the fluid. The usual findings are those of an acute purulent meningitis with increased pressure and a large number of polymorphonuclear leu-

kocytes and intracellular gram-negative diplococci in the gram-stained smear. There are relatively fewer numbers of bacteria in the stained smear than in pneumococcal meningitis.

3. Cerebrospinal fluid can be tested for the presence of antigens to several organisms (meningococcus, pneumococcus, *H. influenzae*) by counterimmunoelectrophoresis. This is a sensitive test giving rapid results in meningitis.[84, 310]

Treatment

The drug of choice is penicillin G. Treatment should be continued for four days after symptoms have subsided and the patient is afebrile. The treatment of septicemia and shock is discussed on page 402.

Sulfadiazine was an effective prophylactic against systemic meningococcal disease until the emergence of sulfonamide-resistant strains of meningococci in 1963. Penicillin is not an effective prophylactic agent, and there has been only limited success in the short-term control of meningococcal disease in military recruits using rifampin and minocycline. There is some indication that future prophylaxis will be carried out with vaccines and that new vaccines for meningococcal meningitis may soon be available for immunization procedures in childhood.[193]

Meningitis Due to Other Organisms of the *Neisseria Group*

Occasionally, there are reports of an acute purulent meningitis due to *N. catarrhalis* or *N. gonorrhoeae*. *N. catarrhalis* is frequently found in the upper respiratory tract, and meningitis usually develops as a complication of otitis media or paranasal sinusitis. Gonococcal meningitis usually follows acute gonococcal urethritis in young males but may occur in newborn infants who acquire the organism at birth from maternal infection. The meningitis is similar to meningococcal meningitis. The diagnosis of gonococcal meningitis should be suspected in a patient with meningitis with clinical signs or past history of gonococcal infection.[270, 305]

Treatment

Treatment consists of penicillin G, 10 to 40 million units a day for 21 days.

Clostridium perfringens Meningitis

The organism of gas gangrene usually enters the meninges as a complication of contaminated and penetrating head wounds. Most cases of meningitis have occurred among military casualties. A few cases have been reported in civilian practice following relatively mild puncture wounds to the scalp. Meningitis has also been reported following *Clostridium perfringens* septicemia without head trauma.[283]

The symptoms are those of an acute purulent meningitis, with typical changes in the cerebrospinal fluid including increased pressure, polymorphonuclear pleocytosis, elevated protein, and decreased glucose content. The organism can be identified following anaerobic culture.

Treatment

Scalp wounds, no matter how trivial, should receive prompt treatment with removal of all necrotic material. Hyperbaric oxygenation has been reported to produce dramatic improvement in tissues infected by gas gangrene organisms.[25] Large doses (40 million units daily) of penicillin G are most effective, and anti-gas gangrene serum is probably unnecessary.[107]

Klebsiella pneumoniae Meningitis

Klebsiella pneumoniae (Friedländer's bacillus) is a rare cause of meningitis. The majority of patients give a history of antecedent infection, such as otitis media, pneumonia, or sinusitis, and many have diabetes mellitus or other debilitating diseases. The pathologic findings are those of an acute meningitis with a jelly-like, slightly greenish exudate lying over the cerebral hemisphere and in the basal cisterns.

The clinical features are those of an acute purulent meningitis. The cerebrospinal fluid shows a pleocytosis with 90 per cent polymorphonuclear leukocytes, and *Klebsiella pneumoniae* is usually obtained on culture. This is usually a fulminating meningitis with a mortality of 50 per cent.[294]

Treatment

Treatment consists of systemic and intrathecal administration of gentamicin and colistin. Gentamicin administration is described under *E. coli* meningitis (Table 7–2). Colistin should be given in 1 mega units IM every four hours and 50,000 units twice daily for two days followed by once daily intrathecally.[249]

Listeria monocytogenes Meningitis

Listeria monocytogenes is a rare cause of meningitis, and most cases have been reported in adults who are suffering from an underlying illness and altered host resistance. Treatment with steroids or cytotoxic agents may also affect host resistance, and infection by *Listeria monocytogenes* may be regarded as an opportunistic infection under such circumstances.[285] Maintenance immunosuppression following organ transplantation also increases the risk of infection by this organism.[89]

The disease produces a fulminating meningoencephalitis in infants, and the usual signs of neck stiffness and a positive Kernig's sign may be absent.

The infection may present in three forms in the adult:

1. A classic purulent meningitis.
2. A subacute infection with fluctuating episodes of stupor and clear sensorium, with delusions, illusions, or hallucinations in some cases. Seizures and focal cranial nerve palsies may occur with dystonic movements and myoclonic jerks.
3. A chronic process of progressive dementia and signs resembling normal pressure hydrocephalus.[135]

The cerebrospinal fluid shows a pleocytosis, predominantly of polymorphonuclear leukocytes which are usually less than 1,000 per cubic millimeter. The protein content is elevated and the glucose content depressed, although the latter may be normal in some cases. Culture reveals gram-positive rods, frequently mistaken for diphtheroids. Rapid identification is possible, using a fluorescent antibody technique.[91, 327]

Treatment

The drug of choice is penicillin. Ampicillin and erythromycin have been used with equal success.

Vibrio fetus Meningitis

The microorganism *Vibrio fetus* causes abortion in cattle and sheep and occasionally causes meningoencephalitis in infants and adults.[346] It may also cause an arteritis and cerebral infarction or subarachnoid hemorrhage in adults without signs of meningeal involvement.[125]

Infection may be severe in the neonatal period, with fulminating meningoencephalitis and death within a few days. Adults tend to develop a nonspecific illness with fever and arthralgia. Some two weeks later, localizing infection including septic arthritis, pericarditis, endocarditis, cerebral thrombosis, subarachnoid hemorrhage, or meningoencephalitis, may occur.

In meningoencephalitis of both infants and adults, the cerebrospinal fluid shows a predominantly polymorphonuclear pleocytosis. The vibrios may be seen by dark-field illumination or after anaerobic culture on MacConkey's agar or blood agar.

Treatment

The drug of choice is ampicillin.

Meningitis Due to Unknown Organisms

The widespread use of antibiotics in the early stages of any febrile illness has resulted in admission to the hospital of cases of acute meningitis that have already received antibiotics. This has resulted in a marked increase in cases of acute meningitis of "unknown etiology." These cases have the typical changes in the cerebrospinal fluid suggesting an acute purulent meningitis, but the antibiotics inhibit the growth of the organisms on attempted culture from the CSF. Under these circumstances, further antibiotics must be used that are effective against a wide spectrum of organisms.

Treatment

Penicillin G and gentamicin are recommended for both adults and children. See Table 7–2 for dosage and duration.

Tuberculous Meningitis

There has been a radical change in the prognosis for patients with tuberculous meningitis since the introduction of streptomycin in 1947. Before the use of streptomycin this disease was invariably fatal, with a course seldom exceeding three months. While the disease remains serious, complete recovery can be anticipated if treatment is instituted at an early stage.

Tuberculous meningitis has a worldwide incidence and occurs equally in both sexes and at any age. The incidence is higher in poorer communities, where overcrowding and poor hygiene are prevalent and public health facilities are poor. As the standard of living rises, the incidence of tuberculous meningitis in a community tends to fall.

The disease was formerly considered to be a disease of childhood but this view is no longer tenable. Tuberculous meningitis is usually a complication of primary tuberculosis, so that the incidence is similar to that of primary infection. The occurrence of primary tuberculosis in both the United States and Great Britain is now more common in the second and third decades of life with a corresponding increase in the ages at which the maximal incidence of tuberculous meningitis occurs. In Asian countries, however, the disease still occurs predominantly in infants and children.[263]

Pathology

Tuberculous meningitis is usually found to be associated with primary tuberculous infection elsewhere in the body, particularly in the lungs. It also occurs as a complication of miliary tuberculosis with seeding of the meninges or microembolism of the brain and passage through the walls of small arteries. When it occurs following a primary infection, it is transmitted to the meninges and brain as part of a tuberculous bacteremia. This results in a few foci in the meninges and brain, with the development of meningitis following the rupture of one or more of these foci and the dissemination of infected material into the ventricles or the subarachnoid space.

Occasionally, tuberculous meningitis occurs during the course of a chronic tuberculosis as a complication of bacteremia or as an extension directly into the subarachnoid space from an extradural abscess complicating a tuberculous osteomyelitis of the spine (Pott's disease). It may also result from the rupture of a tuberculoma into the subarachnoid space. The meningeal reaction appears to depend on two types of inflammatory reaction, the first a chronic inflammatory or granulomatous response and the second due to an acute "tuberculin" reaction throughout the subarachnoid space and ventricular systems. This second type of response varies a great deal in severity from individual to individual. The resultant inflammatory exudate is thick and heavy and tends to be marked at the base of the brain. Consequently, cranial nerve involvement is a prominent feature of tuberculous meningitis. The thick exudate may also block the aqueduct of Sylvius, the foramina in the roof of the fourth ventricle, and the subarachnoid space around the midbrain, producing hydrocephalus, papilledema, and increased intracranial pressure.

After two to three months there is fibroblastic proliferation in the subarachnoid space. At first, this was thought to be a reaction to the use of intrathecal agents, but it is now evident that since patients on chemotherapy live longer, time is allowed for the fibroblastic reaction to develop.

The arteries crossing the subarachnoid space show a characteristic arteritis with marked inflammation of the adventitia and media. Many become thrombosed, resulting in multiple small infarcts of the brain, particularly in the cortex. Both superficial and perforating arteries are involved, producing scattered infarcts of the cerebral cortex, brainstem, and basal ganglia. This is probably responsible for the marked cerebral edema found in some cases of tuberculous meningitis.

Clinical Features

The onset of tuberculous meningitis is insidious and there are no distinguishing features, at first, other than low-grade fever, headache, and stiff neck. The diagnosis should be considered in all cases of low-grade pyrexia with headache and stiff neck. Infants and children present with listlessness, fatigue, irritability, poor appetite, vomiting, and a low-grade fever. Adults often complain of malaise, weight loss, myalgia, backache, low-grade fever, and mental confusion.

Careful history often reveals that the patient has had exposure to the disease. A positive tuberculin or PPD skin test should enhance suspicion of tuberculous meningitis. In any case, a lumbar puncture should be performed.

In the infant, a further sign of meningeal involvement is fullness of the anterior fontanel. In children and adults, the first obvious clinical sign of meningeal irritation is usually stiffness of the neck, but in some children, the first symptom may be focal motor seizures followed by postictal (Todd's) paralysis.

The fully developed picture of tuberculous meningitis consists of mental confusion often accompanied by "psychotic behavior" with hallucinations, delusions, and excitement. The patient becomes obtunded but is frequently irritable when aroused. Characteristic signs at this stage are papilledema and paralysis of the third, fourth, and sixth cranial nerves, sometimes accompanied by mild hemiparesis and seizures.

Diagnostic Procedures

1. The cerebrospinal fluid is frequently under increased pressure and the fluid appears clear. Occasionally, the fluid may be ground-glass in appearance, greenish, or xanthochromic. A fine fibrin coagulum usually develops when the cerebrospinal fluid is allowed to stand or if the specimen is centrifuged; this web should be used when staining for the organisms. The cell count is usually between 50 and 400 cells

per cubic millimeter but there may be few cells early in the disease. Occasionally an exaggerated "tuberculin" reaction in the subarachnoid space produces cell counts of more than 1,000 cells per cubic millimeter. Lymphocytes predominate except in acute and severe cases, when polymorphonuclear leukocytes may be abundant. Chemical analysis usually shows a glucose content of less than 40 mg per cent, chlorides below 600 mg per cent, and total protein content between 80 and 400 mg per cent. A protein content of 1,000 mg per cent is occasionally seen, particularly in cases with a partial or complete spinal subarachnoid block. The centrifuged material or the web that appears on standing should be stained by the Ziehl-Neelsen method and the diagnosis will be confirmed if it is positive for *Mycobacterium tuberculosis*. The percentage of positive identification increases with the experience of the examiner and the amount of time spent examining the smear.

Diligent examination of the smear is most important because growth of the bacteria in culture or after inoculation of a guinea pig may not be positive for six weeks.

2. There may be considerable difficulty in the diagnosis of tuberculous or viral meningitis in early cases presenting as a lymphocytic meningitis with absence of acid-fast bacilli in the cerebrospinal fluid. The radioactive bromide partition test[204] is valuable in such cases where the increased permeability of the meninges in tuberculous meningitis results in a low serum/spinal fluid ratio of less than 1.6 with higher values in viral meningitis.

3. Computed tomography will reveal diffuse ventricular dilatation in patients with hydrocephalus due to obstruction of flow of the cerebrospinal fluid around the brainstem and through the basal cisterns.

4. Cerebral arteriography shows narrowing or "spasm" of the intracranial portion of the carotid artery and proximal segments of the major cerebral vessels[329] (Fig. 7–3).

5. A therapeutic trial of antituberculous therapy is justified in some cases of suspected tuberculous meningitis with cerebrospinal fluid findings compatible with the diagnosis but where confirmation is lacking after several smears and cultures have been made. When the therapeutic trial is initiated, there may be a fluctuation in the cell content of the cerebrospinal

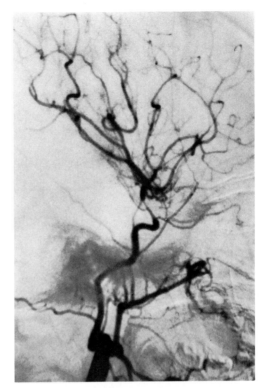

FIGURE 7–3. Arteriogram in a case of basal meningitis. There is marked narrowing of the supraclinoid portion of the internal carotid artery. This abnormality is not unusual in tuberculous meningitis and in other forms of basal meningitis.

fluid with a progressive rise in protein during the first four weeks of therapy. By the sixth week, however, if the diagnosis is correct, there should be clinical signs of improvement and a decrease in the cell count and protein content of the cerebrospinal fluid.

Treatment

Streptomycin and Isonicotinic Acid Hydrazide. Most satisfactory drugs in the treatment of tuberculous meningitis have been streptomycin and isonicotinic acid hydrazide (INAH), which should always be used in combination to prevent the development of streptomycin-resistant tuberculous bacilli. The dose of streptomycin in infants and children is 20 to 30 mg per kilogram by intramuscular injection daily for two weeks and then two to three times weekly for the duration of therapy (usually two years). This may be supplemented by intrathecal streptomycin in doses of 10 to 25 mg daily, although this is not necessary in most cases. In adults, the recommended dose of streptomycin is 1.0 gram daily by intramuscular injection. This used to be supplemented by intrathecal injection of 50 mg daily, but this is no longer recommended. Streptomycin should be continued as recommended above. The recommended dose of isonicotinic acid hydrazide (INAH) to be combined with streptomycin is 3 to 5 mg/kg daily by mouth in infants and children and 400 mg daily by mouth in adults. Vestibular and auditory function (by audiogram) should be repeatedly tested during administration of streptomycin and treatment should be discontinued if toxic damage to the eighth nerve appears.

Other Drugs. Para-aminosalicylic acid (PAS), ethionimide, and rifampicin[112] should be reserved for cases showing toxic reactions to streptomycin or INAH (Table 7–4), or where the organism appears to be resistant to these drugs. There is no evidence that steroids are helpful in the initial therapy of tuberculous meningitis.[110a, 118a]

Complications

The subarachnoid space or the ventricular system may be blocked by exudate, with the production of hydrocephalus. A ventriculoatrial shunt may be necessary in such cases. The effects of tuberculosis elsewhere may also endanger the patient's life, and special treatment should be instituted as required. Seizures may occur during the active phase of the illness or as a late complication of the disease. Seizures should be controlled by anticonvulsant drugs. Intellectual impairment, persistent cranial nerve palsies or hemiparesis,

TABLE 7–4

**Complications of
Tuberculosis Chemotherapy**

Streptomycin	Skin rash
	Bone marrow depression
	Labyrinthine damage
	Deafness
Isoniazid	Convulsions
	Optic neuritis
	Peripheral neuritis
	Psychosis
Para-aminosalicylic acid	Fever
	Nausea
	Vomiting
	Diarrhea
	Arthritis

and hypopituitarism have all been observed in patients treated for tuberculous meningitis.[181, 282]

Prognosis

The Medical Research Council of Great Britain has classified tuberculous meningitis into three groups, which serve considerable usefulness when prognosis is estimated.

Group I. This includes patients who are fully conscious and rational, with signs of meningeal irritation but no focal neurologic signs or signs of hydrocephalus.

Group II. This includes patients who are mentally confused and/or have focal neurologic signs such as extraocular paralysis or hemiparesis.

Group III. This includes those patients who are unresponsive or inaccessible due to stupor or delirium and/or have a complete hemiplegia or paraplegia.

Patients in group I may be expected to show complete recovery on adequate antituberculous therapy. More than 80 per cent of the patients in group II make a good recovery, but the survival rate in group III is less than 50 per cent and many cases show permanent brain damage. The prognosis is particularly bad at the extremes of age, with a relatively higher mortality in infants and the elderly patients. The overall mortality in centers treating large numbers of cases of tuberculous meningitis is now well below 50 per cent.

Tuberculoma

Tuberculomas may be found in any part of the brain where they may mimic other types of space-occupying lesions.[62,208a] Tuberculomas are usually found in the supratentorial region where they are multiple in about 60 per cent of patients. Cerebellar tuberculomas tend to be singular lesions.

The pathology and clinical features of the tuberculoma are similar to those of the syphilitic gumma (p. 417).

Diagnostic Procedures

1. Computed tomography will show one or more areas of increased density with displacement of surrounding brain. Calcification is the end result of the disease process and does not occur in an active tuberculoma.

2. Arteriography shows displacement of blood vessels by an avascular mass.[63] The absence of hypertrophied vessels from the external carotid system is useful in differentiating tuberculoma from a meningioma.

Treatment

Tuberculomas causing neurologic symptoms are usually excised, and the diagnosis is confirmed by microscopic examination. The patient should be given a full course of antituberculous treatment after surgery.

Neurosyphilis: General Considerations

A considerable number of clinical conditions were mistakenly believed to be due to syphilis and were erroneously classified under the term "neurosyphilis" in the late nineteenth century. Many of the conditions are now known to be unrelated to syphilis owing to the positive identification of *Treponema pallidum* as the causative agent of syphilis in 1905 and the development of serologic tests for syphilis after 1906.

Primary Syphilis

In the primary stage of syphilis, there is rapid dissemination of the *Treponema* throughout the body, including some involvement of the central nervous system, which is usually asymptomatic. Occasionally symptoms of neurologic involvement appear during this early stage, with headache, nuchal rigidity, and pleocytosis. It has been estimated that an increase in cells in the cerebrospinal fluid may be found in about 20 per cent of symptomatic cases of primary syphilis. It is possible that such cases show a higher incidence of clinical neurosyphilis in later stages of the disease.

Secondary Syphilis and Syphilitic Meningitis

Acute syphilitic meningitis is seen most frequently in the secondary stage but has also been described in congenital syphilis and during the tertiary stage many years after the primary infection.

Pathology

At necropsy, a few cases have shown diffuse meningitis with lymphocytic infiltration of the meninges. In such cases, there is marked perivascular cuffing of the penetrating blood vessels of both brain and spinal cord with astrocytic and microglial reaction in the cerebral cortex. There is an endarteritis with inflammatory changes in all layers of the vessel walls as well as endothelial proliferation.

Clinical Features

The symptoms are those of acute meningitis, with fever, headache, nausea, vomiting, clouding of consciousness, cranial nerve palsies, nuchal rigidity, and occasionally increased deep tendon reflexes and extensor plantar responses. Cases showing marked mental changes including delirium and confusion may be inferred to be suffering from encephalitis and arteritis in addition to meningitis.

Diagnostic Procedures

1. The blood serologic test for syphilis is positive.
2. Lumbar puncture reveals clear or cloudy, or sometimes xanthochromic, cerebrospinal fluid with moderate elevation in pressure. There is lymphocytic pleocytosis with cell counts ranging from 50 to 2,000 per cubic millimeter, and elevated total protein. The serologic test for syphilis is positive in the cerebrospinal fluid.

Tertiary Syphilis

Some 6.5 per cent of people with untreated primary or secondary syphilis develop neurosyphilis, with a 2:1 ratio of males to females. Chronic basal meningitis and meningovascular syphilis account for 38 per cent of cases, general paresis 32 per cent, tabes dorsalis 27 per cent, and gumma of the brain about 3 per cent. Although there appears to be a steady decline in the incidence of neurosyphilis, it remains a serious public health problem and accounts for about 4,000 deaths annually in the United States. Neurosyphilis is rare in patients who contract the primary disease after the age of 40 years.

Syphilis of the Brain

Chronic Basal Meningitis with Cranial Nerve Paralysis

Acute syphilitic meningitis of the secondary stage occasionally develops into chronic basal meningitis, but the latter condition usually occurs during the tertiary stage of syphilis.

Pathology

There is marked thickening of the meninges at the base of the brain, particularly around the brainstem and roof of the fourth ventricle. Obstruction of the foramina in the fourth ventricle and meningitis of the basal cisterns may produce hydrocephalus. The basilar artery and the cranial nerves may become embedded in thick, granulomatous tissue, and the floor of the fourth ventricle may become covered by overgrowth of neuroglial cells, with obliteration of the normal anatomic landmarks.

Microscopically, the meninges show diffuse fibrosis and infiltration with lymphocytes and plasma cells. Numerous small miliary gummas may be present

Clinical Features

Chronic syphilitic basal meningitis usually presents with the sudden onset of diplopia due to paralysis involving the third and sixth cranial nerves. This may be followed by paralysis of any of the other cranial nerves. Involvement of the fifth and seventh nerves may produce trigeminal neuralgia and bilateral facial palsy; involvement of the eighth nerve may result in tinnitus, vertigo, and deafness; and if the tenth and twelfth nerves are involved, dysphagia, dysarthria, and wasting of the tongue may also occur. Extension of meningitis rostrally may produce syphilitic optic atrophy.

Diagnostic Procedures

1. The blood serologic test for syphilis is usually positive.
2. The cerebrospinal fluid shows a lymphocytic pleocytosis with an elevated protein content. Gamma globulin is significantly increased.
3. The serologic tests for syphilis are positive in the cerebrospinal fluid.

Treatment

See discussion of treatment of patients with neurosyphilis (p. 425).

The basal meningitis is rapidly arrested by penicillin, but cranial nerve palsies may persist. Hydrocephalus may result from adhesive arachnoiditis despite treatment and require surgical relief by a ventriculoatrial shunt.

Meningovascular Syphilis

This condition presents a combination of chronic basal meningitis and syphilitic arteritis.

Pathology

The meninges show chronic granulomatous thickening typical of syphilitic meningitis. There are inflammatory changes in the blood vessels involving the adventitia and media but the internal elastic lamina is preserved and the intima shows endothelial proliferation. The inflammatory changes may begin in the subarachnoid space and spread along the Virchow-Robin spaces into the arteries penetrating the brain substance. Thrombosis of the penetrating arteries is not infrequent, and occasionally weakening of the vessel wall may occur with the formation of a fusiform aneurysm, which usually does not rupture. In addition, there may be syphilitic endarteritis with endothelial proliferation and fibrous thickening of the intima of the smaller vessels within the brain.

Clinical Features

Symptoms are due to occlusive thrombosis of blood vessels and infarction in the brain or brainstem. Syphilitic hemiplegia may occur with infarction in the distribution of the middle cerebral artery or in the distribution of the paramedian branches of the basilar artery supplying the brainstem. Occlusion of the middle cerebral artery due to syphilis usually presents with contralateral hemiplegia, homonymous hemianopia, and aphasia or apraxia, particularly if there is involvement of the dominant hemisphere. The possibility of meningovascular syphilis should always be considered when a stroke or seizure occurs in a relatively young person.[145, 333] Vertebral-basilar artery insufficiency and brainstem infarction are frequently seen in meningovascular syphilis with the development of infarction of the medulla, pons, or midbrain often preceded by recurrent symptoms suggesting vascular insufficiency. Psychosis occurs in some cases, usually presenting with intermittent episodes of impaired judgment owing to involvement of the frontal lobes. This may be associated with excitement, delirium, delusions, and hallucinations or clouding of consciousness and disorientation. Spontaneous improvement usually occurs but some degree of dementia remains. Other patients may develop slowly progressive neurologic signs suggesting an intracranial neoplasm.[76]

Extrapyramidal Symptoms. Infarction or vascular insufficiency involving the deeper structures of the brain or brainstem may result in an acute syndrome similar to Parkinson's disease or hemi-chorea. Interruption of the cerebellar connections to the red nucleus results in a marked cerebellar intention tremor with hypotonia and dysmetria or rubral tremor. Infarction in or near the subthalamic nucleus occasionally results in hemiballismus.

Diagnostic Procedures

1. The blood and cerebrospinal serologic tests for syphilis are positive and usually there is a lymphocytic pleocytosis of the spinal fluid with increased protein content.
2. Arteriography may demonstrate irregular constriction and dilatation of cerebral arteries due to syphilitic arteritis. There may be occlusion of major vessels.[318]

Treatment

See discussion of treatment of neurosyphilis (p. 425).

The meningovascular process is promptly arrested by penicillin but residual symptoms due to infarction may remain. In early cases, particularly in cases with cerebrovascular insufficiency, cessation of symptoms may be seen within a few days of beginning treatment.

Gumma of the Brain

Large solitary gummas of the meninges are rare but when they occur they are usually situated superficially over the surface of the brain or cerebellum. Occasionally they become embedded in the brain and behave as a deep tumor.

Pathology

A gumma consists of a central area of necrosis surrounded by epithelioid cells, plasma cells, and giant cells enclosed in a layer of dense fibroglial tissue. It is grossly indistinguishable from a tuberculoma. A gumma may occasionally occur in association with widespread syphilitic granulomatous meningitis.

Clinical Features

The symptoms depend on the site of the gumma. The most frequent location is over the convexity of the hemisphere, producing a contralateral hemiparesis often accompanied by focal seizures. However, a meningeal gumma may present as an expanding mass located anywhere in the central nervous system.

Diagnostic Procedures

1. The blood serologic tests (Reiter protein, complement fixation, treponemal immobilization, fluorescent treponemal antibody, VDRL, etc.) for syphilis are positive.
2. The cerebrospinal fluid will show positive serologic tests in 50 per cent of cases along with increased pressure, a lymphocytic pleocytosis, and elevated protein content. In about 50 per cent of cases, the CSF serology has been normal but the blood serology has been positive.
3. The electroencephalogram shows changes compatible with a focal structural lesion in gummas located within the cerebral hemispheres.
4. Computed tomography shows an area of increased density with displacement of the underlying brain. There may be some enhancement with injection of contrast material.
5. Arteriography will usually show displacement of blood vessels by a mass, particularly in gummas involving the erebral hemispheres. The mass is usually avascular but may have a diffuse hypervascular blush.[318]

Treatment

Gummas present as intracranial space-occupying lesions, and the diagnosis is often made following surgical removal of the mass.

The patient should also be given a full course of penicillin (see discussion of treatment of neurosyphilis, p. 425).

General Paresis

General paresis does not appear to have been clearly described prior to the Napoleonic wars and the first clinical descriptions have been thought by some to indicate that the disease may have originated in northern France during this period. It is their belief that there was a rapid spread throughout Europe with later spread to the Americas. Those believing in such a recent origin of the disease quote such evidence to indicate a mutant form of the *Treponema pallidum* possessing neurotropic properties. The disease in all probability, however, has been present since the history of man. Neurosyphilis was thought to represent an inadequate immune response by the host toward the organism. However, the recent Oslo study clearly shows that the pathologic effects are due to viable treponemes.

Pathology

General paresis is essentially a subacute encephalitis with diffuse thickening of the meninges, atrophy of the brain, and compensatory dilatation of the ventricular system. The ventricular system frequently exhibits a granular ependymal lining, known as "granular ependymitis." Microscopic examination shows diffuse infiltration of the meninges with lymphocytes and plasma cells. The gray matter of the brain shows loss of neurons, with proliferation of astrocytes and an increase in microglial cells, which have a rod-shaped appearance and tend to orientate themselves perpendicular to the brain surface. These migratory microglia often have a deposition of iron granules. The diffuse syphilitic arteritis is characterized by perivascular cuffing of the meningeal vessels with endothelial proliferation throughout most of the smaller vessels. Spirochetes may be demonstrated in the brain substance by special staining techniques using silver carbonate.

Clinical Features

The clinical picture of general paresis is characterized by progressive mental deterioration, which may be abrupt or insidious in onset.[23]

History. The history usually can be obtained only from the family and the changes described are usually typical of organic dementia. They consist of:

LOSS OF OPERATIONAL JUDGMENT. There is deterioration in performance at work with loss of ability to make correct decisions. Patients may become accident-prone when driving an automobile.

CHANGES IN TEMPERAMENT. There may be loss of common courtesies, which are replaced by overt rudeness. Obscenities may be used and these may be blurted out loudly and inappropriately.

LOSS OF RECENT MEMORY. The patient may resort to note taking in order to counter this situation of forgetting names, dates, and places.

CHANGES IN PERSONALITY. Initially the patient may show increased irritability, which may be followed by emotional lability, outbursts of excitement, and manic episodes. As the behavior deteriorates the appearance becomes slovenly.

CHANGES IN AFFECT. The patient progresses to a state of apathy and mental dullness occasionally interspersed with periods of excitement.

DISORIENTATION AND DELUSIONS. Further deterioration results in disorientation often accompanied by paranoid delusions or hallucinations. These may be responsible for outbursts of destructive violence. Delusions of grandeur are infrequent.

Physical Signs. Tremor is a very common sign of general paresis. The patient develops a coarse tremor involving the eyes, tongue, labial muscles, and fingers. The tremor of the outstretched hands may be rapid and reminiscent of thyrotoxicosis. The classical Argyll Robertson pupils develop at an early stage in about 90 per cent of cases of general paresis and can be assumed to be present, invariably, in advanced cases. There is usually an increase of the deep tendon reflexes with loss of the superficial abdominal reflexes. The speech becomes progressively slurred and eventually dysarthia becomes so severe that the speech is unintelligible.

The writing also deteriorates and eventually becomes unintelligible. There may be varying degrees of dysgraphia, with omission of words and syllables and frequent misspelling of words. Seizures may occur at any stage in general paresis; they are a common complication and may be the first symptom of the disease. Seizures may be generalized or focal and are often followed by a prolonged period of postictal confusion.

LISSAUER'S TYPE OF GENERAL PARESIS. This clinical variety of general paresis is rare and is characterized by the onset of seizures and focal signs including hemiplegia, hemianopia, and dysphasia.

Diagnostic Procedures

1. The blood serologic tests for syphilis are positive in 95 per cent of cases. The percentage is higher if the *Treponema* immobilization test or the fluorescent *Treponema* antibody absorption test is used.
2. The cerebrospinal fluid shows a lymphocytic pleocytosis and increased protein content. The serologic test for syphilis is positive.
3. Serial electroencephalography shows progressive loss of alpha activity with an increase of slow activity over both hemispheres.
4. Computed tomography shows symmetric ventricular dilatation, particularly in the frontal

horns. Advanced cases show diffuse cortical atrophy.

Treatment

Treatment with penicillin is outlined under treatment of neurosyphilis (p. 425).

The majority of cases of general paresis can be diagnosed at an early stage and show an excellent response to penicillin therapy.[207] Cases diagnosed at a later stage may have residual dementia. The patients are often able to return to work but at a less responsible level.[175a] A few patients in whom treatment is instituted only after severe deterioration may require permanent institutional care. A few cases may relapse despite adequate penicillin therapy and will require a second course of treatment.[72, 150]

Asymptomatic Tertiary Neurosyphilis

A number of patients receiving routine follow-up care following apparent recovery from primary or secondary syphilis develop changes in the cerebrospinal fluid indicating central nervous system infection. The usual findings are a lymphocytic pleocytosis, increased protein content, and positive serologic test for syphilis. These patients show a prompt response to penicillin with disappearance of the CSF abnormalities. The prognosis is excellent but further follow-up with repeated lumbar punctures every 12 months is recommended.

Syphilitic Primary Optic Atrophy

Primary optic atrophy occurs in about 0.5 per cent of cases of untreated syphilis and is frequently associated with tabes dorsalis.

Pathology

The pia surrounding the optic nerve shows a chronic inflammation with the presence of lymphocytes or plasma cells. The inflammatory reaction is marked around the nutrient blood vessels that penetrate the nerve in the intraneural septa and these vessels show both arteritis and thrombosis. Degeneration of nerve fibers begins at the periphery of the nerve and extends toward the center, so that there is eventually complete loss of nerve fibers and total demyelination of the nerve with secondary gliosis. The retina shows simple atrophy of nerve cells.

Clinical Features

There is progressive constriction of the visual fields, which often begins in one eye. The constriction of the visual field progresses and eventually involves the central visual field with total blindness. Involvement of the other eye may not occur for some months or years, but the usual course results in total blindness within ten years. The optic fundi show progressive pallor and loss of the small vessels, and eventually they become paper white. Optic atrophy is commonly associated with tabes dorsalis.

Diagnostic Procedures

The serologic test for syphilis is usually positive, but some cases have negative reactions in the blood. If syphilitic optic atrophy is suspected, a *Treponema* immobilization test, Reiter protein complement fixation test, or a fluorescein *Treponema* antibody absorption test should be performed in blood and CSF. These tests give a higher percentage of positive reaction.[291]

Treatment

The most effective treatment is penicillin therapy, as outlined under treatment of neurosyphilis (see p. 425).

The condition will be arrested if penicillin therapy is given at an early stage. In advanced cases, the drug may not prevent the development of blindness.[83]

Syphilitic Secondary Optic Atrophy

Primary syphilitic optic atrophy has to be differentiated from syphilitic secondary optic atrophy. This latter condition may occur owing to external pressure on the optic nerve, caused by chronic syphilitic basal meningitis, or to increased intracranial pressure from hydrocephalus, caused by syphilitic meningitis or meningeal gumma.

Congenital Neurosyphilis

Infection of the developing fetus by *Treponema pallidum* does not occur before the fourth month of intrauterine life, and adequate treatment of the mother before the sixteenth week of pregnancy will prevent fetal infection.[41]

A child with congenital syphilis may be still-born, survive but show the stigmata of congenital syphilis, or be apparently normal at birth but later develop signs of neurosyphilis. These include mental retardation, syphilitic meningitis, chronic basal meningitis, and juvenile general paresis. Tabes dorsalis is rarely seen in congenital syphilis. General paresis usually occurs during the second decade and is rapidly progressive. The pathologic changes in the brain are similar to those seen in the adult except for the frequent occurrence of binucleated Purkinje cells in the cerebellum.

The symptoms of juvenile general paresis are progressive dementia in a child or young adolescent usually associated with the stigmata of congenital syphilis including interstitial keratitis, nerve deafness, Hutchinson's teeth, saddlenose, a high arched palate, and signs of periostitis and osteochondritis as seen by roentgenograms of the long bones.

Diagnostic Procedures

1. The serologic tests for syphilis are usually positive in the blood.
2. The cerebrospinal fluid shows a positive serologic test for syphilis and shows evidence of inflammation in active neurosyphilis.

Treatment

The routine use of a reliable serologic test should lead to detection of the syphilitic mother at early stages of the pregnancy. Institution of penicillin therapy at this stage will prevent transplacental infection of the fetus. If any doubt exists, the mother should be given a course of penicillin on an elective basis. A child born with congenital syphilis should be treated immediately with aqueous penicillin G, 50,000 units/lb of body weight given in ten equally divided doses daily by intramuscular injection.

Syphilis of the Spinal Cord

Acute Syphilitic Transverse Myelitis

This is a rare complication that may occur at any time in the tertiary stage of syphilis.

Pathology

The term "transverse myelitis" is a misnomer since the condition results from infarction of the spinal cord due to syphilitic arteritis involving the anterior spinal artery and the penetrating branches of this vessel.

Clinical Features

The onset is sudden with the rapid development of a flaccid paraplegia associated with paralysis of bladder function and a sensory loss below the level of the cord infarction. The paralysis is flaccid at first, becoming spastic after four to six weeks. The sensory loss involves pain and temperature sensations with some loss of touch, but position and vibration sense are preserved (anterior spinal artery syndrome).

Diagnostic Procedures

1. The blood serologic tests for syphilis are positive.
2. The cerebrospinal fluid is usually under normal pressure with a lymphocytic pleocytosis, increased protein content, and positive serologic test for syphilis. Occasionally the spinal fluid may be normal, although the blood serologic test for syphilis is positive.

Diffuse Syphilitic Meningomyelitis

The spinal cord may be involved by chronic syphilitic meningitis as an isolated phenomenon or in association with chronic cerebral basal meningitis.

Pathology

These is an inflammatory thickening of the pia-arachnoid with obstruction of the subarachnoid space, which may contain pockets of yellow cerebrospinal fluid. The meninges show infiltration with lymphocytes and plasma cells and occasionally multiple small gummas. There is syphilitic arteritis with small infarcts of the cord.

Clinical Features

The onset is usually insidious with a progressive spinal paraparesis.[94a] Root pains are frequent owing to involvement of the posterior nerve roots with sensory loss in the chest or abdomen. There is loss of sphincter control and the sensory loss becomes more widespread with patchy hypalgesia and hypersthesia involving both limbs and trunk. Involvement of the anterior nerve roots and the anterior horns eventually results in muscle wasting and fasciculations.

Diagnostic Procedures

1. The blood serologic test for syphilis is positive.
2. Lumbar puncture will usually reveal evidence of subarachnoid block with low cerebrospinal fluid pressure and no pressure change during the Queckenstedt test. The spinal fluid is xanthochromic with a marked elevation in protein content and a positive serologic test for syphilis.

Treatment

The most effective treatment is penicillin therapy (see discussion of treatment for neurosyphilis). If there is a regional block on myelography, surgical therapy with decompression may be considered.

Penicillin therapy arrests the active syphilitic process but the results of spinal cord and nerve root compression may be permanent with marked disability.

Pachymeningitis Cervicalis Hypertrophica

This is a rare complication of tertiary syphilis due to a localized thickening of the meninges, which are firmly adherent to the cervical portion of the spinal cord. The cervical cord and the emerging nerve roots are atrophic owing to compression or ischemia resulting from compression of blood vessels.

Clinical Features

The condition begins with slowly progressive paraparesis, accompanied by loss of sphincter control and a patchy sensory loss below the cervical area. Pressure on the anterior nerve roots produces muscle atrophy affecting the shoulder girdles, arms, and small muscles of the hands. Pressure on the cervical cord or roots may produce a bilateral Horner's syndrome.

Diagnostic Procedures

1. The blood serologic test for syphilis is positive.
2. Lumbar puncture demonstrates a complete block of the subarachnoid space with a low opening pressure and negative Queckenstedt test. The fluid may be xanthochromic and a Froin's syndrome may be present. The serologic test for syphilis in the cerebrospinal fluid is positive.

Treatment

Penicillin therapy, as outlined in the treatment of neurosyphilis (p. 425), should be instituted. Surgical decompression after cervical laminectomy has been reported to be beneficial.

Penicillin therapy will arrest the active syphilitic process but there is usually only minimal recovery of neurologic deficit.

Syphilitic Amyotrophy

This is a very rare form of syphilis that was diagnosed more frequently in the past when syphilis was a more common disease.

Pathology

There is a progressive loss of neurons in the ventral horns due to a syphilitic arteritis involving the penetrating branches of the anterior spinal artery.

Clinical Features

This condition mimics amyotrophic lateral sclerosis. There is progressive wasting involving the small muscles of the hands and other muscle groups in upper and lower limbs accompanied by fasciculations. The corticospinal tracts are involved in the lateral funiculus of the cord, producing increased tone, hyperreflexia, and extensor plantar responses.

Diagnostic Procedures

1. The blood serologic test for syphilis is positive.
2. In order to make a diagnosis of syphilitic amyotrophy the cerebrospinal fluid should show a lymphocytic pleocytosis, increased protein content, and positive serologic test for syphilis.

Electromyography of the denervated muscles will show the presence of fibrillations and a poor interference pattern typical of a lower motor neuron lesion. The nerve conduction velocities are normal.

Treatment

Penicillin therapy is indicated, as outlined in the treatment of neurosyphilis (p. 425).

Penicillin therapy arrests the amyotrophy but there may be little improvement in the strength of the affected muscles.

Spinal Gumma

Spinal gummas are rare and resemble extramedullary tumors of the spinal canal.

Clinical Features

The patient presents with progressive spastic paraparesis followed by sphincter impairment and sensory loss below the level of the lesion.

Diagnostic Procedures

1. The blood serologic test for syphilis is positive.
2. The lumbar puncture may reveal evidence of a subarachnoid block with elevated protein content and a positive serologic test for syphilis.
3. Myelography will demonstrate the level of the lesion and indicates extramedullary compression of the spinal cord.

Treatment

Surgical removal of a spinal gumma should be followed by adequate penicillin therapy. There is usually marked improvement following removal of the gumma and only minimal neurologic deficits remain.

Tabes Dorsalis

About 25 per cent of cases of neurosyphilis develop tabes dorsalis. Although the frequency of new cases is declining, many patients are still seen with persisting severe disability. This is because survival of patients with this form of neurosyphilis is much longer than in general paresis.

Pathology

The disease affects both the dorsal nerve roots and the posterior columns of the spinal cord. The spinal cord shows thickening of the meninges, particularly in the dorsal regions, and both the dorsal nerve roots and posterior columns are thin and atrophic.

The degenerative changes begin in the midportion of the posterior columns in the lumbar area. This area is believed to carry proprioceptive fibers, which may account for the profound ataxia seen in tabes dorsalis. As the disease progresses, the posterior columns show degenerative changes in the lumbar area with some involvement of the funiculus gracilis in the cervical area. In extreme cases, the posterior columns show severe degeneration throughout the length of the spinal cord.

Atrophy of the dorsal nerve roots also begins in the lumbar area and extends into thoracic and eventually cervical areas. There is a loss of both axons and myelin sheaths with a marked reduction in the ganglia cells in the dorsal root ganglia.

Pathogenesis

The early impression that tabes dorsalis was a primary degenerative condition involving the posterior columns has now been discarded in view of the marked degeneration seen in the dorsal nerve roots which precedes the cord changes. The primary lesion is believed to begin where the posterior nerve root penetrates the pia and enters the spinal cord (Obersteiner-Redlich area). It has been postulated that inflammatory changes in the pia (possibly allergic in nature to the *Treponema pallidum*) may lead to strangulation of the nerve fibers of the posterior nerve roots, but these changes are now felt to be the direct result of viable spirochetes. Inflammatory changes have also been described around the posterior nerve root lying between the dorsal root ganglion and the subarachnoid space with degeneration of nerve fibers.

Clinical Features

Lightning Pains. These are almost pathognomonic of tabes dorsalis. There is a history of recurrent and paroxysmal lightning pains in almost all patients with tabes, which often extends for many years prior to the development of other neurologic symptoms.[279] The pains are usually described as being in the lower limbs in the distribution of the lumbosacral nerve roots and are frequently termed "rheumatic" by the patients who note that they are worse in damp and cold weather. Occasionally the pains may appear in girdle fashion around the abdomen or thorax and less frequently in the face, where they may resemble tic douloureux. The pains are severe and lancinating, particularly in the limbs, but their onset is rapid and the duration very brief, hence the term "lightning pains." They have usually disappeared by the time the patient reaches down to massage the affected region.

Tabetic Crises. These are also characteristic of tabes dorsalis. They consist of sudden attacks of epigastric pain, nausea, and vomiting, which last from a few hours to several days. The symptoms of a gastric crisis may resemble those of a perforated peptic ulcer.[1] However, there is hyperesthesia of the abdominal wall without deep tenderness, and the boardlike rigidity of the abdomen typical of a ruptured abdominal viscus is lacking. Nevertheless, diagnostic roentgenograms of the abdomen should be made to exclude these conditions if there is any doubt. It should be remembered that abdominal visceral disease may occur in tabes dorsalis, and the presence of Argyll Robertson pupils should not lead to the automatic diagnosis of gastric crisis. Other forms of tabetic crisis may also occur, including laryngeal crisis with paroxysmal coughing and dyspnea and rarely rectal, vesicle, uterine, and genital crises.

Locomotor Ataxia. This is also highly characteristic of tabes dorsalis.

The majority of tabetics develop ataxia before the diagnosis is established and most complain of an increase in ataxia in the dark. Some patients become helpless without visual clues to maintain balance and may fall suddenly when they close the eyes to wash the face.

Sensory Loss and Paresthesias. These are common in tabes. Many patients with ataxia complain of loss of sensation in the feet and describe walking as though they were stepping on cotton. In addition, numbness or tingling may occur in other areas of the body and face, particularly in the perioral area. Hyperesthesia on contact with clothing or shoes may also occur.

Bladder Disturbances. These are so common that the descriptive term "tabetic type" is commonly used. Involvement of the posterior nerve roots in the sacral area results in loss of bladder sensation and loss of reflex contraction of the bladder. There is a painless distention of the bladder, which can become extremely large. A gradual increase in intravesicular pressure finally overcomes the tone of the internal sphincter and results in incontinence. Examination reveals a constant dribbling of urine and a huge, distended, insensitive bladder.

Loss of Libido. Loss of libido due to the loss of sensation and reflex activity of the genital organs occurs in both males and females.

Complications

Syphilitic optic atrophy (see p. 419) is not uncommon in tabes dorsalis, so that the untreated condition may be complicated by blindness. Involvement of the cranial nerves due to syphilitic basal meningitis occurs in tabes with ptosis, ocular palsies, and weakness of the oral and pharyngeal muscles. Loss of joint sensation due to degeneration of the posterior nerve roots leads to painless injuries to the articular surfaces and ligaments, resulting in Charcot's joints (Fig. 7–4). There is progressive destruction of the articular surfaces with new bone formation, laxity of ligaments, and effusion into the joints. The joint shows increased mobility and instability. The ankle, knee, and hip joints are most frequently involved, but the arthropathy may occur in the spine, in the shoulder, and occasionally in the smaller joints of the hands and feet.

Lack of cutaneous sensation, particularly in the feet, leads to painless destruction of skin and superficial tissues with the development of painless

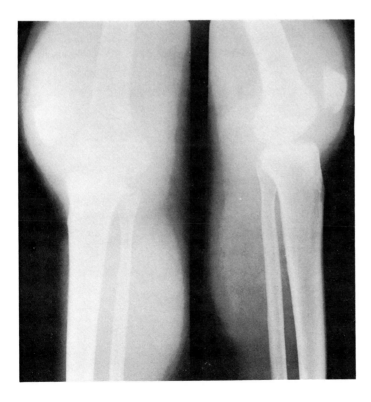

FIGURE 7–4. Roentgenographs of both knees in a case of tabes dorsalis showing bilateral Charcot joints. The joints are swollen, and there are painless destructive changes.

"trophic" ulcers. The ulcers are commonly seen over the heels or over the head of the first metatarsal bone, with involvement of the tarsometatarsal joints by osteomyelitis. The viscera become insensitive to pain, and silent perforation of a peptic ulcer or inflamed appendix may occur.

The diagnosis of tabes is usually not difficult because of certain outstanding neurologic signs. The Argyll Robertson pupil should be regarded as the hallmark of neurosyphilis and usually develops at an early stage in tabes. There may be a period when the pupils are unequal and irregular with a sluggish reaction to light before the development of the classic miotic pupil, which fails to react to light. Sometimes, the pupil may be irregular and dilated but fails to react to light. The reaction to near vision is preserved but may be difficult to demonstrate if the pupil is miotic. The Argyll Robertson pupil may be found in a number of other conditions as well as neurosyphilis (p. 24). The visual field may be constricted and the optic disks pale owing to syphilitic optic atrophy, which is not uncommon in tabes dorsalis. Advanced cases of tabes dorsalis frequently develop a rather characteristic facial appearance, with bilateral ptosis and prominent nasolabial folds. Cranial nerve palsies are common, and paralysis of any of the cranial nerves may occur, but the oculomotor nerves are most commonly involved owing to associated syphilitic basal meningitis.

Passive movement of the limbs, particularly the lower, reveals marked hypotonia, presumably due to denervation of the muscle spindles secondary to the atrophy of the posterior nerve roots. There is usually areflexia of the lower limbs but the plantar response remains flexor. The loss of proprioceptive impulses from the lower limbs and trunk results in a wide-based station, and the gait is highly characteristic with a wide-based stamping of the feet, termed "locomotor ataxia." The ataxia is increased if the patient closes his eyes or is blindfolded, and the Romberg test is positive.

Degeneration of the posterior columns produces marked loss of vibration and position sense beginning in the lower limbs and later involving the upper limbs. In addition, the tabetic develops areas of hypalgesia (Hitzig's zones). These are usually seen in a butterfly distribution over the nose and cheeks, down the ulnar distribution in the forearms, around the nipples, along the medial aspect of the thighs, and over the lateral aspect of the legs.

Other important confirmatory signs include a nontender, distended bladder, Charcot joints, and trophic ulcers.

Diagnostic Procedures

The blood serologic test for syphilis is positive in the early stages of the disease but may be negative in more chronic stages. A *Treponema* immobilization test or fluorescein *Treponema* antibody absorption test should be performed in such cases. The cerebrospinal fluid shows a lymphocytic pleocytosis, elevated protein content, a first- or medium-zone colloidal gold curve, and a positive serologic test for syphilis during the early active phase of tabes, but may be normal in chronic spontaneously healed or "burnt-out" cases.

Treatment

Penicillin therapy is recommended as outlined in the section on treatment of neurosyphilis (see p. 425).

In early cases complete recovery with penicillin is the rule. A number of chronic cases continue to have symptoms or actually show further deterioration despite adequate penicillin therapy. Repeated courses of penicillin have little effect on the course of such cases, and the progression is not due to any active syphilitic process but probably due to increasing fibrosis and gliosis in posterior nerve roots and posterior columns. Without treatment, chronic incapacitation results, with death occurring after 10 to 20 years owing to urinary tract infection or other intercurrent disease.

Treatment of Complications

Lightning Pains.   Those patients who experience persistence of lightning pains may be treated with diphenylhydantoin (Dilantin)[119] or carbamazepine (Tegretol).[86] Carbamazepine has been most effective in the control of lightning pains. Some intractable cases may still require cordotomy.

Gastric Crises.   The majority of cases can be controlled with intravenous fluids and adequate doses of barbiturates or phenothiazines.

Charcot Joints.   Adequate external support by bracing or orthopedic fusion may help considerably.

Urinary Retention with Overflow Incontinence. Many patients benefit from a transurethral resection of the prostate or resection of the hypertro-phied bladder neck. Such restoration of function is to be preferred to a permanent indwelling ure-thral catheter. Should an indwelling urethral catheter be necessary, it must be changed fre-quently under conditions as aseptic as possible. An ileal loop procedure will reduce the risk of repeated urinary tract infection.

Trophic Ulcers. The removal of weight bear-ing on the area by elevating the shoe may help. Careful dressing of the ulcer with antibiotic oint-ments will tend to promote healing, which is, however, a slow process.

Treatment of Patients with Neurosyphilis

The recommended treatment is outlined in Ta-ble 7–5.[151, 287, 296] If the patients show severe sensitivity to penicillin, use of erythromycin is recommended. This is usually given in 0.5-gm doses every six hours for 20 days.

The Jarisch-Herxheimer Reaction

This is a rare complication of therapy consist-ing of fever, chills, headaches, and muscle and joint pains occurring several hours after the first injection of penicillin. Since it was also encoun-tered with the use of bismuth and arsenical prepa-

TABLE 7–5

Treatment of Patients with Syphilis
(Recommended by Center for Disease Control, Atlanta, Georgia)

Type of Syphilis	Benzathine Penicillin G	Aqueous Procaine Penicillin G
Primary, secondary, and latent syphilis of less than 1 year's duration	2.4 million units by intramuscular injection at a single session	4.8 million units total: 600,000 by intramuscular injection daily for 8 days
	Patients who are allergic to penicillin: Tetracycline hydrochloride, 500 mg 4 times a day by mouth for 15 days, or erythromycin, 500 mg 4 times a day by mouth for 15 days	
Syphilis of more than 1 year's duration including latent syphilis, asymptomatic neurosyphilis, and neurosyphilis	7.2 million units total, 2.4 million units by intramuscular injection weekly for 3 successive weeks	9.0 million units total, 600,000 units by intramuscular injection daily for 15 days
	Patients who are allergic to penicillin: Tetracycline hydrochloride, 500 mg 4 times a day by mouth for 30 days, or erythromycin, 500 mg 4 times a day by mouth for 30 days	
Congenital syphilis	Aqueous crystalline penicillin G, 50,000 units/kg intramuscularly or intravenously daily in two divided doses for a minimum of 10 days, or	
	Aqueous procaine penicillin G, 50,000 units/kg intramuscularly for a minimum of 10 days	
Follow-up early syphilis	Congenital syphilis quantitative or treponeme test at 3, 6, and 12 months after treatment	
Follow-up syphilis of more than 1 year	Repeat serology at 24 months	
Follow-up neurosyphilis	Repeat serology every 6 months for 3 years Repeat lumbar puncture every 6 months for 3 years	
Retreatment: a. If cerebrospinal fluid abnormal b. If clinical signs of syphilis persist c. If sustained fourfold increase in titer of nontreponemal test d. If an initially high nontreponemal test fails to show fourfold decrease within a year		

Note: Dosages recommended for treatment of neurosyphilis are minimal since there is evidence that penicillin levels on the cerebrospinal fluid are extremely low after recommended doses of benzathine penicillin G have been given.[2] *Treponema pallidum* has been isolated from the cerebrospinal fluid after treatment with recommended doses of benzathine penicillin G.[3]

rations, it is not a reaction to penicillin. It is not related to the dose of the drug given and is not an indication for a reduction is the amount of penicillin.[95, 207] The symptoms subside in about 24 hours.

Seronegative Neurosyphilis

A certain proportion of cases of the more chronic forms of neurosyphilis, particularly syphilitic optic atrophy and tabes dorsalis, give a negative serologic test for syphilis. Many of the same cases will give a positive *Treponema* immobilization test (TPI) or fluorescein treponema antibody test (FTA-ABS). In view of this, all cases with a negative serologic test for syphilis that present with one or more of the following should have a TPI or FTA-ABS test:

1. Optic atrophy
2. Argyll Robertson pupils
3. Signs and symptoms suggesting tabes dorsalis

Sarcoidosis

Although sarcoidosis is an inflammatory disease, its infectious nature remains unproved. There is some disagreement about the incidence of sarcoidosis involving the nervous system, but this condition probably occurs in about 4 per cent of cases with sarcoidosis and it may be higher in cases with signs of diffuse systemic involvement. The condition is rare and frequently runs a benign course, although cases with cerebral involvement may prove fatal, and optic, cranial, and peripheral nerve involvement is sufficiently disabling to warrant treatment.

Etiology and Pathology

The majority of authors consider sarcoidosis as a chronic "anergic" response to the tubercle bacillus or some other antigenic agent. Although the relationship of sarcoidosis to the tubercle bacillus has been postulated in some cases, it certainly cannot be established in all. The condition is best characterized as a pathologic entity in which the tissues show a nonspecific inflammatory response without caseation necrosis but with giant cell and epithelioid cell hyperplasia possibly resulting from tuberculosis and other agents.

Cases with central nervous system involvement usually show similar granulomatous inflammation in other organs, such as the lung, liver, kidney, and spleen (Fig. 7–6). There are two major changes in the central nervous system: (1) a diffuse granulomatous leptomeningitis, most marked over the base of the brain, or (2) circumscribed granulomatous lesions involving the pia-arachnoid, ependyma, brain, and spinal cord.

The thickened meninges have a nodular appearance, and the cranial nerves are buried and difficult to identify at the base of the brain and over the brainstem. Scattered nodules in the brain are most frequent over the pial surface and in the ventricles and appear to extend into the cortical parenchyma from the meninges or ependyma. The hypothalamus shows the most involvement, followed by the pons,[140] and small cortical infarcts have been described in some cases.

Microscopic examination shows the typical appearance of noncaseating granulomas containing epithelioid cells and giant cells, with a varying degree of fibroblastic reaction at the periphery. There may be some additional inflammatory response due to lymphocytes and plasma cells. The changes in the spinal cord are of a similar type with a variable degree of granulomatous infiltration of the arachnoid and some extension of the granulomatous process into the parenchyma of the spinal cord.[65] The dorsal and ventral nerve roots and the peripheral nerves may show similar noncaseating granulomatous involvement.

Clinical Features

The clinical features show considerable variation.[68] Encephalopathy may occur as a structural or metabolic complication of sarcoidosis. Granulomatous changes in the brain or meninges may present with psychosis, drowsiness, unilateral or bilateral corticospinal tract signs, focal or generalized seizures, dementia, and dysphasia. Occasionally, focal signs are prominent owing to the presence of a focal granulomatous lesion that mimics a brain tumor. Focal or generalized seizures are occasionally the presenting symptom of neurologic sarcoidosis.

Metabolic encephalopathy can also occur in sarcoidosis with involvement of other organ systems. Sarcoidosis of the kidneys, liver, or lungs may produce metabolic changes resulting in uremia, hepatic encephalopathy, or pulmonary insufficiency with CO_2 narcosis, respectively. The hypercalcemia of sarcoidosis can cause neuropsychiatric symptoms, and granulomatous destruction of the pituitary gland may result in panhypopituitarism and encephalopathy.

Meningeal sarcoidosis is one of the most common neurologic manifestations of the disease. The condition is a chronic basal meningitis with multiple cranial nerve involvement, hypothalamic and pituitary involvement, and hydrocephalus.

The hypothalamus and pituitary gland are the most common sites of intracranial involvement in sarcoidosis. Symptoms of hypothalamic involvement include somnolence, obesity, changes in appetite, weight gain or weight loss, hyperthermia or hypothermia, and diabetes insipidus. Pituitary granulomata may produce partial or total pituitary failure.

Cranial nerve involvement occurs as a symptom of chronic basal meningitis or peripheral neuropathy. Optic nerve involvement can present as papilledema, optic atrophy, or retrobulbar neuritis. Isolated optic neuritis or retrobulbar neuritis may be the only manifestation of systemic sarcoidosis or occasionally the first symptom of the disease occurring without evidence of sarcoidosis elsewhere. Many cases develop unilateral or bilateral facial nerve palsy of sudden onset. The paralysis may be followed by complete recovery, although some cases develop facial spasms or contractures. Involvement of the eighth nerve results in unilateral deafness and occasionally vertigo. Bilateral paralysis of the vagus will produce dysarthria and bulbar palsy.

Brainstem and cerebellar involvement results in unilateral or bilateral cerebellar signs including nystagmus, truncal and limb ataxia, and dysmetria. There may be direct involvement of the spinal cord or spinal cord atrophy, secondary to chronic meningitis and arachnoiditis.

Sarcoidosis of the peripheral nerves can present as a mononeuropathy, polyneuropathy, or symmetric peripheral neuropathy. Sudden isolated mononeuropathies with areas of sensory loss or pain are not uncommon in sarcoidosis. These changes may occur in the limbs or in the intercostal distribution and are often transient. Muscle weakness and wasting of muscles supplied by the affected nerve can occur in some cases.

Sarcoidosis of muscle may present as an acute myositis with marked proximal muscle weakness or as a chronic myopathy with stiffness, weakness, and atrophy of the limbs and girdle musculature. Local muscle tenderness with palpable nodules in the muscle has occasionally been described.

Diagnostic Procedures

1. The usual signs of systemic sarcoidosis are usually present, including chronic uveitis, parotid gland enlargement, lymphadenopathy, hepatomegaly, and hilar lymphadenopathy or pulmonary infiltration shown by roentgenograms of the chest.

2. Skin tests usually reveal a negative reaction to tuberculin or PPD. The Kveim test is of limited practical value since at least six weeks is necessary for the development of the characteristic nodule of the skin.

3. There may be depressions or elevations or serum calcium and lowered serum albumin with elevation of serum globulin. Recent studies have shown that hypercalcemia is infrequent.[116]

4. The diagnosis may be established by biopsy of an enlarged lymph node or by liver biopsy.

5. The scalene node biopsy is often positive if there is no evidence of lymphadenopathy elsewhere.

6. In sarcoid encephalopathy, roentgenograms of the skull, electroencephalography, and a CT scan are necessary to demonstrate the presence of a space-occupying lesion or hydrocephalus.

7. A lumbar puncture should be performed in all cases with suspected meningeal involvement once a space-occupying lesion has been ruled out. The cerebrospinal fluid is often under increased pressure and shows a lymphocytic pleocytosis with elevated protein and decreased glucose content, negative cytology, and negative cultures for bacteria and fungi.

8. A skeletal muscle biopsy may be useful as a diagnostic method in systemic sarcoidosis or in the diagnosis of sarcoidosis of muscle.

9. Nerve conduction velocities and electromyography are indicated in cases with peripheral nerve involvement.

10. Appropriate endocrine studies should be performed in cases with suspected hypothalamic or pituitary gland dysfunction.

Treatment

1. Corticosteroids are the only effective treatment of sarcoidosis but do not produce arrest of the process in all cases. This may be owing to too short a trial of steroids. Longer periods of treatment should be tried, particularly with large doses every 48 hours. Our experience with steroid therapy has been remarkably good in the cerebral forms of sarcoid. The initial dosage is 96 mg of methyl prednisolone every other day.

2. Diabetes insipidus can be treated successfully with posterior pituitary extract, and adequate substitution therapy is necessary in patients with anterior pituitary failure.
3. A ventriculoatrial shunting procedure should be considered in patients with hydrocephalus.
4. Rare cases of sarcoidosis presenting with intracerebral mass lesions require surgical removal of the mass.

Adhesive Arachnoiditis

Etiology and Pathology

Adhesive arachnoiditis has been described as a sequel to head trauma; acute bacterial meningitis, subacute meningitis including tuberculous and syphilitic meningitis; myelography particularly after the use of water-soluble contrast agents;[155] intrathecal injection of drugs including spinal anesthesia, penicillin, streptomycin; and the accidental injection of toxic materials.[64] The latter may result when glass vials filled with anesthetic solutions for spinal anesthesia are placed in potentially toxic sterilizing solution. A crack or leak in the vial may permit the sterilizing solution to mix with the anesthesia, which is then injected into the subarachnoid space. In many cases, the chronic inflammatory changes appear to be due to drug sensitivity or represent an allergic reaction of the meninges. Adhesive arachnoiditis has also been reported to follow traumatic and spontaneous subarachnoid hemorrhage, particularly in cases with recurrent bleeding into the subarachnoid space, and not infrequently results as a delayed complication of surgical procedures on the spinal canal.

In established cases, there are loculated areas containing cerebrospinal fluid, and the meninges are thickened and infiltrated with lymphocytes, plasma cells, and proliferating fibroblasts. The changes are usually marked at three sites: (1) around the optic chiasm, (2) in the posterior fossa involving the roof of the fourth ventricle, and (3) in the spinal canal. The changes in the spinal cord appear to be ischemic in nature and may result in cystic changes in the cord reminiscent of syringomyelia.

Clinical Features

Adhesive arachnoiditis involving the optic chiasm produces loss in the visual fields which sometimes presents as a bitemporal hemianopia.

There may be steady progression to complete blindness with optic atrophy.

When the condition occurs in the posterior fossa, obstruction of the foramina in the roof of the fourth ventricle produces hydrocephalus.

Spinal cord involvement is the most common form and results in progressive spastic paraparesis and impairment of bladder function. The sensory loss varies in severity, but some patients complain of girdle-like pains or constricting pains in the limbs. Complete paraplegia may result.

Diagnostic Procedures

1. The cerebrospinal fluid pressure is low in spinal adhesive arachnoiditis and the Queckenstedt test is negative. Occasionally it is impossible to obtain cerebrospinal fluid by lumbar puncture and a cisternal tap is necessary. The fluid is often xanthochromic and the protein content increased.
2. Myelography will demonstrate nerve root obliteration, meningeal thickening, narrowing of the subarachnoid space, or complete blockage of the subarachnoid space in some cases (Fig. 7–7). Loculated arachnoid cysts and intramedullary cavitation are present in severe cases.[250]
3. There is failure to fill the ventricular system with air on attempting a pneumoencephalogram when the roof of the fourth ventricle is blocked by adhesions. The chiasmatic cistern cannot be outlined in cases with arachnoiditis involving the optic chiasm.
4. Computed tomography can be used to demonstrate basal arachnoiditis in the region of the circle of Willis and basal cisterns.[88]

Treatment

Suspected infections such as syphilis and tuberculosis require adequate treatment with appropriate antibiotics.[163] The use of corticosteroids may reduce the inflammatory reaction in cases of syphilis and in other cases, particularly where there has been an unusual or allergic reaction to a drug or iodized oil and following surgery. Localized compression of the spinal cord due to the adhesions may be relieved by laminectomy and lysis of the arachnoid adhesions. Surgical lysis of adhesions may improve vision in cases with optic nerve or chiasmatic involvement.[154] Hydrocephalus is treated by a ventriculoatrial shunt.

Tetanus

The powerful exotoxin of the tetanus bacillus has a unique effect on the anterior horn cells of the spinal cord, resulting in the muscle spasms characteristic of this disease. Tetanus is best defined as an acute infectious process characterized by tonic spasms of skeletal muscle.

Etiology and Pathology

The infectious agent is *Clostridium tetanus,* an anaerobic, gram-positive, sporebearing organism normally found in the intestinal tract of animals and man. It multiples only in the depth of wounds, where there are likely to be anaerobic conditions. During growth it produces and releases an exotoxin into the systemic circulation and peripheral nerves. The disease is particularly prevalent in agricultural communities, following wounds in battles, and in contaminated puncture wounds. Less frequent causes include self-induced and septic abortions, contaminated vaccinations, and intramuscular infections or surgical procedures using inadequately sterilized equipment. The essential lesion in each case is a deep and contaminated wound in which the organism can multiply anaerobically. The exotoxin reaches the central nervous system via the systemic circulation and/or peripheral nerves where it depresses the activity of inhibitory synapses at the anterior horn cells[152a] and damages inhibitory interneurons.[36] The alpha motor neurons become highly reactive to excitatory stimuli and discharge periodically in response to stimuli producing tonic muscular contractions.

Clinical Features

Symptoms usually appear five to eight days after the infection. The patient experiences tingling or pain in the area of the wound. This is followed by restlessness, mild pyrexia, and stiffness of the masseter muscles with tightening of the jaw. The limb and axial muscles are the next to become involved, and the patient suffers from repeated tonic muscular spasms, which are intensely painful and produce opisthotonus. These are often initiated by slight noise or tactile stimuli. Involvement of the facial muscles results in a characteristic expression, with wrinkling of the forehead, elevation of the eyebrows, and drawing out of the corners of the mouth, the "risus sardonicus" or sardonic smile (Fig. 7–5). Spasm of the

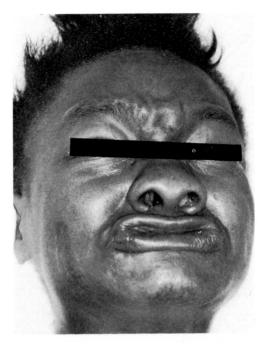

FIGURE 7–5. A patient suffering from severe tetanus. The trismus of the jaw and sardonic smile (risus sardonicus) are characteristic of this condition.

respiratory muscles produces periods of apnea and cyanosis. Death can occur from anoxic damage to the central nervous system, pneumonia, dehydration and electrolyte imbalance, hypotension, and shock.[144, 203]

Tetanus is a serious disease and the prognosis depends on the previous physical condition of the patient as well as the speed with which treatment is given. Those cases with a short incubation period have an unfavorable outlook. If the incubation period is six days or longer, there is an 80 per cent chance of recovery, but it is less than 50 per cent in cases with a short incubation period of less than six days.

Treatment

All children should be immunized with tetanus toxoid (contained in triple vaccine against diphtheria, whooping cough, and tetanus). This confers a high degree of immunity and should be repeated with a booster dose every five years.

Mild Cases. Those without cyanotic episodes can be treated with promazine, 90 to 180 mg every six hours, and barbiturates in sufficient amounts to reduce spasms yet not depress respiration.

Severe Cases.   Treatment is as follows:

1. All cases should be treated by a team of nurses and physicians in an intensive care unit.
2. A low-pressure, cuffed endotracheal tube should be inserted. The tube should be cleared of secretions by gentle suctioning once every hour.
3. Curare should be given in sufficient amounts to prevent tetanus spasms for two hours. This means that the patient is completely paralyzed and has to be treated with assisted respiration. The respirator should be managed by those thoroughly familiar with the use of the machine, that is, by a physician specializing in respiratory diseases, an anesthesiologist, or a physician who has received special training in the management of the machine.
4. The patient is turned every two hours, and attention is given to all pressure areas. The risk of conjunctivitis is high, and eye toilet is performed every two hours.
5. A nasogastric tube is passed, and the patient is given a high-calorie diet. Fluid requirements are often high, up to 6,000 ml/day in some cases.
6. The bladder is catheterized and irrigated, using a neomycin-polymyxin solution and a three-way system. An accurate intake-and-output record is kept.
7. Daily serum electrolytes, blood urea, and blood gases are obtained.
8. The chest roentgenogram is taken every morning.
9. In time, the effect of the curare lasts longer and the patient can be weaned off the drug. The endotracheal tube can then be removed when the vital capacity is satisfactory.

Tetanus remains a major public health problem in rural areas of developing countries. The following method of treatment is applicable in areas where elaborate equipment is not available.[268]

1. Sedation: 50 mg of promazine and 10 mg diazepam should be given to all adults by intramuscular or intravenous injection as soon as the diagnosis of tetanus is made. Supplementary injections of 10 mg of diazepam may be given every two hours as necessary with 25 mg promazine every six to eight hours.
2. Corticosteroids: 8 mg betamethasone IV should be given initially followed by 8 mg every 12 hours.
3. Antitetanic serum:
   a. 750 units of antitetanic serum intramuscularly or intravenous each day for three days.
   b. 200 units of antitetanic serum injected intrathecally.
4. Treatment of wounds: All wounds should be cleaned and dressed.
5. Antibiotics: 800,000 units procaine penicillin should be given intramuscularly every 12 hours until normal respiratory function returns. Treat any infection with appropriate antibiotic therapy.
6. General management: The patient should be nursed in a quiet area with minimal handling. Oral feeding should be maintained if possible but intravenous or rectal infusions may be used if necessary.

Cerebral Brucellosis

Three types of *Brucella* organisms, *abortus, melitensis,* and *suis,* produce clinical infections in man, with a wide variety of symptoms and signs including neurologic disorders that are often difficult to diagnose. Infection is acquired by occupational contact with cattle, goats, or pigs or by the ingestion of infected cows' or goats' milk. The incidence is high in areas where there are large farming communities, and 40 per cent of cases in the United States have been reported from the state of Iowa.[94]

The clinical picture is that of an acute febrile illness (undulant fever), with severe headache, muscle pains, considerable prostration, and weakness. The chronic manifestations of brucellosis include *Brucella* spondylitis and a number of neurologic complications.[106]

Pathology

Involvement of the nervous system by *Brucella* organisms is said to be rare, and pathologic changes in the central and peripheral nervous system may be due to the action of an endotoxin.[71] There are chronic inflammatory changes in the meninges associated with perivascular cuffing and loss of neurons in the superficial layers of the cortex. Meningomyelitis may result, with similar changes involving the spinal meninges and spinal cord. Rarely, brucellosis may produce a mycotic aneurysm of the cerebral arteries secondary to arteritis. Brucellosis may also cause a peripheral neuritis of the "mononeuritis multiplex" type. Rarely, chronic brucellosis may produce spondylitis with extradural abscess and spinal cord compression.

Clinical Features

Meningoencephalitis occasionally presents as a fulminating infection, with severe headache, nuchal rigidity, and rapid progression to stupor and coma. More frequently the condition is subacute with long-standing headaches complicated later by focal signs such as seizures or hemiparesis. The condition may mimic brain tumor. Those cases with meningomyelitis present as a progressive spastic paraparesis with incontinence due to loss of control of micturition. Those cases with mycotic aneurysms that rupture may present with subarachnoid hemorrhage mimicking ruptured saccular aneurysm (p. 575). *Brucella* neuritis presents as a peripheral nerve paralysis often with considerable pain. *Brucella* spondylitis may lead to extradural abscess with pain in the back, root pains in the distribution of thoracic or lumbar nerves, and a progressive spastic paraparesis with bladder involvement.

Diagnostic Procedures

1. Lumbar puncture may show xanthochromic fluid under increased pressure if there is meningoencephalitis. The spinal fluid usually shows a moderate pleocytosis with a mixture of polymorphonuclear leukocytes and lymphocytes with high protein and low glucose content.
2. The organisms may take several weeks to culture from blood or spinal fluid.
3. Serologic tests, in particular the antihuman globulin and complement-fixation tests, are the most helpful in establishing a diagnosis, especially if a rising titer of brucella antibodies can be demonstrated.[334]
4. *Brucella* spondylitis produces typical roentgenographic changes, with narrowed disk spaces, erosion of the vertebral margins, areas of bone rarefaction, and collapse and wedging of vertebral bodies.

Treatment

The persistence of live *Brucella* organisms within the cells of the reticuloendothelial system is a major problem when treating chronic brucellosis. Cotrimoxazole, three tablets three times a day for eight weeks, may be effective but repeated courses are often required at four- to six-week intervals. Intramuscular gentamicin, 120 mg every eight hours for five days, has given encouraging results in patients with normal renal function who are unable to tolerate cotrimoxazole.[288]

Prophylaxis

All milk for human consumption should be pasteurized. Vaccination should eliminate the disease from cattle and pigs.

The prognosis is good if the condition is diagnosed prior to irreversible damage to the nervous system.

Psittacosis (Chlamydiosis)

The organism causing psittacosis has recently been reclassified as a bacterium called *Chlamydia psittaci*. Psittacosis may be acquired through contact with infected birds, particularly the parrot, although it is recognized that the bacteria may be transmitted by a wide variety of wild and domestic birds, including the pigeon and turkey. There have been several recent outbreaks of human psittacosis in employees of turkey-processing plants in Texas, Nebraska, and Missouri.[73, 79] The disease presents as a severe penumonia, but meningitis and encephalitis may complicate the disease.[44]

Diagnostic Procedures

In psittacosis, the organisms may be isolated through the intraperitoneal injection of infected material (blood sputum and throat washings) into mice. A rise in antibodies should be demonstrable between sera drawn in the acute and convalescent stages of the disease. *Chlamydia psittaci* may be isolated from the diseased or dead birds suspected as the carriers.

Treatment

Psittacosis responds to the tetracycline group of antibiotics.

Fungal Infections of the Central Nervous System

Aspergillosis

There are approximately 350 species of aspergillosis but relatively few are pathogenic to man. Aspergillosis occurs primarily in patients whose occupation brings them into contact with dust, grain, birds, and animals, and it affects all ages. Cerebral aspergillosis is rare and usually complicates disseminated aspergillosis. It often appears as a complication of primary lesions in the lungs, skin, or paranasal sinuses. Occasionally, a more chronic infection may enter the cranial cavity by direct spread to the meninges from the paranasal sinuses or the orbit.[136] There may be a history of a chronic debilitating disease that has been treated with antibiotics for a long time, or with antimetabolites and steroids, which lower resistance to infection. There has been an increase in the number of cases of disseminated aspergillosis reported since 1963, and it appears likely that the increase is due to this form of combined therapy. Intravenous drug abuse has been reported in some cases of disseminated and cerebral aspergillosis.[174]

Clinical Features

The acute disseminated form of the disease may result in rapid deterioration and death with few signs of meningeal involvement. In such reported cases the diagnosis was recognized only at autopsy. This fulminating form of the disease tends to occur in infants. In other cases the signs of a rapidly developing meningoencephalitis were followed by death within a few days.[177]

The more chronic forms of cerebral aspergillosis present with symptoms and signs suggesting a brain tumor or brain abscess.[6] A chronic basal meningitis has also been described with headache, neck pain, and cranial nerve involvement. Aspergillosis arteritis produces mycotic aneurysms and subarachnoid hemorrhage[217a] or thrombosis of the internal carotid or middle cerebral arteries with cerebral infarction.[149, 319]

Diagnostic Procedures

1. In the acute form of the disease the cerebrospinal fluid shows an increased pressure and pleocytosis predominantly composed of polymorphonuclear cells. The spinal fluid glucose content is decreased, and the protein and gamma globulin content is elevated.[239] The diagnosis can be established by growth of the organism on Saboraud's medium.
2. It may be possible to obtain evidence of aspergillosis from other sites, including the sputum, or from skin lesions.
3. The more chronic cases may show an increased cerebrospinal fluid protein content.

Treatment

Drug of Choice.   In those cases where the diagnosis can be established, immediate therapy with intravenous and intrathecal amphotericin B is recommended. This disease, in both acute and chronic forms, carries a high mortality rate.

Actinomycosis

Mycotic infection of the central nervous system by the genus *Actinomyces* is rare. The most common site of infection is the cervicofacial region, followed in frequency by pulmonary and visceral disease. Actinomycosis of the lung may spread into the left atrium of the heart, resulting in systemic dissemination of the fungus. The organism may also enter the bloodstream from carious teeth, with the production of remote infections.

Infection of the central nervous system may occur either from direct extension from cervicofacial actinomycosis or by hematogenous spread to the brain or meninges from pulmonary lesions or from carious teeth.

The fungus may produce several types of lesions in the central nervous system, including acute purulent meningitis, brain abscess, meningoencephalitis, a solitary granuloma simulating brain tumor, and a granuloma of the third ventricle simulating a third ventricular cyst.

In the case of brain abscess and granuloma the pathologic changes are essentially those of a granulomatous inflammation with marked fibroblastic reaction. In actinomycotic brain abscess, this is followed by central necrosis with pus formation.

Clinical Features

The symptoms are usually those of a cerebral abscess but occasionally the disease presents as an acute meningitis.[35] Solitary granulomas of the meninges may produce focal seizures and contralateral hemiparesis. Granulomas of the third ventricle may produce intermittent hydrocephalus characterized by severe paroxysmal headache with vomiting. Generalized convulsions and vertigo may also be a prominent feature of such lesions.[241]

Diagnostic Procedures

1. There may be evidence of cervicofacial actinomycosis, or roentgenograms of the chest may reveal an opacity suggesting tumor of the lung.
2. Lumbar puncture reveals a markedly purulent fluid if there is meningeal actinomycosis, although a cerebral abscess may result in mild pleocytosis with normal glucose and protein content. The organism requires an anaerobic

culture medium (e.g., dextrose-agar), and this must be used in any case where suspicion of actinomycosis exists.

3. Roentgenograms of the skull may reveal evidence of displacement of the pineal gland, and arteriograms may reveal displacement of the anterior or middle cerebral arteries if there is a brain abscess. Pneumoencephalography may also indicate a shift of the midline structures or a third ventricular mass producing a filling defect of the third ventricle.

Treatment

The drug of choice is aqueous penicillin G (e.g., 20,000,000 to 30,000,000 units intravenously per day). If there is a brain abscess, surgical drainage is advised followed by long-term penicillin therapy. This will produce healing in some cases, but excision of the abscess may be required if there is recurrence of infection.

Cryptococcal Infections

Cryptococcus neoformans is a yeastlike organism formerly called *Torula histolytica*. It produces infection of the lungs, kidneys, lymph nodes, and central nervous system in man. Cryptococcal meningitis was almost invariably fatal prior to the introduction of amphotericin B in 1956. The organism is probably inhaled with dust and enters the body through the respiratory system. Birds probably act as a reservoir and the organism has been isolated in droppings from sparrows and pigeons.

Pathology

Respiratory infection results in chronic granulomatous inflammation of the lungs, which is usually localized and is only slowly progressive. Infected lymph nodes occasionally show histologic changes resembling Hodgkin's disease.

Cryptococcal meningitis may occur secondary to chronic granulomatous changes in the lungs but it does occur without evidence of lung involvement. It is frequently found in association with chronic debilitating diseases such as diabetes mellitus and Hodgkin's disease.

At necropsy, there is diffuse opacity of the meninges, which have a slippery feeling to the touch. Small granular or tubercle-like nodules are often found in the interpeduncular fossa and along the major sulci. On sectioning of the brain, small perivascular cysts may be seen, which open onto the cortical surface by a thin neck. Occasionally, these small cysts develop into large multicystic or coalesced lesions.

There is granulomatous thickening of the meninges on microscopic examination, with lymphocytes, plasma cells, and occasional giant cells containing cryptococci. The Virchow-Robin spaces are distended with inflammatory cells and cryptococci. However, the subcortical cysts are thin-walled and often show surprisingly little inflammatory or glial reaction, although they contain numerous organism.

Clinical Features

The onset is insidious, with headache usually accompanied by nausea and vomiting. Early symptoms include unsteadiness of gait, photophobia, blurred vision, and retrobulbar pain. Personality changes, impaired memory, agitation, and occasionally psychotic behavior are also early manifestations, but fever and neck stiffness may occur in only 50 per cent of cases at this stage. Papilledema, cranial nerve involvement, and long tract signs are late findings.[42, 85, 117]

Diagnostic Procedures

1. The cerebrospinal fluid may be clear or turbid, with a lymphocytic pleocytosis, elevated protein content, and depressed glucose and chloride content. Normal glucose levels may be obtained in some cases, or the glucose content may be elevated in patients with diabetes mellitus.
2. The encapsulated organisms can be seen on direct smear in an India ink preparation in 60 per cent of cases.
3. Diagnosis can be confirmed by culture and mouse inoculation in the majority of the remaining cases.
4. There should be no hesitation in the performance of cisternal puncture in suspected cases of cryptococcal meningitis when the cerebrospinal fluid obtained by lumbar puncture fails to show organisms in the Indian ink preparation or on culture. Cisternal puncture frequently produces viable organisms.[31]
5. Cryptococcal antibody may be detected in the serum and CSF by indirect fluorescent antibody and agglutination tests.[118]
6. Cryptococcic antigen can be detected in the CSF by later agglutination tests (titers of 1.8 or more). This may be the only means of achieving a diagnosis during life in some cases.[293]

7. A specific pattern for cryptococcal meningitis has been described following cerebrospinal fluid analysis by electron capture gas liquid chromatography.[273]
8. Cryptococci may be cultured from the urine, blood, lymph nodes, and bone marrow.
9. Computed tomography may show the presence of cryptococcal abscesses, which appear as multiple areas of increased density in both white and gray matter (Fig. 7–6).

Treatment

The antibiotic of choice is amphotericin B.[269] Amphotericin B should be given in doses of 0.25 to 1 mg/kg of body weight in 500 ml of 5 per cent dextrose in water over a six-hour period on alternate days for at least four weeks (see Table 7–6). A similar course should be given if there is a relapse within a few months of treatment. Pyrexia, nausea, and vomiting during infusion can be reduced by thorough mixing of the infusion bottle by shaking every 15 minutes.

This drug is fungistatic and allows the development of adequate immunity, which arrests further infection. Tests of renal function, such as blood urea nitrogen, serum creatinine, and glomerular filtration measured by creatinine clearance, should be performed at frequent intervals during the administration of this drug to anticipate nephrotoxicity. Rises in BUN or serum creatinine and falling creatinine clearance levels are an

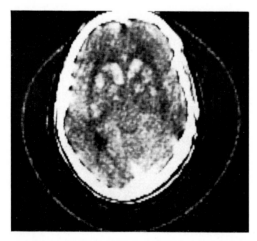

FIGURE 7–6. Computed tomography in a case of cryptococcosis. There are many areas of increased density in this contrast-enhanced study. These areas represent cryptococcal abscesses. The anterior horns of the lateral ventricles are also involved.

TABLE 7–6

Amphotericin B in Treatment of Fungal Meningitis

Dosage	Complications
1. Alternate day infusion of 0.25 mg/kg increasing to a dose of 1 mg/kg*	1. Fever, chills
2. Alternate day intrathecal injection of 0.5 mg dissolved in 10 ml of cerebrospinal fluid	2. Progressive anemia due to bone marrow depression
	3. Renal impairment due to tubular damage

* The infusion should be carried out through a Y tube with a bottle of 5 per cent dextrose in water attached to the other stem of the tubing. The infusion of amphotericin B should be stopped if chills and fever occur and the infusion switched temporarily to 5 per cent dextrose in water. Since amphotericin B disintegrates when exposed to sunlight, the infusion bottle containing it should be shaded.

The amphotericin should be dissolved in 500 ml of 5 per cent dextrose in water and the flask should be agitated frequently during the infusion. The addition of 25 mg of diphenhydramine hydrochloride may reduce the frequency of febrile reactions, while the addition of 20 mg of heparin will reduce any tendency to phlebothrombosis at the site of infusion.

† The frequency of fever and chills during the infusion of amphotericin B may be reduced by giving 10 gr of acetylsalicylic acid and 50 mg of diphenhydramine hydrochloride orally 30 minutes prior to infusion.

indication for reduction of the dosage of amphotericin B.

The use of amphotericin B has altered the outlook in cryptococcic meningitis from a disease that was almost invariably fatal within a period of three years to one in which recovery can now be anticipated. The relapse rate has been reported to be as high as 30 per cent, and careful follow-up of patients with regular examination of the CSF for at least three years is recommended in order to recognize and treat relapsing cases.

Candida albicans Meningitis

Meningitis due to *Candida albicans* is rare but may occur in the newborn infant as a complication of gastroenteritis treated by broad-spectrum antibiotics.[180] It may occur in narcotic addiction, in patients treated with ventriculoatrial shunts, or during the treatment of a systemic disease with corticosteroids, immunosuppressive drugs, or antibiotics. Indwelling central, venous, or bladder catheters are also probable predisposing factors to *Candida* infections.[21]

The illness presents with high fever, headache, and nuchal rigidity, but findings in the cerebrospinal fluid are likely to vary a great deal from case to case. There may occasionally be no cells in the CSF, with normal glucose and protein levels. In such a situation the diagnosis may be established at autopsy or by cerebrospinal fluid culture. Cultures of the CSF should be observed for three weeks in suspected cases before being interpreted as negative.

Treatment

The drug of choice in treating *Candida albicans* meningitis is amphotericin B.

The majority of cases were fatal prior to the introduction of amphotericin B. Although only a few cases of this rare condition have been treated with amphotericin B, there are an increasing number of reports of recovery.

Histoplasmosis

Infection by the yeast *Histoplasma capsulatum* is common in certain regions of the United States but the majority of cases are asymptomatic. Pulmonary and disseminated histoplasmosis are usually found in the southern, midwestern, and western United States, Central and South America, and southern Africa and Australia, and a few cases have been reported from Europe. The disease is believed to be spread by birds since the organism has been isolated from pigeon droppings, which may be inhaled in contaminated dust. Most commonly, lesions are confined to the lungs, but when disseminated histoplasmosis occurs, there is about a 25 per cent risk of central nervous system involvement.[58]

Pathology

In cases of meningitis due to histoplasmosis, microscopic examination of the brain shows the yeast organisms inside histiocytes contained within the meninges. The infection may also produce perivenous miliary granulomatosis with small, noncaseating granulomas within the substance of the brain. These may enlarge as coalescent parenchymatous granulomatosis, with multiple necrotic granulomas within the cerebrum, cerebellum, and brainstem. The most common lesion is a basal meningitis with a thick granulomatous exudate in the basal cisterns and around the brainstem.[109, 322] An isolated histoplasmoma is relatively rare.[121]

Clinical Features

Disseminated histoplasmosis produces fever, weight loss, hepatomegaly, splenomegaly, and lymphadenopathy. Neurologic signs do not occur until there is extensive brain damage[171] that results in predominantly cranial nerve and brainstem dysfunction, with diplopia, nystagmus, pupillary irregularity, facial paralysis, dysarthria, and cerebellar ataxia. Corticospinal tract involvement results in increased tone, clonus, increased tendon reflexes, and bilateral extensor plantar responses. Neck stiffness and a positive Kernig's sign may not be present. Focal seizures and hemiparesis may indicate spread of the lesions of the cerebral cortex. The course is usually one of steady deterioration, with raised intracranial pressure producing obtundity, stupor, coma, and death within a period of several months following the onset of the disease.

Diagnostic Procedures

1. At lumbar puncture the cerebrospinal fluid usually shows increased pressure, mild lymphocytic pleocytosis, and an elevated protein content. Glucose levels vary from case to case but tend to be reduced. The organism is not usually seen in the smear. There have been reports of normal cerebrospinal fluid findings in cases of cerebral histoplasmosis demonstrated at necropsy.
2. The histoplasmin skin test is unreliable and may be negative in cerebral histoplasmosis.
3. A positive complement-fixation test strongly supports the diagnosis of cerebral histoplasmosis.
4. Bone marrow biopsy or bone marrow culture is usually positive in disseminated histoplasmosis. The test should be performed in cases of suspected cerebral histoplasmosis. A lymph node biopsy or a biopsy of an ulcerating lesion may also show *Histoplasma capsulatum.* Visualization of the yeast within monocytes is facilitated by a carbohydrate stain (e.g., periodic acid Schiff).

Treatment

The drug of choice is amphotericin B. Treatment should be given by both intravenous and intrathecal routes since amphotericin B passes the blood-CSF barrier with difficulty. Histoplasmoma may occasionally present as a brain tumor, in which case surgical removal is indicated.

Disseminated histoplasmosis with involvement of the central nervous system was invariably fatal prior to amphotericin B therapy. The combination of systemic and intrathecal therapy is effective in many cases, and prolonged arrest or cure may be obtained.

Mucormycosis

Mucormycosis is the most acutely fatal mycosis of man, and fortunately it is a rare condition. Infection is caused by one of the fungi belonging to the class Phycomycetes, which are saprophytic fungi forming the fluffy molds on foodstuffs.

Mucormycosis usually occurs as a complication of debilitating diseases such as diabetes mellitus, leukemia, Hodgkin's disease, carcinoma, and myelomatosis, or following burns. However, mucormycosis has been described in otherwise healthy children[299] and following open head trauma and craniotomy.[152] Cerebral infection usually enters the cranial cavity following infection of the paranasal sinuses.[251, 257] The fungi proliferate within communicating blood vessels entering the orbit and the brain. This results in cerebral arteritis and phlebitis with widespread thrombosis and infarction.

The symptoms are those of a fulminating meningoencephalitis with the rapid onset of coma occurring in a chronically debilitated patient often with ketoacidosis in the diabetic. Cavernous sinus thrombosis is a frequent complication. The cerebrospinal fluid is usually clear and cultures are negative. A bloody nasal discharge with black-appearing nasal turbinates is a characteristic sign of mucormycosis. Roentgenographic evidence of destruction of the bony walls of bony sinuses suggests the diagnosis of mucormycosis, which can be confirmed by biopsy of the mucosa.[3]

Treatment

The drug of choice in mucormycosis is amphotericin B. Alternate-day therapy should be started as soon as possible because of the rapid and fatal course of mucormycosis.[30] There are a few reports of recovery following amphotericin B therapy, but the disease is still a dangerous and often lethal condition.[41a]

Cerebral Nocardiosis

Infection by *Nocardia asteroides* resembles actinomycosis, but the fungus is aerobic and usually produces a brain abscess and rarely produces a marked meningeal reaction. Cerebral nocardiosis usually results as a complication of systemic infection disseminated from infection of the pharynx or lung and usually in association with some chronic, debilitating illness,[328] intensive antibiotic therapy, treatment with corticosteroids, or use of immunosuppressive agents.[198]

The clinical picture of cerebral nocardiosis is that of a cerebral abscess with fever, headache, nuchal rigidity, seizures, and signs of a focal cerebral lesion.

Diagnostic Procedures

The cerebrospinal fluid may show mild polymorphonuclear pleocytosis with normal glucose levels, and the electroencephalogram usually shows a delta focus in the region of the abscess. The presence of the abscess can be confirmed by computed tomography (p. 392).

Treatment

The diagnosis is frequently made following surgical drainage of a brain abscess. The organism is gram-positive with branching filaments, which have a tendency to fragmentation. They are found in the purulent material or in a biopsy specimen taken from the wall of the abscess. The organism does not produce "sulfur granules," which are commonly seen in the purulent drainage of actinomycosis. Diagnosis is confirmed by aerobic culture of the abscess material on a blood agar plate. The fungus is sensitive to sulfonamides, and it has been recommended that a sulfonamide should be inserted in the abscess cavity at operation.[320] This should be followed by a long course of oral sulfonamides lasting several months.[248]

Coccidioidomycosis

Infection by *Coccidioides immitis* occurs in areas with low precipitation and high temperatures and is prevalent in the southwest United States, Mexico, and parts of Central America. The majority of infections are subclinical, although primary coccidioidomycosis may present as an upper respiratory tract infection or pneumonia. About 1 per cent of primary coccidioidomycosis is complicated by the disseminated forms of the disease, including lesions of the central nervous system.

Pathology

The fungus usually produces a chronic granulomatous meningitis, frequently obstructing the fourth ventricle and causing hydrocephalus. A coccidioidal osteomyelitis of the cervical vertebrae may produce spinal cord compression.

Clinical Features

Coccidioidal meningitis presents as a low-grade meningeal infection with headache, nuchal rigidity, nausea, and vomiting, progressing to stupor and death within two to three months. Coccidioidal osteomyelitis of the cervical spine produces progressive spastic quadriparesis with loss of bladder control and sensory loss below the level of the compressive lesion.[159]

Diagnostic Procedures

1. The intradermal skin test for coccidioidomycosis is unreliable and may become negative in disseminated coccidioidomycosis.
2. A positive complement-fixation test is obtained in virtually all cases of disseminated coccidioidomycosis.
3. Lumbar puncture reveals a spinal fluid under increased pressure with both lymphocytes and polymorphonucleocytes present. The glucose content is low, with increased protein content and positive complement-fixation tests for coccidioidomycosis. *Coccidioides immitis* is obtained by culture in less than 25 per cent of cases.
4. In cases with coccidioidal osteomyelitis and cervical cord compression, the usual changes indicating a subarachnoid block will be obtained at lumbar puncture.
5. There may be signs of disseminated infection elsewhere, e.g., coccidioidal arthritis, which may afford the opportunity for culture.
6. Roentgenographic examination of the spine may reveal lytic lesions due to coccidioidal osteomyelitis in cases with cord compression.[61]
7. Pneumoencephalography may show irregular and asymmetric accumulations of air over the cerebral hemispheres (soap bubble effect), which are seen in chronic granulomatous meningitis.[242] Absence of ventricular filling will occur if there is obstructive hydrocephalus.

Treatment

The drug of choice in the treatment of coccidioidomycosis is amphotericin B. Combined intravenous and intrathecal treatment is indicated in coccidioidal meningitis (p. 434).

Intrathecal amphotericin B may be administered via the lumbar route or by cisternal puncture. Intraventricular administration can also be carried out via an indwelling subcutaneous capsule of silicone rubber, which fits into a cranial burr hole and is connected to a ventricular catheter.[338]

Patients with coccidioidal vertebral osteomyelitis and cord compression may require laminectomy and surgical decompression of the spinal cord. These patients should also receive both intravenous and intrathecal amphotericin B.

The prognosis in coccidioidal meningitis is usually good following amphotericin B therapy, but intrathecal therapy must be continued until the complement-fixation test in the cerebrospinal fluid has been negative for two to three months.[335] Signs of relapse should be watched for and regular follow-up examinations of patients should be carried out for a period of at least three years.

There are encouraging reports of the use of the antifungal agent miconazole in the treatment of systemic mycosis, including coccidioidomycosis. The drug appears to have low toxicity and may be a useful addition to the therapy of human mycosis.[303]

A ventriculoatrial shunt will be required in cases developing hydrocephalus and will prevent the development of severe neurologic manifestations due to this complication.

Toxoplasmosis of the Central Nervous System

A large proportion of adults have been infected at some time by the protozoan organism *Toxoplasma gondii,* judging by the frequency of positive skin reactions and various serologic tests to *Toxoplasma* in populations tested in many areas of the world. The majority of adult infections are asymptomatic, but the organism may be transmitted through the placenta when the infection is acquired during pregnancy, producing congenital toxoplasmosis, which can result in severe damage to the developing brain.

Congenital Toxoplasmosis

Fetal infection by *Toxoplasma gondii* results when a nonimmune pregnant woman acquires a subclinical infection. The parasites enter the bloodstream, infect the placenta, and establish a focus from which the fetus is infected.

Pathology

In fatal cases, the pia-arachnoid is inflamed and thickened and there are numerous areas of cortical softening. There are also many miliary granulomas scattered throughout the brain, and occasional larger granulomas are found with central necrosis. The granulomas tend to be more numerous around the lateral ventricles and form zones of confluent necrosis there. Many granulomas show early calcification. The fundi usually show chorioretinitis with granulomatous inflammation of the choroid, retina, and ciliary bodies.

Clinical Features

About 25 per cent of children with congenital toxoplasmosis are born prematurely and there is a 20 per cent mortality rate in this group. The disease should be suspected in infants who show signs of encephalitis and hydrocephalus with a rash, jaundice, enlargement of the liver and spleen, and chorioretinitis shortly after birth. Children who survive with congenital toxoplasmosis may show mental retardation, microcephaly, chorioretinitis, and seizures.[93]

Diagnostic Procedures

1. In infants with severe congenital toxoplasmosis, lumbar puncture may reveal xanthochromic cerebrospinal fluid with a lymphocytic pleocytosis and elevated protein content.
2. Roentgenograms of the skull may reveal intracerebral calcifications, which tend to take the form of curvilinear streaks.
3. A positive Sabin-Feldman dye test with titers in excess of 1:1,000 may be found within the first few weeks of life in infants with congenital toxoplasmosis.
4. Complement-fixation antibodies appear later in congenital toxoplasmosis, and the test may not be positive during the first month of life. A titer exceeding 1:32 is an indication of a recent infection.

Treatment

There is no treatment for congenital toxoplasmosis at this time. The majority of children with congenital toxoplasmosis survive but commonly have some degree of brain damage and mental retardation. The mother of a child with congenital toxoplasmosis may be assured that she is immune to further infection and that transplacental infection of any subsequent children will not occur.

While the great majority of acquired childhood and adult toxoplasmosis is subclinical, occasional symptomatic infections have been reported and include the following.[308]

"Glandular" Toxoplasmosis

This is a febrile illness with generalized lymphadenopathy and the presence of abnormal mononuclear cells in the peripheral blood resembling infectious mononucleosis. This illness is relatively benign.

Miliary Toxoplasmosis

This is an acute febrile illness with a maculopapular rash resembling Rocky Mountain spotted fever. Lung involvement results in bronchopneumonia, and myocardial lesions produce tachycardia, arrhythmia, decreased exercise tolerance, and heart failure. Signs of pericarditis may also be present. Widespread muscle weakness may be due to toxoplasmic polymyositis.[120] Involvement of the central nervous system may appear with symptoms of diffuse meningoencephalitis.

Localized Toxoplasmosis

Chorioretinitis in the adult is probably the most common manifestation of localized toxoplasmosis, but isolated pulmonary lesions, myocarditis, pericarditis, polymyositis, hepatitis, and a localized cerebral toxoplasmosis have been described.[258]

Toxoplasmosis Meningoencephalitis

This occurs as a complication of miliary toxoplasmosis with the development of signs and symptoms suggesting involvement of the central nervous system. These include headache, nuchal rigidity, changes in personality, intellectual deterioration, seizures, cataplexy, narcolepsy, and focal signs of paralysis with asymmetric reflexes. If a localized toxoplasmic granuloma is present in the brain, it produces signs typical of a space-occupying intracranial lesion.[34, 182] Toxoplasmosis meningoencephalitis is usually an opportunistic infection occurring in patients who are receiving immunosuppressive therapy.[312]

Diagnostic Procedures

1. Lumbar puncture may reveal increased pressure, xanthochromia, lymphocytic pleocytosis, and increased content of protein.
2. Serial Sabin-Feldman dye tests or complement-fixation tests may show a progressive rise in antibody titers.
3. A bone marrow biopsy may be positive for *Toxoplasma gondii* on microscopic examination.

4. The organism may be cultured from the cerebrospinal fluid, blood, urine, lymph nodes, bone marrow, or muscle biopsies.

Treatment

Both sulfadiazine and pyrimethamine have been reported to be effective in the treatment of toxoplasmosis.

Other Protozoan Infections of the Central Nervous System

Cerebral Amebiasis

The central nervous system is rarely invaded by *Entamoeba histolytica* or *Iodamoeba buetschlii,* owing to hematogenous dissemination from intestinal, hepatic, or pulmonary lesions. This type of involvement should be distinguished from primary amebic meningoencephalitis caused by free-living amebae of the genera *Naegleria.* Pathogenic *Naegleria* enter the nose and paranasal sinuses during swimming in contaminated water and spread from there to the subarachnoid space, producing an acute and frequently fatal meningoencephalitis.[301]

Clinical Features

The first symptoms are lethargy, headache, and some nasal congestion, occurring a day or so after swimming. This is followed by fever, vomiting, severe headache, and nuchal rigidity. There is a rapid progression to stupor, seizures, respiratory arrest, and death within several days in *Naegleria* infections.

Diagnostic Procedures

The cerebrospinal fluid is cloudy with a predominantly polymorphonuclear pleocytosis and cell counts ranging from several hundred to 20,000. The protein content is elevated but the glucose level is variable. Amebae can usually be found in the fluid, but identification may be difficult since they are easily confused with macrophages.[230]

Treatment

Primary amebic meningoencephalitis carries a high mortality. There have been some reports of temporary improvement and an occasional cure with amphotericin B.[9, 77] If amebic meningoencephalitis is suspected despite the absence of pathogenic *Naegleria* in the cerebrospinal fluid,

treatment with amphotericin B should be started and the lumbar puncture repeated in 12 hours.[332] Intraventricular amphotericin B should be added once amebae are identified.

Cerebral Malaria

The cerebral form of malaria is a well-recognized complication of infection by the malarial parasite *Plasmodium falciparum.* It is a dramatic and potentially fatal condition that occurs in 1 to 2 per cent of cases of *falciparum* malaria. Complete recovery can be expected in most cases with adequate therapy, and permanent neurologic sequelae are unusual.

Etiology and Pathology

The parasite *Plasmodium falciparum* enters the bloodstream following the bite of the mosquito vector. The parasites proliferate within the red cells, which are destroyed, releasing fatty acids and other lytic agents into the circulation causing hemolysis of nonparalyzed cells. The released substances also damage the capillary endothelium in the brain, and there is an inflammatory response with proliferation of microglial cells surrounding the capillaries. Cerebral malaria is in fact a vasculitis compounded by anoxia already present from the anemia and by shock, which occurs in the terminal stages of the disease.[274] Fatal cases show diffuse perivascular hemorrhages due to capillary necrosis, and there is marked cerebral edema.[310a]

Clinical Features

The cerebral form of malaria usually develops in patients who have had symptoms of *falciparum* malaria for more than a week. Some cases have received what is apparently adequate antimalarial therapy and have reached a stage of convalescence when they show a dramatic relapse. The onset is abrupt, with high fever and the development of organic mental symptoms including disorientation, impairment of judgment and insight, and confusion and clouding of consciousness. The symptoms are occasionally heralded by a generalized seizure. Personality changes with paranoid delusions or hallucinations may be prominent in other cases.[183] The course can progress through stupor to coma, but some patients develop severe choreiform movements associated with restlessness and hyperactivity and frequent irregular myoclonic jerks. Focal signs, including hemiparesis, hemisensory loss, or unilateral increase in deep tendon reflexes, are an additional feature in some cases.

Diagnostic Procedures

1. The malarial parasites can be readily identified in blood smears.
2. Inconsistent changes in the cerebrospinal fluid have been reported. The fluid may be normal or under increased pressure with a pleocytosis and increased protein content.

Treatment

Patients with mild or early symptoms of cerebral malaria should be treated with quinine sulfate, 650 mg every eight hours orally for 14 days. This should be supplemented by pyrimethamine, 25 mg three times a day for three days, and sulfadiazine, 500 mg four times a day for seven days.

Severely ill patients with stupor or coma require intravenous quinine, while the pyrimethamine and sulfadiazine can be given through a nasogastric tube.

Drug therapy should be supplemented by low-molecular-weight dextran intravenously. This is given in 10 per cent solution in dextrose beginning with a loading dose of 500 ml in one hour and followed by 500 ml every 12 hours. The risk of cerebral edema is reduced by giving dexamethasone, 4 mg every eight hours.

Parasitic Infections of the Brain

Cysticercosis

Cysticercosis is a global disease, and although public health measures have made it uncommon in North America and most European countries, it is still common in many parts of the world.

Etiology and Pathology

Cysticercosis occurs when man ingests the ova of the tapeworm *Taenia solium.* The ova hatch in the gastrointestinal tract, and the liberated oncospheres pass into the bloodstream to be carried to various tissues, including the central nervous system. The oncosphere then develops a hooked scolex and short neck. An extension of the neck forms a fluid-filled bladder that surrounds the scolex, forming a cysticercus cyst. Cysticercosis can occur anywhere in the central nervous system.[179]

Clinical Features

The interval between infection and the appearance of symptoms varies from a few months to 20 years. Patients may present with:

1. Seizures, which often are partial motor seizures with spread of activity (jacksonian seizures).[4a]
2. Hydrocephalus with headache, vomiting, and ataxia due to the presence of a cysticercus cyst lying in the ventricular system.[67]
3. Hydrocephalus due to the development of chronic basal meningitis due to the presence of cysticercosi in the subarachnoid space.[124]
4. Focal neurologic deficits and raised intracranial pressure due to one or more large parenchymal cysts.[82]
5. Progressive paraparesis or quadriparesis due to cysticercosis of the spinal canal or spinal cord.[43, 225, 259]

Diagnostic Procedures

1. Computed tomography will show the presence of calcified ventricular cysts, subarachnoid cysts, or hydrocephalus.[179]
2. The cerebrospinal fluid is often xanthochromic with a mononuclear pleocytosis, low glucose, and a marked elevation in protein content in cases with meningeal involvement. The indirect hemagglutination test for cysticercosis is usually positive in the cerebrospinal fluid. False negative results may occur in about 15 per cent of patients.
3. Cerebral cysts can be demonstrated by means of a specific radioimmunoscan.[286]
4. Myelography will demonstrate cysts in the spinal canal in some cases or a complete blocking of the subarachnoid space due to the presence of intramedullary or intraspinal cysts.

Treatment

Dexamethasone can be used to provide temporary reduction in intracranial pressure. Hydrocephalus should be relieved by removal of intraventricular cysts or by performing a ventriculoatrial shunt. Large parenchymal cysts should be excised after they have been located accurately by CT. Pressure on the spinal cord should be relieved by laminectomy and removal of the cyst to prevent permanent neurologic deficits. Patients with seizures often require anticonvulsants for an indefinite period.

Infections of the Spinal Canal and Spinal Cord

Under this heading all infections of the spinal cord and related structures will be discussed except spinal forms of syphilis, which are discussed under the heading Neurosyphilis. Viral infections of the spinal cord will be discussed under the heading Viral Encephalitides and Viral Infection of the Central Nervous System.

Spinal Epidural Abscess

The dura mater is separated posteriorly by loose connective tissue from the bones of the vertebral canal. This potential space permits the invasion by infecting organisms resulting in a spinal epidural abscess, which may be large, extending over almost the entire length of the spinal epidural space.

There may be a history of prior back trauma, diabetes mellitus, or intravenous drug abuse in some cases. Occasionally an abscess develops after a penetrating wound or lumbar puncture. Probable sources of infection include furunculosis, upper respiratory tract infections, dental extraction, operative wounds, decubitus ulcers, and abscesses at other sites.[14] The infection is usually due to *Staphylococcus aureus*, which produces an osteomyelitis involving the vertebral body, lamina, or pedicle, although this focus of infection may be minute and escape detection. The pus collects predominantly posterior to the spinal cord and, because of the loose attachment of the dura mater, usually spreads over several segments and may extend to the lumbar sac.[15]

Clinical Features

The spinal epidural abscess usually produces pain at the site of the infection, which is exacerbated by movement and which is associated with spasm of the erector spinae muscles. The pain is severe and the patient usually seeks medical advice within 24 hours. Root pains usually develop on the second or third day around the chest or in the distribution of the sciatic nerve if the lumbar area is involved. There is tenderness on pressure over the affected vertebra. As the abscess develops, it produces pressure on the spinal cord with rapid progression from paraparesis to paraplegia. There is marked neck stiffness and a positive Kernig's sign. The deep tendon reflexes are usually depressed, and there is a bilateral extensor plantar response. A patchy sensory loss occurs below the level of the lesion, with urinary retention and overflow incontinence.[272]

Acute spinal epidural abscess may simulate poliomyelitis, acute transverse myelitis, or postinfectious polyneuropathy when the paralysis of the lower limbs develops quickly. Profound paraparesis occurring within a 24-hour period is more likely to be due to transverse myelitis.[10]

Chronic epidural abscess differs from the acute process in that the neurologic deficits develop over a period of weeks or months. However, the pain is severe at the site of infection and nerve root pains develop within a week of the initial backache. Chronic epidural abscess must be differentiated from extramedullary tumors and a herniated intervertebral disk.

Diagnostic Procedures

1. The fasting blood glucose may show the patient to be diabetic.
2. Lumbar puncture must be performed with care and suction applied constantly to the needle on insertion since the abscess may have spread to the lumbar sac. Aspiration of pus is diagnostic and under these circumstances the needle should not be allowed to enter the subarachnoid space.

   Usually the spinal needle passes into the subarachnoid space without incident, and the cerebrospinal fluid may be xanthochromic with decreased opening pressure and little or no response to compression of the jugular veins in the neck should the block be nearly complete. If the block is incomplete, the fluid shows all the features of an aseptic meningeal reaction with a pleocytosis of polymorphonuclear leukocytes and an elevated protein content but normal glucose and chloride levels. In chronic cases, the cerebrospinal fluid may show few abnormalities unless there is a partial or complete block (see Froin's syndrome, p. 655) at higher levels. Culture of the spinal fluid will be sterile.
3. Roentgenograms of the spine may reveal osteomyelitis involving the vertebral body or its pedicles and lamina. In cases with tuberculosis there may be widespread destruction of the vertebral body.
4. Myelography should be performed in all cases with signs of nerve root or spinal cord compression at the time of lumbar puncture. The demonstration of a block or epidural mass on myelography should be followed by laminectomy without delay.

Treatment

Surgical drainage of an epidural abscess and any related osteomyelitis should be performed as an emergency measure, particularly if there is evidence of a spinal cord compression. The appropriate antibiotic, usually penicillin G or methicillin, should be administered in adequate dosage. This may require confirmation from culture and sensitivity tests obtained at surgery. The suggested dose is 30 million units of penicillin G by vein and 1 gm of methicillin every three hours intramuscularly. After sensitivity studies, one or the other may be discontinued. This dosage should be continued for three weeks.

It should be emphasized that acute spinal epidural abscess with cord compression is a surgical emergency, and the prognosis will depend on the speed of surgical decompression. Delay for more than a few hours may result in irreversible damage to the spinal cord with permanent spastic paraparesis or paraplegia.[80]

Spinal Subdural Empyema

This condition is rare and, like the epidural abscess, is usually observed in diabetic patients with focal infection elsewhere, such as furunculosis. The clinical features include fever, stiffness and rigidity of neck and spine, backache, root pain, lack of vertebral column percussion tenderness, and signs of spinal cord or cauda equina pressure.[98] The cerebrospinal fluid shows a pleocytosis, elevated protein, and low glucose content. There is no roentgenographic evidence of osteomyelitis, which frequently occurs in spinal epidural abscess. Myelography shows a block with a "paintbrush" appearance, as seen in an epidural mass with irregular collections of contrast material at more rostral levels, which are not seen in epidural abscess.

Treatment

Investigation of a patient with a suspected paraspinal infectious process should proceed rapidly and be followed by surgical drainage and antibiotic therapy if severe permanent neurologic deficit is to be avoided.

Acute Intramedullary Abscess of the Spinal Cord

This is a rare condition but it may result from infection by a wide variety of bacteria if they gain access to the spinal cord. The abscess may be primary, with a remote focus of infection such as pneumonia, endocarditis, or septic abortion. Secondary abscesses may result from direct spread of infection via an epidural abscess, sacrococcygeal fistula, or introduction of infection by a stab wound.[341] Occasionally, cases of intra-

medullary abscess are reported without any demonstrable primary focus of infection.

Pathology

The infection begins in the central portion of the spinal cord and may spread over a number of segments. There is softening of the cord, with pus formation and surrounding edema. Microscopic examination shows central necrosis surrounded by an area of acute inflammation often with organisms identifiable in the exudate.

Clinical Features

The abscess may occur as a complication of a fulminating septicemia.

Such patients are acutely ill with high fever and have known suppurative lesions or bacterial endocarditis when they develop a rapidly progressive paraparesis with paralysis of the bladder and a severe or complete sensory loss below the level of the lesion. This may occur in patients who have been given inadequate antibiotic therapy.

Diagnostic Procedures

1. The white blood count usually shows polymorphonucleocytosis in acute cases.
2. Lumbar puncture may reveal evidence of subarachnoid block with low spinal fluid pressure and negative Queckenstedt test. A few inflammatory cells may be present in the fluid, but the culture is likely to be sterile. Marked elevation in protein content of the spinal fluid may be anticipated.
3. Myelography will demonstrate a complete or partial block with evidence of widening of the cord just below the level of the block.

Treatment

The appropriate antibiotic should be given immediately if results of culture are available from the primary focus of infection. In cases where bacterial cultures are not available, early use of a broad-spectrum antibiotic such as ampicillin is recommended. Laminectomy with decompression and drainage of the abscess should be performed as soon as possible.

In patients who survive, the recovery of neurologic function is often surprisingly good following drainage of an intramedullary abscess. There may be useful motor function in the lower limbs and adequate sphincter control in patients who were totally paraplegic at the height of the illness.[81]

Chronic Spinal Epidural Infections

The most common cause of chronic epidural infections if the tuberculous cold abscess secondary to tuberculous osteomyelitis of the vertebral bodies (Pott's disease). Syphilis also causes a granulomatous thickening of the meninges (pachymeningitis cervicalis hypertrophica) and granulomatous arachnoiditis. Coccidioidomycosis, brucellosis, and cryptococcosis are other rare causes of granulomatous inflammation involving the epidural space. Chronic inflammation has been induced by discharge of the contents of a spinal epidermoid in the lumbar area.[326]

Tuberculous cold abscesses usually occur in the mid- or upper thoracic region and may extend over several segments, pass through the intravertebral foramina and track external to the pleura or peritoneum, and present anteriorly as a fluctuant mass. A psoas abscess presenting in the inguinal area is caused by a cold abscess passing through the intervertebral foramina and tracking down the psoas sheath.

Pathology

The accumulation of granulomatous tissue of a cold abscess in the spinal epidural space produces pressure on the spinal cord. In Pott's disease, damage to the cord is due to a combination of four factors:

1. Pressure from the cold abscess
2. Ischemia due to pressure on the spinal arteries
3. Tuberculous endarteritis of spinal arteries at the level of spinal block
4. Occasional narrowing of the spinal canal due to angulation following collapse of the diseased vertebral body

Clinical Features

The clinical picture resembles that of an extradural tumor. Initial symptoms are usually of root pains radiating around the chest or abdomen, followed by the development of a slowly progressive paraparesis, with weakness, spasticity, clonus, hyperreflexia, and bilateral extensor plantar responses in the lower limbs. Urgency of micturition may be followed by incontinence. There is often a patchy sensory loss below the level of the lesion and a band of hyperthesia around the chest or abdomen at the level of the lesion. There may be no deformity of the spine in the early stages, and tenderness on percussion at the level of the lesion may also be absent.

Diagnostic Procedures

1. Lumbar puncture should be performed with care since the needle may enter a cold abscess that has tracked down to the lumbar area. The cerebrospinal fluid pressure will be low, with a negative Queckenstedt test, if the pressure of the abscess has produced a complete block. Under these circumstances, the protein content may be very high and the fluid may clot spontaneously (Froin's syndrome).
2. Roentgenographic examination of the spine may reveal a destructive process involving the vertebral body or collapse of a diseased vertebral body.

Treatment

1. Tuberculous infections should be treated with adequate doses of streptomycin and isoniazid.
2. Fungal infections respond to amphotericin B.
3. Orthopedic measures and eventual laminectomy may be necessary to relieve pressure on the spinal cord.

Chronic Spinal Intradural Infections

Intradural infections may be extramedullary or intramedullary but the conditions are usually indistinguishable clinically. The most common cause of chronic spinal intradural infections is tuberculosis, but intradural granulomas due to syphilis, actinomycosis, aspergillosis, coccidioidomycosis, and schistosomiasis have been described.

Chronic Intramedullary Abscess

This is an unusual condition that presents difficulties in diagnosis and treatment. It may follow purulent meningitis[32] or develop following hematogenous spread from a distant focus of infection.

Clinical Features

There may be absence of signs of infection and a fluctuating course of paraparesis, retention of urine, and urinary incontinence. Eventually there are signs of bilateral lower limb spasticity, increased reflexes, and bilateral plantar extensor response with a sensory disturbance bilaterally, up to the level of the lesion.[206]

Diagnostic Procedures

1. Roentgenograms may show a widening of the spinal canal, suggesting a space-occupying lesion.

2. The cerebrospinal fluid is xanthochromic, and the Queckenstedt test is negative.
3. Myelography will reveal a partial or complete block at the level of the lesion with widening of the medullary shadow, characteristic of an intramedullary mass.

Treatment

The spinal cord is exposed by total laminectomy, and the abscess is incised. The mass can then be removed from the cord by dissection. The pus should be cultured, and the appropriate antibiotic given for two weeks.

Intradural Spinal Tuberculomas

In contrast to extradural tuberculosis of the spinal cord, which is usually secondary to Pott's disease, intradural spinal cord lesions are hematogenous.[244] The extramedullary tuberculoma may encase the spinal cord or produce an arachnoiditis around the cord, resulting in pressure on the cord and subarachnoid block.[184] Intramedullary tuberculomas are also frequently associated with an arachnoiditis with partial or complete subarachnoid block.

Clinical Features

Intradural tuberculomas usually occur in patients with pulmonary tuberculosis. This may, however, be undiagnosed or minimal, so that it is not immediately detected. There is usually a period of vague ill health and weight loss followed by backache and pain from inflamed nerve roots. Weakness and spasticity of the lower limbs follow, with numbness or paresthesias below the level of the lesion and impairment of sphincter control.[161] Symptoms of meningitis may occur if the infection spreads into the subarachnoid space.

Diagnostic Procedures

1. A rise in sedimentation rate and positive tuberculin test in a patient with pulmonary tuberculosis and the recent onset of a progressive lesion of the spinal cord should suggest the possibility of intradural tuberculoma of the spinal cord.
2. Lumbar puncture usually reveals partial or complete subarachnoid block, with xanthochromic cerebrospinal fluid and elevated protein content. Tubercle bacilli may be obtained by culture.

Treatment

Antituberculous therapy should be started as soon as the diagnosis of tuberculosis is made (see p. 413). Unless symptoms of cord compression are mild and the response to antituberculous therapy is rapid, laminectomy and decompression should be considered. If laminectomy is performed for an intradural mass that is subsequently proved to be a tuberculoma, antituberculous therapy should be started immediately, both to cure the lesion and to prevent tuberculous meningitis.

The combination of antituberculous therapy and laminectomy has produced satisfactory results in tuberculomas of the spinal cord and intradural space.

Viral Encephalitides and Viral Infections of the Central Nervous System

The viral encephalitides are a group of diseases characterized by inflammation of the parenchyma of the brain and its surrounding meninges in response to infection by virus or viral-like (psittacosis) organisms. Since the isolation of the virus of St. Louis encephalitis from the brain in 1933, numerous types of viruses have now been isolated and identified as the etiologic agents for other forms of encephalitis. At the present time, identification of the virus can be accomplished in the majority of cases of encephalitis by serologic tests and tissue culture methods.

Viruses consist of a core of either DNA (deoxyribonucleic acid) or RNA (ribonucleic acid), but not both, and can be regarded as living organisms with the properties of self-reproduction. They are obligatory intracellular organisms that can only grow and multiply within the tissue cells of the host. The term "viral encephalitis" or "viral encephalomyelitis" implies invasion of cells of the brain and spinal cord by virus. In certain virus diseases, cellular invasion is followed by the development of inclusion bodies in the nucleus or cytoplasm of the cell. Intranuclear inclusion bodies are of two types:

1. Type A intranuclear inclusions are single amorphous structures surrounded by a clear "halo" which displaces the nucleolus. They occur in herpes simplex encephalitis and in subacute sclerosing panencephalitis and may be seen in neurons and oligodendroglial cells. In

cytomegalic inclusion disease they are also seen in the subependymal astrocytes.

2. Type B intranuclear inclusions are smaller structures that may be multiple but do not displace the nucleolus. They are seen in the anterior horn cells in poliomyelitis.

Virus infections of the brain may produce two distinct syndromes: aseptic meningitis or encephalitis.

All neurotropic viruses, with the exception of rabies, produce either of these conditions. In aseptic meningitis, the inflammatory process is confined to the meninges and choroid plexus, which become hyperemic and infiltrated with lymphocytes. The pathologic picture in viral encephalitis includes destruction or damage to neurons, the presence of intranuclear inclusion bodies, and edema and inflammation of the brain and spinal cord with perivascular cuffing by polymorphonuclear leukocytes and lymphocytes. There is an angiitis of small vessels, with thrombosis and proliferation of astrocytes and microglia. There may also be widespread destruction of white matter by the inflammatory process and by thrombosis of perforating vessels.

Diagnostic Procedures

1. The cerebrospinal fluid is clear or opalescent and may show increased pressure. There is usually a pleocytosis of from 50 to 500 (sometimes 1,000) white cells per cubic millimeter. The cells are often polymorphonuclear in the early stages, followed by the appearance of lymphocytes within a few days Chemical analysis shows moderate elevation in the levels of protein to between 80 and 100 mg/ml. Spinal fluid glucose and chloride contents are normal.

2. Virus may be cultured using suitable animal cells or human cell tissue cultures, but positive results may not be obtained for several weeks after inoculation. It is important to inoculate specimens (CSF, blood, urine, feces, and throat swab) for tissue culture as soon as possible. If there is a short delay in inoculating specimens, they should be kept at 4°C, but they must be stored at −70°C if the delay is more than a few hours. In suspected cases of viral encephalitis coming to autopsy, half the brain should be placed in a deep-freeze unit for virologic examinations.

3. Serologic tests are used for the following purposes: to positively identify a virus isolated by tissue culture, to confirm the nature of a viral encephalitis by demonstrating a rise in titer of antibodies against a specific virus, and to diagnose the nature of a suspected viral encephalitis by testing acute and convalescent sera against several virus types and demonstrating the rise in titer against one of these types.

When testing is being done for antibody titers in acute and convalescent sera, the specimens should be obtained as soon as possible after the patient is first examined and some two to three weeks later.

4. A rapid diagnosis of encephalitis by immunofluorescent examination of cerebrospinal fluid cells is available in some hospitals. In this test, cells obtained from fresh CSF are stained for specific viral antigens by an indirect immunofluorescent technique or for immunoglobulins (IgG and IgM) by a direct method using fluorescein-conjugated anti-IgG or anti-IgM. Immunoglobulin-containing cells are found in the CSF some 48 hours after the onset of clinical viral encephalitis.[66]

Classification

It is convenient to classify the virus encephalitides into those transmitted by arthropod vectors and those transmitted by other means. The arthropod-borne animal viruses (arboviruses) are subclassified into groups according to their serologic reactions,[55] but only groups A and B appear to infect man (Table 7–7). They have the properties of causing a viremia in the vertebrate host, of multiplying in the arthropod vector, and of being transmitted by the arthropod during feeding.

Aseptic Meningitis

"Benign lymphocytic choriomeningitis" and "nonparalytic poliomyelitis" have often been used synonymously with aseptic meningitis. However, the syndrome of aseptic meningitis can result from infection by a wide variety of viruses, and the term "aseptic meningitis" should be used for any suspected viral inflammation of the central nervous system, with lymphocytes in the cerebrospinal fluid, but whose cause remains unproved.[2]

The illness probably begins as a viremia followed by localization of the virus in the meninges and choroid plexus, resulting in a mild inflamma-

TABLE 7–7

Classification of Virus Encephalitides

1. *Anthropod-borne animal viruses (arboviruses)*

	Virus	Vector
Group A	Western equine encephalitis	Mosquito
	Eastern equine encephalitis	Mosquito
	Venezuelan equine encephalitis	Mosquito
Group B	St. Louis encephalitis	Mosquito
	Japanese B encephalitis	Mosquito
	West Nile encephalitis	Mosquito
	Ilheus	Mosquito
	Murray Valley (Australian X)	Mosquito
	Yellow fever	Mosquito
	Dengue	Mosquito
	Tick-borne encephalitis	Tick
	Louping ill	Tick
	Colorado tick fever	Tick
Unclassified	California encephalitis	Mosquito

Nongrouped

2. Rabies	11. Lymphocytic choriomeningitis
3. Poliomyelitis	12. Encephalomyocarditis (E.M.C.)
4. Coxsackie A	13. Infectious mononucleosis
5. Coxsackie B	14. Influenza
6. Herpes simplex	15. Psittacosis—lymphogranuloma venereum
7. Herpes zoster	16. Cytomegalovirus (C.M.V.)
8. ECHO	17. Infectious hepatitis
9. Mumps	18. *Mycoplasma pneumoniae*
10. Measles	

Slow virus encephalitides
Chronic progressive panencephalitis
   a. Subacute sclerosing panencephalitis (SSPE)
   b. Rubella panencephalitis
   c. Russian spring-summer panencephalitis
Spongiform encephalopathies
   a. Kuru
   b. Jakob-Creutzfeldt disease
Progressive multifocal leukoencephalopathy

tory response that is predominantly lymphocytic in type. It is likely that any of the viruses with neurotropic properties (with the exception of rabies) may give rise to aseptic meningitis, but Coxsackie B, mumps, ECHO, and lymphocytic choriomeningitis viruses are the most common offenders. It should be noted that *Leptospira* may produce an identical picture and should be regarded as the chief nonviral agent responsible for the syndrome of aseptic meningitis.[321]

Clinical Features

The onset of aseptic meningitis may be sudden or gradual and may be associated with pleurodynia or myalgia in Coxsackie B infections. There is moderate elevation of temperature, headache, stiff neck, vomiting, and generalized malaise, which usually lasts about ten days, but exceptionally may last longer. The patients do not appear toxic or seriously ill but show mild pharyngitis and neck stiffness with a positive Kernig's sign. The white blood cell count is usually normal, with a relative lymphocytosis, while the cerebrospinal fluid may show a slight increase in pressure and pleocytosis of up to 1,000 white blood cells per cubic millimeter, with lymphocytes accounting for 90 per cent of the cells present. The glucose and chloride levels are normal, but the protein may show a slight elevation above normal.

Diagnostic Procedures

Isolation of virus from throat, feces, or urine is suggestive. The diagnosis may be established by isolation of virus from CSF or the demonstration of a fourfold rise in specific neutralizing or complement-fixing antibody in acute and convalescent sera. In view of the frequency of leptospiral infections as a cause of aseptic meningitis, blood urine and spinal fluid cultures should always be taken for *Leptospira*. A culture for tubercle bacilli should also be routine.

Treatment

There is no specific treatment for aseptic meningitis. The headache may be distressing in the early stages and should be controlled with analgesics and bed rest, while intravenous fluids may be necessary if vomiting is a prominent feature of the illness. This should be followed by a light fluid diet with gradual resumption of normal diet as the symptoms subside.

This condition is benign with full recovery within a period of a few days to a few weeks. Occasionally, some patients complain of undue fatigue and malaise for a few months after the attack, but this is unusual. It should be noted, however, that the early stages of tuberculous meningitis may mimic aseptic meningitis. This diagnosis should be considered in any case showing persistence of symptoms for two weeks, particularly with deterioration in the clinical condition.

Equine Encephalitides

Equine encephalitides are caused by three varieties of virus: western, eastern, and Venezuelan equine encephalitis virus. The three types of equine encephalitis caused by group A arbovirus were first isolated from outbreaks of encephalitis in horses and later were identified in man. The virus of western equine encephalitis was isolated in 1930[213] from the brain of a horse in California and was recognized as a cause of human disease in 1938.[150] Since that time cases have been recognized in nearly all parts of the United States and western Canada, and the virus is probably widely disseminated in the North American continent. Eastern equine encephalitis was first recognized as a viral infection during an outbreak among horses in the eastern United States in 1933.[111] It was established as a cause of encephalitis in man in 1938.[96] The virus seems to be localized to the eastern part of the United States, the West Indies, and the eastern seaboard of South America. The virus of Venezuelan equine encephalitis was isolated during an outbreak of encephalitis in horses in Venezuela in 1938[22] and recognized as a cause of human encephalitis in 1943.[45]

While the viruses of these three forms of encephalitis are closely related antigenically, they have distinct antigenic properties, which permit their separate identification. The reservoir of infection is believed to be small rodents and wild birds that develop asymptomatic viremia. Transmission is by the bite of the mosquito,[130] and the natural life cycle is between the mosquito, the rodent, and the wild bird population. Man and horses are accidentally infected by mosquitoes during periods when, for some reason, the mosquito feeds on vertebrates other than its natural host.

Clinical Features

Western Equine Encephalitis. This is an illness affecting both children and adults beginning with fever and severe headaches followed by vomiting, mental obtundity, and nuchal rigidity. Convulsions are common, particularly in children, and stupor or coma is seen in a high proportion of cases. Recovery usually occurs within five to ten days in the majority of cases and fatalities are rare. Permanent sequelae are relatively rare, but postencephalitic parkinsonism has been described.[275]

Eastern Equine Encephalitis. This is a more severe form of encephalitis than the western variety and predominantly affects infants and young children. The onset is abrupt, with high fever, headache, nuchal rigidity, convulsions, and rapid development of stupor or coma. The mortality rate is high, and surviving children usually show evidence of permanent damage to the central nervous system, while adults who survive usually make complete recovery.

Venezuelan Equine Encephalitis. Infection by the virus of Venezuelan equine encephalitis usually produces a mild systemic illness with fever, headache, and myalgia. Some outbreaks of encephalitis have occurred in epidemic proportions in South America and more recently in Central America, where severe encephalitis and death have been reported in children.[97]

Apparently, the three viruses of equine encephalitis may produce asymptomatic or unrecognized mild febrile infections in a large proportion of the population in endemic areas, as judged from serologic surveys carried out in North and South America.[137]

Diagnostic Procedures

1. The virus may be isolated by tissue culture from the brain in fatal cases and from brain biopsies in living cases.
2. Inoculation of blood into tissue culture may be of some value in early cases of encephalitis.
3. Nasopharyngeal swabs or washing may yield virus in tissue culture.
4. Diagnosis may be confirmed by demonstration of a fourfold rise in specific complement-fixing or neutralizing antibody titer in acute and convalescent sera.

Prophylaxis

Control of the mosquito population in endemic areas may reduce the incidence of human infections. Vaccines are available for protection of horses but are not suitable for human inoculation.

Treatment

No specific treatment is available for treatment of equine encephalitis. Good nursing care and symptomatic treatment should be given as indicated.

Viral Encephalitis Due to Group B Arbovirus

Only those viruses commonly causing encephalitis in man will be discussed.

St. Louis Encephalitis

St. Louis encephalitis is the most common form of viral encephalitis in the United States, and outbreaks of epidemic proportions occur from time to time in the southwestern, south central, and southeastern states.[137] The virus was isolated in 1933 following an epidemic of encephalitis that was thought to be transmitted by the mosquito in St. Louis and Kansas City, Missouri. This was confirmed by isolation of the virus from the mosquito in 1941. Since that time the disease has been recognized throughout the United States, the West Indies, and Central and South America. The virus has been classified with the group B arboviruses and is closely related antigenically to the viruses of Japanese B and West Nile encephalitis. The natural cycle appears to be between wild rodents or wild birds and the mosquito. Man is an accidental host infected during the height of the mosquito season in late summer and early fall.

The pathologic findings in St. Louis encephali-

tis are typical of those of a viral encephalitis, although focal necrosis is said to be infrequent, which may account for the lower incidence of permanent sequelae when compared with equine encephalitides or Japanese B encephalitis.

Clinical Features

There is a high incidence of subclinical infections in man, as judged by the high percentage of the population showing neutralizing antibodies to St. Louis encephalitis during epidemics. Mild systemic illnesses are also quite common during epidemics, with fever and headache lasting for a few days followed by complete recovery.

Encephalitis occurs in the minority of people exposed to infection and is frequently seen in elderly patients. The illness begins abruptly, with fever, myalgia, and headache associated with drowsiness, irritability, mental confusion, nausea, vomiting, and seizures. Cranial nerve involvement occurs in about 20 per cent of cases. Tremors and rigidity of the extrapyramidal type are common.[295] Nuchal rigidity and a positive Kernig's sign are usually present. The illness resolves in about seven days with complete recovery. The mortality rate is low in those under 40 years of age. However, the mortality shows a marked increase in patients with arteriosclerosis and hypertensive vascular disease. In some cases, convalescence may be prolonged for some months due to generalized weakness, fatigue, and poor intellectual performance, but permanent sequelae are uncommon.

Diagnostic Procedures

1. The white blood count may be normal or show a mild polymorphonuclear leukocytosis.
2. Lumbar puncture usually shows clear spinal fluid with slight increase in the opening pressure. The cell count shows slight pleocytosis and the protein may be moderately elevated.
3. Confirmation of St. Louis encephalitis may be obtained by demonstrating a rise in specific antibodies in acute and convalescent sera.

Treatment

Prophylaxis depends on adequate mosquito control in endemic areas. Treatment of the encephalitis is symptomatic.

Japanese B Encephalitis

This disease was first studied in Japan in 1924 and given the name "Japanese B encephalitis" to distinguish it from type A encephalitis of Von Economo. The virus was isolated from the human brain in 1935, and the belief that the disease was mosquito-borne was confirmed by isolation of the virus from mosquitoes in 1941.

The virus of Japanese B encephalitis is related antigenically to the group B arboviruses of St. Louis encephalitis and West Nile encephalitis. It is now known to exist in many areas in the Far East, including Japan, Korea, China, Eastern Siberia, Taiwan, Malaya, Singapore, and Guam. The arthropod vector is the mosquito, and the animal reservoir includes wild birds and pigs. Human and equine infections are accidental and break the cycle of viral development.

The pathologic changes are typically those of viral encephalitis, with marked neuronal degeneration and intense neuronophagia in the cerebral cortex and involving the Purkinje cells of the cerebellum. Patchy areas of necrosis may be seen in the cerebral cortex, thalamus, striatum, brainstem, cerebellum, and spinal cord. In chronic cases these areas show reactive gliosis.

Clinical Features

Japanese B encephalitis is a disease of the summer months when the mosquito population is most numerous. The majority of infections appear to be subclinical, or a mild systemic febrile illness may occur without the development of encephalitis.[127]

The onset of encephalitis, when it occurs, is usually abrupt but may occasionally follow a mild febrile illness. The temperature rises rapidly, with intense headache, lethargy, and occasionally stupor or coma. Masklike facies, extrapyramidal rigidity, and tremors are common, while convulsions and focal motor weakness are indicative of brainstem involvement. Death occurs in fatal cases, usually within the first week. Recovery occurs by lysis of fever and gradual convalescence, which may take several weeks or months during which time the patient experiences headache, fatigue, lethargy, tremors, and mental dullness. Permanent sequelae, consisting of poor orientation, impaired recent memory, and gross dementia in some cases, occur in about 40 per cent of cases.[176]

Diagnostic Procedures

1. The white blood count may be as high as 30,000 per cubic millimeter with a relative neutropenia and a lymphocytosis.
2. The cerebrospinal fluid is clear with a moderate elevation in pressure and up to 400 cells per cubic millimeter. These may be predominantly polymorphonuclear cells in the early stages, but lymphocytes predominate after the first few days.
3. Virus may be cultured and identified serologically from brain biopsy or brain specimens in fatal cases.
4. Acute and convalescent sera show a rise in specific antibodies.

Treatment

Control of mosquito vectors has been effective in reducing the incidence of Japanese B encephalitis. A vaccine is now available and appears to be effective in protecting the population in endemic areas.

Treatment of the encephalitis is symptomatic.

Although figures vary following studies of various epidemics, approximately 10 per cent of cases are fatal, 40 per cent show permanent sequelae, and about 50 per cent make a full recovery.

Tick-Borne Encephalitis

The term "tick-borne encephalitis" covers a group of viral encephalitides with close antigenic relationships. These are the encephalitides termed Far Eastern, Russian spring-summer, Czechoslovakian, central Europe, and louping ill. Actually, only subtle differences are detected on culture and antigenic evaluation among viruses isolated in any of these conditions. Tick-borne encephalitis was first recognized in the far eastern regions of the U.S.S.R. in 1934 and later in the western Soviet Union. Czechoslovakia, and other central European countries. Louping ill has been recognized as a disease of sheep in the British Isles for many years and, more recently, as an occasional cause of aseptic meningitis or a poliomyelitic type of illness in man.

The host range of the tick-borne viruses is wide, including rodents, birds, domestic sheep, cattle, and goats. Transmission to man is accidental due to the bite of an infected tick or by drinking infected goat's milk.

Clinical Features

Infection occurs in the months between late spring and early autumn when ticks are active. All types may give rise to subclinical infections or mild febrile illnesses, and serologic surveys have shown a high percentage of infection in populations from areas of central Europe and the

U.S.S.R. The tick-borne virus, including louping ill, may also be the cause of aseptic meningitis or a mild meningoencephalitis with complete recovery. The Far Eastern, Russian spring-summer, Czechoslovakian, and central European varieties may cause severe meningoencephalitis, with high fever, severe headache, obtundity, stupor, or coma, nuchal rigidity, epileptic seizures, and bulbar or bulbospinal paralysis. Other clinical types include hemiparetic, bulbar, poliomyelitic, and ascending parlaytic forms. In fatal cases, death usually occurs within seven days of the onset and the fatality rate may be as high as 40 per cent. The disease is more severe in children than in adults. Residual paralysis or diffuse brain damage may occur in survivors. In those who recover, convalescence may be prolonged, with complaints of chronic fatigue and emotional disturbances.

Diagnostic Procedures

Tick-borne encephalitides should be suspected in cases presenting with symptoms of encephalitis in endemic areas between late spring and early autumn. The virus may be isolated from the brain by tissue culture in fatal cases, and a rising titer of antibodies can be demonstrated in acute and convalescent sera in survivors.

Treatment

Protective clothing should be given to those exposed to infection in endemic cases, and insect repellents should be used. Control may be achieved by spraying tick-infected areas with insecticides and by vaccination of the exposed population. Milk-borne infection can be prevented by adequate pasteurization of milk.

Antiencephalitic globulin, 6 ml IM daily for three days, is effective in reducing the extracellular activity of the virus. Pancreatic ribonuclease (specific RNase activity 7×10^6 units/gm), 30 mg IM every four hours for six days, is believed to be the most effective treatment available for tickborne encephalitis at this time.[113]

Other Types of Encephalitis Due to Group B Arbovirus

There are at least five other forms of encephalitis due to group B arboviruses. All are mosquito-borne infections but there is some variation in the capacity of different viruses to produce encephalitis. The usual clinical picture is that of a febrile illness with systemic features. This is occasionally followed by encephalitis, particularly among children, during epidemics. The virus of Murray Valley encephalitis (Australian X disease) has the most potent neurogenic properties and is closely related antigenically to Japanese B virus. The disease has been studied during a number of epidemics in Australia and New Guinea and has a clinical course similar to that of Japanese B encephalitis.

Infection by the West Nile virus or the virus of dengue usually produces a febrile illness, and encephalitis is uncommon but has been described in both cases. In South America, encephalitis may also occur as a rare complication of infection by the virus of ilheus. Similarly, a few cases of encephalitis have been described during an epidemic of yellow fever. In the case of dengue and yellow fever, however, encephalitis is a most unusual occurrence.

Unclassified Arbovirus: Colorado Tick Encephalitis

Colorado tick fever has been recognized as "mountain fever" since the middle of the nineteenth century, and the virus was isolated from the blood of patients in 1944 and from the tick vector in 1950.

The virus is an unclassified member of the arbovirus group, and the natural reservoir includes squirrels and other small rodents. Man acquires the disease following a bite from an infected tick, and the infection is endemic in the western United States.

Clinical Features

Mild or subclinical infections are common. The usual signs of clinical infection are the appearance of sudden febrile illness with systemic symptoms lasting two or three days followed by apparent recovery for one or two days and then a second attack of fever lasting about 24 hours. This denguelike illness is followed by complete recovery. Encephalitis occurs in about 15 per cent of infected children. They develop fever, with a short episode of headache, nuchal rigidity, somnolence, and severe muscle tenderness. A maculopapular rash may appear on the trunk and extremities, sparing the hands and the soles of the feet. A period of delirium with convulsions and coma may occur within 48 hours in severe cases, but the illness does not usually last more than five days, with a rapid fall in temperature and recovery.

Diagnostic Procedures

1. The white blood count shows a leukopenia throughout the illness.
2. The virus may be isolated from the blood or spinal fluid during the febrile illness.
3. Antibodies may be detected in the convalescent sera, although their appearance may be delayed for as long as six weeks after the febrile episode.

Treatment

Protective clothing should be worn to prevent tick bites in areas where the condition is endemic. Repeated inspection and removal of ticks should be carried out in those persons exposed to infection. The treatment of encephalitis is symptomatic.

The prognosis is good with a low mortality rate and absence of sequelae.

California Arbovirus Encephalitis

The virus of California encephalitis was identified in California in 1943 and has subsequently been isolated in the central and eastern states and in Canada. It is transmitted by mosquitoes, and closely related viruses have been isolated from mosquitoes in South America, Trinidad, Africa, and Europe.

Clinical Features

The majority of cases occur in children during the months of July, August, and September, the infection presenting as an aseptic meningitis or encephalitis. Nearly all cases make a full recovery, and permanent neurologic sequelae are unusual.[54]

Diagnostic Procedures

1. The white blood count is often elevated, with a polymorphonucleocytosis.
2. The spinal fluid shows a lymphocytic pleocytosis. The protein content is usually normal but may be slightly elevated.
3. Neutralizing and hemagglutination-inhibition antibodies appear in the serum within a few days of the onset of symptoms. The appearance of complement-fixing antibodies is delayed until after the tenth day, with the highest titers noted at 30 days.

Treatment

Treatment of the encephalitis is symptomatic.

Rabies

References to hydrophobia, or rabies, and the association of this disease with the bite of rabid dogs may be found in writings of great antiquity, for epidemics of rabies have waxed and waned in various parts of the world for more than 2,000 years.[170]

Transmission of rabies by the inoculation of saliva from a rabid dog into a noninfected animal was demonstrated early in the nineteenth century. This led to public health measures in certain European countries, with the destruction of stray dogs and quarantining of domestic dogs entering the country,[143] leading to the elimination of rabies in Great Britain, Scandinavia, Iceland, Cyprus, Spain, and Portugal.[202]

Pasteur and his associates were able to reduce the incubation period of the disease by serial intracerebral passage of infected material in the rabbit. The modified virus was called "fixed" virus to distinguish it from the naturally occurring "street" virus. However, further intracerebral passage of the "fixed" virus led to the loss of pathogenicity with inability to infect dogs. Pasteur was then able to produce a vaccine by drying rabbit spinal cord infected with "fixed" virus, which protected dogs against inoculation by the natural or "street" virus.[245, 246] The vaccine was soon found to be effective in the protection of humans bitten by rabid dogs, and the Pasteur treatment was introduced on a worldwide scale. Several modifications of the vaccine were made, culminating in the phenol-treated tissue virus suspension of Semple in 1919.

It is probable that the virus exists in asymptomatic form in a variety of wild animals and is spread by infected saliva, introduced by bites. Man is usually infected by saliva following a bite from a rabid dog, but bats, weasels, skunks, wolves, mongooses, cats, jackals, foxes, squirrels, raccoons, and ermine have all been shown to infect man. Airborne rabies is rare and has been reported in laboratory accidents and in individuals exploring bat caves.[57] The virus passes through the peripheral nerves to reach the central nervous system, producing an encephalomyelitis. Inflammatory changes are present throughout the brain and spinal cord but tend to be particularly intense in the jugular, gasserian, and dorsal root ganglia. The dentate nucleus, lower medulla, locus ceruleus, hypothalamus, and tuberal nuclei are also highly infected. There is chromatolysis of nerve cells, which is more marked in the highly infected areas, and inclusion bodies (Negri bodies) are seen as sharply defined cytoplasmic inclusions, particularly in areas showing relatively less inflammation, such as the cerebral cortex, hippocampus, and Purkinje cells of the cerebellum.[78]

In the paralytic type of rabies described in Trinidad following bites of the feet from vampire bats, there is intense inflammation and necrosis of the lower spinal cord, which decreases progressively in the upper segments of the cord.

Clinical Features

The incubation period usually lasts 21 to 60 days (range six days to 14 months).[214]

There may be prodomal fever and general malaise for a few days associated with pain and paresthesias at the site of the bite. This is followed by symptoms of anxiety and a general overreaction to sensory stimuli or so-called "stimulus-sensitive myoclonus" in response to stimuli such as noise or light touch. This is associated with increases of sympathetic activity characterized by excessive sweating, salivation, lacrimation, and constriction of the pupils. As anxiety increases, the classic symptom of forceful expulsion of water occurs when an attempt is made to drink fluid owing to spasmodic contraction of the pharyngeal muscles on contact with fluid. This may be followed later by similar spasmodic contractions of both pharyngeal and respiratory muscles at the sight, sound, or even mention of water. Periods of respiratory arrest and cyanosis may occur; seizures are common and death may occur at this stage. In the majority of cases, however, the stage of excitement is followed by apathy, stupor, and usually coma and death.

In some cases, progressive muscle weakness may be a prominent feature with less evidence of sympathetic overactivity and excitement. Patients with this form of predominantly spinal cord involvement are similar to those described in Trinidad and present with an ascending paralysis and terminal respiratory paralysis.

Diagnostic Procedures

1. The white blood count shows a polymorphonucleocytosis often as high as 25,000 cells per cubic millimeter.
2. Lumbar puncture usually reveals a clear fluid with a slight increase of opening pressure. There is mild lymphocytic pleocytosis, slight elevation in protein, and normal sugar and chloride content.
3. Rabies antibodies can be measured in 24 hours. The presence of antibody in a nonimmunized individual or high serum neutralizing antibody titers or antibody levels in the cerebrospinal fluid indicate rabies infection.
4. The diagnosis may be established by immunofluorescence following brain biopsy.[323a]

Prophylaxis

1. In countries where dog rabies is still the major problem, rabies can be controlled by adequately vaccinating the dog population and by destroying stray dogs. All pet dogs should receive prophylactic vaccination.
2. First aid treatment should be carried out immediately. The wound should be thoroughly cleansed with soap and water.
3. Treatment by or under the direction of a physician:
   a. The wound should be thoroughly cleansed immediately with soap solution.
   b. Tetanus prophylaxis and measures to control bacterial infection should be given as indicated.
4. When a patient is bitten by an animal known to be rabid, he should be treated with rabies hyperimmune horse serum and given a course of injections of duck embryo vaccine.

A rabid animal may be defined as an animal showing clinical signs of rabies or an animal showing Negri bodies in the brain at autopsy or an unidentified animal that escapes after biting in an area where rabies is prevalent. The rabies antiserum may be omitted in the case of mild exposure (a lick on abrased skin or a single bite not on the head, face, neck, or arm).

If a person is bitten by a domestic animal and the animal is apprehended, it should be kept under observation and given adequate food and water for ten days. At the end of that period, if the animal is still healthy, it can be assumed that it is not suffering from rabies. Under these circumstances, the person bitten does not require vaccination. If the animal develops clinical signs of rabies during the ten-day period, the exposed patient should be vaccinated.

Two types of vaccine, the Semple vaccine and the duck embryo vaccine, have been used extensively. The Semple vaccine is a 20 per cent suspension of rabbit brain tissue infected with fixed virus and is given daily in 2-ml doses subcutaneously in the abdominal wall. Sensitivity to the Semple vaccine may produce a severe and diffuse demyelination involving the central nervous system and the peripheral nerves. Post-rabies-vaccine encephalomyelitis is usually a devastating and severe disease, and the residual neurologic disability may be incapacitating. Duck embryo vaccine is the only vaccine licensed in the United States and the United Kingdom. It does not contain myelin, and postvaccinal leukoencephalopathy does not occur following the use of this preparation. Minor vaccine reactions may occur but can usually be treated by aspirin. Serious reactions are extremely rare, and, since duck embryo vaccine appears to be as effective as the Semple vaccine, it should be given whenever the possibility of exposure to rabies exists.[208, 260] It is given in a single dose by subcutaneous injection (one ampule) daily for 14 days into the abdominal wall. Confirmation of satisfactory levels of neutralizing antibodies may be obtained through state health laboratories in the United States.

Certain patients have a higher risk of developing rabies. The risk is higher following multiple bites over the body and after single bites on the face, head, or neck. Persons bitten by wild animals have a much higher risk of rabies than those bitten by domestic animals and should receive rabies antiserum plus vaccination with duck embryo vaccine. These higher-risk patients should be given two doses daily of the vaccine for seven days, followed by a single dose daily for another seven days. Since antiserum may interfere with the production of antibodies, booster doses of vaccine should be given 10 and 20 days after completion of the initial course of vaccination.

The duck embryo vaccine or the Flury HEP live virus vaccine may be used for preexposure vaccination of persons who are exposed to a higher risk of contracting rabies such as laboratory workers who handle live vaccine or veterinarians practicing in regions where the disease is prevalent.

Treatment

Rabies has been regarded as invariably fatal, but the use of intensive support care has led to prolonged survival and recovery in some cases.[133]

Herpes Simplex Encephalitis

Herpes simplex or herpes hominis encephalitis constitutes about 10 per cent of cases of viral encephalitis in the United States. It occurs in nonepidemic form and at any age. The infecting virus, *Herpes virus hominis,* was first isolated from the brain in 1941 at which time the typical intranuclear inclusion bodies within nerve cells were also described.[292] Since that time a positive viral diagnosis has been established with increasing frequency both at autopsy and during life. Untreated, severe cases of herpes simplex encephalitis carry a mortality rate in excess of 80 per cent.

Pathology

In fulminating and acute cases, the brain is edematous, while in severe cases dying after an interval of several weeks to three months, the brain shows areas of necrosis with or without hemorrhage and cavitation scattered throughout the cerebral hemispheres and the pontine portion of the brainstem. There may be evidence of uncal herniation due to brain swelling. The microscopic appearance is that of a viral encephalitis with marked perivascular accumulation of lymphocytes. In addition, there are scattered areas of nerve cell loss, necrosis, and zones of hemorrhage, or the so-called "lakes of blood." Type A inclusion bodies are found in both neurons and astrocytes.

Clinical Features

The clinical picture of herpes simplex encephalitis varies considerably from a mild aseptic meningitis to the more common fulminating and fatal encephalitis. Those cases presenting with symptoms of aseptic meningitis have fever, headache, and nuchal rigidity, but there is no major neurologic deficit on examination and the disease may resolve in a few days without residual neurologic disorder.

The usual course is one of severe encephalitis. Such patients develop headache, lethargy, myalgia, anorexia, nausea, vomiting, irritability, and sore throat. This is followed by marked confusion, deterioration of memory, disorientation, and eventually stupor or coma. Myoclonic jerks as well as focal and generalized seizures are extremely common. There may be conjugate deviation of the eyes with hemiparesis, quadriparesis, and diffuse rigidity. Herpetic stomatitis may be present in a few patients, and a history of recurrent herpes labialis is obtained in a high proportion of cases. This observation has led some to conclude that herpes simplex encephalitis is due to a reactivation of a latent infection rather than an infection of the brain de novo.[188] The encephalitic process usually terminates in death within a few weeks (in about 80 per cent) and rarely after several months. If recovery should occur, there are usually marked neurologic deficits.

There are reports of herpes encephalitis presenting with symptoms of bizarre psychotic behavior several days before the onset of clear signs of encephalitis.[337] The disease may also run a relapsing course where patients present with recurrent neurologic deficits, often with good recovery[216] or with recurrent episodes of psychosis with changes in personality, confusion, disorientation, and memory deficits. There is usually evidence of cumulative and permanent brain damage between attacks.[281] Herpes simplex is the occasional cause of a severe brainstem encephalitis with a surprisingly good recovery.[87]

The most severe cases of herpes simplex encephalitis have the rapid onset of brain necrosis (acute necrotizing hemorrhagic encephalitis) associated with signs of encephalitis.[132] These fulminating cases complain of headache and vomiting.[165] There are often papilledema, retinitis, memory deficit, dysphasia, dysarthria, facial palsies, and hemiparesis. The occurrence of early neurologic signs is characteristic of herpes simplex encephalitis and frequently suggests the possibility of brain abscess or brain tumor. This type carries the highest mortality rate, with death usually occurring within a few days.

Diagnostic Procedures

1. An increase in the titer of neutralizing or complement-fixing specific antibodies for herpes simplex virus of more than fourfold is strongly suggestive of herpes simplex encephalitis. Complement-fixing antibodies increase earlier than neutralizing antibodies in herpes simplex encephalitis. An increase in the complement-fixing:neutralizing antibody ratio is an early diagnostic sign.[189, 233]
2. The spinal fluid may show none or a pleocytosis of up to 1,000 mononuclear cells per cubic millimeter with variable numbers of polymorphonuclear leukocytes. Xanthochromia with several thousand red cells may occur in some cases. The glucose level is usually normal but may be depressed.[160]
3. Immunofluorescent antibodies may be demonstrated in the cerebrospinal fluid within 24 hours.
4. The herpes virus may be cultured from pharyngeal swabs in a few cases but the majority are negative.
5. If brain biopsy material is obtained from a heavily injected area of the brain, it may show the presence of intranuclear eosinophilic inclusion bodies in the neurons.[166]
6. The virus can be cultured from brain biopsies within 48 to 96 hours, using tube cultures of human embryonic lung or human epithelial line cells.[166]
7. Brain biopsy material may show the presence of fluorescent antibodies after staining with monkey antiherpes simplex fluorescent conjugate.

   Rapid identification of herpes simplex virus antigen in brain biopsy material can be accomplished with a simple immunoperoxidase technique.[29]
8. The electroencephalogram may show loss of alpha activity and diffuse slowing in the theta range over both hemispheres.

   In some cases distinctive high-voltage periodic sharp waves recurring every two to three seconds are seen over one temporal lobe appearing within one week after the onset of the illness. This EEG abnormality may indicate the best site for brain biopsy that will give maximal yield of herpes simplex virus.[51]
9. Computed tomography shows areas of decreased density in both temporal lobes, which is often asymmetric and extends into the frontal and parietal areas. There may be a shift of the midline structures away from the side of maximal involvement.[309]
10. In cases coming to autopsy the herpes virus may be isolated from the brain. Since the life of the virus is very short (four hours at 37°C), isolation depends on obtaining material shortly after death.

Treatment

1. Administration of pooled human gamma globulin is probably of no benefit.
2. Repeated lumbar punctures and drainage of cerebrospinal fluid may reduce acute cerebral edema.
3. Dexamethasone, 4 mg every six hours, may produce clinical improvement, probably by reducing cerebral edema.[323]

4. Surgical decompression may be indicated in cases with rapid rise in intracranial pressure.[186] This also affords opportunity for brain biopsy and excludes the diagnosis of brain abscess.

5. The use of antiviral agents in the treatment of herpes simplex encephalitis is controversial, and both idoxuridine and cytosine arabinoside have been abandoned as therapeutic agents.[5, 304] There are reports of success with adenine arabinoside (Ara A) in the treatment of severe herpetic infections. This drug has undergone successful clinical trials in the treatment of herpes simplex encephalitis. Adenine arabinoside is administered intravenously in doses of 10 mg/kg of body weight per day over a 12-hour period.[138] Side effects of Ara A include nausea and vomiting, weight loss, weakness, megaloblastosis in the erythroid series of the bone marrow, tremors beginning five to seven days after the start of therapy, and thrombophlebitis at the intravenous site.[256]

6. Surviving patients frequently show residual brain damage. Children often require speech therapy and special education after an attack of herpes encephalitis.[340] Some may require institutional care owing to dementia or uncontrolled involuntary movements.

Herpes Simplex Type 2 Encephalitis

Type 2 herpes simplex virus produces a recurrent local cutaneous eruption in adults. The virus is retained in the vagina for many years, and there is a high risk of neonatal infection during passage through the birth canal. The infection can cause a generalized herpetic papulovesicular skin eruption, which may be followed by acute encephalitis in neonates. Surviving infants often have recurrent vesicular skin eruptions and severe cerebral damage, which can be demonstrated by computed tomography.[289]

Diagnostic Procedures

Immunofluorescence provides a rapid means of identification of a herpes simplex type 2 virus infection.[40] The virus may be cultured from skin vesicles.

Treatment

Treatment is the same as for herpes simplex encephalitis. Adenine arabinoside (Ara A) therapy appears to be effective in neonatal herpes simplex virus encephalitis.[52]

Herpes Simiae Virus Encephalomyelitis

Fatal cases of encephalomyelitis have been reported following contact with monkeys. Most of these infections occurred in laboratory workers, but the virus may be transmitted by apparently healthy animals and has occurred following handling of pets. Special protective clothing should be worn by laboratory workers handling monkeys, and contact with secretions should be avoided.

Herpes Zoster and Varicella

Varicella (chickenpox) and herpes zoster are believed to represent different clinical manifestations of infection by a single virus. It is possible that herpes zoster is the result of a latent reactivation of an earlier attack or exposure to varicella or that it represents an infection by the virus in a partly immune patient.

Clinical Features

A full description of herpes zoster is given in Chapter 10. The nervous system may be involved during or following varicella or herpes zoster, as follows:[123]

1. A viral encephalomyelitis[209]
   a. Cerebral type occurring one day to three weeks after the rash with lethargy, seizures, headache, and nuchal rigidity. The mortality is 35 per cent. The CSF shows a lymphocytic pleocytosis with normal or elevated protein content.
   b. Cerebellar type with lethargy, headache, ataxia, nystagmus, scanning speech, and nuchal rigidity. The prognosis is excellent in this type.[167]
2. Aseptic meningitis
3. Postinfectious leukoencephalitis
4. Postinfectious polyneuropathy

Treatment

The treatment is the same as outlined for herpes simplex encephalitis. There have been some preliminary reports of the efficacy of adenine arabinoside in the treatment of zoster and varicella infections.[50, 53]

Measles Encephalitis

Neurologic complications develop in about 1 in 1,000 cases of measles, but involvement of the central nervous system may be more common since 50 per cent of patients with measles have been reported to have an abnormal electroencephalogram.[240] Encephalitis may be the result of direct invasion of the brain by measles virus or a postinfectious leukoencephalitis of "autoimmune" type. Probably both situations exist, and the isolation of measles virus in acute measles encephalitis confirms the direct viral etiology in at least some cases.

Symptoms of encephalitis usually appear on the fourth or fifth day following the onset of the rash. There is a return of fever, headache, cranial nerve palsies, dystonic movements of several types, and cerebellar and long tract signs. The mortality is about 10 per cent, and many survivors show evidence of central nervous system damage including seizures.

Infectious Mononucleosis

Infectious mononucleosis or glandular fever is probably a virus infection and is almost certainly caused by Epstein-Barr (EB) virus.[230a, 249a] However, a number of cases of infectious mononucleosis with a negative heterophil antibody test are caused by cytomegalovirus or acute acquired toxoplasmosis.[168] The disease presents as a mild, febrile illness with sore throat and lymphadenopathy. Occasionally an erythematous rash and splenomegaly are also present. Diagnosis depends on the demonstration of typical mononucleosis cells in the blood smear and heterophil antibodies in the serum.

Neurologic complications of infectious mononucleosis occur in about 5 per cent of cases, although asymptomatic pleocytosis may occur in about 25 per cent of cases. Aseptic meningitis appears to be the most common symptomatic complication, but polyneuritis, mononeuritis, encephalitis, and encephalomyelitis have also been reported.[284]

Encephalitis may be the sole manifestation of infectious mononucleosis[101] and develop abruptly with seizures, stupor, coma, and focal signs of hemiplegia, aphasia, and involuntary movements. Brainstem signs with cranial nerve palsies, vertigo, nystagmus, dysarthria, and cerebellar ataxia may also occur.[13] Spinal cord involvement may lead to paraplegia.

The diagnosis of encephalitis due to infectious mononucleosis depends on the presence of the typical blood picture and the demonstration of

heterophil antibodies. The prognosis is good and complete recovery is to be anticipated.

Treatment

There is no specific treatment for infectious mononucleosis, but bed rest, nursing care, adequate diet, and maintenance of fluid balance are essential.

Coxsackie Virus Infections

Two serologically distinct groups of Coxsackie viruses may be responsible for infections in man that occur predominantly in children. Both groups may produce neurologic signs and symptoms due to infections involving the central nervous system.

Viruses of the group A type characteristically produce herpangina, a febrile disease with discrete herpetiform lesions involving the tonsils and pharynx resulting in cervical lymphadenopathy. Group A viruses can also cause aseptic meningitis, acute cerebellar ataxia in children,[93a] and hemiconvulsions and hemiplegia followed by a permanent motor deficit and epilepsy in infants and young children (HHE syndrome).[48, 255]

Viruses of the group B type cause epidemic pleurodynia (epidemic myalgia. Bornholm disease, p. 730) frequently associated with benign pericarditis in children and adults, but the pericarditis and myocarditis in the newborn may be severe.[178] Aseptic meningitis and an infection clinically indistinguishable from poliomyelitis also results from infection by Coxsackie B group virus. A fatal encephalomyelitis with meningoencephalitis, myocarditis, adrenal necrosis, and hepatic necrosis has been reported in infants due to Coxsackie B virus. The central nervous system shows diffuse lymphocytic meningitis, perivascular cuffing, neuronophagia, and microglial proliferation in the anterior horn cells of the cervical cord and the brainstem.[219]

Diagnostic Procedures

1. The cerebrospinal fluid shows a lymphocytic pleocytosis with normal protein and glucose content.
2. The Coxsackie virus may be isolated from the nasopharynx.

Treatment

Most patients improve rapidly. Treatment is symptomatic.

Cytomegalovirus Infections

Cytomegalovirus, or salivary gland virus, derives its names from the changes produced in the cells of infected organs as well as a tendency to involve the salivary glands. The virus produces a characteristic enlargement of the infected cell, and the nucleus develops a prominent type A intranuclear inclusion body.

Cytomegalic virus infection produces a systemic disease of newborn infants resulting in severe brain damage and microcephaly. The infant may be infected in utero since the virus passes through the placenta, and cytomegalic cells have been demonstrated in the chorionic villi. The child is usually premature but if born at full term usually fails to thrive. If the child survives to the age of six months, it is evidently retarded and often microcephalic. Chorioretinitis, microphthalmia, optic atrophy, and perivascular calcifications in the brain may also occur. Other systemic manifestations of the infection include hepatomegaly, splenomegaly, and jaundice.

The possibility of cytomegalic inclusion disease should be considered in all microcephalic infants since in one series, cytomegalovirus antibody was demonstrated in the sera of 44 per cent of microcephalic infants and children (p. 78).[90, 131]

Cytomegalovirus infection may produce a heterophil-antibody–negative infectious mononucleosis, and the virus is a rare cause of aseptic meningitis encephalitis and acute polyneuritis in children and adults.[46]

Treatment

Since cytomegalovirus is a DNA herpes group virus, treatment with adenine arabinoside (Ara A) might be considered for cytomegalovirus disease of infants and for the encephalitis occurring in children and adults.

Poliomyelitis

This disease, which was formerly called infantile paralysis, was a major public health problem. There were epidemics almost yearly in the temperate zones of the world until the introduction of the poliomyelitis vaccines in 1953.[264] Since that time there has been a dramatic reduction in the incidence of poliomyelitis but sporadic cases are still occasionally seen in the summer months.

Poliomyelitis is caused by three immunologically distinct viruses but immunity to one does not confer immunity to the other two. Serologic surveys have shown that although infection with the three types of poliomyelitis virus occurs in tropical and arctic areas as well as in temperate zones, the majority of individuals show no clinical signs of infection and become silently immunized during infancy and early childhood. The spread of the virus is thought to be primarily through fecal contamination of food or water supplies, although the virus has been isolated in flies, which may act as carriers.

The virus can be obtained after pharyngeal swabbing of exposed individuals, which suggests that spread may also occur by droplet infection. Once the virus has been ingested, it multiplies in the regional lymph nodes and enters the circulation, causing a viremia. The virus will then invade the central nervous system unless it is blocked by antibodies present in the bloodstream.

Pathologic Changes

When the virus reaches the meninges, there is an initial inflammatory response with changes resembling an aseptic meningitis. The infection may subside at this stage, but in some cases the virus enters the nervous tissue showing a marked predilection for motor neurons of the spinal cord, brainstem, and hypothalamus. There are usually marked inflammatory changes involving the anterior horns of the spinal cord; the motor nuclei of the brainstem; the neurons of the substantia nigra, hypothalamus, and cerebellar nuclei; and occasionally and to a lesser extent the precentral gyri of the frontal lobes.

Microscopically, those patients dying in the acute stage show diffuse infiltration of the anterior horns of the spinal cord with inflammatory cells. The initial response may be polymorphonuclear, but lymphocytes and monocytes predominate after a few days. There may be marked perivascular cuffing, but in some cases the inflammatory cells are so numerous that they cover the neurons and mask any changes in these cells. The damage to the neurons varies. Some may show necrosis and neuronophagia, while others are less severely damaged and exhibit central chromatolysis or show type B intranuclear inclusions. At a later stage there is proliferation of microglial cells, which may become distended with lipid and ingested material from necrotic neurons. As the inflammation and edema subside, the area within the anterior horn becomes shrunken and scarred with secondary gliosis and even cyst formation.

Clinical Features

Prior to the widespread use of immunization, poliomyelitis was an epidemic disease of late summer and autumn months. Fortunately, it is seldom seen now except in sporadic forms.

The virus produces subclinical infection in 95 per cent of those infected, systemic infection in 3 per cent, aseptic meningitis in 1 per cent, and paralytic poliomyelitis in 1 per cent.

Subclinical infections with poliomyelitis virus are important because they lead to immunization of those infected against that particular virus type. The virus, however, may be excreted in the feces for as long as three months after infection, so that those who are infected should be regarded as carriers.

Systemic infection with poliomyelitis produces fever, malaise, nausea, and occasionally diarrhea and vomiting. The condition usually subsides in three or four days or it may be followed by aseptic meningitis (p. 445). In addition to the usual signs of fever, headache, drowsiness, and meningeal irritation, there may be acute muscle pain with tenderness, particularly in the muscles of the back and proximal limbs. There appear to be certain factors that predispose to the development of paralytic poliomyelitis. These include recent tonsillectomy, pregnancy, inoculations, and physical exertion.

The high incidence of poliomyelitis following tonsillectomy led to the suspension of this type of surgery during the late summer months in many areas of the United States prior to the era of vaccination. Tonsillectomy performed on a carrier has been followed by bulbar poliomyelitis within two weeks of the operation.

There is also a higher incidence of poliomyelitis in pregnant women and particularly women with families of young children, which presumably increases the exposure to infection.

Recent inoculations of diphtheria toxoid, pertussis vaccine, and tetanus toxoid appear to predispose individuals to poliomyelitis within one month of the inoculation. There was also definite correlation between the site of inoculation and the site of paralysis.

Strenuous exercise during the incubation period may predispose to paralytic poliomyelitis with severe paralysis, particularly in young adults.

Paralytic Poliomyelitis. In children the paralytic stage of poliomyelitis usually follows an initial febrile illness corresponding to the systemic infection. Often, there may be apparent recovery from the systemic infection with a reduction in body temperature to normal followed by a secondary fever during the paralytic stage. This "dromedary" type of temperature response used to be a characteristic feature of epidemic poliomyelitis. The secondary fever is accompanied by nuchal rigidity together with the symptoms already described for the aseptic meningeal stage of poliomyelitis. The paralysis usually appears as the temperature falls. The prodromata are less apparent in adults, and the paralysis usually follows a period of malaise and slight temperature. The disease is however, more severe in adults, with a higher incidence of quadriplegia, respiratory paralysis, and death. A combination of the spinal and bulbar types is also more common in adults.

Paralytic poliomyelitis may be classified as spinal when the paralysis involves the skeletal muscles supplied by spinal nerves. A temporary paralysis of the bladder with urinary retention was common in this form. Paralytic poliomyelitis is classified as bulbar when there is involvement of muscles supplied by the ninth, tenth, and twelfth cranial nerves resulting in pharyngeal, laryngeal, and lingual paralysis. Respiratory paralysis or paralysis of the respiratory and vasomotor centers in the medulla was common in this type. Paralytic poliomyelitis is classified as bulbospinal when there is a combination of bulbar and spinal paralysis.

Respiratory paralysis may occur in all three types of paralytic poliomyelitis. In spinal poliomyelitis it is due to paralysis of the diaphragm, intercostal, and abdominal muscles. This decreases respiratory excursion and the ability to cough up mucous secretions. The respirations are regular but shallow, and the patients appear apprehensive and cyanotic. Bulbar poliomyelitis produces respiratory paralysis owing to involvement of the respiratory center. This is further complicated by pharyngeal paralysis permitting pooling of secretions in the pharynx and obstruction of the airway. The respirations are irregular, with a rising pulse rate before cyanosis appears. Bulbar poliomyelitis may be further complicated by involvement of the vasomotor center resulting in tachycardia and elevated blood pressure followed by circulatory collapse and shock. Bulbospinal cases may show a combination of intercostal paralysis and central respiratory collapse.

Sensory loss is rare in poliomyelitis but occasional involvement of the neurons in the posterior root ganglia produces sensory disturbances in this disease.[277]

Differential Diagnosis

Paralytic poliomyelitis is not usually difficult to diagnose, but since the condition is now uncommon, diagnosis depends on maintaining an awareness that there may be an occasional case. Other viruses, particularly of the Coxsackie and ECHO groups, may produce a transient or mild paralysis. Paralysis may also be a feature of encephalitis due to the arboviruses, but the encephalitic symptoms are the dominant features in these cases. Post-infectious polyneuropathy (Guillain-Barré syndrome) is more likely to cause problems in differential diagnosis, but the absence of cells in the spinal fluid and a rise in protein content if serial specimens are examined should help in differentiating these cases.

Diagnostic Procedures

1. The differential white blood cell count may be normal or show a moderate leukocytosis.
2. The cerebrospinal fluid is clear and pressure is usually normal or may be slightly elevated. There is a mild pleocytosis of from 10 to 200 cells, which are often predominantly polymorphonuclear in the early stages but change to lymphocytes within a few hours. The protein content may be slightly elevated with normal glucose and chloride levels.
3. The virus may be isolated by tissue culture from throat swabbings during the acute phase and from the feces both during the acute phase and for some months after the acute illness.
4. Neutralizing and complement-fixation antibodies may be high when paralysis occurs, but a fourfold rise in titer is diagnostic in sera taken at intervals of ten days.

Prophylaxis

The introduction of an effective vaccine against poliomyelitis has abolished epidemics in many countries. The infrequent appearance of vaccine-associated paralysis is a minor hazard when compared to the enormous benefit of vaccination programs in the United States.[146] There are two vaccines available: *The Salk vaccine,* which was introduced in 1953, consists of formalin-inactivated virus. This preparation is given by injection of two doses at monthly intervals followed by a booster dose at six months and a supplementary dose at six or seven years of age. It stimulates the production of antibodies, which prevent invasion of the central nervous system but do not prevent the viremic stage of the disease. The killed virus vaccine is safe and is probably the most effective method of immunization against poliomyelitis.[265] *The Sabin vaccine* consists of live attenuated virus that is given orally. Infection by this virus simulates subclinical infection and immunization against poliovirus.[261, 262] There have been occasional reports of paralytic poliomyelitis apparently caused by the live attenuated virus. The vaccine is given in trivalent form, two or three drops in a lump of sugar at two-month intervals for three doses. Children should receive a booster dose at 18 months and on entering school.

Treatment

Acute Paralytic Poliomyelitis. The patient should be kept at rest in bed during the acute or febrile stages with maintenance of adequate fluid intake and electrolyte balance. Analgesics may be necessary to reduce muscle pains and hot packs to the limbs, or a heating pad over the lumbar area may also relieve the myalgia. The development of deformities in paralyzed limbs should be prevented by use of sandbags, splints, and footboards, and all joints in paralyzed limbs should be put through a full range of movement at least twice a day.

Respiratory failure requires the use of an intermittent positive pressure respirator. The chest should be examined by percussion and auscultation daily in all cases whether or not respiratory failure is evident, and roentgenograms should be obtained if pneumonia or atelectasis is suspected. Pneumonia should be treated with the appropriate antibiotics as indicated by gram stain and culture of the sputum. Oxygen may be administered by nasal catheter through the respirator if pneumonia is severe. If atelectasis occurs, bronchoscopy may be required to remove the secretions obstructing the bronchi.

In cases with respiratory paralysis requiring a respirator, the vital capacity should be frequently measured early in convalescence in order to indicate when the patient may be weaned from the respirator. This may be started with the use of a rocking bed, which assists respiration temporarily while the patient gains confidence in independent breathing and his respiratory muscle function improves.

Transient retention of urine may occur during the acute stage of the disease, and catheterization is almost always necessary. However, permanent paralysis of the bladder does not occur in poliomyelitis.

The treatment of residual paralysis requires optimum development of remaining strength by physical and occupational therapy. Sometimes surgical procedures such as tendon transplantation are indicated. Rehabilitation is often a long-term process, beginning with passive movements in the acute phase but evolving into a program designed to obtain the maximum efficiency of surviving muscles, including the ability to function for others that remain paralyzed. Patients who survive the acute phase with residual paralysis should be encouraged to enter rehabilitation and physical therapy programs. Improvement in muscle strength may be expected to continue for two years from the onset of weakness. Much can be done even for severely paralyzed patients. Reeducation, rehabilitation, and a positive approach to their special problems by the team of medical, nursing, and ancillary personnel allows even the most severely paralyzed patient to serve a useful function in a restricted environment.

Adequate care in the acute phase plus the use of assisted respiration has reduced the mortality to below 5 per cent in centers adequately equipped to deal with poliomyelitis.

ECHO Virus Infections

There are now over 40 types of ECHO viruses that have been identified. The majority have been implicated in various types of human infection. Infants and children are particularly susceptible to ECHO viruses, which have been causally related to infantile diarrhea, upper respiratory infections, and a febrile illness with or without a generalized maculopapular rash.[20] Many of the ECHO viruses have been isolated from cases of aseptic meningitis,[221] and from a disease closely resembling paralytic poliomyelitis. Pseudo-poliomyelitis infections also resemble infections by the Coxsackie virus and usually have a good prognosis. Some cases of encephalitis in children are not uncommon during epidemics of ECHO virus infections.[7] The virus appears to have a predilec-

tion for the brainstem and cerebellum, so that cerebellar signs and ataxia are characteristic features of these illnesses. The usual course is one of recovery after a 14-day period of neurologic signs.

Encephalomyocarditis

The encephalomyocarditis group of viruses has been reported to cause aseptic meningitis and encephalomyelitis as well as a condition resembling paralytic poliomyelitis in man. The myocarditis is not characteristic of human infections but commonly occurs in infected laboratory animals.

Mumps

The virus of mumps usually produces an infection of the salivary glands about 18 to 21 days after exposure to the virus. In addition, the virus may infect the testes, epididymis, prostate, ovaries, thyroid, pancreas, and nervous system. Subclinical infection of the nervous system presenting as an asymptomatic meningitis with pleocytosis of the cerebrospinal fluid probably occurs in about 65 per cent of patients with mumps parotitis.[16] A much smaller percentage of cases develop symptomatic aseptic meningitis with headache, stiff neck, and mild confusion. About 50 per cent of these patients have parotitis with the development of neurologic symptoms about three days later.[191] Mumps encephalitis is rare and has a good prognosis.[11] However, aqueductal stenosis and hydrocephalus have been reported as rare sequelae of mumps encephalitis.[297] Occasionally, it may produce a clinical picture resembling paralytic poliomyelitis. In addition, neuritis of the optic, trigeminal, and facial nerves may occur as a complication of mumps. However, both aseptic meningitis and encephalitis may occur independently of parotid gland involvement.

A presumptive diagnosis of mumps with aseptic meningitis or encephalitis is not difficult in the presence of the classic parotitis. The diagnosis is more difficult when salivary gland involvement is absent clinically. In such cases of meningeal or encephalitic infection by the mumps virus, the diagnosis may be confirmed by demonstrating an increase in complement-fixation antibodies measured in two specimens of serum taken at an interval of two weeks.

Treatment

There is no specific treatment for mumps encephalitis.

Lymphocytic Choriomeningitis

The virus of lymphocytic choriomeningitis readily infects lower animals, particularly mice, producing a severe or fatal encephalitis. It is usually transmitted to man by house mice, which are carriers of the virus. Dwellings are then contaminated by their excretions and secretions. It is possible that the final mode of infection may be house dust.

The resulting type of infection in man is an influenza-like illness that resolves in a few days. A few patients, however, develop symptoms of aseptic meningitis with typical meningeal irritation, stiff neck, and lymphocytic pleocytosis characteristic of that condition. Complete recovery occurs within two weeks. Encephalitis is a rare complication of infection by this virus.[192]

Diagnostic Procedures

The spinal fluid shows 100 to 5,000 lymphocytes. Inoculation of mice with the spinal fluid may allow isolation of the virus, and the blood will show a rising titer in specimens of serum drawn at intervals of two weeks.

Treatment

There is no specific treatment for the viral infection in man, but prevention by adequate rodent control will prevent human infection.

Mycoplasma pneumoniae Infections

Mycoplasma pneumoniae has been related to a variety of diseases in man, including tracheobronchitis, atypical pneumonia, pericarditis, and hemolytic anemia. Neurologic complications include aseptic meningitis, meningoencephalitis, transverse myelitis, and acute postinfectious polyneuropathy (Guillain-Barré syndrome).[290] The meningoencephalitis may present as an acute cerebellar ataxia in children,[298] or with multiple cranial nerve palsies.[158] In other cases, symptoms have been severe with focal seizures, decerebration, and coma.[222] There is a 25 per cent mortality in such cases, but survivors tend to make a complete recovery.

Diagnostic Procedures

1. The cerebrospinal fluid shows a pleocytosis with variable percentages of polymorphonuclear leukocytes and monocytes. The protein content is increased, but the glucose levels are normal.[307]

2. A fourfold or greater rise in the complement-fixation test titer is diagnostic of *Mycoplasma pneumoniae* infection.
3. Cold agglutinins are usually present in the serum.
4. *Mycoplasma pneumoniae* can usually be cultured from the pharynx.

Treatment

There is no specific treatment for *Mycoplasma pneumoniae* infections.

Rickettsial Infections of the Central Nervous System

The rickettsial diseases that are associated with involvement of the nervous system may be classified as follows:

Disease	Rickettsia	Vector
1. Epidemic typhus	*R. prowazekii*	Louse
2. Murine typhus	*R. mooseri*	Rat flea
3. Rocky Mountain spotted fever	*R. rickettsii*	Tick
4. Scrub typhus (tsutsugamushi)	*R. tsutsugamushi*	Mite

Involvement of the central nervous system is almost invariable in epidemic typhus, Rocky Mountain spotted fever, and scrub typhus as well as in the more severe forms of murine typhus. The initial lesion of the brain and spinal cord begins in the endothelium of small blood vessels, which become swollen, and there is thrombosis of the lumen. This is followed by the appearance of leukocytes and microglial cells around the thrombosed blood vessel, forming a typhus nodule. Occlusion of the blood vessels leads to microinfarction, with degenerative changes in nerve cells in proximity to the typhus nodule. Recovery is followed by astrocytic proliferation and the formation of glial scars scattered throughout the nervous system.[215]

Clinical Features

In typhus, severity of the systemic infection may mask signs of encephalitis, but severe headache, mental dullness, delirium, stupor, coma, and nuchal rigidity are the rule. Seizures, involuntary movements, hemiplegia, and deafness result from the focal lesions in the brain and brainstem. While most neurologic signs resolve and there is apparent recovery, mental dullness and neurotic symptoms often remain.

Rocky Mountain spotted fever is becoming more frequent and is now found throughout the United States. Patients, of whom two thirds are children, present with fever, rash, headache, gastrointestinal symptoms, prostration, and myalgia. The rash usually appears on the third or fourth day, beginning on the ankles and wrists, then spreading to the palms and soles, then extending proximally, and finally involving the face. It has a maculopapular appearance but later becomes petechial. Neurologic symptoms consist of headache and neck stiffness resembling meningitis, followed by stupor, seizures, and coma. Focal signs, including hemiplegia, paraplegia, and hyperreflexia, and bilateral extensor plantar responses can occur. Papilledema with retinal exudates has been described, even in the presence of normal spinal fluid pressure.[26]

Diagnostic Procedures

1. An increase in specific antibodies to the rickettsiae is found in sera taken in the first week, second week, and fourth week after the onset of the fever.
2. The Weil-Felix reaction is positive. This is performed by testing the patient's serum for the presence of agglutinins against the OX19, OXK, and OX2 types of *Proteus vulgaris*. A cross-immunity results from the rickettsial infection.

Treatment

Persons entering areas where there is a risk of rickettsial infection should be immunized against the rickettsial agent. Protective clothing, the use of insect repellents and insecticides, strict attention to personal hygiene, and daily inspection of clothing for lice, fleas, ticks, and mites prevent these diseases.

Rickettsial diseases respond to chloramphenicol or one of the tetracycline group of antibiotics, but adequate supportive therapy, including fluid and electrolyte balance, treatment of shock, and control of severe headache, is still important. A combination of antibiotic and steroid therapy is said to be more beneficial than the use of antibiotics alone.

The use of chloramphenicol and the tetracyclines has altered the clinical picture.[325] The previous high mortality seen in the rickettsial diseases has now been reduced, although rickettsial infection remains a serious and potentially dangerous disease.

Infections of the Meninges and Central Nervous System of Uncertain Cause

Cat Scratch Disease

This infectious disease, which is believed to be caused by a virus, usually presents with fever, cutaneous lesions, and regional lymphadenitis. There is usually a history of close contact with a pet cat. Encephalitis is an uncommon but recognized complication which follows the initial symptoms by one to five weeks. The onset is usually abrupt with seizures and coma. Recovery occurs in about one week and is usually complete, although some minor neurologic abnormalities may persist for several months.[201]

Diagnostic Procedures

1. The cerebrospinal fluid shows a pleocytosis with elevation of the protein content.
2. The electroencephalogram shows diffuse showing, and minor abnormalities in the record may remain for several months.

Treatment

There is no specific treatment for cat scratch disease.

Uveomeningoencephalic Syndrome

A rare neuro-ophthalmologic syndrome characterized by uveitis, meningoencephalitis, pigmentary loss of the skin and hair, and impaired hearing has been described by a number of authors and is often referred to as the Vogt-Koyanagi syndrome or the syndrome of Harada. The condition has also been described as the oculosubcutaneous syndrome of Yuge, uveoencephalitis, idiopathic uveoneuritis, and preferably as the uveomeningoencephalitic syndrome.[254, 306]

The cause of the syndrome has never been proved although it is supposed to be related to virus infection, chronic brucellosis, tuberculosis, chronic viral, rickettsial, and mycotic infections. It may also occur during the course of a chronic malignancy, and it has even been suggested that the syndrome is due to some antibody reaction to pigmented cells.

The pathologic changes consist of thickening of the arachnoid over the base of the skull with lymphocytic and histiocytic infiltration of the meninges. The temporal lobes may be necrotic, with loss of neurons, secondary gliosis, and a perivascular cuffing of lymphocytes and histiocytes.

Clinical Features

Neurologic Signs. The onset may be abrupt with low-grade fever, headache, and meningeal irritation. This is followed by symptoms of a subacute meningoencephalitis, with persistent headache, confusion, and personality changes. Focal signs include seizures, monoparesis, and hemiparesis. Involvement of the brainstem may produce diplopia, cerebellar ataxia, and nystagmus. Eighth-nerve involvement results in vertigo, tinnitus, and impairment of hearing. Spinal cord involvement is suggested by the occurrence of a progressive spastic paraparesis and loss of sphincter control.

Ophthalmologic Signs. A progressive uveitis usually begins a few weeks after the initial meningeal phase. This is complicated by retinal hemorrhages, retinal detachment, glaucoma, optic neuritis, decrease in visual acuity, and, in some cases, blindness.

Dermatologic Signs. Patchy loss of hair from the scalp (alopecia areata) and eyelashes (poliosis) occurs after several weeks of illness. Areas of pigmentary loss in the skin (vitiligo) and hair may also occur.

Endocrine Signs. Diabetes insipidus has occurred in some cases.

The cerebrospinal fluid usually shows an excess of mononuclear cells with a moderate elevation of the protein content. The glucose and chloride levels are normal.

Treatment

If the infecting organism can be identified, this should be treated, if possible. Steroid therapy has been reported to be of value but results have not been consistent in patients so treated. Every effort should be made to prevent blindness by management of glaucoma and the prevention of synechia.

Behçet's Disease

A recurrent disease characterized by iridocyclitis, aphthous ulcers of the mouth and genitalia, and involvement of the nervous system by a presumed generalized viral infection was described by Behçet in 1937.[24] Since that time many other lesions have been described in what is essentially a systemic disorder. Recurrent involvements of the nervous system occur in about 20 per cent of cases with signs of meningoencephalomyelitis.

Etiology and Pathology

The cause is not known but Behçet's disease has been regarded as a viral infection, an allergic reaction, a vasculitis, or similar to experimental allergic encephalomyelitis.[217] The presence of autoantibodies and lymphocytic sensitization to mucosal antigens has been described. When the brain is involved, there are atrophic changes with numerous areas of softening in the gray and white matter and some perivascular infiltration. The fusion of small areas of softening produces neuronal loss in the gray matter and areas of demyelination in the white matter.

Clinical Features

The initial symptoms are a low-grade fever and aphthous ulcers of the mouth followed by ulcerated lesions of the genitalia, involvement of the eye, and cutaneous lesions including papules, vesicles, pustules, furuncles, and erythema nodosum-like lesions. These symptoms usually subside in about ten days but recur within a week or up to two months. The interval between attacks gradually increases, and they may cease after 15 to 20 years.

Involvement of the eye may produce iritis, iridocyclitis, uveitis, glaucoma, atrophy of the lens, and hypopyon. Periarteritis and thrombophlebitis of the retinal vessels may occur, with retinal hemorrhages and retinal detachment. Optic neuritis and optic atrophy have also been described. It is usual to have bilateral involvement of the eyes, and the incidence of blindness is high.

Other manifestations include erythema nodosum, cuneiform lesions, furunculosis, subungual infarction, and a recurrent migratory polyarthritis. Recurrent gastrointestinal symptoms suggesting pancreatitis or ulcerative colitis have also been described. Bronchitis, viral pneumonia, and lobar pneumonia have all occurred in Behçet's disease.[234] Recurrent episodes of superficial and deep thrombophlebitis occur in some patients. Superficial thrombophlebitis may follow venepuncture, and both superior and inferior vena canal obstruction have been reported.

Involvement of the central nervous system is often fatal and usually produces permanent damage. Symptoms vary from aseptic meningitis to severe meningoencephalomyelitis. Meningoencephalitis due to Behçet's disease is characterized by drowsiness and obtundity, which may progress to delirium and coma. Seizures and focal signs including deviation of the eyes, hemiparesis, or dysphasia may occur. Meningeal signs include nuchal rigidity and a positive Kernig's sign. Brainstem involvement with paralysis of cranial nerves, cerebellar signs, spastic quadriparesis, dysarthria, and dysphagia has been frequently reported. Involvement of the spinal cord may produce spasticity, particularly in the lower extremities, with loss of bladder function and a sensory loss below the level of the lesion. Other neurologic signs include intellectual impairment, spastic quadriparesis, peripheral neuropathy, involuntary "pseudobulbar" laughing and crying, and cerebellar ataxia. Some cases have shown progressive dementia and signs similar to those of Parkinson's disease.

Diagnostic Procedures

The cerebrospinal fluid usually shows increased pressure, with a lymphocytic pleocytosis and elevated levels of protein. Glucose and chloride contents are normal. Routine bacterial cultures are sterile.

Treatment

Clinical observations suggest that corticosteroids are effective in reducing or preventing damage to the central nervous system if given early in the course of Behçet's disease.[235] The recommended dosage is 60 mg of prednisone daily. Immunosuppressive therapy has been tried on the assumption that Behçet's disease is an autoimmune condition, but results have been equivocal.[126] There have been recent reports of improvement following treatment with transfer factor, and further studies are indicated.[339] Other forms of therapy that have had some beneficial effect include blood or plasma transfusion and fibrinolytic drugs.[47]

Slow Virus Infections (SSPE)

A "slow virus infection" is a condition in which the infecting viral agent continues to multiply within the host, producing progressive disability over a period of many months or years. These infections were first demonstrated in animals and are now recognized in man.[103] The presence of slow virus infections in man was established by the demonstration that the neurologic disease kuru, which is confined to the Fore people of the Eastern Highlands of New Guinea, is due to a slow virus infection of the brain. Kuru is a disease producing widespread neuronal degeneration, and intracerebral inoculation of a brain suspension obtained from patients dying from kuru into chimpanzees has resulted in the development of a kuru-like syndrome in the majority of these animals within 18 to 30 months. Inoculation of brain suspensions obtained from these chimpanzees into healthy animals has resulted in second passage of the disease with the development of a similar kuru-like syndrome with an unusually rapid course.

Similar inoculation experiments have demonstrated that Jakob-Creutzfeldt disease[104] can also be transmitted from human patients to chimpanzees, with incubation periods of 11 to 14 months. On second passage in chimpanzees the incubation period has not changed.

The importance of these inoculation experiments lies in the possible connection between other neuronal degenerative conditions in man and slow virus infections, and in the fact that the prescribed dementias, such as Alzheimer's disease or possibly amyotrophic lateral sclerosis, may be of viral etiology.

A third slow virus infection of the brain, subacute sclerosing panencephalitis (SSPE), is known to be a "slow measles encephalitis."

Subacute Sclerosing Panencephalitis

The isolation of measles or measles-like virus from the brain of patients with subacute sclerosing panencephalitis (SSPE) has established this condition to be an unusual encephalitic response to a virus infection.[147, 148, 212, 247] Electron microscopic studies have documented the presence of tubular structures similar to the nucleocapsid of measles virus, and immunofluorescent staining of biopsy material by direct and indirect techniques has revealed the presence of measles antigen and gamma globulin in the brain.[162]

Pathology

The pathologic picture is one of a diffuse inflammatory reaction in gray and white matter. There is perivascular cuffing by monocytes, and the leptomeninges are infiltrated by lymphocytes, eosinophils, and plasma cells. The gray matter shows neuronal loss, neuronophagia with proliferation of astrocytes, and microglia in the form of rod cells. There is a patchy loss of myelin in the white matter with vacuolated areas surrounded by large astrocytes with abundant cytoplasm.

The neurons show Alzheimer's neurofibrillary changes[205] and three types of inclusion bodies. Small intranuclear inclusion bodies are a feature of the early stages of SSPE. Large multitubular inclusions that nearly fill the nucleus are seen at a later stage. Cytoplasmic inclusions that resemble multitubular inclusions are also seen in some cases. Measles virus or measles-like virus has been recovered from the brain in SSPE using the technique of coculture of brain tissue and HeLa cells. Measles-specific lgG has been eluted from the brain in SSPE.[210a]

The nuclei of the neurons and, in some cases, the oligodendrocytes contain Cowdry type A inclusion bodies. Material studies by electron microscopy show intranuclear nucleocapsid filaments similar in appearance to the nucleocapsid of measles virus.[238] The neuronal perikaryon also shows an aggregate of electron-dense granular material resembling pseudomyxovirus particles.[157]

Clinical Features

This condition has a reported incidence of one per million. It occurs at an early age (mean age 7.2 years), with a male-to-female ratio of 3.3:1 and a history of early measles infection under two years of age in more than half of the patients.[156]

Stage 1. The earliest symptoms are personality changes, irritability and abnormal behavior, failing memory, and lethargy. Inappropriate affect, dysarthria, and impairment of vision owing to macula degeneration occur in some patients.[8, 228]

Stage 2. Myclonic jerks, which are mild at first but gradually increase in severity, appear some two months after the onset. In addition, choreoathetosis, ballism, rigidity, dystonia, and spasticity may occur. Generalized seizures are usually present.

Stage 3. There is an increase in spasticity, episodic opisthotonus, and gradual deterioration into coma. Irregular respiration with periods of cyanosis and temperature fluctuations with intermittent flushing and sweating indicate hypothalamic dysfunction.

Stage 4. The severe hypertonia gradually decreases and the myoclonus lessens. Terminal flaccidity may occur. Optic atrophy is seen in some cases.

Duration of Illness. Mean duration to death is nine months from the onset of the disease. Some cases show a more protracted course with a chronic deterioration interspersed by periods of apparent arrest or recovery. Remission may last several years, giving a spurious impression of apparent recovery, but this does not exclude the possibility of a relapse some years later.[75,254a]

Diagnostic Procedures

1. In most cases, well-defined periodic paroxysmal discharges occur in the EEG. The background rhythm is normal in the early stages but is replaced by low-voltage activity occurring between the paroxysmal high-voltage diphasic delta bursts, which are sometimes preceded by or associated with spikes. The interval between discharge is usually three to five seconds (burst suppression). The periodic discharges show poor correlation with the myoclonic jerks.[157, 197]

2. Measles complement-fixing, neutralizing, hemagglutinating, and fluorescent antibody titers are elevated in the serum and cerebrospinal fluid of all patients.[278] The mean time between measles infection and the development of SSPE is about six years.[28]

3. The cerebrospinal fluid protein content and cell count may be normal or slightly increased with a lymphocytic pleocytosis. Electrophoresis reveals elevated gamma globulin, which is more than 20 per cent of the total protein. Immunoelectrophoresis shows that the gamma globulin is predominantly I_gG.

4. CT scan (Fig. 7–7).

5. Brain biopsy shows perivascular infiltration with inflammatory cells and the pathognomonic type A intranuclear inclusion bodies within the neurons.

Treatment

There is no effective treatment for SSPE at this time. There are reports that isoprinosine has produced clinical improvement in a few cases and further studies of isoprinosine are needed.[302] The incidence of SSPE may be reduced or the disease may be eliminated with the increasing use of vaccination against measles.[4]

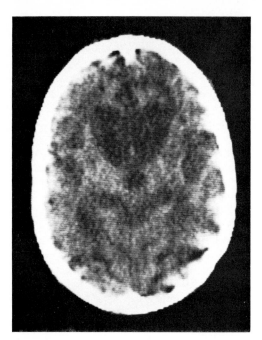

FIGURE 7–7. Computed tomography in subacute sclerosing panencephalitis. There are numerous areas of decreased density throughout the white matter. The ventricular system is diffusely and symmetrically dilated.

Rubella Panencephalitis

Acute rubella encephalitis is a rare condition usually presenting as a postinfectious leukoencephalitis and showing a prompt response to corticosteroid therapy.[226]

A chronic form of rubella panencephalitis has been described to children born with defects consistent with congenital rubella infection.

Rubella panencephalitis is a slow virus disease with persistence of the rubella virus in the central nervous system. The brain shows a widespread panencephalitis mainly affecting the white matter with loss of myelin, fragmentation of axons, and widespread gliosis.[314] There is a diffuse neuronal loss in the cortical gray matter.

Clinical Features

Children with rubella panencephalitis have signs of congenital rubella infection including deafness, microcephaly, cataracts, and cardiac anomalies. There is no further sign of infection until the second decade when the affected child shows a progressive illness with intellectual dete-

rioration, seizures, ataxia, and spasticity, culminating in death after several years.[313]

Diagnostic Procedures

The cerebrospinal fluid shows an elevated protein and gamma globulin content. There are increased antibody titers to rubella virus in the serum and cerebrospinal fluid.

Treatment

The condition is rare. Treatment is symptomatic and there is no specific therapy for rubella panencephalitis.

Russian Spring-Summer Panencephalitis

There are several reports of a chronic progressive panencephalitis occurring about 14 years after an acute attack of Russian spring-summer panencephalitis. Examination of the brain showed chronic inflammation of the white matter, cortex, and meninges without inclusion bodies. High titers of hemagglutination inhibition antibody against Russian spring-summer panencephalitis were found in serum and cerebrospinal fluid.[22]

Mollaret's Meningitis

A benign, recurrent meningitis of unknown etiology was first described by Mollaret in 1944. There are other causes of recurrent meningitis from which this condition must be differentiated (Table 7–8).

Clinical Features

The onset is sudden, with fever, myalgia, nuchal rigidity, nausea, vomiting, and occasionally seizures. The condition reaches a peak within 12 hours, and then subsides rapidly with complete recovery after two or three days. Subsequent attacks produce a similar clinical picture and occur at intervals of weeks to months following the initial illness. Complete recovery occurs after each attack. As many as six attacks have been recorded before the patient finally recovers.[134, 139]

Diagnostic Procedures

1. Lumbar puncture may reveal cerebrospinal fluid under increased pressure with several thousand polymorphonuclear leukocytes and lymphocytes. The characteristic finding is a large, so-called endothelial cell in the stained smear, which disappears from the cerebrospinal fluid within a few hours following the onset of the illness. The polymorphonuclear leuko-

TABLE 7–8

Possible Causes of Recurrent Meningitis

Type	Diagnosis
1. *Recurrent acute purulent meningitis*	
a. Due to congenital defects	Presence of meningocele, midline dermal fistula, or deficit of the cribriform plate of the ethmoid
	Organism cultured from cerebrospinal fluid
b. Nontraumatic *E. coli*	Organisms cultured from cerebrospinal fluid, inadequate therapy
B. melitensis	
Leptospiral	
Recurrent otitis media	
Recurrent sinusitis	
Chronic debilitating disease (malignancy, leukemia, Hodgkin's disease)	
c. Traumatic Any organism	Organism cultured from cerebrospinal fluid
	Localization and demonstration of fistula or fracture of skull or spine
2. *Subacute meningitis*	
a. Tuberculosis	Organism cultured from cerebrospinal fluid
b. Sarcoidosis	Other signs of sarcoidosis (uveitis, lung infiltrates or lymphadenopathy)
	Positive lymph node biopsy
c. Due to fungi or yeasts if inadequately treated	Organism cultured from cerebrospinal fluid
3. *Meningeal reaction*	
a. Recurrent otitis media	Clinical and roentgenographic evidence of primary condition
b. Recurrent sinusitis	Cerebrospinal fluid culture is sterile
4. *Behçet's disease*	Recurrent aphthous ulceration of mouth and genitalia, iritis, uveitis; recurrent encephalitis or meningoencephalitis
5. *Recurrent aseptic meningitis*	Viral cultures positive from cerebrospinal fluid
	Antibody titers increase in serum
6. *Hydatid disease*	Presence of intracranial mass
	Positive skin test
7. *Dermoid cysts*	Presence of intracranial mass
8. *Mollaret's meningitis*	Benign rapid resolution
	Complete recovery between attacks
	No evidence of focal infection
	Cerebrospinal fluid culture is sterile

cytes are no longer present after 24 hours, and the fluid then contains lymphocytes, which gradually disappear over the next few days. The protein content of the fluid shows a moderate elevation but glucose and chloride are normal. Both bacterial and viral cultures are negative.

2. All other studies, including roentgenograms of the skull, paranasal sinuses, and chest, and blood cultures, are negative.

Differential Diagnosis

There are many conditions that may give rise to recurrent meningitis, all of which should be considered and excluded before making a diagnosis of Mollaret's meningitis (Table 7–8).

Treatment

Mollaret's meningitis subsides within a few days, and there is no treatment that affects the course of this disease.

Cited References

1. Abdominal pain, shock and history of gastric crisis: Clinicopathologic conference. *Am. J. Med.,* **40:**110–118, 1965.
2. Adair, C. V.; Gault, R. L.; and Smadel, J. E.

Aseptic meningitis, a disease of diverse etiology; clinical and etiologic studies on 854 cases. *Ann. Intern. Med.,* **39:**675–704, 1953.

3. Addlestone, R. B., and Baylin, G. J. Rhinocerebral mucormycosis. *Radiology,* **115:**113–17, 1975.

4. Addy, D. P. Subacute sclerosing panencephalitis: Microbiological aspects. *Dev. Med. Clin. Neurol.,* **19:**69–71, 1977.

4a. Ahuja G. K.; Roy S. et al. Cerebral cysticercosis. *J. Neurol. Sci.,* **35:**365–74, 1978.

5. Alford, C. A., Jr., and Whitley, R. J. Treatment of infections due to herpes virus in humans. A critical review of the state of the art. *J. Infect. Dis.,* **113:**suppl. 101–107, 1976.

6. Amromin, G. D., and Gildenhorn, V. B. Massive cerebral aspergillis abscess in a leukemic child: Case report. *J. Neurosurg.,* **35:**491–94, 1972.

7. Anderson, S.-V.; Bjorksten, B.; and Burman, L. A. A comparative study of meningoencephalitis epidemic caused by Echo virus type 7 and Coxsackie virus type B5. Clinical and virological observations during two epidemics in northern Sweden. *Scand. J. Infect. Dis.,* **7:**233–37, 1975.

8. Andriola, M. Maculopathy in subacute sclerosing panencephalitis. *Am. J. Dis. Child.,* **124:**187–89, 1972.

9. Apley, J.; Clarke, S. K. R.; Roome, A. P. C. H.; Sandry, S. H.; Sayr, G.; Silk, B.; and Warhurst, D. C. Primary amebic meningoencephalitis in Britain. *Br. Med. J.,* **1:**596–99, 1970.

10. Attrocchi, P. H. Acute spinal epidural abscess vs. acute transverse myelopathy. *Arch. Neurol.,* **9:**17–25, 1963.

11. Azimi, P. H., and Shaban, S. Mumps encephalitis. Prolonged abnormality of cerebrospinal fluid. *J.A.M.A.,* **234:**1161–62, 1975.

12. Baird, D. R.; Whittle, H. D.; and Greenwood, B. M. Mortality from pneumococcal meningitis. *Lancet,* **2:**1344–46, 1976.

13. Bajada, S. Cerebellitis in glandular fever. *Med. J. Aust.,* **1:**153–56, 1976.

14. Baker, A. S.; Ojemann, R. G.; et al. Spinal epidural abscess. *N. Engl. J. Med.,* **293:**463–68, 1975.

15. Baker, C. J. Primary spinal epidural abscess. *Am. J. Dis. Child.,* **121:**337–39, 1971.

16. Bang, N. O., and Bang, J. Involvement of the central nervous system in mumps. *Acta Med. Scand.,* **113:**487–606, 1943.

17. Barkin, R. M.; Greer, C. C.; et al. *Haemophilus influenzae* meningitis. An evolving therapeutic regimen. *Am. J. Dis. Child.,* **130:**1318–21, 1976.

18. Barnes, B. D., and Winestock, D. P. Dynamic radionuclide scanning in the diagnosis of thrombosis of the superior sagittal sinus. *Neurology* (Minneap.), **27:**656–61, 1977.

19. Barrett, F. F.; Taber, L. H.; Morris, C. R., et al. A 12 year review of the antibiotic management of *Hemophilus influenzae* meningitis. Comparison of ampicillin and conventional therapy, including chloramphenicol. *J. Pediatr.,* **81:**370–77, 1972.

20. Barton, L. L. Febrile neonatal illness associated with Echo virus type 5 in the cerebrospinal fluid. *Clin. Pediatr.,* **16:**383–85, 1977.

21. Bayer, A. S.; Edwards, J. E.; et al. Candida meningitis. Report of seven cases and review of the English literature. *Medicine,* **55:**477–85, 1976.

22. Becker, L. E. Slow infections of the central nervous system. *J. Can. Neurol. Sci.,* **4:**81–88, 1977.

23. Beerman, H., and Schamberg, I. L. Diagnosis and treatment of late syphilis. *Geriatrics,* **18:**64–72, 1963.

24. Behçet, H. A propos d'une entité morbide due probablement à un virus spécial donnant lieu a une infection généralisée se manifestant par des pousses récidivants en trois régions principales et occasionnant en particular des iritis répétés. *Bull. soc. franc. dermat. syph.,* **46:**674–87, 1939.

25. Behke, A. R., and Saltzman, H. A. Hyperbaric oxygenation. *N. Engl. J. Med.,* **276:**1478–84, 1967.

26. Bell, W. E., and Lascari, A. D. Rocky Mountain spotted fever. Neurological symptoms in the acute phase. *Neurology* (Minneap.), **20:**841–47, 1970.

27. Bell, W. E., and Silber, D. L. Meningococcal meningitis: Past and present concepts. *Milit. Med.,* **136:**601–11, 1971.

28. Bellman, M. H., and Dick, G. Register of cases of subacute sclerosis panencephalitis. *Br. Med. J.,* **1:**430–31, 1977.

29. Benjamin, D. R., and Ray, C. G. Use of immunoperoxidase on brain tissue for the rapid identification of herpes encephalitis. *Am. J. Clin. Pathol.,* **64:**472–76, 1975.

30. Berger, C. J.; Disque, F. C.; and Topazian, R. G. Rhinocerebral mucormycosis, diagnosis and treatment. Report of two cases. *Otol. Surg.,* **40:**27–33, 1975.

31. Berger, M. P., and Paz, J. Diagnosis of cryptococcal meningitis. *J.A.M.A.,* **236:**2517–18, 1976.

32. Betty, M., and Loober, J. Intramedullary abscess of the spinal cord. *J. Neurol. Neurosurg. Psychiat.,* **26:**236–40, 1963.

33. Bhandari, Y. S., and Sarkari, N. B. S. Subdural empyema. *J. Neurosurg.,* **32:**35–39, 1970.

34. Bobowski, S. J., and Reed, W. G. Toxoplasmosis in an adult presenting as a space occupying lesion. *Arch. Pathol.,* **65:**460–64, 1958.

35. Bolton, C. F., and Ashenhurst, E. M. Actinomycosis of the brain: Case report and review of the literature. *Can. Med. Assoc. J.,* **90:**922–28, 1964.

36. Bratzlavsky, M., and Vander Eecken, H. Medullary actions of tetanus toxin. An electrophysiological study in man. *Arch. Neurol.,* **33:**783–85, 1976.

37. Brewer, N. S.; MacCarty, C. S.; and Wellman, W. C. Brain abscess: A review of recent experience. *Ann. Intern. Med.,* **82:**571–76, 1975.

38. Brismar, G., and Brismar, J. Thrombosis of the intraorbital veins and cavernous sinus. *Acta Radiol.,* **18:**145–52, 1977.

39. Brotchi, J., and Bonnal, J. Surgical treatment of subdural effusions in infants. *Acta Neurochir.,* **33:**59–67, 1976.

40. Brown, R. S. Herpes simplex virus encephalitis in the newborn. *Dev. Med. Child Neurol.,* **19:**407–409, 1977.

41. Brown, W. J., and Moore, M. B. Congenital syphilis in the United States. *Clin. Pediatr.,* **2:**220–22, 1963.

41a. Burrow, G.; Salmon, R.; and Nolan, J. Successful treatment of mucormycosis with amphotericin B. *J.A.M.A.,* **183**:370–72, 1963.

42. Butler, W. T.; Alling, D. W.; Speckard, A.; and Utz, J. P. Diagnostic and prognostic value of clinical laboratory findings in cryptococcal meningitis: Follow-up of forty patients. *N. Engl. J. Med.,* **270**:59–67, 1964.

43. Carmalt, J. E.; Theis, J.; and Goldstein, E. Spinal cysticercosis. *West. J. Med.,* **123**:311–13, 1975.

44. Carr-Locke, D. L., and Mair, H. J. Neurological presentation of psittacosis during a small outbreak in Leicestershire. *Br. Med. J.,* **2**:853–54, 1976.

45. Casals, J.; Curnen, E. C.; and Thomas, C. Venezualan equine encephalomyelitis in man. *J. Exp. Med.,* **77**:521–30, 1943.

46. Causey, J. O. Spontaneous cytomegalovirus mononucleosis-like syndrome and aseptic meningitis. *South. Med. J.,* **69**:1384–87, 1976.

47. Chajek, T., and Fainaru, M. Behçet's disease: Report of 41 cases and a review of the literature. *Medicine,* **54**:179–94, 1975.

48. Chalhub, E. G.; Devivo, D. C.; et al. Coxsackie A9 focal encephalitis associated with acute infantile hemiplegia and porencephaly. *Neurology* (Minneap.), **27**:574–79, 1977.

49. Chemotherapeutic routes in meningitis. *Br. Med. J.,* **1**:977–78, 1976.

50. Chemotherapy for varicella-zoster infections. *Br. Med. J.,* **2**:1466–67, 1976.

51. Ch'ien, L. T.; Boehm, R. M.; et al. Characteristic early electroencephalographic changes in herpes simplex encephalitis. *Arch. Neurol.,* **34**:361–64, 1977.

52. Chi'en, L. T.; Whitley, R. J.; et al. Antiviral chemotherapy and neonatal herpes simplex virus infections: A pilot study—experience with adenine arabinoside. *Pediatrics,* **55**:678–85, 1975.

53. Ch'ien, L. T.; Whitley, R. J.; et al. Adenine arabinoside for therapy of herpes zoster in immunosuppressed patients: Preliminary results of a collaborative study. *J. Infect. Dis.,* **133**: suppl. 184–91, 1976.

54. Chun, R. W. M.; Thompson, W. H.; Grabow, J. D.; and Mathews, G. G. California arbovirus encephalitis in children. *Neurology* (Minneap.), **18**:369–75, 1968.

55. Clarke, D. H. Further studies on antigenic relationships among viruses of the group B tick borne complex. *Bull. WHO,* **31**:45–46, 1964.

56. Coleman, R. W.; Robboy, S. J.; and Minna, J. D. Disseminated intravascular coagulation (DIC): An approach. *Am. J. Med.,* **52**:679–89, 1972.

57. Conomy, J. P.; Lubovitz, A.; et al. Airborne rabies encephalitis: Demonstration of rabies virus in the human central nervous system. *Neurology* (Minneap.), **27**:67–69, 1977.

58. Cooper, R. A., Jr., and Gotstein, E. Histoplasmosis of the central nervous system: report of two cases and review of the literature. *Am. J. Med.,* **35**:45–57, 1963.

59. Cooper, R. M., and Noble, R. C. Bacterial meningitis. A review of the pathophysiology, diagnosis and treatment. *J. Ky. Med. Assoc.,* **74**:393–401, August, 1976.

60. Coorod, J. D., and Dons, P. E. Subdural empyema. *Am. J. Med.,* **53**:85–91, 1972.

61. Dalinka, M. K., and Greendyke, W. H. The spinal manifestations of coccidioidomycosis. *J. Can. Assoc. Radiol.,* **22**:93–99, 1971.

62. Damergis, J. A.; Leftwich, I.; et al. Tuberculosis of the brain. *J.A.M.A.,* **239**:413–15, 1978.

63. Danziger, J.; Bloch, S.; et al. Cranial and intracranial tuberculosis. *S. Afr. Med. J.,* **50**:1403–1405, 1976.

64. Davidson, S. Cryptococcal spinal arachnoiditis. *J. Neurol. Neurosurg. Psychiat.,* **31**:76–80, 1968.

65. Day, A. L., and Sypert, G. W. Spinal cord sarcoidosis. *Ann. Neurol.,* **1**:79–85, 1977.

66. Dayan, A. D., and Stokes, M. Rapid diagnosis of encephalitis by immunofluorescent examination of cerebrospinal fluid cells. *Lancet,* **1**:177–79, 1973.

67. DeFeo, D.; Foltz, E. L.; and Hamilton, A. E. Double compartment hydrocephalus in a patient with cysticercosis meningitis. *Surg. Neurol.,* **4**:247–51, 1975.

68. Delaney, P. Neurologic manifestations of sarcoidosis. Review of the literature with a report of 23 cases. *Ann. Intern. Med.,* **87**:336–45, 1977.

69. DeLouvois, J.; Gortvai, P.; and Hurley, R. Bacteriology of abscesses of the central nervous system: A multicentre prospective study. *Br. Med. J.,* **2**:981–84, 1977.

70. DeLouvois, J.; Gortvai, P.; and Hurley, R. Antibiotic treatment of abscesses of the central nervous system. *Br. Med. J.,* **2**:985–87, 1977.

71. Desai, B. T., and Toole, J. F. Polyneuropathy as a feature of brucellosis. *South. Med. J.,* **70**:259, 1977.

72. Dewhurst, K. Atypical serology in neurosyphilis. *J. Neurol. Neurosurg. Psychiat.,* **31**:496–500, 1968.

73. Dickerson, M. S.; Bilderback, W. R.; and Pessarra, L. W. Ornithosis (chlamydiosis) outbreaks in Texas. *Tex. Med.,* **72**:57–61, 1976.

74. Donald, G., and McKendrick, W. The treatment of pyogenic meningitis. *J. Neurol. Neurosurg. Psychiat.,* **31**:528–31, 1968.

75. Donner, M.; Waltimo, O.; Porros, J.; Forsus, H.; and Saukkonen, A. L. Subacute sclerosing panencephalitis as a cause of chronic dementia and relapsing brain disorder. *J. Neurol. Neurosurg. Psychiat.,* **35**:180–85, 1972.

76. Drusen, L.; Singer, C.; et al. Infectious syphilis mimicking disease. *Arch. Intern. Med.,* **137**:156–60, 1977.

77. Duma, R. J.; Rosenblum, W. I.; McGehee, R. F.; Jones, M. M.; and Nelson, E. C. Primary amebic meningoencephalitis caused by Naegleria. Two new cases. Response to amphotericin B and a review. *Ann. Intern. Med.,* **74**:923–31, 1971.

78. Dupont, J. R., and Earle, K. M. Human rabies encephalitis; study of forty-nine fatal cases with a review of the literature. *Neurology* (Minneap.), **15**:1023–34, 1965.

79. Durfee, P. T. Psittacosis in humans in the United States in 1974. *J. Infect. Dis.,* **132**:604–605, 1975.

80. Dus, V. Spinal paripachymeningitis (epidural abscess); report of 8 cases. *J. Neurosurg.,* **17:**972–83, 1960.

81. Dutton, J. E. M., and Alexander, G. L. Intramedullary spinal abscess. *J. Neurol. Neurosurg. Psychiat.,* **17:**303–307, 1954.

82. Dyck, P.; Ramseyer, J. C.; and Doyle, J. B. Cysticercus cyst of temporal lobe presenting as a tentorial pressure cone. *West. J. Med.,* **125:**317–20, 1976.

83. Earl, C. J., and Zillcha, K. J. Syphilitic visual failure. *Br. J. Ophthalmol.,* **48:**630–32, 1964.

84. Edwards, E. A.; Muehl, P. M.; and Peckenpaugh, R. O. Diagnosis of bacterial meningitis by counter-immunoelectrophoresis. *J. Lab. Clin. Med.,* **80:**449–54, 1972.

85. Edwards, V. E.; Sutherland, J. M.; and Tyrer, J. H. Cryptococcosis of the central nervous system. Epidemiological clinical and therapeutic features. *J. Neurol. Neurosurg. Psychiat.,* **33:**415–25, 1970.

86. Ekbom, K. Tegretol, a new therapy for tabetic lightning pains; preliminary report. *Acta Med. Scand.,* **179:**251–52, 1966.

87. Ellison, P. H., and Hanson, P. A. Herpes simplex: A possible cause of brain stem encephalitis. *Pediatrics,* **59:**240–43, 1977.

88. Enzmann, D. R.; Norman, D.; et al. Computed tomography of granulomatous basal arachnoiditis. *Radiology,* **120:**341–44, 1976.

89. Etheridge, E. E.; Light, J. A.; et al. Listeria monocytogenes meningitis in a transplant recipient. *J.A.M.A.,* **234:**78–79, 1975.

90. Etiologic factors in microcephaly (editorial). *N. Engl. J. Med.,* **275:**502, 1966.

91. Eveland, W. O. Demonstration of *Listeria monocytogenes* in direct examination of spinal by fluorescent antibody technique. *J. Bacteriol.,* **85:**1448–50, 1963.

92. Feigin, R. D.; Stechenberg, B. W.; et al. Prospective evaluation of treatment of Hemophilus influenzae meningitis. *J. Pediatr.,* **88:**542–48, 1976.

93. Feldman, M. A., and Miller, L. T. Congenital human toxoplasmosis. *Ann. N.Y. Acad. Sci.,* **64:**18–84, 1956.

93a. Feldman, W., and Larke, R. Acute cerebellar ataxia with isolation of coxsackie virus type A9. *Can. Med. Assoc. J.,* **106:**1104–1107, 1972.

94. Fincham, M. A.; Sahs, A. L.; and Joynt, R. J. Protean manifestations of nervous system brucellosis. *J.A.M.A.,* **184:**269–75, 1963.

94a. Fisher, M., and Poser, C. M. Syphilitic meningomyelitis. *Arch. Neurol.,* **34:**785, 1977.

95. Fiumara, N. J. The treatment of syphilis, current concepts. *N. Engl. J. Med.,* **270:**1185–88, 1964.

96. Fothergill, L. D.; Dingle, J. H.; Farber, S.; and Connerley, M. L. Human encephalitis caused by the virus of the Eastern variety of equine encephalomyelitis. *N. Engl. J. Med.,* **219:**411, 1938.

97. Franck, P. T., and Johnson, K. M. An outbreak of Venezualan equine encephalomyelitis in Central America. Evidence for exogenous source of a virulent virus subtype. *Am. J. Epidemiol.,* **94:**487–95, 1971.

98. Fraser, R. A. R.; Ratzan, K.; Wolpert, S. M.; and Weinstein, L. Spinal subdural empyema. *Arch. Neurol.,* **28:**235–38, 1973.

99. French, L. A., and Chou, S. N. Osteomyelitis of the skull and epidural abscess in cranial and intracranial suppuration, E. S. Gurdjian (ed.). Thomas, Springfield, Ill., 1969, pp. 59–72.

100. French, L. A., and Chou, S. N. Treatment of brain abscesses. In Thompson, R. A., and Green, J. R. (eds.). *Advances in Neurology,* Vol. 6. Raven Press, New York, 1974, pp. 269–75.

101. Friedland, R., and Yahr, M. D. Meningoencephalopathy secondary to infectious mononucleosis. Unusual presentation with stupor and chorea. *Arch. Neurol.,* **34:**186–88, 1977.

102. Furey, W.; Cirac, I.; and Porter, R. H. Monitoring of intrathecal polymyxin B dosage during treatment of pseudomonas meningitis. *Ill. Med. J.,* **139:**507–11, 1971.

103. Gajdusek, D. C. Slow virus diseases of the central nervous system. *Am. J. Clin. Pathol.,* **56:**320–32, 1971.

104. Gajdusek, D. C., and Gibbs, C. J., Jr. Transmission of two subacute spongiform encephalopaties of man (Kuru and Creutzfeldt-Jacob disease) to New World monkeys. *Nature,* **230:**588–91, 1971.

105. Galbraith, J. G., and Barr, V. W. Epidural abscess and subdural empyema. In Thompson, R. A., and Green, J. R. (eds.). *Advances in Neurology,* Vol. 6. Raven Press, New York, 1974, pp. 257–67.

106. Ganado, W. Human brucellosis: Some clinical observations. *Scott. Med. J.,* **10:**451–60, 1965.

107. Ganchrow, M. I., and Bref, D. K. A case of meningitis secondary to *Clostridium welchii. J. Trauma,* **11:**444–46, 1971.

108. Garfield, J. Management of supratentorial intracranial abscess: A review of 200 cases. *Br. Med. J.,* **2:**7–11, 1969.

109. Gerber, H. J.; Schoonmaker, F. W.; and Vazquez, M. D. Chronic meningitis associated with *Histoplasma* endocarditis. *N. Engl. J. Med.,* **275:**74–76, 1966.

110. Gettelfinger, D. M., and Kokmen, E. Superior sagittal sinus thrombosis. *Arch. Neurol.,* **34:**2–6, 1977.

110a. Ghosh, S.; Seshardi, R.; and Jarn, K. C. Evaluation of corticosteroids in treatment of tuberculous meningitis. *Arch. Dis. Child.,* **46:**51–54, 1971.

111. Giltner, L. T., and Stahan, M. S. The 1933 outbreak of infectious equine encephalomyelitis in the Eastern states. *N. Am. Vet.,* **14:**25–27, 1933.

112. Girling, D. J. Adverse reactions to rifampicin in antituberculosis regiments. *J. Antimicrob. Chemother.,* **3:**115–32, 1977.

113. Glukhov, B. N.; Jerusalimsky, A. P.; et al. Ribonuclease treatment of tick-borne encephalitis. *Arch. Neurol.,* **33:**598–603, 1976.

114. Goldman, J. A., and Eckerling, B. Intracranial dural sinus thrombosis following intrauterine instillation of hypertonic saline. *Am. J. Obstet. Gynecol.,* **112:**1132–33, 1972.

115. Goldman, J. A.; Eckerling, B.; and Gans, B. Intracranial venous sinus thrombosis in pregnancy

and the puerperium: report of 15 cases. *J. Obstet. Gynaecol. Br. Commonw.,* **71:**791–96, 1965.

116. Goldstein, R. A.; Israel, H. L.; and Becker, K. L. The infrequency of hypercalcemia in sarcoidosis. *Am. J. Med.,* **51:**21–30, 1971.

117. Gonyea, E. F., and Heilman, K. M. Neuro-ophthalmic aspects of central nervous system cryptococcosis. Internuclear and supranuclear ophthalmoplegia. *Arch. Ophthalmol.,* **87:**164–68, 1972.

118. Goodman, J. S.; Kaufman, L.; and Koenig, M. G. Diagnosis of cryptococcic meningitis: Value of immunologic detection of cryptococcic antigen. *N. Engl. J. Med.,* **285:**434–36, 1971.

118a. Gordon, A., and Parsons, M. The place of corticosteroids in the management of tuberculous meningitis. *Br. J. Hosp. Med.,* **7:**651–55, 1972.

119. Green, J. B. Dilantin in the treatment of lightning pains. *Neurology* (Minneap.), **11:**257–58, 1961.

120. Greenlee, J. E.; Johnson, W. D., Jr.; et al. Adult toxoplasmosis presenting as polymyositis and cerebellar ataxia. *Ann. Intern. Med.,* **82:**367–71, 1975.

121. Greer, H. D.; Geraci, J. E.; Corbin, K. B.; Miller, R. H.; and Weed, L. A. Disseminated histoplasmosis presenting as a brain tumor and treated with amphotericin B. Report of a case. *Mayo Clin. Proc.,* **39:**490–94, 1964.

122. Gregory, D. H.; Messner, R.; and Zinneman, H. H. Metastatic brain abscesses: A retrospective appraisal of 29 patients. *Arch. Intern. Med.,* **119:**25–31, 1967.

123. Griffith, J. F.; Salan, M. N.; and Adams, R. D. The nervous system diseases associated with varicella. *Acta Neurol. Scand.,* **46:**279–300, 1970.

124. Gubbay, S. S., and Matz, L. R. Meningeal cysticercosis diagnosed in western Australia. *Med. J. Aust.,* **1:**523–25, 1977.

125. Gunderson, C. H., and Sark, G. E. Neurology of *Vibrio* fetus infection. *Neurology* (Minneap.), **21:**307–309, 1971.

126. Haim, S. Behcet's disease: Etiology and treatment. *Dermatologica,* **150:**163–68, 1975.

127. Halstead, S. B., and Grosz, C. R. Subclinical Japanese encephalitis. I. Infection of Americans with limited residence in Korea. *Am. J. Hyg.,* **75:**190–201, 1962.

128. Haltalin, K. C., and Smith, J. B. Re-evaluation of ampicillin therapy for *Hemophilus influenzae* meningitis. *Am. J. Dis. Child.,* **122:**328–36, 1971.

129. Hambleton, G., and Davies, P. A. Bacterial meningitis. Some aspects of diagnosis and treatment. *Arch. Dis. Child.,* **50:**674–84, 1975.

130. Hammor, W. M.; Reeves, W. C.; Brookman, B.; and Izumi, E. M. Isolation of the viruses of Western equine and St. Louis encephalitis from *Culex tarsalis* mosquitoes. *Science,* **94:**328–30, 1941.

131. Hanshaw, J. B. Cytomegalovirus complement fixing antibody in microcephaly. *N. Engl. J. Med.,* **275:**476–79, 1966.

132. Harland, W. A.; Adams, J. H.; and McSeveney, D. Herpes simplex particles in acute necrotizing encephalitis. *Lancet,* **2:**581–82, 1967.

133. Hattwick, M. A. W.; Weiss, T. T.; et al. Recovery from rabies: A case report. *Ann. Intern. Med.,* **76:**931–42, 1972.

134. Haynes, B. F.; Wright, R.; and McCracken, J. P. Mollaret meningitis. A report of three cases. *J.A.M.A.,* **236:**1967–69, 1976.

135. Heck, A. F.; Hameroft, S. B.; and Hornick, R. B. Chronic *listera monocytogenes* meningitis and normotensive hydrocephalus. *Neurology* (Minneap.), **21:**263–70, 1971.

136. Hedges, T. R., and Leung, L.-S. E. Parasellar and orbital apex syndrome caused by aspergillosis. *Neurology* (Minneap.), **26:**117–20, 1976.

137. Henderson, B. E.; Pigford, C. A.; Work, T.; et al. Serologic survey for St. Louis encephalitis and other group B arbovirus antibodies in residents of Houston, Texas. *Am. J. Epidemiol.,* **91:**87–98, 1970.

138. Hermans, P. E. Antiviral agents. *Mayo Clin. Proc.,* **52:**683–86, 1977.

139. Hermans, P. E.; Goldstein, N. P.; and Wellman, W. E. Mollaret's meningitis with differential diagnosis of recurrent meningitis. *Am. J. Med.,* **52:**128–40, 1972.

140. Herring, A. B., and Urch, H. Sarcoidosis of the central nervous system. *J. Neurol. Sci.,* **9:**405–22, 1969.

141. Hitchcock, E., and Andreddis, A. Subdural empyema, review of 29 cases. *J. Neurol. Neurosurg. Psychiat.,* **27:**422–34, 1964.

142. Hodges, G. R., and Perkins, R. L. Acute bacterial meningitis: An analysis of factors influencing prognosis. *Am. J. Med. Sci.,* **270:**427–40, 1975.

143. Hole, N. H. Rabies and quarantine. *Nature,* **224:**244–46, 1969.

144. Holloway, R. Fluid and electrolyte status in tetanus. *Lancet,* **2:**1278–80, 1970.

145. Hooshmand, H. Seizure disorders associated with neurosyphilis. *Dis. Nerv. Syst.,* **37:**133–36, 1976.

146. Hopkins, C. C.; Dismukes, W. E.; Glick, T. H.; and Warren, R. J. Surveillance of paralytic poliomyelitis in the United States; 1966–1967 cases and 1965–1967 cases associated with oral poliovirus vaccine. *J.A.M.A.,* **210:**694–700, 1969.

147. Horta-Barbosa, L.; Fucullo, D. A.; Hamilton, R.; Traub, R.; Ley, A.; and Sever, J. L. Some characteristics of SSPE measles virus. *Proc. Soc. Exp. Biol. Med.,* **134:**17–21, 1970.

148. Horta-Barbosa, L.; Fucullo, D. A.; London, W. T.; Jabbour, J. T.; Zeman, W.; and Sever, J. L. Isolation of measles virus from brain cell cultures of five patients with subacute sclerosing panencephalitis. *Proc. Soc. Exp. Biol. Med.,* **132:**272–77, 1969.

149. Horten, B. C.; Abbott, G. F.; and Porro, R. S. Fungal aneurysms of intracranial vessels. *Arch. Neurol.,* **33:**577–79, 1976.

150. Howitt, B. Recovery of the virus of equine encephalomyelitis from brain of a child. *Science,* **88:**455–56, 1938.

151. Idsøe, O.; Guthe, T.; and Willcox, R. R. Penicillin in the treatment of syphilis. *Bull. WHO,* suppl. 47, 1972.

152. Ignelzi, R. J., and Vanderark, G. D. Cerebral

mucormycosis following open head trauma. Case report. *J. Neurosurg.,* **42:**593–96, 1975.

152a. Illis, L., and Taylor, F. Neurologic and electroencephalographic sequelae of tetanus. *Lancet,* **1:**826–30, 1971.

153. Ingham, H. R.; Selkan, J. B.; and Roxby, C. M. Bacteriological study of otogenic cerebral abscesses: Chemotherapeutic role of metronidazole. *Br. Med. J.,* **2:**991–93, 1977.

154. Iraci, G.; Pellone, M.; et al. Posttraumatic optochiasmatic arachnoiditis. *Ann. Ophthalmol.,* **8:**1313–28, 1976.

155. Irstam, I.; Sundstron, R.; and Sigstedt, B. Lumbar myelography and adhesive arachnoiditis. *Acta Radiol.,* **15:**356–68, 1974.

156. Jabbour, J. T.; Duenas, D. A.; Sever, J. L.; Krebs, H. M.; and Horta-Barbosa, L. Epidemiology of subacute sclerosing panencephalitis (SSPE). A report of the SSPE Registry. *J.A.M.A.,* **220:**959–62, 1972.

157. Jabbour, J. T.; Garcia, J. H.; Lemmi, H.; Ragland, J.; Duenos, D. A.; and Sever, J. L. Subacute sclerosing panencephalitis. A multidisciplinary study of eight cases. *J.A.M.A.,* **207:**2248–54, 1969.

158. Jachuck, S. J.; Gardner-Thorpe, C.; et al. A brainstem syndrome associated with mycoplasma pneumoniae infection. A report of two cases. *Postgrad. Med. J.,* **51:**475–77, 1975.

159. Jackson, F. E.; Kent, D.; and Clare, F. Quadriplegia caused by involvement of cervical spine with *Coccidioides immitis;* symptomatic cure after operation and amphotericin-B treatment. *J. Neurosurg.,* **21:**512–15, 1964.

160. Jacoby, G. A. J.; Blenerhaset, J. B.; and Richardson, E. P., Jr. Fulminant central nervous system disease with lowering of cerebrospinal fluid glucose. *N. Engl. J. Med.,* **284:**1023–31, 1971.

161. Jenkins, R. B. Intradural spinal tuberculoma with genitourinary symptoms. *Arch. Neurol.,* **8:**539–43, 1963.

162. Johannes, R., and Sever, J. Subacute sclerosing panencephalitis. 589–607, 1975.

163. John, J. F., and Douglas, R. G., Jr. Tuberculous arachnoiditis. *J. Pediatr.,* **86:**235–37, 1975.

164. Johnsen, S. D. Some important pitfalls in the diagnosis and treatment of bacterial meningitis in children. *Clin. Pediatr.,* **14:**191–200, 1975.

165. Johnson, B. L., and Wisotzkey, H. M. Neuroretinitis associated with herpes simplex encephalitis in an adult. *Am. J. Ophthalmol.,* **83:**481–89, 1977.

166. Johnson, K. R.; Rosenthal, M. S.; and Lerner, P. I. Herpes simplex encephalitis: The course in five virologically proven cases. *Arch. Neurol.,* **27:**103–108, 1972.

167. Johnson, R., and Milbourn, P. E. Central nervous system manifestations of chickenpox. *Can. Med. Assoc. J.,* **102:**831–34, 1970.

168. Jordan, M. C. Nomenclature for mononucleosis syndromes. *J.A.M.A.,* **234:**45–46, 1975.

169. Joubert, M. J., and Stephanov, S. Computerized tomography and surgical treatment in intracranial suppuration. Report of 30 consecutive unselected cases of brain abscess and subdural empyema. *J. Neurosurg.,* **47:**73–78, 1977.

170. Kaplan, M. M. Epidemiology of rabies. *Nature,* **221:**421–25, 1969.

171. Karalakulasingam, Rajah; Arora, K. K.; et al. Meningoencephalitis caused by *Histoplasma capsulatum. Arch. Intern. Med.,* **136:**217–20, 1976.

172. Karandanis, D., and Shulman, J. A. Factors associated with mortality in brain abscess. *Arch. Intern. Med.,* **135:**1145–50, 1975.

173. Kaufman, D. M., and Leeds, N. F. Computed tomography (CT) in the diagnosis of intracranial abscesses: Brain abscess, subdural empyema and epidural empyema. *Neurology* (Minneap.), **27:**1069–73, 1977.

174. Kaufman, D. M.; Thal, L. J.; and Farmer, P. M. Central nervous system aspergillosis in two young adults. *Neurology* (Minneap.), **26:**484–88, 1976.

175. Kazner, E. Effects of computerized axial tomography on the treatment of cerebral abscess. *Neuroradiology,* **12:**57–58, 1976.

175a. Kelly, R. The treatment of neurosyphilis. *Practitioner,* **192:**90–95, 1964.

175b. Kennedy, D. H., and Fallon, R. J. Tuberculous meningitis. *J.A.M.A.,* **241:**264–68, 1979.

176. Ketel, W. B., and Ognibene. Japanese B encephalitis in Vietnam. *Am. J. Med. Sci.,* **26:**271–79, 1971.

177. Khoo, T. K.; Sugal, K.; and Leong, T. K. Disseminated aspergillosis: case report and review of world literature. *Am. J. Clin. Pathol.,* **45:**697–703, 1964.

178. Kibrick, S., and Benirschke, K. Acute aseptic myocarditis and meningoencephalitis in the newborn child infected with Coxsackie virus group B, type 3. *N. Engl. J. Med.,* **255:**883–89, 1956.

179. King, J. S., and Hosobuchi, Y. Cysticercus cyst of the lateral ventricle. *Surg. Neurol.,* **7:**125–29, 1977.

179a. Kingsley, D. P. E.; Kendall, B. E.; and Moseley, I. F. Superior sagittal sinus thrombosis: An evaluation of the changes demonstrated on computed tomography. *J. Neurol. Neurosurg. Psychiatry,* **41:**1065–68, 1978.

180. Klein, J. D.; Yamouchi, T.; and Horlick, S. P. Neonatal candidiasis meningitis and arteritis: observations and a review of the literature. *J. Pediatr.,* **81:**31–34, 1972.

181. Kocen, R. S., and Parsons, M. Neurologic complication of tuberculosis: Some unusual manifestations. *Q. J. Med.,* **39:**17–30, 1970.

182. Koeze, T. H., and Klingon, G. H. Acquired toxoplasmosis: Case with focal neurologic manifestations. *Arch. Neurol.,* **11:**191–97, 1964.

183. Koranyi, F. K. Two cases of malaria presenting with psychiatric symptoms. *Biol. Psychiat.,* **11:**445–49, 1971.

184. Kosen, R. S. Neurological complications of tuberculosis: some unusual manifestations. *Q. J. Med.,* **39:**17–30, 1970.

185. Krayenbuhl, H. A. Abscess of the brain. *Clin. Neurosurg.,* **14:**25–44, 1966.

186. Laha, R. K.; Saunders, F. W.; and Huestis, W. S. Herpes simplex encephalitis: Treatment with surgical decompression and cytosine arabinoside. *Can. Med. Assoc. J.,* **115:**236–37, 1976.

187. Law, J. D.; Lehman, R. A. W.; et al. Diagnosis and treatment of abscess of the central ganglia. *J. Neurosurg.,* **44:**226–32, 1976.

188. Leider, W.; Magoffin, R. L.; Lennette, E. H.; and Leonards, L. N. R. Herpes simplex virus encephalitis: its possible association with reactivated latent infection. *N. Engl. Med.,* **273:**341–47, 1965.

189. Lerner, A. M.; Bailey, E. J.; and Nolan, D. C. Complement requiring neutralizing antibodies in herpes virus hominis encephalitis. *J. Immunol.,* **104:**607–15, 1970.

190. Lerner, P. I. Selection of antimicrobial agents in bacterial infections of the nervous system. In Thompson, R. A., and Green, J. R. (eds.). *Advances in Neurology,* Vol. 6. Raven Press, New York, 1974, pp. 169–203.

191. Levitt, L. P.; Rich, T. A.; Kinde, S. W.; Lewis, A. C.; Gates, E. H.; and Bond, J. O. Central nervous system mumps: Review of 64 cases. *Neurology* (Minneap.), **20:**829–34, 1970.

192. Lewis, J. M. Orchitis, parotitis and meningoencephalitis due to lymphocytic choriomeningitis virus. *N. Engl. J. Med.,* **265:**776–80, 1961.

193. Lipow, M. L., and Gold, R. Current status of vaccines against the meningococcus. *Prevt. Med.,* **3:**449–55, 1974.

194. Liske, E., and Weikers, N. J. Changing aspects of brain abscess: review of cases in Wisconsin, 1940 through 1962. *Neurology* (Minneap.), **14:**294–300, 1964.

195. Lloyd, G. A. S. The localization of lesions in the orbital apex and cavernous sinus by frontal venography. *Br. J. Radiol.,* **45:**405–14, 1972.

196. Loeser, E., Jr., and Scheinberg, L. Brain abscesses: Review of ninety-nine cases. *Neurology* (Minneap.), **7:**601–609, 1957.

197. Lombroso, C. T. Remarks on the EEG and movement disorder in SSPE. *Neurology* (Minneap.), **18:**69–75, 1968.

198. Lope, E. S., and Gutierrez, D. C. Nocardia asteroides primary cerebral abscess and secondary meningitis. *Acta Neurochir.,* **37:**139–45, 1977.

199. Lorinez, A. B., and Moore, R. Y. Puerperal cerebral venous thrombosis. *Am. J. Obstet. Gynecol.,* **83:**311–19, 1962.

200. Lyon, L. W. Neurologic manifestations of cat-scratch disease. Report of a case and review of the literature. *Arch. Neurol.,* **25:**23–27, 1971.

201. Lott, T.; El Gammal, T.; et al. Evaluation of brain and epidural abscesses by computed tomography. *Radiology,* **122:**371–76, 1977.

202. Macrae, A. D. Rabies. *Br. Med. J.,* **1:**604–606, 1973.

203. Macrae, J. Tetanus. *Br. Med. J.,* **1:**730–32, 1973.

204. Mandal, B. K.; Evans, D. I. K.; Oronside, A. G.; and Pullan, B. R. Radioactive bromide partition test in differential diagnosis of tuberculous meningitis. *Br. Med. J.,* **4:**413–15, 1972.

205. Mandybur, T.; Nagpaul, A.; et al. Alzheimer's neurofibril changes in subacute sclerosing panencephalitis. *Ann. Neurol.,* **1:**103–107, 1977.

206. Manfredi, M.; Bozzao, L.; and Frasconi, F. Chronic intramedullary abscess in the spinal cord. *J. Neurosurg.,* **33:**352–55, 1970.

207. Martin, J. P. Conquest of general paralysis. *Br. Med. J.,* **3:**159–60, 1972.

208. Mathison, D. A. Active rabies immunization in an individual sensitive to duck embryo vaccine. *J. Allerg. Clin. Immunol.,* **50:**246–51, 1972.

208a. Mayers, M. M.; Kaufman, D. M.; and Miller, M. H. Recent cases of intracranial tuberculomas. *Neurology* (Minneap.), **28:**256–60, 1978.

209. McCormick, W. F.; Rodnitzky, R. L.; Schochet, S. S., Jr.; and McKee, A. P. Varicella-zoster encephalomyelitis: Morphologic and virologic study. *Arch. Neurol.,* **21:**559–70, 1969.

210. McDonald, R. Purulent meningitis in newborn babies. *Clin. Pediatr.,* **11:**450–54, 1972.

210a. Mehta, P. D.; Kane, A.; and Thormar, H. Further characterization of bound measles-specific IgG eluted from SSPE brains. *Ann. Neurol.,* **3:**552–55, 1978.

211. Melamed, E.; Rachmilewitz, E. A.; et al. Aseptic cavernous sinus thrombosis after internal carotid arterial occlusion in polycythemia vera. *J. Neurol. Neurosurg. Psychiat.,* **39:**320–24, 1976.

212. Meulen, V. ter; Katz, M.; Köchell, Y. M.; Barbanti-Brodano, G.; Koprowski, H.; and Lennette, E. H. Subacute sclerosing panencephalitis: In vitro characterization of viruses isolated from brain cells in culture. *J. Infect. Dis.,* **126:**11–17, 1972.

213. Meyer, K. F.; Haring, C. M.; and Howitt, B. Etiology of epizootic encephalomyelitis in horses in the San Joaquin Valley. *Science,* **74:**227–28, 1930.

214. Miller, A., and Nathanson, N. Rabies: Recent advances in pathogenesis and control. *Ann. Neurol.,* **2:**511–19, 1977.

215. Miller, J. O., and Price, T. R. Involvement of the brain in Rocky Mountain spotted fever. *South. Med. J.,* **65:**437–39, 1972.

216. Milstein, J. M., and Biggs, H. E. Recurrent encephalitis with elevated titers for herpes simplex. *Arch. Neurol.,* **34:**434–36, 1977.

217. Miyakawa, T.; Murayama, E.; et al. Neuro-Behcet's disease showing severe atrophy of the cerebrum. *Acta Neuropathol.,* **34:**95–103, 1976.

217a. Mohandas, S.; Ahaya, G. K.; et al. Aspergillosis of the central nervous system. *J. Neurol. Sci.,* **38:**229–33, 1978.

218. Mohr, J. A.; Griffith, W.; et al. Neurosyphilis and penicillin levels in cerebrospinal fluid. *J.A.M.A.,* **236:**2208–2209, 1976.

219. Moossy, J., and Geer, J. C. Encephalomyelitis myocarditis and adrenal cortical necrosis in Coxsacki B3 virus infection; distribution of the central nervous system lesions. *Arch. Pathol.,* **70:**614–22, 1960.

220. Morganroth, J.; Deisseroth, A.; Winokur, S.; and Schein, P. Differentiation of carcinomatous and bacterial meningitis. *Neurology* (Minneap.), **22:**1240–42, 1972.

221. Mukhopadhyay, D.; Clark, T.; Spencer, L.; and Marlis, M. I. Aseptic meningitis due to echovirus type 9. *Can. J. Public Health,* **63:**157–60, 1972.

222. Murray, H. W.; Mansur, H.; et al. The protean manifestation of Mycoplasma pneumoniae infection in adults. *Am. J. Med.,* **58:**229–42, 1975.

223. Myhre, E. B. Rapid diagnosis of bacterial men-

ingitis. Demonstration of bacterial antigen by counterimmunoelectrophoresis. *Scand. J. Infect. Dis.,* **6:**237–39, 1974.

224. Nager, G. T. Mastoid and paranasal sinus infection and their relation to the central nervous system. *Clin. Neurosurg.,* **14:**288–313, 1966.

225. Natarajan, M.; Ramasubramanian, K. R.; and Muthu, A. K. Intramedullary cysticercosis of spinal cord. *Surg. Neurol.,* **6:**157–58, 1976.

226. Naveh, Y., and Friedman, A. Rubella encephalitis successfully treated with corticosteroids. *Clin. Pediatr.,* **14:**286–87, 1975.

227. Nelson, K. E.; Levin, S.; Spies, H. W.; and Lepper, M. H. Treatment of *Hemophilus influenzae* meningitis, a comparison of chloramphenicol and tetracycline. *J. Infect. Dis.,* **125:**459–65, 1972.

228. Nelson, D. A.; Warner, A.; Yanoff, M.; and dePeralta, J. Retinal lesions in subacute sclerosing panencephalitis. *Arch. Ophthalmol.,* **84:**613–21, 1970.

229. New, P. F. J.; Davis, K. R.; and Ballantine, H. I. J. Computed tomography in cerebral abscess. *Radiology,* **121:**641–46, 1976.

230. Ng, Khye Weng; Wagner, W.; and Parker, J. C. Primary amebic meningoencephalitis: A potential problem in the Southeastern United States. *South. Med. J.,* **64:**691–94, 1971.

230a. Niederman, J.; McCollum, R.; Henle, G.; and Henle, W. Infectious mononucleosis: Clinical manifestations in relation to E virus antibodies. *J.A.M.A.,* **203:**205–209, 1968.

231. Nielson, H., and Gyldensted, C. Computed tomography in the diagnosis of cerebral abscess. *Neuroradiology,* **12:**207–17, 1977.

232. Nielson, H., and Halaburt, H. Cerebral abscess with special reference to the angiographic changes. *Neuroradiology,* **12:**73–78, 1976.

233. Nolan, D. C.; Carruthers, M. M.; and Lerner, A. M. Herpes virus hominis encephalitis in Michigan. Report of 13 cases, including 6 treated with idoxuridine. *N. Engl. J. Med.,* **282:**10–13, 1970.

234. O'Duffy, J. D.; Carrey, J. A.; and Deodbar, S. Behcet's disease. *Ann. Intern. Med.,* **75:**561–70, 1971.

235. O'Duffy, J. D., and Goldstein, N. P. Neurologic involvement in seven patients with Behcet's disease. *Am. J. Med.,* **61:**170–78, 1976.

236. Olafsson, M.; Lee, Y. C.; and Abernathy, T. S. Mima polymorpha meningitis. Report of a case and review of the literature. *N. Engl. J. Med.,* **258:**465–70, 1958.

237. Oldendort, W. H.; Cornford, M. E.; and Brown, W. J. The large apparent work capability of the blood-brain barrier: A study of mitochondrial content of capillary endothelial cells in brain and other tissues of the rat. *Ann. Neurol.,* **1:**409–17, 1977.

238. Oyanagi, S.; Rorke, L. B.; Katz, M.; and Koprowski, H. Histopathology and electron microscopy of 3 cases of subacute sclerosing panencephalitis. *Acta Neuropathol.* (Berl.), **18:**58–73, 1971.

239. Palo, J.; Haltia, M.; and Uutela, T. Cerebral aspergillosis with special reference to cerebrospinal fluid findings. *Eur. Neurol.,* **13:**224–31, 1975.

240. Pampiglione, G. Prodromal phase of measles: Some neurophysiological studies. *Br. Med. J.,* **2:**1296–1300, 1964.

241. Pantazopoulos, P. E. Actinomycosis of brain manifested by vestibular symptoms. *Arch. Otolaryngol.,* **80:**309–12, 1964.

242. Papatheodorou, C. A., and Teng, P. Pneumoencephalographic findings in coccidioidal meningitis. *Calif. Med.,* **101:**479–81, 1964.

243. Pardridge, W. M., and Oldendorf, W. H. Transport of metabolic substances through the blood brain barrier. *J. Neurochem.,* **28:**5–12, 1977.

244. Parsons, M., and Pallis, C. A. Intradural spinal tuberculomas. *Neurology* (Minneap.), **15:**1018–22, 1965.

245. Pasteur, L.; Chamberland, C.; and Roux, P. P. E. Nouvelle communication sur la rage. *C. R. Acad. Sci.,* **98:**457–63, 1884.

246. Pasteur, L. Méthode pour prévenir la rage après morsure. *C. R. Acad. Sci.,* **101:**765–72, 1885.

247. Payne, F. E.; Baublis, J. V.; and Itabashi, H. N. Isolation of measles virus from cell culture of brain from a patient with subacute sclerosing panencephalitis. *N. Engl. J. Med.,* **281:**585–89, 1969.

248. Poretz, D. M.; Smith, M. N.; and Park, C. H. Intracranial suppuration secondary to trauma. Infection with Nocardia asteroides. *J.A.M.A.,* **232:**730–31, 1975.

249. Price, D. J. E., and Sleigh, J. D. *Klebsiella* meningitis, report of nine cases. *J. Neurol. Neurosurg. Psychiat.,* **35:**903–908, 1972.

249a. Pullen, H. A new look at infectious diseases: Infectious mononucleosis. *Br. Med. J.,* **2:**350–53, 1973.

250. Quencer, R. M.; Tenner, M.; and Rothman, L. The postoperative myelogram. Radiographic evaluation of arachnoiditis and dural/arachnoidal tears. *Neuroradiology,* **123:**667–79, 1977.

251. Reeves, D. L.; Dickson, D. R.; and Benjamin, E. L. Phycomycosis (mucormycosis) of the central nervous system; report of a case. *J. Neurosurg.,* **23:**82–84, 1965.

252. Richards, D. J. Case of superior longitudinal sinus thrombosis in pregnancy. *Postgrad. Med. J.,* **41:**702–705, 1965.

253. Richter, R. W., and Braest, J. C. M. Pneumococci meningitis at Harlem Hospital. *N.Y. State J. Med.,* **71:**2747–54, 1971.

254. Riehl, J. L., and Andrews, J. M. The uveomeningencephalic syndrome. *Neurology* (Minneap.), **16:**603–609, 1966.

254a. Risk, W. S.; Haddad, F. S.; and Chemali, R. Substantial spontaneous long-term improvement in subacute sclerosing panencephalitis. Six cases from the Middle East and a review of the literature. *Arch. Neurol.,* **35:**494–502, 1978.

255. Roden, V. J.; Cantor, H. E.; et al. Acute hemiplegia of childhood associated with Coxsackie A9 viral infection. *J. Pediatr.,* **86:**56–58, 1975.

256. Ross, A. V.; Julia, A.; and Balakrishnan, C. Toxicity of adenine arabinoside in humans. *J. Infect. Dis.,* **133:** suppl. 192–198, 1976.

256a. Rotheram, E. G., Jr., and Kessler, L. A. Use of computerized tomography in nonsurgical management of brain abscess. *Arch. Neurol.,* **36:**25–26, 1979.

257. Rowe, P. B., and Payne, W. H. Rhino-cerebral mucormycosis. *Med. J. Aust.,* **51:**960–61, 1964.

258. Rowland, L. P., and Greer, M. Toxoplasmic polymyositis. *Neurology* (Minneap.), **11:**367–70, 1961.

259. Roy, R. N.; Bhattacharya, M. B.; et al. Spinal cysticercosis. *Surg. Neurol.,* **8:**129–31, 1976.

260. Ruben, R. H.; Mattwick, M. A. W.; Jones, S.; Gregg, M. B.; and Schwartz, V. D. Adverse reaction to duck embryo vaccine, range and incidence. *Ann. Intern. Med.,* **78:**643–49, 1973.

261. Sabin, A. B. Oral poliovirus vaccine: recent results and recommendations for optimum use. *Roy. Soc. Health J.,* **2:**51–59, 1962.

262. Sabin, A. B. Properties of attenuated poliovirus and their behavior in human beings. *N. Y. Acad. Sci. Special Publ.* No. 5, 1957, pp. 113–27.

263. Saksena, P. N., and Anand, J. S. Study of 224 cases of tubercular meningitis in children with particular reference to its symptomatology and prognostic features. *Indian J. Child Health,* **12:**563–66, 1963.

264. Salk, J. E. Principles of immunization as applied to poliomyelitis and influenza. *Am. J. Public Health,* **43:**1384–98, 1953.

265. Salk, J., and Salk, D. Control of influenza and poliomyelitis with killed virus vaccines. *Science,* **195:**834–47, 1977.

266. Salmon, J. H. Ventriculitis complicating meningitis. *Am. J. Dis. Child.,* **124:**35–40, 1972.

267. Samson, D. S., and Clark, K. A current review of brain abscess. *Am. J. Med.,* **54:**201–10, 1973.

268. Sanders, R. K. M.; Joseph, R.; et al. Intrathecal antitetanus serum (horse) in the treatment of tetanus. *Lancet,* **1:**974–77, 1977.

269. Sarosi, G. A.; Parker, J. D.; Doto, I.; and Tosh, F. E. Amphotericin B in cryptococcic meningitis. Long term. Results of treatment. *Ann. Intern. Med.,* **71:**1079–87, 1969.

270. Sayeed, Z. A.; Bhaduri, U.; Howell, E.; and Meyers, M. L. Gonococcal meningitis, a review. *J.A.M.A.,* **219:**1730–31, 1972.

271. Scheidemandel, V.; Campbell, C. W.; and Curtin, J. A. *Escherichia coli* meningitis—treatment with gentamicin sulphate. *Med. Ann. D.C.,* **40:**85–87, 1971.

272. Schiller, F., and Shadle, O. W. Extrathecal and intrathecal suppuration; report of two cases and discussion of the spinal subdural space. *Arch. Neurol.,* **7:**33–36, 1962.

273. Schlossberg, D.; Brooks, J. B.; and Shulman, J. A. Possibility of diagnosing meningitis by gas chromatography: Cryptococcal meningitis. *J. Clin. Microbiol.,* **3:**239–45, 1976.

274. Schmid, A. H. Cerebral malaria. On the nature and significance of vascular changes. *Eur. Neurol.* **12:**197–208, 1974.

275. Schultz, D. R.; Barthal, J. S.; and Garrett, G. Western Equine encephalitis with rapid onset of parkinsonism. *Neurology* (Minneap.), **2:**1095–96, 1977.

276. Schwartz, G. A.; Blumenkrantz, M. J.; and Sundmäher, W. L. H. Neurologic complications of malignant external otitis. *Neurology* (Minneap.), **21:**1077–84, 1971.

277. Seggey, J.; Ohry, A.; et al. Sensory loss in poliomyelitis. *Arch. Neurol.,* **33:**664, 1976.

278. Sever, J. L., and Zeman, W. Serological studies of measles and subacute sclerosing panencephalitis. *Neurology* (Minneap.), **18:**95–97, 1968.

279. Shamberg, I. L., and Beerman, H. Clinical emphasis on the diagnosis and management of syphilis. *Med. Clin. North Am.,* **46:**689–705, 1962.

280. Shaw, M. D. M., and Russell, J. A. Cerebellar abscess. A review of 47 cases. *J. Neurol. Neurosurg. Psychiat.,* **38:**429–35, 1975.

281. Shearer, M. L., and Finch, S. M. Periodic organic psychosis associated with recurrent herpes simplex. *N. Engl. J. Med.,* **27:**494–97, 1964.

282. Sherman, B. M.; Gordon, P.; and DeChen, G. Postmeningitis selective hypopituitism with suprasella calcification. *Arch. Intern. Med.,* **128:**600–604, 1971.

283. Sikorski, J. B.; Gilroy, J.; and Meyer, J. S. *Clostridium perfringes* (gas bacillus) septicemia and acute purulent meningitis. *Harper Hosp. Bull.,* **21:**38–40, 1963.

284. Silverstein, A.; Steinberg, G.; and Nathanson, M. Nervous system involvement in infectious mononucleosis. *Arch. Neurol.,* **26:**353–58, 1972.

285. Simpson, J. F. *Listeria monocytogenes* meningitis: an opportunistic infection. *J. Neurol. Neurosurg. Psychiat.,* **34:**657–63, 1971.

286. Skromme-Kaddubik, G.; Celis, C.; and Ferez, A. Cysticericosis of the nervous system: Diagnosis by means of specific radioimmunoscan. *Am. Neurol.,* **2:**343–44, 1977.

287. Slatkin, M. H. Trends in the diagnosis and treatment of syphilis. *Med. Clin. North Am.,* **49:** 823–42, 1965.

288. Smith, C. C. Treatment of human brucellosis. *Scott. Med. J.,* **21:**132–33, 1976.

289. Smith, J. B.; Groover, R. V.; et al. Multicystic cerebral degeneration in neonatal herpes simplex virus encephalitis. *Am. J. Dis. Child.,* **131:**568–72, 1977.

290. Smith, C., and Sunster, G. *Mycoplasma pneumoniae* meningoencephalitis. *J. Infect. Dis.,* **4:**69–71, 1972.

291. Smith, J. L., and Taylor, W. H. The FTA-ABS test in ocular and neurosyphilis. *Am. J. Ophthalmol.,* **60:**653–58, 1965.

292. Smith, M. G.; Lennette, E. M.; and Reames, H. R. Isolation of the virus of herpes simplex and demonstration of intracellular inclusions in cases of acute encephalitis. *Am. J. Pathol.,* **17:**55–68, 1941.

293. Snow, R. M., and Dismukes, W. E. Cryptococcal meningitis. Diagnostic value of cryptococcal antigen in cerebrospinal fluid. *Arch. Intern. Med.,* **135:**1155–57, 1975.

294. Soscia, J. L.; Di Benedetto, R.; and Crocco, J. *Klebsiella pneumoniae* meningitis. *Arch. Intern. Med.,* **113:**569–72, 1964.

295. Southern, P. M., Jr.; Smith, J. W.; Luby, J. P.; Barnett, J. A.; and Sandford, J. P. Clinical and laboratory features of epidemic St. Louis encephalitis. *Ann. Intern. Med.,* **71:**681–89, 1969.

296. Sparling, P. F. Diagnosis and treatment of syphilis. *N. Engl. J. Med.,* **284:**642–53, 1971.

297. Spataro, R. F.; Lin, S.-R.; et al. Aqueductal stenosis and hydrocephalus: Rare sequalae of mumps virus infection. *Neuroradiology,* **12:**11–13, 1976.

298. Steele, J. C.; Gladstone, R. M.; Thanasophon, S.; and Fleming, P. C. Acute cerebellar ataxia and concomitant infection with *Mycoplasma pneumoniae. J. Pediatr.,* **80:**467–69, 1972.

299. Stefani, F. H., and Mehraein, P. Acute rhino-orbito-cerebral mucormycosis. *Ophthalmologica,* **172:**38–44, 1976.

300. Stevens, J., and Robinson, K. Chronic cavernous sinus thrombosis. Discussion and report of a case. *J. Oral Surg.,* **35:**136–39, 1977.

301. Strauss, R. A. Primary amebic meningoencephalitis. *Chicago Med. Sch. Q.,* **31:**30–39, 1972.

302. Streletz, L. J., and Cracco, J. The effect of isoprinosine in subacute sclerosing panencephalitis (SSPE). *Am. Neurol.,* **1:**183–84, 1977.

303. Sung, J. P.; Grendahl, J. G.; and Levine, H. B. Intravenous and intrathecal miconazole therapy for systemic mycoses. *West. J. Med.,* **126:**5–13, 1977.

304. Taber, L. H.; Greenberg, S. B.; et al. Herpes simplex encephalitis treated with vidarabine (adenine arabinoside). *Arch. Neurol.,* **34:**608–10, 1977.

305. Taubin, H. L., and Landsberg, L. Gonococcal meningitis. *N. Engl. J. Med.,* **285:**504–505, 1971.

306. Tay Chon Hai. The uveomeningoencephalitic syndrome (Vogt-Koyargi-Harada syndrome). *Far East Med. J.,* **6:**314–18, 1970.

307. Taylor, M. J.; Burrow, G. N.; and Horstmann, D. M. Meningoencephalitis associated with pneumonitis due to *Mycoplasma pneumoniae. J.A.M.A.,* **199:**813–16, 1967.

308. Theologides, A., and Kennedy, B. J. Clinical manifestations of toxoplasmosis in the adult. *Arch. Intern. Med.,* **117:**536–40, 1966.

309. Thomson, J. L. G. The computerized axial tomography in acute herpes simplex encephalitis. *Bri. J. Radiol.,* **49:**86–87, 1976.

310. Tobu, B. M., and Jones, D. M. Immunoelectrosinophoresis in the diagnosis of meningococcal infections. *J. Clin. Pathol.,* **25:**583–85, 1972.

310a. Toro, G., and Romain, G. Cerebral malaria. A disseminated vasculomyelinopathy. *Arch. Neurol.,* **35:**271–75, 1978.

311. Towbin, A. The syndrome of latent cerebral venous thrombosis: Its frequency and relation to age and congestive heart failure. *Stroke,* **4:**419–30, 1973.

312. Townsend, J.; Wolinsky, J.; Baringer, J.; and Johnson, P. Acquired toxoplasmosis: A neglected cause of treatable nervous system disease. *Arch. Neurol.,* **32:**335–43, 1975.

313. Townsend, J. J.; Baringer, J. R.; et al. Progressive rubella panencephalitis. Late onset after congenital rubella. *N. Engl. J. Med.,* **292:**990–93, 1975.

314. Townsend, J. J.; Wolinsky, J. S.; and Baringer, J. R. The neuropathology of progressive rubella panencephalitis of late onset. *Brain,* **99:**81–90, 1976.

315. Tramont, E. C. Persistence of *Treponema palli-dum* following penicillin G therapy. *J.A.M.A.,* **236:**2206–2207, 1976.

316. Tramont, E. C. Management of bacterial meningitis. *Milit. Med.,* **141:**589–94, 1976.

317. Tsai, Y.; Schilp, A. O.; and Leo, J. S. Angiographic findings with an intracranial gumma. *Neuroradiology,* **13:**1–5, 1977.

318. Treatment of cerebral abscesses. *Br. Med. J.,* **2:**978, 1977.

319. Tueten, L.; Loken, C.; and Hauge, T. Aspergillosis cerebri: Report of a case. *Acta Neurol. Scand.,* **130:**149–56, 1965.

320. Turner, E., and Whitby, J. L. Nocardial cerebral abscess with systemic involvement successfully treated by aspiration and sulphonamides. *J. Neurosurg.,* **31:**227–29, 1969.

321. Turner, L. N. Leptospirosis. A new look at infectious diseases. *Br. Med. J.,* **1:**537–40, 1973.

322. Tynes, B. G.; Crutcher, J. G.; and Utz, J. P. *Histoplasma* meningitis. *Ann. Intern. Med.,* **59:**619–21, 1963.

323. Upton, A. R. M.; Barwick, D. D.; and Foster, J. B. Dexamethasone treatment of herpes simplex encephalitis. *Lancet,* **1:**290–91, 1971.

323a. Vallat, J. M.; Vital, C.; et al. Clinical and ultrastructural study of a case of human rabies. *Rev. Neurol.,* **133:**637–46, 1977.

324. Van Alphen, H. A. M., and Dreissen, J. J. R. Brain abscess and subdural empyema. Factors influencing mortality and results of various surgical techniques. *J. Neurol. Neurosurg. Psychiat.,* **39:**481–90, 1976.

325. Vianna, N. J., and Hinman, A. R. Rocky Mountain spotted fever on Long Island. *Am. J. Med.,* **51:**725–30, 1971.

326. Vijayen, N., and Dreyfus, P. M. Chemical epidural abscess. Case report. *J. Neurol. Neurosurg. Psychiat.,* **34:**297–99, 1971.

327. Villella, R. L.; Halling, L. W.; and Biegelersen, J. Z., Jr. A case of listerosis of the newborn with fluorescent antibody histologic studies. *Am. J. Clin. Pathol.,* **40:**151–56, 1963.

328. Viroslav, J., and Williams, T. W., Jr. Nocardial infection of the pulmonary and central nervous system. Successful treatment with medical therapy. *South. Med. J.,* **64:**1382–85, 1971.

329. Wadia, N. H., and Singhal, B. S. Cerebral arteriography in tuberculous meningitis. *Neurol. India,* **15:**127–32, 1967.

330. Waite, C. L., and Kline, A. H. *Mima polymorpha* meningitis: report of a case and review of the literature. *Am. J. Dis. Child.,* **98:**379–84, 1959.

331. Weiss, W.; Figueroa, W.; Shapiro, W. H.; and Flippin, H. F. Prognostic factors in pneumococcal meningitis. *Arch. Intern. Med.,* **120:**517–24, 1967.

332. Wellings, F. M. Amoebic meningoencephalitis. Editorial. *J. Fla. Med. Assoc.,* **64:**327–28, 1977.

333. Wetherill, J. H.; Webb, H. E.; and Cotterall, R. D. Syphilis presenting as an acute neurological illness. *Br. Med. J.,* **1:**1157–58, 1965.

334. Williams, E. Brucellosis. *Br. Med. J.,* **1:**791–93, 1973.

335. Williams, T. W., Jr. Meningitis: Special tech-

niques in treatment. *Mod. Treat.,* **7**:606–15, 1970.

336. Wilson, F. M., and Lerner, A. M. Etiology and mortality of purulent meningitis at the Detroit Receiving Hospital. *N. Engl. J. Med.,* **27**:1235–40, 1964.

337. Wilson, L. G. Viral encephalography mimicking functional psychosis. *Am. J. Psychiat.,* **133**:165–70, 1976.

338. Witorsch, P.; Williams, T. W., Jr.; Ommaya, A. K.; and Utz, J. P. Intraventricular administration of amphotericin B; use of subcutaneous reservoir in four patients with mycotic meningitis. *J.A.M.A.,* **194**:699–702, 1965.

339. Wolf, R. E.; Fundenberg, H. H.; et al. Treatment of Behcet's syndrome with transfer factor. *J.A.M.A.,* **238**:869–71, 1977.

340. Wolman, B., and Longson, M. Herpes encephalitis. *Acta Paediatr. Scand.,* **66**:243–46, 1977.

341. Wright, R. L. Intramedullary spinal cord abscess; report of a case secondary to stab wound with good recovery following operation. *J. Neurosurg.,* **23**:208–10, 1965.

342. Wright, R. L., and Ballantine, H. T. Management of brain abscesses in children and adolescents. *Am. J. Dis. Child.,* **114**:113–22, 1967.

343. Yeung, C. Y. Intrathecal antibiotic therapy for neonatal meningitis. *Arch. Dis. Child.,* **51**:686–90, 1976.

344. Yoshikawa, T. T., and Goodman, S. J. Brain abscess. *West. J. Med.,* **121**:207–19, 1974.

345. Young, L. S.; LaForce, F. M.; Head, J. J.; Feeley, J. C.; and Bennett, J. V. A simultaneous outbreak of meningococcus and influenza infections. *N. Engl. J. Med.,* **287**:5–9, 1972.

346. Zelinger, K. S., and Vargas, R. D. Central nervous system infection by Vibrio fetus. *Neurology* (Minneap.), **28**:968–71, 1978.

8 TRAUMATIC INJURIES TO THE BRAIN AND SPINAL CORD

Injuries to the Brain

Modern society has an appalling number of traumatic injuries, most of which result from the widespread use of the automobile[111] and the hazards of industry. There has also been a steady rise in the number of children treated for head injury in the last 20 years.[42] At least 7 per cent of industrial injuries associated with permanent functional impairment are due to craniocerebral trauma. The increase in automobile accidents in the United States has led to legislation governing the building of automobile safety features, many of which are directed toward the prevention of head injury. Severe head injuries and spinal injuries have been reduced in some countries following the introduction of seat belt legislation.[185] However, it is still not generally recognized that the unprotected head is prone to serious injury

in industrial accidents, in automobile and motorcycle accidents, and in many sports. The wearing of protective headgear is now commonly required in industry because management, encouraged by compensation laws, has become aware of the importance of prevention. However, protective headgear is often neglected by drivers and passengers in automobiles, on motorcycles, and in many hazardous sports.

Mechanisms of Injury

Forces which act upon the head at the time of injury may produce deformation due to acceleration, deceleration, or rotation of the skull and its contents. The forces injure the craniocerebral mass by (1) compression (pushing the tissues together), (2) tension (tearing the tissues apart), or (3) shearing (sliding of portions of tissues over other portions). Compression, tension, and shearing operate simultaneously or in succession.[88]

Deformation of the Skull. A blow to the head results in a temporary deformation of the cranial vault, which is greater in the relatively fixed head than in the freely moving head. Deformation leads to a decrease in volume and temporary rise in cerebrospinal fluid pressure. If the velocity of the impacting force is high, it may produce a depressed fracture or perforation of the skull. Impacts of low velocity tend to produce linear fractures.

ACCELERATION. In acceleration injuries, which result from linear or angular acceleration, the slower moving contents of the cranial cavity are damaged by sudden contact with bony prominences or the edge of dural membranes. There may be bruising or contusion of the brainstem, the undersurface of the occipital lobes, or the superior surface of the cerebellum against the edge of the tentorium cerebelli. The upper surface of the corpus callosum can be damaged by the free edge of the falx cerebri. The tips of the frontal and temporal lobes are particularly vulnerable to injury when they move in an anteroposterior and superoinferior direction because they strike the bony ridges dividing the anterior and middle cranial fossae anteriorly.

An accompanying factor which causes acceleration injuries is the effect of the pressure wave that traverses the skull from the point of impact. The highest pressure occurs at this point, with the lowest pressure, often a negative pressure, directly opposite. Theoretically, if the negative pressure reaches vapor pressure, cavitation occurs with tearing of tissue and the production of contrecoup injuries.

DECELERATION. When the moving head strikes a fixed and solid object, there is rapid deceleration of the skull and the development of coup and contrecoup injuries. A fall on the back of the head results in contusion of the frontal and temporal lobes due to inertia of the cranial contents. The development of a pressure wave with negative pressure in the area of injury and rotation of the cranial contents so that the frontal and temporal lobes abut against bony prominences are also important factors in this type of injury.[174] The midbrain may be damaged by striking the clivus as a result of the same type of injury. Blows over the lateral aspect of the freely movable head result in contusion of the

opposite temporal lobe. A fall on the frontal region has a somewhat different effect, and contrecoup injuries to the occipital lobes are rare,[173] probably owing to the smooth contour and absence of bony projection in the occipital area. However, a blow to the frontal region with acute hyperextension of the head may produce partial or complete tearing of the brainstem at the pontomedullary junction.[16]

ROTATION AND SHEARING. The energy which enters the head on impact produces skull distortion, linear movement of the head (acceleration or deceleration), and rotation of the head. Rotation occurs as a result of hyperflexion, hyperextension, lateral flexion, and turning movements of the head on the neck, which produce shearing forces in the brain and tearing of tissue. This mechanism is probably the major cause of contrecoup injuries to the brain.[173]

Movements of the brain within the cranial cavity also set up shearing forces within the brain substance. These shearing forces can act at any site in the brain, producing damage to blood vessels and to the brain, including fractures or rupture of axons in the white matter.[232]

Types of Injury

Skull Fracture. The type of skull fracture depends on the velocity of the object striking the skull and the force applied to the skull. The skull is a remarkably strong structure, and it can withstand a great deal of force and energy without fracturing. However, severe or even fatal intracranial damage can occur in the absence of a skull fracture. Thus, the presence of a skull fracture alone without neurologic abnormalities is of limited clinical significance.[97] In general, high-velocity objects produce perforation of the skull or depressed fractures, while low-velocity objects tend to produce comminuted or linear fractures. About 70 per cent of skull fractures are of the linear type. This results from an inbending of the skull at the site of the impact and an outbending of the bone around this area. The tensile stresses in the outbending area initiate the linear fracture, which extends toward the point of impact and in the opposite direction toward the base of the skull. There are also remote effects of impact due to deformation of the skull. A blow to the occipital or temporal bone may produce a fracture in the anterior cranial fossa, usually involving the orbital roof.[104]

The inbending of the skull at the point of impact can cause contusion of the brain surface and meninges. A linear fracture can produce laceration of meningeal blood vessels and extradural hemorrhage or traumatic aneurysms of the middle cerebral artery.[205] A similar fracture extending into the base of the skull can tear the internal carotid artery or weaken its wall with the subsequent development of an aneurysm.[114] Blood from a ruptured carotid artery may enter the paranasal sinuses and result in epistaxis, or it may enter the middle ear and exit through the eustachian tube or the external ear. A posttraumatic aneurysm that ruptures into the cavernous sinus produces an arteriovenous fistula with exophthalmos, paralysis of extraocular movements, and a loud murmur over the eye and orbit.[247] The venous sinuses are occasionally torn by a skull fracture, and the resulting acute subdural hematoma carries a high mortality rate.

Depressed fractures decrease the volume of the cranial cavity and may produce uncal herniation or herniation of the lower brainstem and cerebellum through the foramen magnum. All the cranial nerves are vulnerable to direct trauma by skull fracture, although nerve palsies are probably the result of shearing forces rather than bony displacement in the majority of cases.

Fractures involving the cribriform plate or middle ear may result in cerebrospinal fluid rhinorrhea or otorrhea with the risk of pneumocephalus or intracranial infection.

Closed Head Injury Without Fracture. The majority of individuals who sustain a minor head injury without skull fracture experience no more than transitory symptoms of neurologic dysfunction with complete recovery within a short period of time. However, a patient with a closed head injury without a fractured skull may sustain severe and irreversible brain damage.[2]

The injuries resulting from closed head injury are of six main types:

1. Primary brainstem damage
2. Diffuse brain damage
3. Traumatic injury to blood vessels
4. Secondary brainstem damage
5. Damage to cranial nerves
6. Traumatic cerebrospinal fluid rhinorrhea

PRIMARY BRAINSTEM DAMAGE. In the majority of cases of head injury, the traumatic event produces acceleration or deceleration of the head. The maximum tolerance of the brain to deceleration is in the range of 188 to 230 Gs with a time duration of 310 to 400 milliseconds.[192] The application of stresses beyond this range may have its greatest effect at the level of the brainstem with the passage of a pressure wave toward the spinal canal. The skull is unable to sustain pressure in this area owing to the presence of the foramen magnum, and the pressure wave will be dissipated in the spinal canal. The result is a sudden downward movement of the brainstem with injury to its contents. Neuronal changes in the upper reticular activating system in the midbrain have been demonstrated in the monkey following experimental head injury.[35] Thus, mild head trauma may produce minor injury to the brainstem, which may be irritative, causing the mild concussive effects of "seeing stars." However, more severe head injury may result in degrees of loss of reticular activation that produce clinical states ranging from transitory depression of cerebral function to irreversible coma. This hypothesis is supported by the demonstration of microglial scars in the periaqueductal gray matter of the midbrain in patients with irreversible coma.[37, 175]

DIFFUSE BRAIN DAMAGE. A number of patients experience sudden loss of consciousness after severe closed head injury and die without evidence of elevation of intracranial pressure. These cases show diffuse damage to white matter with severance of axons due to shear forces applied to the brain at the time of impact.[223] The brain may appear to be normal at autopsy, but detailed examination shows focal lesions in the corpus callosum and the dorsolateral quadrant of the midbrain and microscopic evidence of diffuse damage to white matter. It is possible that there is a gradation of clinical findings following head injury which correspond to the degree of diffuse brain damage produced by the injury.[172] This concept supports an increasing acceptance of the importance of diffuse brain damage in patients with head injuries.[119]

TRAUMATIC INJURY TO BLOOD VESSELS. Posttraumatic arteriospasm is a rare complication of head injury and may result in cerebral infarction.[8] Mass movement of the brain at the moment of impact can cause damage to arterial walls with subsequent formation of a traumatic aneurysm.[9] The vessel may be damaged and weakened by contact with the edge of the falx cerebri or tentorium cerebelli, or by contact with a bony prominence. Damage to the internal carotid artery as it enters the base of the skull is probably the most common form of injury to an intracranial artery following head injury.[109] Traumatic aneurysm produced by this type of injury may eventually rupture into the cavernous sinus producing a traumatic carotid cavernous sinus fistula. The basilar artery is susceptible to injury during fracture of the clivus with thrombosis and basilar infarction of the pons[218] or formation of a traumatic aneurysm. The development of traumatic aneurysms has been reported on all major intracranial arteries and their branches and presents a high risk of subarachnoid hemorrhage in the posttraumatic period in affected individuals.[39] Posttraumatic thrombotic occlusion of the middle cerebral artery is rare compared to traumatic occlusion of extracranial vessels but can occur at any age, sometimes after relatively minor head trauma.[193] The mechanism of thrombus formation is not clear, but arterial spasm, embolism, or dissecting aneurysm arising in damaged carotid arteries in the neck should be considered.[110] Tearing of penetrating intracerebral arteries or veins by shearing may produce subarachnoid hemorrhage or a traumatic intracerebral hematoma at any site in the brain. The cortical veins have relatively little capacity for movement at the point of entry into a venous sinus and may be torn by sudden movements of the brain following head trauma, producing a subdural hematoma. Damage to capillaries is extremely common in head injury and produces the minor degrees of subarachnoid hemorrhage seen after relatively trivial blows to the head. Contact by the moving brain often produces considerable capillary rupture over the tips of the frontal or temporal lobes as they strike bony prominences and results in the bruising in these areas that is commonly seen in head injuries. Capillaries may also be injured by shearing forces within the brain parenchyma or may be damaged by hypoxia after head injury with production of petechial hemorrhages and edema.

SECONDARY BRAINSTEM DAMAGE. The development of cerebral edema following head injury may be a direct effect of damage to the brain or may be due to the effects of hypoxia and/or hypotension, which will produce additional injury to the brain. In either case there will be an increase in the volume of the supratentorial contents and increased intracranial pressure. The expanded volume and increased pressure may be further increased by intracranial hemorrhage including extradural, subdural, and intracerebral hemorrhage. The supratentorial contents are contained within a rigid structure, and there is limited capacity to compensate for any increase in volume. A continuing increase in supratentorial mass results eventually in three major complications.

1. Cingulate herniation. This occurs when there is a relative increase in volume of one hemisphere. There is restricted lateral movement of the expanding hemisphere, which produces a herniation of the cingulate gyrus beneath the falx cerebri. This has the effect of compressing the anterior cerebral vessels producing cerebral ischemia, cerebral infarction, and increasing edema, which further enhances the supratentorial volume.

2. Central or transtentorial herniation with progressive dysfunction of the brainstem. This condition occurs when the expanding supratentorial contents displace the diencephalon and upper midbrain through the tentorial notch. There is a decrease in the angle between the diencephalon and the midbrain, and the diencephalon eventually compresses the anterior aspect of the midbrain. The displacement of the brainstem stretches the penetrating arteries arising from the basilar artery, which is tethered to the circle of Willis. This results in brainstem ischemia followed by arterial necrosis and brainstem hemorrhage.[65] Stretching of the posterior cerebral arteries over the free edge of the tentorium cerebelli also produces ischemia and infarction in the occipital lobes. This adds to the supratentorial edema and supratentorial volume. Progressive brainstem dysfunction due to increased intracranial pressure is also discussed in Chapter 10, page 614.

3. Temporal lobe or uncal herniation. Increased supratentorial pressure with asymmetric involvement will eventually lead to a movement of the midline structures away from the side of the lesion and a movement of the medial aspect of the temporal lobe toward the midline. This movement places the uncus of the temporal lobe over the free edge of the tentorium cerebelli, and increased supratentorial pressure causes herniation of the uncus over the edge of the tentorium displacing the midbrain and compressing it against the edge of the tentorium cerebelli. The effect of uncal herniation is to compress the third nerve and the posterior cerebral artery on the side of the herniation and to compress the midbrain. Further increase in supratentorial pressure

displaces the herniated uncus and the brainstem downward and produces the changes described under central or transtentorial herniation.

DAMAGE TO CRANIAL NERVES. All of the cranial nerves are susceptible to injury by shearing forces that result from cerebral trauma. Damage to cranial nerves is discussed in detail on page 504.

CEREBROSPINAL FLUID RHINOR-RHEA. Sudden increase of intracranial pressure or shearing forces accompanying head trauma occasionally give rise to cerebrospinal fluid rhinorrhea in closed head injury without fracture. This is one of the many causes of cerebrospinal fluid rhinorrhea, which is discussed on page 507.

Penetrating Wounds of the Skull and Brain. This type of injury is usually due to gunshot and mortar wounds and is most frequently seen under conditions of warfare. Similar wounds are not infrequent in civilian practice due to accident, attempted suicide, or homicide. Penetration of the skull by metallic fragments also occurs as the result of industrial accidents. In its mildest form, penetration involves the skull and dura without damage to the brain. There may be an associated linear fracture of the skull, which carries the risk of an extradural hemorrhage if it passes across the middle meningeal artery.

Further penetration of metallic and bone fragments into the brain is often followed by a rapid rise in intracranial pressure. At the same time the pressure waves set up by the missile produce a profound change in brainstem function and there is a fall in systemic blood pressure. The combination of raised intracranial pressure and falling systemic blood pressure produces a marked reduction in cerebral perfusion pressure. However, there is a loss of autoregulation with a reduction in cerebrovascular resistance, and the net effect is a sudden increase in cerebral blood volume which sustains the raised intracranial pressure. This may be augmented by bleeding in the missile track producing tamponade that compresses cerebral veins and further increases cerebral blood volume. The loss of autoregulation transfers the full effect of arterial blood pressure to the capillary bed leading to transudation of fluid and cerebral edema. If the injury is severe, the intracranial pressure will continue to rise and death occurs. When the injury is less severe, the brainstem centers begin to function again, sys-

temic blood pressure rises, and autoregulation is restored, although increased intracranial pressure may remain high due to increasing cerebral edema.[44]

Traumatic Injury to Extracranial Blood Vessels. The internal carotid artery may be damaged by gunshot wounds, a blow to the neck, injury to the face, or stretching over the bony prominence of the atlas when the head is hyperextended. Injuries may result in thrombosis[140] or the development of a traumatic carotid-jugular fistula.[143] Carotid insufficiency or cerebral infarction may occur in such cases.

Vertebral artery injury has been reported in association with chiropractic manipulation,[157] head trauma, cervical traction, voluntary movement, or sudden hyperextension or rotation of the neck.[87] Symptoms of brainstem infarction may occur,[216] and reversible signs of brainstem dysfunction have been reported due to spasm of the vertebral basilar system after head injury.[149]

Craniospinal Injuries. The increasing exposure of humans to injury in high-speed vehicles has led to the recognition that both head and neck trauma play an important role in fatal accidents.[45] Concomitant skull fracture or brain injury and damage to the upper cervical cord occur in some 60 per cent of fatal traffic accidents. The association of head injury with fractures or dislocations of the upper cervical spine, particularly at the C_1-C_2 level, is not uncommon.[220]

A severe head injury causing unconsciousness may mask the neurologic findings of a spinal cord injury. This possibility should be considered in all patients with head injury and loss of consciousness, particularly following a traffic accident.

Pathologic Sequelae of Head Injury

A minor degree of head injury or concussion is by definition a totally reversible neurologic deficit due to a transient loss of brain function. This implies that concussion does not produce structural damage to the brain. However, there is a point in the spectrum of head injury where permanent damage to the brain occurs, although this does not necessarily correlate with clinical findings. It is possible and not infrequent for an individual to suffer severe focal damage to the brain with tissue destruction without loss of consciousness, particularly following penetrating wounds of the frontal lobes. Diffuse damage to the brain with prolonged loss of consciousness is followed by the development of microglial scars in the white matter at the numerous sites of axon fracture. Whether there is also focal neuronal damage and neuronal loss in the brainstem periaqueductal gray matter is still debated between those who believe loss of consciousness is due to diffuse damage to the brain and those who believe that it is due to focal neuronal dysfunction in the brainstem. In either case, severe head trauma is likely to be followed by some neuronal loss in the cortical mantle and deeper gray matter, and the combination of neuronal loss, axonal degeneration, and loss of white matter may present as diffuse brain atrophy (Fig. 8–1). The condition is associated with ventricular dilatation of a compensating nature (hydrocephalus ex vacuo), but hydrocephalus also occurs as a sequel to head injury and the increased pressure in the cerebrospinal fluid may contribute to further brain damage. Hydrocephalus can occur after traumatic subarachnoid hemorrhage, which produces an inflammatory response in the subarachnoid space and is followed by the formation of scars that obliterate the space

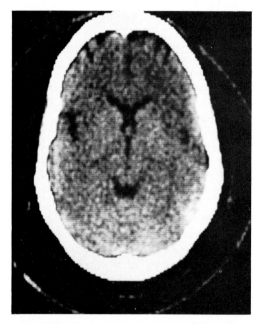

FIGURE 8–1. Computed tomography taken three years after head injury of sufficient degree to produce loss of consciousness followed by right-sided weakness and impairment of memory. The scan shows evidence of cortical atrophy with enlargement of the sulci over both frontal lobes and in the left sylvian region.

and prevent the free circulation of cerebrospinal fluid. A similar picture may occur following minor degrees of brainstem compression with recovery. Damage and kinking of the aqueduct in the midbrain are followed by the formation of scar tissue with narrowing of the channel and obstruction to the flow of cerebrospinal fluid. Atrophy of one hemisphere sometimes occurs when this hemisphere has borne the brunt of the head trauma and may also occur beneath a chronic subdural hematoma with incomplete recovery following removal of the hematoma.

Contusion of the brain in man may be recognized grossly because of rupture of capillaries in the cortex and white matter and destruction of tissue. These lesions heal as golden-brown scars or "plaque jaunes." These lesions are particularly common in the region of the frontal and temporal poles and around the orbital surface of the frontal lobe owing to angular acceleration of the brain and abutment against bony projections, as already discussed. The dead tissue, which includes neurons, astrocytes, and blood elements, is removed by the phagocytic action of microglial cells. There is proliferation of surviving astrocytes with the eventual formation of a glial scar or meningocerebral cicatrix. This scar may contain surviving neurons, which suffer an alteration in blood supply and metabolism and frequently develop the tendency to release spontaneous electrical discharges. This abnormal neuronal activity constitutes the focus causing posttraumatic seizures.

Focal destruction of the brain also occurs in regions of cerebral infarction or intracerebral hemorrhage when these events have occurred after head trauma. The dead tissue is slowly removed by microglia with incomplete replacement by proliferation of astrocytes so that irregular cavities may be formed within the brain substance.

Clinical Aspects of Head Injury in Man

Head Injury Without Loss of Consciousness. It is quite possible for head injury to occur without loss of consciousness, i.e., without concussion, but with some minor or even major degree of contusion or laceration of the brain. The immediate effect is a soreness of the scalp, a short period of feeling "dazed" with mild confusion, lightheadedness, and generalized motor weakness. Transitory cortical blindness with rapid recovery can occur.[72] In the majority of cases, the cerebral injury is mild, but headache is usually experienced for a few days after the injury and the patient complains of irritability, poor concentration, poor memory, and insomnia (post-head-injury syndrome or postconcussion syndrome, see p. 502). These symptoms gradually resolve to complete recovery, although this may take many months. Patients with cerebral laceration and subarachnoid bleeding usually complain of neck stiffness and occipital headache.

Head Injury with Loss of Consciousness. The patient with posttraumatic unconsciousness loses awareness immediately after the impact to the head. In mild concussion, recovery is rapid and occurs within a few minutes. In moderate and severe injury, recovery may be more prolonged. There are five stages in recovery.

STAGE 1: COMA. In mild to moderate posttraumatic unconsciousness, this stage is usually of short duration. There is complete paralysis of all cerebral function with preservation of reflex medullary activity, permitting the pulse, blood pressure, and respirations to be maintained, but there is no response to painful stimulation. The pupils react to light, and reflex eye movements in response to head movements are preserved. In severe posttraumatic unconsciousness, respirations may be stertorous, and this stage may persist for several hours.

STAGE 2: SEMICOMA. With return of some reflex activity, the patient begins to respond to painful stimuli by withdrawal. Vomiting may occur owing to irritation of the vomiting center in the medulla, with the risk of aspiration if the stomach is full.

STAGE 3: STUPOR. The patient becomes restless but is at first mute. He then responds to simple commands but is irritable and resents disturbance. Some patients may become violent or delirious, particularly at night.

STAGE 4: OBTUNDITY. The restlessness and delirium gradually give way to a stage of quiet confusion. The patient responds to the examiner but is disoriented, with defective judgment, insight, and retention. The patient may appear to be elated and often talks excessively with a tendency to confabulate.

STAGE 5: FULLY CONSCIOUS. There is a gradual change over a period of days or hours to full recovery. This usually begins with recovery of orientation followed by insight and ability to retain facts and remember recent events. The severity of head injury may be judged long after the injury by testing the length of *retrograde am-*

nesia. Testing is achieved by asking the patient if he remembers the impact and, if not, what he does remember last. In concussion, the events immediately preceding the blow will be remembered, but in severe head injury, the events for one hour or even the whole day preceding the blow will not be recalled.

Concussion should last a relatively short time, and impaired consciousness should not exceed 12 to 24 hours. Prolongation of unconsciousness beyond this stage or any delay in improvement signifies a more severe head injury. Relapse with regression to an earlier stage suggests the possibility of an intracranial hematoma and is an indication for further investigation. Following concussion, as after other forms of head injury, there may be irritability, poor concentration, and difficulty with reading and memory similar to the symptoms described under the Post-Head-Injury Syndrome. These symptoms may persist for many months but eventual recovery is the rule.

Juvenile Head Trauma Syndrome. This benign syndrome occurs in children who have had relatively trivial head injury and causes considerable distress to parents. The child is known to have suffered relatively minor head trauma producing no more than crying and often followed by return to normal activities. After an interval of several minutes to several hours, there are somnolence, irritability, pallor, vomiting, and headache. This is followed by confusion and even coma in some cases or the appearance of focal neurologic deficits, including cortical blindness in others. The episode may terminate at that point with recovery over a period of several hours, or the child may have a focal or generalized seizure followed by postictal focal paresis and recovery.[91, 169] The episodes that terminate without seizures often present as a severe attack of migraine, and some patients continue to have attacks of classic migraine at intervals after minor head trauma.[132]

Severe Head Injury with Prolonged Coma. It should be recognized that extensive open wounds of the brain may occur with little change in the conscious state. The patient with a severe head injury with unconsciousness passes through the same five stages of recovery discussed under Head Injury with Loss of Consciousness. But there is associated cerebral contusion and/or laceration; hence, each stage tends to be of longer duration and recovery is often incomplete. On examination, a skull fracture may be suspected if there are bluish discolorations around the mastoid, around the orbits, or behind the eardrum (the latter indicates a basal skull fracture). A depressed skull fracture can usually be palpated through the scalp.

There is commonly immediate loss of consciousness, with coma following the injury, although some patients progress into coma over an interval of several hours. Severe head trauma with brain damage produces a critically ill patient with signs of increasing intracranial pressure and shock with hypotension. Poor pulse volume, tachycardia, and a subnormal temperature do not usually occur.[1] When a state of shock is observed, it should raise the question of the presence of a severe internal injury to other organs of the body. The usual sign of severe cerebral contusion is deep coma, with dilated pupils, a sluggish light reflex, and absence of reflex eye movements on head turning, indicating damage to the brainstem.

In severe head injury the body temperature may be persistently subnormal or steadily increase to 104° or 105°F. Both situations carry a poor prognosis. Deep coma of this type, lasting more than three hours, carries a mortality rate of about 20 per cent. The outlook is much better if the patient survives for more than 24 hours without signs of brainstem injury or persisting and prolonged coma. Survivors may remain in a semicomatose state for several days or even weeks before recovery. During the next stage of recovery from cerebral contusion there is restlessness, irritability, and traumatic delirium, which may be prolonged for days or weeks. The neurologic examination often varies from day to day or even hour to hour because of alteration in brain swelling and the general state of the patient. Aphasia, dysphasia, apraxia, and hemiparesis are common. Recovery is frequently incomplete and residual signs of brain damage (see p. 500) are common. These include poor judgment, impaired insight, poor memory, and emotional lability with outburst of temper. Focal signs, including impairment of eye movements, hemiparesis, and ataxia due to brainstem involvement, are not infrequent. Headache and dizziness are usually not complaints of patients who suffer severe head injury but frequently follow more minor trauma.

Diagnostic Procedures

Roentgenographic Examination of the Skull, Cervical Spine, and Chest in Cases of Head Injury. Although the introduction of newer techniques of investigation has decreased the importance of the radiographic examination in the evaluation of the patient with head injury,[187] the roentgenogram remains the first procedure of choice in centers not equipped to perform computerized tomography or arteriography.

THE PATIENT WHO IS UNCONSCIOUS. The patient with head injury who is still unconscious by the time he is seen in the emergency room of a hospital is likely to have a severe head injury. Roentgenograms should be performed as soon as possible after assuring an adequate airway together with proper supervision during transportation to and from the radiology department.

THE PATIENT WHO WAS UNCONSCIOUS BUT SHOWS RAPID RECOVERY. If the duration of unconsciousness was brief, the period of amnesia is insignificant, and the neurologic examination appears to be normal, immediate roentgenograms of the skull are not necessary. The patient should be observed carefully and the vital signs recorded every 15 minutes. If there are any signs of deterioration suggesting an extradural hematoma, the skull roentgenograms should be obtained immediately. Even patients who show rapid neurologic recovery should always have skull and cervical spine roentgenograms at a convenient time within 48 hours of admission to hospital.

THE PATIENT WHO NEVER WAS UNCONSCIOUS. Patients with mild concussion who appear to be neurologically intact should always have a skull roentgenogram when convenient for future reference should their condition deteriorate.

Many patients with severe penetrating injuries may present without loss of consciousness, even though severely injured. These patients all require immediate skull, cervical spine, and chest roentgenograms. This also applies to patients with clinical signs of skull fracture or those who have signs of a progressive neurologic abnormality, even though there has been no loss of consciousness.

Great care should be taken during the transportation of patients with head injury. Unnecessary movement of the cervical spine may lead to injury to the cervical cord so that transportation should be carried out on suitably designed stretchers and the patient should be lifted with adequate support to the head so that the neck is neither flexed nor extended.

SPECIAL CONSIDERATIONS RE-

GARDING ROENTGENOGRAMS OF THE SKULL. Although anteroposterior and lateral views of the skull are usually sufficient for examination of patients with minor head injury without loss of consciousness, cases with neurologic signs require more extensive roentgenographic studies, and a neurologist should become expert in their interpretation. A stereoscopic lateral and separate right and left lateral views of the skull show considerably more detail than a single lateral exposure. Frontal exposures should include the Caldwell projection to examine the orbits and the frontal and ethmoid sinuses. The Waters projection is useful for showing the maxillary sinuses and the floor of the orbit. The occipital (Towne's) projection and the submentovertical projection permit adequate visualization of the base of the skull. Oblique and tangential views may be required to clarify abnormalities seen in the other projections. These special projections should be ordered after consultation with the radiologist.

Skull fractures vary according to the age of the patient and the type of forces exerted on the skull. The soft bones of the infant or young child often bend like a ping-pong ball beneath the area of trauma. The depression usually persists without a clearly defined fracture line owing to impaction of the bone edges and may contuse or compress the underlying brain.

Linear fractures of the skull are usually not of great importance unless they pass through the course of the middle meningeal artery or involve the middle ear or one of the paranasal sinuses. They do indicate, however, that the skull has been struck with considerable force, and hence there is the possibility of intracranial injury, despite the fact that the patient may not have neurologic complaints at the time of examination. The recent linear fracture is sharply defined, appearing as a dark line with jagged margins that taper toward the periphery and finally blend with the normal bone. There are usually angular changes in its course, which help to differentiate it from vascular markings. The relationship of the fracture line to vascular channels is of particular importance in the temporal and parietal areas. Almost all cases of epidural hematoma show a linear fracture in the temporoparietal area crossing the meningeal vascular markings. Old fractures of long standing tend to be blurred at the edges and less distinct.

In general, there is little difficulty in determining or recognizing linear fractures involving the cranial vault, but fractures at the base of the skull are difficult to recognize roentgenographically. Many small fractures at the base are not visualized in routine roentgenograms of the skull, and fractures of the base that are evident at autopsy or are suspected from physical examination (such as blood and spinal fluid emerging from the ears) may not be recognized from roentgenograms of the skull.

Comminuted fractures of the skull are usually the result of injuries of high velocity. The majority occur over the cranial vault and are rarely seen at the base of the skull. There is usually some depression of comminuted fragments, some of which usually enter the brain. There may be one or more linear fractures extending out in radial fashion ("cartwheel fractures"). Stereoscopic views and special tangential films may be necessary to define the amount of depression of bone fragments. Depression of bone fragments by more than 0.5 cm should be considered to be associated with laceration of the dura and underlying brain and to be an indication for surgical decompression.

A compound fracture of the skull, by definition, is present when some communication exists with the outside air. This usually occurs through the scalp but may result if the fracture extends into the middle ear or paranasal sinuses. The threat of a compound fracture is intracranial infection with the possibility of osteomyelitis of the skull and intracerebral abscess. All compound fractures should be treated by surgical removal of any foreign material, including hair and bone fragments. The wound should be closed and antibiotic therapy administered.

Certain associated abnormalities may be observed in roentgenograms of the skull which should suggest the presence of a skull fracture. Soft tissue swelling of the scalp should suggest the possibility of underlying skull fracture, although this may have already been noted on clinical examination. Decreased air or fluid in the mastoid air cells or a fluid level in the sphenoid sinus following head injury is highly suggestive, and the presence of intracranial air is virtually diagnostic of skull fracture.

About 80 per cent of normal adults have calcification of the pineal gland, which can usually be recognized from roentgenograms of the skull. The choroid plexus is also sufficiently calcified to be seen in about 30 per cent of individuals. The pineal gland is usually displaced in unilateral space-occupying lesions, including sub- and epidural hematomas. Hemorrhage or hematoma into the contents of the posterior fossa may produce elevation of the pineal gland in lateral views of the skull, which can be measured due to its relation to standard points of reference in the skull such as the foramen magnum and the sella turcica. Calcification of the choroid plexus usually appears as symmetric curvilinear and paramedian shadows in the anteroposterior view. Loss of such symmetry suggests displacement by a space-occupying lesion such as an intracranial hematoma.

Practical clinical considerations concerning roentgenographic examination of the cervical spine will be discussed later when injuries of the spine and spinal cord are considered (p. 513). But it should be borne in mind that associated injury to the cervical spine and spinal cord is common following injury to the head, and roentgenograms of the cervical spine are indicated in such cases.

Roentgenograms of the chest are also useful since they permit later comparison with other films if pneumonia or atelectasis due to aspiration should develop. Unsuspected intrathoracic injury or atelectasis following aspiration of blood or vomiting may be revealed.

Computed Tomography in Head Injury. The use of computed tomography has sharply reduced the need for other procedures in the management of head-injured patients, and the CT scan and skull roentgenogram are the first procedures performed in many major centers.[159] The CT scan can be performed without anesthesia in many cases, although restless patients may require intubation and general anesthesia to obtain an adequate scan.[68] The high-density areas produced by intracerebral or acute subdural hematomas may be distinguished early in most cases and enhanced by the use of iodinized contrast material.[160] Cerebral edema presents as an area of low density, and multiple areas of abnormality can often be seen in a single study. Sequential CT scanning should be employed in all cases who fail to improve or who deteriorate[5] to detect the development of complications such as subdural hematoma or hydrocephalus. Serial scans are also useful in monitoring the treatment of cerebral edema.[127] In addition to hematomas and cerebral edema, depressed skull fractures and intracranial air are readily detected by computed tomography.[38] The herniation of intracranial contents into the ethmoidal, frontal, or sphenoidal sinuses

can usually be demonstrated by the CT scan. Injuries to the orbit, including damage to the optic nerves and frontobasal fractures, can be seen in most cases. The presence of posttraumatic infection in the paranasal sinuses or in the brain may be detected by sequential scanning when there is a possibility of traumatic communication between the sinuses and the cranial cavity.

The Use of Echoencephalography in Head Injury. The term "echoencephalography" refers to the use of ultrasound in examining the intracranial contents. It is a useful and simple technique, when employed as a screening method in the emergency room following head injury. The principle of the method requires that echos be recorded after transmitting ultrasonic impulses through the skull and its intracranial structures. The echos are displayed on a cathode ray screen, and normally those derived from the scalp, the outer and inner tables of the skull, and the walls of the third ventricle in the midline are easily recognizable. A shift of the midline echo derived from the third ventricle of more than 2 mm indicates displacement of the third ventricle due to a space-occupying lesion such as a hematoma. A fluid collection next to the outer and inner tables representing a subdural or epidural hematoma and, in more chronic cases, a subdural hygroma or leptomeningeal cyst can be registered by this method. An abnormal echoencephalogram, when reported by an experienced individual, should be considered as an indication for computed tomography.

Electroencephalography in Cerebral Trauma. The EEG is useful in the investigation of head injury, particularly when serial records are taken at intervals of 24 hours during the acute phase and at longer intervals for the follow-up investigation (Fig. 8–2). The electroencephalographer should consider a number of factors when interpreting the records. For example, it is rare to have a "control" tracing taken before the injury for comparison with the recordings made after injury. Furthermore, it is often difficult to obtain recordings free of artefacts in patients who are restless or uncooperative or who are receiving intensive care. Symmetry of electrode placement is often impossible because of lacerations, swelling, or hematomas of the scalp or a skull defect due to penetrating wounds. Pulsation artefact,

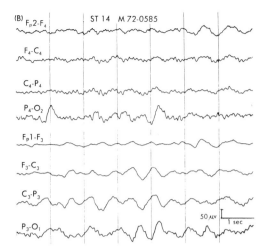

FIGURE 8–2. Electroencephalogram recorded following acute head injury. This EEG shows marked suppression of normal activity on the side of the injury with the presence of moderate- to high-voltage 2-cps delta activity and the recording of phase reversal from C_3 and P_3 leads. The suppression of activity and marked slowing in these areas are due to underlying cerebral contusion and infarction. The isoelectric activity in the occipital areas is probably due to occipital lobe contusion or ischemia in the posterior cerebral arterial distribution due to compression of these arteries. The low-voltage delta activity noted on the right side may be due to compression of these arteries. The low-voltage delta activity noted on the right side may be due to either cerebral ischemia or contusion of the right hemisphere. Electrode positions: F_p, frontopolar; *F*, frontal; *C*, central; *P*, parietal; *O*, occipital. Even numbers, right hemisphere. Odd numbers, left hemisphere.

transmitted through cranial defects, can also mimic delta activity.

The following recommendations are made for the management of patients with head injury, particularly when CT scanning is not available.

1. The first EEG record should be obtained as soon as possible after injury, with serial recordings at intervals of 24 hours if the patient is comatose or stuporous. If the patient has recovered consciousness and the record shows minor abnormalities, it is still advisable to repeat the EEG at least twice in the next 48-hour period before discharge from the hospital, since unexpected deterioration could occur during that period. This precaution reduces the risk of delay in detecting a complication

such as a progressive increase in intracranial pressure due to extradural hematoma, subdural hematoma, or brain edema. After the patient is discharged from the hospital, arrangements should be made to repeat the EEG after three or four weeks to rule out the development of chronic subdural hematoma.

2. Initial improvement in the EEG, followed by deterioration with the appearance of a generalized, localized, or lateralized abnormality, suggests the presence of a subdural hematoma. Improvement of the background activity on one side with deterioration over the other hemisphere is often due to a rapidly progressive subdural hematoma or progressive focal edema occurring in an area of infarction, severe cerebral contusion, or intracerebral hematoma. The delayed appearance of diffuse slowing may be due to cerebral edema.

3. Older patients with significant cerebrovascular disease and a marginal arterial circulation may show deterioration in the EEG owing to further impairment of the cerebral circulation in the presence of raised intracranial pressure. It is possible to record maximal slowing on the side opposite a subdural hematoma, cerebral contusion, or intracerebral hematoma in such cases when there is a severe stenosis of internal carotid artery or middle cerebral artery on the side of maximal slowing.

4. Auditory, tactile, and painful stimuli should be applied during the EEG recording and noted on the record.

Many EEG abnormalities have been encountered following head injury. When the injury is mild, the EEG may be normal. Serial records in head injury with a small cerebral contusion have shown that there is usually alpha asymmetry with a return to normal over a period of weeks or months. Occasionally there is the development of high-amplitude alpha activity on the side of the injury.

The EEG is always abnormal in severe head injuries. The immediate changes are due to cerebral contusions, extracerebral or intracerebral hematomas, or infarction. The patients have some degree of impairment of consciousness at the time of recording, and it is possible to demonstrate some correlation between the level of consciousness and the degree of EEG abnormality. Patients who are obtunded or stuporous may show diffuse theta activity, while more severe cases of head injury who are semicomatose or comatose will have diffuse delta activity. If the background activity improves on painful stimulation with the appearance of some alpha activity, the prognosis is better. Occasionally, the background activity presents as diffuse alpha activity in all leads in the presence of deep coma. Such cases carry a poor prognosis, and the EEG shows rapid deterioration over the next few days. This change probably reflects the presence of severe trauma to the midbrain or pons with relative sparing of the cortical structures in the period immediately following head injury. The deeply comatose patient with a severe and focal head injury usually presents with diffuse high amplitude delta activity in the acute phase. The amplitude may progressively decrease, and some focal abnormality of slower delta activity may be seen. Irreversible brain damage is indicated by a persistently flat EEG recorded at high gains (see p. 488). In severe head injury with survival, focal abnormalities usually appear after a few days, and the amplitude and frequency of these focal changes progressively increase. An electroencephalographic pattern resembling sleep may occasionally be recorded after head injury with symmetric sleep spindles over both hemispheres. This is also replaced by diffuse theta activity followed by the gradual development of alpha activity on recovery.

The occurrence of focal slowing in an EEG that has a generalized slowing of background activity following head injury may indicate contusion; epidural, subdural, or intracerebral hematoma; or cerebral infarction. These patients require neurosurgical consultation and further investigation. The presence of a subdural hematoma should be suspected if there is asymmetric or unilateral slowing, or if the alpha is suppressed over one hemisphere. An increase in slow activity appearing in serial records with bilateral and progressive loss of alpha activity is strongly suggestive of bilateral subdural hematoma. In cases of large subdural hematomas and brainstem compression, there may be episodic bilateral and synchronous slowing in both anterior head regions. In such cases, stimulation may cause increase in frequencies over one hemisphere only or focal slowing may be recognized intermittently on the side of the hematoma.

Visual, Auditory, and Somatosensory Evoked Potentials in Head Injury.

Data obtained from evoked potential studies in comatose patients with severe head trauma indicate that these electrophysiologic procedures may be useful in the determination of the extent of head injury and prognosis.[81, 133] Abnormalities in visual, auditory, and somatosensory evoked potentials indicate that decortication or decerebration depends on cerebral hemisphere dysfunction rather than brainstem dysfunction. The majority of patients with lesser degrees of abnormality in multimodality evoked potentials recover consciousness and have a much better prognosis than those with severe disturbances recorded early after injury.[80]

Arteriography in the Evaluation of Cerebral Trauma.

Computed tomography has replaced arteriography as the method of choice in the evaluation of head injury in most centers. However, arteriography remains important when a CT scan is not available, and some neurosurgeons still prefer to perform arteriography even if they have a CT scan in cases with a suspected intracranial hematoma. The methods employed in arteriography vary, but selective catheterization of the cervical vessels, using a transfemoral approach and series films taken at one-half-second intervals with a biplane apparatus, is probably the best technique.

Characteristic changes produced in the arteriogram by subdural, epidural, and intracerebral hematomas will be discussed later. In brief, if the anterior cerebral artery is displaced to the side opposite the lesion, it is an indication of herniation of the frontal lobe under the falx. The middle cerebral vessels are displaced away from the skull by subdural and epidural hematomas. The branches of the middle cerebral artery are distorted by intracerebral hematomas.

The Spinal Fluid in Head Injury.

Lumbar puncture is rarely performed in the evaluation of an acute head-injured patient, since the examination of the cerebrospinal fluid adds little to the knowledge gained by the use of more sophisticated techniques. It is possible that determination of CSF enzyme activity may be of prognostic value in the assessment of head injury in the future, since elevated enzyme levels appear to correlate with the degree of brain damage.[164] However, lumbar puncture is probably only of value at this time in the detection of early infection of the subarachnoid space following head injury with skull fracture.

Treatment

Emergency Treatment of Closed Head Injury. The majority of closed head injuries are the result of automobile accidents, although falls, industrial accidents, and certain sports add to the problem. Severe injuries in which there has been sufficient force to crush the skull are usually fatal within a few minutes of impact. Less severe and nonfatal blows causing closed head injury may result in concussion, intracranial hematomas, contusion, and laceration of the brain, depending on the severity and type of injury. The detection of intracranial hematomas depends on careful examination and continued observation of the patient thereafter for changes in the level of consciousness and the development of focal neurologic abnormalities. During the period of observation, facilities for emergency care should be arranged and a diagnostic program should be planned.[231]

When a patient arrives in the emergency ward, the first concern should be the establishment of an unobstructed airway for respiratory exchange.[59, 188, 214] The mouth and larynx should be cleared of secretions. If there is nasopharyngeal bleeding or the accumulation of mucus that cannot be removed by suctioning, a low-pressure, cuffed endotracheal tube should be inserted to ensure free respiratory exchange. If cardiovascular shock occurs following a head injury, it is usually due to blood loss from other areas of the body rather than directly due to cerebral trauma. Circulatory shock should be treated with intravenous fluids, plasma, blood transfusions, and vasopressor agents. Drawing of blood samples for immediate typing and cross-matching is required for those patients requiring transfusion. The patient should then receive a rapid but complete examination to determine the extent of injury.[243] Bleeding from scalp wounds may cause sufficient blood loss to cause circulatory shock, but the possibility of hemothorax and intra-abdominal bleeding should always be considered.

Once a satisfactory airway has been established and any necessary treatment for shock has been instituted, detailed neurologic examination can be performed to ascertain the extent of head injury. Scalp wounds should be noted and the underlying skull palpated with the fingertips to detect any depressed fracture. The presence of blood in the external auditory canal or behind the eardrum suggests a basal skull fracture involving the middle cranial fossa. An ecchymosis over the mastoid process (Battle's sign) indicates a fracture of the base of the skull. Epistaxis may also result from fractures of the base of the skull involving the perinasal sinuses, particularly the sphenoid sinus. Drainage of clear fluid from the nose or ear, termed "cerebrospinal fluid rhinorrhea" or "otorrhea" (p. 506), also indicates a fracture involving the paranasal sinuses or ear.[233]

The neurologic examination should be carefully recorded so that the neurologic status can be compared from hour to hour. The pulse, blood pressure, and respirations should be recorded at intervals of 15 minutes during the first 24 hours since they are sensitive indicators of dangerous increase in intracranial pressure.[48] If intracranial pressure compresses the brainstem, the blood pressure rises, the respirations become periodic, and the pulse slows. If the vasomotor center becomes irreversibly damaged or compressed, the blood pressure falls and death is a possibility as a result of vasomotor collapse. Roentgenograms of the skull and cervical spine should be obtained at an early stage, followed immediately by computed tomography, but they should be obtained with as little movement of the patient as possible.

In all cases of severe head injury, the neurosurgeon should be called in consultation since he may elect to perform emergency craniotomy after arteriography to evacuate any demonstrated hematoma and to reduce increased intracranial pressure.

Medical Management of Patients with Head Injury: General Considerations. The majority of patients with head injury do not require surgery, and medical treatment therefore would follow that outlined under emergency care. The patient who is comatose or stuporous requires the same treatment as that outlined for the treatment of other conditions causing impaired consciousness. The patient should be turned from side to side every two hours to improve pulmonary exchange and to drain dependent parts of the lungs as well as to prevent the formation of decubitus ulcers.[53] Suctioning of the bronchi should be performed with sterile plastic catheters to reduce the risk of infection. If there is any infection, cultures should be made of the aspirated material. Although the use of prophylactic antibiotics is justified, the detection and identification of the pathogens and resistant strains of bacteria are important not only in the treatment of the patient but also to prevent spread of infection to other patients in the intensive care unit. Intermittent positive pressure respiration may be necessary to treat atelectasis and to improve ventilation. In such cases, determination of arterial P_{CO_2}, P_{O_2}, and pH levels is useful in assessing respiratory function.[89]

Many patients with head injury develop impairment of control of temperature regulation owing to hypothalamic injury and are prone to develop hyperthermia. This can be treated in most cases by covering the patient with a single sheet and maintaining the room temperature at 68°F. More severe cases will require a hypothermic mattress. The temperature should be recorded rectally every two hours, and the patient should be treated by intramuscular chlorpromazine if the temperature rises above 101°F.

Continuous cardiac monitoring should be carried out during the first four days after severe head injury because of the occurrence of some form of cardiac arrhythmia in a significant number of cases.[58]

Physical therapy should be instituted at an early stage.[194] Passive movement of the joints through a full range of motion prevents contractures, which are disabling and painful and impede functional recovery.

The comatose patient requires catheterization of the bladder on admission. Catheterization should be performed, using aseptic technique, and the catheter should be changed at weekly intervals. The incidence of urinary tract infection can be reduced to a minimum by the use of careful asepsis while changing the catheter and irrigation of the bladder with a neomycin-polymyxin solution twice daily.

There is usually a retention of fluid in the comatose head-injured patient during the first few days. In adults fluids should be restricted to 1,000 ml/day during this period unless the patient is receiving dexamethasone, in which case the requirement will be higher, i.e., about 2,000 ml/day. Fluids may be given intravenously or by nasogastric tube. It is essential to monitor daily fluid intake and output and daily serum sodium chloride, potassium, and blood urea nitrogen levels during this period to prevent dehydration and to detect inappropriate secretion of antidiuretic hormone. This condition is not uncommon after head injury and can be detected by the progressive development of oliguria with the osmolality of the urine exceeding the osmolality of the serum. Most cases respond to fluid restriction.

The recovery of the patient with head injury is usually associated with a period of restlessness, combativeness, and confusion. These symptoms can be treated by the use of phenothiazine drugs or by paraldehyde given rectally or through a nasogastric tube. Opiates and other narcotics should be avoided because they depress respirations and worsen the neurologic status.

As already mentioned, hypotensive episodes are usually due to causes other than head injury. If hemorrhage at other sites and impaired cardiac failure are excluded, the possibility that the hypotension may be due to hypothalamic injury with disturbance of pituitary function should be considered, and steroids may be given.

A number of centers now use continuous ventricular, subarachnoid, or extradural pressure monitoring in the management of head injuries.[52, 235] These methods will detect early increase in intracranial pressure due to cerebral edema, intracranial hematoma, or hydrocephalus and indicate the need for computed tomography. Mild cases of cerebral edema often respond to restricted fluid intake. If cerebral edema is severe, the most effective therapy appears to be the intramuscular injection of dexamethasone, 10 mg initially followed by an additional 4 mg every eight hours.[121] The intravenous use of diuretic agents, which cause plasma hyperosmolality, such as intravenous urea or mannitol, is also effective in reducing severe cerebral edema. Mannitol is administered as an intravenous infusion of a 25 per cent solution at the rate of 5 gm/minute in doses of 0.25 gm/kg of body weight.[150] The continuous monitoring of intracranial pressure will detect the response to mannitol infusion and the "rebound" after several hours. This return of increased intracranial pressure can be prevented by further infusion of mannitol, and the relatively low dosage of 0.25 gm/kg body weight reduces the risk of severe dehydration and electrolyte imbalance if serial infusions of mannitol are used to control intracranial hypertension.

Bifrontal decompressive craniotomy may be necessary in cases with massive cerebral edema who fail to respond to glucocorticoids or hyperosmotic agents.[125]

The majority of patients with minor nonpenetrating injuries to the head followed by a short period of coma are able to leave the hospital and return home within an interval of one to two weeks. The more severely injured require more prolonged care and transfer to a rehabilitation unit followed by a period of ambulatory treatment on an outpatient basis. Specific defects such as dysphasia, dysarthria, incoordination, and difficulties with gait can be treated effectively by suitable rehabilitation. Consideration should also be given to vocational rehabilitation if a patient is unable to return to his former occupation as a result of injury to the brain. A program of this type requires the cooperation of the neurosurgeon, neurologist, physiatrist, physical therapist, speech therapist, social worker, and vocational rehabilitationist.

Treatment of Penetrating Injuries of the Skull and Brain. All penetrating injuries involving the skull require prompt neurosurgical treatment. They are usually caused by gunshot and mortar wounds, so that they become of major importance in wartime.[32] They also occur in civilian practice from accidents involving sharp instruments or objects moving at high velocity. A penetrating wound of the scalp should be thoroughly explored to exclude the possibility of an underlying injury to the skull. Prompt treatment of a penetrating wound is the best means of preventing infection, for the use of antibiotics will not prevent intracranial sepsis unless all foreign bodies and devitalized or necrotic tissue are removed from the brain.[43, 55] Another aim of early neurosurgical treatment of penetrating wounds of the brain is to control increased intracranial pressure by the removal of intracranial hematomas and to reduce cerebral edema by evacuation of severely injured brain substance. Certain penetrating injuries such as the passage of a foreign body into or through the ventricular system or the rupture of major blood vessels are likely to have a fatal outcome unless they are treated within a few hours of injury.

Adequate neurosurgical care assumes that all necessary measures will be taken to prevent systemic complications following the surgical procedure. High standards of medical, neurologic, and nursing care are required during the postoperative period.

With such standards of care in mind, the following steps are recommended for treatment of penetrating wounds of the skull and brain:

1. All layers of the scalp, including the periosteum, should be excised around the edges of the wound.
2. All depressed and comminuted bone fragments should be removed.
3. The dural edges should be identified and excised at the site of penetration.
4. Careful exploration of the missile track should be made with resection of all devitalized tissue and removal by suction of all macerated cerebral tissues.
5. Fragments of metal and bone and other foreign bodies should be removed from the surrounding brain. Failure to remove bone fragments and nonmetallic foreign bodies usually leads to the development of a brain abscess.
6. Intracranial hematomas are common following penetrating wounds of the brain and require removal and hemostasis.
7. It is particularly important to remove foreign bodies from transventricular wounds because ventricular infection and bleeding are fatal. Bleeding from the choroid plexus should be controlled by resection or coagulation.
8. Wounds involving the dural sinuses may cause air embolism, so that considerable care should be exercised in the removal of blood clots near the sinuses. A lacerated sinus can often be sutured without occlusion.
9. The danger of fatal cerebral edema in the postoperative period can be reduced by the use of steroids, intravenous mannitol or urea, and repeated lumbar puncture.

Following penetrating wounds of the skull, the majority of patients are acutely ill and often are comatose or stuporous, so that the ultimate success of the surgical treatment will depend on the standards of postoperative medical and nursing care that have already been outlined in the care of closed head injury. Intubation with a low-pressure, cuffed endotracheal tube and frequent suctioning of secretions will prevent atelectasis or aspiration pneumonia. Any impairment of pulmonary function may be fatal by causing retention of carbon dioxide, which increases cerebral blood flow and may increase cerebral edema and intracranial pressure. The patient's chest should be examined daily. Clinical signs of dullness on percussion and diminished breath sounds on auscultation suggest atelectasis, which should be confirmed by roentgenograms of the chest and treated by bronchoscopy and removal of mucous plugs in the bronchi as soon as possible.

Disseminated Intravascular Coagulation in Head Injury. Many patients with moderate or severe head injury have destruction of brain tissue which may be followed by the release of tissue emboli[136] or thromboplastin in the systemic circulation.[234] Disseminated intravascular coagulation can be triggered by thromboplastin and has been reported shortly after head injury.[124] The circulating thromboplastin activates the coagulation mechanism, and fibrin thrombi form in small vessels throughout the body. The process incorporates platelets and several clotting factors that are depleted with a resulting bleeding diathesis. The disturbance of coagulation may increase intracranial bleeding or prolong hemorrhage from traumatic lesions in other parts of the body.[74] Disseminated intravascular coagulation will also increase the difficulty of performing neurosurgical procedures because of severe bleeding.

Disseminated intravascular coagulation probably occurs more frequently than previously suspected after head injury, and coagulation studies should be performed in patients with massive cerebral trauma or if there is excessive or uncontrolled bleeding from venous or arterial puncture sites. Abnormalities in the coagulation profile include a low platelet count, decreased serum fibrinogen, excess fibrinogen split products, increased prothrombin time, increased thrombin time, and failure of clot formation in the euglobulin clot lysis test.[153]

Heparin has been recommended in the treatment of disseminated intravascular coagulation, but heparin should probably not be used when there are open wounds or when surgical procedures may be contemplated. Replacement therapy with fibrinogen, platelet concentrates, or plasma factor concentrates is usually effective.

Traumatic Meningeal Hemorrhage

Hemorrhages into the epidural, subdural, and subarachnoid space are frequent complications following head injury, and are important causes of death and disability. Acute epidural hemorrhage usually causes death within 24 hours and should be regarded as a surgical emergency requiring prompt treatment. Acute subdural hematoma usually accompanies severe damage to the brain and carries a high mortality. Subarachnoid hemorrhage is occasionally associated with epidural and subdural hematomas.

Epidural Hemorrhage

Epidural hemorrhage has been defined as an acute hemorrhage with accumulation of blood between the skull and the dura. This condition occurs in about 1 to 3 per cent of patients with severe head injuries. This is usually due to tearing of the middle meningeal vessels by disruption from a linear fracture of the skull.

Etiology and Pathology

The middle meningeal artery enters the skull through the foramen spinosum and divides into the anterior and posterior branches, which run in shallow grooves over the inner surface of the bones of the cranial vault. Each branch is accompanied by two or more thin-walled veins. Either the arteries or veins or both may be torn as a result of a skull fracture that crosses the path of the middle meningeal artery or one of its branches. This often results in a combination of arterial and venous bleeding. Blood accumulates in the epidural space, between the dura and bone in the temporoparietal area. As the volume of blood increases, the brain is subjected to pressure and distortion. This usually is fatal often within 24 hours unless the epidural clot is removed and bleeding controlled.

Epidural hemorrhage has occasionally been reported to result from traumatic rupture of a dural sinus or traumatic laceration of the internal carotid artery at the base of the skull.[240] Bleeding from the superior sagittal sinus produces a hematoma overlying the upper frontoparietal area,[36] while rupture of the transverse sinus results in a rare type of epidural hematoma occurring in the posterior fossa. Epidural hematomas have occurred without evidence of a skull fracture, predominantly in patients under the age of 30.[67]

The epidural clot has a discoid shape on section and the underlying brain often shows evidence of contusion, laceration, or intracerebral hematoma, particularly of the temporal lobe. Fatal cases show displacement of the brain to the opposite site across the midline, with brain edema, uncal herniation, and secondary venous hemorrhages in the midbrain and pons.

Clinical Features

The classic history of head injury followed by unconsciousness (the concussive effects) followed by recovery, a lucid interval, then drowsiness, stupor, and deepening coma occurs in about 50 per cent of cases. The initial period of unconsciousness is usually short, but the lucid interval may vary from 15 minutes to several hours and, very rarely, may last for as long as 30 days. It should be remembered that a number of patients do not have any initial loss of consciousness, but following the head injury, they exhibit progressive drowsiness, obtundity, stupor, and coma over a period of several hours. Others remain drowsy throughout and develop nuchal rigidity and well-marked focal signs, particularly contralateral hemiparesis. Another pattern consists of alternating periods of stupor and mental clarity occurring over a period of several days, particularly in epidural hematoma of the posterior fossa.[179] Those with severe head injury and an associated intracerebral hematoma may remain unconscious from the time of the accident but develop deepening coma under observation. Use of alcohol, drugs, or a history of seizures prior to head injury may delay diagnosis.[131]

Patients with epidural hemorrhage are usually young adults, but the condition can occur at any age, including infancy. There is usually some degree of nuchal rigidity unless the patient is in deep coma, and papilledema has occurred in some cases within a few hours of injury. Focal signs include edema of the scalp over the site of injury, contralateral hemiparesis, and occasionally focal motor seizures. There is progressive deepening of stupor and coma, with increased intracranial pressure and signs of uncal herniation, including unilateral dilatation of the pupil, Cheyne-Stokes respirations followed by a loss of reflex eye movements, and decerebrate rigidity, which may be episodically present or elicited by painful stimulation. At this stage, plantar stimulation results in extensor plantar responses; the pulse is slow (40 to 55 per minute); there is central pontine hyperventilation; and the blood pressure usually shows progressive elevation.

Diagnostic Procedures

Almost all cases of epidural hemorrhage show radiographic evidence of a linear fracture in the temporoparietal area, crossing the meningeal vascular markings. Displacement of the pineal gland to the opposite side is usually noted if the pineal gland is calcified.

Acute epidural hemorrhage is easily seen on computed tomography because of the high density of the fresh blood clot.[13] The hemorrhage appears as an area of increased density that separates the brain from the inner table of the skull. There may be enhancement of the area with the use of contrast material when the contrast material passes into the epidural space. Selective external carotid arteriography is indicated in cases with delayed onset of symptoms since bleeding may occur from a traumatic false aneurysm on one of the branches of the middle meningeal artery.[102] Vertebral angiography should be performed in cases with occipital skull fracture and suspected posterior fossa hematoma.[128, 184]

Treatment

If there has been time to perform computed tomography with verification of the location of the hemorrhage, surgical exploration is usually performed on an emergency basis. In extremely ill patients, surgical exploration may have to be made before diagnostic procedures can be carried out, in which case the openings in the skull should be made along the site of the fracture. Hematomas in the temporal region are usually treated by subtemporal decompression, while those over the convexity require a bone flap. After the clot is evacuated, the dura should be opened to exclude any associated subdural hematoma. Hemostasis is then secured and the wound closed. Postoperative complications are infrequent unless there has been brainstem compression or associated intracerebral hematoma, in which case the mortality rate is higher.

Subdural Hematoma: General Considerations

The subdural hematoma, particularly the chronic subdural hematoma, is the most common type of meningeal hemorrhage in neurologic practice. It is one of the most common remediable lesions which is misdiagnosed and passes untreated to the necropsy table. *Because subdural hematoma is often misdiagnosed, it is considered to be a subject of the utmost importance.* There is a marked difference in the semeiology and prognosis of acute and chronic forms of subdural hematoma. Three forms are recognized, acute, subacute, and chronic, each of which will be discussed separately.

Acute Subdural Hematoma

Etiology and Pathology

An acute subdural hematoma may be defined as an acute venous hemorrhage into the subdural space following head injury due to rupture of emissary and bridging veins as they cross the subdural space to enter the sagittal, sphenoparietal, lateral, or superior petrosal sinuses. In rare cases, contusion or laceration of the surface of the brain and the overlying pia and arachnoid may lead to accumulation of blood in the subdural space. The volume of the acute subdural hematoma often amounts to 150 ml. The blood usually clots after a short period of time and hemolyzes later.

There are associated contusions, lacerations, and hematoma formations in the brain, particularly in the frontal and temporal poles, and a skull fracture may be present in some cases. While the majority of acute subdural hematomas follow head injury, a certain number result from rupture of congenital saccular aneurysms, bleeding from an arteriovenous malformation, or as rare complications of anticoagulant therapy and blood dyscrasias.

The acute subdural hematoma is infrequent in the posterior fossa except in infants, due to birth injury. This produces tearing of the transverse sinus or great vein of Galen, with acute and often fatal subdural hemorrhage.

Clinical Features

The majority of patients with acute subdural hematoma have suffered a severe head injury with loss of consciousness. They remain unconscious and have a progressively deteriorating course. The minority present with symptoms typical of those described when discussing "classic" epidural hemorrhage. They suffer an initial period of unconsciousness followed by a lucid interval and then deterioration with drowsiness progressing to stupor and coma. In some cases the history is that of a conscious patient who shows a slowly deteriorating course.

A certain number of cases show venous engorgement of the retina and papilledema due to increased intracranial pressure, but this is often absent. Unilateral dilatation of the pupil is an ominous sign, indicating brainstem compression due to uncal herniation. Some 50 per cent of patients develop a contralateral hemiparesis and another 20 per cent an ipsilateral hemiparesis. The ipsilateral hemiparesis is due to compression of the corticospinal tract in the midbrain against the opposite tentorial edge. Signs of brainstem compression (p. 614) can develop within a few hours, with decerebration and bilateral extensor plantar responses.

Diagnostic Procedures

1. Roentgenograms of the skull may reveal a fracture or displacement of the calcified pineal gland to the opposite side.
2. Computed tomography will readily demonstrate the high-density, acute subdural hematoma lying between the inner table of the skull and the surface of the brain. The midline structures are displaced to the opposite side, and there is often evidence of damage to the brain with associated intracerebral hemorrhage and edema.[135] Quicker diagnosis by computed to-

mography may contribute to reduced mortality and morbidity in patients who have a reversible injury and subdural hematoma.[202]
3. Many neurosurgeons prefer to perform arteriography after the CT scan to confirm the site and extent of the hematoma and to demonstrate damage to or extravasation from laceration of major vessels.

Treatment

The acute subdural hematoma should be drained as soon as possible, and the condition, like the epidural hemorrhage, should be regarded as a surgical emergency.

Many neurosurgeons prefer to remove the subdural hematoma by craniotomy[197] rather than through burr holes, since recurrence is less likely following craniotomy.[105] The mortality remains above 50 per cent in many series despite postoperative treatment with corticosteroids and dehydration agents, which is an indication of the severity of the underlying brain damage in the majority of patients with acute subdural hematoma.[62]

Subacute Subdural Hematoma

There are also cases of subdural hematoma that have a subacute course and carry a much better prognosis than the acute form. They usually arise as a sequel to a more trivial head injury, and the venous bleeding is slower. The subdural space contains a mixture of blood and cerebrospinal fluid.

Clinical Features

Some 60 per cent of cases have a lucid interval following head injury, which is followed by drowsiness, stupor, and coma. However, the patient does not show a steady, deteriorating course; and the condition appears to become stable for a number of days. This period is followed by fluctuating signs of drowsiness and generalized rigidity with increasing intracranial pressure. Death results unless the subdural hematoma is relieved.

The diagnosis is established by computed tomography. This procedure should be carried out with enhancement with intravenous contrast material, since there is a progressive decrease in absorption values in a hematoma so that the absorption value may be the same as that of the brain by CT scan (isodense) some 7 to 14 days after onset. However, there is usually an enhanced medial border to the hematoma following the injection of contrast material. Bilateral isodense subacute subdural hematomas without midline shift on CT scan will require arteriography for definitive identification of the extracerebral blood clot.

Treatment

The contents of the subdural space should be drained through burr holes or by craniotomy.[201] The mortality rate is about 25 per cent in the postoperative period, but only about one third of survivors are able to return to their previous occupation.

Chronic Subdural Hematoma

The diagnosis of chronic subdural hematoma is often one of the most difficult neurologic diagnoses to make, and frequently the correct diagnosis depends on a high index of suspicion. This is because the preceding head trauma is often trivial or has been forgotten by the patient and the family. The elderly patient or apparently demented or alcoholic patient[196] with a history of chronic progressive neurologic deficit of uncertain cause should be considered to have a chronic subdural hematoma until proved otherwise and should receive appropriate diagnostic studies to exclude this diagnosis. Such an approach is justifiable, since the untreated condition is potentially fatal, and the prognosis following surgical evacuation of the fluid from the subdural space is excellent and one of the most gratifying therapeutic experiences in neurology.[134]

Etiology and Pathology

Although often recorded as being minor, the head injury that caused the subdural hematoma must be of sufficient magnitude to produce sudden movement of the brain within the cranial cavity. This is the type of injury that commonly occurs in the alcoholic, the elderly, and the demented. One or more veins are torn as they cross the subdural space to reach the dural sinuses, and there is a slow accumulation of venous blood within the subdural space. An initial period of clotting is followed by hemolysis. The lysed blood attracts cerebrospinal fluid by osmosis through the arachnoid, which acts as a semipermeable membrane between the cerebrospinal fluid and the hemolyzed clot in the subdural space.

As the subdural hematoma increases in size, there is further tearing of capillaries at the periphery. This tearing produces fresh bleeding into the subdural space, which further increases the osmotic pressure of the subdural hematoma and leads to a further increase in size as more fluid passes from the subarachnoid space into the subdural space.[246]

After two weeks the fibroblasts in the dura and arachnoid surrounding the subdural hematoma begin to proliferate, with the gradual production of a membrane. After several months, this may become quite thick and rigid, particularly on the dural surface, and may even calcify in the more chronic cases.

Clinical Features

There is usually a history of head injury and, in the alcoholic, there are often multiple head injuries. However, many elderly and debilitated patients are confused and suffer from poor memory. Furthermore, the subdural hematoma itself impairs memory, so that often there is no historic report of a head injury. Younger patients frequently have a history of being involved in an automobile accident or having received a head injury sufficient to produce loss of consciousness or concussion. The vast majority of patients are conscious on admission to the hospital or when seen in the office unless the condition has been allowed to progress to severe brainstem compression.

Many complain of generalized dull but persistent headaches. Others are obtunded and disoriented and show lack of judgment and insight with impairment of retention and recent memory, mimicking dementia. A subdural hematoma lying over the left hemisphere may produce intermittent dysphasia suggesting a transient ischemic attack.[158] The course is later characterized by a waxing and waning of the level of consciousness and, finally, coma and death. In some cases inappropriate secretion of antidiuretic hormone and hyponatremia may contribute to the picture of apathy, stupor, and eventually coma.[147, 196]

In the early stages, there may be a hemiparesis of mild degree on the opposite side of the body, with increased deep tendon reflexes and an extensor plantar response. The majority of cases, however, simply show progressive dementia and rigidity. Uncal herniation eventually develops as the hematoma increases in size and may be on the ipsilateral or contralateral side. This produces unilateral dilatation of the pupil and, occasionally, a homonymous hemianopia due to compression of the posterior cerebral artery. The patient sometimes shows papilledema, ptosis, and other signs of third-nerve compression, with bilateral signs of corticospinal tract involvement including bilateral extensor plantar responses. Further signs of brainstem compression (p. 614) appear unless the condition is relieved surgically.

Diagnostic Procedures

1. Roentgenograms of the skull may show a shift of a calcified pineal gland or evidence of skull fracture in about 25 per cent of cases of subdural hematoma. This is more frequent in the alcoholic and the younger patient who has suffered an automobile accident.
2. Computed tomography will usually show an area of decreased density in the subdural space between the inner table of the skull and the surface of the brain (Fig. 8–3). Since blood clots eventually assume the same density as brain tissue, there is a risk of missing the isodense subdural hematoma, which can be reduced by contrast enhancement. The use of contrast material usually produces an area or rim of contrast enhancement on the inner aspect of the subdural hematoma clearly defining the hematoma and the brain surface. A unilateral chronic subdural hematoma will produce a shift of the midline structures of the brain. However, this may be absent if there are bilateral hematomas.
3. The electroencephalogram usually shows increased slow activity in the theta and delta

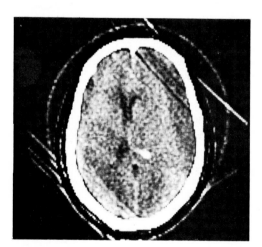

FIGURE 8–3. Computed tomography in a case of chronic subdural hematoma. There is an area of decreased density in the right frontoparietal area, representing a large subdural hematoma. The ventricular system is displaced to the left because of the right-sided mass.

range and decreased voltage on the side of the subdural hematoma. The decrease in voltage is probably because the subdural "insulates" the electrical activity of the underlying brain. Serial records are useful in doubtful cases when the development of this pattern can be seen over a period of several days or weeks (see p. 488).

4. The cerebrospinal fluid is seldom under increased pressure but is almost invariably xanthochromic, with increased protein content in 75 to 80 per cent of cases. It is important to be aware that a clear CSF without xanthochromia may be reported in subdural hematoma, possibly because slight degrees of xanthochromia often are missed unless examined by an experienced individual who compares the spinal fluid with water.
5. Arteriography may be needed if computed tomography is equivocal. The arteriogram shows a characteristic biconvex shape because the brain underlying the hematoma has undergone pressure atrophy. There should always be suspicion of a subdural hematoma on the opposite side when the displacement of the anterior cerebral arteries in the anteroposterior view is less than 50 per cent of the width of the subdural hematoma. These cases should have bilateral arteriographic studies.

Treatment

The subdural hematoma may be drained through burr holes or slowly decompressed by twist drill craniostomy and closed-system drainage.[224] Thickened membranes may require removal by craniectomy to prevent reaccumulation of fluid. Chronic calcified subdural hematomas should be removed if the patient shows a significant progressive neurologic disorder or progressive dementia.[237]

Subdural Hygroma in Adults

Traumatic subdural hygroma in the adult mimics chronic subdural hematoma, and the diagnosis is usually made at operation.

Etiology and Pathology

The most likely mechanism appears to be tearing of the arachnoid following head injury with escape of cerebrospinal fluid into the subdural space. The tear may act as a one-way valve with passage of fluid during coughing, sneezing, or straining. In other cases, it is possible that the accumulation of small amounts of blood in the subdural space results in increased osmotic pressure and the passage of cerebrospinal fluid into the subdural space without further bleeding.

Clinical Features

The clinical picture is indistinguishable from chronic subdural hematoma.

Diagnostic Procedures

See Chronic Subdural Hematoma.

Treatment

The fluid is drained through burr holes. The mortality rate is approximately 30 per cent.

Subdural Hematoma in Infants and Children

Subdural hematoma is a common complication of head injury in infancy as at any other age. The etiology is almost invariably traumatic, but the history of head injury may be trivial or the condition may occur following sudden acceleration or deceleration of the head in a "whiplash injury."[90]

The symptoms are lethargy, poor appetite, vomiting, and failure to thrive. The head circumference may be enlarging more rapidly than expected, and bulging of the anterior fontanel is frequently present.

Diagnostic Procedures

1. Transillumination may show a difference in the extent of the light glow when comparing the two sides of the head.
2. Roentgenograms may show widening of the sutures or a skull fracture.
3. A subdural tap through the lateral angle of the anterior fontanel should be performed when there is suspicion of a subdural hematoma and the subdural tap establishes the diagnosis.
4. The diagnosis can be confirmed by computed tomography.

Treatment

Repeated subdural taps should be performed whenever the child is lethargic or when there is bulging of the anterior fontanel. Craniotomy is rarely required.

Subdural Hygroma in Infants and Children

The mechanism of subdural hygroma in infants and children is the same as in adults following

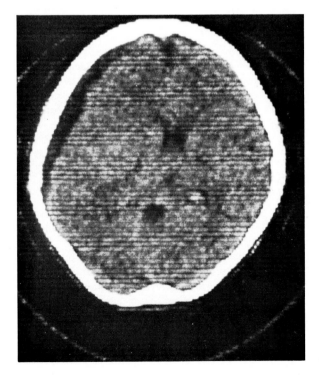

FIGURE 8–4. Computed tomography in a case of subdural hygroma. The hygroma presents as an area of decreased density in the left frontal area. The ventricular system is displaced to the right side.

traumatic injury. A similar condition occurs in association with meningitis in infancy and is called a subdural effusion.

Etiology and Pathology

There is an accumulation of clear or xanthochromic fluid in the subdural space following head injury. Accumulation may be due to passage of cerebrospinal fluid through a ball valve tear in the arachnoid.[95]

Subdural effusion occurs at the height of the inflammatory response in infants with meningitis. The fluid accumulates as a loculated subdural effusion or hygroma after the meningitis has been controlled and the infection eliminated.

Clinical Features

The condition should be suspected in infants who do not show a normal recovery following head injury or meningitis. There is poor feeding, drowsiness, vomiting, and bradycardia, usually without focal neurologic abnormalities.

Diagnostic Procedures

Such infants suspected of having a subdural effusion should receive a diagnostic subdural tap by passing a needle through the anterior fontanel. If clear or xanthochromic fluid is obtained, the cyst may be outlined by the injection of a small volume of air. A subdural hygroma appears as an area of low density over the superior surface of the brain on computed tomography (Fig. 8–4).

Treatment

Repeated aspiration may be necessary to clear the subdural hygroma. Surgery is indicated when the effusion persists. The results are good unless there is underlying damage to the brain.[155]

Intracerebral and Intracerebellar Hematoma

Between 1 and 2 per cent of patients with severe head injury have an intracerebral or, less frequently, an intracerebellar hematoma.

Etiology and Pathology

Movements of the brain within the skull and shearing forces within the brain substance produced by head injury result in laceration and tearing of blood vessels with hemorrhage into the parenchyma. Intracerebral hematomas occur commonly in the temporal lobes, in the frontal lobes, and in the centrum semiovale.[15] Cerebellar hematomas rarely occur and are usually due to direct blows to the suboccipital regions.

Clinical Features

Some patients with traumatic intracerebral hematomas are comatose from the onset, but a hemiplegia or hemiparesis may be demonstrated in those who respond to painful stimuli. Others have a lucid interval before lapsing into coma, and occasionally there may be several days' delay in the onset of symptoms following head injury.[11, 165] The stuporous or obtunded patient commonly shows dysphasia when there is involvement of the dominant hemisphere, and in temporal lobe hematomas, this is often of the receptive type. Cerebellar hematomas exert pressure on the brainstem, with headache, vomiting, and associated unilateral or bilateral cerebellar signs.

Diagnostic Procedures

The investigation of patients with intracerebral hematoma is essentially the same as outlined under Subdural Hematoma. More than 50 per cent of these patients have roentgenographic evidence of skull fracture. Computed tomography shows the hematoma as an area of increased density. Displacement of the ventricles, acute hydrocephalus, or rupture of the hematoma into the ventricular system is also apparent on the CT scan.

Treatment

The hematoma can be explored and removed through a large burr hole or after turning a bone flap. Patients who are unconscious at the time of surgery have a significantly higher mortality rate.[112] A few show permanent neurologic disability, such as hemiparesis, dysphasia, and seizures; but in general, in young individuals who survive, there is a good recovery of neurologic function after removal of a hematoma.

Outlook Following Head Injury

There has been a steady decline in the mortality rate of head injury in recent years and the mortality is now under 4 per cent in most major medical centers. Although many factors may be involved in this process, it is clear that recognition of avoidable factors that may contribute to death plays a major role in improved survival. These factors include early recognition and treatment of intracranial hematomas, better control of early posttraumatic seizures, avoidance of status epilepticus, control of intracranial infections, prompt treatment of hypoxia, early treatment of increased intracranial pressure, and prevention of hypotension.[200] Although it is apparent from the low mortality that head injury produces an eminently recoverable lesion, about 6.5 per cent of patients who experience prolonged unconsciousness may have permanent brain damage.[139]

During recovery from head injury with loss of consciousness, the patient usually passes through the stages of coma and traumatic delirium before recovering consciousness. The duration of the retrograde amnesia, that is, the memory for events leading up to the accident, is a good indication of the severity of the head injury. In the acute stages, the retrograde amnesia may shorten, but it remains as a permanent feature in virtually all cases. In severe cerebral contusions, there may be a period of a Korsakoff-like psychosis, with confabulation, a short memory span, and disorientation to time and place. However, the impairment of retention and recent memory is the outstanding neurologic defect. In such cases, there is often prolonged retrograde amnesia, and there may be ideational dyspraxia, but remote memory is intact. The majority recover over a period of several weeks.

Adults may show posttraumatic changes in personality and temperament, which are evident to the family and friends. There may be periods of puerile behavior, with impulsiveness, irritability, and temper outbursts or explosive rage[56] interspersed with periods when the patient appears to be depressed, dull, and apathetic and lacks initiative. Emotional lability is marked in some cases with bilateral cerebral or brainstem injury, so that they are easily provoked into anger, tears, or laughter. When symptoms persist for more than six months, the patients should be investigated for normal pressure hydrocephalus. A ventriculoatrial shunt may be followed by improvement in some cases.[209]

Permanent signs of a focal nature (e.g., hemiparesis, dysphasia, dyscalculia) may occur as a result of head injury and are related to localized damage to specific parts of the brain. However, other neurologic complaints due to more diffuse disorders of the brain are often seen after head injury. Patients with posttraumatic amnesia show slowness of thought, inaccurate memory, disturbance of perception,[84] changes in personality, difficulty in concentrating and reading, and loss of self-confidence in solving problems and occupational activities. Definition of the degree of deterioration of mental status of a patient following head injury may be extremely difficult since there is usually no record of the pretraumatic mental status. The history supplied by relatives and friends is often biased and inaccurate. However, the school, college, military, and work records are likely to be more reliable.

Neuropsychologic testing of head-injured individuals shows that patients with posttraumatic amnesia have low scores in both verbal and performance tests in the immediate postinjury period with significantly lower scores and slower improvement in performance tests.[145, 146] Patients with dysphasia tend to make a good recovery in most cases.[230]

Children usually show symptoms of restlessness and impulsive, antisocial, and infantile behavior during the recovery stage from coma. In some cases, these changes in mental status may become permanent, and there is a linear correlation between duration of coma and measured intelligence after head injury in children.[27] However, children with severe head injuries have the capacity to show recovery over an extended period of time,[126] and few show intellectual loss even though neurologic abnormalities are permanent.

Traumatic Encephalopathy of Boxers

The "punch-drunk" boxer is still encountered in the professional boxing world, although the use of headguards during sparring practice and better medical examination of boxers prior to professional bouts has probably decreased the incidence of this condition. This form of traumatic encephalopathy can occur in any sport resulting in multiple cerebral injuries.

The syndrome of "punch-drunkenness" usually appears in professional boxers after more than 30 contests in which they have taken considerable punishment. When the syndrome appears, there is diminished tolerance to further blows to the head with a visible motor retardation in defensive maneuvers, which leads to a succession of further injuries with the development of the flat nose and "cauliflower" ears so characteristic of the veteran boxer. These injuries are followed by impairment of judgment, retention, and memory and the development of a staring expression and dysarthria. The fully developed picture consists of mental deterioration, marked dysarthria, parkinsonian-like features, titubation of the head, tremors of the hands, and ataxia of gait.[120]

Posttraumatic Neurosis and Postconcussion Syndrome

The occurrence of psychoneurotic symptoms after head injury is also common and may be difficult to separate from true organic symptoms already discussed under "post-concussive" effects. From a medicolegal point of view, the question of whether the symptoms are psychoneurotic or not becomes somewhat academic, if the symptoms are disabling and clearly can be causally related to the head injury.

Etiology and Pathology

Because the condition often occurs after concussion, it is not clearly related to gross structural changes in the central nervous system, although microscopic changes in nerve cells have been described following concussion. Psychoneurotic features also occur in patients with chronic residual brain damage as an additional feature owing to depression, loss of self-confidence, and feelings of dependency. Those with significant initial and residual neuropsychologic deficits experience greater emotional distress than those with negligible difficulties.[50]

The postconcussion syndrome occurs at any age in adult life but is not seen in children.[162] Any changes in mentation or psychoneurotic features show some correlation with the pretraumatic personality of the patient. For example, the anxious, neurotic, and dependent type of individual is more likely to develop psychoneurotic features after head injury than the self-reliant individual. There is also a higher incidence of prior mental disturbance in patients who develop psychoneurotic features following head injury. The presence of pretraumatic stress in family relationships, occupation, religion, and socioeconomic conditions also appear to be contributory factors to the incidence of psychoneurotic symptoms. Patients who have a dangerous occupation, such as firemen, policemen, and military personnel, have a high incidence of posttraumatic neurosis.

Almost all individuals have an understandable concern or fear of impaired cerebral function following head injury. The brain is generally regarded as the most important endowment we have, and there often follow deep-seated fears that there may be some damage to the brain even after relatively trivial head injuries. This may lead to overt anxiety and depression and deterioration of performance, which initiates a vicious circle of disability.

Clinical Features

Typically, cases of postconcussion syndrome complain of highly stereotyped symptoms that differ little from one patient to another. The history is often that of minor head trauma with little or no loss of consciousness.[12] The complaints consist of headache, irritability, easy fatigue in both mental and physical spheres, inability to concentrate, and "dizziness," usually precipitated by assuming the upright posture.[123] The latter is a descriptive term covering vague lightheadedness or a feeling of unsteadiness with ataxia; syncope rarely occurs. Vertigo is unusual and suggests damage to the inner ear, eighth nerve, or brainstem. Other rare symptoms include photophobia and sensitivity to noise. Occasionally there may be frank conversion hysteria, including visual defects, loss of hearing, ataxia, paresis of one or more limbs, and vague complaints of sensory loss.

In cases with psychoneurotic features the neurologic examination is normal or inconsistent with the symptoms, since the signs are bizarre and do not conform to an organic lesion of the brain. Symptoms of a conversion reaction are occasionally seen following a head injury, but frank malingering, which is a conscious exaggeration or pretense of signs and symptoms, is rare.

Treatment

The physician can accomplish a great deal to minimize disability due to the postconcussion syndrome by reassuring those patients who are likely to develop anxiety following head injury. The symptoms are often improved by explaining to the patient the nature and extent, if any, of his injuries; answering his questions with understanding and reassurance that the brain is not irreparably damaged, if the latter appears to be the case; and outlining the future with an optimistic outlook toward recovery and resumption of previous activities.

This necessitates that the physician be prepared to spend time at the initial and follow-up examinations, in order to discuss with the patient the many problems that the injury has created for him. In addition, the judicious use of phenothiazines or propranolol[57] may be useful to control severe anxiety or belligerent behavior. The depressed patient may benefit from the so-called "psychic energizer" drugs. Early ambulation often tends to prevent the development of neurotic symptoms, and patients with minor head injuries should be allowed to dress and become mobile and self-dependent as soon as possible. More severely injured patients, who are confined to bed for prolonged periods because of additional complications such as fractured limbs, benefit by physical therapy and occupational therapy.

Concern about pending compensation tends to prolong convalescence.[22] Those who are able should return to work as soon as possible. Undue delay on the part of the attending or the industrial physician may enhance rather than allay anxiety, particularly if there is a financial loss resulting from loss of work. Above all, the patient who returns to work has little time to ruminate on his real or supposed disability.

Posttraumatic Seizures

Posttraumatic seizures may begin as early as a week after injury in some cases and as late as ten years or more after injury in others. Penetrating wounds due to high-velocity missiles have a much higher incidence of posttraumatic seizures than closed head injury[41] (Fig. 8–5). Consequently, there is a higher incidence of seizures following head injury as a result of warfare than in civilian practice. The different methods of classifying injuries have led to the publication of variable figures for the incidence of posttraumatic sei-

zures. In general, if the follow-up extends long enough, it appears that in cases of casualties during wartime there is a 20 per cent liability to seizures when the wound does not penetrate the dura and a 50 per cent incidence of seizures when there is penetration of the dura. In civilian practice, the incidence of seizures following closed head injury with loss of consciousness exceeding 24 hours is probably less than 20 per cent.

Factors increasing the liability to posttraumatic seizures are as follows:

1. Injuries due to high-velocity missiles are followed by seizures three times as frequently as those due to blunt injuries.
2. Wounds that penetrate the dura have a much higher incidence of seizures than those in which the dura remains intact.
3. The presence of foreign bodies within the brain, such as metallic pieces, bone fragments, hair, and clothing, and complications, such as brain abscess, meningitis, and intracerebral hematoma, increase the incidence of posttraumatic seizures.
4. Patients with a short period of coma have a lower incidence of seizures than those with prolonged unconsciousness.
5. Those with residual neurologic deficits, particularly with marked focal abnormalities, have a higher incidence of posttraumatic seizures.

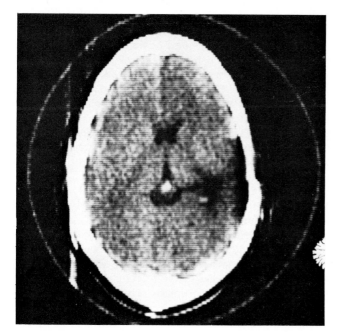

FIGURE 8–5. Computed tomography following a gunshot wound to the right temporal area. A craniotomy had been performed with removal of blood clot and necrotic brain. The patient subsequently developed psychomotor seizures. The scan shows an area of decreased density in the right posterior temporal lobe, representing scarring and cavity formation. A metallic fragment can be seen in the center of the affected area.

6. Wounds involving the precentral gyri carry the highest incidence of subsequent seizures.

About 7 per cent of patients with closed head injury and depressed skull fracture have seizures within the first 24 hours of injury and 10 per cent have seizures within the first week. There is no recurrence of seizures in about half of these patients. Late-onset seizures occurring after the first week affect 15 per cent of patients with depressed skull fractures. The onset is delayed for more than a year in about half of these cases and for more than four years in a fifth of the cases.[118] Early seizures occurring in the first week have been reported to carry a good prognosis,[163] but they do influence the late onset of epilepsy. This applies particularly to children under the age of five years who have an early seizure following relatively trivial head injury that is uncomplicated by a depressed fracture or intracranial hematoma, who would be expected to have a low risk of late-onset seizures.[117]

The delayed onset of seizures is associated with the development of a meningocerebral cicatrix, cerebral cicatrix, or cerebral cyst as a result of the injury.[181] The nerve cells bordering the injury become highly epileptogenic. The presence of a foreign body or walled-off abscess may also be the cause of posttraumatic seizures.

An early onset of posttraumatic seizures occurs more commonly with closed craniocerebral injuries rather than missile injuries, and the late onset is characteristic of penetrating missile wounds. The seizures may be generalized or partial in nature at the onset, but partial motor or partial sensory seizures frequently terminate as a generalized attack. Partial seizures of the psychomotor type occur in about 10 per cent of cases.

Approximately 50 per cent of posttraumatic seizures cease spontaneously within ten years of the injury, and the great majority can be controlled by adequate anticonvulsant medication. Patients with frequent seizures carry a poorer prognosis than those with less frequent attacks prior to treatment. In general, the onset of epilepsy in a patient who has had a head injury with penetration of the brain suggests that a surgically remediable condition, such as a cicatrix or foreign body, may be present. Such patients should receive a diagnostic evaluation, including computed tomography and arteriography, to define the nature of the injury unless the seizures are readily and completely controlled by anticonvulsant medication.

Damage to the Cranial Nerves in Head Injury

Involvement of the cranial nerves following head injury may occur owing to the following conditions:

1. Direct trauma to the nerve by a missile or penetrating object in penetrating wounds.
2. Damage within the brainstem by a traumatic hematoma.
3. Avulsion or contusion by the displaced bone fragments in fractures of the skull.
4. Damage secondary to meningitis or increased intracranial pressure.

The Olfactory Nerve

About 5 per cent of patients with head injury develop unilateral or bilateral anosmia or impairment of olfaction. The majority of cases are due to fracture of the cribriform plate, but the olfactory nerve filaments may be shorn off following trauma to the occipital or parietotemporal areas.[92]

The Optic Nerve

The optic nerve is usually damaged by blows to the frontal area of the skull. The trauma may not be severe enough to cause loss of consciousness, and only a relatively small number of patients have a fracture of the orbit and optic foramen. The majority of such injuries probably result from sudden movement of the brain with contusion of the optic nerve against the side of the optic foramen or from injury to the blood vessels supplying the nerve. The visual loss is maximal immediately after the injury, and if there is blindness in the affected eye, this will be associated with loss of the direct light reflex, but preservation of the consensual reflex.

Some degree of recovery of vision, if it is to occur, should be expected over a period of about one month following injury with little chance of further improvement expected after a month's time. There is gradual development of optic atrophy, which begins about one month after the injury. Damage to the optic chiasm may result in a bitemporal field defect. An injury involving one optic nerve and the chiasm produces blindness on one side and a temporal field defect in the other eye.

Severe impairment of vision may also result following occipital lobe contusion. The light reflex is preserved, and there is often good recovery of vision in these cases. Those with permanent residual homonymous field defects have injuries that are largely confined to the area surrounding one calcarine fissure. Episodic blindness owing to inhibitory visual seizures has been reported as a late complication of occipital lobe trauma.[130]

The Third, Fourth, and Sixth Cranial Nerves

The majority of cases of head injury resulting in involvement of the third, fourth, or sixth nerves have suffered injury to the frontal area of the skull resulting in orbital hemorrhage or a fracture involving the bones of the orbit with peripheral injury to those nerves. Direct trauma to the brainstem or uncal herniation usually results in difficulties with conjugate eye movements, although paralysis of individual nerves follows in some patients. Impairment of conjugate movement commonly results in difficulties of upward gaze, poor convergence, and occasionally an inability to completely move the eyes to one side. The eye movements may exhibit irregular jerking on lateral gaze (coarse saccadic movements) but are otherwise intact.

A unilateral third-nerve palsy with a widely dilated pupil may rarely persist following uncal herniation. As might be expected from anatomic considerations, a variety of combinations of third-, fourth-, and sixth-nerve palsies can be expected when there is injury to the nerves at the superior orbital fissure. Sometimes diplopia may be due to displacement of individual muscles following a fracture of the orbit or displacement of the pulley arrangement of the superior oblique.

The Fifth Cranial Nerve

This nerve is usually involved in its extracranial course in head injuries. The supraorbital nerve may be severed in scalp wounds or compressed by fractures involving the supraorbital margin. Injury is occasionally followed by the development of hyperesthesia, paresthesias, and an unpleasant neuralgic type of pain in the forehead and scalp on the affected side. The infraorbital nerve is occasionally contused or compressed by fractures of the maxilla, with anesthesia of the cheek and upper lip.

Complete fifth-nerve damage is rare but has been reported following basal fractures involving the foramen ovale.

The Seventh Cranial Nerve

The great majority of cases with peripheral facial paralysis following head injury result from fracture of the petrous portion of the temporal bone. The facial nerve is damaged in the facial canal, and there is usually associated bleeding into the middle ear or from the external canal. About 50 per cent of cases show an immediate facial paralysis, indicating direct and usually severe traumatic damage to the seventh nerve. In spite of the severity of the injury, the prognosis is fairly good, with slow recovery over a period of months as the nerve regenerates. The remaining 50 per cent develop a delayed facial palsy two to seven days after injury. This probably represents edema of the nerve in the facial canal, and recovery occurs within a few days as the edema subsides.

The Eighth Cranial Nerve

Loss of hearing following head injury is not uncommon and is usually due to fracture extending through the middle ear, although fractures of the petrous bone not uncommonly contuse or sever the eighth nerve. Permanent deafness will result if the nerve is severed. In those cases of deafness due to hemorrhage into the middle ear, some degree of recovery can be expected as the blood clot is absorbed. Recovery also is the rule in cases of edema and contusion of the eighth nerve. Inner ear deafness may be total and associated with loss of vestibular function. There is usually an associated seventh-nerve paralysis in all these types of injury. Many patients develop tinnitus following injury to the inner ear and the eighth nerve, which usually resolves over a period of several months. Vertigo is particularly distressing and is presumably due to edema or hemorrhage into the labyrinth. Vertigo is associated with nausea and vomiting on movement of the head, and the patient may prefer to lie immobile in bed. There may be some relief from the intramuscular use of a phenothiazine. The condition usually resolves over a two- or three-week interval, although the patient may feel lightheaded and ataxic and have nystagmus[208] for some months after the injury.[183]

The Ninth, Tenth, Eleventh, and Twelfth Cranial Nerves

One or more of the last four cranial nerves may be involved in injuries of the lower brainstem, fractures of the posterior fossa, or hematomas at the base of the skull. A patient with a severe head injury, with prolonged coma and partial recovery, sometimes shows signs of lower brainstem damage. In such cases there is a marked cerebellar ataxia, rarely palatal nystagmus, and more commonly paralysis of the lower cranial nerves. Fractures of the posterior fossa involving the jugular foramen are likely to involve the ninth, tenth, and eleventh nerves. The paralysis is unilateral in such cases. A hematoma occurring at the base of the skull following fracture may produce unilateral paralysis of all of the last four cranial nerves.

Cerebrospinal Fluid Rhinorrhea

About 2 per cent of head injuries severe enough to require admission to the hospital are complicated by cerebrospinal fluid rhinorrhea. Cerebrospinal fluid rhinorrhea can also occur without head trauma, and it is possible to recognize two major groups: the more common traumatic and the less frequent nontraumatic group (Table 8–1).

Etiology and Pathology

Traumatic Cerebrospinal Fluid Rhinorrhea. Fractures through the posterior wall of the frontal sinus with tearing of the dura and arachnoid are the most common cause.[78] In cases of head injury without fracture or with a remote fracture of the skull (e.g., in the parietal or occipital area), cerebrospinal fluid rhinorrhea probably results from a congenital weakness or defect of the cribriform plate or rupture of an arachnoid sleeve passing through the cribriform plate. The rupture of the meninges presumably results from the sudden wave of pressure passing through the cerebrospinal fluid immediately following the blow to the head.

Nontraumatic Cerebrospinal Fluid Rhinorrhea. Some cases result from increased intracranial pressure, and in these cases cerebrospinal fluid rhinorrhea is probably the result of a congenital defect in the cribriform plate of the ethmoid.[77] Rarely, tumors may erode through

TABLE 8–1

Cerebrospinal Fluid Rhinorrhea

Traumatic	Fracture involving posterior wall of the frontal sinus
	Associated with remote fracture of the skull
	Associated with relatively minor head trauma without skull fracture
Nontraumatic	Associated with raised intracranial pressure
	Associated with normal cerebrospinal fluid pressure

the paranasal sinuses and cause cerebrospinal fluid rhinorrhea. Another possible cause is rupture of a congenital encephalocystocele that extends from the frontal lobe through the cribriform plate of the ethmoid. A rare cause is rupture of a persistent embryonic olfactory ventricular lumen that communicates with the ventricles.[103]

There is a group of nontraumatic or "spontaneous" cases of spinal fluid rhinorrhea without obvious cause.[170] These cases almost always show the presence of a fistula through or congenital defect of the cribriform plate of the ethmoid. The precipitating mechanism is often similar to that described under increased intracranial pressure. During sneezing and coughing there is a sudden rise in cerebrospinal fluid pressure, which may cause rupture of the arachnoid in a congenitally weak area of the cribriform plate.

Clinical Features

In traumatic cases, the presence of persistent or intermittent clear fluid draining from the nose should arouse suspicion of cerebrospinal fluid rhinorrhea. The flow is increased by flexing the head forward, coughing, or straining. In nontraumatic cases, the presence of a clear nasal discharge in patients with increased intracranial pressure may be an indication of cerebrospinal fluid rhinorrhea. In those cases with normal intracranial pressure, there is often a history of sneezing, coughing, or straining preceding the initial appearance of the discharge.

Rarely, patients with cerebrospinal fluid rhinorrhea show progressive intellectual deterioration and headache resulting from pneumocephalus (a pocket of air in the brain) caused by the passage of air through the cribriform plate into the ventricular system. This is usually caused by coughing or sneezing.

Cases of "nontraumatic" or spontaneous cerebrospinal fluid rhinorrhea are often referred to the neurologist because of recurrent meningitis, which results from the passage of organisms from the nose into the subarachnoid space. Any patient with two or more attacks of meningitis should be suspected of having cerebrospinal rhinorrhea and should be investigated accordingly.[138]

Diagnostic Procedures

1. The identification of the nasal discharge as cerebrospinal fluid and the demonstration of the fistula may be accomplished as outlined in Table 8–2.

TABLE 8-2

Diagnosis of Cerebrospinal Fluid Rhinorrhea

Identification of spinal fluid draining from the nose.

1. Positive test for glucose.
2. Protein content the same as CSF obtained at lumbar puncture.
3. Roentgenograms of skull and paranasal sinuses may show fracture or an intracranial mass or air in brain tissue or in the ventricles. Congenital defects of the cribriform plate of the ethmoid may be demonstrated by tomography.[63]
4. Injection of indigo carmine into the lumbar sac during lumbar puncture may show the dye appearing in the nostril on the affected side.
5. Myelography, with passage of pantopaque into the anterior fossa, may demonstrate the fistula by fluoroscopy.
6. The intrathecal injection of radionuclides or metrizamide followed by scintillation scanning or C.T. of the head may detect a narrow channel of leaking CSF from the subarachnoid space through the cribriform plate to the nasal cavity. Exact location of the leak may be obtained by superimposition of the scan and roentgenograms of the skull. A swab taken from the nose of the involved side shows increased radioactivity.[4, 49]

2. Many patients with an intermittent nasal discharge are able to produce cerebrospinal fluid from the nose by flexion of the head ("teapot sign"). The flow can be increased temporarily by the Queckenstedt maneuver or by having the patient strain so that sufficient fluid can be collected in a sterile test tube or sterile jar for cellular and chemical examination.
3. Computed tomography will readily demonstrate even small amounts of air in the cranial cavity because of the low density (low attenuation) of air as compared to other tissues. Potentially serious complications such as a tension pneumocephalus are readily identified.[176]
4. There is a serious risk of meningitis in all cases. Lumbar puncture should be performed if there is the slightest suspicion of nuchal rigidity. The cerebrospinal fluid draining from the nose should also be cultured. If the culture is positive, sensitivity tests should be performed and an appropriate antibiotic administered.[144]

Treatment

The majority of cases of cerebrospinal rhinorrhea respond to medical treatment. The patient should be placed in a semi-Fowler position and instructed not to cough, sneeze, or strain. Antibiotics should be administered during the period of cerebrospinal fluid drainage.[76]

Further Treatment as Dependent on the Cause. Further treatment is as follows:

1. In cases of nontraumatic cerebrospinal fluid rhinorrhea with increased intracranial pressure the patient should be treated for any identifiable cause, such as tumor or hydrocephalus.
2. Normal pressure leaks should be treated medically for two weeks. Leaks that fail to resolve should have surgical repair of the fistula. A tissue adhesive such as isobutyl-2-cyanoacrylate may help to produce a watertight seal.[152]
3. Surgical treatment is indicated in all cases with meningitis after successful treatment with antibiotics.[199]
4. Immediate surgical treatment is recommended for all traumatic cases with frontal fractures below the hairline.[115]
5. Persistent cerebrospinal fluid rhinorrhea following failure of intracranial surgery may respond to a lumboperitoneal shunt.[82]

Traumatic Pneumocephalus

Traumatic injury and fracture to the frontal area with involvement of the paranasal sinuses may be followed by the passage of air into the cranial cavity. In severe trauma the air may enter the ventricular system and there may be a rapid increase in intracranial pressure. Less severely injured patients usually have air in the subdural or subarachnoid space and cerebrospinal fluid rhinorrhea. The diagnosis is established by computed tomography which shows the presence of intracranial air.

Treatment

Traumatic pneumocephalus with increased intracranial pressure requires immediate surgery with closure of the fistula.[26] Patients with subdural or subarachnoid air can be treated as cases of cerebrospinal fluid rhinorrhea.

Traumatic Injuries to the Brain at Birth

The role of trauma as a cause of brain damage during parturition has probably been overestimated. Nevertheless, brain injury at birth is responsible for about 10 per cent of deaths in infancy, although the percentage is decreasing with steady improvement in obstetric techniques.

Etiology and Pathology

Certain factors that predispose to birth injury are listed in Table 8–3. Primiparity is associated with a high incidence of head trauma because of the tendency to prolonged labor and increased use of forceps. Abruptio placentae, placenta praevia, and other conditions causing severe hemorrhage require prompt and sometimes hurried treatment, including obstetric maneuvers that can lead to head injury.[23, 24]

Multiple pregnancies are commonly associated with abnormal presentation, and the latter is also associated with a high incidence of trauma to the head. The main causes of head injury during parturition include abnormal presentations, precipitate delivery, prolonged labor, the use of obstetric procedures such as internal and external version, and the premature or unnecessary use of obstetric forceps. The major postnatal factor complicating neonatal head injury is anoxia. Many of the conditions thought to arise from birth injury in the past appear now to be the sequel of anoxia at birth or occurring during the first few days of life. Trauma to the head of the newborn may result in depression of the medullary respiratory center, with delayed onset of respirations, irregular respirations, or periods of apnea. Subsequent cerebral damage is often due to resulting anoxia rather than the direct effect of trauma.

There are two main types of trauma that can result in injury to the head during labor. The first is direct trauma from the application of forceps or other injurious obstetric maneuvers. The second is excessive compression or moulding of the head within the birth canal during labor. In either case, injury can occur to the scalp, skull, or meninges, including the venous sinuses, or the brain.

Cephalhematoma. Subperiosteal hematomas can lead to deformity of the skull unless they are treated shortly after birth. They are usually unilateral and occur in the parietal area. The blood clot elevates the periosteum, leading to new bone formation beginning at the edge of the clot. The pressure of the clot can cause a depression of the skull. This is occasionally associated with absorption of bone leading to exposure of the dura. This should be treated by aspiration, or the clot may be evacuated through a small incision.

Skull Fracture. Skull fracture is usually due to the use of forceps or excessive pressure to the head during breech extraction. Any of the bones of the vault may be involved, but fractures of the base of the skull are unusual and nearly always fatal. The fracture may be linear or depressed. Symptoms depend on the extent of the associated brain damage.

Infants or children who have focal neurologic deficits with marked swelling of the scalp have probably suffered a dural laceration and may have brain herniation through the fracture site which may or may not show posttraumatic depression.[229] If dural tears are not repaired, the fracture site becomes filled with dense scar tissue and there is damage to the underlying brain with unilateral ventricular dilatation.[137] However, some fractures are unrecognized at birth but give rise to a local area of scarring in the arachnoid or brain, which may act as an epileptic focus later in life. The majority of fractures, whether linear or depressed, do not require any specific treatment.

Indications for surgery include brain herniation at the fracture site, the presence of a dural tear, bone fragments in the cerebrum, increased intracranial pressure, and the presence of cerebrospinal fluid beneath the galea.[142]

Epidural Hemorrhage. Epidural hemorrhage is rare in the newborn and results from a linear fracture of the skull with tearing of the middle meningeal vessels. The infant becomes stuporous with a bulging fontanel and focal seizures. Death

TABLE 8–3

Factors Predisposing to Brain Injury at Birth

1. Primipara
2. Abruptio placentae, placenta praevia, and uterine hemorrhage during parturition
3. Abnormal position of the fetus, multiple pregnancies
4. Precipitate delivery
5. Prolonged labor
6. The use of version maneuvers
7. Premature use of forceps

occurs within 24 to 48 hours unless the clot is evacuated and the bleeding is controlled.

Subdural Hemorrhage. Subdural hemorrhage in the newborn is always acute and tends to occur in full-term infants who have suffered severe birth trauma. The usual cause is a tear in the tentorium cerebelli with bleeding from venous sinuses or the great vein of Galen. Tearing of cerebral veins at the junction with the superior longitudinal sinus is occasionally encountered.

The condition is not always fatal but many children present with shock, irregular respirations, generalized convulsions, and a bulging fontanel. Hemiparesis can result if there is an accumulation of blood over one hemisphere. The diagnosis may be established by a subdural tap through the lateral angles of the anterior fontanel. Computed tomography may show displacement of the fourth ventricle and the presence of one or more areas of high density at the periphery and within the substance of the cerebellum. Treatment consists of repeated subdural taps, with aspiration of blood[155] or craniotomy and removal of the clot, particularly in cases with bleeding into the posterior fossa.[34]

Subarachnoid Hemorrhage. Mild subarachnoid hemorrhage is extremely common in the newborn. It is asymptomatic and the blood is absorbed during the first three weeks of life. More severe subarachnoid bleeding occurs in infants with subdural hemorrhage or cerebral contusion. Anoxia with or without trauma is also cited as one of the most common causes of subarachnoid hemorrhage in the first few days of life. When the condition occurs alone, the prognosis is good and most infants make a full recovery.

Intracerebral Hemorrhage. Large intracerebral hemorrhages are uncommon in the newborn and usually result from severe head trauma. Small subependymal hemorrhages are the result of anoxia rather than trauma. Intraventricular hemorrhages due to rupture of the angular veins are also due to hypoxia rather than trauma.

Computed tomography scans show crescent-shaped parasagittal areas of increased density in cases of intraventricular hemorrhage. Subependymal hemorrhages appear as small, dense areas along the lateral borders of the ventricles.[186]

The Sequelae of Injury to the Brain at Birth

The majority of children who survive traumatic brain injury at birth develop normally, and in the past there has been a tendency to overemphasize this factor as a cause of "cerebral palsy," "slow learning," or "minimal brain damage." Nevertheless, traumatic hemorrhage in the neonate may result in the formation of porencephalic cysts and is probably one of the major causes of this condition. These cysts are lined by glial scar tissue and usually have a thin roof of cerebral cortex. They may communicate with the ventricular system or the subarachnoid spaces or both. Symptoms vary with the site of the porencephalic cyst, but there are frequently some degree of mental retardation and focal signs, including hemiparesis or partial seizures of the jacksonian type. Delay in speech development with some elements of dysphasia can result from a porencephalic cyst in the temporal lobe. The diagnosis is established by computed tomography. Seizures should be controlled by adequate anticonvulsant therapy. Refractory cases may show improvement if the roof of the cyst is removed.

Another cause of partial seizures that is related to birth trauma is the development of glial scars within the medial aspects of the temporal lobe. This condition of sclerosis of Ammon's horn or incisural sclerosis has been reported to result from excessive molding of the head during passage through the birth canal. This results in temporary herniation of the medial aspect of the temporal lobe over the free edge of the tentorium cerebelli, which reduces itself when the child is born. The damaged area undergoes gliosis and may act as an epileptic focus. Some cases of partial seizures of "psychomotor" or "temporal lobe" type that begin in childhood or adolescence are possibly the result of this form of cerebral trauma.

Fat Embolism of the Brain

It is probable that some entry of fat emboli into the bloodstream regularly occurs following fractures involving long bones, but this is rarely of sufficient magnitude to produce symptoms. In symptomatic cases, however, the mortality is high.

Etiology and Pathology

Most cases of fat embolism occur following fracture of a long bone with involvement of the fatty marrow. Rarer causes include concussion of bones, trauma, necrosis, infection, burns, and crushing injuries involving adipose tissue. The fat globules enter the bloodstream and are trapped in the capillaries of the lung. This is a temporary phenomenon, and many globules pass into the systemic circulation, where they form aggregates that block the smaller arterioles and capillaries in many organs including the brain.

Following obstruction of the vessels, the fat globules are hydrolysed and release highly toxic unsaturated fatty acids.[168] The brain becomes edematous, with numerous petechial hemorrhages and ecchymoses scattered throughout the white and gray matter.

Clinical Features

There is a latent period of 48 to 60 hours following the injury prior to the development of symptoms of fat embolism. The latent period is followed by a stage in which cough, dyspnea, chest pain, and restlessness denote the presence of fat emobli in the pulmonary circulation. The development of cerebral fat emboli is heralded by confusion, delirium, and seizures with progression to stupor, often with signs of focal weakness, decerebrate rigidity, coma, and death.[228] The "cerebral stage" usually lasts from 24 to 96 hours, and recovery, in untreated cases, is rare.

Diagnostic Procedures

The development of neurologic symptoms after a latent period following traumatic injury with fractures of the long bones should arouse suspicion of fat embolism. The diagnosis is frequently missed, however, and revealed at autopsy. Suspected cases of fat embolism may show petechial hemorrhages over the chest, neck, and conjunctivae; fat emboli in the optic fundi; roentgenographic evidence of pulmonary embolism; the presence of fat droplets in the blood[86] and urine; and an unexplained drop in hemoglobin levels.

The electroencephalogram shows generalized paroxysmal slowing with a gradual return to normal appearance over a period of several days in those who recover.[155]

Treatment

As soon as the diagnosis is established, the patient should be treated with inhalation of 5 per cent carbon dioxide in 95 per cent oxygen. This treatment produces cerebral vasodilatation and facilitates the passage of fat emboli through the cerebral capillary bed into the venous circulation.

Infusion of low-molecular-weight dextran should inhibit the plugging of smaller vessels by aggregations of platelets, which appear to be activated in this condition.[19]

Air Embolism of the Brain

The passage of air into the general circulation is fortunately uncommon, but has been reported during cardiac surgery,[113] cerebral arteriography, cardiac catheterization, thoracic surgery, and neurosurgical procedures on highly vascular tumors.[219]

The entry of air into the venous circulation is usually followed by cardiac embarrassment and death if the volume of air exceeds 30 cc. When air enters the pulmonary vein or arterial system, emboli will occur in many organs including the brain, and cerebral symptoms are prominent. If conscious, the patient complains of lightheadedness, vertigo, and respiratory difficulties. There is pallor and, in some cases, cyanosis. The condition may resolve within a few minutes or progress to stupor and coma and is often associated with a major epileptic seizure. Death can occur at this stage or recovery may result with confusion and focal neurologic signs such as dysphasia and hemiparesis. The usual course is one of steady improvement with full recovery in a period of two or three weeks, but permanent and irreversible encephalopathy may result.

Treatment

The transcutaneous monitoring of both carotid arteries using Doppler ultrasonic flow detectors may permit the early detection of air embolism during open-heart surgery.[148] If cerebral air embolism should occur, the following procedures are recommended:

1. Anesthesia should be discontinued.
2. Severe cases require anticonvulsants and supportive measures to combat shock.
3. The patient should be ventilated with 5 per cent CO_2 and 95 per cent oxygen to increase cerebral blood flow and assist passage of small air bubbles out of the cerebral circulation.
4. When neurologic deficits are present, the patient should be placed in a hyperbaric chamber. Hyperbaric therapy at 6 atmospheres absolute will reduce the volume of the air bubbles. If therapy is continued with the use of 100 per cent oxygen at 3 atmospheres absolute, the denitrogenation of the tissues will improve the

rate of diffusion of nitrogen from the bubble.[31, 245]

Electrical Injury

Accidental electrical shock from power lines and naturally occurring lightning results in more than 1,000 deaths in the United States every year. Actual statistics of accidental electrical injury are unreliable since some electrical shocks, particularly those that occur in the home and some that occur in industry, are rarely reported.[61]

Etiology and Pathology

Electricity is a form of energy that is capable of damaging living tissue. The human body can act as a conductor and as in nonliving conductors the current always flows by the shortest path of least resistance from the point of contact to point of exit. The brain, spinal cord, and peripheral nerve are particularly liable to injury if they happen to lie within the route taken by the current. There is little diffusion of current, although multiple groundings will result in multiple pathways that pass simultaneously through different parts of the body.

A current sufficient to cause tissue damage usually produces burning of tissue, particularly at the points of entry or exit. The heat generated by the current also passes into deeper tissues, often damaging blood vessels and resulting in inflammation of the vessel wall and thrombosis. Such vascular damage may result in delayed infarction of tissue due to interruption of the blood supply.

A number of changes can result from electrical injury to the brain.

1. An electrical current passing through the respiratory center may produce respiratory arrest and death. In such cases, the brain is often normal in appearance both grossly and microscopically, since there is insufficient time for the development of signs indicating tissue damage.
2. If the current produces respiratory arrest followed by restoration of respiration after several minutes, changes of anoxic encephalopathy (p. 241) may occur throughout the central nervous system.
3. If passage of the electrical current through the brain does not result in immediate death, inflammatory changes in the blood vessels of the meninges and brain tissue usually result. These

may be followed by subarachnoid hemorrhage or thrombosis of vessels and infarction of tissue.
4. The cerebral neurons are particularly susceptible to direct injury by the electric current, with necrosis, neuronophagia, proliferation of microglial cells, and replacement by gliosis.

Changes in the spinal cord after electrical injury can be either focal or diffuse. Severe focal changes result in a "transverse myelitis." More diffuse changes include neuronal loss and gliosis.

Electrical injury to peripheral nerves produces a wallerian degeneration with loss of axons and myelin.

Clinical Features

A current traversing the brain and involving the respiratory center frequently results in sudden death. Survivors who have had a respiratory arrest for more than six minutes usually show changes of anoxic encephalopathy (p. 241). When the passage of the current does not involve the respiratory center, there is immediate disturbance of neuronal function, with generalized seizures followed by coma. If the current is of insufficient strength to produce gross tissue damage (as occurs in therapeutic electroconvulsive therapy), full recovery occurs after the patient passes through a period of excitement and confusion resembling the recovery from cerebral contusion. Tissue damage, including damage to blood vessels and neurons, may be followed by the delayed appearance of subarachnoid hemorrhage and evidence of focal abnormalities including dysphasia and hemiparesis. A residual organic dementia from frontal or temporal lobe involvement has also been reported.

Permanent damage to the brainstem nuclei can result in focal paralysis, loss of taste, loss of sensation over the face, and deafness or atrophy of the tongue with fasciculations. Symptoms of parkinsonism have been reported in some cases due to involvement of the substantia nigra, and choreoathetosis has been described in patients with neuronal loss in the basal ganglia.

The passage of an electric current through the spinal cord may result in a temporary flaccid paraplegia or quadriplegia,[222] but complete recovery is the rule. Permanent tissue damage results in the gradual development of wasting owing to anterior horn cell involvement[106] with spacticity below the level of tissue damage, impairment of sphincter control, and variable loss of sensation.[71]

Peripheral nerve injury is not uncommon when the damage is confined to one limb. This may result in a painful brachial neuropathy if there is damage to the nerves of the upper limb. In other cases, muscular weakness with fasciculations and atrophy, loss of reflexes, and a sensory loss corresponding to the distribution of certain damaged nerves have been reported.[61]

Treatment

Comatose patients should receive immediate artificial respiration if respirations cease, since there is no means of detecting irreversible damage to the respiratory center. If there is cardiac arrest, external cardiac massage should be given. This usually prevents changes of anoxic encephalopathy in survivors. Survivors should be treated in a manner similar to that described for the care of acute head injury (p. 491) or injury to the spinal cord (p. 518).

Radiation Injury

Adverse effects of irradiation have been reported in both the brain and spinal cord following high-voltage radiation treatment of tumors. Injury can follow irradiation to tissues in the pharynx, larynx, neck, lungs, mediastinum, or abdomen.

Etiology and Pathology

The damage to the central nervous system does not seem to be related to irradiation dosage. The brain and spinal cord show signs of atrophy[244] with loss of neurons, proliferation of astrocytes, and the presence of macrophages filled with lipid material. The white matter shows demyelination with relative preservation of axons. The blood vessels are thickened with increased collagen and endothelial proliferation, which may obliterate the lumen.[198]

Occasionally the brain shows a focal reaction, particularly at the site of an irradiated tumor, and there is marked astroglial proliferation resulting in a tumor-like mass.[225]

Clinical Features

Signs of brain involvement include progressive dementia, spasticity, and rigidity. Focal signs of hemiparesis, dysphasia, and seizures are often delayed and are probably the result of vascular changes and ischemia.[178] Focal radionecrosis

may present as a recurrent brain tumor with focal signs and increased intracranial pressure. Irradiation damage to the brainstem may result in progressive hemiparesis or quadriparesis, dysarthria, and ataxia.

Four types of spinal cord involvement are recognized.[116, 191]

Early Transient Form. This occurs after a latent interval of about three months and consists of subjective mild sensory symptoms. The symptoms resolve after three months.

Lower Motor Neuron Disease. This is presumably due to selective damage to anterior horn cells and can affect upper or lower extremities, according to the level of irradiation.

Acute Paraplegia or Quadriplegia. This probably results from acute cord infarction secondary to vascular changes following radiation therapy.

Chronic Progressive Radiation Myelopathy. This is the most common form of spinal cord involvement. There is progressive loss of spinal cord function with increasing spasticity, hyperreflexia, extensor plantar response, sensory loss, and impaired bladder function, which may progress to complete loss of function below the level of the lesion.[30]

Diagnostic Procedures

Computed tomography of the brain shows a low-density area which may appear to have mass effect with a shift of the ventricular system. There is irregular contrast enhancement, and it is not possible to differentiate between regrowth of a tumor and radiation necrosis by computed tomography.[161]

Treatment

There is no specific treatment for the cerebral or spinal cord syndrome.

Decompression Sickness (Caisson's Disease)

Decompression sickness was originally described in caisson workers who worked under increased atmospheric pressure and suffered symptoms at the end of a shift following rapid decompression. Decompression sickness may occur under any situation involving rapid decompression whether it be from increased pressure to normal atmospheric pressure (as occurs with divers) or from relatively normal atmospheric pressure to a decreased pressure (as occurs with aviators and astronauts at high altitude). Nowadays, the latter situation is more likely to occur at high altitude when there is mechanical failure of pressurized aircraft and space vehicles.

Etiology and Pathology

The pathologic changes result from the sudden release of gaseous nitrogen, which is normally dissolved in the plasma and tissues, following sudden decompression. The formation of bubbles in the plasma alters the rheologic characteristics of the blood, which shows increased viscosity, an increased hematocrit, and erythrocyte aggregation.[238]

The spinal cord is particularly prone to involvement. The epidural vertebral venous system becomes obstructed by bubble emboli, which cause obstruction of the venous drainage of the cord, resulting in spinal cord infarction.[93] The zones of infarction consist of multiple areas of necrosis with pericapillary diapedesis and hemorrhage that apparently affect the white matter more than the gray matter.

The brain shows laminar infarction in the cortex in the boundary zones between territories supplied by major cerebral arteries.[25]

Clinical Features

The upper thoracic segments of the spinal cord are most frequently involved although the spinal cord may have numerous areas of infarction. Usually, ischemia results in the rapid onset of paraplegia, with loss of sensation below the level of the lesion and sphincter paralysis. In the majority of cases, symptoms may be temporary, but sometimes they are permanent. Alteration in cerebral circulation may result in seizures, hemiparesis, aphasia, and visual field defects. Brainstem involvement is quite common, with vertigo and impairment of hearing. Cerebral edema with papilledema and optic atrophy may also occur.

In the acute phase of decompression sickness, there may be symptoms involving other organs besides the brain and spinal cord. Abdominal pain is not uncommon (the bends), while other persons develop dyspnea (the chokes), joint pains, and generalized pruritus due to the collection of nitrogen bubbles beneath the skin.

Treatment

The ability of the tissues to compensate for excessive amounts of nitrogen gas released from solution following rapid reduction of air pressure is limited. In general, in deep-water diving, it may be stated that the limit of tolerance is a rapid reduction of pressure by 1.25 atmospheres. Any rapid change greater than this will result in the formation of nitrogen bubbles. The threshold for tolerance during ascent to high altitude is different, but in decompression at high altitudes when the atmospheric pressure rapidly falls toward zero, the formation of gas bubbles in the tissues becomes a serious problem.

In the case of the deep-water diver, an ascent from a depth of approximately 40 ft of water can be made without the necessity of decompression. When divers work at depths greater than 40 ft, sufficient time should be allowed for decompression at intervals of 1.25 atmospheres. Public health authorities in most countries have protective rules regarding the hazards of working under increased pressure particularly concerning the rate of decompression of those working at more than 1.25 atmospheres of pressure.

If decompression sickness occurs, recompression should be carried out as soon as possible.[46] Recompression is preferably done in a recompression chamber, which is usually effective in most cases. The patient should be placed in a chamber that has pressure equal to the previous working depth or that is maintained at 10 to 15 lb higher than the previous working pressure. Decompression is then carried out slowly. Oxygen and oxygen-helium mixtures administered to the patient in the chamber are valuable in the treatment of decompression sickness. Complete recovery can be expected in about 90 per cent of cases. There is a mortality rate of less than 1 per cent.

Injuries to the Spinal Cord

Mechanisms causing spinal cord injury differ from those discussed under traumatic injuries of the brain. Indirect forces play a more important part in injuries to the spinal cord, often as a result of fractures or dislocations of the vertebral column that damage the cord. Direct injury to the cord is usually caused by gunshot wounds and is commonly encountered under conditions of warfare and, less commonly, in civilian practice. In civilian practice, stab wounds of the back may cause direct trauma to the spinal cord.

Etiology and Pathology

Injury to the spinal cord varies, and concussion, laceration, compression, extramedullary hemorrhage, or hematomyelia may occur, depending on the extent and force of the injury.

Experimental injury to the spinal cord has shown that there is an immediate and marked reduction in blood flow in both gray matter and white matter after injury.[210] In mild or moderate degrees of injury the white matter blood flow shows a gradual return to normal levels at 24 hours followed by a period of hyperemia,[211] but the gray matter remains ischemic. Severe injury produces permanent reduction in blood flow in both white and gray matter. Examination of traumatized spinal cords has shown that there is an initial leakage of erythrocytes into the perivascular space surrounding the thin-walled vessels in the ischemic central gray matter[236] followed by extension and coalescence of the hemorrhagic areas within two hours.[129] The neurons in the central gray matter show chromatolysis and evidence of ischemic damage.[10, 60] The surrounding white matter shows edema[51] and hemorrhages with fragmentation of axons and loss of myelin extending out from the gray matter to the periphery.

These morphologic changes are accompanied by biochemical changes including a rise in tissue lactate levels at the site of spinal cord trauma.[141] However, reported increased levels of norepinephrine[177] have not been confirmed,[14, 203] and the use of agents that reduce tissue norepinephrine does not alter the marked reduction in blood flow in the ischemic gray matter.[204] Damage to blood vessels and reduction in blood flow in the traumatized cord is more likely to be mechanical than due to release of norepinephrine.[54] Therefore, agents that increase oxygen diffusion and provide an increase in oxygen at the level of the capillary endothelium may be useful in reducing the effects of spinal cord trauma.[66]

Mechanisms of Injury

Dislocation of the Vertebral Column. Dislocation of the vertebral column usually occurs in the cervical area between C_1 and C_2 and most commonly between C_5 and C_6. Dislocations occasionally occur in the lower thoracic area, in particular T_{11} or T_{12}, but dislocations are rare in other sites.

The dislocation may be momentary and slight with rapidly reversible damage to the spinal cord (concussion of the cord)[17] or it may persist with narrowing of the spinal canal. The severity of the dislocation, however, does not necessarily parallel the degree of damage to the spinal cord. Complete transection of the spinal cord can occur with reversible subluxations of the cervical or thoracic areas,[29, 73] while temporary paralysis with recovery is not uncommon with cervical dislocation. The extent of the damage is influenced by other factors such as preexisting degenerative changes in the cervical spine,[28] damage to the blood vessels supplying the cord, and swelling and disruption of the anterior longitudinal ligament. In the most severe injuries, there is usually associated rupture of the posterior longitudinal ligament.

A number of other structures are prone to injury as a result of spinal dislocation. There may be damage to nerve roots, rupture of intervertebral disks,[216] injury to arteries and veins,[87, 221] and extra- or intramedullary hemorrhage. The nucleus pulposus, as a result of damage to the intervertebral disk, may be displaced into the spinal canal or intervertebral foramina, producing compression of the spinal cord or nerve roots. Injury to the intervertebral disks may lead to healing with bony spur formation and degenerative arthritic changes (see Cervical Spondylosis, p. 224).

Fracture of Vertebrae. Fractures can occur without displacement or with displacement, as fracture dislocations. These may involve the vertebral bodies, laminae, pedicles, and transverse or spinous processes. In severe trauma, bony fragments may be driven into the spinal canal and impinge on, compress, or transfix the spinal cord and/or nerve roots.

Spinal Epidural Hematoma. Acute epidural spinal hemorrhage is usually the result of bleeding following trauma but can occur in patients with a coagulation defect following the use of anticoagulant therapy, in sepsis, and has been reported following epidural anesthesia.[100] Occasionally there is no apparent cause.[18, 207]

There are immediate signs of radicular pain at the site of the hemorrhage with progressive paraparesis over a short period of time. When paraplegia occurs, spinal epidural hemorrhage is a surgical emergency, and pressure on the spinal cord must be relieved as soon as possible if permanent paralysis is to be avoided.[224]

Spinal Subdural Hematoma. This condition is one of the rarer causes of acute spinal cord compression. Spinal subdural hematoma may follow relatively minor trauma, and symptoms are dramatic with rapid onset of a severe flaccid paraparesis.[7] Myelography, which should be performed as an emergency procedure, will demonstrate a complete block at the level of the hematoma. Laminectomy and decompression by evacuation of the hematoma should be performed as soon as possible.

Indirect Trauma to the Spinal Cord. The spinal cord is susceptible to injury from indirect forces generated by blows to the head, frequently owing to automobile accidents.[45] The injury results from the transmission of energy along the brainstem and spinal cord, producing hemorrhages in the gray matter of the upper cervical region.[75, 213] Similar injuries may occur after a fall onto the feet or buttocks,[195] or following an explosion. If the injury is of low energy, there may be a temporary disturbance of spinal cord function lasting for a few seconds, minutes, or hours, with complete recovery presumably indicating concussion of the cord. Injuries of higher energy result in contusion of the cord with incomplete recovery of function. In the latter cases hemorrhages within the gray matter are associated with edema in the white matter. The white matter shows patchy wallerian degeneration, but there is permanent loss of neurons with neuronophagia in the anterior horns. Neuronal loss is followed by a proliferation of microglial cells and astrocytes and the eventual formation of a glial scar.

Laceration of the Spinal Cord. Severe injury to the spinal cord may result in its laceration. Common causes are stabbing or gunshot wounds and fracture dislocations of the vertebrae. The changes are much the same as those described under contusion of the cord except that there is disruption of the continuity of the cord substance with hemorrhage and edema of the meninges and cord followed by necrosis and gliosis.

Hematomyelia. Any type of injury can produce a spindle-shaped hemorrhage within the substance of the cord located primarily in the gray matter. It can occur as a complication of fracture dislocation, whiplash injuries, or following indirect injuries such as those which follow explosions or falls onto the feet and buttocks. Hematomyelia, which is reported as a complication of lifting heavy objects or during heavy labor, probably results from preexisting small angiomatous malformations of the spinal cord.

At necropsy, in cases of hematomyelia, the cord is usually swollen in the area of the hemorrhage, which extends over several segments. It is spindle-shaped, tapering off in its rostral and caudal parts. The hemorrhage apparently begins in the central gray matter and extends laterally, anteriorly, and posteriorly on both sides of the cord. The gray matter tends to be more severely affected than the white matter, although the hemorrhage may dissect along the fiber tracts in the posterior column in some cases. The microscopic appearance consists of an area of hemorrhage and infarction surrounded by petechiae. There is patchy necrosis of tissue in the white and gray matter around the central blood-filled cavity. The hemorrhage and necrosis are followed by phagocytosis and eventual gliosis.

Compression of the Spinal Cord. Fracture dislocation of the vertebral column is the most common cause of acute cord compression, but this also results from epidural and subdural hemorrhages. A fracture dislocation should be treated as soon as possible to relieve pressure on the spinal cord since compression of the cord (with complete block) for more than a few hours will usually result in permanent and severe neurologic defects.[107] In the initial stages of compression, there is collapse of the meningeal and spinal vessels, with reversible ischemia of the cord and potential recovery if surgical decompression is prompt. If the ischemia is untreated, infarction of the cord results, and edema and necrosis develop. There are loss of neurons in the gray matter and wallerian degeneration of the white matter. These are followed by microglial proliferation, phagocytosis, and the eventual development of a glial scar in the area of compression.

Clinical Features

Injury to Nerve Roots. Relatively minor degrees of injury to the spinal cord may result in compression of nerve roots without any damage to the spinal cord. Nerve root compression is frequently associated with herniation of an intervertebral disk (p. 521). The symptoms consist of radiating pain in the distribution of the affected root; muscle weakness, wasting, and occasional fasciculations in the muscles supplied by the affected anterior root; and sensory loss in the appropriate dermatomes of the compressed posterior nerve root. High-speed road accidents can cause lumbosacral nerve root avulsion with formation of a traumatic meningocele, which can be demonstrated by myelography.[156]

Compression of Nerve Roots and Spinal Cord.
In this type of injury, the symptoms of root compression are associated with signs of spinal cord compression. There are radiating pain, muscle weakness, and wasting due to root compression at the level of the lesion, but there is flaccid paresis or paralysis of the limbs below this level. This is followed by the gradual development of spastic paresis or paralysis, which usually begins after four weeks.

The deep tendon reflexes are initially absent below the lesion but reappear and become hyperactive with clonus and extensor plantar responses. There is retention of urine immediately after the traumatic episode, with distention of the bladder. After several weeks a small spastic bladder develops with reflex emptying. The degree of sensory loss depends on the extent of the compression. In severe cases, there is a complete sensory loss below the affected level with a narrow zone of hyperesthesia separating the anesthetic area from that of normal sensation. Incomplete traumatic transection of the cord produces various patterns of sensory loss.

Lateral injuries of the cord that spare the posterior columns leave touch, vibration, and position sense intact. Compression of the lateral spinothalamic tracts above the lumbar level often results in loss of pain and temperature in the sacral and lumbar segments before the thoracic segments, owing to the segmental distribution of fibers in this tract, and this gives rise to possible errors in diagnosis of the level of injury. Some cervical cord injuries produce distal sensory loss in the limbs, which poses as a peripheral neuropathy.

Transection of the Spinal Cord.   This is followed by complete flaccid paralysis below the level of the lesion. There is retention of urine, with painless distention of the bladder and eventual overflow as the pressure overcomes the reflex closure of the bladder sphincters. The state of flaccidity or spinal shock lasts for about four weeks and is followed by gradual return of tone and the eventual development of a spastic paralysis with increased deep tendon reflexes, clonus, and extensor plantar responses. Involuntary spasms of the lower limbs may appear on stimulation and sometimes develop into severe flexor spasms with piloerection, sweating, and evacuation of the bowel and bladder, the so-called "mass reflex." After several months, in neglected cases, flexor spasms decrease with the development of a stage of paraplegia in flexion. Patients who receive adequate physical therapy do not develop this stage of generalized flexion of the lower limbs but remain in a state of paraplegia in extension.

Hemisection of the Spinal Cord.   This usually occurs in gunshot or knife wounds of the cord. The clinical picture (the Brown-Séquard syndrome) consists of flaccid paralysis below the level of the lesion on the same side, followed by the eventual development of spasticity, increased deep tendon reflexes, and an extensor plantar response on the involved side. There is a loss of vibration and position sense on the same side as the lesion owing to posterior column involvement and a loss of pain and temperature on the opposite side, beginning two segments below the level of the lesion, owing to involvement of the spinothalamic tract.

Hematomyelia.   The occurrence of an acute hemorrhage into the central gray matter of the cord following trauma is followed by loss of function below the level of the lesion, which often suggests that complete transection of the cord has occurred. As edema subsides and the clot is slowly absorbed, there is a return of function in the posterior and lateral white columns, with the emergence of a clinical picture typical of hematomyelia. The patient usually has a flaccid paralysis and muscular atrophy in muscles supplied by anterior horn cells at the level of the lesion. There is a gradual development of spastic paresis below this level, with loss of pain and temperature sensation occurring over those segments affected by the blood clot. Pain and temperature are preserved below the level of the hematomyelia, and posterior column function is normal.

Syringomyelia.   A late progressive form of syringomyelia has been reported following injury to the cervical cord by fracture dislocation. The initial injury causes few and transient sensory symptoms with rapid recovery, but typical signs of syringomyelia (p. 221) begin several years later.[239]

Compression of the Conus Medullaris. This follows a compression fracture of the first lumbar vertebra. The injury results in contusion and hemorrhage with damage to the sacral segments of the cord. There is usually no persistent motor involvement, but sensory loss occurs in the sacral segments, particularly in the "saddle area" of the buttocks and perineum. This predisposes to the development of bed sores. Destruction of the sacral cord which innervates the bladder produces retention with overflow. There is usually complete loss of sexual function in the male due to impotence.

Compression of the Cauda Equina. The symptoms depend on the extent of involvement of the nerve roots in the cauda equina. There is a flaccid paralysis and wasting of the involved muscles and sensory loss corresponding to the involved dermatomes. Partial destruction of nerve roots results in pain and hyperesthesia. Compression of the nerve roots of S_2, S_3, and S_4 produces disturbance of bladder function with retention of urine and loss of voluntary control of the bladder. Disturbances of sexual function and fecal incontinence are also common in lesions involving the same sacral nerve roots.

Symptoms Associated with Lesions at Specific Levels. Fracture dislocation of the atlanto-occipital joint is rare and is apparently caused by violent hyperextension of the upper cervical spine. This usually produces signs of damage to the spinal cord and acute downward traction and injury to lower cranial nerves.[64]

Fracture or congenital dislocation of the odontoid process may follow relatively trivial trauma. Symptoms are mild and usually consist of pain in the neck, often in the distribution of the greater occipital nerve.[212] The incidence of nonunion is high despite adequate treatment, and there is a risk of severe damage to the spinal cord if the patient suffers further trauma. Fracture of the odontoid usually occurs after traffic accidents in children where satisfactory union and stability can usually be obtained by simple skull traction.[83]

Fracture dislocation of the second cervical vertebra is produced by acute hyperextension of the neck and symmetric fractures of the pedicles of C_2. This permits the forward dislocation of C_2 and C_3 and is the cause of death in judicial hanging, giving rise to the term "hangman's fracture." This type of fracture dislocation sometimes occurs in children or in adults who suffer acute hyperextension of the neck in a head-on automobile collision.[217] There are relatively few symptoms apart from a stiff and painful neck and spasm of the cervical muscles. The condition requires immediate immobilization of the head and neck and may require surgical fusion.[154]

Lesions of the cervical cord from C_3 to C_7 result in two distinct syndromes. The first is a centromedullary syndrome and is due to contusion, edema, and hemorrhages in the central portion of the cord. It consists of tetraparesis, loss of sphincter control, and impairment of temperature and pain sensation below the level of the lesion. There is usually progressive improvement. The second, a more severe syndrome, is due to acute protrusion of a cervical disk and damage to the anterior spinal artery. It consists of tetraplegia, loss of sphincter control, and complete loss of sensation below the level of the lesion. There is little improvement in these cases. Loss of sensation over the face due to involvement of the spinal tract of the trigeminal nerve occurs with high cervical cord lesions, and Horner's syndrome may occur if there is interruption of the descending sympathetic fibers.[108] Bladder sensation may be preserved following transection of the cord below T_{11}, and there may be painful retention of urine.

Lesions of the lower thoracic and lumbar segments inhibit intestinal peristalsis and result in a temporary paralytic ileus.

Diagnostic Procedures

Lumbar Puncture. The lumbar puncture is useful in the acute phase following spinal cord injury. A slow rise of the cerebral spinal fluid in the manometer and a negative Queckenstedt test are indicative of a severe degree of edema of the cord, sufficient to block the spinal canal and occlude the subarachnoid space.

Roentgenograms of the Spine. Anteroposterior and lateral views of the suspected site of injury will reveal the extent of fracture involving the vertebrae and whether dislocation has occurred (Fig. 8–6).

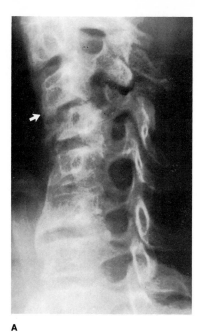

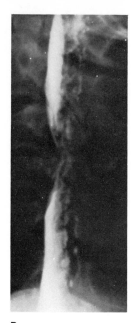

A   **B**

FIGURE 8–6. *A.* Cervical spine roentgenograms in a patient with subluxation of C_3 vertebra on C_4 and cervical spondylosis following an old traumatic injury to the neck. *B.* Myelogram in the same case to show compression of the cervical cord resulting in spastic quadriparesis.

Multidirectional Tomography. Multidirectional tomography should be performed in cases with a suspected fracture that is not shown by conventional radiography.[206]

Myelography. There does not seem to be any indication for this procedure following acute injury to the spinal cord. However, it is advisable to perform a myelogram in patients recovering from a fracture involving the lumbar spine because of the high incidence of associated herniation of the intervertebral disks, which may cause chronic nerve root compression. Failure to recognize that herniation has occurred may be followed by disabling symptoms, even though the fracture has been treated satisfactorily.

Cystometrograms. Patients who are unable to reestablish adequate voluntary control of the bladder following the return of function of the lower limbs may require urologic consultation and cystometrograms to ascertain the condition of the bladder.

Treatment

Fracture dislocation of the vertebral column with cord compression is a surgical emergency requiring prompt care and expert handling.

Emergency Treatment of Fractures of the Cervical Spine. There is always the danger of increasing spinal deformity by movement and transportation of the patient after fracture dislocation in this area. Patients should, therefore, not be moved more than is absolutely necessary, and this should be done with great care. They should be transported lying supine with the neck in slight hyperextension. If lifting is necessary, it should be performed by three people, one exerting slight traction on the head by grasping the chin and occiput, the second applying traction to the ankles, and the third lifting the shoulders and hips to maintain the cervical spine in slight hyperextension.

Whenever possible, a patient should be rolled rather than lifted onto a stretcher and transported on a firm surface with a roll behind the shoulders to maintain hyperextension. Upon the patient's arrival in the emergency room of the hospital or the casualty clearing center, a cervical brace should be fitted and any further transportation performed with the brace supporting the neck. Many patients require analgesics, such as morphine for pain, and this should be given as soon as possible and in adequate dosage. There is acute retention of urine, which requires catheterization with a Foley catheter in the bladder for intermittent drainage (see p. 520).

Emergency Treatment of Fractures of the Lumbar Spine. The same principle should be applied to the immediate treatment of fracture dislocation of the lumbar spine as outlined for fracture of the cervical spine. Persons with suspected fractures of the spine should not be moved any more than is absolutely necessary. The patient should lie supine on a hard surface with a roll under the lumbar area to maintain extension of the lumbar spine and should be transported to the hospital in a prone position, which prevents flexion of the spine.

Management of Fractures of the Odontoid Process. All undisplaced odontoid fractures should be treated by external immobilization, and all fractures displaced more than 4 mm should be treated by operative fusion.[99]

Management of Cervical Cord Injuries. The cervical cord may be contused at the time of injury by subluxation of the cervial spine with compression of the cord followed by spontaneous realignment of the vertebral bodies. During the next few days, there is edema of the cord.

There does not seem to be any benefit from spinal cord decompression in patients with complete paralysis and sensory loss below the level of the lesion.[98] Attention should be diverted toward reduction and stabilization of fracture dislocations in patients with nonprogressive partial neurologic deficits and the dura should not be opened. Decompressive procedures should be reserved for those with progressive neurologic deficits. In view of this, the condition is usually treated by bed rest, intravenous injection of hypertonic solutions such as mannitol, and prompt administration of corticosteroids to reduce edema of the cord. Dexamethasone can be given in doses of 8 mg intramuscularly three times daily followed by 4 mg three times a day intramuscularly or orally after three days, with gradual reduction of the dose over the next seven days.

Management of Hematomyelia. The presence of a central blood clot within the cord substance is rarely diagnosed clinically in the acute stages since the early symptoms suggest complete transection of the cord. By the time that the clinical findings suggest hematomyelia, cord swelling has subsided and attempts to evacuate the clot are not indicated.

Management of Compression of the Spinal Cord Due to Fracture of the Dorsal Arch. This is a rare injury due to a direct blow to the dorsal arch. Depressed bony fragments compressing the cord should be removed surgically.

Management of Fracture Dislocation of the Cervical Spine. Any operative procedure to correct a fracture dislocation of this type, in the acute stages of spinal cord injury, carries the risk of further injury to the cord. The majority of cases are best treated by traction, using Crutchfield tongs applied to the skull for a period of six to ten weeks. The patient should not be permitted to ambulate for another 12 weeks and should be placed in a plastic collar for six months. Edema of the cord is often present in the early stages and can be treated with intravenous mannitol and corticosteroids.

Management of Fracture with Dislocation of the Thoracic Vertebrae. The incidence of transection of the cord is high in this type of injury. Incomplete acute traumatic myelopathies should be treated with surgical decompression by way of a transthoracic approach.[180] Unstable fractures of the thoracolumbar area should be treated with posterior stabilization of the spine and anterior decompression of the cord carried out at the same operation.[241]

Management of Fractures of the Lumbar Spine. This type of injury is usually a compression fracture with little or no dislocation. The patient should be placed on a firm mattress over a fracture board with a rolled blanket between the mattress and the board at the level of the injury. This produces hyperextension with gradual reduction of the bony deformity. A lumbar myelogram is advised after the fracture is healed since many patients suffer a concomitant herniation of a lumbar disk with compression of nerve roots.

Management of Penetrating Wounds of the Spinal Canal. Patients with complete or very severe lesions should be treated conservatively, and surgery should be reserved for cases with gross contamination of the wound. Patients with less severe injuries such as a mild or moderate paraparesis and incomplete sensory loss or a Brown-Séquard syndrome require surgery only if there are signs of a progressive neurologic deficit.[101]

If the patient is in circulatory shock, it is likely that he has suffered associated injury to the thoracic or abdominal cavity with bleeding. The shock and hemorrhage require emergency treatment before laminectomy is considered.

Penetrating wounds of the spinal canal require laminectomy with removal of all bony fragments, foreign bodies, and dead tissue. Defects in the dura should be repaired, if possible, before closure of the wound. The risk of meningitis and osteomyelitis is greatly reduced by adequate removal of dead tissue and foreign material, primary closure, and the liberal use of antibiotics in the postoperative period.

General Considerations of Treatment Common to the Majority of Spinal Cord Injuries. Many of the conditions discussed in this section require a protracted period of bed rest. The nursing care is important, and where available, the skilled services provided by a neurologic or neurosurgical unit should be utilized. Every effort should be made to prevent the development of decubiti during the period of immobilization and paralysis by turning the patient at frequent intervals to prevent prolonged pressure on bony prominences. Turning may be accomplished mechanically in some centers, but whether turning is mechanical or manual, the prescribed position and posture of the spine must be maintained.

Bed sores are particularly likely to occur in areas of sensory loss. The lack of sensation allows the development of pressure necrosis, skin abrasions, ulceration, and burns without the patient's knowledge, so that nursing personnel should be instructed and trained to inspect all pressure areas every day in such patients. The heels, knees, buttocks, elbows, and shoulders are the common sites of pressure necrosis. Inflamed areas can be protected by special padding and by special posturing. Pressure on the heels can be prevented by using a second short mattress on top of the regular mattress so that the heels can dangle free, supported by the calves. If decubiti develop, infection must be controlled by topical antibiotics and all dead tissue must be cut away. Skin grafting can be performed at a later date in selected cases. The clinical efficiency of a neurologic unit can usually be assessed by the care which is taken to prevent bed sores.

Patients with upper cervical cord injuries suffer diaphragmatic paralysis and impairment of respiratory exchange predisposing to atelectasis and pneumonia. The risk of pneumonia is reduced by frequent turning, which allows drainage of the dependent parts of the lung. Deep breathing and percussion of the chest, with drainage of secretions, are useful in patients who show a tendency to the accumulation of mucous plugs. The early use of antibiotics may prevent pneumonia in suspected atelectasis. Rarely, in patients with high cervical cord injuries, hypoventilation may lead to carbon dioxide retention, with CO_2 narcosis (see p. 246). Such patients require endotracheal intubation, which must be performed with extreme care since the head cannot be hyperextended to facilitate this maneuver.[122] Treatment should be continued in an extensive care unit using a mechanical respirator.

Paralytic ileus commonly occurs for the first few days following injuries to the cervical or thoracic cord. This may require limitation of oral fluids, supplemental intravenous fluids, or the use of gastric suction through a nasogastric tube if vomiting occurs. Fluid intake and output and serum electrolyte levels should be recorded and noted carefully during this period so that early parenteral correction of fluid or electrolyte imbalance can be instituted. Paralytic ileus resolves spontaneously after a few days if these precautions are observed.

Pain and painful muscular spasms are often a major complaint in the period immediately following injury. If severe, they may require the use of narcotics (morphine, ¼ gr, or meperidine hydrochloride, 100 to 150 mg in the adult male) every four to six hours. The action of the narcotic can be potentiated by the use of simultaneous parenteral phenothiazines.

Bladder care and prevention of urinary tract infection should also be a major consideration following severe cord injury. During the initial period of retention, urinary drainage should be maintained by means of a Foley catheter, which can be clamped and released at intervals of two hours. This prevents the development of a small, contracted irritable bladder (the so-called "spastic bladder"). Irrigation with 250 ml of antibiotic solution (neomycin, 100 mg, and polymyxin, 25 mg, in 1,000 ml of water) twice daily is useful in preventing infection and prevents the formation of adhesions or pressure ulcers in the bladder and around the catheter.

Patients who show signs of return of function in the lower limbs should have the catheter removed at an early stage so that bladder control may be reestablished. Those with paraplegia or quadriparesis can be trained to develop reflex emptying of the bladder. This sometimes can be initiated by stimulation of the lower abdominal wall. The development of this spinal reflex is aided by prevention of bladder infection and early training. It requires removal of the Foley catheter as soon as reflex movements can be demonstrated in the paraplegic limbs and the gradual development of reflex bladder emptying.

Patients who remain completely incontinent should have an ileal loop conduit constructed. This facilitates management of urinary excretion and lowers the risk of debilitating urinary tract infections.

Many patients with paraparesis or paraplegia develop severe reflex spasms (usually flexor spasms) in the lower limbs. These may even be initiated by cutaneous stimuli and may involve sudden contraction of all muscle groups in the lower limbs, with associated reflex emptying of the bowel and bladder (mass reflex). The condition can be reduced or abolished by the use of Baclofen, 10 mg four times a day, slowly increasing the dosage until flexor spasms are abolished. Diazepam is also useful in doses of up to 20 mg four times daily, a somewhat higher dose than that usually recommended for other conditions. Intractable cases of adductor and flexor spasms may require obturator neurectomy or blocking of the anterior nerve roots of the lumbosacral plexus by intrathecal phenol. The latter procedure carries some risk of increasing bladder paralysis and probably should only be performed if all control of micturition is lost.

The patient who shows return of motor function following cord injury benefits enormously from a planned program of rehabilitation. The help and advice of the physiatrist are invaluable in the treatment of patients with spinal cord injury. The planned program should include occupational and, later, vocational rehabilitation.

Herniation of the Intervertebral Disks

Low-back pain and pain radiating in the distribution of the sciatic nerve owing to herniation of an intervertebral disk in the lumbosacral area are commonly encountered in neurologic practice. They are usually related to injury to the spine or excessive strain, such as is caused by lifting heavy weights. The preponderance of herniated disks are in the lumbar area, but it should be borne in mind that herniated disks can occur at almost any level of the spinal cord. Herniated disks are also common in the cervical area but are rare in the thoracic zone. They are extremely rare in children and adolescents but the incidence increases with age after the twenties.

Etiology and Pathology

The intervertebral disks are situated between opposing surfaces of the vertebral bodies. They act as joints of the symphysis type, thereby imparting mobility to the spinal column. The disk surfaces are firmly adherent to thin plates of hyaline cartilage covering the bony surfaces of the vertebral bodies. The disk is a fibrocartilaginous structure consisting of an outer circumferential annulus fibrosus made up of dense, interwoven, collagenous fibers and an inner gelatinous nucleus pulposus. The annulus fibrosus is thicker anteriorly and thinner posteriorly, is firmly attached to the periosteum of the vertebral bodies, and blends with the anterior and posterior longitudinal ligaments. The nucleus pulposus consists of loose connective tissue and cartilage cells and has a high water content. It acts as a fluid medium, and since it is incompressible, it becomes flatter and broader under pressure and distends the annulus fibrosus.

Herniation of a portion of the nucleus pulposus through the annulus fibrosus occurs as a result of sudden compressive forces above and below the spinal vertebra which are sufficient to rupture the fibers of the annulus. Additional factors are involved, the most important of which are degenerative changes and loss of elasticity of the annulus fibrosus.[227] This facilitates herniation since the annulus can no longer sustain sudden compressive forces of the vertebrae that had previously been tolerated.

Since the annulus fibrosus is thinner posteriorly, the herniation occurs posteriorly or posterolaterally into the spinal canal. The herniated material usually consists of nucleus pulposus, which often fragments when extruded. As a result, some fragments may lie free in the spinal canal as isolated cartilaginous bodies. This material forms the so-called "chondromata" of the spinal canal described in surgical texts during the first quarter of this century.

All protrusions are not necessarily composed of the nucleus pulposus, and occasionally, there is protrusion of the annulus fibrosus itself. This appears to result from loss of water content in the nucleus pulposus, which narrows the disk and results in an outward protrusion of the annulus fibrosus in all directions. This may reach sufficient proportions to cause pressure on structures within the spinal canal.

The protrusion of disk material posteriorly or posterolaterally results in pressure on the spinal cord, cauda equina, or the spinal nerves as they pass anterolaterally to exit through the intervertebral foramina. Degenerative changes in the cord or nerves giving rise to symptoms may occur intermittently and over a long period of time, depending on the degree and nature of the compressive forces. Once herniation has occurred, symptoms are likely to occur and continue until the herniation is reduced or removed.

Clinical Features

Herniated Cervical Disks. The most common site of herniation in the cervical region involves the disk between the vertebral bodies of C_5 and C_6, followed in frequency by that between C_4 and C_5 or C_6 and C_7. The protrusion is usually posterolateral, producing pressure on the nerve root as it leaves the spinal canal on the affected side. This produces radicular pain, which is usually the earliest symptom and is referred to the appropriate dermatome.

There are usually associated pain and stiffness in the neck. The pain may radiate down to the shoulder and into the dermatome of C_5 or C_6 or to the anterior chest wall in some cases, posing as angina due to myocardial ischemia. The development of muscle weakness is usually delayed for some time after sensory symptoms, but occasionally appears within a few days of development of pain. Midline herniation with compression of the spinal cord results in progressive difficulties in gait due to spasticity in the lower limbs. There may be urgency of micturition and complaints of paresthesias in both legs.

On examination, the neck is stiff owing to spasm of the neck muscles, and there is pain on passive movement. The normal anterior convexity of the cervical spine is lost. The pain may be exacerbated by movements of the neck or by compression of the cervical vertebra by gently striking the top of the head downward with the palm of the hand. Such movements may precipitate shooting radicular pain in the affected dermatome. The muscles innervated by the compressed nerve root (rhomboids, supraspinatus, deltoid by C_5; biceps, brachioradialis by C_6; triceps by C_7) begin to show some degree of wasting after several weeks,

and fasciculations confined to these muscles are occasionally seen. There may be hypalgesia and hypesthesia of the involved dermatome. Depression of the affected deep tendon reflexes is a useful indication of the level of nerve root compression, with reduction or absence of the biceps reflex when the disk is at the level C_5 to C_6 or triceps reflex when it affects the C_7 root. In severe cases with cord compression there may be an increased resistance to passive movement in the lower limbs and ankle clonus. This may be more marked on the side of maximal herniation. If the disk is untreated, the gait becomes spastic, with increased tendon jerks in the lower limbs and extensor plantar responses. In such neglected cases, patchy hypalgesia may be present in the periphery of the lower limbs or a sensory level may extend up to the chest. The posterior columns are usually spared, so that vibration and position sense remain intact.

Herniation of Thoracic Intervertebral Disks. This is uncommon and usually occurs at the lower four thoracic disk spaces. The symptoms consist of radicular pain at the level of the lesion with disagreeable paresthesias below the level of the lesion on one or both sides of the body and weakness of the lower limbs owing to progressive spastic paraparesis.[33] Occasionally, the onset is sudden with a complete paraplegia, which imitates transverse myelitis. Herniation at the first thoracic disk level is rare but produces a specific syndrome of hand weakness, Horner's syndrome, and pain radiating along the medial aspect of the upper extremity.[70]

Herniation of Lumbosacral Intervertebral Disks. Herniation of a disk in the lumbar area is the most common site of disk herniation, and this usually involves the disks between L_4 and L_5 or between L_5 and S_1, although lesions at other lumbar levels occur less frequently and there are often multiple protrusions.

A posterolateral protusion compresses the lumbar nerve roots as they pass to the intervertebral foramen at the level of the lesion. A posterior protrusion, toward the cauda equina, tends to affect the nerve descending to the next intervertebral foramen below the level of the lesion.

There is a history of trauma to the back in more than 50 per cent of patients.[20] This may be dramatic with the report of "something giving way" or a "click" in the lumbar area followed by the development of low-back pain. The next complaint is usually the development of sciatic pain radiating down the buttock to the posterior aspect of the thigh and sometimes extending down to the dermatome of the compressed nerve root.[182]

The pain in the lumbar area and over the sciatic nerve is usually constant and severe, but the sensation in the affected dermatome is one of discomfort or paresthesias. The lumbar and sciatic pain are exacerbated by certain movements and certain postures, so that the patient tends to assume an attitude of slight flexion of the trunk and lateral flexion in order to obtain some degree of relief. Some patients obtain relief by flexing the knees and thighs. There may be quite severe exacerbation on sudden movements such as coughing, sneezing, straining at stool, and when lifting objects. All these maneuvers produce compression of the vertebral column with further displacement of the disk compressing the sensitive nerve root resulting in a sudden increase in the pain.

Muscle weakness is usually not a prominent feature as a result of lumbar disk protrusion, although this does occur and unilateral or bilateral foot drop may result. The usual picture is, however, that of a slowly developing weakness and wasting of the affected muscles, which may not even be noticed by the patient. Urgency of micturition with incomplete emptying of the bladder and impotence are rare complications owing to pressure on the cauda equina.[3, 6, 85]

Examination of the patient with an acute herniated lumbar disk usually reveals an individual with an abnormal posture who is suffering from pain. There is marked restriction of movement in the lumbar spine, a loss of lumbar lordosis, unilateral or bilateral spasm of the spinal muscles, and a scoliosis with a pelvic tilt away from the side of the lesion. Percussion in the lumbar area at the level of herniation may produce local pain or a sudden shooting pain down the affected sciatic nerve.

The gait is frequently abnormal owing to flexion of the spine, pelvic tilt, and a limp in the affected lower limb. The patient should be requested to walk on his heels and on his toes, to reveal any weakness of the leg muscles. Weakness of dorsiflexion of the great toe or plantar flexion of the second through fifth toes is not unusual in the absence of demonstrable weakness of other muscles in the leg. The tendon jerks are depressed or absent on the affected side in a manner appropriate to the level of the lesion (knee jerk, L_4; ankle jerk, L_5, S_1). Sensory loss is often patchy, with some irregular areas of hypesthesia and hypalgesia in the affected dermatomes. The diagnosis is confirmed by performing the straight-leg-raising test with flexion of the hip in the affected side. The test shows marked restriction of leg raising due to stretching of the sciatic nerve with pain and reflex spasm. Another useful test is carried out with the patient prone. The knee is flexed on the thigh with the production of pain in the back or sciatic distribution on the affected side.[69]

Diagnostic Procedures

Anteroposterior and lateral or oblique roentgenograms of the spine may reveal narrowing of the intervertebral space in suspected cases of disk herniation. This finding sometimes occurs in asymptomatic individuals, however, and should be interpreted as significant only when the narrowing corresponds to the level of the suspected lesion based on clinical findings.

Lumbar diskography is now used in many hospitals in the diagnosis of lumbar disk lesions and has increased the accuracy of diagnosis and knowledge of the extent of disk involvement.[96, 190]

Electromyography is an important procedure in the evaluation of root lesion owing to protruded intervertebral disk. In experienced hands, EMG is positive in about 90 per cent of cases.[21] This is significant since lumbar myelography may be negative in about 25 per cent of patients who are subsequently shown to have a herniated lumbosacral intervertebral disk at surgery.

It is important to keep in mind that fibrillations appear only two to three weeks after the onset of the lesion. In the first few days the only abnormality will be a reduction in the number of motor units in the appropriate root distribution. Fibrillations appear earlier in the more proximal muscles. Lumbosacral paraspinal muscles should be sampled routinely at several places in addition to examining the limb muscles. In long-standing cases polyphasic motor unit potentials of more than 10-millisecond duration would indicate reinnervation. EMG can also be helpful in determining whether there has been a new root lesion in a person known to have previous root involvement. It is essential not only to show evidence of denervation in a particular root distribution but also to show that the roots above and below the level of the lesion are not involved.

Myelography is of great value in the accurate localization and diagnosis of herniated disks, particularly in the detection of multiple lesions (Fig. 8–7). The test is performed by injecting 9 to 12 ml of iophendylate injection U.S.P. (Pantopaque) into the lumbar sac after lumbar puncture. The needle is left in place and the patient placed prone on the tilt table. The dye is allowed to flow into the cervical area under fluoroscopic control by tilting the patient, head down, on an electrically operated table. Suspicious areas of obstruction to the flow or distortion of the dye column are seen on fluoroscopy and are recorded permanently by roentgenograms taken at the time of examination. After the dye has been allowed to flow as high as the foramen magnum, it is returned to the lumbar sac by tilting the patient, feet down, and

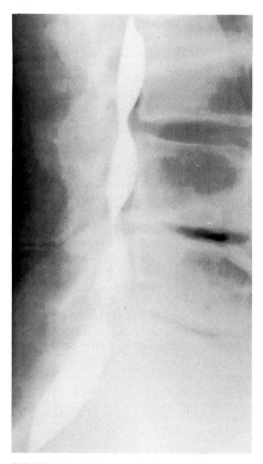

FIGURE 8–7. Myelogram to show multiple herniated disks at L_3–L_4, L_4–L_5, L_5–S_1. There are defects in the contrast media at the levels of each of these disks.

removed by gentle suction via the spinal needle. The procedure is occasionally followed by headache, but this can be minimized by laying the patient in a prone position in bed for six hours, followed by the supine position for another 12 hours, and forcing fluids. If postspinal headache is severe, an intravenous infusion of 5 per cent dextrose in 0.2 N saline over an eight-hour period is of value or inhalation of 5 per cent CO_2 and oxygen intermittently will also afford relief.

Myelographic abnormalities should always be assessed in the light of the clinical findings. Minor filling defects are sometimes seen when there are no symptoms to suggest the presence of a lesion in that region. The complete study includes anteroposterior, lateral, and oblique views of the dye column, which allow some assessment of the position and extent of any defect produced by a herniated disk. Whenever a myelogram is performed, even in cases of suspected lumbar disk herniation, the entire spinal cord and roots should be examined up to and including the cervical area.

A posterolateral herniation of a disk produces a filling defect in the dye column by indentation of the lateral border. Since the arachnoidal sleeve covering the nerve root is also compressed, there is usually absence of filling of the appropriate root sleeve at the level of the lesion. Lateral herniations result in a normal dye column, with absence of filling of the affected nerve root sleeve as the only abnormality. Midline lesions may produce an "hourglass" deformity in the lumbosacral area owing to displacement of the nerve roots of the cauda equina laterally, allowing the dye to flow over the dome of the herniation. This type of protrusion produces striking indentations of the dye column in the lateral view.

Treatment

Herniated Cervical Disks. When symptoms are mild without muscle weakness and the only signs consist of limitation of neck movement and depression of one or more of the deep tendon reflexes, a trial of ambulatory treatment is justified. The arm should be supported by a sling, a plastic neck collar should be worn, and the pain should be controlled by analgesics for a four-week period. If the condition does not resolve within that time, the patient should be treated by bed rest with cervical traction using a halter over the chin and occipital area and 5 to 15 lb of weight.

The patient who is seen during the first attack with severe pain, muscle weakness, and depressed deep tendon reflexes requires a two-week trial of bed rest in the hospital. Pain should be controlled as soon as possible with liberal use of analgesics. The time until return of pain following a dose of an analgesic should be determined, and the patient should be given doses of the analgesic at regular time intervals to prevent any recurrence of pain. Dry heat should be applied to the neck using an electrical heating pad, and the patient should receive an effective soporific to induce sleep and thus avoid insomnia and restlessness at night. This regimen can be augmented by the use of corticosteroids in daily doses on a reducing scale over a ten-day period (see Treatment of Herniated Lumbar Intervertebral Disks).

If symptoms persist without improvement after two weeks of treatment, a myelogram should be performed to define the lesion and a neurosurgical opinion requested.

Surgical treatment is indicated in patients who fail to respond to medical treatment and in those who show signs of cord compression or severe motor defect. A number of procedures are used including foraminectomy and removal of herniated disk material[189] or anterior cervical diskectomy with or without interbody bone graft.[94, 151]

Herniated Lumbar Intervertebral Disks. THE MEDICAL TREATMENT. Conservative treatment should be used in patients who are experiencing their first attack of disk herniation unless there is obvious and severe compression of the nerve root with marked muscle weakness. Medical treatment may also be used in recurrent cases with mild symptoms of low-back pain and paresthesias in the affected dermatome or in those patients who refuse surgical treatment or in whom surgery is contraindicated because of associated disease.

Effective medical treatment requires a period of *complete* bed rest with the patient lying on his back using one pillow. Bathroom privileges should be restricted for bowel movements only. The mattress must be firm, and any tendency to sagging can be prevented by the use of a fracture board or some other wooden board between the mattress and the bed springs.[96]

Adequate doses of analgesics are necessary to control pain. This requires regular administration of analgesics in amounts and at time intervals sufficient to prevent return of pain (see Treatment, Herniated Cervical Disks).

The patient should lie on an electric heating pad, which should be regulated to supply heat to the lumbar area in comfort. An eight-day course of corticosteroids in gradually reducing dosage often produces rapid improvement. The corticosteroids can be given as methylprednisolone, 64 mg on the first day, reducing by 8 mg each morning for eight days, or as dexamethasone, 40 mg on the first day, reducing by 5 mg each morning.[79]

Patients who recover within three weeks may be gradually ambulated after they have been fitted with an orthopedic corset or lumbosacral brace, which should be worn for at least six months. Those who fail to respond to medical treatment should have myelography and may require surgical treatment.

SURGICAL TREATMENT. The operative procedure consists of partial hemilaminectomy and removal of as much of the herniated disk material as possible. Postoperative pain may require narcotics during the first day or two, but the patient should be out of bed for progressive intervals as soon as possible and started in a program of physical therapy.[166] Complete ambulation can usually be achieved within ten days after surgery, and patients with sedentary occupations may be permitted to return to work after six weeks. Those engaged in heavy work should not resume full activity for six months after the operation.

Lumbar disk surgery is usually successful but may fail to provide adequate relief from pain in 8 to 25 per cent of cases.[135] These patients should have careful reassessment before further surgery, and a convincing myelographic defect should be present to justify reoperation, since only about 25 per cent of cases will benefit from a second operation.

"Whiplash Injury" of the Cervical Spine

The cervical spine is susceptible to injury by sudden hyperextension and flexion of the neck, and this type of injury is referred to as "whiplash injury." There has been a remarkable increase in injuries of this type owing to the widespread use of the automobile. The injury usually results from rear-end collisions and is a frequent cause for litigation.[215]

Etiology and Pathology

Sudden and violent hyperextension and flexion of the neck are capable of producing damage to the strap muscles of the neck, the ligaments of the cervical spine, the intervertebral disks, the nerve roots, and the spinal cord in the cervical region. In addition, the vertebral arteries passing through the foramina in the transverse processes are likely to be injured, particularly if they are arteriosclerotic. This may lead to stenosis or occlusion of these vessels, with acute or chronic ischemia of the brainstem and occipital lobes. The linear acceleration produced by this movement may also result in concussion and contusion of the brainstem and brain.[171]

Clinical Features

The patient is usually dazed and pale immediately after the impact but loss of consciousness is rare. There is a feeling of weakness and unsteadiness, and some patients experience ataxia, vertigo, and vomiting after a short interval. These symptoms are probably due to ischemia of the brainstem due to injury of the vertebral arteries or to concussive effects on the brainstem. Most patients develop occipital headache, which may spread to the temporal regions within minutes or hours after the accident.

Headache and neck pain are the most common and troublesome complaints that follow a whiplash injury. The headache and neck pain are usually associated with stiffness in the neck and pain radiating down into the arms and occasionally the forearms.

Examination of the patient shortly after the accident reveals an apprehensive patient with tachycardia and slight elevation of blood pressure. There may be tenderness on palpation over the cervical spine and quite marked restriction of neck movements. Apart from this, the general physical and neurologic examination is usually within normal limits. The pain and tenderness in the neck usually resolve after a few days' rest in bed, but the headache may persist for weeks or even months after the accident before finally resolving.

Most cases recover satisfactorily without residual abnormalities, but a small number of patients show persistent symptoms and signs indicating damage to the brainstem or compression of the nerve roots in the neck. Persistent pain in the neck which radiates into one of the upper limbs, paresthesias in the distribution of the involved dermatome, and depression of the tendon reflexes in one upper limb are suggestive of cervical nerve root compression, possibly due to an acute herniation of a cervical disk. It is also possible that the injury may precipitate cervical spondylosis

(see p. 224). Older patients who already have some degree of cervical spondylosis may have their symptoms exacerbated by this type of accident, with pain in the distribution of nerve roots and signs of cord compression. If the vertebral arteries are arteriosclerotic, they may be damaged, with resultant thrombosis and the development of brainstem infarction. The symptoms in such cases usually resemble those of a lateral medullary syndrome (p. 565).

Diagnostic Procedures

1. Patients with a history of whiplash injury should have roentgenograms of the skull and cervical spine with anteroposterior, lateral, and oblique views immediately following the accident.
2. Myelography may be indicated at a later date in those patients who have signs suggesting herniation of an intervertebral disk or where there has been exacerbation or initiation of signs and symptoms of cervical spondylosis.
3. The occasional occurrence of brainstem infarction following neck injuries should be investigated and treated as recommended for the acute stroke (p. 568).

Treatment

Many patients have suffered some degree of concussion and should be treated with bed rest for two or three days. The pain in the neck and headache can be treated with adequate analgesics and the application of hot packs to the neck. Drugs that relax muscles in spasm are of questionable value. A plastic neck collar should be worn for a number of weeks after the accident to prevent aggravation of the inflamed or bruised structures in the neck by head turning or sudden movements of the head. Patients with exacerbation of symptoms owing to cervical spondylosis should be treated as outlined on page 224.

Cited References

1. Adams, J. H., and Connor, R. C. R. The shocked head injury. *Lancet,* **1:**263–64, 1966.
2. Adams, J. M.; Mitchell, D.; et al. Diffuse brain damage of immediate impact type. *Brain,* **100:**489–502, 1977.
3. Aho, A. J.; Auranen, A.; and Pesonen, K. Analysis of cauda equina symptoms in patients with lumbar disc prolapse. *Acta Chir. Scand.,* **135:**413–20, 1969.
4. Alker, G. J.; Glasauer, F. E.; and Leslie, E. V. Long-term experience with isotope cisternography. *J.A.M.A.,* **219:**1005–10, 1972.

5. Ambrose, J.; Gooding, M. R.; and Uhley, D. EMT scan in management of head injuries. *Lancet,* 1:847–48, 1976.

6. Amelar, R. D. Impotence in low back syndrome. *J.A.M.A.,* 216:520, 1971.

7. Anagnostopoulos, D. I., and Gortvai, P. Spontaneous spinal subdural haematoma. *Br. Med. J.,* 1:30, 1972.

8. Arseni, C.; Maretsis, M.; and Horvath, L. Posttraumatic intracranial arterial spasm. Report of three cases. *Acta Neurochir.,* 24:25–35, 1971.

9. Asari, S.; Nakamura, S.; et al. Traumatic aneurysm of peripheral cerebral arteries. Report of two cases. *J. Neurosurg.,* 46:795–803, 1977.

10. Assenmacher, D. R., and Ducker, T. B. Experimental traumatic paraplegia: The vascular and pathological changes seen in reversible and irreversible spinal cord lesions. *J. Bone Joint Surg.,* 53:671–80, 1971.

11. Baratham, G., and Dennyson, W. G. Delayed traumatic intracerebral haemorrhage. *J. Neurol. Neurosurg. Psychiat.,* 35:698–706, 1972.

12. Bennett, A. E. Psychiatric and neurologic problems of head injury with medico-legal implication. *Dis. Nerv. Syst.,* 30:314–17, 1969.

13. Bergstrom, M.; Ericson, K.; et al. Computed tomography of cranial, subdural and epidural hematomas. Variation of attentuation related to time and clinical events such as rebleeding. *J. Comput. Assist. Tomography,* 1(4): 449–55, 1977.

14. Bingham, W. G.; Ruffolo, R.; and Fredman, S. J. Catecholamine levels in the injured spinal cord of monkeys. *J. Neurosurg.,* 42:174–78, 1975.

15. Bishara, S. N. Intracerebral haemorrhage in closed head injury. *Br. J. Surg.,* 58:437–41, 1971.

16. Bortt, R. H.; Heck, M. K.; and Hamilton, R. D. Traumatic locked-in syndrome. *Ann. Neurol.,* 1:590–92, 1977.

17. Bovill, E. G.; Eberle, C. F.; and Day, L. Dislocation of the cervical spine without spinal cord injury. *J.A.M.A.,* 218:1288–90, 1971.

18. Boyd, H. R., and Pear, B. C. Chronic spontaneous spinal epidural hematoma. Report of two cases. *J. Neurosurg.,* 36:239–42, 1972.

19. Bradford, D. S.; Foster, R. R.; and Nossel, H. L. Coagulation alterations hypoxemia and fat embolism in fracture patients. *J. Trauma,* 10:307–21, 1970.

20. Bradford, D. S., and Garcia, A. Herniations of the lumbar intervertebral disk in children and adolescents. A review of 30 surgically treated cases. *J.A.M.A.,* 210:2045–51, 1969.

21. Brady, L. P.; Parker, L. B.; and Vaughan, J. An evaluation of the electromyogram in the diagnosis of the lumbar-disc lesion. *J. Bone Joint Surg.,* 51:539–47, 1969.

22. Bremmer, D. N., and Gillingham, F. J. Patterns of convalescence after minor head injury. *J. R. Coll. Surg. Edinb.,* 19:94–97, 1974.

23. Bresnan, M. J. Neurologic birth injuries, I. *Postgrad. Med.,* 49:199–205, 1971.

24. Bresnan, M. J. Neurologic birth injuries, II. *Postgrad. Med.,* 49:202–206, 1971.

25. Brierley, J. B., and Nicholson, A. N. Neuropathological correlates of neurological impairment following prolonged decompression. *Aerospace Med.,* 40:148–52, 1969.

26. Briggs, M. Traumatic pneumocephalus. *Br. J. Surg.,* 61:307–12, 1974.

27. Brink, J. D.; Garrett, A. L.; Hale, W. R.; Woo-Sam, J.; and Nickel, V. L. Recovery of motor and intellectual function in children sustaining severe head injury. *Dev. Med. Child Neurol.,* 12:565–71, 1970.

28. Burke, D. C. Hyperextension injuries of the spine. *J. Bone Joint Surg.,* 53:3–12, 1971.

29. Burke, D. C. Spinal cord trauma in children. *Paraplegia,* 9:1–14, 1971.

30. Burns, R. J.; Jones, A. N.; and Robertson, J. S. Pathology of radiation myelopathy. *J. Neurol. Neurosurg. Psychiat.,* 35:888–98, 1972.

31. Calverley, R. K.; Dodds, W. A.; Trapp, W. G.; and Jenkins, L. C. Hyperbaric treatment of cerebral air embolism. A report of a case following cardiac catheterization. *Can. Anaesthet. Soc. J.,* 18:665–74, 1971.

32. Carey, M. E.; Young, H. F.; and Mathis, J. L. The neurosurgical treatment of craniocerebral missile wounds in Vietnam. *Surg. Gynecol. Obstet.,* 135:386–89, 1972.

33. Carson, J.; Gumpert, J.; and Jefferson, A. Diagnosis and treatment of thoracic intervertebral disc protrusions. *J. Neurol. Neurosurg. Psychiat.,* 34:68–77, 1971.

34. Carter, L. P., and Pittman, H. W. Posterior fossa subdural hematoma of the newborn. *J. Neurosurg.,* 34:423–26, 1971.

35. Chason, J. L.; Hardy, W. G.; Webster, J. E.; and Gurdjian, E. S. Alterations in cell structure of the brain associated with experimental concussion. *J. Neurosurg.,* 15:135–39, 1958.

36. Cjruszkiewicz, J.; Doran, Y.; and Peyser, E. Frontal extradural hematomas. *Surg. Neurol.,* 5:122–28, 1976.

37. Clark, J. M. Distribution of microglial clusters in the brain after head injury. *J. Neurol. Neurosurg. Psychiat.,* 37:463–74, 1974.

38. Clausen, C. D.; Lohkamp, F. W.; and Krastel, A. Computed tomography of trauma involving brain and facial skull (craniofacial injuries). *J. Comput. Assist. Tomography,* 1(4):472–81, 1977.

39. Cockrill, H. H.; Jimmez, J. P.; and Gorse, J. A. Traumatic false aneurysm of the superior cerebellar artery simulating posterior fossa tumor. Case report. *J. Neurosurg.,* 46:377–80, 1977.

40. Coin, C. G., and Chan, Y. S. Computed assisted myelography in disk disease. *J. Computerized Tomogr.,* 1:398–404, 1977.

41. Courjon, J. A longitudinal electro-clinical study of 80 cases of post traumatic epilepsy observed from the time of trauma. *Epilepsia,* 11:29–36, 1970.

42. Craft, A. W.; Shaw, D. A.; and Cartlidge, N. E. F. Head injuries in children. *Br. Med. J.,* 4:200–203, 1972.

43. Craigmile, T. K. Operative treatment of acute craniocerebral injuries. *Surg. Clin. North Am.,* 49:1425–34, 1969.

44. Crockard, H. A.; Brown, F. D.; et al. Physiological

consequences of experimental cerebral missile injury and data analysis to predict survival. *J. Neurosurg.,* **46:**784–94, 1977.

45. Davis, D.; Bohlman, H.; Walker, A. E.; Fisher, R.; and Robinson, R. The pathological findings in fatal craniospinal injuries. *J. Neurosurg.,* **34:**603–13, 1971.

46. Davis, J. C.; Tager, R.; Polkovitz, H. P.; and Workman, R. D. Neurological decompression sickness: Report of two cases at minimal altitudes with subsequent seizures. *Aerospace Med.,* **42:**85–88, 1971.

47. Davis, K. R.; Poletti, C. E.; et al. Conplementary role of computed tomography and other neuroradiologic procedures. *Surg. Neurol.,* **8:**437–46, 1977.

48. De Vivo, D. C., and Dodge, P. R. The critically ill child: Diagnosis and management of head injury. *Pediatrics,* **48:**129–38, 1971.

49. Di Chiro, G.; Ommaya, A. K.; Ashburn, W. L.; and Briner, W. H. Isotope cisternography in the diagnosis and follow-up of cerebrospinal fluid rhinorrhea. *J. Neurol. Neurosurg. Psychiat.,* **28:**522–29, 1968.

50. Dikeman, S., and Reitan, R. M. Emotional sequelae of head injury. *Ann. Neurol.,* **2:**492–94, 1977.

51. Dohrmann, G. J.; Wagner, F. C.; and Bucy, P. C. Transitory traumatic paraplegia: electron microscopy of the early alterations in myelinated nerve fibers. *J. Neurosurg.,* **36:**407–15.

52. Dorsch, N. W. C., and Simon, L. A practical technique for monitoring extradural pressure. *J. Neurosurg.,* **42:**249–57, 1975.

53. Dowman, C. E. Early management of head injuries in children. *South. Med. J.,* **63:**992–97, 1970.

54. Doyle, T. F., and Martins, A. N. Local spinal cord blood flow in experimental traumatic myelopathy. *J. Neurosurg.,* **42:**144–49, 1975.

55. Duffy, G. P., and Bhandari, Y. S. Intracranial complications following transorbital penetrating injuries. *Br. J. Surg.,* **56:**685–88, 1969.

56. Elliott, F. A. The neurology of explosive rage. *Practitioner,* **217:**51–59, 1976.

57. Elliott, F. A. Propranolol for the control of belligerent behavior following acute brain damage. *Ann. Neurol.,* **1:**489–91, 1977.

58. Evans, D. E.; Alter, W. A., III; et al. Cardiac arrhythmias resulting from experimental head injury. *J. Neurosurg.,* **45:**609–16, 1976.

59. Evans, J. P. Acute trauma to the head. Fundamentals of management. *Postgrad. Med.,* **39:**27–30, 1966.

60. Fairholm, D. J., and Turnbull, I. M. Microangiographic study of experimental spinal cord injuries. *J. Neurosurg.,* **36:**277–86, 1971.

61. Farrell, D. F., and Starr, A. Delayed neurological sequelae of electrical injuries. *Neurology,* **18:**601–606, 1968.

62. Fell, D. A.; Fitzgerald, S.; et al. Acute subdural hematoma. Review of 144 cases. *J. Neurosurg.,* **42:**37–42, 1975.

63. Floyd, H. L.; Pribham, H. F. W.; and Velo, A. G. Primary cerebrospinal fluid fistula. *Am. J. Roentgenol.,* **110:**88–91, 1970.

64. Freun, A. H., and Pirotte, T. P. Traumatic antlanto-occipital dislocation. *J. Neurosurg.,* **46:**663–66, 1977.

65. Friede, R. L., and Roessmann, U. The pathogenesis of secondary midbrain hemorrhages. *Neurology,* **16:**1210–16, 1966.

66. Gainer, J. V. Use of crocetin in experimental spinal cord injury. *J. Neurosurg.,* **46:**358–60, 1977.

67. Galbraith, S. L. Age distribution of extradural hemorrhage without skull fracture. *Lancet,* **1:**1217–18, 1973.

68. Galbraith, S.; Teasdale, G.; and Blaiklock, C. Computerised tomography of acute traumatic intracranial haematoma: reliability of neurosurgeon's interpretations. *Br. Med. J.,* **2:**1371–73, 1976.

69. Gardner, R. C. New test for intervertebrae disc disease. *Ann. Intern. Med.,* **75:**480–81, 1971.

70. Gelch, M. M. Herniated thoracic disc at T1–2 level associated with Horner's syndrome. Case report. *J. Neurosurg.,* **48:**128–30, 1978.

71. Gerhard, L., and Spanken, E. Chronic spinal cord lesion following electric injury. *Acta Neuropathol.* (Berl.), **20:**357–62, 1972.

72. Gjerris, F., and Mellerngaard, L. Transitory cortical blindness in head injury. *Acta Neurol. Scand.,* **45:**623–31, 1969.

73. Glasauer, F. E., and Cares, H. L. Traumatic paraplegia in infancy. *J.A.M.A.,* **219:**38–41, 1972.

74. Goodnight, S. H.; Kenoyen, G.; et al. Defibrination after brain tissue destruction. Serious complication of head injury. *N. Engl. J. Med.,* **290:**1043–47, 1974.

75. Gosch, H. H.; Gooding, E.; and Schneider, R. C. Cervical spinal cord hemorrhage in experimental head injuries. *J. Neurosurg.,* **33:**640–44, 1970.

76. Gotham, J. E.; Meyer, J. S.; Gilroy, J.; and Bauer, R. B. Observations on cerebrospinal fluid rhinorrhea and pneumocephalus. *Ann. Otol.,* **74:**215–33, 1965.

77. Grahne, B. Spontaneous cerebrospinal fluid rhinorrhea. *Acta Otolaryngol.,* **70:**383–91, 1970.

78. Grahne, B. Traumatic cranionasal fistual persistent cerebrospinal fluid rhinorrhea and their repair with frontal sinus osteoplasty. *Acta Otolaryngol.,* **70:**392–400, 1970.

79. Green, L. N. Dexamethasone in management of symptoms due to herniated lumbar disc. *J. Neurol. Neurosurg. Psychiat.,* **38:**1211–17, 1975.

80. Greenberg, R. P.; Becker, D. P.; et al. Evaluation of brain function in severe human head trauma with multimodaility evoked potentials. Part 2. Localization of brain dysfunction and correlation with posttraumatic neurologic conditions. *J. Neurosurg.,* **47:**163–77, 1977.

81. Greenberg, R. P.; Mayer, D. J.; et al. Evaluation of brain function in severe human head trauma with multimodality evoked potentials. Part 1. Evoked brain-injury potentials, methods and analysis. *J. Neurosurg.,* **47:**150–62, 1977.

82. Greenblatt, S. H., and Wilson, D. H. Persistent cerebrospinal fluid rhinorrhea trachea by lumbo-peritoneal shunt. *J. Neurosurg.,* **38:**524–26, 1973.

83. Griffiths, S. C., Fracture of odontoid process in children. *J. Pediatr. Surg.,* 7:680–83, 1972.

84. Gronwall, D., and Wrightson, P. Delayed recovery of intellectual function after minor head injury. *Lancet,* 2:605–608, 1974.

85. Grynderup, V. Cauda equina lesion from lumbar disc prolapse. *Acta Neurol. Scand.,* Suppl **43,** **46:**267–68, 1970.

86. Gurd, A. R. Fat embolism: an aid to diagnosis. *J. Bone Joint Surg.,* **52B:**732–37, 1970.

87. Gurdjian, E. S.; Hardy, W. G.; Lindner, D. W.; and Thomas, L. M. Closed cervical cranial trauma associated with involvement of the carotid and vertebral arteries. *Laryngoscope,* 81:1381–87, 1971.

88. Gurdjian, E. S.; Thomas, L. M.; Hodgson, V. R.; and Patrick, L. M. Impact head injury. *GP,* **37:**78–87, 1968.

89. Gurdjian, E. S., and Thomas, L. M. Neurosurgical problems in trauma. *AORN J.,* 9:71–75, 1969.

90. Guthkelch, A. N. Infantile subdural haematoma and its relationship to whiplash injuries. *Br. Med. J.,* 2:430–31, 1971.

91. Haas, D. C.; Pineda, G. S.; and Lourie, H. Juvenile head trauma syndromes and their relationship to migraine. *Arch. Neurol.,* 32:727–30, 1975.

92. Hagan, P. J. Post-traumatic anosmia. *Arch Otolaryngol.,* 85:107–11, 1967.

93. Hallenbeck, J. M.; Bove, A. A.; and Elliott, D. H. Mechanisms underlying spinal cord damage in decompression sickness. *Neurology* (Minneap.), 25:308–16, 1975.

94. Hankinson, H. L., and Wilson, C. B. Use of operating microscope and anterior cervical diskectomy without fusion. *J. Neurosurg.,* 43:452–56, 1976.

95. Hansson, O.; Hugosson, R.; and Tonnby, B. The management of chronic subbdural effusion in infancy. *Dev. Med. Child Neurol.,* 14:813–14, 1972.

96. Hartman, J. T.; Kendrick, J. I.; and Lorman, P. Discography as an aid in evaluation for lumbar and lumbosacral fusion. *Clin. Orthop.,* 81:77–81, 1971.

97. Harwood-Nash, D. C.; Hendrick, E. B.; and Hudson, A. R. The significance of skull fracture in children: A study of 1,187 patients. *Radiology,* 101:151–55, 1971.

98. Heiden, T. S.; Weiss, M. H.; et. al. Management of cervical spinal cord trauma in Southern California. *J. Neurosurg.,* 43:732–36, 1975.

99. Heiden, J. S.; Weiss, M. H.; et al. Acute fracture of the odontoid process: An analysis of 45 cases. *J. Neurosurg.,* **48:**85–91, 1978.

100. Helperin, S. W., and Cohen, D. D. Hematoma following epidural anesthesia. Report of a case. *Anesthesiology,* 35:641–44, 1971.

101. Herden, J. S.; Weiss, M. H.; et al. Penetrating gunshot wounds of the cervical spine in civilians. Review of 38 cases. *J. Neurosurg.,* 42:575–79, 1975.

102. Higazi, I.; El-Banhawy, A.; and El-Nady, F. Importance of angiography in identifying false aneurysm of the middle meningeal artery as a cause of extradural hematoma. *J. Neurosurg.,* 30:172–76, 1969.

103. Hinggorani, R. K. Cerebrospinal fluid rhinorrhea. *J. Laryngol. Otol.,* 85:999–1006, 1971.

104. Hirsh, C. A., and Kaufman, B. Contrecoup skull fractures. *J. Neurosurg.,* 42:530–34, 1975.

105. Hoff, J.; Grollmus, J.; et al. Clinical arteriographic and cisternographic observations after removal of acute subdural hematoma. *J. Neurosurg.,* 43:27–31, 1975.

106. Holbrook, L. A.; Beach, F. X. M.; and Silver, J. R. Delayed myelopathy: A rare complication of severe electrical burns. *Br. Med. J.,* 4:659–60, 1970.

107. Holdsworth, F. Fractures, dislocations and fracture-dislocations of the spine. *J. Bone Joint Surg.,* 52:1534–51, 1970.

108. Itzchaki, M., and Hemshanu, T. Dislocation of the cervical spine with Horner's syndrome and a lesion of the spinal trigeminal tract. *J. Neurol.,* **217:**139–43, 1977.

109. Jackson, F. E.; Gleave, J. R. W.; and Janon, E. Traumatic cranial and intracranial aneurysms. *Med. Counterpoint,* 6:44–56, 1974.

110. Jacques, S.; Shelden, H.; et al. Posttraumatic bilateral middle cerebral artery occlusion. Case report. *J. Neurosurg.,* 42:209–11, 1975.

111. Jamieson, K. G. Extradural and subdural hematomas. Changing patterns and requirments of treatment in Australia. *J. Neurosurg.,* 33:632–35, 1970.

112. Jamieson, K. G., and Yellard, J. D. N. Traumatic intracerebral hematoma-report of 63 surgically treated cases. *J. Neurosurg.,* 37:528–32, 1972.

113. Janke, W. H., and Esfahani, A. A. Air embolism following open heart surgery. *Mich. Med.,* 69:761–62, 1970.

114. Janon, E. A. Traumatic changes in the internal carotid artery associated with basal skull fractures. *Radiology,* 96:55–59, 1970.

115. Jefferson, A., and Reilly, G. Fracture of the floor of the anterior cranial fossa: the selection of patients for dural repair. *Br. J. Surg.,* 59:585–92, 1972.

116. Jellinger, K., and Sturm, K. W. Delayed radiation myelopathy in man. Report of twelve necropsy cases. *J. Neurol. Sci.,* 14:389–408, 1971.

117. Jennett, B. Early traumatic epilepsy. Incidence and significance after non-missile injuries. *Arch. Neurol.,* 30:394–98, 1974.

118. Jennett, B.; Miller, J. D.; and Brookman, R. Epilepsy after non-missile depressed skull fracture. *J. Neurosurg.,* 41:208–16, 1974.

119. Jennet, B., and Plum, F. Persistent vegetative state after brain damage. *Lancet,* 1:734–37, 1972.

120. Johnson, J. Organic psychosyndromes due to boxing. *Br. J. Psychiat.,* 115:45–53, 1969.

121. Jolley, F. L. The management of head injuries in adults. *South. Med. J.,* 63:989–91, 1970.

122. Kapp, J. P. Endotracheal intubation with fractures of the cervical spine. *J. Neurosurg.,* 42:731–32, 1975.

123. Kay, D. W. K.; Kerr, T. A.; and Lassman, L. P. Brain trauma and the postconcussional syndrome. *Lancet,* 2:1052–55, 1971.

124. Keimowitz, R. M., and Annis, B. L. Disseminated intravascular coagulation associated with massive brain injury. *J. Neurosurg;* 39:178–80, 1973.

125. Kjellberg, R. N., and Prieto, A. Bifrontal decom-

pressive craniotomy for massive cerebral edema. *J. Neurosurg.,* **34:**488–93, 1971.

126. Klonoff H.; Low, M. D.; and Clark C. Head injuries in children: A prospective five year follow up. *J. Neurol. Neurosurg. Psychiat.,* **40:**1211–19, 1977.

127. Kobrine, A. I.; Timmins, E.; et al. Demonstration of massive traumatic brain swelling within 20 minutes after injury. Case report. *J. Neurosurg.,* **46:**256–58, 1977.

128. Koch, R. L., and Glickman, M. G. The angiographic diagnosis of extradural hematoma of the posterior fossa. *Am. J. Roentgenol. Radium Ther. Nucl. Med.,* **112:**289–95, 1971.

129. Koenig, G., and Dohrmann, G. J. Histopathological variability in "standardized" spinal cord trauma. *J. Neurol. Neurosurg. Psychiat.,* **40:**1203–10, 1977.

130. Kooi, K. A. Episodic blindness as a late effect of head trauma. Electrophysiological study of 3 cases. *Neurology* (Minneap.), **20:**569–73, 1970.

131. Lake, P. A., and Pitts, F. W. Recent experience with epidural hematomas. *J. Trauma,* **11:**397–411, 1971.

132. Lance, J. W. *Migraine in the Mechanism and Management of Headache,* 2nd ed. Butterworth and Company, London, 1973, pp. 91–94.

133. Larson, S. J.; Sances, A. J.; et al. Non-invasive evaluation of head trauma patients. *Surgery,* **74:**34–40, 1973.

134. Lavy, S., and Herishianu, Y. Chronic subdural haematoma in the aged. *J. Am. Geriatrics Soc.,* **17:**380–83, 1969.

135. Law, J. D.; Lehman, R. A. W.; and Kirsch, W. M. Reoperation after lumbar intervertebral disc surgery. *J. Neurosurg.,* **48:**259–63, 1978.

136. Legier, J., and Rivaldi I. Gross pulmonary embolization with cerebral tissue following head trauma: Case report. *J. Neurosurg.,* **39:**109–13, 1973.

137. Lends, R. A. Enlarging skull fractures of childhood. *Neuroradiology,* **7:**119–24, 1974.

138. Levin, S.; Nelson, K. E.; Spies, H. W.; and Lepper, M. H. Pneumococcal meningitis: the problem of the unseen cerebrospinal fluid leak. *Am. J. Med. Sci.,* **262:**319–27, 1972.

139. Lewin, W. Changing attitudes to the management of severe head injuries. *Br. Med. J.,* **2:**1234–39, 1976.

140. Little, J. M.; May, J.; Vanderfield, G. R.; and Lamond, S. Traumatic thrombosis of the internal carotid artery. *Lancet,* **2:**926–30, 1969.

141. Locke, G.; Yashon, D.; Feldman, R. A.; and Hunt, W. E. Ischemia in primate spinal cord injury. *J. Neurosurg.,* **34:**614–17, 1971.

142. Loeser, J. D.; Kilbison, H. L.; and Jolley, T. Management of depressed skull fracture in the newborn. *J. Neurosurg.,* **44:**62–64, 1976.

143. Loré, J. M.; Grisanti, A.; and Kane, A. Traumatic carotid jugular fistula. *Laryngoscope,* **82:**2153–59, 1972.

144. MacGee, E. E.; Cauthen, J. C.; and Brackett, C. E. Meningitis following acute traumatic cerebrospinal fluid fistula. *J. Neurosurg.,* **33:**312–16, 1970.

145. Mandelberg, I. A. Cognitive recovery after severe head injury. 2. Wechsler Adult Intelligence Scale during posttraumatic amnesia. *J. Neurol. Neurosurg. Psychiat.,* **38:**1127–32, 1975.

146. Mandelberg, I. A., and Brooks, D. N. Cognitive recovery after severe head injury. 1. Serial testing on the Wechsler Adult Intelligence Scale. *J. Neurol. Neurosurg. Psychiat.,* **38:**1121–26, 1975.

147. Maroon, J. C., and Campbell, R. L. Subdural hematoma: With inappropriate antidiuretic hormone secretion. *Arch. Neurol.,* **22:**234–39, 1970.

148. Maroon, J. C.; Edmonds-Seal, J.; and Campbell, R. L. An ultrasonic method for detecting air embolism. *J. Neurosurg.,* **31:**196–201, 1969.

149. Marshall, L. F.; Bruce, D. A.; et al. Vertebrobasilar spasm: A significant cause of neurological deficit in head injury. *J. Neurosurg.,* **48:**560–64, 1978.

150. Marshall, L. F.; Smith, R. W.; et al. Mannitol dose requirements in brain injured patients. *J. Neurosurg.,* **48:**169–72, 1978.

151. Martins, A. N. Anterior cervical diskectomy with and without interbody bone graft. *J. Neurosurg.,* **44:**290–95, 1976.

152. Maxwell, J. A., and Goldware, S. I. Use of tissue adhesive in surgical treatment of cerebrospinal fluid leaks: Experience with isobutyl 2-cyanoacrylate in 12 cases. *J. Neurosurg.,* **39:**332–36, 1973.

153. McGauley, J. L.; Miller, C. A.; and Penner, J. A. Diagnosis and treatment of diffuse intravascular coagulation following cerebral trauma. *J. Neurosurg.,* **43:**374–76, 1975.

154. McGrory, B. E., and Fenichel, G. M. Hangman's fracture subsequent to shaking in an infant. *Ann. Neurol.,* **2:**82, 1977.

155. McLaurin, R. L.; Isaacs, E.; and Lewis, H. P. Results of nonoperative treatment in 15 cases of infantile subdural hematoma. *J. Neurosurg.,* **34:**753–59, 1971.

156. McLennan, J. E.; McLaughlin, W. T.; and Skillcorn, S. A. Traumatic lumbar nerve root meningocele: Case report. *J. Neurosurg.,* **39:**528–32, 1973.

157. Mehalis, T., and Farhat, S. M. Vertebral artery injury from chiropractic manipulation of the neck. *Surg. Neurol.,* **2:**125–29, 1974.

158. Melowed, E.; Lavy, S.; et al. Chronic subdural hematoma simulating transient cerebral ischemic attack. Case report. *J. Neurosurg.,* **42:**101–103, 1975.

159. Merrino-de Villasante, J., and Taveras, J. Computerized tomography (CT) in acute head trauma. *Am. J. Roentgenol.,* **126:**765–78, 1976.

160 Messina, A. V. Computed tomography: contrast media within subdural hematomas. A preliminary report. *Radiology,* **119:**725, 1976.

161. Mikhael, M. A. Radiation necrosis of the brain: Correlation between computed tomography, pathology and dose distribution. *J. Computerized Tomogr.,* **1:**71–80, 1978.

162. Miller, H., and Cartlidge, N. Simulation and malingering after injuries to the brain and spinal cord. *Lancet,* **1:**580–85, 1972.

163. Mises, J.; Lerique-Koechlin, A.; and Rimbot, B. Post-traumatic epilepsy in children. *Epilepsia,* **11:**37–39, 1970.

164. Moas, A. I. E. Cerebrospinal fluid enzymes in

acute brain injury. 2. Relation of CSF enzyme activity to extent of brain injury. *J. Neurol. Neurosurg. Psychiat.,* **40:**666–67, 1977.

165. Morin, M. A., and Pitts, F. W. Delayed apoplexy following head injury (traumatiche Spät-apoplexie). *J. Neurol. Neurosurg. Psychiat.,* **33:**542–47, 1970.

166. Moyes, P. D. Protruded lumbar intervertebral discs with special reference to surgical technique and preoperative and postoperative management. A clinical essay. *Can. J. Surg.,* **13:**382–86, 1970.

167. North, J. B. On the importance of intracranial air. *Br. J. Surg.,* **58:**826–29, 1971.

168. O'Higgins, J. W. Fat embolism. *Br. J. Anaesth.* **42:**163–68. 1970.

169. Oka, H.; Kako, M.; et al. Traumatic spreading depression syndrome—review of a particular type of head injury in 37 patients. *Brain,* **100:**287–98, 1977.

170. Ommaya, A. K.; Di Chiro, G.; Bladwin, M.; and Pennybacker, J. B. Non-traumatic cerebrospinal fluid rhinorrhea. *J. Neurol. Neurosurg. Psychiat.,* **31:**214–25, 1968.

171. Ommaya, A. K.; Faas, F.; and Yarnell, P. Whiplash injury and brain damage. *J.A.M.A.,* **204:**285–89, 1968.

172. Ommaya, A. K., and Gennarelli, T. A. Cerebral concussion and traumatic unconsciousness: Correlation of experimental and clinical observations in blunt head injuries. *Brain,* **97:**633–54, 1974.

173. Ommaya, A. K.; Grubb, R. L.; and Naumann, R. A. Coup and contrecoup cerebral contusions. An experimental analysis. *Neurology* (Minneap.), **20:**388–89, 1970.

174. Ommaya, A. K.; Grubb. R. L.; and Naumann, R. A. Coup and contre-coup injury: Observations on the mechanics of visible brain injuries in the rhesus monkey. *J. Neurosurg.,* **35:**503–16, 1971.

175. Oppenheimer, D. R. Microscopic lesions in the brain following head injury. *J. Neurol. Neurosurg. Psychiat.,* **31:**299–306, 1968.

176. Osborn, A. G.; Daines, J. H.; et al. Intracranial air on computerized tomography. *J. Neurosurg.,* **48:**355–59, 1978.

177. Osterholm, J., and Mathews, G. Altered norepinephrine metabolism following experimental spinal cord injury I. Relationship to hemorrhagic necrosis and post-wounding neurological deficits. *J. Neurosurg.,* **36:**386–94, 1972.

178. Painer, M. J.; Chutorian, A. M.; and Halil, S. K. Cerebrovasculopathy following irradiation in childhood. *Neurology* (Minneap.), **25:**189–94, 1975.

179. Parkinson, D.; Hunt, B.; and Shields, C. Double lucid interval in patients with extradural hematoma of the posterior fossa. *J. Neurosurg.,* **34:**534–36, 1971.

180. Paul, R. L.; Michael, R. G.; et al. Anterior transthoracic surgical decompression of acute spinal cord injuries. *J. Neurosurg.,* **43:**299–307, 1975.

181. Payan, H.; Toga, M.; and Berard-Badier, M. The pathology of post-traumatic epilepsies. *Epilepsia,* **11:**81–94, 1970.

182. Pearce, J. The lumbar disc syndrome. *Postgrad. Med. J.,* **45:**278–84, 1969.

183. Pearson, B. W., and Barber, H. O. Head injury. Some otoneurologic sequelae. *Arch. Otolaryngol.,* **97:**81–84, 1973.

184. Perlmutter, I.; Dooley, D. M.; and Auld, A. W. Vertebral angiography in the presence of an extradural hematoma of the posterior fossa. *South. Med. J.,* **64:**245–46, 1971.

185. Petty, P. G. Influence of seat belt wearing in incidence of severe head injury. *Med. J. Aust.,* **2:**768–69, 1975.

186. Pevsner, P. H.; Garera-Bunuel, R.; et al. Subependymal and intraventricular hemorrhage in neonates: Early diagnosis by computed tomography. *Radiology,* **119:**111–14, 1976.

187. Piazza, G., and Corsti, G. Role of radiographic skull examination in emergency evaluation of intracranial expanding lesions following closed head injuries. *Neuroradiology,* **6:**101–103, 1973.

188. Potter, J. M. Emergency management of head injuries. *Br. Med. J.,* **2:**1477–78, 1965.

189. Raaf, J. E. Surgical treatment of patients with cervical disc lesions. *J. Trauma,* **9:**327–38, 1969.

190. Raynor, R. B. Discography and myelography in acute injuries of the cervical spine. *J. Neurosurg.,* **35:**529–35, 1971.

191. Reagan, T. J.; Thomas, J. E.; and Colby, M. Y., Jr. Chronic progressive radiation myelopathy, Its chronical aspects and differential diagnosis. *J.A.M.A.,* **203:**106–10, 1968.

192. Reid, S. E.; Tarkington, J. A.; Epstein, H. M.; and O'Dea, T. J. Brain tolerance to impact in football. *Surg. Gynecol. Obstet.,* **133:**929–36, 1971.

193. Reisner, H.; Drofanter, W.; and Reisner, Th. Cerebral vascular thrombosis after closed head injury. *Wien. Klin. Wochenschr.* **88:**162–65, 1976.

194. Relander, M.; Troupp, H. A. F.; and Bjorkesten, G. Controlled trial of treatment for cerebral concussion. *Br. Med. J.,* **4:**777–79, 1972.

195. Reynolds, B.; Balsano, N. A.; and Reynolds, F. X. Falls from heights: A surgical experience of 200 cases. *Am. Surg.,* **174:**304–308, 1971.

196. Richards, D. E.; White, R. J.; and Yashon, D. Inappropriate release of ADH in subdural hematoma. *J. Trauma,* **11:**758–62, 1971.

197. Richards, T., and Hoff, J. Factors affecting survival from acute subdural hematoma. *Surgery,* **75:**253–58, 1974.

198. Rivett, J. D. Paraplegia due to radiation myelitis following the treatment of carcinoma of the bronchus by radiotherapy. Report of two cases. *Paraplegia,* **9:**65–72, 1971.

199. Robinson, R. G. Cerebrospinal fluid rhinorrhea, meningitis and pneumocephalus due to non-missile injuries. *Aust. N.Z. J. Surg.,* **39:**328–34, 1970.

200. Rose, J.; Valtonen, S.; and Jennett, B. Avoidable factors contributing to death after head injury. *Br. Med. J.,* **2:**615–18, 1977.

201. Rosenorn, J., and Gjerris, E. Long-term followup review of patients with acute and subacute subdural hematomas. *J. Neurosurg.,* **48:**345–49, 1978.

202. Rovit, R. L., and Ransohoff, J. Hemicraniectomy.

1. Treatment of acute subdural hematoma—reappraisal. *Surg. Neurol.,* **5:**25–28, 1976.

203. Rowe, S. E.; Roth, R. H.; et al. Norepinephrine levels in experimental spinal cord trauma. Part 1. Biochemical study of hemorrhagic necrosis. *J. Neurosurg.,* **46:**342–49, 1977.

204. Rowe, S. E.; Roth, R. H.; and Collins, W. F. Norepinephrine levels in experimental spinal cord trauma. Part 2. Histopathological study of hemorrhagic necrosis. *J. Neurosurg.,* **46:**350–57, 1977.

205. Rumbaugh, C. A.; Bergeron, R. J.; Talalla, A.; and Kurze, T. Traumatic aneurysms of the cortical cerebral arteries. Radiographic aspects. *Radiology,* **96:**40–54, 1970.

206. Russin, L. D., and Guinto, C., Jr. Multidirectional tomography in cervical spine injury. *J. Neurosurg.,* **45:**9–11, 1976.

207. Russman, B. S., and Kazi, K. H. Spinal epidural hematoma and the Brown Séquard syndrome. *Neurology* (Minneap.), **21:**1066–68, 1971.

208. Sabin, T. D., and Poche, J. A. Pure tortional nystagmus as a consequence of head trauma. *J. Neurol. Neurosurg. Psychiat.,* **32:**265–67, 1969.

209. Salmon, J. H. Surgical treatment of severe posttraumatic encephalopathy. *Surg. Gynecol. Obstet.,* **133:**634–36, 1971.

210. Sandler, A. N., and Tator, C. Effect of spinal cord compression on regional spinal cord blood flow in primates. *J. Neurosurg.,* **45:**660–76, 1975.

211. Sandler, A. N., and Tator, C. H. Review of the effect of spinal cord trauma on the vessels and blood flow in the spinal cord. *J. Neurosurg.,* **45:**638–46, 1976.

212. Schatzker, J.; Rorabeck, C. H.; and Waddell, J. P. Fractures of the dens (odontoid process). An analysis of 37 cases. *J. Bone Joint Surg.,* **53:**392–405, 1971.

213. Schneider, R. C. Concomitant craniocerebral and spinal trauma with special reference to the cervicomedullary region. *Clin. Neurosurg.,* **17:**266–309, 1969.

214. Schulhof. L. A.; Rivet, R.; and Maroon, J. C. Severe head injuries: A retrospective review of 100 consecutive cases, Marion General Hospital. *J. Ind. State Med. Assoc.,* **65:**739–46, 1972.

215. Schutt, C. H., and Dohan, F. C. Neck injury to women in auto accidents. A metropolitan plague. *J.A.M.A.,* **206:**2689–92, 1968.

216. Selecki, B. R. Cervical spine and cord injuries. Mechanisms and surgical implications. *Med. J. Aust.,* **1:**838–40, 1970.

217. Seljekog, E. L., and Chou, S. N. Spectrum of the hangman's fracture. *J. Neurosurg.,* **45:**3–8, 1976.

218. Shaw, C. M., and Alvord, E. R., Jr. Injury of basilar artery associated with closed head trauma. *J. Neurol. Neurosurg. Psychiat.,* **35:**247–57, 1972.

219. Shenkin, H., and Goldfedder, P. Air embolism from exposure of posterior cranial fossa in prone position. *J.A.M.A.,* **210:**726, 1969.

220. Shrago, G. G. Cerebral spine injuries: Associated with head trauma: Review of 50 patients. *Am. J. Roentgenol. Radium Ther. Nucl. Med.,* **118:**670–73, 1973.

221. Simeone, F. A., and Goldberg, H. I. Thrombosis of the vertebral artery from hyperextension injury to the neck, case report. *J. Neurosurg.,* **29:**540–44, 1968.

222. So, S. C., and Lee, M. L. K. Spastic quadriplegia due to electric shock. *Br. Med. J.,* **2:**590, 1973.

223. Strich, S. J. Lesions in the cerebral hemispheres after blunt head injury. *J. Clin. Pathol.,* **23:**suppl. 4, 154–65, 1970.

224. Tabaddor, K., and Shulman, K. Definitive treatment of chronic subdural hematoma by twist-drill craniostomy and closed-system drainage. *J. Neurosurg.,* **46:**220–26, 1977.

225. Takeuchi, J.; Hanakita, J.; et al. Brain necrosis after repeated radiotherapy. *Surg. Neurol.,* **5:**89–93, 1976.

226. Tarlov, I. M. Acute spinal cord compression paralyses. *J. Neurosurg.,* **36:**10–20, 1972.

227. Taylor, T. K. F., and Akeson, W. H. Intervertebral disc prolapse: A review of morphologic and biochemic knowledge concerning the nature of prolapse. *Clin. Orthop.,* **76:**54–79, 1971.

228. Thomas, J. E., and Ayyar, D. R. Systemic fat embolism. A diagnostic profile of 24 patients. *Arch. Neurol.,* **26:**517–23, 1972.

229. Thompson, J. B., and Mason, T. H. Surgical management of diastalic linear skull fractures in infants. *J. Neurosurg.,* **39:**493–97, 1973.

230. Thomsen, I. V. Evaluation and outcome of aphasia in patients with severe closed head trauma. *J. Neurol. Neurosurg. Psychiat.,* **38:**713–18, 1975.

231. Tindall, G. T., and Meyer, G. A. Head injury. Diagnostic and therapeutic management. *Tex. Med.,* **67:**56–63, 1971.

232. Tomlinson, B. E. Brain-stem lesions after head injury. *J. Clin. Pathol.,* **23:**suppl. 4, 154–65, 1970.

233. Torres, H., and Ferguson, L. Acute head injuries. *Am. Fam. Physic.,* **2:**88–98, 1970.

234. Vecht, Ch. J.; Smit Subinga, C. Th.; and Minderhound, J. M. Disseminated intravascular coagulation and head injury. *J. Neurol. Neurosurg. Psychiat.,* **38:**567–71, 1975.

235. Vires, J. K.; Becker, D. P.; and Young, H. F. Subarachnoid screw for monitoring intracranial pressure: Technical note. *J. Neurosurg.,* **39:**416–19, 1973.

236. Wagner, F.; Dohrmann, G.; and Bucy, P. Histopathology of transitory traumatic paraplegia in the monkey. *J. Neurosurg.,* **35:**272–86, 1971.

237. Watts, C. Management of intracranial calcified subdural hematomas. *Surg. Neurol.,* **6:**247–50, 1976.

238. Wells, C. H.; Bond, T. P.; guest, M. M.; and Barnhart, C. C. Rheologic impairment of the microcirculation during decompression sickness. *Micro. Vasc. Res.,* **3:**162–69, 1971.

239. White, J. C.; Kneisley, L. W.; and Rossner, A. B. Delayed paralysis after cervical fracture-dislocation. *J. Neurosurg.,* **46:**512–16, 1977.

240. Whitehurst, W. R., and Christensen, F. K. Epidural hemorrhage from traumatic laceration of internal carotid artery. *J. Neurosurg.,* **31:**352–54, 1969.

241. Whitesides, T. E., and Shah, S. G. A. On the man-

agement of unstable fractures of the thoracolumbar spine. *Spine,* **1:**99–107, 1976.

242. Wilson, C. B., and Markesbery, W., Traumatic carotid-cavernous fistula with fatal epistaxis. *J. Neurosurg.,* **24:**111–13, 1966.

243. Wilson, C. B., and Norrell, H. A. Management of head injuries. *Minn. Med.,* **50:**177–84, 1967.

244. Wilson, G. H.; Byfield, J.; and Hanafee, W. N. Atrophy following radiation therapy for central nervous system neoplasms. *Acta Radiol. (Ther.),* **11:**361–68, 1972.

245. Winter, P. M.; Alvis, H. J.; and Gage, A. A. Hyperbaric treatment of cerebral air embolism during cardiopulmonary bypass. *J.A.M.A.,* **215:**1786–92, 1971.

246. Zulch, K. J. Neuropathology in intracranial haemorrhage. *Prog. Brain Res.,* **30:**151–65, 1968.

9 CEREBROVASCULAR DISEASE

Cerebrovascular disease is the third most common cause of death in the United States. The magnitude of this as a public health problem is compounded further by the fact that cerebrovascular disease is a major cause of chronic disability and affects not only the elderly but also many individuals in their forties and fifties who are still active contributors to family and community life. The exact number of persons chronically disabled from cerebrovascular disease in the United States is unknown but is probably in the neighborhood of 2 million.

Diagnosis, treatment, and prevention of cerebrovascular disease require familiarity with the anatomy and physiology of the cerebral circulation, which are different in many respects from those of other organs of the body. The pathogenesis of the clinical and pathologic changes that occur in cerebrovascular disease will be discussed

first in terms of disturbance of anatomy and physiology of the cerebral circulation.

Anatomy of the Cerebral Vessels

In order to recognize cerebrovascular disorders of the nervous system and to interpret angiograms, precise knowledge of the anatomy of the cerebral vessels is essential (Fig. 9–1).

The blood supply to the brain depends on four major conducting arteries in the neck: the two internal carotid arteries anteriorly and the two vertebral arteries posteriorly.

The Carotid System

The right common carotid artery arises from the brachiocephalic trunk and the left common carotid artery from the aortic arch. Both internal carotid arteries arise at the bifurcation of the com-

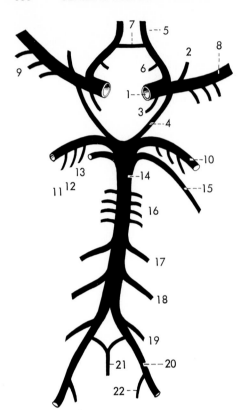

1 Internal carotid a.
2 Ophthalmic a.
3 Anterior choroid a.
4 Posterior communicating a.
5 Anterior cerebral a.
6 Recurrent artery of Huebner
7 Anterior communicating a.
8 Middle cerebral a.
9 Lenticulostriate aa.
10 Posterior cerebral a.
11 Posteromedial branches post. cerebr. a.
12 Thalamogeniculate a.
13 Posterior choroid a.
14 Basilar a.
15 Superior cerebellar a.
16 Pontine branches basilar a.
17 Internal auditory a.
18 Anterior inferior cerebellar a.
19 Posterior inferior cerebellar a.
20 Vertebral a.
21 Anterior spinal a.
22 Posterior spinal a.

FIGURE 9–1. Diagram of the major cerebral vessels and circle of Willis.

mon carotid artery in the neck at the level of the upper border of the thyroid cartilage. Each vessel then runs perpendicularly upward in front of the transverse processes of the upper three cervical vertebrae to enter the carotid canal in the petrous temporal bone. The vessel has an unusual **S**-shaped course in the carotid canal, which tends to dampen the pulsatile thrust of each cardiac systole. The vessel ascends for a short distance, and after passing forward and medially, it enters the skull. The internal carotid artery enters the cavernous sinus, then passes upward, lateral to the posterior clinoid process, and turns anteriorly past the side of the body of the sphenoid bone to the medial aspect of the anterior clinoid process. The vessel then ascends once more and pierces the dura. The terminal portion passes between the optic nerve and the oculomotor nerve, immediately lateral to the anterior clinoid process and inferior to the anterior perforated substance, where it divides into the anterior and middle cerebral arteries.

The cervical portion of the internal carotid artery has no branches, but there are two small branches in the carotid canal. The first is the caroticotympanic artery, which enters the middle ear and supplies a portion of its mucosa before anastomosing with branches of the internal maxillary artery. A second small vessel, the artery of the pterygoid canal, also anastomoses with branches of the internal maxillary artery after entering the pterygoid canal. The cavernous portion of the internal carotid artery supplies cavernous branches to the walls of the cavernous sinus, branches to the trigeminal ganglion, hypophyseal branches to the pituitary gland, and the anterior meningeal artery, which supplies the dura of the anterior fossa before anastomosing with the posterior ethmoidal artery. The most important branch of the cavernous portion of the internal carotid artery is the ophthalmic artery, which arises medial to the anterior clinoid process and passes forward with the optic nerve through the optic foramen into the orbit. The ophthalmic artery has numerous branches in the orbit, including the central artery of the retina and a number of important anastomotic connections with branches of the external carotid system. This anastomosis should be remembered as a potential source of rich collateral circulation via the ophthalmic artery, following occlusion of the internal carotid artery in the neck.

All the branches of the terminal cerebral portion of the internal carotid artery are important and consist of the posterior communicating, the anterior choroidal, the anterior cerebral, and the middle cerebral arteries.

Posterior Communicating Artery

This arises from the internal carotid artery and passes posteriorly to anastomose with the posterior cerebral artery about 1 cm lateral to the terminal division of the basilar artery. It shows marked variation in size, may be absent, and is frequently larger on one side. Branches enter the base of the brain to supply the genu and anterior one third of the posterior limb of the internal capsule, the anterior one third of the thalamus, and the walls of the third ventricle.

Anterior Choroidal Artery

This usually arises from the terminal portion of the internal carotid immediately above the posterior communicating artery. Occasionally, it originates from the proximal part of the middle cerebral artery. From its origin it passes along the optic tract and around the cerebral peduncle as far as the lateral geniculate body.

The vessel gives off numerous small branches in its course to supply the optic tract, the cerebral peduncle, and the lateral portion of the lateral geniculate body. Perforating branches supply the posterior two thirds of the posterior limb of the internal capsule and the infra- and retrolenticular portion of the internal capsule, including the optic radiation. The artery also supplies the choroid plexus in the inferior horn of the lateral ventricle after traversing the choroidal fissure, the tail of the caudate nucleus, and the amygdala. There is some variation in the nuclear structures supplied by this vessel, and branches which supply the globus pallidus have been described in some anatomic preparations.

Anterior Cerebral Artery

This arises as one of the two terminal branches of the internal carotid artery. It passes anteromedially lying dorsal to the optic chiasm and then curves around the corpus callosum to supply the medial aspect of the cerebral hemisphere as far back as the parieto-occipital fissure, where it anas-

tomoses with branches of the posterior cerebral artery. A number of small branches, which arise near the origin of the vessel, pierce the anterior perforated substance to supply the rostrum of the corpus callosum, the septum pellucidum, and the lamina terminalis. A larger recurrent branch (the recurrent artery of Huebner or medial striate artery) takes a backward course through the anterior perforated substance to supply the anterior limb of the internal capsule, the lower part of the head of the caudate nucleus, and the lower part of the anterior portion of the putamen and globus pallidus.

The cortical branches of the anterior cerebral artery supply the major portion of the mesial aspect of each hemisphere. The orbital branches supply the orbital surface of the frontal lobe as well as the olfactory bulb and tract. The frontopolar branches pass forward toward the frontal pole of the frontal lobe, supply the anterior portion of the superior frontal gyrus on its medial aspect, and extend to its lateral surface to supply a rim of the cortex of both superior and middle frontal gyri. The main part of the anterior cerebral artery continues posteriorly on the superior surface of the corpus callosum and is called the pericallosal artery, which supplies the corpus callosum, the adjacent cingulate gyrus, and the medial aspect of the parietal lobe. One other important branch of the anterior cerebral artery, the callosomarginal, supplies most of the cingulate gyrus as well as the adjacent portion of the superior frontal and cingulate gyri and the paracentral lobule.

Anterior Communicating Artery

This connects the two anterior cerebral arteries immediately anterior to the anterior perforated substance, and from this point the two anterior cerebral arteries lie in close proximity on the genu of the corpus callosum. Occasionally, one of the anterior cerebral arteries is much smaller, or a single anterior cerebral artery supplies both mesial frontal lobes.

Middle Cerebral Artery

This is the largest of the two terminal branches of the internal carotid artery and may be considered the anatomic extension of the internal carotid artery in its intracranial course. The middle cerebral artery runs laterally deep within the lateral (sylvian) fissure, over the surface of the insula, and then divides into a number of radiating branches that supply most of the lateral surface of the hemisphere.

Immediately beyond the origin of the middle cerebral artery, it gives rise to a series of perforating branches called the lenticulostriate arteries, which enter the substance of the brain to supply the superior portion of the head and body of the caudate nucleus as well as the major portion of the putamen and globus pallidus. The internal capsule above the level of the globus pallidus is supplied by these branches of the middle cerebral artery.

The radiating cortical branches of the middle cerebral artery consist of the orbitofrontal, frontal, prerolandic, postrolandic, anterior parietal, and posterior parietal branches, all of which emerge from the lateral fissure and ascend to the frontal and parietal lobes. The parieto-occipital branch may be regarded as the terminal branch of the middle cerebral artery and has a horizontal course. Finally, the posterior, middle, and anterior temporal branches of the middle cerebral artery radiate inferiorly over the surface of the temporal lobe.

The Vertebral-Basilar System

The posterior portions of the brain (hindbrain) including the brainstem, cerebellum, major portions of the diencephalon, and occipital lobes are supplied by the vertebral-basilar system.

Vertebral Artery

This arises as the first branch of the first portion of the subclavian artery. Rarely (in about 1 per cent of cases) the left vertebral artery arises directly from the arch of the aorta. The vessel is divided anatomically into four portions in its course from the subclavian artery until it joins the opposite vertebral artery to form the basilar artery. *The first portion* passes posteromedially from its origin to the level of the sixth cervical vertebra, where it usually turns to enter the foramen in the transverse process of this vertebra. Occasionally, it may enter at higher levels. *The second portion* consists of that part of the vessel which passes vertically within the foramina of the transverse processes of the sixth to second cervical vertebrae. *The third portion* curves backward around the lateral mass of the atlas and behind its superior articular process to enter the vertebral canal beneath the posterior atlanto-occipital membrane. *The fourth and final portion* of the artery pierces the dura and arachnoid and passes medially through the rootlets of the twelfth cranial nerve, on the ventral surface of the medulla to join the opposite vertebral artery in front of the lower border of the pons to form the basilar artery.

There are no branches from the first portion of the vertebral artery, but in its second portion, it gives rise to segmental spinal branches at the level of each vertebral body. These branches pass medially to supply the nerve roots and meninges around the spinal cord and anastomose with the branch from the opposite side on the posterior surface of the vertebral bodies. There may be only one, or occasionally two, major anastomotic connections between the vertebral artery and the anterior spinal artery in the cervical area. The fourth portion of the vertebral artery gives rise to a meningeal branch, which supplies the meninges of the posterior fossa, including the falx cerebelli.

Posterior Spinal Arteries

These arise from the vertebral artery on either side or from the posterior inferior cerebellar arteries. The two vessels pass backward over the medulla and descend in a parallel course ventral to the posterior nerve roots of the spinal nerves, to the level of the cauda equina. Each vessel receives anastomotic branches from the vertebral, intercostal, and lumbar vessels and has numerous communications with its companion vessel and with the anterior spinal artery. The posterior spinal arteries supply the white matter of the posterior columns together with the posterior horns of gray matter throughout the spinal cord.

Anterior Spinal Artery

This is a single vessel lying in the anterior ventral median fissure of the spinal cord. It arises near the termination of the fourth portion of the vertebral arteries as two vessels that descend ventromedially over the surface of the medulla to join at its lower border. As a result of this junction, the single vessel called the anterior spinal artery descends the entire length of the spinal cord, has several segmental anastomotic vessels at the cervical, thoracic, and lumbar levels, and finally terminates as a tiny vessel on the filum terminale.

This important artery supplies the medullary pyramids and the midline structures of the medulla including the medial lemniscus, medial longitudinal fasciculus, hypoglossal nucleus, and hypoglossal nerve. As it descends in the ventral median fissure of the spinal cord the anterior spinal artery supplies the anterior two thirds of the spinal cord, including the anterior horns of gray matter, the corticospinal tracts, and the spinothalamic tracts. It does not supply the dorsal columns.

Posterior Inferior Cerebellar Artery

This also arises near the termination of the vertebral artery. Rarely, as an anomaly, a small vertebral artery may terminate as the posterior inferior cerebellar artery. The vessel passes posteriorly over the olive and the inferior cerebellar peduncle and divides into two branches on the inferior surface of the cerebellum. The medial branch supplies the choroid plexus of the fourth ventricle, while the lateral branch supplies the inferior surface of the cerebellum and anastomoses with branches of the anterior inferior and superior cerebellar arteries. This artery supplies a variable amount of the lateral medulla. The structures usually supplied include the inferior cerebellar peduncle, the lateral spinothalamic tract, the descending spinal tract of the trigeminal nerve, the nucleus ambiguus, the nucleus and tract of the tractus solitarius, the caudal part of the inferior vestibular nucleus, the fibers of the vagus and accessory nerves, and part of the reticular substance containing the descending sympathetic fibers from the hypothalamus.

Basilar Artery

This is formed by the union of the two vertebral arteries at the lower border of the pons and ascends in a median groove in the midline to terminate by dividing into the two posterior cerebral arteries at the upper border of the pons. It gives off a series of median branches, which supply the basilar portion of the pons, and a series of short and long circumferential branches. The short circumferential vessels supply the antero- and posterolateral areas of the pons, including the motor and main sensory nuclei of the fifth cranial nerve, the nuclei of the seventh and eighth cranial nerves, the superior olive, the lateral lemniscus, and the middle cerebellar peduncle. There are three long circumferential branches named the auditory artery, anterior inferior cerebellar, and superior cerebellar arteries.

Auditory Artery

This accompanies the seventh and eighth cranial nerves into the internal auditory meatus and supplies these nerves and most of the inner ear.

Anterior Inferior Cerebellar Artery

This arises from the lower part of the basilar artery and runs laterally over the sixth, seventh, and eighth nerves to the inferior surface of the cerebellum. It supplies the lower pons, upper lateral medulla, inferior and middle cerebellar peduncles, and a variable amount of the inferior surface of the cerebellum where it anastomoses with the posterior inferior verebellar artery.

Superior Cerebellar Artery

This arises immediately below the termination of the basilar artery and passes laterally around the pons, separated from the posterior cerebral artery by the oculomotor nerve, on to the superior surface of the cerebellum. The superior cerebellar artery supplies the upper pons, the middle and superior cerebellar peduncles, the inferior colliculus, the superior surface of the cerebellar hemisphere, and the vermis and then anastomoses with the posterior inferior cerebellar artery.

Posterior Cerebral Arteries

These are the two terminal branches of the basilar artery, which arise at the upper border of the pons. Each vessel passes laterally around the cerebral peduncle, receiving the posterior communicating artery from the internal carotid artery. The artery then continues to the medial surface of the temporal and occipital lobes where it divides into its terminal branches. This vessel supplies a number of small posteromedial central branches, which enter the posterior perforated substance to supply the median and paramedian structures in the midbrain including the oculomotor and trochlear nuclei and nerves, the periaqueductal gray, the medial longitudinal fasciculus, and the nuclei of Cajal and Darkschewitsch. The medial aspect of the cerebral peduncle, substantia nigra, and red nucleus may also be supplied by these vessels. As the posterior cerebral artery passes around the midbrain, it gives off a number of small penetrating branches that supply the cerebral peduncle, the lateral and posterolateral portions of the midbrain, and the superior and inferior colliculi in the quadrigeminal plate. The terminal cortical branches of the posterior cerebral artery include the anterior and posterior temporal branches supplying the inferior and medial surfaces of the temporal lobe and the calcarine branch, which supplies the medial surface (visual area) of the occipital lobe.

Thalamogeniculate Arteries

These important branches of the posterior cerebral artery supply the posterior two thirds of the thalamus.

Posterior Choroidal Artery

This arises as a branch of the posterior cerebral artery and passes beneath the splenium of the corpus callosum to supply the choroid plexus of the third and lateral ventricles.

Circle of Willis

This forms a unique anastomotic system at the base of the brain between the internal carotid and vertebral-basilar systems. There is considerable variation in diameter and development of the participating vessels, particularly the posterior communicating arteries, but the circle is complete in the majority of cases. The anterior portion of the circle of Willis consists of the terminal portions of the internal carotid arteries and the two anterior cerebral arteries united by the anterior communicating artery. The posterior portion consists of the terminal portion of the basilar artery and its two branches, the posterior cerebral arteries. The circle is completed by the two posterior communicating arteries, which pass from the internal carotid artery to the posterior cerebral artery on each side. Structures surrounded or related to the circle of Willis include the optic chiasm, infundibulum, tuber cinereum, and mammillary bodies.

The Cerebral Venous System

The venous blood leaving the brain drains into a system of thin-walled veins lying in the subarachnoid space. These vessels ultimately cross the subdural space to enter the venous sinuses, which lie between two layers of dura and drain into the internal jugular vein. Almost all the venous blood from the brain leaves via the confluence of sinuses (torcular) and the internal jugular veins, although there may be a small amount of shunting via a series of emissary veins that form connections between the intracranial veins and the veins of the scalp.

The cerebral veins are divided into two separate groups, the superficial external and deep internal veins, which function as separate systems with little, if any, collateral connections.

The superficial cerebral veins lie in the sulci of the brain, and although there is considerable variation in the pattern of venous drainage in man, certain vessels can usually be identified.

Superior Cerebral Veins

These consist of about 12 vessels that drain the upper lateral portion of the hemisphere and empty into the superior longitudinal sinus at an angle that is opposed to the blood flow of this vessel.

Superficial Middle Cerebral Vein

This drains the major portion of the lateral surface of the hemisphere. It passes forward in the posterior limb of the lateral fissure to empty into the cavernous sinus. There is a communication between the posterior part of the superficial middle cerebral vein and the superior longitudinal sinus via the superior anastomotic vein of Trolard. It also communicates with the transverse sinus via the inferior anastomotic vein (Labbé).

Inferior Cerebral Veins

These drain the orbital surface of the frontal lobe as well as the lateral aspect of the temporal and occipital lobes. They empty into the cavernous and transverse sinuses.

Deep Middle Cerebral Vein

This drains the insula and passes anteriorly deep in the lateral fissure to join the basal vein.

Basal Vein (Rosenthal)

This arises in the anterior perforated substance by the union of the anterior cerebral vein and anterior veins of the corpus callosum, both of which drain the medial surface of the hemisphere. From its origin the basal vein passes posteriorly, lying medial to the uncus and hippocampus to turn around the midbrain and empty into the great cerebral vein beneath the splenium of the corpus callosum.

Deep Internal Group of Cerebral Veins

These veins have some importance because they may be visualized in the venous phase of a cerebral angiogram, and abnormalities may indicate a displacement of the midline structures of the brain, the presence of a lesion in the thalamus or perithalamic area, as well as accurate estimation of the size of the ventricles.

Terminal or Thalamostriate Vein

This arises in the inferior horn of the lateral ventricle and follows the tail of the caudate nucleus into the body of the ventricle to lie between the caudate nucleus and thalamus. It drains both structures and passes forward to the interventricular foramen, where it contributes to the formation of the internal cerebral vein.

Anterior Caudate Vein

This drains the head of the caudate nucleus and proceeds posteriorly to the interventricular foramen.

Septal Vein

This drains the septum pellucidum and runs posteriorly to the region of the interventricular foramen.

Choroidal Vein

This arises in the choroid plexus in the inferior horn of the lateral ventricle and runs the whole extent of the plexus to the interventricular foramen.

Internal Cerebral Vein

This arises at the interventricular foramen by the union of the anterior caudate, septal, choroidal, and terminal veins. It turns posteriorly onto the roof of the third ventricle forming the venous angle and then passes along the roof of the ventricle through the velum interpositum to join with the opposite internal cerebral vein to form the great cerebral vein of Galen.

Great Cerebral Vein of Galen

This receives the basal veins at its origin and, after a short course, is joined by the inferior sagittal sinus to form the straight sinus. It also receives the posterior vein of the corpus callosum, the internal occipital veins draining the medial surface of the occipital lobe, and veins from the tentorium cerebelli and the superior surface of the cerebellum.

Venous Drainage of the Cerebellum

The veins from the superior surface of the cerebellum pass into the straight and transverse sinuses. A few pierce the tentorium cerebelli to enter the great cerebral vein. The veins draining the inferior surface of the cerebellum pass into the superior petrosal and sigmoid sinuses.

Intracranial Venous Sinuses

The venous sinuses are endothelial-lined vessels lying within the dura. The walls are formed by the fibrous tissue of the dura. They are valveless structures and do not collapse like systemic veins.

Superior Longitudinal (Sagittal) Sinus

This arises at the foramen caecum anteriorly and passes posteriorly in the attached edge of the falx cerebri to end at the internal occipital protuberance usually by turning to the right transverse sinus. The sinuses receive the superior cerebral veins throughout their course. The wall of the sagittal sinus contains pacchionian granulations, which are probably the most important site for absorption of cerebrospinal fluid into the venous system.

Inferior Longitudinal (Sagittal) Sinus

This lies in the posterior half of the free border of the falx cerebri. It begins anteriorly by the union of a number of veins running in the falx and runs posteriorly to enter the straight sinus at the junction of the falx cerebri with the tentorium cerebelli.

Straight Sinus

This is formed by the junction of the great cerebral vein and the inferior longitudinal sinus and passes posteriorly within the dural canal formed by the falx cerebri at its union with the tentorium cerebelli. The straight sinus usually turns to the left side at the internal occipital protuberance and ends in the left transverse sinus.

Transverse Sinus

This begins at the internal occipital protuberance and runs anteriorly in the edge of the tentorium cerebelli to end at the base of the petrous portion of the temporal bone, where it curves downward to become the sigmoid sinus, which drains into the internal jugular vein. It receives the superior petrosal sinus at its termination and some of the inferior cerebral and cerebellar veins.

Sigmoid Sinus

This is a direct continuation of the transverse sinus, which begins at the base of the petrous temporal bone and curves downward and medially to end in the internal jugular vein at the jugular foramen. It forms a deep groove in the mastoid portion of the temporal bone and is separated from the mastoid air cells by a thin layer of bone.

Occipital Sinus

This is a small venous sinus lying on the floor of the posterior fossa at the attachment of the falx cerebelli. It is formed by veins that run from the margins of the foramen magnum and passes posteriorly to the confluence of the sinuses.

Confluence of Sinuses (Torcular Herophili)

This is the confluence or junction of the superior longitudinal, straight, and occipital sinuses with the transverse sinuses. Although there is free communication with good mixing between all these vessels at this point, the blood from the superior longitudinal sinus theoretically drains into the right transverse sinus, while the straight sinus is supposed to drain into the left transverse sinus.

Cavernous Sinus

This is a relatively short but important structure that lies alongside the body of the sphenoid bone from the superior orbital fissure anteriorly to the apex of the petrous temporal bone posteriorly, where it divides into the superior and inferior petrosal sinuses. It receives the ophthalmic veins anteriorly, and there is a communication with the angular vein of the face through the superior ophthalmic vein. The cavernous sinus also receives blood from the sphenopalatine sinus, a small venous sinus lying on the undersurface of the lesser wing of the sphenoid, as well as from some of the inferior cerebral veins. There are communications with the opposite cavernous sinus through the two intercavernous sinuses, with the transverse sinus through the superior petrosal sinus and with the internal jugular vein through the inferior petrosal sinus. Emissary veins pass through the foramina ovale and lacerum between the cavernous sinus and the pterygoid plexus of veins.

The lateral wall of the cavernous sinus contains the oculomotor and trochlear nerves as well as the ophthalmic and maxillary divisions of the trigeminal nerve. The medial wall contains the S-shaped internal carotid artery with the abducens nerve immediately inferior.

Superior Petrosal Sinus

This arises from the cavernous sinus at the apex of the petrous temporal bone and passes along the edge of the tentorium cerebelli to end in the transverse sinus. It receives some of the inferior cerebral and cerebellar veins and those from the middle ear and mastoid air cells.

Inferior Petrosal Sinus

This begins at the apex of the petrous temporal bone, where it leaves the cavernous sinus and passes in a groove lying in the junction of the petrous temporal and occipital bones to end in the jugular bulb of the internal jugular vein. In its course it receives some of the inferior cerebellar veins, the internal auditory vein, and veins from the pons and medulla. The two petrosal sinuses are joined by an interlacing network of veins lying on the basilar part of the occipital bone, which constitute the basilar plexus. This plexus has connections with the anterior vertebral plexus.

The Venous System of the Spinal Cord

External Vertebral Venous Plexus

This consists of an anterior external plexus lying in front of the vertebral bodies and a posterior external plexus lying on the posterior surface of the vertebral arches and on the transverse and spinous processes.

Internal Vertebral Venous Plexus

This consists of an anterior internal plexus lying on the posterior surface of the vertebral bodies and a posterior internal plexus lying in the vertebral canal in front of the vertebral arches.

The anterior external plexus communicates with the anterior internal plexus through large tortuous veins, the basivertebral veins, which pass through foramina in the vertebral bodies. The anterior and posterior plexuses communicate through a series of venous rings opposite each vertebral body, and there is a free anastomosis between the posterior internal and posterior external plexuses through the ligamenta flava. Thus, all four of these plexuses are in free communication. There is also free communication between the vertebral plexus and the occipital sinus and basilar plexus through the foramen magnum. Because the anterior external plexus is in free communication with the pelvic veins, the vertebral plexus constitutes a potential pathway for spread of metastases, infection, and embolization from the pelvis into the spinal cord and intracranial venous sinuses. However, it is doubtful that this anastomosis is important in the metastatic spread of pelvic tumors or abscesses to the central nervous system.

Veins of the Spinal Cord

These consist of two median longitudinal veins, one lying anteriorly in the ventral median fissure and the other posteriorly in the posterior sulcus. There are also four longitudinal veins running behind the anterior and posterior nerve roots on each side of the cord. The frequent communications between the longitudinal veins form a tortuous venous plexus running the whole length of the spinal cord. The venous blood from the cord drains into the vertebral plexus through a series of intervertebral veins that accompany the spinal nerves. There is, in addition, communication through the foramen magnum into the inferior cerebellar veins and inferior petrosal sinuses.

Regulation and Adjustment of Cerebral Blood Flow

Under physiologic conditions cerebral blood flow in man usually amounts to 50 to 60 ml/100 gm of brain per minute, or a total flow of 700 to 840 ml/minute. This represents about 17 per cent of the cardiac output and illustrates the very high metabolic requirements of the brain. Under normal conditions each internal carotid artery contributes approximately one third of the total cerebral blood flow, and the remaining one third is derived from the vertebral-basilar system.

Factors Regulating Cerebral Blood Flow

Extrinsic Factors

The circulation of blood through an organ depends on the perfusion pressure and the regional resistance.[124, 126]

This principle applies to cerebral blood flow, where the perfusion pressure is equal to the difference between the systemic arterial blood pressure and the cerebral venous pressure. Under normal circumstances the cerebral venous pressure is quite small (5 mm Hg) and the systemic arterial blood pressure represents the perfusion pressure of the cerebral circulation. The cerebral venous pressure may, however, become significantly elevated when there is increased intracranial pressure, when gravitational forces are applied from the feet toward the head, or when there is obstruction of venous return via the jugular system to the right side of the heart. Other factors that are external to the brain but also influence the perfusion pressure and vascular resistance will be considered.

Maintenance of Systemic Blood Pressure. The single most important factor in maintaining cerebral blood flow is the arterial perfusion pressure or blood pressure. The systemic arterial blood pressure depends on the efficiency of the heart as a pump (cardiac output) and the peripheral vasomotor tone or resistance. The sympathetic and parasympathetic control of the heart and peripheral vascular tree are governed principally by the vasomotor center in the medulla, which undergoes almost constant modification in an effort to maintain optimum levels of blood pressure despite changes in the internal and external environment.

The vasomotor center is influenced by impulses from the baroreceptors within the carotid sinus and aortic arch, which function in an inhibitory fashion when there is an increase in systemic blood pressure. This constant monitoring action of the baroreceptors results in appropriate variation in inhibitory impulses from the vasomotor center to maintain constant blood pressure.

Variations in systemic arterial blood pressure do not produce changes in cerebral blood flow in young, healthy individuals with intact cerebral autoregulation (see next section). Autoregulation is extraordinarily efficient under normal circumstances, until the mean arterial blood pressure falls to levels about half of normal (circa 50 mm Hg). A fall in blood pressure below this level may be accompanied by some decrease in cerebral blood flow, but because more oxygen is extracted from the blood, consciousness is usually maintained, even in severe shock.

A rise in mean arterial blood pressure is also compensated by cerebral autoregulation, which is probably effective in the range of 50 to 200 mm Hg.

Changes in Cardiac Output. There is no change in cerebral blood flow over a wide range of changes in cardiac output. Cerebral blood flow is maintained by autoregulatory mechanisms until there is a marked fall in cardiac output accompanied by a fall in systemic arterial pressure below a critical level. When the combination of reduced pressure and volume can no longer be met by autoregulation, the cerebral blood flow will decrease precipitously.

Intrinsic Factors

Certain factors that arise within the brain itself and may regionally influence the cerebrovascular resistance will now be considered.

Autoregulation Due to Changes in Intraluminal Pressure. The cerebral vessels function in a manner similar to other hollow organs possessing a wall containing smooth muscle. The vessels adjust their diameter in such a way as to maintain constant flow to the brain despite changes in perfusion pressure, a phenomenon termed "autoregulation." They constrict when there is an increase in intraluminal pressure and dilate when intraluminal pressure decreases. This effect (known as the Bayliss effect) is a sensitive and rapidly reacting mechanism that constantly alters vascular resistance in response to changes in systemic arterial blood pressure.

In the healthy individual, the response of such autoregulation begins within a few seconds and is effective within a wide range of pressure changes. Thus, in healthy individuals the cerebral blood flow is able to adapt without significant change unless the blood pressure falls below 50 mm Hg, whereupon cerebral blood flow decreases. Similarly, cerebral blood flow remains more or less constant in hypertension until high levels, exceeding 200 mm Hg systolic and 110 to 120 mm diastolic, are reached. When blood pressure exceeds these levels, there is loss of autoregulation with dilatation of cerebral vessels and a sharp increase in cerebral blood flow, which is pressure-dependent.[68, 171]

Autoregulation normally provides the mechanism that maintains constant cerebral blood flow despite variations in arterial blood pressure as a result of various factors such as alterations in posture and changes in blood flow through other organs. Such autoregulation may be regional within the brain by adjustment of the regional vascular resistance.

The circle of Willis and its supplying arteries have the capacity to alter blood flow from one hemisphere to the other and to reverse the direction of flow between the carotid and basilar arterial systems. This function is provided by an autoregulatory mechanism of sufficient flexibility such that the arteries of the circle of Willis and the arteries distal to the circle can dilate and contract independently.[98]

Autoregulation, which is a pressure-controlled autoregulatory mechanism, operates independently but synergistically with intrinsic biochemical factors released regionally by the brain. These biochemical factors are concerned with the regional control of cerebral blood flow in order to meet the brain's metabolic requirements.

Biochemical Factors

Carbon Dioxide. Inhalation of carbon dioxide in man or animals produces marked cerebral vaso-dilatation, and the cerebral blood flow increases as the cerebrovascular resistance rapidly decreases.

The hypercapnic flow increase may be attributed to periarteriolar acidosis[185] or may be dependent upon neurogenic reflex mechanisms with central connections in neurons of the brainstem.[166] A reduction in partial pressure of carbon dioxide in the blood (e.g., during hyperventilation) results in cerebral vasoconstriction and a rapid decrease in cerebral blood flow. Either mechanism causes a change in cerebral blood flow within a few seconds. The vasodilator effect of carbon dioxide, as well as the constrictor response to hyperventilation, decreases with age and probably with cerebral arteriosclerosis, although some degree of responsiveness is found in patients with cerebral arteriosclerosis and cerebral ischemia.

In normal subjects, local increase in cerebral blood flow result from regional increases in carbon dioxide tension in order to provide a mechanism whereby regional blood supply may meet increased regional metabolic demands.[94] Normally the metabolism of the brain is dependent almost entirely on complete oxidation of glucose and consequent production of carbon dioxide. Regional or total increases in cerebral metabolism result in increased carbon dioxide production, cerebral vasodilatation, increased cerebral blood flow, and an increase in oxygen and glucose supply to the brain.

Oxygen. Reduction of arterial oxygen tension by hypoxia or anoxia from any cause produces cerebral vasodilatation and an increase in cerebral blood flow. This may be regional or generalized. Conversely, increases in arterial oxygen tension cause cerebral vasoconstriction and a reduction in cerebral blood flow. Despite this effect, inhalation of 100 per cent oxygen increases the amount of oxygen available to an ischemic area of brain by increasing the gradient between capillaries and tissues.

The vasoconstrictor action of oxygen on the cerebral vessels is independent of decreased carbon dioxide levels. Also, within physiologic limits, the vasomotor effects of changes in oxygen tension are not as remarkable as those of carbon dioxide tension. During severe hypoxia, however, the vasodilator effect of decreased oxygen tension becomes much greater, and vasodilatation will occur even in the presence of hypocapnia. This suggests that the response to cerebral hypoxia may be mediated via an intracerebral autonomic pathway.[149]

Hydrogen Ion Concentration (pH). When pH of the blood is changed in animals or man by the intravenous injection of an acid, such as lactic acid, there is an increase in cerebral blood flow. The increase in flow is probably independent of accompanying increases in carbon dioxide tension. Acidemia produces an increase in cerebral blood flow, while alkalemia tends to produce a decrease. In general, carbon dioxide appears to be more important than pH in the control of cerebral blood flow. In either event, it appears that ultimately the intracellular pH of the smooth muscle fibers of the cerebral arterioles is the important factor controlling vasomotor tone.[61]

Autonomic Control of Cerebral Blood Flow

The autonomic nervous system appears to function by maintaining vasomotor tonus.[29] Usually the vasodilator action of the parasympathetic and beta-adrenergic systems is in balance with the vasoconstrictor action of the alpha-adrenergic system. Under certain situations, such as autonomic blockade by drugs or circulatory shock, the autonomic tonus may be altered in favor of vasoconstriction of dilatation.[65]

The Sympathetic System

The postganglionic fibers from the stellate and cervical sympathetic ganglia supply fibers to the carotid and vertebral arteries. The internal carotid nerves arise from the superior cervical ganglion and enter the carotid canal via the petrous portion of the temporal bone to form the internal carotid and cavernous plexuses. Fibers from both plexuses accompany the anterior and middle cerebral arteries, anterior communicating artery, and ophthalmic artery. The external carotid nerves also arise from the superior cervical ganglion and innervate the external carotid artery and its major branches.

Stimulation of the cervical sympathetic system has been reported to have no effect on cerebral blood flow in some studies.[21, 130] Other reports indicate that cervical sympathetic stimulation produces vasoconstriction of cerebral vessels and decreased blood flow.[65] Removal of the superior cervical ganglion decreases sympathetic tone in the cerebrovascular bed and increases cerebral blood flow.[69] The removal of sympathetic influences on the cerebral vessels also appears to

decrease the autoregulatory response[200] and the sensitivity to changes in P_{CO_2}.[175] The central connections for sympathetic reflex activity are not yet clearly defined but are probably located in the brainstem where they are subject to supranuclear influences from the hypothalamus and the fastigial nucleus of the cerebellum.[114]

The Parasympathetic System

Cholinergic nerve fibers have been shown to innervate cerebral vessels down to 20 μm in size.[78, 137] These vasodilator fibers probably arise from central catecholaminergic neurons in the brainstem,[77] exit in the facial nerve, and pass via the petrosal nerve to the internal carotid plexus and intracerebral vessels. Stimulation of the cut end of the facial nerve or of certain regions in the brainstem and diencephalon causes widening in the diameter of pial vessels and increased blood flow.[88, 126] The cholinergic system is believed to be important in the facilitation of cerebrovascular reactivity to carbon dioxide.[4, 166]

Organic Factors That Influence Cerebral Blood Flow

The blood flow through any organ may be influenced by three factors.

1. Changes in blood viscosity
2. Changes in the vessel walls
3. Changes outside the blood vessels

Changes in Blood Viscosity

Any alteration in the viscosity of the blood will alter the blood flow through an organ, provided the perfusion pressure remains constant. There is an increase in cerebral blood flow in anemia because of the decrease in the cerebrovascular resistance due to decreased blood viscosity. The increased blood viscosity of polycythemia causes increased cerebrovascular resistance and produces a marked reduction in cerebral blood flow.

Changes in the Vessel Walls

Total cerebral blood flow is dependent primarily on the volume of blood delivered to the brain via the internal carotid and vertebral arteries. The application of Poiseuille's law governing volume flow through small tubes to the cervical vessels would predict that marked narrowing of these vessels must be present in order to reduce cerebral blood flow.

However, Poiseuille's law is not applicable to

man, since it assumes that perfusion pressure and peripheral resistance are constant, conditions that do not occur in the living organism under physiologic conditions. Subjects with atherosclerosis frequently show wide fluctuations in systemic arterial blood pressure and increased cerebrovascular resistance. Thus, the application of the results of flow studies made in individual vessels in dogs following experimental narrowing to stenotic lesions in the cerebral vessels of man is almost certainly invalid.

Flowmeter studies have been performed in man during surgical exposure of the carotid arteries in the neck and application of an adjustable clamp. In these cases significant reduction of blood flow did not occur above the site of the occlusion until the size of the lumen had been reduced by 70 to 90 per cent. Such results are also subject to criticism since they were obtained in subjects with cerebral aneurysm whose other vessels were free of occlusive disease and who were supine under anesthesia with the systemic blood pressure (and therefore perfusion pressure) kept within a narrow range. There is a good deal of evidence that a decrease in cerebral blood flow results with lesser degrees of stenosis in the presence of diffuse arteriosclerosis of the small cerebral vessels and multiple involvement of the cervical vessels, conditions that are often present in patients with symptoms of cerebrovascular insufficiency. Cerebral arteriosclerosis impairs the cerebral circulation, particularly during the marked fluctuations of blood pressure that occur in the arteriosclerotic patient.[112]

If plaques at the origin of the carotid and vertebral arteries undergo ulceration, which they commonly do, they may give rise to emboli and hence impair the circulation in the cerebral vessels in a manner that bears no relation whatsoever to the degree of stenosis of the lumen by the plaque itself.

The most common cause of stenosis of the cerebral vessels in the neck is an atheromatous plaque located at the origin of internal carotid and vertebral arteries. The cerebral arteries are also subject to more diffuse and irregular narrowing owing to arteriosclerosis, particularly in association with long-standing hypertension. Disease of the cervical and intracranial vessels supplying the brain is usually complementary. The effects of arteriosclerotic stenosis may also be accentuated by kinking of diseased vessels in the neck during head turning or by osteophytic compression of the vertebral arteries because of cervical spondylosis. The caroticovertebral arteries may also be subject to diffuse or localized disease following thrombosis, giant cell arteritis, or syphilis and by external compression from tumors, and scarring in the neck.

Cerebral arteriosclerosis is associated with increased cerebrovascular resistance and reduced cerebral blood flow. Cerebral blood flow measurements in patients with cerebrovascular disease, including those manifested by transient ischemic attacks, progressive stroke, or completed stroke, have shown reduction of cerebral blood flow and metabolism.

Cerebrovascular resistance is also measurably increased in meningovascular syphilis and in other types of arteritis affecting the cerebral vessels. Severe spasm also reduces cerebral blood flow. This is a frequent occurrence following rupture of an intracranial aneurysm with subarachnoid hemorrhage and in severe or malignant hypertension. The spasm that occurs after subarachnoid hemorrhage appears to be due to increased sensitivity of the alpha-adrenergic system to vasoconstrictor agents present in the blood and platelets, such as serotonin, norepinephrine, and prostaglandins.

Changes Outside the Blood Vessels

Cerebral edema and increased intracranial pressure increase cerebrovascular resistance and decrease cerebral blood flow. Local pressure from cerebral abscesses, tumors, intracerebral hematomas, or subdural hematomas will also produce a local decrease in cerebral blood flow.

In contrast, there is marked reduction in cerebrovascular resistance in the case of an intracerebral arteriovenous malformation or a carotid cavernous fistula with considerable increase in cerebral blood flow (Fig. 9–2).

Regional Regulation of Cerebral Blood Flow

The general principles discussed here concerning the regulation of blood flow apply to regulation of regional blood flow as well. If regional metabolism is increased, such as occurs in the occipital lobe during intense visual activity or during a focal seizure discharge, regional increases in P_{CO_2} and reduction in P_{O_2} will increase regional cerebral blood flow. Such a regional system is self-regulating and reduces regional flow when metabolism decreases.

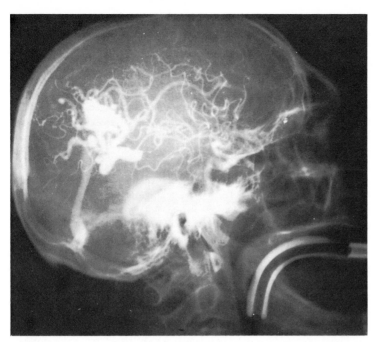

FIGURE 9–2.   Arteriovenous malformation of the parieto-occipital area. Measurement of cerebral blood flow showed greatly increased flow (more than twice normal). Following successful surgical excision of the malformation, the measurements of cerebral blood flow were restored to normal.

In regional cerebral ischemia following occlusion of a cerebral vessel, CO_2 and lactate accumulate in the ischemic zone and regional oxygen tension falls. This stimulates the collateral circulation to increase the flow to the ischemic area.[122, 125]

Cerebrovascular Insufficiency

Almost all cases of cerebrovascular insufficiency are the result of cerebrovascular atherosclerosis. Infrequent causes include repeated embolism of insufficient degree to cause infarction in patients with rheumatic heart disease and prolapsed mitral valve or other cardiac abnormalities. Other unusual conditions associated with cerebrovascular insufficiency include the several types of arteritis and sickle cell disease. In general, however, the prevention of cerebrovascular insufficiency and of cerebral infarction lies in the understanding and prevention of atherosclerosis.

Atherosclerosis of the cerebral vessels is usually a chronic degenerative process beginning at an early age and progressing throughout several decades. The process appears to be accelerated by a number of factors, three of which, hypertension, heart disease, and diabetes mellitus, are the most significant. More than 80 per cent of patients with cerebrovascular disease suffer from, give a history of, or show evidence of hypertension. Cerebrovascular insufficiency and cerebral infarction are from two to four times as frequent in hypertensive individuals as in comparable normotensives. The risk of cerebrovascular disease is not suddenly increased in hypertensive individuals whose blood pressure is elevated beyond certain levels. However, there does seem to be a steady linear relationship between increased risk of cerebral infarction and elevation of both systolic and diastolic blood pressure. Adequate medical treatment of hypertension has been shown to significantly reduce the incidence of cerebrovascular disease.[190]

At least 60 per cent of patients with cerebrovascular disease have accompanying heart disease, and about 10 per cent of those with acute strokes have associated myocardial infarction. The association is not unexpected since both conditions are the result of atherosclerosis, and individuals with necropsy evidence of myocardial infarction also show a high prevalence of severe atheroma in the carotid arteries.[109] Furthermore, following myocardial infarction, mural thrombi in the heart may be a source of embolism,[59] and in many types of heart disease atrial thrombi may be thrown off as emboli to the brain.

Some 30 per cent of patients with cerebral atherosclerosis have diabetes mellitus. This figure may be increased to 40 to 50 per cent if patients with mild or subclinical diabetes whose metabolic defect is revealed only by special tests such as the glucose tolerance test are included. Since the metabolic disorder leading to vascular complications of mild or subclinical diabetes mellitus may be unrelated to the disorder of glucose metabolism, the inclusion of mild or subclinical cases of diabetes mellitus as a factor predisposing to cerebral atherosclerosis will probably be eventually justified.[40, 116-119]

It is apparent that lipid metabolism plays a major role in cerebral atherogenesis. The incidence of occlusive cerebrovascular disease is increased in familial and nonfamilial hyperlipidemias, particularly type 4 hyperlipidemia. Patients with type 4 hyperlipidemia and cerebral infarction also have a higher incidence of extracranial occlusive disease when compared to patients without lipid abnormalities or those with other types of hyperlipidemia.[103a] Elevated serum cholesterol and triglyceride values have frequently been associated with accelerated atherosclerosis, and high triglyceride values have been associated with a high risk of cerebral infarction occurring before the age of 50.[48] Other factors that should be considered in the pathogenesis of accelerated cerebral atherosclerosis include excess body weight,[86] smoking, hypothyroidism, hyperuricemia, and platelet disease.

Hypotheses on the pathogenesis of atherosclerosis are undergoing rapid change, but certain basic facts have achieved some stability in current concepts. The initial event appears to be endothelial injury[173] that results from hemodynamic stress such as hypertension or turbulence of blood at the bifurcation of the arteries. This is followed by the deposition of platelets on the damaged endothelium and the release of a number of substances including serotonin, epinephrine, and histamine which may injure the vessel wall.[136] The platelets also release a growth factor that stimulates proliferation of smooth muscle cells at the site of endothelial damage. The smooth muscle cells are also stimulated to proliferate by exposure

to lipoproteins that have access to the cells because of endothelial damage. The proliferated smooth muscle cells then synthesize connective tissue elements, including collagen, elastin, and mucopolysaccharides. The mechanism of hydrolysis and removal of cholesterol esters by lysosomes is also deranged, and there is an accumulation of cholesterol esters, possibly influenced by increased synthesis of protaglandin PGE_2 in the vessel wall.[177] This early stage of atherosclerosis is followed by the release of lipids from the damaged cells into the area of proliferating connective tissue and the gradual development of an atherosclerotic plaque.[90] This lesion has three effects: (1) the production of narrowing and stenosis of the lumen, probably the result of repeated mural thrombosis on the plaque and the incorporation of the thrombus into the plaque; (2) the destruction of the surface endothelium, the formation of an ulcerated plaque, and the liberation of atheromatous material and clot in the form of emboli; and (3) the formation of thrombi on the surface of the plaque, which act as the nidus for progressive thrombosis and occlusion of the vessel.[148]

The development of atherosclerotic plaques tends to occur at certain predictable sites in the cervical vessels, e.g., the origin of the internal carotid and vertebral arteries (Fig. 9–3). The process tends to be more generalized, however, in the intracranial vessels, probably because of their more frequent branching. When the atherosclerotic process involves both large and small vessels, there is an increased tendency to develop symptoms.[71]

Three major effects of cerebrovascular atherosclerosis may result: (1) transient ischemic attacks, resulting from cerebrovascular insufficiency; (2) regional infarction in the brain with a focal neurologic defect persisting for 24 hours or longer; and (3) arteriosclerotic dementia due to multiple areas of microinfarction (multi-infarct dementia).

Transient Ischemic Attacks (T.I.A.s)

Transient ischemic attacks are brief neurologic deficits lasting a few minutes but not longer than 24 hours. The symptoms and signs of T.I.A.s will be described in detail later, but when they appear to be attributed to the carotid or vertebral territory, the term "carotid insufficiency" or "vertebral-basilar insufficiency" is used. These terms are intended to describe the regional system of vessels within which the circulating disorder gives rise

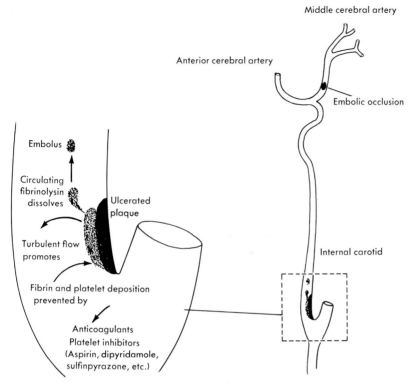

FIGURE 9–3. Diagram showing how a plaque in the internal carotid artery may give rise to recurrent cerebrovascular symptoms. Deposits of fibrin and platelets may occur on the plaque due to turbulence and hypercoagulable states of the blood. Fragments may break off and be carried to the middle cerebral artery as emboli, where they are lysed by fibrinolysins. If the thrombus progresses, the carotid artery may become occluded.

to symptoms. This does not imply any functional independence of these systems in health since they are highly integrated and interdependent. There is a rich potential collateral circulation between the two systems, which varies a great deal from one individual to another. When symptoms of cerebral circulatory insufficiency occur, they are the result of the transient failure of compensatory mechanisms (Fig. 9–4). Although symptoms suggest that the cerebral ischemia is occurring within the territory of one of the two systems, from a hemodynamic point of view, blood flow is altered in both systems, and a decrease in one is unable to be compensated by an increase in the other. Similar regional alterations in the small cerebral vessels less commonly give rise to transient ischemic atacks.[134, 135]

There are a number of predisposing factors that may give rise to transient ischemic attacks.

1. Emboli may be released intermittently from ulcerated plaques in cervical vessels.[111] These bear no relation to posture and give rise to well-defined focal neurologic defects frequently in a stereotyped manner. This is because emboli from the same source frequently tend to follow the same pathway and involve the same territory of supply (Fig. 9–5).

2. Attacks may occur following a sudden transient hypotensive episode, particularly if there is postural hypotension. Here the signs and symptoms are more diffuse and generalized and tend to be less focal than in (1). Systemic and postural hypotension are probably more important in transient ischemic attacks affecting the vertebral-basilar system which shows impaired autoregulation in patients with vertebral-basilar insufficiency.[136a]

3. Attacks may be precipitated when the neck

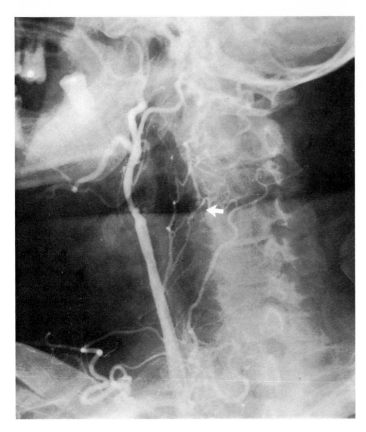

FIGURE 9–4. Left carotid arteriogram in a case of occlusion of the proximal vertebral artery. There is filling of the distal vertebral artery (see arrow) via the cervical collateral vessels. The left internal carotid artery is also occluded at its origin.

vessels, in particular the vertebral arteries, are compressed and temporarily occluded by turning of the head.[127]

4. Attacks may be precipitated by sudden and transient reduction in cardiac output due to arrhythmias or incomplete heart block.[108]

5. Attacks may occur because of atherosclerosis and occlusion of small intracerebral arteries in the brains of chronic hypertensive patients.[159]

The clinical importance of transient ischemic episodes and strokes of brief duration (longer than 24 hours) but with recovery (reversible ischemic neurologic deficits) cannot be overemphasized. Any patient with these symptoms is a potential candidate for a major stroke and deserves full evaluation as outlined later in this chapter, unless there are striking medical contraindications.

Estimates of the percentage of patients who have transient ischemic attacks preceding cerebral infarction range from 4 per cent to 75 per cent.[51] There is a similar uncertainty about the natural history of transient ischemic attacks and the evidence of cerebral infarction in patients who have symptoms of cerebrovascular insufficiency. However, in a recent series of patients with transient ischemic attacks, there was a 36 per cent incidence of cerebral infarction in a 45-month period of observation.[187] Thus there is no doubt that patients who have transient ischemic attacks carry an appreciable risk of cerebral infarction, but the degree of risk remains to be defined. There is some suggestion that the majority of patients with symptoms of carotid insufficiency and about half the patients with vertebral basilar insufficiency who subsequently develop infarction do so after only one or two transient ischemic attacks.[103] Nevertheless, some patients continue to have transient ischemic attacks for many years without the development of cerebral infarction,[201] although there is presumably an increased risk that this event may occur. In another group the attacks cease probably due to the development of an adequate collateral circulation[8] or spontaneous cessation of emboli. It must also be emphasized that many patients with transient ischemic attacks succumb to myocardial infarction. Consequently, a

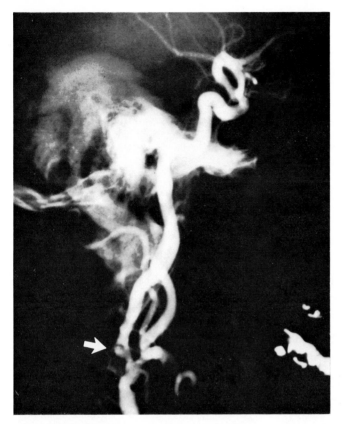

FIGURE 9–5. Carotid arteriogram showing severe stenosis at the origin of the internal and external carotid arteries. There is an ulcerated plaque (arrow) just beyond the origin of the internal carotid artery.

transient ischemic attack is a warning for cardiac as well as cerebrovascular disease.[188a]

Carotid Insufficiency

Transient ischemic episodes due to insufficiency within the carotid system occasionally produce recurrent attacks of dimness of vision or blindness on the side of the involved vessel (amaurosis fugax) owing to embarrassment of circulation within the ophthalmic artery. There may be episodic homonymous hemianopia, hemiparesis, and hemisensory loss on the side opposite the diseased vessel, lasting from a few minutes to several hours. If the dominant hemisphere is involved, transient dysphasia, dyslexia, and dyscalculia may occur. Some patients develop unilateral or generalized headache after an attack.

One characteristic of transient ischemic episodes is that from a clinical viewpoint there is complete recovery between attacks. When examined, the patient may show few abnormal neurologic signs. Some patients may show minimal contralateral weakness with slight increase in deep tendon reflexes and, occasionally, an extensor plantar response for 24 hours after they have experienced symptoms. A considerable number have a loud murmur (bruit)* on auscultation over the origin of the internal carotid artery in the neck where the presence of a stenotic plaque in the vessel causes turbulence of blood flow.[57]

Vertebral-Basilar Insufficiency

Symptoms of vertebral-basilar insufficiency usually appear for the first time in patients in the sixth decade or older. They occur with equal frequency in either sex and may continue for many years, the frequency varying from several every 24 hours to one attack in several months.

Attacks are frequently associated with occipital headaches, which may persist for several days. The headaches are probably caused by congestion of collateral vessels. When the insufficiency involves the posterior cerebral vessels, there is dim-

---

* Murmurs of significance are loud and coarse, particularly if they are heard in both systole and diastole, and should not be confused with soft functional murmurs and venous hums.

ness of vision or transient blindness. The patient may experience attacks of "flashing lights" in the visual fields, and transient altitudinal or homonymous hemianopia may appear. Certain segments of the brainstem may be affected, and this may result in diploplia, ptosis, transient facial weakness, tinnitus, vertigo, nausea and vomiting, dysphagia, and dysarthria. Facial paresthesias, especially in the perioral area, are commonly encountered. Temporary cerebellar dysfunction results in ataxia, while involvement of the corticospinal tracts may cause sudden collapse with or without temporary loss or impairment of consciousness or transient hemiparesis. In vertebral artery insufficiency (Fig. 9–6) sudden collapse without loss of consciousness (the "drop attack") is highly characteristic.[168]

The neurologic examination is often normal between attacks, but variable signs may be found if the patient is examined during the episode. These include impaired visual acuity, diplopia, ptosis, facial weakness, poor elevation of the palate, dysarthria, cerebellar ataxia and intention tremor, hemiparesis, and hemihypalgesia. There may be inequality of deep tendon reflexes and extensor plantar responses, which revert to normal.

Transient Global Amnesia Syndrome

This syndrome is included with cerebrovascular disease since it seems evident that some cases are due to a form of transient cerebrovascular insufficiency.[17, 45, 104, 169, 174]

Clinical Features

The condition occurs in middle-aged and elderly patients (42 to 92 years of age) who develop sudden, brief episodes of total amnesia for recent events. During an attack they are able to carry out functions such as dressing or driving an automobile, but there is complete amnesia during the episode. Patients may be unable to remember talking to the examiner if he leaves the room and returns within a few minutes, or they may be unable to remember why they have left home and are driving a car. Remote memory appears to

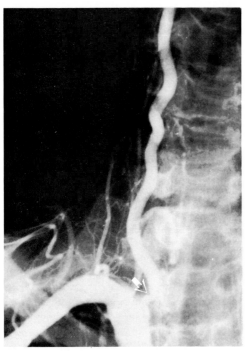

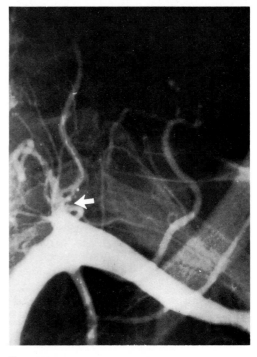

A

B

FIGURE 9–6. *A.* Right vertebral arteriogram showing stenosis at origin of the vertebral artery (indicated by arrow). The patient suffered from vertebral artery insufficiency. *B.* Left vertebral arteriogram showing occlusion of the left vertebral artery at its origin (indicated by arrow).

be intact; the memory gap extends in retrograde fashion over a period of a day or occasionally as long as several days to a week. Recovery gradually occurs over a period of hours or after the patient has fallen asleep. After repeated attacks permanent dementia usually supervenes.[104]

Electroencephalographic abnormalities of nonspecific type have been described, including episodic theta activity in one or both temporal lobes.

A transient disturbance of recent memory with intact immediate and remote memory suggests a temporary disturbance of hippocampal function. The attacks are often interspersed with attacks of vertebral-basilar insufficiency, and arteriography shows occlusive or stenotic lesions in the vertebrobasilar system in the majority of cases.

Diagnostic Procedures

Patients with transient ischemic attacks and reversible deficits should have an adequate diagnostic evaluation since it may be possible to offer definitive medical and/or surgical therapy with improvement or alleviation of symptoms and control of risk factors.

Complete Blood Count. Both anemia and polycythemia may contribute to cerebrovascular insufficiency and stroke. If either is found, further investigations and treatment are indicated.

Elevated hemoglobin values are not uncommon in elderly dehydrated patients. Polycythemia occurs in association with cerebellar hemangioblastoma and kidney disease, particularly renal tumors. The diagnosis of polycythemia vera is made by measurement of total blood volume and examination of the bone marrow.

An elevated white blood count with a polymorphonucleocytosis usually indicates an infection. The platelet count is elevated in polycythemia vera. Increased platelet aggregability has been described in young patients with transient ischemic attacks.[28, 81, 198]

Erythrocyte Sedimentation Rate. A moderate elevation of the erythrocyte sedimentation rate is not unusual in patients with anemia. However, marked elevation occurs in cranial arteritis and occasionally in malignant disease, which may present with neurologic symptoms.

Serologic Tests for Syphilis. These should be obtained on blood and on the cerebrospinal fluid if a lumbar puncture is performed. If there is a past history of syphilis, the fluorescein *Treponema* antibody absorption test should be obtained.

Blood Glucose. A two-hour postprandial blood glucose is a reliable screening test for diabetes mellitus. Those patients with an abnormal two-hour glucose level or those with a strong family history of diabetes mellitus should have a five-hour glucose tolerance test performed after three days on a high-carbohydrate diet.

Blood Urea Nitrogen, Serum Creatinine, and Urinalysis. It is important to exclude renal disease in patients with cerebrovascular insufficiency since the planning of treatment may be influenced by the presence of renal insufficiency. In addition, the presence of abnormal renal function may indicate a renal cause for chronic hypertension in a patient with cerebrovascular insufficiency.

Serum Uric Acid Levels. There is an association between elevated serum uric acid levels and the presence of atheromatous plaques in the internal carotid and vertebral arteries.

Serum Cholesterol and Triglyceride Levels. Both elevated cholesterol and elevated triglyceride levels have been identified as risk factors in cerebrovascular disease. Elevated lipid levels are common in diabetes mellitus and occasionally occur in pancreatitis and alcoholism. If the level of either cholesterol or triglyceride is abnormal, further studies should be performed using lipoprotein electrophoresis to determine the lipid phenotype.

Electrocardiography. Between 60 and 80 per cent of patients with cerebrovascular disease have abnormal electrocardiograms. The changes include evidence of myocardial ischemia, old and recent myocardial infarction, bundle branch block, and left ventricular hypertrophy in long-standing hypertension. Dysrhythmias are also commonly recorded.

Evaluation of the cardiac status is important in the patient with cerebrovascular disease, and if heart failure is suspected, a venous pressure estimation and sodium dehydrocholate (Decholin) circulation time should be obtained.

Cardiac abnormalities, particularly chronic atrial fibrillation, are important causes of transient cerebral ischemia and strokes,[196a] and continuous electrocardiographic monitoring by the

Holter technique is indicated in most patients. The Holter technique will reveal brief changes in rhythm; episodic dysrhythmias, including brief episodes of atrial fibrillation or flutter; premature atrial or ventricular contractions; or intraventricular conduction abnormalities that may coincide with neurologic symptoms.[113] The cardiac monitor may reveal previously undetected cardiac abnormalities that can be alleviated by treatment and result in disappearance of the cerebral symptoms.[96]

A patient with a transient ischemic episode who does not show significant extracranial or intracranial atherosclerotic disease should have cardiac monitoring and echocardiographic studies to rule out recurrent embolism from a prolapsed mitral valve.[9, 59]

Roentgenograms of Skull, Cervical Spine, and Chest. These may reveal a shift of a calcified pineal gland in the case of an unsuspected brain tumor or subdural hematoma that poses as a stroke. The intramural portions of the carotid arteries are sometimes calcified in long-standing arteriosclerosis. Cervical spondylosis can cause compression of the vertebral arteries in the neck when the head is turned with obstruction to the flow of blood and the production of symptoms of vertebral-basilar insufficiency. The chest roentgenogram should be a routine investigation in the neurologic evaluation. It provides an estimation of heart size and may reveal the presence of unsuspected pulmonary congestion or tumor.

Blood Pressure. This should be recorded every hour for 24 hours. If hypertensive episodes occur, treatment with hypotensive agents is indicated. Severe paroxysmal hypertension requires further evaluation to exclude pheochromocytoma or renal artery stenosis.

Hypotensive Episodes. When these occur under mild stress or in relation to changes in posture, they require investigation for Shy-Drager syndrome[128] or possible pituitary-adrenal insufficiency. Tests of autonomic function should be made. Serum corticoid levels, urinary 17-hydroxyketosteroids, and 17-ketogenic steroids should be measured.

Hypothyroidism. A small percentage of patients with cerebral arteriosclerosis have hypothyroidism, and a few have hyperthyroidism, as judged by clinical tests.

Serum triiodothyronine, T3, and total thyroxine, T4, estimations are adequate screening tests.

Electroencephalography. It is not unusual to find a normal EEG or occasionally some focal or diffuse brief bursts of moderate-amplitude slow activity in the electroencephalogram in cases of cerebrovascular insufficiency.[186, 188] A history of a stroke may account for focal slowing, but the presence of persistent focal high-amplitude slowing in a patient who has had symptoms only of cerebrovascular insufficiency should raise the question of a possible brain tumor. A subdural hematoma usually produces slowing and reduction in voltage over the site of the hematoma, which is seldom seen in stroke.

Computed Tomography of the Brain. The CT scan should be normal in cerebrovascular insufficiency[85] but is useful in excluding unsuspected cerebral infarction, cerebral hemorrhage, brain tumor, or subdural hematoma. Some patients may show evidence of previous undocumented infarction or cortical atrophy.

Doppler and Real Time Ultrasound Techniques. The Doppler and real time ultrasonic techniques are valuable noninvasive screening tests in the assessment of carotid artery and ophthalmic artery hemodynamics. The techniques provide an accurate means of detecting carotid occlusion[16] and are rapid, safe, and inexpensive techniques for the evaluation of carotid bruits. However, they are not as accurate as the arteriogram in assessing the degree of carotid stenosis.[18]

Ophthalmodynamometry. This procedure is another useful noninvasive screening test for internal carotid artery disease. Ophthalmodynamometry is a method for the measurement of blood pressure in the eye and can be performed rapidly and with little discomfort.[170] Reduction in blood pressure in one eye may indicate reduced internal carotid artery pressure on that side.[143] The test may be positive in ophthalmic artery stenosis and negative when the ophthalmic artery arises from the external carotid system or when there is a well-developed collateral circulation from that source.

Radionuclide Imaging. The static radionuclide brain scan has been superceded by computed tomography, which has the advantage of increased accuracy and the ability to distinguish between cerebral infarction and hematoma.[52]

The dynamic rapid serial scintigraph, which utilizes a scintillation (gamma) camera, usually provides sufficient information to distinguish between arteriovenous malformation, infarction, or neoplasm and is therefore useful in the evaluation of cerebrovascular insufficiency. The technique also gives information on cerebral perfusion and is useful in detecting impaired passage of the indicator through a carotid artery.[64]

Lumbar Puncture.   The development of newer techniques in the investigation of cerebrovascular insufficiency has made lumbar puncture unnecessary in most cases. Lumbar puncture is indicated when the diagnosis of cerebrovascular insufficiency is in doubt or if there is evidence for intracranial hemorrhage. Such a situation can occur in chronic meningitis, mild encephalitis, or a minor degree of bleeding from an arteriovenous malformation. The opening and closing pressure should be recorded during the procedure, and the cerebrospinal fluid should be examined for cell count, differential count, glucose, and protein content. A serologic test for syphilis should be obtained and the fluid cultured for bacteria. A smear should be stained with Gram's stain in all cases of suspected infection. Examination for the presence of tumor cells is useful in cases of possible brain tumor.

Miscellaneous Studies.   Accelerated partial thromboplastin time, increased plasma fibrinogen levels, elevated plasma plasminogen, and increased soluble fibrin monomer may be useful in the diagnosis of cerebrovascular insufficiency and to detect patients who have a high risk of cerebral infarction.[147]

Facial thermography has been used to detect carotid artery insufficiency based on the lowering of forehead temperature on the affected side.[161] Echoencephalography is useful in the detection of an unsuspected shift of midline structures due to tumor or subdural hematoma.

Arteriography.   Improvement in diagnoses, diagnostic procedures, and the introduction of computed tomography of the brain have reduced the need for arteriography in the evaluation of cerebrovascular insufficiency. Since the performance of cerebral angiography carries a small but defi-

nite risk,[40a] the decision to advise arteriography should be based on:

1. The possibility of the demonstration of a surgically treatable lesion.
2. The possibility that the diagnosis of cerebrovascular insufficiency is incorrect and that arteriography will contribute to the correct diagnosis (e.g., brain tumor or abscess or subdural hematoma).

Using these guidelines, arteriography is indicated in patients who have had symptoms of transient cerebrovascular insufficiency if adequate investigation has been carried out to exclude concomitant conditions that might increase the risk of arteriography (see above) or if any identified abnormalities have been treated. The performance of arteriography in patients with asymptomatic midcervical carotid bruits remains controversial. The detection and removal of asymptomatic stenotic plaques in the carotid arteries are probably justified before performing major surgery elsewhere, particularly peripheral vascular surgery.

Cerebral angiography is contraindicated in patients with recent myocardial infarction, severe pulmonary disease, or blood dyscrasias.

A high proportion of patients with transient ischemic attacks show arteriographic evidence of arteriosclerosis in the extra- or intracranial vessels. The carotid system is frequently involved at the origin of the internal carotid artery, which may be the site of stenosis due to plaque formation (Fig. 9–7). There may be elongation, kinking, or tortuosity of this vessel in the neck and more diffuse arteriosclerotic plaques in the area of the carotid siphon and occasionally of the intracerebral branches. Stenosis occurs at the origin of the vertebral arteries from the subclavian arteries in the neck. These vessels may show stenosis in the fourth portion proximal to or at the junction with the basilar artery.

Diffuse arteriosclerosis produces tortuosity and kinking of the vertebral artery as it passes through the foramina of the transverse processes of the cervical vertebrae. The vessel may be occluded on head turning by compression owing to osteophyte formation in cervical spondylosis. If the condition is suspected because of the history, arteriography should be performed with head turning to demonstrate this.

Occasionally, filling of one vertebral artery is followed by retrograde flow of the contrast mate-

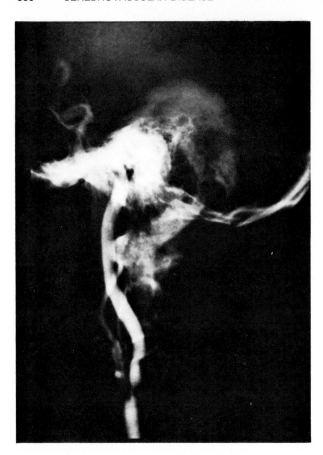

FIGURE 9-7. Carotid arteriogram showing a very severe stenosis at the origin of the internal carotid artery. The dye appears as a threadlike opacity at the site of the stenosis.

rial down the contralateral vertebral artery into the subclavian artery. This is associated with a proximal stenosis of the subclavian artery, and because it results in the flow of blood away from the basilar artery into the stenosed subclavian artery, the term "subclavian steal" has been given to this condition (Fig. 9–8).

Treatment

Control of hypertension is probably the most important factor in the treatment of transient ischemic attacks. This alone will reduce the incidence of strokes. Many patients respond to oral diuretics such as hydrochlorothiazide, 50 mg daily. Others require the addition of other drugs such as alpha-methyldopa, 250 to 500 mg tid, or propranolol, beginning 10 mg qid and gradually increasing the dosage until it is effective. When using propranolol care should be taken to avoid bradycardia or heart block.

All other associated medical conditions such as heart disease, diabetes mellitus, hyperlipid-

emia, obesity, anemia, polycythemia, hypoglycemia, hypothyroidism, idiopathic thrombocytosis, and hyperuricemia should be treated.[97, 171] Patients who suffer hypotensive episodes may benefit from small doses of oral steroids (fludrocortisone acetate, 0.1 mg twice daily) and should have intravenous corticosteroids immediately prior to arteriography to prevent hypotension from the stress of this procedure.

In many cases transient ischemic attacks are the result of fibrino-platelet emboli arising from roughened or ulcerated atheromatous plaques in the major cervical vessels or having origin in the heart. This suggests that attacks may be controlled or reduced by the use of drugs that inhibit platelet aggregation or by the use of anticoagulants.

The value of antiplatelet therapy is now established, and the safety and low incidence of side effects have resulted in widespread use of these agents. Aspirin therapy is most effective,[23a] but a combination of dipyridamole (Persantine), 25

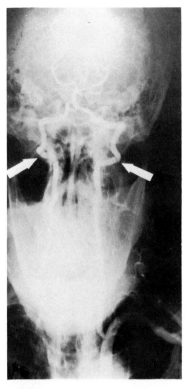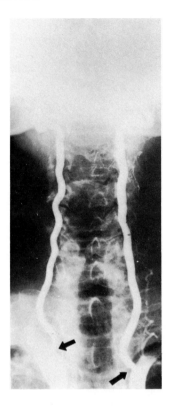

A

FIGURE 9–8.   Left brachial arteriogram in a patient with right subclavian steal and symptoms of vertebral basilar insufficiency exacerbated by turning the head. The entire vertebral basilar system fills by left brachial artery injection of dye, and because the right subclavian is occluded, this vessel steals blood from the vertebrobasilar system. When the head was rotated to either side, the vertebral arteries became kinked at the points marked by black and white arrows.

mg qid, with aspirin, 1,000 mg (gr 15), at night has been recommended for the treatment of transient ischemic attacks. Sulphinpyrazone, 200 mg qid, is also believed to be an effective antiplatelet agent.[121]

Anticoagulants.   The value of anticoagulants in the treatment of patients with transient ischemic attacks remains an unproven hypothesis.[20] The many studies carried out in the last two decades show a marked difference in their conclusions, which range from unequivocal support for anticoagulants[132] to outright rejection.[144] The difference is due in part to the fact that all of the studies to date lack either randomized controls or statistical significance. However, since some studies do indicate trends that suggest some benefit from anticoagulants in patients with transient ischemic attack, some physicians will choose to use these drugs. Patients with cerebrovascular insufficiency who are to receive anticoagulant therapy should meet rigid criteria before treatment. Severe hypertension should be treated, there should be no potential site of bleeding such as a peptic ulcer, and the patient and family should be of sufficient intelligence to understand the function of anticoagulants and the necessity for strict adherence to the prescribed dosage. The oral dose of sodium warfarin should be adjusted in the hospital so that the prothrombin time is two to two and one-half times the control. Thereafter the dose is managed after discharge by bimonthly examination and measurements of prothrombin time.

There is no general agreement among advocates on the duration of anticoagulant therapy. The recommendations range from one to two months[195] to the advice that patients receive life-long anticoagulant treatment.[51] This situation would suggest that each patient must be followed closely and the decision to continue or withdraw anticoagulants must be made based on clinical assessment at each examination.

Patients who have a significant degree of stenosis of the internal carotid or vertebral arteries in the neck, due to atherosclerotic plaques, should be considered for surgical reconstruction of the vessels (Fig. 9–9).

The most suitable case is the patient with transient ischemic attacks, but without a severe and permanent neurologic deficit, who has a stenosis of one carotid artery exceeding 50 per cent or an ulcerated plaque. Candidates for surgery may be rejected because of severity of neurologic deficit, advanced occlusive arterial disease involving multiple cranial vessels, and associated diseases such as myocardial infarction or congestive heart failure.[12]

All patients who are being considered for surgery must have adequate treatment of associated medical conditions prior to arteriography. This reduces the risk of complications at the time of arteriography and the morbidity of the surgical procedure. Patients with complete occlusion of one or both carotid arteries in the neck or with intracranial stenosis or occlusion of an internal carotid artery or with proximal stenosis of a middle cerebral artery should be recommended for a superficial temporal to middle cerebral artery bypass procedure[24, 95a, 152] (Fig. 9–10).

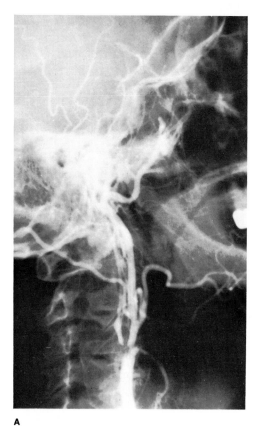 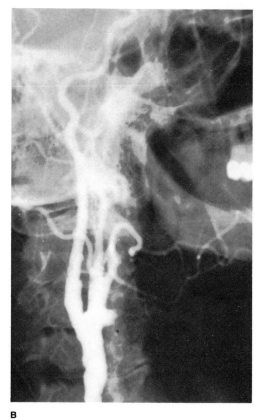

A   B

FIGURE 9–9. Carotid arteriograms in a patient with symptoms of carotid insufficiency. *A.* There is marked stenosis of the internal and external carotid arteries with poor filling of the intracranial cerebral vessels. *B.* Three months after carotid endarterectomy, filling of the intracranial vessels is improved.

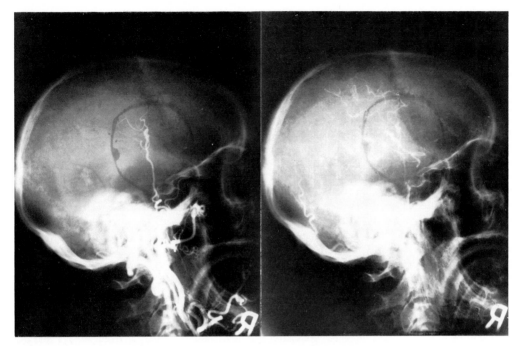

FIGURE 9–10. Early- and late-phase serial arteriograms in a patient with occlusion of the right internal carotid artery following a superficial temporal to middle cerebral artery bypass procedure. The middle cerebral artery filling is clearly demonstrated.

Infarction of the Brain Due to Thromboembolism

The most common type of stroke is due to infarction of an area of the brain secondary to arterial occlusion by thrombosis or embolism of a major vessel with insufficient collateral circulation.

Etiology, Pathogenesis, and Pathology

The blood flow to any organ depends on three factors: (1) condition of the blood vessels, (2) composition of the blood, and (3) perfusion pressure.

Condition of the Blood Vessels. The majority of strokes due to infarction occur in the atherosclerotic patient. The arteries may show diffuse narrowing due to atherosclerosis or focal stenosis in a number of places, but the most common sites are at the origin of the internal carotid and vertebral arteries. Less frequently, the arteries may be compressed externally by tumors or by fibrous bands in the neck. The vessels are also subject to kinking on head turning and to compression by the lateral mass of the atlas. Arterial narrowing

due to fibromuscular dysplasia is a rare occurrence.[156] The vertebral and carotid vessels in the neck and their intracranial vessels may be involved by arteritis, particularly due to syphilis. In any of these conditions the tendency for thrombus formation and vascular occlusion is increased. In addition, both healthy and diseased vessels may be occluded by emboli, arising at a distant site and lodging within the carotid, vertebral, and cerebral vessels. Possible sources of emboli are listed in Table 9–1 in the section on cerebral embolism.

Many of these may give rise to infarction and the typical clinical picture of a stroke. It is often difficult to distinguish clinically between a stroke due to thrombosis and one due to embolism.[121]

Composition of the Blood. There is an increased tendency for the blood to clot in patients who have suffered a stroke (hypercoagulable state),[54] and it seems evident that these alterations in the composition of the blood are present prior to the event.[40] These include an increase in the adhesiveness of platelets and elevation of fibrinogen levels.[184] The thrombotic tendency is also enhanced in primary and secondary polycythemia and may be influenced by a reduction in the oxygen tension of the blood. Low arterial oxygen tensions are regularly found in stroke patients, probably owing to poor pulmonary function. The latter factor may become exaggerated by heart failure and from other causes such as atelectasis, hypostatic and aspiration pneumonia, chronic bronchitis, emphysema, bronchiectasis, and lobar pneumonia.

Perfusion Pressure. Adequate perfusion pressure is particularly important in the atherosclerotic patient for the maintenance of adequate cerebral blood flow. The patient with cerebrovascular disease is subject to wide variations in systemic blood pressure for reasons that are not entirely clear at this time. Possible factors include defective baroreceptors, myocardial fibrosis, pituitary adrenal insufficiency, and loss of elasticity of the vascular bed. A sudden hypotensive episode may be sufficient to produce a critical decrease in cerebral blood flow in an already impaired cerebral circulation. Fluctuations in perfusion pressure also occur in heart disease, particularly when associated with attacks of cardiac dysrhythmia. There is often severe impairment of cardiac output following myocardial infarction, and cerebral autoregulatory mechanisms that are impaired by cerebral atherosclerosis may be unable to compensate during the reduction in perfusion pressure.

There is considerable variation in the frequency and distribution of infarcts in the brain when autopsied cases of ischemic stroke are compared. This can be related to two factors: (1) the efficiency of the collateral circulation in the brain and (2) the pattern of atherosclerosis and stenosis of large and small cerebral vessels.

The site of infarction will depend on its cause. When it is due to occlusion of a vessel with a well-defined territory of supply, whether the occlusion is due to embolism or thrombosis, the infarct will be in the center of the territory supplied, the bordering areas being spared.

When infarction is due to a fall in blood pressure, the peripheral areas of supply tend to be involved. However, occlusion of a major vessel may be accompanied by a hypotensive episode so that infarction can occur in any area of the territory supplied by the occluded vessel, depending on the degree of impairment of collateral circulation and the extent of the atherosclerotic process in the smaller cerebral arteries.

It is apparent that some cerebral infarcts tend to occur at the extreme periphery of a vascular territory. They are more common in those parts of the brain lying between the areas supplied by the middle and posterior cerebral arteries on the surface of the brain. The region of the internal capsule, lying between the territories supplied by the recurrent artery of Huebner and the lenticulostriate branches of the middle cerebral artery, is also a particularly vulnerable site. Presumably, the vessels of these two systems become progressively narrowed with reduction of vasomotor capacitance in the artherosclerotic patient. If the supply from one of these systems is suddenly reduced or occluded, the metabolic needs of the tissue cannot be met through the other vessels (as they would in the healthy individual), and infarction results. In other words, the collateral supply is insufficient.

It is evident that the boundaries of an autonomous vascular area are not fixed but may be altered by cerebral atherosclerosis. As an example, should the circulation be reduced by a marked stenosis at the origin of the middle cerebral artery or by severe atherosclerotic changes in the proximal portion of that vessel, the volume of blood reaching the periphery may be reduced and the supply augmented by the flow through collaterals from the posterior cerebral artery. This means, in effect, that if the collateral is adequate, the vascular area supplied by the middle cerebral artery is reduced and that supplied by the posterior cerebral artery is increased. The most critical area will be that area of the brain supplied by the most peripheral branches of the two adjacent systems—the so-called watershed area. This area will be abnormally close to the main trunk of a proximally stenosed middle cerebral artery because of the restricted middle cerebral circulation and will be the area of infarction if perfusion falls below the critical level necessary for tissue survival. This may account for the development of infarction in the posteroinferior portion of the frontal lobe or in the superior temporal gyrus in patients with atherosclerotic changes in the middle cerebral artery and a well-developed anterior cerebral or posterior cerebral collateral circulation.

Infarcts show marked variation in size, but all acute infarcts have a central area of tissue necrosis with surrounding edema. From a functional aspect, this means that there is an area of dead and nonfunctioning tissue surrounded by an area of nonfunctioning but potentially viable tissue.

Treatment should be directed toward the recovery of this zone of viable tissue, which will minimize the neurologic deficit caused by the stroke.

The earliest changes in an infarct occur in gray matter, with Nissl degeneration and pyknosis of neurons, which stain eosinophilic with hematoxylin and eosin. In any infarct there is central coagulation necrosis with a surrounding area in which there is disintegration of nerve cells, axons, myelin sheaths, and oligodendroglial cells and some damage to astrocytes.

The blood vessels are necrotic in the center of the infarct but are preserved and widely dilated with damaged endothelium toward the periphery of the infarct. Autoregulation is lost, and subsequent changes depend on the efficiency of the collateral circulation, changes in systemic blood pressure, and lysis of thrombi or emboli or their movement into smaller branches of the main vessel. Under these circumstances persistent hypertension or an episode of hypertension may lead to rupture of necrotic blood vessels and hemorrhage in the necrotic area, producing a hemorrhagic infarction. At the same time there is leakage of red cells through the damaged endothelium of the vessels in the periphery of the infarct and the development of perivascular hemorrhages. Hypotensive episodes may also have a detrimental effect in cerebral infarction where there is impairment of cerebral autoregulation.[179] A sudden fall in blood pressure will result in a profound fall in regional cerebral blood flow in the infarcted area and further extension of the area of impaired brain function.[5] The dilated blood vessels also contain numerous polymorphonuclear cells in the first 24 hours, many of which pass into the perivascular spaces. In the case of superficial cortical or periventricular infarcts these polymorphonuclear cells may enter the cerebrospinal fluid, which may show a polymorphonuclear pleocytosis in the early stages of cerebral infarction.

By the fourth day, the blood vessels at the borders of the infarct and their perivascular spaces are packed with mononuclear cells, and there is active microglial proliferation with phagocytosis of degenerative products of cellular disintegration and myelin breakdown. Many of these cells contain lipid material and stain with sudanophilic dyes (gitter cells). There is also astrocytic proliferation at the periphery of the infarcted area as repair processes are initiated.

The process of removal of the infarcted material proceeds over a period of months, with the gradual formation of a cystic space surrounded by glial tissue containing hypertrophied astrocytes. Eventually, a cyst remains containing clear or xanthochromic fluid lined by astrocytes and glial fibers.

Infarction of white matter follows a similar pattern, beginning with disintegration of axons, myelin sheaths, and oligodendroglial cells. There is active phagocytosis by microglial cells and eventual replacement of the infarcted area by a glial scar or cystic area.

Clinical Features

Since brain infarction tends to occur more frequently in certain sites, a number of types of stroke may be recognized by the constellation of symptoms peculiar to each type.[43, 44] This has led to the identification of the stroke by the use of the name of the blood vessel supplying the involved area, by the area of the brain involved, or by the use of an eponym. The latter type of syndromic neurology has been carried to absurdity partly due to competitive efforts by neurologists of the last century to lay claim to numerous syndromes occurring with brainstem infarction.[99] Some of them are exceedingly rare while some have never even been confirmed at necropsy. In any event it seems more important to understand the pathogenesis of cerebrovascular symptoms rather than to memorize a series of symptoms and their eponym. It is proposed to describe the more common type of stroke, using only those names that appear to be widely used.

Internal Carotid Artery Occlusion. Thrombosis of an internal carotid artery in a patient with cerebral arteriosclerosis is usually followed by the development of an infarction in the area supplied by the middle cerebral artery. However, the result depends on the efficiency of the collateral circulation from the contralateral carotid system through the anterior communicating artery, from the vertebral basilar system through the posterior communicating artery, via the pial collaterals, and from the ipsilateral external carotid artery through the ophthalmic artery to the carotid siphon.

If the collateral circulation is efficient, thrombotic occlusion of an internal carotid artery may be asymptomatic.[38] At the other end of the scale, when the collateral circulation is poor and the occluded carotid system supplies the territory of the ipsilateral posterior cerebral artery and both anterior cerebral arteries, the resulting infarction may involve the whole of one hemisphere and the mesial frontal lobe of the opposite hemisphere.

Although the term "internal carotid artery occlusion" is used to describe the syndromes referred to above, similar symptoms and signs may also occur in association with a severe degree of internal carotid artery stenosis but without complete occlusion of this vessel. Furthermore, from the clinical signs and symptoms, it is not always possible to differentiate occlusion of the internal carotid artery from middle cerebral artery occlusion or a small capsular hemorrhage.

In the majority of cases, occlusion of the internal carotid artery is due to thrombus formation at the origin of this vessel from the common carotid artery in the neck. Occasionally, the thrombus develops in the carotid siphon and rarely in the petrous portion of the vessel. The most common site of plaque formation is at the origin of the internal carotid artery in the neck.

Stenosis at this site may be associated with marked arteriosclerotic changes throughout the carotid system.

There is good evidence that the effect of the stenosis is not entirely dependent on the degree of the occlusion of the vessel. The length of the stenosed segment is important, and a stenosis of 1 cm or more in length will result in a much greater degree of reduction of blood flow than more localized narrowing of the vessel. Similarly, the compounded effect of a stenosis at the origin of the internal carotid artery and narrowing of the carotid siphon (stenosis in tandem) produces about twice the reduction in flow through that vessel as would occur with a single lesion. Another factor that produces a significant reduction of blood flow through a stenotic vessel is a fall in the perfusion pressure. This frequently occurs in the patient with diffuse atherosclerosis and arteriosclerotic heart disease with paroxysmal dysrhythmias or myocardial infarction.

Since the possible hemodynamic effects of carotid occlusion are so variable, it is not surprising that the clinical picture should be equally variable. The patient may remain asymptomatic; a number develop a slow, progressive picture of neurologic deterioration, similar to brain tumor or multi-infarct dementia, and the majority eventually develop symptoms of acute stroke following episodes of transient ischemic attacks.

At least 50 per cent of patients with carotid occlusions as a cause of acute stroke have had obvious prodromal symptoms before the major event. In the remainder, the onset is catastrophic without obvious antecedents, but a careful history will frequently reveal less obvious warning episodes preceding the catastrophe, such as transient monocular blindness. In any event, prodromal symptoms are common and, although of a relatively minor nature, may precede the catastrophic stroke for weeks or even months and should be considered as warning signs indicating that treatment should be instituted. If patients with warning signs are investigated and treated at this stage thrombosis will be prevented in many cases. The clinical signs of carotid insufficiency are described on page 551. Unfortunately, many patients neglect to seek advice when they have transient ischemic episodes and proceed to develop a major stroke.

When infarction occurs, the onset is abrupt and the symptoms often are present on awakening. The patient frequently becomes stuporous or comatose and develops a flaccid hemiplegia with decreased deep tendon reflexes usually present on the affected side.

Impaired consciousness, hemiplegia, and forced deviation of the eyes with failure of conjugate gaze usually indicate infarction involving the whole of the middle cerebral artery territory. There is usually a unilateral and sometimes a bilateral extensor plantar response (Babinski sign). This type of cerebral infarction is often associated with fatal cerebral edema.[141]

The less severely affected and conscious patient with involvement of the dominant hemisphere usually has various admixtures of dysphasia, contralateral homonymous hemianopia, facial weakness, flaccid hemiparesis or hemiplegia, hemisensory loss, depressed deep tendon reflexes, and a unilateral extensor plantar response. The usual course is one of slow and partial recovery with some improvement in language function, persistence of the homonymous hemianopia, and a greater degree of functional recovery in the lower limb than in the upper.

A large infarction can involve most of the lateral portion of the hemisphere, and cases of complete hemispheric infarction with death are not uncommon. These cases with massive infarction are associated with considerable edema and raised intracranial pressure. This usually produces pressure on the brainstem, uncal herniation, secondary brainstem hemorrhages, and death from respiratory failure.

Middle Cerebral Artery Occlusion. In the majority of cases, it is impossible to differentiate between middle cerebral artery occlusion and internal carotid artery occlusion on clinical grounds. When there have been prodromal symptoms, including transient dimness of vision or blindness of one eye (amaurosis fugax), the stroke is likely to be due to internal carotid artery occlusion. However, emboli may arise from plaques in the internal carotid artery and occlude the middle cerebral artery. Therefore, a preceding amaurosis fugax, while indicating carotid artery disease, may occur prior to middle cerebral artery occlusion. When the stroke occurs in a patient with rheumatic heart disease, the cause is again embolic, for emboli arising from diseased heart valves frequently lodge in the middle cerebral artery.

A stroke with pure motor hemiplegia and absence of other neurologic abnormalities can result from cerebral cortical infarction in the middle cerebral territory (Fig. 9–11) or from infarction in the internal capsule due to thrombosis of the penetrating deep branches of the middle cerebral artery.[47a] In other cases minimal dysphasia, hemiparesis, and a mild hemisensory loss may result from occlusion of one of the branches of the middle cerebral artery or from occlusion of the left internal carotid artery, which has good collateral circulation from the right carotid system through the circle of Willis. When the main trunk of the middle cerebral artery is occluded (Fig. 9–12),

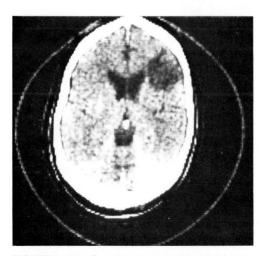

FIGURE 9–11. Computed tomography showing an area of decreased density in the right hemisphere resulting from cerebral infarction. This type of infarction may produce a pure motor hemiplegia with good recovery.

there may be massive hemispheric infarction with death, as also occurs with carotid artery occlusion with poor collateral circulation.

Anterior Cerebral Artery Occlusion. Thrombosis of the proximal portion of both anterior cerebral arteries is uncommon, but the effects are combined infarction of the mesial and anterior portions of both frontal lobes. Occlusion of the recurrent arteries of Huebner may result in infarction of the anterior limb of internal capsule, hypothalamus, and anterior basal ganglia.

The patient with bilateral occlusion of the anterior cerebral arteries presents with alteration in the level of consciousness, which may vary from an apathetic mutism to drowsiness with dysphasia and motor dyspraxia. If the occlusion is unilateral, there will be contralateral hemiplegia with sensory loss involving the lower limb. Thrombosis of the recurrent artery of Huebner, which mainly supplies the anterior limb of the internal capsule, produces a contralateral monoparesis or monoplegia involving the upper limb. Obstruction of the distal portion of the anterior cerebral artery affects the pericallosal and callosal marginal branches, which supply the medial aspect of the frontal lobe and the paracentral lobules. This results in a contralateral monoplegia and sensory loss involving the lower limb but sparing the upper limb. In addition, if the dominant hemisphere is involved, there are varying degrees of dyspraxia and a motor dysphasia with a distinctive hesitation when talking, which results from involvement of the supplementary speech area on the mesial aspect of the superior frontal gyrus.

Anterior Choroidal Artery Occlusion. This artery shows marked variation in size and distribution. It may, however, supply the optic tract, the middle third of the cerebral peduncle, the lateral geniculate body, the internal capsule, and the choroid plexus in the temporal horn of the lateral ventricle. Occlusion of this artery may produce symptoms that resemble middle cerebral artery occlusion. The clinical picture includes contralateral homonymous hemianopia, contralateral hemiplegia, or hemiparesis with a hemisensory loss. There is, however, sparing of language functions in lesions involving the dominant hemisphere.

Brainstem and Cerebellar Infarction. A large number of syndromes have been described due

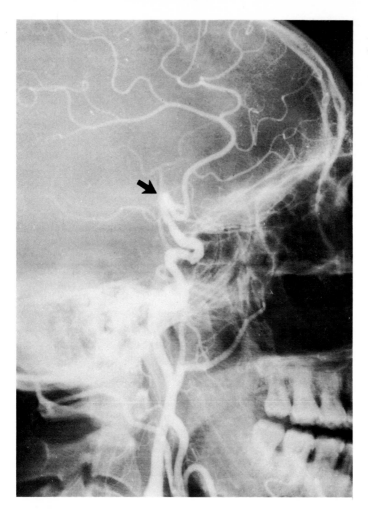

FIGURE 9–12. Right carotid arteriogram showing occlusion of the main trunk of the right middle cerebral artery, indicated by arrow.

to infarction at various levels in the brainstem. Many are rare and hardly deserve recognition as separate entities, while others seldom occur in pure form. The syndromic approach seldom permits pure categorization and if this approach is used, most cases have to be labeled "like the X syndrome," or "a mixture of the X and Y syndromes." This type of categorization is unsatisfactory from a practical therapeutic point of view and is often misleading. A more logical method is to identify the region of the brainstem involved and to describe the lesion in anatomic terms. There is marked variation in the blood supply and collateral circulation to most areas of the brainstem. Therefore, the patterns of infarction vary a great deal, and the most satisfactory descriptions are in terms of correlation with functional neuroanatomy.

Infarction of the Medulla. Infarction involving the lower or caudal portion of one pyramid and the pyramidal fibers, which have crossed from the opposite side, is rare. It does, however, produce a unique clinical picture of paralysis of the upper limb on one side and the opposite lower limb.

Pyramidal infarction involving both pyramids is an uncommon occurrence due to occlusion of the anterior spinal arteries from arteritis or may result from occlusion of the vertebral arteries. The infarcted area involves the medullary pyramids and the medial lemniscus, producing a flaccid quadriplegia of several weeks' duration followed by spastic quadriplegia.

Various combinations of hemiparesis, hemiplegia, tetraparesis, tetraplegia, triparesis, and triplegia may occur in association with paralysis of the lower cranial nerve nuclei. These usually result from vertebral artery occlusion. If the infarction involves the medullary reticular formation, which includes the respiratory and vasomotor centers, disturbances of respiration, blood pressure, and pulse rate may result. These include apneustic or ataxic breathing and automatic respiratory arrest with preservation of voluntary breathing.[30] Involvement of vasomotor and cardiac centers produces episodic hypertension and cardiac arrhythmias.

Infarction involving the region of the inferior olive may result in the development of regular, rhythmic up-and-down or lateral movements of the uvula and soft palate. This unique type of involuntary movement, which has been called "palatal nystagmus" or "palatal myoclonus," also occurs with lesions involving the dentate nucleus, the superior cerebellar peduncle, and the central tegmental bundle. It appears to be more or less pathognomonic of a lesion of the olivary-dentato-tegmental system.

THE LATERAL MEDULLARY SYNDROME (WALLENBERG'S SYNDROME: POSTERIOR INFERIOR CEREBELLAR ARTERY THROMBOSIS). There is considerable variation in the extent of infarction that results in the lateral medullary area when the vertebral or posterior inferior cerebellar artery is occluded, but this is one localization where the term "syndrome" is justified because the clinical findings are highly characteristic and virtually unmistakable.[46]

The majority of cases are due to thrombosis at the site of an atheromatous plaque in the fourth portion of the vertebral artery.[39] Only about 25 per cent are actually due to posterior inferior cerebellar artery thrombosis. Acute medullary infarction has also been reported from vertebral artery occlusion following chiropractic manipulation, yoga exercises, and trauma to the head and neck.[64a] The clinical picture provides a classical exercise in functional correlation with disturbed neuroanatomy (Fig. 9–13). The symptoms may begin with homolateral facial pain or paresthesias due to irritation of the spinal tract of the fifth nerve. Intense vertigo and vomiting due to involvement of the inferior vestibular nucleus and its connections to the medullary "vomiting center" are extremely common and should not be confused with acute labyrinthitis from other causes.

In more extensive infarction there is unilateral paralysis of the palate, pharynx, and vocal cords with dysphagia and a peculiar "brassy" dysarthria due to involvement of the ninth and tenth nerves and their nuclei with paralysis of one vocal cord. Soft palate and pharyngeal paralysis can be particularly troublesome because of the increased risk of aspiration and the need for feeding by gastric tube.[49] Destruction of the lateral spinothalamic tract produces contralateral loss of sensation for pain and temperature over the limbs and trunk. Thus, there is loss of pain and temperature on one side of the face and on the contralateral side of the body.

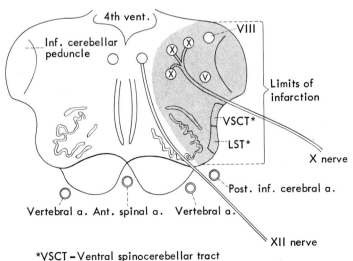

FIGURE 9–13. Diagram of the usual anatomic involvement when there is infarction of the lateral medulla due to occlusion of ipsilateral vertebral or posterior inferior cerebellar artery.

*VSCT – Ventral spinocerebellar tract
*LST – Lateral spinothalamic tract

Involvement of the spinocerebellar tracts and the inferior cerebellar peduncle results in nystagmus, homolateral dysmetria, intention tremor, and ataxia with a tendency to fall toward the side of the lesion. A unilateral Horner's syndrome is almost invariably seen on the side of the lesion owing to destruction of the descending sympathetic fibers in the medullary reticular formation. Less consistent and unusual findings with more extensive infarction include homolateral facial weakness and mild contralateral hemiparesis.

Infarction of the Pons. Basilar artery thrombosis with massive infarction of the pons is usually preceded by multiple small infarcts, which may be scattered in the ventral portion of the pons and other parts of the brainstem, cerebellum, occipital and temporal lobes, and thalamus. Some of these cases are due to repeated embolism arising from atheromatous plaques at the origin of or in the main portion of the vertebral arteries. In other patients infarction occurs in an irregular fashion due to atherosclerosis and occlusion of the small branches of the basilar artery.

Many patients give a history of previous transient ischemic attacks usually consisting of dysarthria, vertigo, ataxia, oculomotor palsies, headache, and syncope.

In about 50 per cent of cases, the onset of the terminal thrombosis results in a sudden catastrophic stroke, while in the other 50 per cent there is a more gradual and progressive course. Patients with a sudden onset are often comatose, with quadriparesis. Brainstem signs include multiple cranial nerve palsies producing dysarthria or anarthria, dysphagia, vertigo, nystagmus, facial paralysis, diplopia, and gaze palsies due to involvement of supranuclear pathways. Bilateral involvement of the basis pontis results in quadriplegia with retention of consciousness (locked-in syndrome).[56] More extensive involvement of the pontine tegmentum may result in the development of a state of akinetic mutism.[83] Signs of occipital lobe infarction include transient or permanent cortical blindness, homonymous hemianopia, and visual agnosia. Recovery after occlusion of the basilar artery is possible.[41]

PARAMEDIAN INFARCTION OF THE PONS. This is the most common form of pontine infarction, which occurs following partial thrombosis or embolism of the basilar artery or occlusion of the paramedian branches. There are scattered infarcts in the paramedian area of the brachium pontis, with spotty involvement of the corticospinal tracts, pontine nuclei, and fibers passing to the middle cerebellar peduncle. The infarction may be predominantly on one side but is usually bilateral, with symptoms of severe hemiparesis, paraparesis, or quadriparesis combined with dysarthria, and dysphagia due to bilateral spasticity of palate, pharynx, and tongue.

LATERAL AND TEGMENTAL INFARCTION OF THE PONS. This is rarer than paramedian infarction. A laterally placed infarct will involve the root of the fifth nerve, the medial lemniscus, and the middle cerebellar peduncle with partial involvement of the corticospinal tract fibers to the lower extremity limb. This will produce homolateral sensory loss over the face, contralateral loss of vibration and position sense, and contralateral hemiparesis with more weakness in the lower than the upper extremity. Cerebellar signs are extremely common and include dyssynergia, dysmetria, and dysdiadochokinesia of the homolateral side. A Horner's syndrome is usually present on the same side as the lesion.

Infarction in the tegmental area of the pons may result in paralysis of the fifth, sixth, and seventh cranial nerves or their nuclei combined with signs of damage to the medial longitudinal fasciculus and superior cerebellar peduncle. As a result, various patterns of paresis of conjugate eye movements, homolateral loss of sensation over the face, and unilateral paralysis of the sixth and seventh cranial nerves are common.

Cerebellar signs, including hypotonia, dysmetria, intention tremor, and dysdiadochokinesis, regularly occur on the same side as the lesion.

Infarction of the Midbrain. Isolated infarction of the midbrain is rare, and the classic syndromes of Weber (ipsilateral third-nerve palsy and contralateral hemiparesis) and Benedikt (ipsilateral third-nerve palsy and contralateral rubral, cerebellar, or parkinsonian-like tremor) are unusual.

Thrombosis of the superior cerebellar artery causes infarction in the origin of the junction of the midbrain and pons, with damage to the superior cerebellar peduncle and superior surface of the cerebellum. As a result, the symptoms may include homolateral cerebellar signs, with rubral tremor or myoclonic jerks in some cases. There frequently is nystagmus, maximal toward the side of the lesion, a homolateral Horner's syndrome, and facial paresis. Involvement of the spinothalamic pathways in the brainstem produces loss of pain and temperature sensation of the opposite side of the body. In addition, there may be mask-like facies and parkinsonian features due to disruption of connections to or from the substantia nigra.

Infarction of the Cerebellum.   The collateral circulation in the cerebellum is well developed, and symptoms due to isolated infarction are rare. Most cases have a history of hypertension and diabetes mellitus and some patients have had previous cerebral infarction. The onset is sudden, and the majority develop some impairment of consciousness with abnormalities of ocular movement and cranial nerve involvement. Cerebellar signs are prominent, and corticospinal tract abnormalities and extensor plantar responses are not unusual. Death may occur from cerebellar edema, brainstem compression, and acute hydrocephalus.[180] Infarction of the cerebellum in the territory of the posterior inferior cerebellar artery results in the acute onset of vertigo, nausea, vomiting, nystagmus, and severe ataxia. This condition is mimicked by acute labyrinthine disease in the absence of brainstem signs.[37]

Posterior Cerebral Artery Occlusion.   The posterior cerebral arteries supply both occipital lobes as well as the upper end of the midbrain, cerebral peduncles, portions of the thalamus, subthalamic area, and portions of the hypothalamus. Embolism of the posterior cerebral artery may give rise to symptoms of infarction of the midbrain (already discussed) as well as hemiballismus if the subthalamic nucleus is involved. Such vascular lesions of the subthalamic nuclei are either hemorrhagic infarcts arising from embolism or slit hemorrhages due to hypertension. The cardinal signs of posterior cerebral artery occlusion are, however, usually homonymous visual field disturbances.

SADDLE EMBOLISM OF THE TERMINAL PORTION OF THE BASILAR ARTERY.   This may result in simultaneous *occlusion of both posterior cerebral arteries.* This condition is not rare. The usual cause is an embolism arising from a mural thrombosis of the myocardium as a result of myocardial infarction, but some cases appear to arise from plaques in the vertebral arteries. As a result, both posterior cerebral arteries become occluded, and cortical blindness results, with preservation of the pupillary

reaction to light and normal appearance of the optic nerves on funduscopy. If the infarction destroys both areas 17 of Brodmann in the calcarine area, the patient will be blind. Fortunately, small islands of visual cortex may be spared, leaving true constricted fields (in contrast to hysterical constriction of the fields, the true constricted fields enlarge appropriately as the patient moves away from the tangent screen). There may be curious patterns in the sparing of the visual fields, including altitudinal hemianopias or sparing of homonymous quadrants.

If areas 18 and 19 are also destroyed, the patients may have anosognosia or denial of blindness. Such patients may confabulate when presented with visual test objects (for example, such patients may describe the examiner's clothing in detail but completely in error). Because of this apparent confusion, the diagnosis is often missed, and the patients are thought to be demented or "confused."

Occlusion of one posterior cerebral artery usually gives rise to a contralateral hemianopia or quadrantanopia. If areas 18 and 19 of the dominant hemisphere are involved, there is also some evidence of visual agnosia. Visuonominal dysphasia may result, with the inability to name objects on inspection. There may be aprosapognosia or the inability to recognize people by their faces. Loss of color vision or abstract revisualization (e.g., recalling what an apple looks like) may be a consequence of small lesions of area 18 and 19. Posterior cerebral artery occlusion may produce infarction of the angular gyrus when the collateral from the middle cerebral artery is poor, resulting in Gerstmann's syndrome, which includes confusion of sides, finger agnosia, acalculia, and agraphia.

In infarction of areas 18 and 19 of the nondominant hemisphere following posterior cerebral artery occlusion, there may be "amorphosynthesis" of the visual field. Objects tend to be ignored within that field. Drawings made by the patient tend to be constricted or incomplete in the affected field, and double, simultaneous visual stimulation will reveal a hemianopia not apparent by usual methods of testing. The patient may also lose the ability to find his way around in familiar surroundings.

Transient ischemic attacks within the posterior cerebral artery may be characterized by spells of blurred vision, graying of vision, attacks of blindness, hemianopia, or visual agnosia, frequently associated with lightheadedness and staggering. Photopsia is a frequent complaint and is reminiscent of migraine. The patient complains of flashing light or streaks of gray and black in one visual field. The attacks are briefer than in migraine and if headache occurs, it is suboccipital and occurs during rather than after the visual symptoms.

Thalamic pain is commonly a consequence of hemorrhagic and ischemic lesions within the distribution of the posterior cerebral artery. At autopsy the lesion is usually in the white matter and not actually within the thalamus. The lesion involves the thalamocortical projection systems to the parietal cortex anywhere from the thalamus to the subcortical fibers in the parietal gyri. The pain usually begins some weeks to months after an acute stroke, with a more or less minor hemiparesis from which there is total or complete recovery. There is, at first, a sensory loss in the affected limbs followed by dysesthesias and spontaneous pains. These are described as "raw" and "burning" in quality, like "stripping the skin from the flesh." The pain is precipitated by squeezing the deep fascia, muscles, and joints of the limbs. Treatment with diphenylhydantoin and phenothiazines may be of help, but the most effective medical treatment is carbamazepine (Tegretol) beginning with 200 mg at night and gradually increasing the dosage until effective but not higher than 400 mg qid.

Sensory strokes may occur in severe hypertensives owing to a lacunar infarct of the posteroventral thalamus. The patient has a permanent neurosensory deficit without motor signs.[47b]

Diagnostic Procedures

The patient should be evaluated as outlined under transient ischemic attacks (p. 553). Computed tomography is abnormal within 24 hours of cerebral infarction showing an area of decreased density due to infarction and edema. There may be enhancement with intravenous iodinated contrast material (Fig. 9–14). This abnormality decreases in size but persists in most cases due to removal of necrotic material in the infarcted area.

Treatment of Cerebral Infarction

Although cerebral infarction is the immediate cause of death in most patients who die within the first week of a stroke, nonneurologic diseases such as pneumonia, heart disease, pulmonary embolism, and urinary tract infections are important causes of mortality.[19] Consequently, the treatment of acute cerebral infarction should include prevention and management of nonneurologic complications.

General Measures for Stuporous or Comatose Patients: Acute Stage. PULMONARY CARE. Respiratory exchange is usually impaired in patients who have suffered an acute stroke and may be further impeded by atelectasis, pneumonia, or bronchitis. Respiratory infections

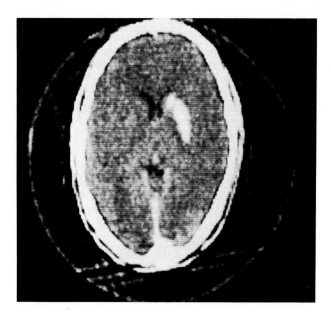

FIGURE 9–14. Computed tomography with enhancement by intravenous iodinated contrast solution in a patient with a recent cerebral infarction. The area of increased density in the right caudate nucleus and internal capsule indicates increased vascularity in the area of infarction.

hinder recovery and are a major cause of mortality. Attention to ventilation is of major importance in the acute stroke, and the chest should be examined by auscultation daily. Care should be taken to prevent aspiration of food and vomitus. Antibiotics should be given if there are signs of infection, and postural drainage is helpful for draining dependent parts of the lungs and preventing atelectasis. The patient should be turned every two hours from the right lateral to the left lateral and then to the supine position, and the upper respiratory tract should be cleared by careful suctioning. Dentures should always be removed.

If secretions accumulate to the degree that suctioning is necessary every ten minutes, a low-pressure, cuffed endotracheal tube should be inserted. This facilitates removal of secretions, improves ventilatory efficiency, and should always be performed before anoxia and cyanosis develop.

BLOOD PRESSURE AND CARDIAC MANAGEMENT. Severe hypertension should be treated cautiously. Once the patient with a stroke is at rest with satisfactory ventilation and bladder drainage, the blood pressure may return to normal levels without specific therapy. In any event, the blood pressure should be measured and charted regularly since injudicious use of antihypertensive drugs can easily precipitate a hypotensive state.

In view of this, the blood pressure should be recorded every hour during the first 24 hours after hospital admission. The aim should be to control the systolic blood pressure between 140 and 160 mm Hg.

Severe sustained hypertension may be controlled by the rapid injection of 300 mg diazoxide intravenously. The patient should be lying flat in bed without elevation of the head and hypotension can be controlled by elevating the foot of the bed. In less urgent situations hypertension can be controlled by the intravenous injection of 15 mg of hydralazine. Moderately severe hypertension usually responds to an oral diuretic such as hydrochlorothiazide, 50 mg every 12 hours, with the addition of alpha-methyldopa, 250 mg every six hours, or propranolol, 40 to 120 mg every eight hours.

Some patients develop hypotension spontaneously or as a result of the improper use of hypotensive and phenothiazine drugs. These patients usually respond readily to pressor agents, but the response may be poor in patients with adrenal insufficiency. All patients with an acute stroke and hypotension who do not show a prompt response to pressor agents should receive steroids intravenously in dosage of 100 mg of hydrocortisone every eight hours for two days, then gradually decreasing the dosage.

Since acute myocardial infarction occurs in about 10 per cent of patients who present with an acute stroke, an electrocardiogram should be obtained in all cases. Those believed to have acute myocardial infarction, or who develop congestive failure or arrhythmias, require immediate treatment. The failure to recognize cardiac complications may delay recovery or result in death from cardiac causes.

BLADDER CARE. The stuporous or comatose patient requires an indwelling catheter. Drainage of a distended bladder may alleviate restlessness and may be followed by a prompt fall in blood pressure from hypertensive levels. If an indwelling catheter is used, the bladder should be irrigated with a suitable urinary antiseptic or a polymyxin-neomycin solution (neomycin, 100 mg, and polymyxin, 25 mg, in 1,000 ml of N saline and irrigating with 250 ml four times daily). After 24 hours, the catheter is clamped, drained, and reclamped every two hours. The catheter should be removed as soon as the patient is conscious and cooperative. There is an unfortunate tendency to forget the proper care of indwelling catheters. A catheter carries with it considerable danger of bladder and renal infection.

POSITIONING. Reference has already been made to the turning of the patient every two hours in relation to pulmonary function. This also helps to prevent the development of decubitus ulcers over "pressure areas." This danger may be further minimized by keeping the skin dry and clean.

Joint deformities due to ankylosis and shortening of muscles and tendons develop rapidly in the hemiplegic. The involved lower limb should be supported in a neutral position and external rotation prevented by the use of a sandbag lying against the thigh or a blanket roll tucked under the greater trochanter. When the limb is flaccid, the foot may be braced against a footboard to prevent contraction of the Achilles tendon. When spasticity occurs, the footboard should be removed and a roll placed under the knee to prevent extensor thrust. The involved arm should be abducted to 90 degrees and a pillow placed in the axilla to prevent adduction. The forearm and elbow are placed on a pillow, with the hand higher than the elbow and the elbow higher than the shoulder. It is important to maintain the hand and wrist in a position of function, with the wrist extended and the fingers lying around a hand roll. All limbs should be placed through full range of passive movement twice daily. As soon as the patient is conscious and cooperative, graded physical therapy should be started.

FEEDING. The comatose or stuporous patient should be given adequate fluids by the intravenous route during the first 24 hours. This requires an infusion of 3,000 ml of 5 per cent dextrose in 0.2 N saline in the average adult. Febrile and dehydrated patients may require more. All cases require accurate recording of intake and output until oral feeding is reestablished. A nasogastric tube can be passed during the second 24 hours and 3,000 ml of water given through the tube in divided amounts (e.g., 250 ml every three hours). The intravenous infusion is then discontinued unless required for specific therapy, in which case the amount given through the nasogastric tube must be reduced according to the volume of the intravenous infusion. During the third 24-hour period and on subsequent days, 2,000 ml of a blender diet plus water to a total of 3,000 ml given in divided amounts every two hours supplies adequate nutrition and water.

Nasogastric feedings are discontinued as soon as the patient has recovered sufficiently to swallow from a feeding cup without danger of aspiration.

General Measures for Conscious Patients: Acute Stage. It is equally important to institute active treatment of the conscious as well as the comatose patient with an acute stroke. Attention should be given to pulmonary care, blood pressure and cardiac management, bladder care, positioning, and feeding as outlined above under the care of the comatose patient. In addition, unless there is evidence of an acute myocardial infarction, the patient should be ambulated at an early stage and a graded course of physical therapy initiated.

Specific Measures in the Treatment of the Acute Stroke. CEREBRAL VASODILATOR DRUGS. The damaged area of the brain consists of a central area of infarction surrounded by a zone of nonfunctioning but potentially viable tissue. The effects of ischemia may be reduced if function is restored to the ischemic zone by increasing the collateral circulation.

Any drug that effectively increases cerebral blood flow may increase collateral circulation to the ischemic area, and from a theoretic point of view this would seem to be a rational form of therapy. However, there is little evidence that treatment with vasodilator drugs has been significantly beneficial to patients with cerebral infarction. Consequently, the use of drugs such as papaverine and the inhalation of carbon dioxide have largely been abandoned.

HYPEROSMOLAR AGENTS IN THE TREATMENT OF CEREBRAL EDEMA. Cerebral edema is maximal three to five days after cerebral infarction, is known to accompany recent cerebral infarction and is a major cause of death in acute stroke. The use of hyperosmolar agents such as mannitol, urea, or glycerol has been recommended for the reduction of cerebral edema during this acute stage of cerebral infarction. Glycerol has probably been used more widely than the other agents, and double-blind studies have shown that in the first few days of acute cerebral infarction, daily intravenous infusions of 50 gm of glycerol mixed in 500 ml of 5 per cent glucose in 0.2 N physiologic saline (1.2 gm/kg of body weight daily) for six days improve the rate and degree of recovery from the neurologic deficit as well as decrease intracranial pressure and increase regional blood flow in the infarcted zone.[72] However, it has also been reported that glycerol infusion produces no significant improvement in patients with early stroke.[93]

CORTICOSTEROIDS IN THE TREATMENT OF CEREBRAL EDEMA. Corticosteroids are believed to reduce cerebral edema and intracranial pressure, thus improving cerebral circulation. However, the results of treatment of acute cerebral infarction with corticosteroids, particularly dexamethasone, have generally not been significant.

Cerebral Embolism

Some 10 per cent of strokes are due to cerebral embolism with impaction of a fragmented thrombus in one of the major vessels supplying the brain. The anatomic structure of the aortic arch and major vessels is such that emboli leaving the left ventricle have a tendency to enter the left common carotid artery more frequently than the right.[11, 121] They lodge in the proximal portion of the internal carotid artery or pass into the middle cerebral artery and its branches (Fig. 9–15).

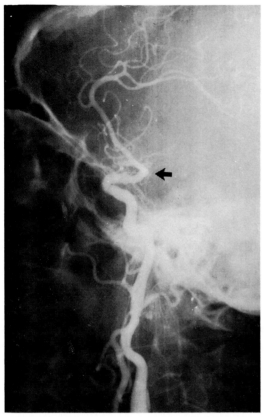
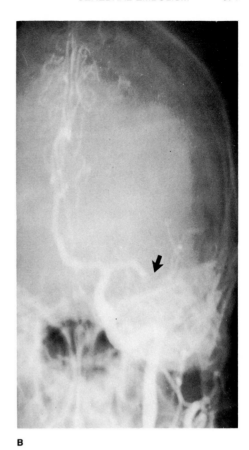

A   B

FIGURE 9-15. Carotid arteriograms in a case of thrombotic occlusion of
the left middle cerebral artery. *A.* Lateral view with arrow indicating the
site of occlusion. *B.* Anteroposterior view showing a thin line of contrast
medium outlining the thrombus.

Here they may be lysed by circulating fibrinolysins or fragment and move distally into the terminal branches and the capillary venous system.

Etiology and Pathology

The common causes of cerebral embolism are
listed in Table 9-1. When a clot lodges in the
internal carotid or middle cerebral arteries, the
effect depends on a number of factors. These include the efficiency of the collateral circulation,
the presence or absence of arteriosclerosis, the
status of the naturally occurring fibrinolytic systems in the blood, and the possible occurrence
of further emboli. If the collateral circulation is
adequate, one of the major vessels may be completely occluded without damage to the brain.

In many cases, however, the collateral circulation is inadequate and occlusion of the vessel is
followed by infarction, usually occurring in the
"watershed area" of the distribution of the middle
cerebral circulation. These infarcts are usually
hemorrhagic since lysis of the clot or the collateral
circulation restores blood flow into the infarcted
area. A second factor is the tendency for the embolus to fragment following the action of circulating fibrinolysins. The fragments pass into the
smaller branches of the middle cerebral artery
and permit the passage of blood into damaged
blood vessels in the infarcted area, often causing
hemorrhagic infarction.

Clinical Features

The symptoms of cerebral embolism are similar
to those already described for occlusion of the

TABLE 9–1

Common Causes of Cerebral Embolism

1. *From cardiac causes*
   a. Congenital heart disease with right-to-left shunt
   b. Rheumatic heart disease, active and old
   c. Subacute bacterial endocarditis
   d. Cardiac arrhythmias, particularly atrial fibrillation
   e. Prolapsed mitral valve
   f. Myocardial infarction
   g. Following heart surgery
   h. Emboli from pulmonary veins in heart failure
   i. Rare causes—systemic lupus erythematosus, paradoxic embolism, myxoma of the heart, endocardial fibrosis, cardiomyopathies

2. *From aortic arch and great vessels*
   a. Emboli arising from plaques at the origin of the internal common carotid, vertebral, brachiocephalic, and subclavian arteries
   b. Trauma to the neck vessels
   c. Emboli from aneurysms of ascending aorta

3. *From systemic causes*
   a. Septic emboli from lung abscess, causing brain abscess
   b. Metastatic cells, causing metastatic brain tumor
   c. Ova and parasites, causing brain abscess, granuloma
   d. Fat embolism
   e. Air embolism
   f. Foreign bodies
   g. Nitrogen embolism in caisson disease

internal carotid or middle cerebral arteries. The onset is usually, but not invariably, abrupt, and diagnosis usually rests on the detection of possible causes for embolism revealed by general physical examination.[47] In fat embolism, there is usually a history of trauma or fracture, and the signs indicate multifocal embolism. Fat globules may be seen on microscopic examination of the urine and sputum.

Diagnostic Procedures

The evaluation of the patient with cerebral embolism is the same as that outlined under Transient Ischemic Attacks (p. 553).

Treatment

An acute stroke due to cerebral embolism should be treated in the same manner as already described for acute stroke from other causes. The use of platelet inhibitors (dipyridamole, sulfinpyrazone, and aspirin) is indicated if the fibrino-platelet emboli arise from atheromatous vessels or prosthetic heart valves.[121] There is an immediate need for anticoagulants to prevent further embolic infarction in cases where larger emboli arise from the heart.[2] The patient should be treated with heparin initially until there is a satisfactory prothrombin level with oral anticoagulants. The possibility of producing severe hemorrhagic infarction by the use of anticoagulants is outweighed by the much higher risk of further cerebral embolization. Therapy is continued for a minimum period of six months.

Patients with subacute bacterial endocarditis, as a cause of cerebral embolism, should have adequate antibiotic therapy after blood cultures have been made. With the widespread use of antibiotics, subacute bacterial endocarditis is now rarely seen as a cause of cerebral embolism. Furthermore, with the prophylactic use of antibiotics in children with rheumatic fever, the incidence of rheumatic heart disease has been reduced, and cerebral embolism from this cause is now also rare.

In fat embolism, heparin therapy is indicated in order to clear the fat from the blood by its lipolytic action.

Chronic Cerebrovascular Insufficiency (Multi-Infarct Dementia)

The concept of multi-infarct dementia has been clouded by the fact that dementias from other causes are common in the elderly and all types have often been lumped together indiscriminately. Careful history taking and examination supplemented by computed tomography and arteriography make accurate diagnosis possible during life (Fig. 9–16). Some question the diagnosis of multi-infarct dementia and suggest that such cases are examples of dementia from other causes (e.g., the neuronal degenerations), which happen to arise in patients with cerebral arteriosclerosis. There are, however, patients who exhibit an episodic intellectual deterioration secondary to cerebral atherosclerosis. There is usually a history of at least one ictus, and the course is usually fluctuating and less steadily progressive than occurs in neuronal atrophies. In multi-infarct dementia there is frequently focal and asymmetric neurologic deficits not usually found in the presenile and senile dementias.[62] These cases should be defined because, theoretically at least, treatment aimed at improved cerebral circulation may lead to arrest of the dementia.

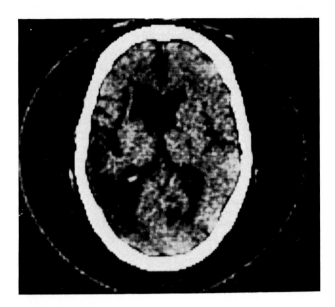

FIGURE 9–16. Computed tomography in multi-infarct dementia. There are several areas of decreased density in the left frontal parietal and occipital regions and in the right occipital area representing many episodes of infarction. The ischemia has also resulted in cortical atrophy and ventricular dilatation.

Etiology and Pathology

Multi-infarct dementia is associated with a marked patchy reduction in cerebral blood flow, since the condition results from multifocal reduction of local blood flow throughout the brain due to arteriosclerosis. Measurement of regional cerebral blood flow is often diagnostic, since multiple patchy areas of reduced flow are seen, whereas in the neuronal atrophies (such as Alzheimer's disease) reduction of flow is mainly in the frontal and temporal regions.[157] Delayed flow is often apparent on angiography where circulation through the small cerebral vessels is delayed. The atherosclerotic process may affect the extracranial vessels, circle of Willis, or its major branches and is often marked at all sites. Irregular beading or narrowing of the smaller cerebral vessels is often apparent. At autopsy, the brain may be underweight, with widening of the sulci and dilatation of the ventricular system. The atrophic process is not uniform but is due to patchy infarction that is found in many parts of the brain (Fig. 9–16). There is a tendency, however, for numerous small infarcts to occur in the so-called watershed areas of the brain. These infarcts are seen, for example, in the parietotemporal areas. In longstanding cases numerous small infarcts are produced in the pons, in the basal ganglia, and less commonly in the cortex, which produce an appearance that has been called the lucunar state, or état lacunaire. Each lacuna occurs around a small sclerotic penetrating vessel, with necrosis of the surrounding tissue producing reactive gliosis.

Clinical Features

The patient with multi-infarct dementia shows three fundamental changes:

1. Signs of dementia, loss of insight and judgment, impaired memory, disorientation, etc.
2. Signs of focal neurologic deficit due to multiple infarcts.
3. Signs of atherosclerosis elsewhere in the body.

The earliest signs of multi-infarct dementia are loss of operational judgment and impairment of memory. If the patient does not hold a responsible position, the impaired judgment may escape attention, but the patient is frequently aware of his failing memory and may resort to copious note taking in an effort to compensate. As time passes, there is general deterioration of intellectual function, eventually with severe dementia. The symptoms and course superficially may seem no different from dementia due to other causes, but careful history taking of the patient with multi-infarct dementia usually reveals history of a stuttering type of progression of dementia and other neurologic deficits.

There may be a history of transient ischemic attacks, particularly due to vertebrobasilar insufficiency.[157] There may be periods of ataxia, dysphasia, or dyspraxia followed by rapid recovery. Episodes of hemiparesis or monoparesis may also occur, which are almost never seen in the senile and presenile dementias. Some patients develop parkinsonian features and rigidity.

The more severely handicapped eventually present with pseudobulbar features including emotional lability, dysarthria, dysphagia, generalized rigidity, and a diffuse but asymmetric increase in deep tendon reflexes with bilateral extensor plantar respones.

Finally, patients with multi-infarct dementia usually show systemic features of generalized atherosclerosis. They have systolic hypertension with a wide pulse pressure and often show wide fluctuations in blood pressure levels including periods of hypotension (particularly if treated with phenothiazine drugs). There may be cardiac enlargement, arrhythmias, and changes in the electrocardiogram. At least 30 per cent have overt or occult diabetes mellitus. Auscultation over the carotid, innominate, and subclavian vessels may reveal loud murmurs due to atherosclerotic narrowing in some cases. Others show absence of or diminished peripheral pulses in the limbs.

Binswanger's Disease

This is a rare form of dementia in which there are multiple infarcts scattered through the white matter of the brain

Etiology and Pathology

Binswanger's disease always occurs in hypertensive individuals and is characterized by atherosclerotic changes in the circle of Willis and diffuse hyalinization of intraparenchymal arteries and arterioles. These changes produce a diffuse ischemia of white matter with loss of myelin and axon and numerous scattered lacunar infarcts.[22]

The condition presents with a history of acute stroke followed by progressive dementia resembling Alzheimer's disease with prominent pseudobulbar signs.[23b] The diagnosis is usually established at autopsy. Serial electroencephalograms show progressive deterioration of background activity and the gradual appearance of delta activity in all leads.

Treatment

There is no known treatment that will affect the course of Binswanger's disease. Ventricular shunting does not alter the course of the dementia.

Bilateral Occlusion of the Internal Carotid Arteries

Although the majority of patients present with a major stroke, about 20 per cent of patients with severe stenosis or bilateral occlusion of the internal carotid arteries present with progressive dementia. The changes in the brain are usually located in the watershed areas of the cortex. It is important to recognize this condition at its inception because of potential treatment by endarterectomy, particularly in those with stenotic lesions of the carotid arteries.

Arteriosclerotic Dilatation of the Basilar Artery

Elongation, dilatation, and tortuosity of the basilar artery may exert pressure on the midbrain producing kinking or backward displacement with narrowing or occlusion of the aqueduct. This may produce hydrocephalus and progressive dementia. Accurate diagnosis is important since the hydrocephalus may be treated surgically by a ventricular shunting procedure. The tube may drain the lateral ventricles into the cisterna magna or into the right atrium via the jugular vein (ventriculoatrial shunt) using a valve. Arteriosclerotic aneurysms of the basilar artery occur in hypertensive individuals and may leak, resulting in subarachnoid hemorrhage. These aneurysms may compress the cranial nerves, producing trigeminal neuralgia and hemifacial spasm (Fig. 9–17).

Subarachnoid Hemorrhage

There are many causes of subarachnoid hemorrhage, and the condition should not be regarded as a disease but rather as a syndrome. The accepted definition of subarachnoid hemorrhage is: a condition in which there is bleeding into the subarachnoid space, occurring alone or in association with bleeding elsewhere in the cranial cavity or vertebral canal.[142]

The most common cause of subarachnoid hemorrhage is trauma, and the most frequent nontraumatic causes are ruptured cerebral aneurysms, vascular malformations, and hypertensive intracerebral hemorrhages. There has been some confusion with the terminology used in subarachnoid hemorrhage, which requires clarification.

Subarachnoid hemorrhage refers to bleeding into the subarachnoid space from any cause.

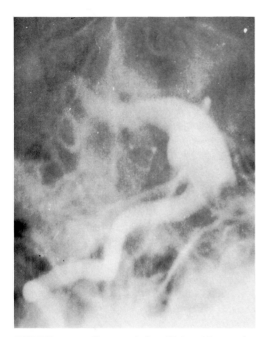

FIGURE 9–17. Retrograde brachial arteriogram in an elderly hypertensive patient with symptoms of vertebral basilar insufficiency. There is a partly thrombosed arteriosclerotic aneurysm of the basilar artery.

While the majority of causes of subarachnoid hemorrhage may be traumatic, the term "spontaneous" is used to denote nontraumatic causes. The term "primary subarachnoid hemorrhage" is used to describe those cases which are not due to trauma and hypertensive intracerebral hemorrhage.

Subarachnoid hemorrhage due to trauma is discussed in Chapter 8, and hypertensive intracerebral hemorrhage will be dealt with later in this chapter.

Etiology, Pathogenesis, and Pathology

The most frequent cause of primary subarachnoid hemorrhage is the rupture of a berry or saccular (congenital) aneurysm into the subarachnoid space. This is followed in frequency by bleeding from an arteriovenous malformation. Other known causes are rare but many are listed in Table 9–2. It should be noted that there are a number of cases with primary subarachnoid hemorrhage in which the cause is unknown, and because of the better prognosis in these cases, they will be considered as a separate group.[192]

TABLE 9–2

Primary Subarachnoid Hemorrhage

1. Ruptured congenital saccular (berry) aneurysm
2. Bleeding from an arteriovenous malformation
3. Developmental defects
   a. Sturge-Weber disease
   b. Hereditary hemorrhagic telangiectasia
   c. Telangiectasia pontis
   d. Pseudoxanthoma elasticum
   e. Ehlers-Danlos syndrome
4. Infectious conditions
   a. Rupture of a mycotic aneurysm
   b. Brain abscess
   c. Tuberculous meningitis
   d. Syphilitic meningovasculitis
   e. Herpes simplex encephalitis
5. Neoplastic conditions
   a. Glioma
   b. Hemangioblastoma
   c. Meningioma
   d. Perivascular sarcoma
   e. Intracranial metastasis
6. Blood dyscrasias
   a. Hemophilia
   b. Aplastic anemia
   c. Leukemia
   d. Hodgkin's disease
   e. Thrombocytopenic purpura
   f. Sickle cell anemia
   g. Pernicious anemia
   h. Anticoagulant therapy
7. Vascular conditions
   a. Polyarteritis nodosa
   b. Disseminated lupus erythematosus
   c. Anaphylactic purpura
   d. Intracranial venous thrombosis
8. Degenerative conditions
   a. Arteriosclerosis
9. Nondemonstrable and miscellaneous causes
   a. "Spontaneous" rupture of an artery
   b. Severe hypertension

Similarly, spinal subarachnoid hemorrhage presents as a distinctive condition and will be discussed separately.

Primary Subarachnoid Hemorrhage from Intracranial, Congenital Saccular (Berry) Aneurysms. These appear as round or oval-shaped, saccular dilatations of cerebral vessels having a berry-like appearance. The incidence of berry or congenital saccular aneurysms varies in autopsy reports from less than 1 to 18 per cent, the latter including minute areas of dilatation on the vessels of the circle of Willis and its major branches. Multiple aneurysms occur in about 15 per cent of cases, and there seems to be a higher incidence of aneurysms in some families of patients with subarachnoid hemorrhage. About 90 per cent of aneurysms occur on the anterior half of the circle of Willis, with 10 per cent arising in the vertebral, basilar, and posterior cerebral arteries. The three most common sites are the terminal portion of the internal carotid artery, the junction of the anterior cerebral and anterior communicating arteries, and the middle cerebral artery at its bifurcation in the lateral sulcus. The most frequent sites in the vertebral-basilar system are at the origin of the posterior inferior cerebellar artery from the vertebral artery and at the origin of the posterior cerebral arteries from the terminal portion of the basilar artery (Fig. 9–18).

The fact that aneurysms arise at the bifurcation of a cerebral vessel suggests that they may be developmental in origin, and the alternative name of "congenital saccular aneurysms" is still used frequently. However, developmental factors cannot be solely responsible since unruptured cerebral aneurysms are rarely found in necropsies of infants, and subarachnoid hemorrhage due to ruptured aneurysm is seldom encountered in infancy and childhood.

An alternative theory is that aneurysms arise at the site of vestigial embryonic vessels, which leave a weakened area in the walls of the circle of Willis and its major branches. This theory has not always been supported by anatomic studies. It seems more likely that aneurysms arise at the bifurcation of a major cerebral vessel and develop at the site of some coexisting defects in the media and internal elastic lamina. There may be additional factors, such as hypertension, occurring in

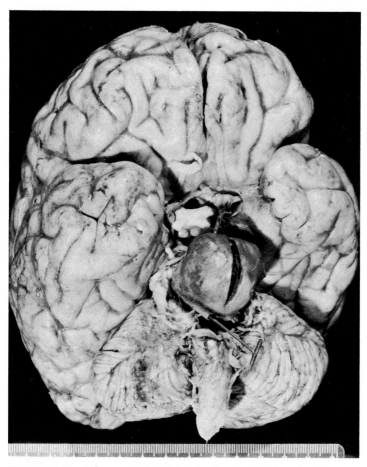

FIGURE 9–18. Autopsy specimen showing huge, partly thrombosed, saccular aneurysm of the basilar artery causing cerebellar and brainstem signs. A probe has been inserted into the basilar artery.

adult life. The progressive weakness of the media at the bifurcation of a vessel may be explained by the increased intraluminal pulsatile pressure.

During embryogenesis, the inner walls of two branches of cerebral arteries immediately beyond a bifurcation are in close apposition, and there is mutual support with little stimulus for the formation of a well-formed media. With the development of the brain, however, the angle between the two branches increases and the two walls no longer support each other. The media in the angle of the V is defective, and there is a potential weakness at this site. The subsequent bulging of the vessel wall at this site with destruction of the internal elastic lamina depends on a number of factors; each of these may act alone or in concert with one or more of the others. These factors will not be considered.

FLOW IN THE CIRCLE OF WILLIS. Cerebral aneurysms are often associated with anomalies in the circle of Willis, the peculiarities of blood flow imposed by these anomalies may cause a strain at the bifurcation of a vessel from the circle of Willis and lead to aneurysm formation.

ATHEROSCLEROSIS. The early intimal changes associated with atherosclerosis may be sufficient to weaken the internal elastic lamina, leading the formation of an aneurysm.

HYPERTENSION. The direct effect of increased blood pressure acting on a weak vessel wall may lead to aneurysm formation or may predispose to early atherosclerosis and the changes already described.

INFLAMMATORY FACTORS. There have been claims that the crucial weakening of the internal elastic lamina at these vulnerable sites is due to focal arteritis. This theory has received little support from histologic examination.

ABSENCE OF INTIMAL "CUSHIONS." It is apparent from autopsy material that defects in the media occur in most individuals. Many of these areas are protected by intimal hyperplasia, which forms intimal cushions lying over the area of the defect. The absence of intimal cushions may permit weakening of the internal elastic lamina owing to the continuous pounding of arterial blood, peculiarities in flow through the cycle of Willis, or atherosclerosis.

OTHER FACTORS. The rupture of a berry aneurysm produces a sudden discharge of blood under high pressure into the surrounding structures. This may be followed by:

1. *Subarachnoid hemorrhage alone,* should the direction of the flow of blood be such that it spurts in the plane of the subarachnoid space.

2. *Subarachnoid hemorrhage and intracerebral hematoma* (meningocerebral hemorrhage), if the blood ruptures into the brain substance.

3. *Subarachnoid hemorrhage and subdural hematoma,* should the direction of the flow go through the arachnoid into the subdural space.

4. *Subarachnoid hemorrhage and hydrocephalus.* This is a relatively common complication and acute hydrocephalus occurs in about 30 per cent of cases. This may be due to erythrocytes blocking the arachnoid villi and interfering with absorption of CSF or to distortion and kinking of the third ventricle or aqueduct caused by unilateral edema or a hematoma. In a small percentage of cases interference with absorption of CSF persists as "normal-pressure" hydrocephalus and requires ventriculo-atrial or lumbar thecoperitoneal shunt procedure to relieve the block.[105]

5. *Spasm of cerebral vessels.* The presence of blood around cerebral vessels commonly causes spasm that may be sufficiently severe to cause cerebral infarction.[27, 92, 202] Spasm of the cerebral vessels may be focal or generalized and is not an immediate response to subarachnoid hemorrhage since it begins three days later.[193] Once established the spasm increases in severity to reach a maximum on the eighth or ninth day after subarachnoid hemorrhage and resolves by the twelvth day. Patients in poor clinical condition tend to have more arterial spasm than those in good clinical condition. The presence of spasm appears to increase morbidity and mortality to a significant degree.

6. *Cerebral edema.* The development of cerebral vascular spasm or the distortion of the circle of Willis by a hematoma causes ischemia and infarction. These conditions are followed by cerebral edema, which is one of the major causes of mortality and morbidity in subarachnoid hemorrhage.

7. *Rupture of an aneurysm on the terminal portion of the internal carotid artery* into the cavernous sinus, with the formation of an internal carotid-cavernous fistula.

8. *Rupture of an aneurysm into the sphenoid sinus,* which is a rare occurrence causing epistaxis.

9. *Rupture of an aneurysm without the production*

of subarachnoid hemorrhage but with bleeding into the parenchyma of the brain or into the subdural space, which occurs only rarely.

The nonruptured aneurysm varies in size from a pinhead to a walnut or even larger. Aneurysms lie within the subarachnoid space, and small aneurysms may escape detection unless the circle of Willis and the major branches are carefully dissected free for examination. On section, an aneurysm is usually spheric in shape, attached to the artery by a neck that varies in development. Large aneurysms may be partly filled with a laminated blood clot, and calcium may be deposited in the wall.

The rupture of an aneurysm and subarachnoid hemorrhage leads to hemorrhagic staining of the brain, which is particularly marked at the base. There may be distortion, compression, or disruption of cranial nerves and brain parenchyma by blood clot or the presence of blood in the subdural space in some cases.

Microscopic examination of an aneurysm shows that the media ends abruptly at the neck of the sac, while the internal elastic lamina passes for a short distance into the wall of the sac, which is composed of fibrous tissue and intima or may have an internal lining of laminated blood clot. Part of the fibrous wall may be degenerated at the site of rupture.

The brain may show areas of disruption and the presence of blood clot within the parenchyma. In patients who have survived for more than a few days, there may be some astrocytic proliferation and microglial reaction. There may be multiple pale ischemic and occasionally hemorrhagic infarcts in the cerebral hemispheres, presumably due to the severe vasospasm associated with subarachnoid hemorrhage or due to compression or distortion of blood vessels or cerebral venous thrombosis. These infarcts are often wedge-shaped, with the base lying in the cortex. Laminar infarcts and irregular infarction of deeper structures, including the basal ganglia and thalamus, are also not uncommon.

Arteriovenous Malformations. Although arteriovenous malformations are second in frequency to berry aneurysms as a cause of primary subarachnoid hemorrhage, they are not an uncommon finding when the hemorrhage has occurred in the second or third decade. They constitute between 2 and 4 per cent of intracranial masses, and many are found at autopsy as an incidental finding. They have been reported in all parts of the brain and spinal cord and are occasionally multiple, but the most common site is in the parietal lobe (Fig. 9–19). About 20 per cent of these malformations occur in the posterior fossa.

They show marked variation in size from small tangles of vessels, which are difficult to detect with the naked eye, to huge collections of abnormal vessels occupying the greater part of one hemisphere. The usual appearance consists of a cone-shaped area, with the base projecting toward the surface of the cerebral cortex, in which there are tangles of abnormal blood vessels of variable caliber. There are one or more large feeding arteries and a number of abnormal draining veins. The surrounding brain may contain areas of old hemorrhage, and the overlying leptomeninges are frequently thickened and stained.

The microscopic appearance shows numerous abnormal vessels without the typical appearance of either arteries or veins. The brain in the affected region shows areas of hemorrhage, gliosis, and astroglial proliferation.

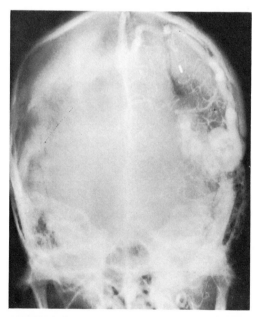

FIGURE 9–19.   Left carotid arteriogram showing huge arteriovenous malformation of left parietal area. One year previously, the patient developed right hemiplegia due to meningocerebral hemorrhage. At operation, the arteriovenous malformation was too large to be excised.

Clinical Features

Ruptured Congenital Saccular (Berry) Aneurysm. Although the onset of subarachnoid hemorrhage is sudden and dramatic, about half these patients have experienced prodromal symptoms, such as episodes of headache and stiff neck, which could have led to an earlier diagnosis of aneurysm if appropriate studies were performed at that stage.

About half the men and two thirds of the women have warning signs, most commonly severe headache preceding the rupture of an intracranial aneurysm.[191] More than 50 per cent of patients with anterior communicating or anterior cerebral aneurysms complain of severe frontal headache, and nearly half of the patients with a middle cerebral aneurysm have the same complaint. Patients with intradural internal carotid aneurysms or posterior communicating aneurysms frequently develop headache on the same side and a unilateral third nerve palsy presenting with ophthalmoplegia, ptosis, dilatation of the pupil, and abduction of the eyes. Other patients may develop focal or generalized seizures, which should always be investigated when the onset is in adult life. There are occasional complaints of recent onset of atypical facial pain in some cases, with aneurysm of the terminal portion of the internal carotid artery.

Whether prodomata have occurred or not, the onset of subarachnoid hemorrhage is sudden in 90 per cent of cases. Some 60 per cent of patients experience a sudden severe headache, while there is a rapid loss of consciousness in 20 per cent. The remaining 20 per cent present with seizures, vomiting, pain in the neck or back, sciatic pain, pain in the limbs, or focal paralysis.

The headache associated with subarachnoid hemorrhage is often described as "severe," "violent," "intense," or "bursting" in character and usually occurs in the occipital area whatever the site of aneurysmal rupture. It is often associated with vomiting and considerable distress if the patient is conscious, requiring narcotics for relief. Although there is almost immediate loss of consciousness in 20 per cent of cases, some 50 per cent of patients have a delayed period of from 6 to 12 hours before the onset of stupor or coma due to raised intracranial pressure. Complaints of photophobia or diplopia are common in conscious patients, and there may be deterioration of vision due to damage to the optic nerve. Retention of urine is not uncommon and may compound the restlessness.

The physical findings show considerable variation. Just about all show a stiff neck unless in profound coma. About one half of patients show some impairment of consciousness on admission to hospital, with one third of this group in coma, one third semicomatosed or stuporous, and one third obtunded. Those without impairment of consciousness frequently exhibit abnormal mentation. Transient dysphasia is not uncommon, and many show excitement, restlessness, and irritability. Others are disoriented, confabulate on questioning, and have impaired retention and recall. Judgment and insight may be poor and there may be deficits of memory. As a result some patients may be erroneously admitted to psychiatric services because of excited and irrational behavior.

On cranial nerve examination, the fundus may show the presence of subhyaloid hemorrhages, which appear like large purple blots on blotting paper, but are actually areas of bleeding between the retina and hyaloid membrane, with a sharp edge, fanning out from the optic nerve. These subhyaloid hemorrhages are pathognomonic of ruptured aneurysms and are usually found with ruptured aneurysms of the anterior communicating or internal carotid arteries but have been reported in association with aneurysms at other sites. Papilledema occurs in some 10 per cent of cases, often developing within a few hours of bleeding. Visual acuity may be reduced, or there may be transient episodes of amblyopia due to pressure on the optic nerve. Unilateral or bilateral optic atrophy may occur owing to chronic pressure on the optic nerve or chiasm by an aneurysm of the internal carotid or anterior cerebral arteries prior to rupture. Damage to the optic chiasm by an enlarging aneurysm results in a bitemporal hemianopia, while bleeding into the optic tract or cerebral hemispheres frequently produces homonymous hemianopia.

The site of the aneurysm governs the development of signs and symptoms that may permit accurate clinical localization. Typical syndromes due to intracranial aneurysms will now be described.

Infraclinoid-Intracavernous Carotid Aneurysms. Clinical features include the following:

1. There may be facial pain of trigeminal neuralgia due to pressure occurring on one or more

divisions of the trigeminal nerve. This may be present before rupture of the aneurysm.

2. The patient may be aware of a noise in the head and occasionally reports temporary relief by pressing on the affected carotid artery in the neck.
3. Paralysis of the third, fourth, and sixth cranial nerves can occur as the aneurysm increases in size or when rupture occurs.
4. A large aneurysm extending into the pituitary fossa mimics a pituitary tumor and produces hypopituitarism.
5. Rupture of the aneurysm may lead to the development of a caroticocavernous fistula.

Supraclinoid Internal Carotid Aneurysms. The aneurysm (Fig. 9–20) develops in the angle between the optic chiasm and the optic nerve medially and the third nerve laterally. Clinical features are as follows:

1. Pressure on the optic nerve produces decreased visual acuity, scotoma, and eventual optic atrophy and blindness.
2. Pressure on the optic chiasm may produce various field defects.
3. Pressure laterally results in an isolated third-nerve paralysis.

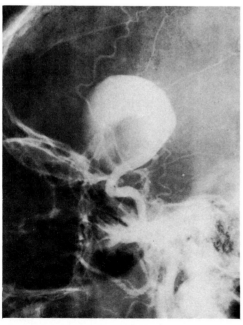

FIGURE 9–20. Huge supraclinoid aneurysm of the right internal carotid artery. This aneurysm simulated a brain tumor by compressing the brain.

Ophthalmic Artery Aneurysms. Aneurysms occurring at this site are uncommon. They tend to project into the optic foramen. Clinical features include:

1. A gradual painless loss of vision and unilateral optic atrophy due to pressure on the optic nerve.[183]
2. Enlargement of the optic foramen on roentgenograms of the orbit.
3. Hypopituitarism, an occasional complication.

Middle Cerebral Artery Aneurysms. Middle cerebral artery aneurysms occur in the lateral fissure and tend to produce bleeding into the brain. Clinical features are as follows:

1. Hemiparesis or hemiplegia is common.
2. Focal motor seizures may occur.
3. Dysphasia or aphasia will occur if there is damage to the dominant hemisphere.
4. Homonymous hemianopia may be present owing to involvement of the optic radiation or an upper homonymous quadrantanopia with bleeding into the temporal lobe.

Syndrome of Anterior Cerebral and Anterior Communicating Artery Aneurysms. These aneurysms (Fig. 9–21) are difficult to localize clinically.

1. Large aneurysms may compress the olfactory tract, producing unilateral anosmia.
2. Pressure on the optic chiasm from above produces bitemporal field defects, which may begin with the lower quadrants.
3. Rupture into the frontal lobes is often bilateral (the butterfly hemorrhage) and produces personality changes and impairment of judgment, insight, retention, and recall. A state of extreme apathy with mutism and little response to the environment, even though the patient is fully conscious, can occur with severe bilateral frontal lobe damage.

Posterior Communicating Artery Aneurysms. These occur at the junction of the internal carotid artery with the posterior communicating artery (Fig. 9–22). Clinical features are as follows:

1. There may be recent onset of severe headache with pain localized to the eye, the orbital region, or the side of the forehead.[172]
2. Third-nerve paralysis occurs before or after rupture of the aneurysm. Patients with oculo-

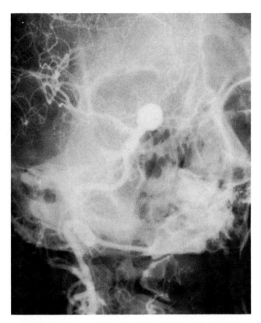

FIGURE 9–21. Right carotid arteriogram (oblique view) showing characteristic appearance of a large saccular aneurysm of the anterior cerebral artery arising at the junction of the anterior communicating artery.

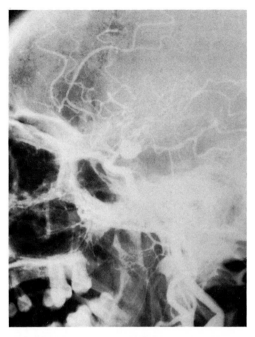

FIGURE 9–22. Left carotid arteriogram showing a ruptured saccular aneurysm at the junction of the posterior communicating artery with the internal carotid artery. The patient presented with a stiff neck, bloody cerebrospinal fluid, and a third-nerve paralysis on the left.

motor nerve paralysis are more likely to have prodromal headache.
3. There is occasional paralysis of the sixth nerve on the same side.

Posterior Cerebral Artery Aneurysms. Posterior cerebral artery aneurysms are rare and occur on the proximal portion of the artery. Reduction of blood flow through the posterior cerebral artery may result in cortical infarction in the occipital lobe and the development of a homonymous field defect. Large aneurysms may compress the midbrain, producing pseudobulbar signs, alteration in the level of consciousness, or akinetic mutism. Increased intracranial pressure and hydrocephalus have been reported.

Basilar Artery Aneurysms. These usually arise at the terminal bifurcation of the basilar artery at the upper border of the pons.[34] This may result in compression of the trigeminal nerve on one side with the development of facial pain or tic douloureux.

Aneurysms also occur at the origin of the superior cerebellar or the anterior inferior cerebellar arteries from the basilar artery and at the verte-brobasilar junction. The superior cerebellar artery aneurysm may compress the third nerve and brainstem, producing ipsilateral oculomotor paralysis and ataxia. Aneurysms located lower in the basilar system can compress the seventh nerve producing a peripheral type of paralysis of the facial muscles. A large aneurysm can produce hydrocephalus owing to pressure on the brainstem and distortion of the cerebral aqueduct. A similar clinical picture occurs in hypertensive subjects with arteriosclerotic aneurysms.[84]

Vertebral Artery Aneurysms. Arising on the surface of the medulla, these produce unilateral paralysis of the lower cranial nerves. Irritation of the eighth nerve may result in intermittent attacks of vertigo, ataxia, nausea, and vomiting.

Arteriovenous Malformations of the Brain. There is a high incidence of abnormal symptoms and signs in patients with arteriovenous malformations prior to subarachnoid hemorrhage.

Arteriovenous malformation is a frequent cause of partial epileptic seizures in young patients.

Both partial and generalized seizures occur, and both types are often found in the same patient. The partial seizures usually present with focal motor manifestations of jacksonian seizures. However, since arteriovenous malformations are often present in the parietotemporo-occipital areas, seizures may begin with sensory, auditory, visual, or psychomotor phenomena.

Some patients present with migraine-like headaches, which are often unilateral and usually occur on the side of the arteriovenous malformation. The diagnosis of an arteriovenous malformation should be considered in patients with headache who present with a bruit or auscultation over the eye, since intracranial bruits are rare with berry aneurysms.

A chronic progressive dementia occurs in some patients with large arteriovenous malformations. This is possibly due to chronic hypoxic changes in cerebral tissue due to an intracranial "steal," which may occur in the presence of large arteriovenous shunts (the blood is shunted away from normal brain). Other important contributing factors are progressive gliosis, secondary to repeated small hemorrhages, and hydrocephalus due to arachnoiditis, which often results from recurrent subarachnoid hemorrhage.

Subarachnoid hemorrhage due to arteriovenous malformation is more common in the second and third decades of life. The bleeding is often venous rather than arterial; hence the symptoms are less severe than those that occur with ruptured berry aneurysm, where the bleeding is arterial. Nevertheless, intracerebral hemorrhage with severe neurologic deficit may occur. Since the mortality with each hemorrhage is less than with ruptured aneurysms, a history of recurrent episodes of subarachnoid hemorrhage associated with seizures is almost pathognomonic of arteriovenous malformation.

Focal neurologic signs are sometimes present in patients with arteriovenous malformation before the occurrence of subarachnoid hemorrhage. These signs include homonymous hemianopia, hemiparesis, and hemisensory loss. Small intracerebral hemorrhages may be followed by the development of dysphasia when the dominant hemisphere is involved. Large arteriovenous malformations with hemispheric atrophy can cause an associated smallness of the skull on the same side as the malformation (Davidoff-Dyke syndrome) and underdevelopment of the opposite side of the body.

There may be communication with extracranial vessels, particularly with the external carotid circulation, with enlargement of these vessels and occasionally the formation of a palpable cirsoid aneurysm of the scalp. In many cases the vessels of the scalp show excessive pulsation and may have a palpable thrill and loud bruit on auscultation. The patient may complain of the bruit. Extension into the orbit produces some degree of exophthalmos. Auscultation over the eye will reveal a bruit in such cases. Auscultation during compression of the internal carotid artery may produce alteration or loss of the bruit and give some indication of the possible origin of the feeding arteries. There is an increase in pulse pressure in the carotid system, which feeds the arteriovenous malformation. This may be seen as an increased pulsation in the retinal vessels on ophthalmoscopic examination. The venous return through the jugular venous system is increased on the side of the malformation, and if both jugular veins are compressed and released simultaneously, the external jugular vein on the side of the venous malformation will fill first.

Rarely, in children, the cerebral arteriovenous malformation may cause cardiac enlargement and heart failure of the high-output type.[60]

Subarachnoid Hemorrhage of Undetermined Etiology. Despite adequate investigation, including arteriography of the entire aortocranial circulation, no aneurysm or malformation will be demonstrated in about 10 per cent of patients with subarachnoid hemorrhage. A few of these patients may be examples of the rare causes of primary subarachnoid hemorrhage listed in Table 9–2. The majority are due to rupture of a small aneurysm or arteriovenous malformation that cannot be demonstrated by angiography.

Diagnostic Procedures

Lumbar Puncture. The cerebrospinal fluid is usually under increased pressure and is grossly bloody in appearance. The quantity of blood is the same in all three tubes, and the supernatant fluid is xanthochromic when the specimen is centrifuged. Xanthochromia appears within four hours of bleeding and persists for about 20 to 30 days. Red cells will, however, disappear within seven days unless there has been fresh hemorrhage. The red cell count is usually above 150,000 cells/cu mm when an aneurysm has ruptured. However, if the bleeding is primarily parenchymatous, the count may be low. This also will occur when there has been a small hemorrhage or "leaking" from an aneurysm or arteriovenous malformation. Initially, the white cell count has the same ratio to the red cell count as in the peripheral blood, but as the products of hemolysis produce meningeal inflammation, there will be an increase in polymorphonuclear cells and lymphocytes within a few days. An increase in monocytes in the spinal fluid may persist for four weeks. The protein content of the fluid is increased and the glucose content is normal.

Radiographic Examination. It is unusual to find any abnormality in roentgenograms of the skull when subarachnoid hemorrhage is due to ruptured aneurysms. However, aneurysms occasionally show calcification of their walls, which appear as a curvilinear shadow. Such calcification looks like an eggshell and is most frequently seen in aneurysms of the internal carotid artery; and consequently, it appears as a parasellar calcification. Aneurysms in this situation may also erode the clinoid processes and cause enlargement of the dorsum sellae. Roentgenographic changes noted within the skull are more frequently encountered in arteriovenous malformations. There may be an increase in vascular markings in the skull unilaterally or calcification within the vessel walls of about 20 per cent of angiomas.

Electroencephalography. The EEG is usually normal in patients with a berry aneurysm prior to the occurrence of subarachnoid hemorrhage, but may show diffuse slowing after severe intracerebral bleeding or focal slowing if there is an intracerebral hematoma.

Large arteriovenous malformations may produce focal slowing in the EEG prior to rupture but are commonly associated with focal spike and slow wave activity. The EEG is abnormal in patients with subarachnoid hemorrhage with cerebral vasospasm, and daily recordings are useful in augmenting the clinical findings and assessing the progress of the patient.

Computed Tomography. Although large aneurysms can be visualized after the infusion of contrast material, it is unusual for aneurysms to be demonstrated by CT scan. However, the scan is useful in the demonstration of intracerebral or subdural hematomas associated with the ruptured aneurysm. There is a tendency for hematomas

visualized on the scan to correlate with the site of the aneurysm. The CT scan also demonstrates acute hydrocephalus, and serial scans can be used to follow the evolution of this condition. There is accurate differentiation between hematoma and edema in a CT scan. Patients with normal CT scans are more likely to have minimal neurologic deficits by clinical examination.[194]

In contrast to the aneurysm, arteriovenous malformations are readily demonstrated by CT scanning and show marked enhancement following intravenous contrast enhancement.

Cerebral Angiography. If the CT scan is not available, cerebral angiography should be performed as soon as possible unless the patient is comatose. The procedure is performed to determine the presence of intracerebral or subdural hematoma or acute hydrocephalus rather than the presence of aneurysm or arteriovenous malformation.[29] This implies that neurosurgical treatment is readily available if emergency surgery is required for evacuation of a hematoma or drainage of the hydrocephalus.[105]

A berry aneurysm may be detected in about 80 per cent of patients with primary subarachnoid hemorrhage by adequate arteriography and the use of seriograms. The latter technique is important since a number of aneurysms do not fill in the initial arterial phase of the arteriogram, presumably due to vasospasm, and may not be seen until the capillary or venous phase. These aneurysms are not visualized by single film exposures. Arterial spasm is quite common in patients with subarachnoid hemorrhage, and although it tends to be more marked in the region of the aneurysm, it may be diffuse in some cases. Aneurysms are multiple in about 15 per cent of cases. The detection of the ruptured aneurysm then depends on the clinical findings and certain indications from angiography. Thus, when spasm is localized, it tends to occur near the ruptured aneurysm (Fig. 9–23). Blood vessels may be stretched or displaced by a hematoma, which also indicates the site of rupture. Rarely, the contrast material may escape through the rupture in the aneurysm wall. A more reliable indicator of the site of rupture is a nipple-like protrusion on the aneurysm. Angiography should be repeated immediately before surgical treatment of an aneurysm to ensure absence of vascular spasm which may have developed in the interval following the initial angiogram.

Arteriovenous malformations are readily dem-

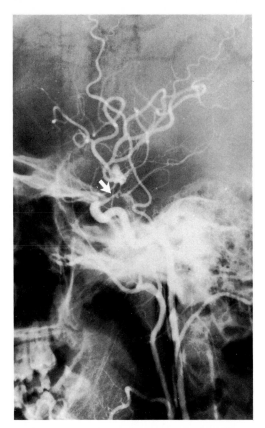

FIGURE 9–23. Left carotid arteriogram showing a ruptured aneurysm of the internal carotid and anterior cerebral arteries. The internal carotid artery (see arrow) proximal to the aneurysm shows intense spasm.

onstrated by angiography. Seriography is again helpful in mapping out the abnormal feeding vessels and detecting the veins draining the area. This facilitates the feasibility of surgical treatment and determines the approach if surgery is contemplated.

About 10 per cent of patients with primary subarachnoid hemorrhage have negative angiographic studies for aneurysm and arteriovenous malformation and no detectable medical cause for bleeding. In some of these cases, aneurysm undoubtedly exists, as has been shown at autopsy.

Treatment of Subarachnoid Hemorrhage Due to Aneurysm

General Measures. The early management of subarachnoid hemorrhage following rupture of a saccular aneurysm is predominantly a medical problem, and most neurosurgeons agree that in-

tracranial surgery should not be performed for seven days to three weeks after the onset of bleeding.[1, 73, 82, 178] The patient should be placed on strict bed rest with constant medical and nursing supervision. The headache should be controlled with adequate doses of meperidine hydrochloride (Demerol) or morphine and restlessness alleviated by regular doses of barbiturates. Excessive movement of the patient increases the possibility of further hemorrhage. If possible, treatment should be provided in a center equipped to give intensive care, including adequate angiographic examination.

All patients should have computed tomography to rule out a subdural hematoma or large intracerebral hematoma. If a CT scan cannot be obtained, angiographic studies are indicated for the same reason unless the patient is in deep coma and is unlikely to tolerate the procedure or be considered for surgery for evacuation of a hematoma.

Patients without neurologic deficits or with minimal neurologic deficits and absence of spasm of the cerebral vessels are usually considered to be ready for surgery after seven days to three weeks of medical treatment. However, medical treatment should be continued under the following circumstances:

1. In a comatose patient or a patient with severe neurologic deficit.
2. In cases without angiographic evidence of berry aneurysm or arteriovenous malformation by angiography.
3. If multiple berry aneurysms are found by angiography without clinical or angiographic evidence as to which one has ruptured.
4. As long as there is severe spasm of the cerebral vessels causing cerebral ischemia.
5. If there is rejection of surgical treatment by the patient or the family.

Medical Treatment. Medical treatment should include the following:

1. Strict bed rest ("coronary-type care" concerning which all the nurses involved should have instruction) must be enforced during the period when the chances of further hemorrhage are high. This means bed rest for a period of three weeks after the bleeding episode, and the necessity for this apparently lengthy confinement should be explained to the patient and his relatives to ensure full

cooperation. He should be turned gently every two hours for skin care and changing the bed when necessary.

2. The mouth and throat should be suctioned frequently in comatose patients and endotracheal intubation performed if secretions accumulate to the extent that respirations are impaired.

3. Conscious patients require adequate doses of analgesics to control headache. This usually requires the use of a narcotic such as meperidine hydrochloride initially, which should be given in adequate doses (100 to 150 mg every four hours as necessary). A phenothiazine helps to prevent vomiting and potentiates the action of the narcotic. When headache begins to subside, codeine given intramuscularly or codeine and aspirin orally are usually adequate to control pain.

4. Restlessness may be reduced by phenobarbital given orally or intramuscularly. This should be continued for three weeks since many patients become restless in the second week of the illness and may attempt to get out of bed under the impression that they have made a full recovery.

5. A distended bladder is an important cause of restlessness and elevated blood pressure. Stuporous and comatose patients require the use of an indwelling catheter, which should be changed and drained every two hours. The risk of a urinary tract infection can be reduced by the use of oral chemotherapy or by irrigating the bladder twice a day, using a suitable irrigating solution containing an antiseptic or antibiotic.

6. The conscious patient may be given a liquid diet but should be fed by a nurse or trained attendant during the first two weeks and remain flat in bed. The stuporous or comatose patient will require 2,500 to 3,000 ml of fluid daily. This may be given intravenously during the first 24 hours but can be given via a nasogastric tube after that period. Once the tube is passed, the fluid may be given as part of a blender diet.

7. Accurate intake of fluids and output of urine must always be charted in all stuporous or comatose patients.

8. In hypertensive patients, the blood pressure should be reduced below 150 mm Hg systolic and maintained at a fairly steady level.[120] This may be accomplished by the use of hydralazine orally or intramuscularly, by the use of oral diuretics, or, in more severe cases, by the use of alpha-methyldopa orally or propranolol orally (or via nasogastric tube).

9. It is essential to avoid constipation and straining, which may increase intracranial pressure. This can be accomplished using softening agents, mineral oil, or mild laxatives.

10. If brain swelling is suspected due to infarction, a course of steroids (Dexamethasone, 12 to 16 mg daily, orally or intramuscularly)[13] during the first two weeks may help reduce edema. Cerebral edema may also be treated by intravenous infusion of 10 per cent glycerol (1 to 2 gm/kg of body weight per day).[185]

11. Hydrocephalus may be treated by daily removal of 25 ml of CSF. A ventricular shunt may be necessary in severe cases of acute hydrocephalus.[150]

12. Rebleeding of a ruptured aneurysm is probably due to lysis of the clot formed at the point of rupture. The peak activity of fibrinolytic substances occurs 7 to 14 days after rupture of the aneurysm and can be reduced by antifibrinolytic therapy during this period.[167] Epsilon aminocaproic acid (EACA) is an effective antifibrinolytic agent and reduces rebleeding in subarachnoid hemorrhage.[138] EACA is given in doses of 36 gm/day by continuous intravenous infusion for ten days. This can be followed by EACA, 3 gm every two hours orally, until the patient is ready for surgery or until a decision has been made to continue medical treatment. Tranexamic acid is likewise effective.[23c]

Surgical Treatment of Berry Aneurysms. There are three basic surgery procedures available in the treatment of berry aneurysms:

1. Extracranial carotid ligation may be employed in patients with an aneurysm involving the terminal portion of the internal carotid artery, particularly for aneurysms arising at the origin of the posterior communicating artery.[115] There is a considerable reduction in mortality following this procedure with a survival rate of 84 per cent in patients followed from 1 to 17 years.[80]

   The occlusion is usually carried out by the application of a ligature to the common carotid artery in the neck. There does not seem to be any advantage in using a clamp and gradually occluding the vessel, but the procedure should not be performed in the presence of cerebral vasospasm. Neurologic complication caused by ischemia of the ipsilateral cerebral hemisphere occurs in less than 20 per cent of cases. The risk of complications is minimized by performing cerebral blood flow determinations before occluding the common carotid artery. The procedure is unsafe if the cerebral blood flow is less than 20 ml/minute/100 gm brain.[131]

2. Direct intracranial correction of the aneurysm is applicable to accessible aneurysms at any site in patients who are considered to be good surgical candidates. The majority of surgeons delay operation for at least a week and often as long as three weeks after rupture of the aneurysm. Surgery is performed only on patients who show absence of or minimal neurologic deficits and who do not have cerebral vasospasm.[74] Patients who do not fit these criteria should continue medical treatment until they are sufficiently improved for surgical treatment.[75] Mortality is increased in patients with a depressed level of consciousness preoperatively, and there is an increased risk in individuals aged 50 years or more.[82] The advantage of surgical obliteration of the aneurysm is that the risk of further bleeding is permanently removed. Current methods include exposure of the aneurysm and applying a clip to its neck, wrapping the aneurysm with fascia or muscle, spraying with plastic material, or injection of a foreign material such as hog hair into the body of the aneurysm to produce thrombosis (pilojection of the aneurysm). The obliteration of the sac by the use of a spring clip seems to be the most widely applicable and useful of these methods. A postoperative angiogram should always be performed to check the results of surgery. More than 10 per cent of cases will still show some filling of the aneurysm, often caused by the surgical clip slipping off the neck of aneurysm.[35]

3. Acute ventricular drainage may be lifesaving in some patients with acute hydrocephalus that develops within a few days of the onset of subarachnoid hemorrhage. Drainage of a subdural hematoma should be carried out as soon as possible if this condition is present in the early angiogram and the patient can tolerate a surgical procedure. A ventriculoatrial, lumbothecoperitoneal, or ventriculoperitoneal shunt may be used in cases with chronic hydrocephalus.

Medical Treatment of Arteriovenous Malformations. Medical treatment is similar to the treatment recommended for subarachnoid hemorrhage following rupture of an aneurysm. Epsilon aminocaproic acid is not recommended in the treatment of arteriovenous malformations.

Surgical Treatment of Arteriovenous Malformations. Excision of an arteriovenous malformation is not always a practical form of therapy. Much depends on the site of the abnormal vessels. However, the introduction of microsurgical techniques now permits the treatment of arteriovenous malformations formerly considered unsuitable for operation by direct surgical approach and excision.[162] Malformations that cannot be excised may be reduced in size or obliterated by superselective internal carotid arteriography and embolization using plastic spheres, silicone polymerization, ferromagnetic silicone, or with a balloon catheter.[33] Embolization has brought significant benefit to patients with cerebral arteriovenous malformations but is still not a substitute for direct surgical excision when this is feasible.[100]

Prognosis

Subarachnoid hemorrhage due to ruptured berry aneurysm carries a mortality rate of 30 per cent within the first 24 hours of the hemorrhage, and about 40 per cent of patients die from the initial bleeding episode, the majority during the first week after hemorrhage. A recurrence of bleeding is likely to occur in 50 per cent of the survivors, with the majority having the second bleeding episode within two weeks of the first. The second episode carries a higher mortality rate than the first, and subsequent recurrences carry a progressively higher mortality. The total mortality seems to be about 60 per cent within six months following the initial subarachnoid hemorrhage due to reputured berry aneurysm.

The mortality is 1 per cent between six months and a year and from 1 to 3 per cent for each yearly interval thereafter up to five years[66] with a total mortality of about 70 per cent at five years.

Subarachnoid hemorrhage due to bleeding from an arteriovenous malformation carries much lower mortality than berry aneurysm. Probably less than 10 per cent of patients die from the initial hemorrhage, and although recurrence rates are high, the mortality remains low. About 20 per cent of the survivors die from recurrent hemorrhages.

In cases with normal arteriograms, the mortality appears to be about one tenth of that associated with proved cases of ruptured aneurysms and one third of that recorded in patients with arteriovenous malformation.

Subarachnoid Hemorrhage from Rupture of Mycotic Aneurysms

These aneurysms are rare but have been seen with increasing frequency in the last decade in drug addicts who repeatedly inject heroin intravenously using contaminated syringes and needles.[55] Mycotic aneurysms usually develop in the branches of the middle cerebral artery in the posterior limb of the lateral fissure. The vessel is occluded by an infected embolus derived from infected vegetations of subacute bacterial endocarditis. This is followed by the development of a local arteritis affecting the adventitia and the media which weakens the vessel wall producing an aneurysm. Recanalization of the vessel may be followed by rupture of the mycotic aneurysm and subarachnoid hemorrhage. The aneurysms are often multiple and occasionally involve both middle cerebral arteries. All drug addicts with subacute bacterial endocarditis who develop focal neurologic abnormalities should have cerebral angiography, which is the only reliable method of demonstrating mycotic aneurysms.

Treatment

The aneurysms regress and sometimes resolve if the patient is given adequate antibiotic therapy in sufficient amounts to cure the subacute bacterial endocarditis. Aneurysmal rupture and subarachnoid hemorrhage require the same treatment as outlined for ruptured saccular aneurysm.

Spinal Subarachnoid Hemorrhage

Primary subarachnoid hemorrhage, arising from lesions in the spinal canal, is rare compared to those arising from intracranial lesions. The main cause is bleeding from an angiomatous malformation of the spinal cord. Spinal artery aneurysms are uncommon, and hemorrhage from this cause is rare. Subarachnoid bleeding may also occur from a hemangioblastoma in the cervical cord or ependymoma of the filum terminale. Systemic diseases such as polyarteritis nodosa or leukemia may also cause spinal subarachnoid hemorrhage. The onset is sudden, frequently following exertion, with the development of severe nerve root pains, followed by the development of pain in the thoracic and lumbar areas. Movements of the spine are excruciatingly painful, Kernig's sign is strongly positive, opisthotonus may occur, and urinary retention is usually present. The hemorrhage may extend into the cranial cavity, with the development of headache and neck stiffness. Flaccid paralysis due to cord damage may present as a manifestation of spinal shock or indicate cord destruction when the patient remains permanently paraplegic.

Transfemoral aortography at the site of the lesion will usually demonstrate the malformation.

Treatment consists of adequate sedation and bed rest as outlined under Medical Treatment of Subarachnoid Hemorrhage. Surgical decompression is helpful in some cases and excludes the possibility of hemorrhage from a tumor.

The development of microsurgical techniques has led to the complete removal of some angiomatous malformations formerly considered inaccessible to surgical treatment.[199] There is, however, no benefit to patients who are completely paraplegic. Embolization of spinal angiomatous malformations is feasible in selected cases but must be performed with extreme caution in nonparaplegic patients.[32] This technique may also be employed to suppress radicular pain in paraplegic patients.

Cerebral Hemorrhage

Hemorrhage into the brain substance may be the result of rupture of an artery, vein, or capillary.

Etiology and Pathology

About 70 per cent of cerebral hemorrhages occur in the area of the internal capsule, 20 per cent occur in the posterior fossa (brainstem or cerebellum), and 10 per cent occur elsewhere in the cerebral hemispheres. Since the hemorrhage invariably destroys the area where the bleeding arose, the cause often remains a matter of conjecture. However, examination of the nonaffected areas of the brain has disclosed changes in the blood vessels that could predispose to rupture and hemorrhage. It is apparent from clinical and pathologic studies that a number of conditions may lead to intracerebral hemorrhage.

Patients with long-standing hypertension develop degenerative changes in the muscle and elastic tissue of the blood vessel walls. These changes are more marked in the penetrating branches of the middle cerebral artery, which supply the lenticular nucleus and internal capsule (lenticulostriate arteries), with the development of small "Charcot-Bouchard" aneurysms.[25] One of these aneurysms may rupture, particularly if there is a sudden elevation of blood pressure. The hemorrhage usually begins in the lenticular nucleus and internal capsule. The bleeding may be confined to the lenticular nucleus (lateral hemorrhage) or to the internal capsule (capsular hemorrhage). In about 10 per cent of cases, the hemorrhage involves the thalamus (medial or thalamic hemor-

rhage), but in severe cases, it may spread through the thalamus, internal capsule, and lenticular nucleus (quadrilateral hemorrhage) and frequently ruptures into the lateral ventricle (Fig. 9–24).

In cases of malignant hypertension, there may be multiple areas of vessel necrosis, that is, a necrotizing arteriolopathy similar to that found in the kidney. These vessels rupture, with hemorrhage into the brain. This is usually preceded by papilledema, seizures, increased intracranial pressure, and transient neurologic deficits called "hypertensive encephalopathy." At this stage, before the occurrence of an intracerebral hemorrhage, the condition is reversible by lowering the blood pressure.

In the more chronic hypertensive patient, lenticulostriate arteries undergo arteriosclerotic changes in chronic hypertension. This may predis-

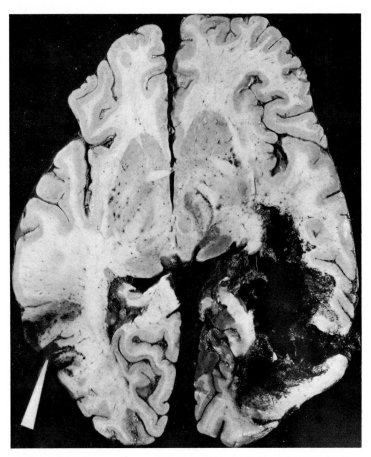

FIGURE 9–24. Horizontal section of an intracerebral hemorrhage in the right cerebral hemisphere. This caused herniation of the brain with compression of the opposite posterior cerebral artery, resulting in hemorrhagic infarction of the opposite parieto-occipital cortex (white arrow).

pose to multiple thromboses and small areas of infarction (lacunar infarcts). The wall of the vessel passing through the infarcted area is likely to be weakened owing to hypoxia. If blood flow is restored by lysis of the clot, rupture with intracerebral hemorrhage may occur.

It is evident that the lenticulostriate arteries are subject to constriction or spasm during severe hypertensive episodes. Possibly this reduces blood flow below the critical levels, with development of small infarcts. Such ischemia also damages the vessel wall, which may rupture.

A small number of brain hemorrhages have been shown to be due to rupture of small angiomatous malformations within the brain substance.

Certain conditions associated with a bleeding tendency may be complicated by brain hemorrhage. Leukemia associated with severe thrombocytopenia is the most common disease in this group,[110] which also includes hemophilia, thrombocytopenia, and long-term anticoagulant therapy.

Bleeding into the brain also occurs as a rare complication of eclampsia and certain of the arteritides such as polyarteritis nodosa. Both the familial and nonfamilial forms of cerebral amyloid angiopathy are rare causes of intracerebral hemorrhage.[101] Hemorrhage is also a rare complication of a rapidly growing malignant brain tumor.

The rupture of an artery is followed by the release of blood into the brain substance under high pressure. There is widespread destruction of tissue in the immediate area, but the blood also dissects along the planes of the nerve tracts. In the case of intracerebral hemorrhage, there is often destruction of the internal capsule, lenticular nucleus, and thalamus, with the possibility of dissection down into the midbrain. Extension into the lateral or third ventricle occurs in many patients, and occasionally, the bleeding may extend laterally through the external capsule, claustrum, and extreme capsule to rupture as a subarachnoid hemorrhage through the cortex of the insula.

Patients who survive the hemorrhage have considerable swelling of the cerebral hemisphere due to the hematoma, with rapid development of edema, which reaches a maximum after four to five days and then subsides. The cerebral edema may produce herniation through the tentorial opening and compression of the brainstem, often with the development of secondary brainstem hemorrhage. The herniation may compress and occlude the posterior cerebral arteries, with infarction of the medial aspects of the occipital lobes.

Clinical Features

Intracerebral Hemorrhage. Patients with hypertension may have premonitory headaches, which are usually worse upon awakening in the morning. The hemorrhage frequently occurs during a period of exertion or excitement, and the occurrence is most common during the day when the patient is active rather than when he is sleeping at night. This is usually the opposite of cerebral infarction. The patient generally complains of severe headache, and there is rapid deterioration into stupor or coma. Examination may reveal a plethoric individual with stertorous respiration. There may be some cardiac enlargement due to chronic hypertensive heart disease, and both systolic and diastolic pressures will be elevated. Funduscopic examination will show grade 2 or 3 hypertensive changes. If the patient is still responding, a homonymous hemianopia can usually be demonstrated by making thrusting movement with the hands from each side toward the patient's eyes and watching for a blink response. The eyes are frequently deviated toward the side of the affected hemisphere, and there is contralateral facial weakness and flaccid hemiplegia. The deep tendon reflexes are decreased, with an extensor plantar response on the side of the hemiplegia.

The majority of patients show a fairly rapid progression, with deepening of coma and signs of brainstem compression, often associated with temporal lobe (uncal) herniation. This produces unilateral dilatation of the pupil due to oculomotor nerve paralysis and Cheyne-Stokes respirations. As pressure increases, reflex movements of the eyes are lost, decerebrate rigidity appears, and the respirations become regular and more rapid, with the development of pontine hyperventilation. This stage may last from a few hours to a few days but is inevitably followed by irregular respirations, falling blood pressure, and death.

Few patients survive an intracerebral hemorrhage, which carries an early mortality of 70 to 80 per cent. In those cases who survive, however, the prognosis for return of some function in the hemiplegic limbs is good. This is probably because the hemorrhage was small and split the tissues rather than destroying much of the deeper structures in the hemisphere. The slow absorption of the clot and disappearance of the edema reduce the pressure on nerve tracts and permit restoration of function.

Medial (thalamic) hemorrhage accounts for about 10 per cent of cases of intracerebral hemorrhage but has a better prognosis than the other types of this condition. The onset is sudden, with clouding of consciousness and dysphasia, if the dominant hemisphere is involved. Oculomotor signs are prominent. The pupils are small, and the reaction to light is sluggish. There is a marked sensory deficit on the opposite side of the body. The bleeding usually extends into the third ventricle, with the development of subarachnoid hemorrhage.

Midbrain Hemorrhage.   This is extremely rare as a primary condition, and the majority of hemorrhages in the midbrain are due to intracerebral hemorrhages with secondary spread to this area. A primary midbrain hemorrhage has been described in the ventral part of the midbrain, producing an ipsilateral paralysis of the third nerve and a contralateral hemiplegia (Weber's syndrome).

Pontine Hemorrhage.   This is usually extensive, producing a sudden loss of consciousness with respiratory arrhythmias, bilateral miosis (pinpoint pupils), ocular bobbing, lack of reflex eye movements on turning the head or irrigating the ear canals with ice water, and bilateral involvement of the corticospinal tracts and cranial nerve nuclei. Hyperpyrexia may occur in some cases because of the interruption of descending autonomic fibers passing from the hypothalamus to the lower brainstem and spinal cord. Although the prognosis is poor, coma is not invariably present and recovery has been reported in an occasional case of pontine hemorrhage.[143a]

Cerebellar Hemorrhage.   Since there are certain special diagnostic and therapeutic considerations regarding cerebellar hemorrhages, this subject will be discussed after general diagnostic and therapeutic considerations of brain hemorrhage.

Diagnostic Procedures

1. Intracerebral hemorrhage is readily diagnosed by computed tomography. The high density of the clotted blood contrasts sharply with the surrounding brain, which may show

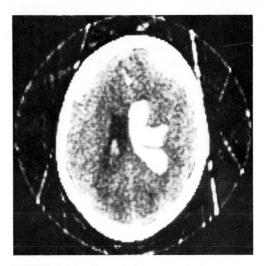

FIGURE 9–25.   Computed tomography in intracerebral hemorrhage. This nonenhanced scan shows an area of increased density in the right hemisphere in the early stages of an intracerebral hemorrhage.

evidence of edema. The majority of intracerebral hemorrhages are seen in the area of the basal ganglia (Fig. 9–25), and intraventricular rupture occurs in about 60 per cent of cases.[195a] The CT scan will also demonstrate smaller hemorrhages in other areas, including the pons. There is a steady decrease in attenuation values of the intracerebral hemorrhage with time, and the involved area may be impossible to distinguish from the surrounding brain for a period of about five days between 5 and 20 days after the bleeding episode.[14] However, the distortion of the ventricular system will indicate the presence of a mass, and the use of contrast material will help to exclude other causes for the dislocation of the midline structures.

2. If lumbar puncture is performed, the procedure should be carried out using a fine-gauge needle if there is any evidence of increased intracranial pressure. The spinal fluid is usually under increased pressure and is frankly bloody in 80 per cent of cases. A further 10 per cent will show xanthochromia. Patients with clear cerebrospinal fluid often show red cell counts in excess of 500 per cubic millimeter.[95] The protein content is elevated, but the glucose content is normal.

3. Roentgenograms of the skull may reveal displacement of the calcified pineal gland when

there is a large hematoma in one hemisphere.

4. A shift of midline structures can often be demonstrated by echoencephalography.

5. The electroencephalograph shows bilateral frontoparietal slowing, often with medium to high voltage, sharp waves, and ipsilateral suppression of background activity in a massive intracerebral hemorrhage. In smaller ganglionic and capsular hemorrhage, the slowing is lateralized to the affected side. A normal or borderline abnormal EEG may be obtained in pontine hemorrhage, even though the patient is comatose.

6. Angiographic studies frequently show a shift of the anterior cerebral vessels to the opposite side and stretching of the middle cerebral group. The distance between the anterior and middle cerebral group of vessels is increased in the anteroposterior study. There may be stretching of the anterior cerebral vessels in the lateral view owing to acute hydrocephalus.

7. As the patient improves, the cardiac status should be ascertained. The chest film usually will demonstrate enlargement of the heart in the chronic hypertensive. Transient electrocardiographic abnormalities are not unusual during the acute phase of intracerebral hemorrhage. These changes consist of various dysrhythmias including frequent premature ventricular contractions and an occasional electrocardiographic record suggesting acute myocardial infarction. Serum creatine phosphokinase (CPK) levels will be elevated in patients who have concomitant myocardial infarction.[31]

8. Renal function is frequently impaired in the chronic hypertensive and may be evaluated by urinalysis, blood urea nitrogen, a creatinine clearance test, and an intravenous pyelography. Renal arteriography should be performed in cases where the hypertension appears to be the result of renal artery stenosis.

9. Patients who have hypertensive crises require screening tests to exclude pheochromocytoma. These include the phentolamine hydrochloride (regitine) and histamine tests, and urinary levels of catecholamines and vanillic mandelic acid.

10. A few cases of brain hemorrhage occur in patients with blood dyscrasias. These may be detected by complete blood and platelet counts together with bleeding, coagulation, and prothrombin times.

Treatment of the Stuporous or Comatose Patient

Ventilation. The patient should be nursed sitting or semirecumbent in bed and turned every two hours from right lateral to left lateral and occasionally with the bed flat in the supine position. Dentures should be removed and pharyngeal secretions aspirated, using a soft sterile catheter. A low-pressure endotracheal tube should be passed if secretions accumulate despite frequent suctioning. The tube should be inserted at an early stage before anoxia and cyanosis have developed.

Management of Hypertension. The early reduction of blood pressure to approximately 160 mm Hg systolic pressure may prevent further hemorrhage while maintaining an adequate perfusion pressure. The blood pressure can be reduced rapidly in the severely hypertensive patient by giving diazoxide, 300 mg intravenously. There is little risk of hypotension if the patient is lying flat in bed without elevation of the head, and hypotension can be effectively controlled by elevating the foot of the bed. The diazoxide can be repeated after 15 to 30 minutes if the blood pressure has not fallen to satisfactory levels. The effect of diazoxide may be enhanced by means of a rapidly acting loop diuretic such as furosemide, 40 to 80 mg intravenously. Intravenous hydralazine, 15 mg, is also effective in controlling severe hypertension. Less critical levels of hypertension may be controlled by propranolol 40 to 120 mg three times a day. If propranolol is not effective, the addition of hydrochlorothiazide, 50 mg daily, usually produces a satisfactory fall in blood pressure. Other useful oral preparations include hydralazine, alpha-methyldopa, and clonidine.

Bladder Care. Bladder drainage, using a Foley catheter, is necessary in stuporous and comatose patients. The catheter should be clamped, drained, and reclamped every two hours. Infection can be minimized or avoided by irrigating with a polymyxin-plus-neomycin antibiotic solution four times a day. An accurate intake-and-output chart should be kept.

Cerebral Edema. The development and treatment of cerebral edema are major problems in cerebral hemorrhage. Neither dexamethasone[182] nor intravenous glycerol[58] appears to reduce edema or affect the course of cerebral hemorrhage.

Feeding. The fluid requirements during the first 24 hours can be met by giving 3,000 ml of 5 per cent dextrose in 0.2 N saline intravenously. After 24 hours, a nasogastric tube should be passed and 250 ml of water given through the tube every two hours to a total of 3,000 ml a day. During the third day, a 2,000-ml blender diet with added water to a total of 3,000 ml may be given, divided into 250 ml every two hours. Oral feeding should be started as soon as possible after the patient regains consciousness.

Avoidance of Pulmonary Infection. The chest must be examined daily as a routine measure. If signs of infection are detected, antibiotics are indicated and postural drainage may be given by elevating the foot of the bed for 20 minutes four times a day.

Early Physical Therapy. The turning of the patient every two hours encourages drainage of the dependent parts of the lungs and prevents the development of decubiti. All limbs should be placed through full range of passive motion twice a day, and external rotation at the hip in the paralyzed lower limb may be prevented by the use of a sandbag. The use of a handroll prevents contractures of the fingers and maintains the hand in a functional position. A pillow in the axilla prevents adduction at the shoulder.

As soon as the patient is conscious and able to cooperate, a physical therapy program is instituted.

Treatment of the Conscious Patient

The conscious patient with an intracerebral hemorrhage is critically ill, and the general treatment follows the same principles as outlined for the comatose patient. In addition, he will require adequate analgesics for headache and sedation for restlessness. Although conscious, he cannot turn himself owing to paralysis and requires turning every two hours.

The risk of pulmonary infection remains high and may require the use of antibiotics and postural drainage. The blood pressure level should be controlled, maintaining systolic pressure in the region of 160 mm Hg. An indwelling urinary catheter is usually required in the acute phase of the illness and should be removed as soon as possible.

Surgical removal of superficially located hematomas is indicated in patients who are conscious or obtunded with relatively minor neurologic deficits.[181] This includes removal of hematomas from the frontal or temporal lobes or those occurring in the external capsule.

Cerebellar Hemorrhage

The general impression that cerebellar hemorrhage is rare appears to be erroneous. Since the condition is compatible with good quality of survival, the subject will be discussed separately. Improvement in diagnostic techniques and increasing interest in cerebellar hemorrhage have shown that it may constitute some 10 per cent of cerebral hemorrhages, which corresponds approximately to the mass of the cerebellum when compared to the total mass of the brain. The main etiologic factor appears to be hypertension, with rupture of a penetrating vessel in the region of the dentate nucleus. Other causes incude intracerebellar bleeding from angiomatous malformation, including hemangioblastoma.

Clinical Features

There appear to be three well-defined clinical pictures associated with cerebellar hemorrhage.

1. In 20 per cent of cases, the onset is catastrophic, with rapid loss of consciousness, absence of focal signs, and death within one to two days. A clinical diagnosis is often impossible in these cases.

2. In the majority of patients (60 per cent), the onset is abrupt, with occipital headache, vomiting, vertigo, and ataxia. Consciousness may be lost a few hours later. At that time, the patient presents with Cheyne-Stokes respirations, marked constriction of the pupils, deviation of the eyes away from the lesion, and contralateral hemiplegia.

3. A group of about 20 per cent of patients present with the gradual onset of symptoms, suggesting a cerebellar lesion. They complain of occipital headache and vertigo. This is followed by nausea, vomiting, ipsilateral gaze palsy, peripheral facial paresis, and signs of cerebellar involvement including clumsiness and ataxia of the limbs and gait ataxia. The eyes may be deviated to the opposite side, and there is nystagmus maximal on attempting to look to the side of the lesion. Nuchal rigidity,

contralateral hemiparesis or hyperreflexia, and extensor plantar responses are occasional findings.[158]

Diagnostic Procedures

1. The blood count may reveal evidence of polycythemia in some cases due to bleeding from a hemangioblastoma.
2. Lumbar puncture will reveal the presence of subarachnoid hemorrhage in 90 per cent of cases.
3. Computed tomography permits rapid and accurate diagnosis of a cerebellar hemorrhage. The CT scan clearly demonstrates the size of the hematoma and the presence or absence of ventricular dilatation.[189]
4. Other studies such as arteriography or ventriculography are required only in the absence of facilities for computed tomography.

Treatment

Recovery from cerebellar hemorrhage is hastened by suboccipital craniotomy and drainage of the hematoma. There is an excellent recovery in many cases, with complete absence of or minimal neurologic disability. Because surgery offers the possibility of recovery in a potentially fatal disease, the early recognition and investigation of possible cases of cerebellar hemorrhage should be encouraged and every effort made to distinguish cases of cerebellar hemorrhage from the more frequent intracerebral hemorrhage.[140]

Rehabilitation of the Stroke Patient: General Considerations

The rehabilitation program should begin as early as possible in the treatment of the stroke patient. Passive movements of paralyzed limbs should be instituted twice daily, as well as measures to prevent the development of deformities in the affected limbs. As some function returns, turning from side to side and lifting the hips from the bed should be encouraged.

The patient should be taught to raise himself to a sitting position with support and to maintain balance unsupported. In the hemiplegic patient, this is accomplished by using the normal hand to grasp the weak arm and place it across the abdomen. The strong foot is then placed under the weak ankle, and both legs are moved to the side of the bed and then dangled over the side.

The patient then turns on his side, grasps the mattress, and pushes with his elbow and forearm until he comes to a sitting position. He then moves his hand to the rear to maintain his position. He should then be sitting on the edge of the bed with his feet on the floor.

Once he is able to sit without support, the patient should practice bending and trunk movements to increase stability. He is then ready to perform activities of self-care, including eating, brushing his teeth, shaving, washing, dressing, and undressing. When there is paresis of the upper limb, these activities should be accomplished using the weak hand as much as possible. However, they may still be accomplished using the nonaffected side in the presence of a total hemiplegia. In such cases, the patient should wear a hemiplegic sling whenever he is out of bed to support the paralyzed upper limb, preventing subluxation at the shoulder joint and traction on the cervical area.

The next logical step in the rehabilitation program of a hemiplegic is the development of mobility. These activities should begin under supervision but will eventually be performed independently. In these activities, the simple rule is that the noninvolved or strong side leads, which affords better control of movement. Usually this is begun with wheelchair mobility. When the patient is transferring from the bed to a wheelchair, the wheelchair is placed on the patient's nonparalyzed side facing the foot of the bed with the wheels locked and the footrests folded up. The patient then comes to a sitting position on the edge of the bed, leans forward, places the strong hand on the edge of the bed, and pushes up to a standing position, keeping the body weight over the strong lower limb. He then reaches for the farthest arm rest of the wheelchair with the strong hand, pivots on the strong leg, and comes to a sitting position in the wheelchair. The procedure is reversed in transferring from the wheelchair back into the bed. The procedure for getting out of a chair is performed by placing both feet firmly on the floor under the body, bending forward, raising up, and taking the weight on the unaffected lower limb.

Ambulation should be encouraged at an early stage unless there are contraindications such as acute myocardial infarction. In the initial stages, temporary splinting may be necessary, but when ankle instability persists, a short leg brace with double upright and spring assist for dorsiflexion may be necessary. If there is knee and ankle instability, a combination long-and-short leg brace may be used, with removal of the upper portion of the brace as knee stability improves.

Many patients tend to scrape the sole of the shoe on the affected side when walking, and the addition of a quarter-inch lift on the sole and heel of the shoe on the opposite side will usually correct this. Graded walking exercises are usually necessary using parallel bars, walkers, and canes as indicated by the progress of the patient. When walking upstairs, the hemiparetic patient should lead with the strong lower limb and then bring the weak limb up to the same step. A similar movement is made when walking up over a curb. On walking downstairs, the patient should be taught to lead with the weak lower limb and then bring the strong limb to the same step. Walking down over a curb, using a cane, is accomplished by placing the cane in the road with the toe on the strong side, extending over the edge of the curb. The weak lower limb is then placed in the road followed by the strong limb.

Skin Care and the Prevention of Bed Sores

Patients who have suffered a severe stroke or those with associated medical conditions that delay ambulation may be bedridden for some weeks, and the care of the skin is of the utmost importance. Turning the patient every two hours with strict insistence on a clean and dry bed is the best prophylaxis against the development of decubitus ulcers. However, the pressure points should be inspected every day, and the patient and the nursing staff should be instructed that movement and even slight changes of posture are helpful.

If areas become red without a break in the skin, turning should be designed to avoid all pressure until the inflammation subsides. Small breaks in the skin are given similar care but should be left exposed to the air as much as possible and treated by painting with merbromin (Mercurochrome) and exposure to ultraviolet light every day. If the area develops into an ulcer, without a necrotic center, bacteriostatic soaks should be applied for two hours twice a day and covered with plastic material to prevent rapid drying of the bacteriostatic agent. Ultraviolet light and Mercurochrome applications should be continued. Deeper areas with necrotic tissue should be treated by the application of proteolytic enzymes following the bacteriostatic soaks until all necrotic tissue has been removed. All dressings used between treatment should be sterile and of the nonadherent type.

Bladder and Bowel Training

Incontinence is not unusual in the early stages of an acute stroke. This may be due to stupor, coma, confusion, or involvement of the higher centers governing the bladder inhibition in the frontal lobe. Fortunately, control of bladder function is recovered in the majority of stroke patients if adequate bladder care is instituted and maintained in the acute phase. An indwelling (Foley) catheter is often needed in the early stages.

A distended bladder commonly causes restlessness and hypertension, while repeated incontinence with wet sheets accentuates the risk of decubitus ulcers. When a urinary catheter is used, however, it increases the risk of genitourinary infection. This can be reduced by irrigation at least twice a day with urinary antiseptics and the use of prophylactic oral sulfonamides. If infection occurs, culture and sensitivity tests should be obtained of the offending organism and the appropriate antibiotic given. When a catheter has been draining for 24 hours, it should be clamped and then drained at two-hour periods until it is removed. This prevents chronic contraction of the bladder secondary to continuous drainage.

As soon as there is improvement in the mental status, a decision should be made to remove the catheter. When this is done, a urinal or bedpan should be offered to the patient every two hours until control is reestablished. Aphasic patients should be encouraged to develop a system of signs to explain their needs, including the desire for a urinal. After control is established, the urinal or bedpan may be offered at less frequent intervals.

Care of bowel function and bowel training programs are also important. When coma persists for more than three or four days, a program of bowel evacuation using enemas every three days should be instituted. All patients with stroke who are bedridden should have a rectal examination every third day to detect impending fecal impaction. When a patient is conscious, a definite time for bowel movements should be aimed at, preferably after a meal. Glycerin or medicated suppositories may be used to assist in the development of regular bowel habits. Food should contain adequate bulk or have a mild laxative effect; e.g., whole-grain cereals, salads, prune juice, and an adequate fluid intake of 2,500 to 3,000 ml per day should be given. If laxatives are required, stool softeners and bulk laxatives are most effective.

Management of Language Disorders

The presence of dysphasia or dysarthria can be a serious disability following a stroke. The services of a speech pathologist, speech therapist, and speech clinic are most valuable if available; however, much can be done by the usually available medical and nursing personnel as well as the patient's family to help promote maximum return of speech function. It is important to talk to the patient whether he has motor or receptive dysphasia. He should hear speech frequently from conversation, radio, or television. When speaking to the patient, the speech should be slow, enunciation clear, and the choice of words simple.

When objects are handed to the patient, they should be named and he should be told their function. Drawing, copying, and tracing letters or geometric designs are also helpful. Since dysphasic patients fatigue easily, such activities should be short in duration, with adequate intervals of rest. This is also important in conversation, which should consist of a few questions or statements made at one time and a break before proceeding further. If dyslexia prevents reading, relatives should be encouraged to read mail, newspapers, and short stories to the patient. With perseverance, improvement may continue for months after the stroke.

Vocational Rehabilitation

Many patients who survive an acute stroke are able to return to useful work. Some require noncompetitive work in a sheltered workshop. Training programs should be a natural extension of a rehabilitation program, and the patient and his family should be guided toward the goal of a return to useful activity throughout the treatment period. At the appropriate time, the patient should be referred to a vocational rehabilitation program that provides counseling, placement, and retraining where necessary.

Inflammatory Disorders of Cerebral Arteries

The cerebral arteritides embrace a heterogenous group of diseases which have in common the presence of inflammation involving the cerebral arteries and perivascular tissues. A number of them, such as systemic lupus erythematosus and polyarteritis nodosa, have been classified as "collagen diseases"; others are rare conditions of unknown etiology.

Systemic Lupus Erythematosus

Many patients with systemic lupus erythematosus (SLE) develop symptoms due to involvement of the central or peripheral nervous system. The disease occurs predominantly in females (80 to 90 per cent) and usually develops during the third decade. It may terminate within a few weeks or run a chronic remitting course of many years' duration.[139]

Etiology and Pathology

The group of autoimmune "collagen diseases" includes systemic lupus erythematosus, in which there appears to be a diffuse fibrinoid degeneration of collagen. The factors involved in the development of an autoimmune state appear to be complex and possibly include exogenous and hereditary mechanisms.

The pathogenesis of the neurologic abnormalities in lupus erythematosus is ill-defined. Pathologic studies often reveal few abnormalities in the central nervous system. It is possible that an immune process occurs within the brain, spinal cord, and peripheral nerves, producing neurologic abnormalities. This is supported by the demonstration of deposits of gamma globulin in the choroid plexus and the demonstration of antibodies to DNA in the cerebrospinal fluid.[146]

Clinical Features

Patients with neurologic symptoms usually present with some of the general manifestations of SLE. The most common manifestation appears to be arthritis or arthralgia, which is likely to be present in more than 90 per cent of cases. There are often marked subjective complaints of arthralgia, with little objective change in the joints, or there may be migratory arthralgia with joint effusions. About 25 per cent develop chronic progressive arthropathy and deformity of the rheumatoid type. However, there is frequently more soft-tissue swelling of the fingers, hands, and wrists in systemic lupus erythematosus, and, in contrast to rheumatoid arthritis, the deformity may be mild despite years of arthritis.[36]

Myalgia is also common in systemic lupus erythematosus and may be diffuse and disabling with little evidence of muscle wasting. Other symptoms include fever, the skin changes of discoid lupus, generalized lymphadenopathy, anemia, gastrointestinal symptoms such as anorexia, nausea, and vomiting, pleurodynia and pleural effusions, and chest pain due to pericarditis and endocarditis.

Since the lesions in the nervous system are multifocal, almost any symptom may occur. "Psychiatric symptoms" are common but analysis shows that these symptoms are, in fact, those of an organic psychosis due to diffuse brain damage. Patients are often described as "confused" but probably have a combination of dysphasia, disorientation, and memory deficits.

Delirium with visual and auditory hallucinations may occur, anxiety and depression are not uncommon, and a "schizophrenia-like" psychosis has been reported. It is felt that these symptoms are due to organic changes in the brain, although the depression may be due to the emotional impact of a chronic debilitating disease.

Seizures are quite common in this condition, particularly in the more chronic cases. Hemiplegia, quadriparesis, and parkinsonian-like features may develop. Choreiform movements have been reported as the initial symptom in SLE and resemble Sydenham's chorea when they occur in younger patients. Involvement of the visual pathways can cause visual hallucinations, homonymous field defects and cortical blindness.

Brainstem involvement produces diplopia, nystagmus, dysarthria, and dysphagia. Acute transverse myelitis is a serious but fortunately unusual complication of this disease.[164] Signs of peripheral neuropathy occur in the majority of patients with neurologic symptoms of SLE. A myasthenia-like picture has been reported in a few cases. Subarachnoid hemorrhage is a rare complication of SLE.

Diagnostic Procedures

1. The blood count may show some degree of anemia. The sedimentation rate is usually elevated but may be normal.
2. Urinalysis frequently reveals pyuria and albuminuria. Renal involvement occurs in about 50 per cent of cases.
3. While abnormalities are common on serum protein electrophoresis, there are no specific changes in systemic lupus erythematosus, and an abnormal pattern is not necessary for the diagnosis.
4. The cerebrospinal fluid may show increased pressure, a mild pleocytosis with excess mono-

nuclear cells, and elevated protein content in about one third of the cases.
5. The fluorescent antinuclear antibody test is positive in almost all untreated patients with active SLE.
6. The LE cell test is positive in about 75 per cent of cases.
7. Antibodies against native DNA are specific for SLE and can be detected by a number of different methods.
8. Computed tomography may show the presence of enlargement of the cortical sulci with or without ventricular enlargement. Infarction or intracerebral hemorrhage can also be seen in some cases.[60a]

Treatment

The benefits of corticosteroid therapy have not been established in SLE although there have been reports of good results in some cases. Since long-term therapy is necessary, a single dose of oral steroid should be given once every 48 hours if steroid therapy is used. This regimen will tend to minimize the development of side effects. The initial dose of 128 mg methylprednisolone qod can be reduced as clinical improvement occurs.

Polyarteritis Nodosa

This, like systemic lupus erythematosus, is a collagen disease that involves the nervous system. It is less common than systemic lupus erythematosus, occurs in slightly older patients, usually in the fourth or fifth decades, and is more frequently encountered in males. Polyarteritis nodosa also tends to run a more acute course than systemic lupus erythematosus, and most patients die within a year, usually from renal failure.

Etiology and Pathology

The etiologic factors are unknown, but the disease is believed to represent an acute response to autoimmune antibodies with multifocal inflammatory lesions involving medium and small arteries throughout the body. The inflammatory response and necrosis of the arterial walls involve all layers, with destruction of the internal elastic lamina. This may be associated with thrombosis and focal infarction in the involved organ, aneurysm formation, or rupture of the vessel with hemorrhage. In the more chronic stages, there is healing, with the development of chronic granulation tissue in the vessel wall, and finally scar formation. One of the characteristics of polyarteritis nodosa is the tendency for acute and chronic lesions to appear in different arteries or in different segments of the same artery.

The arterial lesions produce multiple infarcts in the nervous system. Occasionally, a large infarct occurs when a major vessel such as the middle cerebral artery is occluded. The peripheral neuropathy is due to occlusion of the vasa nervorum. with infarction of peripheral nerves.

Clinical Features

Since polyarteritis nodosa may involve the arteries in any organ, the clinical signs are protean. General features include fever, skin rashes, subcutaneous nodules, and arthralgias and myalgia, particularly in the calves. Gastrointestinal symptoms include anorexia, weight loss, abdominal pain, nausea, and vomiting. There may be diffuse abdominal tenderness and hepatomegaly. Testicular pain and tenderness are not uncommon in the early stages, followed by testicular atrophy. Renal involvement results in hypertension and progressive renal impairment, which frequently is the cause of death.

Lesions of the peripheral nerves are the most common form of neurologic involvement and may present as a mononeuropathy, mononeuropathy multiplex, or symmetric peripheral neuropathy. Central nervous system involvement is usually a late occurrence but has been reported to occur in as many as 46 per cent of cases. The most frequent symptoms consist of headache, blurring of vision, and seizures. There may be organic mental symptoms including confusion, disorientation, intellectual deterioration, memory deficits, hallucinations, delusions, mania, or paranoia. The terminal stages may be marked by fluctuations in the level of consciousness preceding coma and death. Visual involvement produces blurring of vision, sudden unilateral visual loss, homonymous hemianopia, or quadrantanopia. The retina may show exudates, hemorrhages, and occlusion of retinal arteries with retinal infarction and papilledema. Infarction of the brainstem produces diplopia due to involvement of the third-, fifth-, or sixth-nerve nuclei, facial numbness, facial weakness, vertigo, dysarthria, or dysphagia. Motor symptoms include hemiparesis and choreiform movements. Cerebellar ataxia and nystagmus may occur owing to infarction of the cerebellum or cerebellar connections. Infarction of the spinal cord may give rise to anterior spinal artery syndromes with paraplegia and retention of vibration and position sense or central infarction mimicking syringomyelia.

Thrombosis of larger vessels such as the middle cerebral artery may occur in about 10 per cent of cases with the development of an acute stroke due to cerebral infarction. Other acute manifestations include the rapid development of hemiplegia and coma due to intracerebral hemorrhage and the occasional occurrence of subarachnoid hemorrhage.[50]

Diagnostic Procedures

1. The blood count shows anemia, leukocytosis, and an elevated sedimentation rate in the majority of cases.
2. Renal impairment produces albuminuria, with red cells, pyuria, and granular casts in the urine. There is a steady rise in the blood urea nitrogen level with progressive renal impairment.
3. Renal arteriograms show the presence of narrowing, obstruction, and arterial aneurysms in a high percentage of cases (Fig. 9–26).
4. The serum protein electrophoresis is frequently abnormal, with reversal of the albumin:globulin ratio and elevation of one or more of the globulin fractions.
5. Electrocardiographic abnormalities occur in at least 25 per cent of cases.
6. The cerebrospinal fluid may contain mononuclear cells and the protein content may be elevated.
7. The electroencephalogram is abnormal, with local slowing in the presence of large cerebral infarcts. Other patients may show diffuse slowing in the theta range without focal features.
8. Diagnosis depends on the demonstration of polyarteritis by biopsy. Involved tissue such as subcutaneous nodules may be removed for this purpose. If there are no known lesions other than in the nervous system, the highest percentage of positive biopsies have been reported from biopsies of the pectoralis major muscle.

Treatment

The use of corticosteroids in polyarteritis nodosa appears to be of benefit, particularly in those cases without evidence of renal involvement. Long-term therapy is usually required in the treatment of polyarteritis nodosa, and intermittent therapy as outlined for the treatment of systemic lupus erythematosus is recommended.

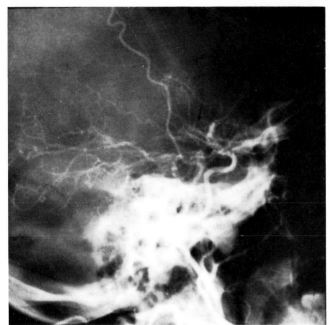

A

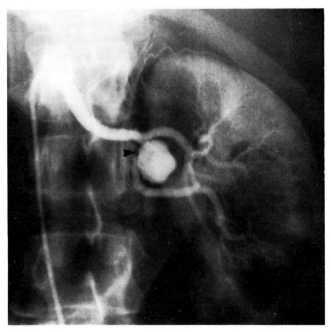

B

FIGURE 9–26. Arteriography in polyarteritis nodosa. The right carotid arteriogram *(A)* shows severe stenosis of the right internal carotid artery from its origin to termination. There is occlusion of the right middle cerebral artery with the development of a collateral circulation (arrow). The renal arteriogram *(B)* shows the presence of an aneurysm on one of the branches of the renal artery.

Polyarteritis with Respiratory Granuloma (Wegener's Granulomatosis, Allergic Granulomatosis)

This diffuse form of granulomatous angiitis differs from classic polyarteritis nodosa because of marked involvement of the respiratory system and a tendency to occur in younger individuals. The pathologic changes consist of a diffuse polyarteritis and the presence of necrotizing granulomas in the lungs and paranasal sinuses. Patients show many of the signs of polyarteritis nodosa with the addition of rhinitis, epistaxis, ulceration of the nasal septum, sinus pain, pulmonary infiltration, and eosinophilia. The neurologic signs are similar to those described in classic polyarteritis nodosa. The cerebrospinal fluid may show a monocytic pleocytosis with elevated protein and normal glucose content.

Treatment

The condition may respond to cyclophosphamide, 50 to 100 mg daily, and single-dose, alternate-day corticosteroid therapy.[6]

Granulomatous Giant Cell Angiitis

A rare but distinct form of angiitis has been described that affects the smaller leptomeningeal and parenchymal arteries of the central nervous system.[72, 123]

Etiology and Pathology

The etiology is unknown but some cases may result from viral or mycoplasma infection, and intranuclear virus-like particles have been identified in glial cells at autopsy.[153] The brain is covered by a gelatinous exudate lying in the subarachnoid space, and there may be some symmetric swelling of the hemispheres. Histologic examination shows that the gelatinous exudate extends deeply into the Virchow-Robin spaces where there is a protein-rich fluid containing some lymphocytes. The cerebral cortex and superficial areas of the brainstem and cerebellum contain numerous small irregular areas of infarction. The essential lesion appears to be a necrotizing angiitis affecting the smaller arteries of precapillary size. This permits the passage of a protein-rich fluid into the Virchow-Robin spaces. The affected vessels are surrounded by a cellular exudate containing lymphocytes and giant cells.

Clinical Features

The clinical picture is nonspecific and presents as a progressive neurologic illness with a headache, mental deterioration, and signs of diffuse involvement of the cerebral hemispheres, brainstem, and cerebellum. The duration varies from three days to two years.

Diagnostic Procedures

There are no specific laboratory tests. The cerebrospinal fluid may show slight elevation in pressure with an excess of mononuclear cells and moderate elevated protein content. The presence of giant cell granulomatous angiitis may be suspected in cases showing beading of the intracranial arteries at angiography.[23]

Treatment

The diagnosis has occasionally has been established during life by brain biopsy. Recovery has been reported following treatment with corticosteroids.[13a, 151]

Giant Cell Arteritis (Takayasu's Disease)

A number of diseases may produce narrowing of the aorta and its major branches, including syphilis, arteriosclerosis, medionecrosis, dissecting aneurysm, and polyarteritis nodosa. When any of these conditions involves the aortic arch, there may be narrowing of the ostia or extension into the major branches producing an aortic arch syndrome with cerebral ischemia and ischemia of the upper extremities.

Giant cell arteritis is another distinct pathologic condition that may produce an aortic arch syndrome, although it is now apparent that this form of panarteritis may involve any part of the aorta or any of its major branches and may extend into the proximal portions of the intracranial arteries. Giant cell arteritis was originally thought to occur almost exclusively in young Japanese women (in whom it is, indeed, relatively common), but it has now been recognized in many parts of the world and in both sexes. This has led to the use of a number of names for this disease, including Takayasu's arteritis. The synonym "pulseless disease" is an unfortunate name since it focuses attention on a late manifestation of this disease, which in its earlier stages is essentially an arteritis.[154, 155, 176]

Etiology and Pathology

Giant cell arteritis occurs predominantly in women and shows many similarities to lupus erythematosus. It is believed to belong to the group of autoimmune collagen diseases.

The aortic arch and its branches are commonly affected, but the process may also affect the proximal portions of the major aortocranial arteries and the celiac, renal, superior mesenteric, inferior mesenteric, and iliac and femoral arteries.[63] There is irregular segmental thickening, and narrowing of the involved arteries and thrombosis may occur. In the acute phase the changes are those of a panarteritis with inflammatory cells, including lymphocytes, plasma cells, and occasional giant cells. Inflammation is followed by a marked proliferation of collagen and the replacement of the elastic tissue and muscle in the intima, media, and adventitia by thick, concentric layers of fibrous tissue. Fibrosis results in irregular narrowing of the affected arteries, with occlusion by thrombosis.

Clinical Features

Early Systemic Phase. Many patients complain of pain and stiffness in the proximal muscles of both upper and lower limbs. These symptoms may be abrupt or gradual in onset and are associated with fever, anorexia, weight loss, and depression. There may also be swelling of the joints, and some patients develop changes resembling rheumatoid arthritis. This syndrome of polymyalgia rheumatica[133] may last from a few weeks to three or more years and resolve spontaneously, or the patient may develop signs of the late phase of giant cell arteritis.

Late Phase. The late manifestations depend on the extent and site of aortic involvement. When the proximal part of the aortic arch is involved, there may be narrowing of the coronary ostia, angina pectoris, and myocardial infarction. Aortic insufficiency may follow the spread of the arteritis proximally into the aortic valve cusps. Narrowing of the ostia of the renal arteries may result in chronic hypertension.

Abdominal complaints including infarction of the bowel and intestinal hemorrhage may occur if there is occlusion of the celiac or mesenteric arteries. Intermittent claudication and reduction or loss of the pulses in the lower limbs are characteristic of giant cell arteritis of the iliac and femoral arteries. Similar involvement of the subclavian arteries results in Raynaud's syndrome, pain in the upper extremities, and loss of the radial and brachial pulses.

The neurologic symptoms associated with giant cell arteritis are due to narrowing or thrombosis of the cervical arteries or the proximal portions of the main intracranial arteries. Reduction in blood flow results in symptoms of carotid or vertebral basilar insufficiency in a relatively young person, usually a female. This is eventually followed by cerebral infarction and recurrent strokes.

Diagnostic Procedures

There is an elevation of the erythrocyte sedimentation rate and an abnormal serum protein electrophoretic pattern. Chest roentgenograms may reveal notching of the ribs due to the pressure of hypertrophied collateral vessels. The diagnosis may be suspected if arteriography shows irregular narrowing of the aorta and similar narrowing or occlusion of its major branches with a well-developed collateral circulation.[87] Confirmation can be obtained by biopsy of an involved artery.

Treatment

Steroid therapy may arrest the course of the disease and should be given in sufficient dosage to restore and keep the sedimentation rate normal. Stenotic lesions in major vessels can be removed and replaced by arterial grafts or treated by the insertion of a bypass.

Temporal Arteritis

The original concept that temporal arteritis is a localized inflammation exclusively affecting the superficial temporal artery or the superficial temporal and ophthalmic arteries is now known to be inaccurate.

The disease is one form of giant cell arteritis which occurs predominantly in the elderly and is therefore a systemic disease.

Etiology and Pathology

The changes in temporal arteritis have all of the features of giant cell arteritis with the changes occurring predominantly in the superficial temporal artery and in the vertebral, ophthalmic, and posterior ciliary arteries. The internal carotid, external carotid, and central retinal arteries are less commonly involved, and the intracranial arteries are spared.[196]

The arteritis affects the intima and media. The intima is infiltrated with lymphocytes and plasma cells. The internal elastic lamina is fragmented, and there is a marked proliferation of fibroblasts and almost complete obliteration of the vessel lumen. A similar inflammatory reaction occurs in the media, with degeneration of the muscle, increase in collagen, and infiltration with lymphocytes, plasma cells, and numerous multinucleated giant cells.

Clinical Features

The disease affects both sexes equally and usually begins after the age of 60. Some patients experience vague symptoms of a systemic disturbance prior to the development of temporal arteritis. Temporal arteritis may masquerade as polymyalgia rheumatica for months or years until the diagnosis is finally established.[89] In other cases, however, the onset is sudden in a previous well individual.

The salient symptoms are headache and visual changes.[26] The headache is severe and classically bitemporal and may be severe enough to interrupt sleep. The scalp over the superficial temporal artery and its branches is exquisitely tender, often with palpable subcutaneous nodules and inflammation of the overlying skin (Fig. 9–27). The pa-

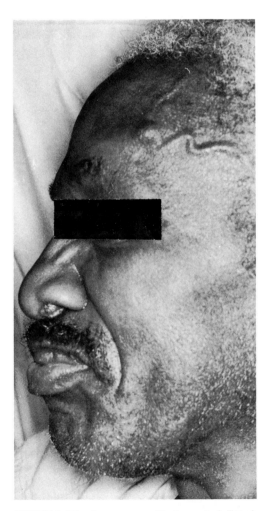

FIGURE 9–27. Appearance of tortuous and dilated temporal arteritis. This patient suffered from headaches that were relieved by surgical excision of the superficial temporal artery. Treatment with oral steroids also provides relief and resolution of the inflammatory swelling of the cranial arteries in temporal arteritis.

tient cannot lie on the affected side or tolerate any pressure on the area. Movement of the temporalis muscle in chewing may be extremely painful. Gentle palpation reveals hard, tender nodular superficial temporal and occipital arteries, often with absence of pulsation.

Involvement of the ophthalmic artery and its branches, including the retinal and posterior ciliary arteries, occurs in about 50 per cent of cases, producing transient blurring of vision or blindness. This may lead to permanent loss of vision in the affected eye. About 25 per cent of patients developed blindness in both eyes before steroid therapy became available. There are white, fluffy exudates and occasional hemorrhages in the retina in the early stages, with occlusion of one or more retinal arteries.

Occasionally, the appearance is that of occlusion of the central retinal artery. The optic disk is edematous initially due to ischemic damage to the optic nerve, and this is followed by optic atrophy. A number of patients experience diplopia, probably due to ischemic necrosis of extraocular muscles.[10]

Patients with temporal arteritis may show other manifestations of giant cell arteritis including myocardial infarction due to involvement of the coronary arteries, signs and symptoms of carotid artery insufficiency, or an aortic arch syndrome when there is more diffuse involvement of the aorta and its major branches. Many patients with temporal arteritis have murmurs on auscultation over the carotid, subclavian, and femoral arteries.

Diagnostic Procedures

The majority of patients have a mild leukocytosis, hypochromic anemia, elevation of the erythrocytic sedimentation rate, and the antinuclear antibody titer may be increased. There is an increase in alpha-2-globulin, decrease in albumin, and occasional increase in gamma globulin on serum protein electrophoresis. The diagnosis may be established by biopsy of the superficial temporal artery, which also has the advantage of relieving pain in many patients. Since the arteritis is segmental, a fairly long segment of the vessel should be obtained to avoid inadvertent biopsy of a normal area. Arteriography may show stenosis of the carotid arteries or the branches of the major vessels at the aortic arch, and in one of our cases the diagnosis was confirmed from the biopsy material obtained during carotid endarterectomy.

Treatment

The dramatic response to steroid therapy is most gratifying in this disease, and symptoms frequently resolve in a matter of hours.[115] Use of intermittent oral steroid therapy is advised, with gradual withdrawal over a period of several months when the sedimentation rate is normal. A number of cases show signs of recurrence and can be controlled promptly by the resumption of steroids.

Thrombotic Thrombocytopenic Purpura (Thrombotic Microangiopathy)

There is a close pathologic relationship between this condition and lupus erythematosus, but the clinical features of thrombotic microangiopathy or multiple platelet thromboses are so unique that it can be classified as a separate entity.

Pathology

The essential lesion appears to be a fibrinoid degeneration of the subintimal tissues in smaller blood vessels. The lesions occur in many organs, including the liver, kidney, heart, and brain, where there is presumably a release of activator substances with the formation of multiple platelet thrombi.

The brain may have a normal appearance or show numerous petechiae. Microscopic examination shows fibrinoid degeneration of subintimal tissue with hyperplasia of the endothelium and occlusion of vessels by platelet thrombi. Small-vessel occlusion results in numerous foci of neuronal damage and glial proliferation.

Clinical Features

The essential features of thrombotic microangiopathy include fever, purpura, hemolytic anemia, thrombocytopenia, microscopic hematuria, and signs of multifocal neurologic involvement. Neurologic signs include headache, intellectual deterioration, seizures, hemiparesis, dysphasia, dysarthria, visual deterioration, and cranial nerve palsies. These signs tend to wax and wane with the appearance of new features at irregular intervals over a period of several weeks. The course is progressive and the outcome fatal. Occasionally, there may be abrupt termination owing to a massive intracerebral hemorrhage.

Diagnostic Procedures

Hemolytic anemia, with numerous irregularly contracted red cells, thrombocytopenia, and microscopic hematuria are usually present and should arouse suspicion of thrombotic microangiopathy in an obscure neurologic illness with multiple levels of involvement.

Treatment

There is no description of successful treatment to date, but the lack of therapeutic endeavor may be related to the rarity of diagnosis during life. Should the diagnosis be established, a trial with high doses of corticosteroids would seem to be worthwhile in view of the belief that the condition may also be a variant of a basic "collagen" disease. Treatment with heparin, anticoagulants, and platelet inhibitors (e.g., sulfinpyrazone) may be of help.[3]

Infarction of the Spinal Cord

Although uncommon, infarction of the spinal cord is occasionally encountered and may arise spontaneously or as a complication of vascular surgery of the aorta.

Arteriosclerotic changes involving the arteries of the spinal cord usually do not reach the severity of those seen in the cerebral vessels. They are generally absent in the first three decades of life, are mild in the fourth and fifth decades, but may become more prominent in the elderly. Atheromatous plaques occur in less than 3 per cent of elderly patients, and arteriosclerotic changes tend to be more extensive in the posterior spinal arteries than in the anterior spinal vessels in this age group.[7, 79, 102]

Infarction of the spinal cord was originally considered to be invariably due to vascular disease of the intrinsic vessels of the cord and meninges, but now more emphasis is placed on disease of the extrinsic cord vessels such as the artery of Adamkiewicz and the major segmental radicular arteries supplying the cord.[42, 70, 197]

Anatomic Considerations

There are considerable anatomic variations in the blood supply to the spinal cord.[102] The anterior spinal artery receives between three and ten radicular branches from both the right and left sides in its course from the foramen magnum to its termination over the filum terminale. The levels of the anastomoses are unpredictable, as is the size of the collateral vessels. However, in the cervical region, the major anterior radicular arteries are most frequently found in the level of

C_3 or C_6 segments. In the thoracic region, T_3, T_4, T_8, or T_9 is usually the site of major radicular arteries whereas the lumbar segments usually receive one other major radicular artery whose level of entry varies. This major artery is usually called the artery of Adamkiewicz. The posterior spinal artery receives a larger number of posterior radicular arteries at numerous segmental levels in their passage down and behind spinal cord.

Etiology and Pathology

Infarction of the spinal cord may be due to involvement of extrinsic vessels, intrinsic vessels, or both.[7, 42, 53, 70, 76, 79, 91, 102, 197]

Involvement of Extrinsic Vessels. This occurs in the following conditions:

1. Aortic aneurysm with occlusion of the origin of the intercostal or lumbar arteries.
2. Thrombosis of the distal aorta.
3. Erosion of atheromatous plaques in the severely arteriosclerotic aorta with repeated embolization.[91]
4. During surgical grafting of aortic aneurysms or following surgical ligation of intercostal or lumbar arteries supplying the cord.
5. Dissecting aneurysm of the aorta with occlusion of intercostal or lumbar arteries.
6. Coarctation of the aorta.
7. Vertebral artery thrombosis with loss of flow through radicular arteries.

Involvement of Both Extrinsic and Intrinsic Vessels. This occurs in the following conditions:

1. Following abdominal aortography.
2. Myocardial infarction with a severe hypotensive episode.
3. Adams-Stokes syndrome with temporary circulating arrest.
4. Emboli arising from cardiac tumors: fibrin emboli from myxoma of the heart.
5. Heroin addiction: "transverse myelopathy," possibly due to spasm of extrinsic or intrinsic arteries.
6. Use of certain drugs therapeutically, such as sulfonamides and arsenicals.
7. Radiation myelopathy: arteritis and fibrosis of extrinsic and/or intrinsic arteries.

Involvement of Intrinsic Vessels. This occurs in thrombosis of anterior or posterior spinal arteries in syphilitic arteritis, diabetes mellitus with arteriosclerosis, or one of the rare arteritides associated with a collagen disease such as polyarteritis nodosa and lupus erythematosus.[145, 165]

Other Considerations. The resulting infarct may involve the entire territory of the anterior spinal artery, which covers the anterior three quarters of the spinal cord but spares the posterior columns. The posterior columns are likely to be involved when infarction occurs in the area supplied by the posterior spinal artery.

Destruction of the complete area of vascular supply, is, however, uncommon, and the extent of the infarction depends on the efficiency of the collateral circulation between the anterior and posterior spinal arteries. An infarct may develop in the "watershed area" between the two circulations in much the same manner as described in the development of infarction in the cerebral hemispheres. In the spinal cord, this results in softening of an intermediate zone involving the central portion of the spinal cord including the posterior portion of the anterior horn and the lateral white funiculus. Finally, patients who are hypertensive and arteriosclerotic may develop focal areas of softening or lacunae in the gray matter of the cord analogous to the lacunae that occur in the gray matter of the cerebral hemispheres.

Clinical Features

A large infarction of the spinal cord produces a flaccid paralysis below the level of the lesion with loss of deep tendon reflexes. There is acute retention of urine and loss of pain and temperature sensation below the level of the lesion. Touch, vibration, and position sense are retained. The prognosis for recovery is poor unless substantial improvement occurs within 24 hours.[67] If the infarction is incomplete, the flaccid state is followed by the gradual development of spastic paraparesis or quadriparesis, according to the level of the lesion, with hyperreflexia and bilateral extensor plantar responses. Bladder function may show partial recovery with some return of pain and temperature sensation.

Intermediate-zone softening presents with flaccid paralysis below the level of the lesion, retention of urine, and loss of pain and temperature sensation with a sharp line of demarcation at the level of the infarct. The degree of recovery is, however, often good, with good return of motor function and bladder control in the presence of hyperreflexia and extensor plantar responses.

The clinical picture associated with lacunar infarction of the spinal cord tends to be more chronic, with muscle wasting and fasciculations due to destruction of anterior horn cells and progressive spastic paraparesis with hyperreflexia and extensor plantar responses. This is particularly common in diabetics and syphilitics with infarction of the lumbosacral cord. Sensation may be normal and the resemblance to amyotrophic lateral sclerosis may be striking, particularly the chronic progressive course of the disease.

Infarction of one posterior column produces numbness and paresthesias below the level of the lesion, with loss of vibration and position sense. If both posterior columns are involved, there will be hypotonia, hyporeflexia, and severe ataxia in addition to the sensory loss.

Treatment

The general principles outlined under treatment of the acute stroke may be applied where appropriate to spinal cord infarction. There is usually generalized arteriosclerosis, which requires full investigation and treatment to prevent further episodes and progressive disability. Sympathectomy and peripheral vasodilator drugs may increase the collateral circulation to the ischemic cord. If the aorta is dissected or occluded, endarterectomy may be successful in restoring the flow. Rehabilitative measures may help to promote return of function in many cases once the initial state of flaccid weakness begins to resolve. It should be recognized that flaccid paraparesis may persist for many weeks, during which period good nursing care and the prevention of bed sores and urinary tract infection are paramount for the survival and ultimate recovery of the patient. Rehabilitation and physical therapy should be started as soon as the general condition of the patient permits.

Cited References

1. Adams, C. B. T.; Loach, A. B.; and L'Laoire, S. A. Intracranial aneurysms: Analysis of results of microneurosurgery. *Br. Med. J.,* **2:**607–609, 1976.
2. Adams, G. F.; Merritt, J. D.; et al. Cerebral embolism and mitral stenosis: Survival with and without anticoagulants. *J. Neurol. Neurosurg. Psychiat.,* **37:**378–83, 1974.
2a. Acosta-Rua, G. J. Familial incidence of ruptured intracranial aneurysms. *Arch. Neurol.,* **35:**675–77, 1978.
3. Amir, J., and Krauss, S. Treatment of thrombotic thrombocytopenia purpura with antiplatelet drugs. *Blood,* **42:**27–33, 1973.
4. Aoyagi, M.; Meyer, J. S.; et al. Central cholinergic control of cerebral blood flow in the baboon. *J. Neurosurg.,* **43:**676–88, 1975.
5. Astrup, J.; Symons, L.; et al. Cortical evoked potentials and extracellular K+ and H+ at cortical levels of brain ischemia. *Stroke,* **8:**51–57, 1977.
6. Atcheson, S. V., and Van Horn, G. Subacute meningitis heralding a diffuse granulomatous angiitis (Wegener's granulomatosis). *Neurology* (Minneap.), **27:**262–64, 1977.
7. Bailey, A. A. Changes with age in spinal cord. *Arch. Neurol. Psychiat.,* **70:**299–309, 1953.
8. Baker, R. N.; Schwartz, W. S.; and Ramseyer, J. C. Prognosis among survivors of ischemic stroke. *Neurology* (Minneap.), **18:**933–41, 1968.
9. Barnett, H. J. M.; Jones, M. W.; et al. Cerebral ischemic events associated with prolapsing mitral valve. *Arch. Neurol.,* **33:**777–82, 1976.
10. Barricks, M. E.; Travieser, D. B.; et al. Ophthalmoplegia in cranial arteritis. *Brain,* **100:**209–22, 1977.
11. Battacharji, S. K.; Hutchinson, E. C.; and McCall, A. J. The circle of Willis—the incidence of developmental abnormalities in normal and infarcted brains. *Brain,* **90:**747–58, 1967.
12. Bauer, R. B.; Gilroy, J.; and Meyer, J. S. A controlled study of surgical treatment of cerebrovascular disease. *Neurology* (Minneap.), **14:**257, 1964.
13. Bauer, R. B., and Tellez, H. Dexamethasone as treatment in cerebrovascular disease. 2. Controlled study in acute cerebral infarction. *Stroke,* **4:**547–55, 1973.
13a. Beresford, H. R.; Hyman, R. A.; and Sharer, L. Self-limiting granulomatous angiitis of the cerebellum. *Ann. Neurol.,* **5:**490–92, 1979.
14. Bergstrom, M.; Ericson, K.; et al. Variations with time of the attenuation values of intracranial hematomas. *J. Computer Assisted Tomogr.,* **1:**57–63, 1977.
15. Birkhead, N. C.; Wagener, H. P.; and Schick, R. M. Treatment of temporal arteritis with adrenal corticosteroids; results in fifty-five cases in which lesion was proved at biopsy. *J.A.M.A.,* **103:**821–27, 1957.
16. Blackwell, E.; Merory, J.; et al. Doppler ultrasound scanning of the carotid bifurcation. *Arch. Neurol.,* **34:**145–48, 1977.
17. Bolwig, T. G. Transient global amnesia. *Acta Neurol. Scand.,* **44:**101–106, 1968.
18. Bone, G. E., and Barnes, R. W. Limitations of Doppler cerebrovascular examination in hemispheric cerebral ischemia. *Surgery,* **79:**577–80, 1976.
19. Brown, M., and Glassenberg, M. Mortality factors in patients with acute stroke. *J.A.M.A.,* **224:**1493–95, 1973.
20. Brust, J. C. M. Transient ischemic attacks: Natural history and anticoagulation. *Neurology* (Minneap.), **8:**701–707, 1977.
21. Burber, B. J.; Martin, J. S.; and Rapela, C. E. Analysis of the effect of bilateral sympathetic

stimulation on cerebral and cephalic blood flow in the dog. *Stroke,* 9:29–34, 1978.

22. Burger, P. C.; Burch, J. G.; and Kunze, U. Subcortical arteriosclerotic encephalopathy (Binswanger disease). A vascular etiology of dementia. *Stroke,* 7:626–31, 1976.

23. Burger, P. C.; Burch, J. G.; and Vogel, F. S. Granulomatous angiitis. An unusual etiology of stroke. *Stroke,* 8:29–35, 1977.

23a. Canadian Cooperative Study Group. A randomized trial of aspirin and sulfinpyrazone in treated stroke. *N. Engl. J. Med.,* 299:53–59, 1978.

23b. Caplan, L. R., and Schoene, W. C. Clinical features of subcortical arteriosclerotic encephalopathy (Binswanger disease). *Neurology* (Minneap.), 28:1206–15, 1978.

23c. Chandra, B. *Ann. Neurol.,* 3:502–504, 1978.

24. Chater, N. Patient selection and results of extra to intracranial anastomosis in selected cases of cerebrovascular disease. *Clin. Neurosurg.,* 23:287–309, 1976.

25. Cole, F. M., and Yates, P. Intracerebral microaneurysms and small cerebrovascular lesions. *Brain,* 90:759–67, 1967.

26. Compton, M. R. The visual changes in temporal (giant-cell) arteritis; report of a case with autopsy findings. *Brain,* 82:377–90, 1959.

27. Compton, M. R. Cerebral infarction following the rupture of cerebral berry aneurysm. *Brain,* 87:263–80, 1964.

28. Couch, J. R., and Hassanein, R. S. Platelet aggregation: Stroke and transient ischemic attacks in middle aged and elderly patients. *Neurology* (Minneap.), 26:888–95, 1976.

29. DeLong, W. B. Diagnostic pitfalls of subarachnoid hemorrhage from intracranial aneurysms. *West. J. Med.,* 123:92–100, 1975.

30. Devereaux, M. W.; Keane, J. R.; and Davis, R. L. Automatic respiratory failure associated with infarction of the medulla: Report of two cases with pathologic study of one. *Arch. Neurol.,* 29:46–52, 1973.

31. Dimant, J., and Grob, D. Electrocardiographic changes and myocardial damage in patients with acute cerebrovascular accidents. *Stroke,* 8:448–55, 1977.

32. Djindjian, R. Embolization of angiomas of the spinal cord. *Surg. Neurol.,* 4:411–20, 1975.

33. Djinddjian, R. Superselective internal carotid arteriography and embolization. *Neuroradiology,* 9:145–56, 1975.

34. Drake, C. G. Ligation of the vertebral (unilateral or bilateral) or basilar artery in the treatment of large intracranial aneurysms. *J. Neurosurg.,* 43:255–74, 1975.

35. Drake, C. G., and Allcock, J. M. Postoperative angiography and the "slipped" clip. *J. Neurosurg.,* 39:683–89, 1973.

36. Dubois, E. L., and Tuffanelli, D. L. Clinical manifestations of systemic lupus erythematosus. *J.A.M.A.,* 190:104–11, 1964.

37. Duncan, G. W.; Parker, S. W.; and Fisher, C. M. Acute cerebellar infarction in the PICA territory. *Arch. Neurol.,* 32:364–68, 1975.

38. Dyken, M. L.; Klatte, E.; et al. Complete occlusion of common or internal carotid arteries: Clinical significance. *Arch. Neurol.,* 30:343–46, 1974.

39. Escourelle, R.; DerAgopian, P.; et al. Bulbar infarctions. Study of vascular lesions in 26 patients. *J. Neurol. Sci.,* 28:103–13, 1976.

40. Ettinger, M. G.; Kusonoki, R.; and Fujishima, H. Coagulation studies in cerebrovascular disease. II. Cooperative study of stroke patients in Minnesota and Japan; preliminary communication. *Neurology* (Minneap.), 17:797–801, 1967.

40a. Faught, E.; Trader, S. D.; and Hanna, G. R. Cerebral complications of angiography for transient ischemia and stroke. Prediction of risk. *Neurology* (Minneap.), 29:4–15, 1979.

41. Fields, W. S.; Ratinov, G.; Weibel, J.; and Campos, R. J. Survival following basilar artery occlusion. *Arch. Neurol.,* 15:463–71, 1966.

42. Fieschi, C.; Gottlieb, A.; and DeCarolis, V. Ischemic lacunae in the spinal cord of arteriosclerotic subjects. *J. Neurol. Neurosurg. Psychiat.,* 33:138–46, 1970.

43. Fisher, C. M. Pure sensory stroke involving face, arm and leg. *Neurology* (Minneap.), 15:76–80, 1965.

44. Fisher, C. M. A lacunar stroke; the dysarthria-clumsy hand syndrome. *Neurology* (Minneap.), 17:614–17, 1967.

45. Fisher, C. M., and Adams, R. D. Transient global amnesia. *Acta Neurol. Scand.,* 40:suppl 9:1–83, 1964.

46. Fisher, C. M.; Karnes, W. E.; and Kubik, C. S. Lateral medullary infarction—the pattern of vascular occlusion. *J. Neuropath. Exp. Neurol.,* 20:323–79, 1961.

47. Fisher, C. M., and Pearlman, A. Nonsudden onset of cerebral embolism. *Neurology* (Minneap.), 17:1025–32, 1967.

47a. Fisher, C. M. Capsular infarcts. The underlying vascular lesions. *Arch. Neurol.,* 36:65–73, 1978.

47b. Fisher, C. M. Thalamic pure sensory stroke. A pathologic study. *Neurology* (Minneap.), 28:1141–44, 1978.

48. Fogelholm, R., and Allo, K. Ischemic cerebrovascular disease in young adults. *Acta Neurol. Scand.,* 49:415–33, 1973.

49. Fogelholm, R., and Aho, K. Characteristics and survival of patients with brain stem infarction. *Stroke,* 6:328–33, 1975.

50. Ford, R. G., and Siekert, R. G. Central nervous system manifestations of periarteritis nodosa. *Neurology* (Minneap.), 15:114–22, 1965.

51. Friedman, G. D.; Wilson, W. S.; et al. Transient ischemic attacks in a community. *J.A.M.A.,* 210:1428–34, 1969.

52. Gado, M. H.; Coleman, R. E.; et al. Comparison of computerized tomography and radionuclide imaging in "stroke." *Stroke,* 7:109–13, 1976.

53. Garland, H.; Greenberg, J.; and Harriman, D. G. F. Infarction of the spinal cord. *Brain,* 89:645–62, 1966.

54. Gaston, L. W.; Brooks, J. E.; et al. A study of blood coagulation following an acute stroke. *Stroke,* 2:81–87, 1971.

55. Gilroy, J.; Andaya, L.; and Thomas V. J. Intercranial aneurysms and subacute bacterial endocarditis. *Neurology* (Minneap.), **23:**1193–98, 1973.

56. Gilroy, J.; Lynn, G. E.; et al. Auditory evoked brainstem potentials in a case of "locked-in" syndrome. *Arch. Neurol.,* **34:**492–95, 1977.

57. Gilroy, J., and Meyer, J. S. Auscultation of the neck in occlusive cerebrovascular disease. *Circulation,* **25:**300–10, 1962.

58. Gilsanz, V.; Rebollar, J. L.; et al. Controlled trial of glycerol dexamethone in the treatment of cerebral edema in acute cerebral infarction. *Lancet,* **1:**1049–51, 1975.

59. Goldberg, A. D.; Raftery, E. B.; and Cashman, P. M. M. Ambulatory electrocardiographic records in patients with transient cerebral attacks or palpitation. *Br. Med. J.,* **4:**569–71, 1975.

60. Gomez, M. R.; Whitten, C.; Nolke, A.; Bernstein, J.; and Meyer, J. S. Aneurysmal malformation of the great vein of Galen causing heart failure in early infancy; report of 5 cases. *Pediatrics,* **31:**400–11, 1963.

60a. Gonzales-Scarano, F.; Lisak, R. P.; et al. Cranial computed tomography in the diagnosis of systemic lupus erythematosus. *Ann. Neurol.,* **5:**158–65, 1979.

61. Gotoh, F.; Tazaki, Y.; and Meyer, J. S. Transport of gases through brain and their extravascular vasomotor action. *Exp. Neurol.,* **4:**48–58, 1961.

62. Hackinsky, V. C.; Lassen, N. A.; and Marshall, J. Multi-infarct dementia. A cause of mental deterioration in the elderly. *Lancet.,* **2:**207–10, 1974.

63. Hamilton, C. R.; Shelley, W. M.; and Tummulty, P. A. Giant cell arteritis: Including temporal arteritis and polymyalgia rheumatism. *Medicine,* **50:**1–27, 1971.

64. Handa, J.; Handa, H.; et al. Serial brain scanning with radioactive xenon and scintillation camera. *Am. J. Roentgenol.,* **109:**701–706, 1970.

64a. Hanus, S. H.; Homer, T. D.; and Harper D. H. Vertebral artery occlusion complicating yoga exercises. *Arch. Neurol.,* **34:**574–75, 1977.

65. Harper, A. M.; Deshmukh, V. D.; et al. The influence of sympathetic nervous activity on cerebral blood flow. *Arch. Neurol.,* **27:**1–6, 1972.

66. Henderson, W. G.; Torner, J. C.; and Nibbelink, D. W. Intracranical aneurysms and subarachnoid hemorrhage—report on a randomized treatment study IVB regulated bed rest statistical examination. *Stroke,* **8:**579–89, 1977.

67. Henson, R. A., and Parsons, M. Ischemic lesions of the spinal cord. An illustrated review. *Q. J. Med.,* **36:**205–22, 1967.

68. Hernandez, M. J.; Brennan, R. W.; and Bowman, G. S. Cerebral blood flow autoregulation in the rat. *Stroke,* **9:**150–55, 1978.

69. Hernandez-Perez, M. J.; Raichle, M. E.; and Stone, H. L. The role of the sympathetic nervous system on cerebral blood flow autoregulation. *Stroke,* **6:**284–92, 1975.

70. Herrick, M. K., and Mills, P. E., Jr. Infarction of spinal cord. Two cases of selective gray matter involvement secondary to asymptomatic aortic disease. *Arch. Neurol.,* **24:**228–41, 1971.

71. Hsieh, H. H. Cerebrovascular disease; comparative study of cerebral and visceral arteries. *Neurology* (Minneap.), **17:**752–62, 1967.

72. Hughes, J. T., and Brownell, B. Granulomatous giant-celled angiitis of the central nervous system. *Neurology* (Minneap.), **16:**293–98, 1966.

73. Hugosson, R. Value of reinforcing intracranial aneurysms with plastic coating. *Acta Chir. Scand.,* **141:**182–86, 1975.

74. Hugosson, R., and Hogstrom, S. Factors disposing to morbidity in surgery of intracranial aneurysms with special regard to deep controlled hypothermia. *J. Neurosurg.,* **38:**561–67, 1973.

75. Hunt, W. E. Prompt surgery reduces cerebral aneurysm deaths. *J.A.M.A.,* **229:**255–59, 1974.

76. Infarction of the spinal cord (editorial). *Lancet,* **2:**143–44, 1967.

77. Itakura, T.; Yamamoto, K.; et al. Central dual innervation of arterioles and capillaries in the brain. *Stroke,* **8:**360–65, 1977.

78. Iwayama. T.; Furness, J. B.; and Burnstock, G. Dual adrenergic and cholinergic innervation of the cerebral arteries of the rat. *Circ. Res.,* **26:**635–46, 1970.

79. Jellinger, K. Spinal cord arteriosclerosis and progressive vascular myelopathy. *J. Neurol. Neurosurg. Psychiat.,* **30:**195–206, 1967.

80. Kak, U. F.; Taylor, A. R.; and Gordon, D. S. Proximal carotid ligation for internal carotid aneurysms. Long-term followup study. *J. Neurosurg.,* **39:**503–13, 1973.

81. Kalendovsky, Z.; Austin, J.; and Steele, P. Increased platelet aggregability in young patients with stroke: Diagnosis and therapy. *Arch. Neurol.,* **32:**13–20, 1975.

82. Kaufman, D. M., and Jabaddor, K. Intracranial surgery for cerebral artery aneurysm—five year experience *J.A.M.A.,* **236:**1707–10, 1976.

83. Kemper, T. L., and Romanul, F. C. A. State resembling akinetic mutism in basilar artery occlusion. *Neurology* (Minneap.), **17:**74–80, 1967.

84. Kerber, C. W.; Margolis, M. T.; and Newton, T. H. Tortuous vertebrobasilar system: A cause of cranial nerve signs. *Neuroradiology,* **4:**74–77, 1972.

85. Kinkel, W. R., and Jacobs, L. Computerized axial transverse tomography in cerebrovascular disease. *Neurology* (Minneap.), **26:**924–30, 1976.

86. Klassen, A. C.; Loewenson, R. B.; and Resch, J. A. Body weight cerebral athersclerosis and cerebral vascular disease. Autopsy study. *Stroke,* **5:**312–17, 1974.

87. Klein, R. G.; Hunder, G. G.; et al. Large artery involvement in giant cell (temporal) arteritis. *Ann. Intern. Med.,* **83:**806–12, 1975.

88. Kobayashi, S.; Waltz, A. G.; and Rhoton, A. L., Jr. Effects of stimulation of cervical sympathetic nerves on cortical blood flow and vascular reactivity. *Neurology* (Minneap.), **21:**297–302, 1971.

89. Kogstad, O. A. Polymyalgia rheumatica and its

relation to arteritis temporalis. *Acta Med. Scand.,* **178:**591–98, 1965.

90. Kottke, B. A., and Subbiah, M. T. R. Pathogenesis of atherosclerosis. Concepts based on animal models. *Mayo Clin. Proc.,* **53:**35–48, 1978.

91. Laguna, J., and Cravioto, H. Spinal cord infarction secondary to occlusion of the anterior spinal artery. *Arch. Neurol.,* **28:**134–36, 1973.

92. Landan, B., and Ransohoff, J. Prolonged cerebral vasospasm in experimental subarachnoid hemorrhage. *Neurology* (Minneap.), **18:**1056–65, 1968.

93. Larsson, O.; Marinovich, N.; and Barber K. Double blind trial of glycerol therapy in early stroke. *Lancet,* **1:**832–34, 1976.

94. Lassen, N. A. Cerebral blood flow and oxygen consumption in man. *Physiol. Rev.,* **39:**183–238, 1959.

95. Lee, M. C.; Heaney, L. M.; et al. Cerebrospinal fluid in cerebral hemorrhage and infarction. *Stroke,* **6:**638–41, 1975.

95a. Lee, M. C.; Ausman, J. I.; et al. Superficial temporal to middle cerebral artery anastomsis. Clinical outcome in patients with ischemia or infarction in internal carotid distribution. *Arch. Neurol.,* **36:**1–4, 1979.

96. Levin, E. B. Use of Holter electrocardiographic monitor in diagnosis of transient ischemic attacks. *J. Am. Geriatr. Soc.,* **24:**516–21, 1976.

97. Levine, J., and Swanson, P. D. Idiopathic thrombocytosis: A treatable cause of transient ischemic attacks. *Neurology* (Minneap.), **18:**711–13, 1968.

98. Levy, L. L.; Wallace, J. D.; et al. Cerebral blood flow regulation: Vascular resistance adjustments in the circle of Willis. *Stroke,* **7:**147–50, 1977.

99. Loeb, C., and Meyer, J. S. *Strokes Due to Vertebro-basilar Disease.* Thomas, Springfield, Ill., 1965.

100. Luenssenhap, A. J., and Presper, J. P. Surgical embolization of cerebral arteriovenous malformation through internal carotid and vertebral arteries. Long-term results. *J. Neurosurg.,* **42:**443–51, 1975.

101. Mandybur, T. I., and Bates, S. R. D. Fatal massive intracerebral hemorrhage complicating cerebral amyloid angiopathy. *Arch. Neurol.,* **35:**246–48, 1978.

102. Mannen, T. Vascular lesions in the spinal cord in the aged. A clinicopathological study. *Geriatrics,* **21:**151–60, 1966.

103. Marshall, J. The natural history of transient ischemic cerebrovascular attacks. *Q. J. Med.,* **33:**309–24, 1964.

103a. Mathew, N. T.; Davis, D.; Meyer, J. S.; and Chandar, K. Hyperlipoproteinemia in occlusive cerebrovascular disease. *J.A.M.A.,* **232:**262–66, 1975.

104. Mathew, N. T., and Meyer, J. S. Pathogenesis and natural history of transient global amnesia. *Stroke,* **5:**303–11, 1974.

105. Mathew, N. T.; Meyer, J. S.; and Hartmann, A. Diagnosis and treatment of factors complicating subarachnoid hemorrhage. *Neuroradiology,* **6:**237–45, 1974.

106. Mathew, N. T.; Meyer, J. S.; Rivera, V. M.; Charney, J. Z.; and Hartmann, A. Double-blind evaluation of glycerol therapy in acute cerebral infarction. *Lancet,* **2:**1327–29, 1972.

107. Matsumoto, G. H.; Baker, J. D.; et al. EEG surveillance as a means of extending operability in high risk carotid endarterectomy. *Stroke,* **7:**554–59, 1976.

108. McAllen, P. M., and Marshall, J. Cardiac dysrhythmia and transient cerebral ischemic attacks. *Lancet,* **1:**1212–14, 1973.

109. McAllen, P. M., and Marshall, J. Cerebrovascular incidents after myocardial infarction. *J. Neurol. Neurosurg. Psychiat.,* **40:**951–55, 1977.

110. McCormick, W. F., and Rosenfield, D. B. Massive brain hemorrhage: Review of 144 cases and examination of their causes. *Stroke,* **4:**946–54, 1973.

111. McDonald, W. I. Recurrent cholesterol embolism as a cause of fluctuating cerebral symptoms. *J. Neurol. Neurosurg. Psychiat.,* **30:**489–96, 1967.

112. McHenry, L. C. Cerebral blood flow studies in middle cerebral and internal carotid artery occlusion. *Neurology* (Minneap.), **16:**1145–58, 1966.

113. McHenry, L. C.; Toole, J. F.; and Miller, H. S. Long-term ECG monitoring in patients with cerebrovascular insufficiency. *Stroke,* **7:**264–69, 1976.

114. McKee, J. C.; Denn, M. J.; and Stone, H. L. Neurogenic cerebral vasodilatation from electrical stimulation of the cerebellum in the monkey. *Stroke,* **7:**179–86, 1976.

115. McKissock, W.; Richardson, A.; and Walsh, L. "Posterior-communicating" aneurysms; a controlled trial of the conservative and surgical treatment of ruptured aneurysms of the internal carotid artery at or near the point or origin of the posterior communicating artery. *Lancet,* **1:**1203–6, 1960.

116. Medical treatment of progressive stroke (editorial). *J.A.M.A.,* **199:**120, 1967.

117. Meyer, J. S. Occlusive cerebrovascular disease; pathogenesis and treatment. *Am. J. Med.,* **30:**577–88, 1961.

118. Meyer, J. S. Ischemic cerebrovascular disease (stroke); clinical investigation and management. *J.A.M.A.,* **183:**237–40, 1963.

119. Meyer, J. S. Acute stroke; biochemical and therapeutic studies. *Minn. Med.,* **47:**265–71, 1964.

120. Meyer, J. S., and Bauer, R. B. Medical treatment of spontaneous intracranial hemorrhage by the use of hypotensive drugs. *Neurology* (Minneap.), **12:**36–47, 1962.

121. Meyer, J. S.; Charney, J. Z.; Riveria, V. M.; and Mathew, N. T. Cerebral embolization: Prospective clinical analysis of 42 cases. *Stroke,* **2:**541–53, 1971.

122. Meyer, J. S.; Fang, H. C.; and Denny-Brown, D. Polarographic study of cerebral collateral circulation. *Arch. Neurol. Psychiat.,* **72:**296–312, 1954.

123. Meyer, J. S.; Foley, J. M.; and Campagna-Pinto, D. Granulomatous angiitis of the meninges in sarcoidosis. *Arch. Neurol. Psychiat.,* **69:**587–600, 1953.

124. Meyer, J. S., and Gilroy, J. Regulation and ad-

justment of the cerebral circulation. *Dis. Chest,* **53:**30–37, 1968.

125. Meyer, J. S., and Gotoh, F. Interaction of cerebral hemodynamics and metabolism. Proc. International Conference on Vascular Diseases of the Brain. *Neurology* (Minneap.), (Suppl.) 11, Part 2, 46–65, 1961.

126. Meyer, J. S., and Schadé, H. P. (eds.). *Progress in Brain Research,* Vol. 35, *Cerebral Blood Flow.* Elsevier, Amsterdam, 1972.

127. Meyer, J. S.; Sheehan, S.; and Bauer, R. B. An arteriographic study of cerebrovascular disease in man. I. Stenosis and occlusion of the vertebral-basilar arterial system. *Arch. Neurol.,* **2:**27–45, 1960.

128. Meyer, J. S.; Shimazu, K.; Fukuuchi, Y.; Ohuchi, T.; Okamoto, S.; Koto, A.; and Ericsson, A. D. Cerebral dysautoregulation in central neurogenic orthostatic hypotension (Shy-Drager syndrome). *Neurology* (Minneap.), **23:**262–73, 1973.

129. Meyer, J. S.; Yoshida, K.; and Sakamoto, K. Autonomic control of cerebral blood flow measured by electromagnetic flowmeters. *Neurology* (Minneap.), **17:**638–48, 1967.

130. Meyer, M. W.; Smith, K. A.; and Klassen, A. C. Sympathetic regulation of cephalic blood flow. *Stroke,* **8:**197–201, 1977.

131. Miller, J. D.; Jawad, K.; and Jennett, B. Safety of carotid ligation and its role in the management of intracranial aneurysms. *J. Neurol. Neurosurg. Psychiat.,* **40:**64–72, 1977.

132. Milliken, C. H. Re-assessment of anticoagulant therapy in various types of occlusive cerebrovascular disease. *Stroke,* **2:**201–208, 1971.

133. Molldrem, N. D., and Olin, R. Polymyalgia rheumatica with temporal and coronary arteritis. *Minn. Med.,* **55:**19–23, 1972.

134. Moossy, J. Cerebral infarction and intracranial arterial thrombosis. *Arch. Neurol.,* **14:**119–23, 1966.

135. Moossy, J. Cerebral infarcts and the lesions of intracranial and extracranial atherosclerosis. *Arch. Neurol.,* **14:**124–28, 1966.

136. Mustard, J. F., and Packham, M. A. Factors influencing platelet function: Adhesion release and aggregation. *Pharmacol. Rev.,* **22:**97–187, 1970.

136a. Naritomi, H.; Sakai, F.; and Meyer, J. S. Pathogenesis of transient ischemic attacks within the vertebrabasilar arterial system. *Arch. Neurol.,* **36:**121–28, 1979.

137. Nelson, E., and Rennels, M. Innervation of intracranial arteries. *Brain,* **93:**475–90, 1970.

138. Nibbelink, D. W.; Torner, J. C.; and Henderson, W. G. Intracranial aneurysms and subarchnoid hemorrhage. A cooperative study: Antifibrinolytic therapy in recent onset subarachnoid hemorrhage. *Stroke,* **6:**622–29, 1975.

139. O'Connor, J. F., and Musher, D. M. Central nervous system involvement in systemic lupus erythematosus. *Arch. Neurol.,* **14:**157–64, 1966.

140. Ott, K. H.; Kase, C. S.; et al. Cerebellar hemorrhage: Diagnosis and treatment. Review of 56 cases. *Arch. Neurol.,* **31:**160–67, 1974.

141. Oxbury, J. M.; Greenhall, R. C. D.; and

Grainger, K. M. R. Predicting the outcome of stroke: Acute stage after cerebral infarction. *Br. Med. J.,* **3:**125–27, 1975.

142. Pakarinen, S. Incidence aetiology and prognosis of primary subarachnoid haemorrhage; a study based on 589 cases diagnosed in a defined urban population during a defined period. *Acta Neurol. Scand.,* **43:**suppl. 29:1–128, 1967.

143. Paulson, E. B. Ophthalmodynamometry in internal carotid artery occlusion. *Stroke,* **7:**564–66, 1976.

143a. Payne, H. A.; Maravilla, K. R.; et al. Recovery from primary pontine hemorrhage. *Ann. Neurol.,* **4:**557–58, 1978.

144. Pearce, J. M. S.; Gubbay, S. S.; and Walton, J. W. Long-term anticoagulant therapy in transient cerebral ischemic attacks. *Lancet,* **1:**6–9, 1975.

145. Penn, A. S., and Rowan, A. J. Myelopathy in systemic lupus erythematosus. *Arch. Neurol.,* **18:**337–49, 1968.

146. Petz, L. D. Neurologic manifestations of systemic lupus erythematosus and thrombotic thrombocytopenia purpura. *Stroke,* **8:**719–22, 1977.

147. Pilgeram, L. O.; Chee, A. N.; and Bussche, G. V.-D. Evidence for abnormalities in clotting and thrombolysis as risk factor for stroke. *Stroke,* **4:**643–56, 1973.

148. Preventive therapy for atherosclerosis (editorial). *J.A.M.A.,* **199:**578, 1967.

149. Radü, E. W., and DuBoulay, G. H. Paradoxical dilatation of the large cerebral arteries in hypocapnia in men. *Stroke,* **7:**569–71, 1976.

150. Raimondi, A. J., and Torres, H. Acute hydrocephalus as complication of subarachnoid hemorrhage. *Surg. Neurol.,* **1:**23–26, 1973.

151. Rajjaub, R. K.; Wood, J. H.; and Ommaya, A. K. Granulomatous angiitis of the brain: A successfully treated case. *Neurology* (Minneap.), **27:**588–91, 1977.

152. Reichman, H. O. Complications of cerebral revascularization. *Clin. Neurosurg.,* **23:**318–41, 1976.

153. Reyes, M. G.; Fresix, R.; et al. Viruslike particles in granulomatous angiitis of the central nervous system. *Neurology* (Minneap.), **26:**797–99, 1976.

154. Riehl, J. L. The idiopathic arteritis of Takayasu; a re-evaluation of its anatomical distribution and neurological implications. *Neurology* (Minneap.), **13:**873–84, 1963.

155. Riehl, J. L., and Brown, W. J. Takayasu's arteritis; an auto-immune disease. *Arch. Neurol.,* **12:**92–97, 1965.

156. Rinaldi, I.; Harris, W. O.; et al. Intracranial fibromuscular dysplasia: Report of two cases, one with autopsy verification. *Stroke,* **7:**511–16, 1976.

157. Rivera, V. M.; Meyer, J. S.; Baer, P. E.; Faibish, G.; Mathew, N. T.; and Hartmann, A. Vertebrobasilar arterial insufficiency with dementia. Controlled trials of treatment with betahistine hydrochloride. *J. Am. Geriatr. Soc.,* **22:**397–406, 1974.

158. Rosenberg, G. A., and Kaufman, D. M. Cerebellar hemorrhage: Reliability of clinical evaluation. *Stroke,* **7:**332–36, 1976.

159. Ross Russell, R. W. How does blood pressure cause stroke? *Lancet,* **2:**1283–85, 1975.
160. Rubino. F. A., and Haller, C. Pure motor hemiplegia due to cerebral cortical infarction. *Arch. Neurol.,* **34:**93–95, 1977.
161. Samuel, E. Thermography—some clinical applications. *Biomed. Eng.,* **4:**15–19, 1969.
162. Sang, U. H., and Wilson, C. B. Surgical treatment of intracranial vascular malformations. *West. J. Med.,* **123:**175–83, 1975.
163. Santambrogio, S.; Martinotti, R.; et al. Is there a real treatment for stroke? Clinical and statistical comparison of different treatments in 300 patients. *Stroke,* **9:**130–32, 1978.
164. Scharf, I.; Nahir, M.; and Hemli, J. Transverse myelitis with systemic lupus erythematosus. *J. Neurol.,* **215:**231–32, 1977.
165. Schrire, V., and Asherson, R. A. Arteritis of the aorta and its major branches. *Q. J. Med.,* **33:**439–63, 1964.
166. Scremin, O. U.; Rubenstein, E. H.; and Sonnenschein, R. R. Cerebrovascular CO_2 reactivity: Role of a cholinergic mechanism modulated by anesthesia. *Stroke,* **9:**160–65, 1978.
167. Sengupta, R. P.; So, S. C.; and Villarejo-Ortega, F. J. Use of e aminocaproic acid (EACA) in the preoperative management of ruptured intracranial aneurysm. *J. Neurosurg.,* **44:**479–84, 1976.
168. Sheehan, S.; Bauer, R. B.; and Meyer, J. S. Vertebral artery compression in cervical spondylosis, arteriographic demonstration during life of vertebral artery insufficiency due to rotation and extension of the neck. *Neurology* (Minneap.), **10:**968–86, 1960.
169. Shuttleworth, E. C., and Morris, C. E. The transient global amnesia syndrome. *Arch. Neurol.,* **15:**515–20, 1966.
170. Sisler, H. A. Optical-corneal pressure ophathalmodynamometer. *Am. J. Ophthalmol.,* **74:**987–88, 1972.
171. Skinhøj, E., and Strandgaard, S. Pathogenesis of hypertensive encephalopathy. *Lancet,* **2:**461–62, 1973.
172. Soni, S. R. Aneurysms of posterior communicating artery and oculomotor paralysis. *J. Neurol. Neurosurg. Psychiat.,* **37:**475–84, 1974.
173. Stehbens, W. E. Cerebral atherosclerosis: Internal proliferation and atherosclerosis in the cerebral arteries. *Arch. Pathol.,* **99:**582–91, 1975.
174. Steinmetz, E. F., and Vroom, F. Q. Transient global amnesia. *Neurology* (Minneap.), **22:**1193–1200, 1972.
175. Stone, H. L.; Raichle, M. E.; and Hernandez-Perez, M. J. The effect of sympathetic denervation on cerebral CO_2 sensitivity. *Stroke,* **5:**13–18, 1974.
176. Strachan, R. W. The natural history of Takayasu's arteriopathy. *Q. J. Med.,* **33:**57–69, 1964.
177. Subbiah, M. T. R. Prostgalandins and the arterial wall: An avenue for research in the pathogenesis of atherosclerosis. *Mayo Clin. Proc.,* **53:**60–62, 1978.
178. Sundt, T. M., Jr. Management of ischemic complications after subarachnoid hemorrhage. *J. Neurosurg.,* **43:**418–25, 1975.
179. Symon, L.; Branston, N. M.; and Strong, A. J. Autoregularion in acute focal ischemia. An experimental study. *Stroke,* **7:**547–54, 1976.
180. Sypert, G. W., and Alvord, E. C. Cerebellar infarction: A clinicopathologic study. *Arch. Neurol.,* **32:**357–63, 1975.
181. Tedeschi, G.; Bernini, P.; and Cerullo. A. Indications for surgical treatment of intracerebral hemorrhage. *J. Neurosurg.,* **43:**590–95, 1975.
182. Tellez, H., and Bauer, R. B. Dexamethasone as treatment in cerebrovascular disease. *Stroke,* **4:**541–46, 1973.
183. Thurd, C.; Rey, A.; et al. Carotid-ophthalmic aneurysm. *Neurochirurgie,* **20:**25–39, 1974.
184. Todd, M.; McDevitt, E.; and McDowell, F. Stroke and blood coagulation. *Stroke,* **4:**400–405, 1973.
185. Tominaga, S.; Strandgaard, S.; et al. Cerebrovascular CO_2 reactivity in normotensive and hypotensive man. *Stroke,* **7:**507–10, 1976.
186. Tomkin, G.; Coe, R. P. K.; and Marshall J. Electroencephalographic abnormalities in patients presenting with strokes. *J. Neurol. Neurosurg. Psychiat.,* **31:**250–52, 1968.
187. Toole, J. F.; Janeway, R.; et al. Transient ischemic attacks due to atherosclerosis. A prospective study of 160 patients. *Arch. Neurol.,* **32:**5–12, 1975.
188. Toole, J. F., and Patel. A. N. *Cerebrovascular Disorders.* McGraw-Blakiston, New York, 1967.
188a. Toole, J. F.; Yuson, C. P.; et al. Transient ischemic attacks: A prospective study of 225 patients. *Neurology* (Minneap.), **28:**746–53, 1978.
189. Tubman, D. E., and Ethier, R. Cerebellar hemorrhage in adults. Diagnosis by computerized tomography. *J. Neurosurg.,* **48:**575–79, 1978.
190. Veterans Administration Cooperative Study Group on Antihypertensive Agents: Effects of treatment on morbidity of hypertension: Results in patients with diastolic blood pressure averaging 90–115 mm Hg. *J.A.M.A.,* **213:**1143–52, 1970.
191. Waga, S.; Ohtsuko, K.; and Handa, H. Warning signs in intracranial aneurysms. *Surg. Neurol.,* **3:**15–20, 1975.
192. Walton, J. N. *Subarachnoid Hemorrhage.* Livingstone, Edinburgh, 1956.
193. Weir, B.; Grave, M.; et al. Time course of vasospasm in man. *J. Neurosurg.,* **48:**173–78, 1978.
194. Weir, B.; Miller, J.; and Russell, D. Intracranial aneurysms: A clinical angiographic and computerized tomographic study. *Can. J. Neurol. Sci.,* **4:**99–105, 1977.
195. Whisnant, J. P.; Matsumoto, N.; and Elveback, L. R. The effect of anticoagulant therapy on the prognosis of patients with transient cerebral ischemic attacks in a community: Rochester, Minnesota, 1955 through 1969. *Mayo Clin. Proc.,* **48:**844–48, 1973.
195a. Wiggins, W. S.; Moody, D. M.; et al. Clinical and computerized tomographic study of hypertensive intracerebral hemorrhage. *Arch. Neurol.,* **35:**832–33, 1978.

196. Wilkinson, I. M. S., and Russell, R. W. R. Arteries of the head and neck in giant cell arteritis. A pathological study to show the pattern of arterial involvement. *Arch. Neurol.,* **27**:378–91, 1972.

196a. Wolf, P. A.; Dawber, T. R.; et al. Epidemiologic assessment of chronic atrial fibrillation and risk of stroke. The Framingham Study. *Neurology* (Minneap.), **28**:973–77, 1978.

197. Wolman, L., and Bradshaw, P. Spinal cord embolism. *J. Neurol. Neurosurg. Psychiat.,* **30**:446–54, 1967.

198. Wu, K. K., and Hoak, J. C. Increased platelet aggregates in patients with transient ischemic attacks. *Stroke,* **6**:521–24, 1975.

199. Yasargil, M. G.; DeLong, W. B.; and Guarnaschelli, J. J. Complete microsurgical excision of cervical extramedullary and intramedullary vascular malformations. *Surg. Neurol.,* **4**:211–24, 1975.

200. Zervas, N. T.; Hori, H.; et al. Neurogenic regulation of cerebral blood flow following ischemia. *Stroke,* **7**:113–18, 1976.

201. Ziegler, D. K., and Hassanein, R. S. Prognosis in patients with transient ischemic attacks. *Stroke,* **4**:666–73, 1973.

202. Zingessen, L. H.; Schecter, M. M.; Dexter, J.; Katzman, R.; and Scheinberg, L. C. On the significance of spasm associated with rupture of a cerebral aneurysm. *Arch. Neurol.,* **18**:520–28, 1968.

CHAPTER 10 TUMORS OF THE CENTRAL NERVOUS SYSTEM

General Considerations

About 10 per cent of tumors that occur throughout the body are located within the central nervous system, its meninges, and related bony structures. Eighty per cent of these occur in the cranial cavity and 20 per cent in the spinal canal. Tumors of the nervous system include a heterogeneous group of primary and metastatic neoplasms. Primary tumors may arise from tissues of the brain and spinal cord as well as their meninges and blood vessels; others arise from the pituitary and pineal glands as well as from embryonic rests. The types of tumors involving the brain and spinal cord are listed in order of frequency in the accompanying table (Table 10–1). The term "glioma" is used in the table to indicate all tumors arising from neuroglia and ependymal tissue. Medulloblastomas are customarily included when considering gliomas although it is recognized that medulloblastomas are probably neuronal in origin.

The incidence of primary tumors of the central nervous system which are of embryonal origin is highest during the first decade of life. Other tumors occur predominantly between the ages of 30 and 70 years with a peak incidence between 55 and 65 years of age.[151] There is a significant increase of primary neoplasms of the brain, pituitary, and spinal cord with increasing age up to 65 years.[129]

Tumors of the central nervous system also show some differences in distribution with age. Cerebellar tumors are more common in children than adults. The most commonly occurring is the cystic astrocytoma, which is a relatively benign tumor uncommon in adult life. The malignant medulloblastomas of the cerebellum are next in order

TABLE 10–1

Frequency of Different Types of Tumors That Involve the Central Nervous System

Those Involving Brain, 80%	Those Involving Spinal Cord, 20%
	Extradural, 17% Intradural but extramedullary, 66% Intramedullary, 17%
1. The gliomas	1. Neurilemmomas
2. Meningiomas	2. Meningiomas
3. Pituitary adenomas	3. The gliomas
4. Neurilemmomas	4. Sarcomas
5. Metastatic tumors	5. Extramedullary hemangiomas
6. Blood vessel tumors	6. Chordomas

of frequency and are exclusively tumors of childhood. Gliomas of the brainstem, particularly the pons, are also more common in childhood than in adult life. However, 50 per cent of gliomas in children occur in the cerebral hemispheres.[104] Metastatic tumors account for about 20 per cent of intracranial tumors. The most common primary sites of metastatic tumors are the lungs, followed by the gastrointestinal tract, breast, and kidneys in that order. They are multiple in 70 per cent of cases.

Etiology

There are few known etiologic factors concerned with the development of tumors of the central nervous system. A number of factors that are usually cited in connection with the development of neoplasia elsewhere in the body should be considered.

Heredity.   The familial occurrence of brain tumors is rare. Meningiomas, astrocytomas, and neurilemmomas occur in von Recklinghausen's disease; cerebellar hemangiomas are found in Lindau-von Hippel disease; and astrocytomas, meningiomas, and ependymomas have been reported in tuberous sclerosis.[78] Meningiomas and gliomas have occasionally been reported in siblings without evidence of familial phakomatoses,[86, 128] and medulloblastomas occur in childhood in twins and siblings.[172]

Embryonic Cell Rests.   The development of intracranial teratomas, craniopharyngiomas, and chordomas may arise from neoplastic change within embryonic cell rests. Brain tumors also may arise from the phakomas or nodules in the brain of persons with tuberous sclerosis.

Inclusion of Cell Rests.   The inclusion of epidermoid elements in the cranial cavity as the skull develops may lead to subsequent development of epidermoid or dermoid cysts, some of which rarely undergo malignant change.

Trauma.   There have been occasional reports of brain tumors, particularly meningiomas, arising at the site of cranial cerebral injury. The evidence for such an etiologic association is extremely tenuous; and in general, it should be considered that trauma is not related to the subsequent development of tumors of the central nervous system.

Radiation.   The tissues in the central nervous system are sensitive to irradiation and develop delayed degenerative changes, but there is no evidence that irradiation can induce the development of a glioma. There are reports of the development of a meningioma many years after irradiation for other lesions of the skull or brain.[17]

Viruses.   Although there may be some association between viral infections and subsequent development of neoplasia (e.g., lymphoma), the relationship between viral infection and development of tumors of the central nervous system is tenuous at this time. Meningioma cells have been shown to possess tumor-specific antigens which may have been virally induced.[159] There is also a significant association between meningioma and breast cancer[150] in which there is some evidence for a chronic virus infection.

Carcinogenic Agents.   A number of carcinogens have been used to produce experimental brain tumors in animals. These agents include polycyclic hydrocarbons, which must be implanted in the brain, and nitroso compounds such as methylnitrosides (MNU), which will induce neoplasms in the nervous system following systemic administration in animals.[171, 195] The ability to induce experimental neoplasia in the central nervous system by the use of carcinogens suggests that carcinogens may play a role in the development of human brain tumors although there is little evidence for this hypothesis at this time.

Pathology

The usual division between benign and malignant tumors is not as well defined in tumors involving the central nervous system as it is elsewhere in the body. The gliomas, which show many features characteristic of malignancy, including the ability to invade normal brain tissue, rarely give rise to metastatic spread outside the central nervous system.[92] On the other hand, any tumor of the central nervous system, including those which are histologically benign, may increase in size and produce damage that is eventually fatal, or an increase in intracranial pressure which results in death. Tumors arising in a particular area such as the posterior aspect of the third ventricle or in the brainstem near the aqueduct of Sylvius may be small but can obstruct circulation of the cerebrospinal fluid, resulting in hydrocephalus with a fatal rise in intracranial pressure (Fig. 10–1). The smallest fatal tumors of the body, as a whole, are those occurring in the region of the cerebral aqueduct.

The histologic diagnosis of tumor of the central nervous system may be facilitated by the following routine considerations when examining surgical biopsy specimens or autopsy material:

1. Is the specimen neoplastic? Differentiation of neoplasm from granulomas, scars, and particularly reactive gliosis is essential since these conditions may have some similarities.
2. If a neoplasm, is it primary or metastatic?
3. If primary, is it a glioma or nongliomatous?
4. If it is a glioma, what is the predominant cell type (e.g., astrocytoma, oligodendroglioma, or ependymoma)?
5. If it is a glioma, what is the grade of malignancy classified in severity from 1 to 4?

Tumors of glial origin may present difficulties in identification of the histologic cell type from which the tumor arose. In any sizable series of brain tumors, a number of glial tumors will re-

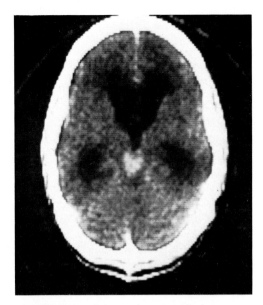

FIGURE 10–1. Computed tomography in hydrocephalus. This enhanced scan shows a discrete area of increased density in the midbrain due to a pinealoma. The tumor has compressed and distorted the cerebral aqueduct, producing hydrocephalus, and the dilated third and lateral ventricles are clearly demonstrated.

main unclassified owing to extreme degrees of anaplastic change. In the majority of cases, however, the cell type can be identified and the tumor classified and graded according to the percentage of differentiated cells (Table 10–2), although features such as vascular and endothelial proliferation as well as necrosis and mitotic activity are also considered.

From a practical and therapeutic point of view, the grade of malignancy is more important than the identification of the cell type of the tumor. The grade of malignancy is closely related to survival following biopsy, diagnosis, and attempts at surgical excision of the tumor, as well as to

TABLE 10–2

Classification of the Gliomas

A. Type of predominant glial cell (e.g., astrocytoma)

B. Grade	Percentage of differentiated cells
1	75 to 100
2	50 to 75
3	25 to 50
4	0 to 25

postoperative radiation therapy or chemotherapy.

A description of the pathologic appearance of individual tumors will be included as each one is discussed later in this chapter.

Intracranial Tumors

Effects Due to Increase in Intracranial Contents

A number of effects common to all enlarging mass lesions of any type will be described.

Increased Intracranial Pressure

The skull is a relatively rigid structure, and the increase in intracranial contents produced by an expanding tumor soon leads to an increase in intracranial pressure. In addition to the space occupied by the tumor, increased intracranial pressure may be enhanced by the occurrence of infarction within the tumor or hemorrhage from neoplastic, thin-walled blood vessels within its substance, producing swelling and rapid increase in its size. The occurrence of edema in the surrounding brain is probably due to metabolic factors and possibly to an inflammatory response following infarction within the tumor or venous obstruction by the tumor. Tumors may also cause rapid increases of intracranial pressure by obstruction of the flow of cerebrospinal fluid at the following sites:

1. The foramen of Monro with enlargement of one lateral ventricle.
2. The posterior portion of the third ventricle with enlargement of both ventricles.
3. The aqueduct of Sylvius with enlargement of both lateral and third ventricles.
4. The fourth ventricle with enlargement of the first three ventricles and the aqueduct.
5. The foramina in the roof of the fourth ventricle with enlargement of all four ventricles.
6. The subarachnoid space with enlargement of all four ventricles and the cisterna magna.

Papilledema

Obstruction of venous return from the optic nerve results in papilledema, with congestion of the veins, edema, elevation of the optic disk, and ultimately venous hemorrhages around the disk.

Separation of the Sutures of the Skull

In children under the age of five years, increased intracranial pressure produces an increase in size of the skull due to separation of the sutures.

Central or Transtentorial Herniation with Progressive Dysfunction of the Brainstem

A rise in supratentorial pressure due to any progressive enlargement of an intracranial mass produces downward displacement and buckling of the brainstem, compression of tissue, and edema. The penetrating branches of the basilar artery are stretched and eventually rupture with the development of midbrain and pontine hemorrhages of different sizes. Damage to the brainstem appears to occur in an orderly fashion in a rostral to caudal direction, i.e., from the midbrain through the pons to the medulla.[79, 115, 130] The medulla is the last to be affected and the most resilient part of the brain to anoxia and ischemic changes. Clinically this results in four distinct stages.

Stage 1: Early Brainstem Compression. There is some impairment of consciousness varying from obtundity to coma. Cheyne-Stokes respirations begin. The pupils become small but still react to light and to the ciliospinal reflex. Lateral conjugate eye movements are still elicited on passive rotation of the head (doll's eye movements). Spontaneous roving, with conjugate or slightly divergent eye movements, may be seen in more stuporous patients.

Caloric stimulation with warm water produces conjugate deviation toward the irrigated side.

There are bilateral signs of motor disorder, which may be more marked on one side. Usually, if there is a tumor mass in one hemisphere, there is contralateral hemiplegia, but the ipsilateral limbs may show slight rigidity with resistance to passive movement (paratonia). The plantar response is extensor bilaterally. There may be some increase in the tone of the neck muscles producing paratonic nuchal rigidity. Painful stimulation may produce decorticate posturing with flexion of both arms and extension of the legs.

Stage 2: Compression of Midbrain and Upper Pons. The respirations change from Cheyne-Stokes respirations to a machine-like hyperventilation. The pupils are moderately dilated and no longer react to light, and the ciliospinal reflex is absent. The doll's eye movement on rotation of the head from side to side becomes sluggish and disappears. Combined caloric testing with rotation of the head may be necessary to elicit any reflex conjugate eye movement.

Spontaneous decerebrate rigidity can occur

when the pressure effect is maximal in the upper midbrain. Painful stimulation is required to produce decerebrate rigidity when the effects of compression have descended to lower midbrain levels, and it becomes progressively more difficult to elicit this reflex activity as compression affects the pons.

Stage 3: Damage to Pons and Upper Medulla. Hyperventilation disappears and there is a return of quiet respiration. The doll's eye movements are unobtainable and there is no response to caloric or combined stimulation. The patient is deeply comatose and flaccid, with no response to painful stimuli. There are bilateral extensor plantar responses. The systolic blood pressure is elevated and the pulse slow and bounding.

Stage 4: Stage of Medullary Damage. Respirations become slow, irregular, and gasping. Periods of apnea occur, and the pupils are widely dilated.'There is a progressive fall in blood pressure, which precedes death.

Temporal Lobe or Uncal Herniation and Progressive Brainstem Dysfunction

An increase in supratentorial pressure from a tumor frequently causes the uncus, or uncinate gyrus of the temporal lobe, on the same side to herniate over the free edge of the tentorium cerebelli into the posterior fossa. This produces distortion and downward displacement of the brainstem. It is possible to recognize five stages of uncal herniation.

Stage 1: Early Compression of the Third Nerve. There is some impairment of consciousness. The pupils are unequal with pupillary dilatation on one side owing to compression of the third nerve against the edge of the falx on the side of the herniation. The pupillary reaction to light becomes sluggish on the side of the third nerve compression and soon disappears. Respirations are quiet and regular. The doll's eye movements are intact on rotation of the head. The motor examination shows hemiparesis on the side opposite the hemisphere containing the tumor, and the plantar response is extensor on that side.

Stage 2: Late Compression of the Third Nerve. The patient now enters into semicoma or coma. The pupil becomes widely dilated on the side of the herniation and is fixed to light. The respirations show progressive increase in rate

and depth. Painful stimuli produce decerebrate posturing on the side opposite the lesion. The plantar response becomes extensor bilaterally.

Stage 3: Compression of the Midbrain and Pons. Both pupils become dilated and nonreactive to light. Respiration becomes deep and machinelike, and the doll's eye response to rotation of the head becomes progressively impaired.

Stages 4 and 5. These two stages are similar to the lower pontine, upper medullary, and medullary stages previously described under progressive brainstem dysfunction associated with increased intracranial pressure.

Herniation of the Cerebellar Tonsils

A tumor in the posterior fossa usually causes herniation of one or both cerebellar tonsils through the foramen magnum, producing pressure on the medulla. This results in severe headache, nuchal rigidity, and spasm of the cervical muscles. If one cerebellar tonsil (usually due to a tumor of the ipsilateral cerebellar hemisphere) is herniated, the occiput is rotated downward and to the side opposite the herniated tonsil, producing a characteristic dystonic posture of the head ("tonsillar tilt").

Cerebellar Herniation Upward and Over the Free Edge of the Tentorium Cerebelli

An increase in the contents of the posterior fossa such as occurs with a cerebellar tumor may cause upward herniation of the medial aspect of the anterior lobe of the cerebellum over the free edge of the tentorium cerebelli. This may produce paralysis of upward gaze, stupor, and signs of brainstem compression similar to those of uncal herniation.

Herniation Beneath the Falx Cerebri

A tumor within the frontal lobe may produce herniation of the cingulate gyrus beneath the free edge of the falx cerebri. The herniation causes compression of the opposite frontal lobe and compression of the anterior cerebral arteries. Such compression may result in infarction of the opposite frontal lobe and bilateral signs of frontal lobe damage (grasping, dementia, apraxia of gait, and quadriparesis).

Compression of Arteries and Veins

Distortion of the cerebral arteries owing to compression by tumor may cause kinking and obstruction of their blood flow. This can result in infarction of areas of brain that may be remote from the tumor (e.g., frontal lobe infarction from compression of the anterior cerebral artery, occipital lobe infarction from compression of the posterior cerebral artery).

Pressure on veins or venous sinuses may impede or obstruct venous drainage, causing cerebral edema, perivenous hemorrhage, and malabsorption of cerebrospinal fluid. In any event, a further increase in intracranial pressure results.

Erosion of Bone

Chronic increased intracranial pressure causes a "hammer-marked" or "beaten-silver" appearance of the skull due to patchy thinning of the calvarium. Meningiomas and, very rarely, superficially located gliomas may erode the skull locally as they increase in size.

Hyperostosis

Some superficial tumors, especially meningiomas, stimulate osteoblastic activity, leading to new bone formation at the site of the tumor in relation to the skull, usually referred to as "hyperostosis."

Symptoms Usually Associated with Intracranial Tumors

Headache

Headache is a common symptom that occurs at some stage of a brain tumor (Table 10–3) and is usually described as "throbbing" or "bursting." The headache is worse upon arising in the morning owing to a rise in the arterial carbon dioxide level during sleep, which produces increased cere-

TABLE 10–3

General Signs and Symptoms Usually Associated with Intracranial Tumors

Symptoms	Signs
Headache	Papilledema
Vomiting	Increased size of the head (hydrocephalus)
Seizures	Slowed pulse and elevated blood pressure
Alteration in level of consciousness	False localizing signs
Mental changes	Respiratory changes
Abnormal sensations in the head	CSF rhinorrhea

bral blood flow, further cerebral venous congestion, and a further increase in intracranial pressure.

The headache of brain tumor is intensified by any action producing a Valsalva maneuver, such as coughing, sneezing, straining at stool, lifting, or sudden exertion. Headache is the first symptom of brain tumor in about 20 per cent of patients. A unilateral headache may occur over the site of a brain tumor. This should be suspected in the absence of papilledema, particularly if there is tenderness on percussion of the skull in the area of the headache. Headache is almost always present with tumors of posterior fossa and usually is located in the occipital and the upper cervical area.

Supratentorial tumors rarely give rise to occipital headaches unless there is tonsillar herniation. The headache associated with tumors acting as a ball valve in the third ventricle may be altered dramatically by changes in the position of the head. For example, the headache may be relieved when the patient is lying prone as the tumor falls away from the aqueduct and hydrocephalus is relieved. Headache is often intermittent in children under the age of five years with brain tumors. This is possibly due to intermittent relief of intracranial pressure by separation of the cranial sutures.

Vomiting

Vomiting may occur in the patient with brain tumor and is due to increased intracranial pressure. It tends to be worse on awakening in the morning and is more common in posterior fossa tumors. Vomiting may also occur intermittently in children with brain tumor and in many textbooks is said to be "projectile." However, vomiting in children is no more "projectile" when due to brain tumors than when due to other causes.

Seizures

A seizure may be the initial symptom of a brain tumor in 15 per cent of patients. The aphorism is justifiable that onset of focal seizures in adults under 50 years of age should be regarded as a symptom of brain tumor until proven otherwise.[3] Changes in behavior, school performance, type and frequency of seizures, neurologic findings, or EEG pattern are of particular significance in children with epilepsy. The possibility of brain tumor in these cases requires immediate investigation.[126]

Generalized seizures usually occur when there is a rapid increase in intracranial pressure and are most commonly seen with grade 3 or 4 astrocytomas rather than in cases with more slowly growing tumors, although seizures are also common with meningiomas and oligodendrogliomas. While generalized seizures probably occur with any type of a tumor in any part of the brain including the posterior fossa, the majority of "cerebellar fits" described by neurologists around the turn of the century were probably intermittent attacks of decerebrate rigidity rather than seizures.

Alterations in Levels of Consciousness

Drowsiness may be an early symptom of brain tumor, and somnolence or stupor is frequently seen in more advanced cases. While somnolence and stupor may be due to pressure on the hypothalamus, they can also occur in downward displacement and kinking of the brainstem due to a supratentorial mass and in diffuse compression of the brain.

Changes in Mentation

Brain tumor may produce symptoms of progressive dementia, with impairment of judgment, lack of insight, apathy, loss of motivation, and impairment of recent memory. Memory loss may be rapid or abrupt in some cases or present as a transient global amnesia.[100, 194] Paroxysmal involuntary laughter has been described in supratentorial and posterior fossa tumors.[1] Repetitive motor movements may be seen, such as forced grasping and groping and rubbing of the nose.

Abnormal Sensations in the Head

Many patients with brain tumors experience abnormal sensations in the head, which they term "dizziness" or "lightheadedness." The sensations are usually vague, often fleeting, and rarely vertiginous. They are probably related to increased intracranial pressure.

Physical Signs Usually Associated with Intracranial Tumors

Papilledema

Papilledema may be caused by increased intracranial pressure or pressure exerted on the optic nerve directly by the tumor. Papilledema does not necessarily bear a relation to the size of the brain tumor, and papilledema is absent in some cases of large chronic tumors due presumably to absence of persistently high intracranial pressure.[175] There may be a difference in the severity of the papilledema in the two eyes particularly if one eye is myopic, and papilledema may appear in one eye a considerable time before the other optic nerve is involved. When there is a rapid rise in intracranial pressure, the papilledema is usually associated with a severe degree of venous congestion of the optic nerve, and the disk looks pink and swollen, often with hemorrhages in and directly around the optic fundus. There may be visual field defects associated with papilledema consisting of enlargement of the blind spot and concentric constriction of the visual fields. Chronic papilledema shows associated gliosis of the optic nerve and a moist, grayish-yellow, and glistening appearance. This is eventually followed by secondary optic atrophy and blindness with extreme pallor of the disk (see p. 17).

Enlargement of the Head in Children

Increased intracranial pressure may lead to progressive separation of the cranial sutures in children under the age of five years, with increase in the size of the head. In children under 18 months, there may be bulging of the anterior fontanel. Some children show venous congestion of the scalp with exophthalmos. Percussion of the scalp produces a characteristic "cracked-pot" sound (Macewen's sign) in infants and children with increased intracranial pressure. A murmur may be heard on auscultation over the skull or the eyes in the case of a vascular tumor or angiomatous malformation.

Bradycardia and Elevation of the Blood Pressure

Increasing intracranial pressure results in bradycardia and progressive elevation in blood pressure due to ischemia or distortion of the medullary vasomotor centers. This is a reflex mechanism that tends to maintain constant cerebral blood flow despite the increased cerebrovascular resistance resulting from compression of the cerebral capillary vessels by the tumor.

Alterations in Respiratory Rate and Depth

Respiration becomes progressively slower and deeper with increasing intracranial pressure prior to the development of uncal herniation or downward displacement of the brainstem. When compression of the brainstem occurs, there is a change in respiratory pattern to the Cheyne-Stokes type. Eventually, hyperventilation results, followed by irregular respiration, apnea, and death. Mechanical respiration at this stage is usually ill-advised for it usually maintains heart and lung action despite cerebral death, which can be documented by the absence of electroencephalographic activity at high gain.

Cerebrospinal Fluid Rhinorrhea and Pneumocephalus

Drainage of cerebrospinal fluid through the cribriform plate may occur following erosion of this area by tumor. Such drainage has also been reported in the presence of increased intracranial pressure due to a tumor elsewhere in the cranial cavity (see p. 506). Pneumocephalus is a condition resulting from cerebrospinal fluid fistula whereby air is driven as in sneezing and coughing into the brain and ventricles through such a fistula.

Skin Changes in Brain Tumors

A persistent severe pruritus of the nose has been described in advanced brain tumors. Generalized itching also occurs in brain tumors and other neoplastic diseases, possibly due to an allergic reaction to tumor-specific antigens.[5] Pigmentary changes including vitiligo and hyperpigmentation of the face have been observed in brain tumor as well as hyperkeratitic changes of the hands and feet.

False Localizing Signs of Intracranial Tumors

Certain signs may be associated with brain tumor due to increased intracranial pressure resulting in displacement and distortion of cerebral structures that are remote from the tumor itself. Because these signs discussed below do not help in the localization of the tumor, they are referred to as false localizing signs.

Cranial Nerve Palsies

Displacement and distortion of the brainstem may produce stretching and paralysis of the cranial nerves. This is particularly common in the case of the third, fourth, and sixth nerves.

Bilateral Extensor Plantar Responses

A tumor in one hemisphere may produce a contralateral extensor plantar response owing to direct involvement of the corticospinal tracts. Lat-

eral displacement of the midbrain may result in compression of the contralateral cerebral peduncle and the production of an extensor response on the same side as the tumor.

Mental Changes

As already stated (p. 617), intellectual impairment and progressive dementia may be associated with any brain tumor due to increased intracranial pressure. The patient usually has little insight into these mental changes, although they are obvious to his relatives or close associates. A history of this change must be obtained from an outside source.

Endocrine Disorders

Chronic increased intracranial pressure with hydrocephalus of the third ventricle may produce changes in hypothalamic or pituitary function, with adiposity and genital atrophy, although the tumor is far removed from the hypothalamus. Pituitary dysfunction is sometimes seen, for example, in children with aqueduct or cerebellar tumors.

Cerebral Infarction

Compression of cerebral arteries due to the expanding tumor or to increased intracranial pressure may result in cerebral infarction in an area remote from the tumor. Infarction will result in the appearance of signs and symptoms unrelated to the site of the tumor, such as hemianopia or even intermittent cortical blindness.

True Localizing Signs of Intracranial Tumors

Frontal Lobe Tumors

Involvement of the Prefrontal Area. The prefrontal area of the brain consists of all the frontal lobe anterior to the precentral sulcus and the orbital surface of the frontal lobe. Tumors involving one or both prefrontal areas produce a constellation of symptoms, which may be modified somewhat by the previous personality of the patient.

MENTAL CHANGES. Some degree of intellectual impairment occurs with some loss of judgment and memory.[7] Unlike the patient with presenile dementia, the patient with a frontal lobe tumor may retain some insight into his condition and recognize that it has deteriorated. In most cases insight is usually sufficiently impaired that the loss of intellectual capability is of little concern; and there may be apathy and a mild degree of euphoria or depression. Some patients exhibit a frivolous and superficial joking and punning attitude, usually directed toward the examiner or those in immediate contact with him *(Witzelsucht)*. There is often lack of foresight and ability to plan for the future. Some patients have limited attention span and become highly distractible. Loss of employment is the rule because of inability to concentrate, impaired judgment and insight, and changes of mood. There may also be a regression in social and moral behavior, with deterioration in speech, manners, and appearance. The speed of evolution of the dementia is usually more rapid than that seen in the dementias.

IMPAIRMENT OF SPHINCTER CONTROL. Tumors situated over the medial aspect of the frontal lobes produce impairment of cortical inhibitory control of the bladder. Initially, urgency and poor control of micturition result, followed by loss of bladder inhibition and, later, urinary incontinence. Extensive involvement of the frontal lobes results in urinary and fecal incontinence, apathy, total lack of concern with grooming, and gross regression of social behavior.

SEIZURES. Frontal lobe tumors are associated with generalized seizures more commonly than partial seizures. Convexity tumors situated at or near Broca's area may produce partial seizures beginning with arrest of speech. The proximity of the motor areas usually leads to contralateral focal motor involvement, often of the jacksonian type. Involvement of the frontal eye field results in a forced deviation of the eyes to the opposite side.

Involvement of the Orbital Surface. Orbital surface tumors may give rise to partial epileptic seizures of psychomotor type with symptoms of autonomic disturbances including alteration in heart rate and paroxysmal atrial tachycardia.[146] This is because there are connections between the orbital surface of the frontal lobe and the temporal lobe through the uncinate fasciculus.

Cranial Nerve Involvement. Medially placed tumors growing into or arising from the olfactory groove usually extend posteriorly and involve the optic nerve. These tumors produce a characteristic triad of signs known as the Foster Kennedy syndrome. These signs consist of:

1. Ipsilateral anosmia due to pressure on the olfactory nerve.[53, 93]
2. Ipsilateral optic atrophy due to pressure on the optic nerve.
3. Contralateral papilledema due to raised intracranial pressure.

Involvement of the Frontal Eye Fields. Connections to the frontal eye fields are frequently affected by frontal lobe tumors, and examination of eye movements may reveal conjugate jerkiness of eye movement in all directions of gaze (coarse pursuit movements). The patient, on request, may also be unable to maintain gaze on an object, and the eyes may tend to return to the position of rest (motor impersistence of gaze). More commonly, the patient on command is unable to deviate the eyes to the side opposite the lesion, although he can do so reflexly (apraxia of gaze).

Involvement of the Motor Pathways. Examination of the motor system may disclose an opposing movement to any motion of the limb initiated by the examiner, which is involuntary and cannot be stopped on request (tonic perseveration or *gegenhalten*). This is usually found in the limbs opposite the involved hemisphere. Later evidence of contralateral hemiparesis, hypertonia, increased deep tendon reflexes, and an extensor plantar response appears owing to involvement of the precentral gyrus of the corticospinal tracts. Unilateral or bilateral grasp and sucking reflexes may occur as release phenomena (e.g., released from cortical inhibition) in frontal lobe tumors.

Involvement of the Precentral Gyrus and the Corticospinal Tract. The precentral gyrus or motor area is located anterior to the central sulcus and includes the area responsible for voluntary movement.

SEIZURES. Seizures may be caused by tumors arising in the precentral area and usually present as partial motor seizures. These may be jacksonian in type beginning with clonic movements in either the opposite thumb, great toe, or face and progressing in an orderly march through contiguous parts. In a matter of seconds or minutes, there is involvement of the whole of the opposite side of the body. The jacksonian march may be followed by a generalized seizure. On the other hand, the spread of the epileptic discharge may be so rapid that the seizure appears from clinical observation to be generalized from the start. In some patients, partial seizures may be confined to one area, usually the thumb, hand, wrist, or face, for hours or days (epilepsia partialis continua). Any type of epileptic seizure may be followed by a transient contralateral hemiplegia or hemiparesis, which may persist for several days up to two weeks (Todd's paralysis, postictal paralysis).

CORTICOSPINAL TRACT. Involvement of the corticospinal tract by tumor growth results in progressive contralateral hemiparesis and finally hemiplegia with increased tone, increased deep tendon reflexes, and an extensor plantar response. A tumor affecting the lower portion of the motor strip may interrupt connections to Broca's area, resulting in motor dysphasia. Involvement of association areas anterior to the motor strip may produce ideomotor or motor dyspraxia of the contralateral limbs.

Involvement of the Paracentral Lobule. The paracentral lobule is on the medial aspect of the cerebral hemisphere, is bisected by the central sulcus, and hence belongs to both frontal and parietal lobes. The frontal portion is a continuation of the motor strip from the lateral convexity of the hemisphere over to the medial surface. This portion of the motor strip is concerned with movements of the leg and foot. The area immediately rostral and inferior to the paracentral lobule, on the medial aspect of the frontal lobe and cingulate gyrus, is the center for cortical control of bladder function. Any tumor arising in the medial aspect of the frontal lobe or in the falx cerebri may act as a midline tumor and produce pressure on the medial aspects of both cerebral hemispheres. The pressure results in bilateral signs of progressive spastic paraparesis, urgency of micturition followed by incontinence, and intellectual deterioration.

Parietal Lobe Tumors

Involvement of the Postcentral Gyri. These areas of the parietal cortex are concerned with the discrimination of texture, weight, size, shape, and identification of objects touched. The primary conception of sensations of touch, pain, temperature, and vibration is at a thalamic level; the interpretative or discriminatory function is within the parietal cortex. Because the motor area of the frontal lobe lies immediately anterior to the parietal lobe, combined frontoparietal tumors tend

to produce signs of motor involvement at an early stage. Because the cortical threshold for seizures is lower in the frontal cortex than in the parietal, motor seizures are more commonly seen than sensory.

The semeiology of parietal lobe tumors includes partial seizures, often of jacksonian type, beginning with a focal sensation of numbness or paresthesias in the face or limbs, which show a stereotyped form of progression. This may be followed or accompanied by partial or generalized motor seizures. Although primary sensation remains intact to touch, pain, temperature, and vibration sense, there is impairment of discriminatory (cortical) sensation. The loss of discrimination results in failure to appreciate touch or pinprick on the contralateral side during bilateral simultaneous stimulation (sensory extinction) and inability to localize touch or pinprick accurately on the contralateral side of the body. There is loss of two-point discrimination on the contralateral side of the body. Astereognosis is present when small objects such as a nickel, dime, and quarter are palpated in the hand contralateral to the parietal lobe tumor. With the eyes closed, there is loss of ability to compare weights of objects (baresthesia) and the texture of objects felt in the contralateral hand, as well as to discriminate numbers written on the fingers (agraphism).

Impairment of visuospatial orientation may result in loss of ability to orient objects in space and to find one's way around the ward or in the environment. There may be irregular jerky movements of the hand and fingers on attempted movement (pseudoathetosis), and the hand may be held with fingers extended and raised (avoiding response). If the parietal lobe tumor is extensive, failure on the part of the patient to identify his own contralateral limbs and their parts (autotopagnosia) may occur, and there may also be a denial of symptoms and signs, such as hemiplegia affecting the contralateral side (anosognosia). Deeper lesions of the parietal lobe produce a contralateral homonymous quadrantanopia involving the lower quadrants, and lesions involving the corona radiata in close proximity to the thalamus may produce "thalamic pain" (p. 620).

Involvement of the Angular Gyrus. Tumors of the angular gyrus or in the parietal or temporal lobes immediately adjacent to the angular gyrus may produce a characteristic group of symptoms (Gerstmann's syndrome) consisting of agraphia, acalculia, contralateral finger agnosia, and confusion of left and right side (allochiria).

Involvement of the Supramarginal Gyrus. Impairment or interruption of function in the supramarginal gyrus may result in ideational apraxia (p. 8).

Occipital Lobe Tumors

The primary visual reception areas are within the medial surfaces of both occipital lobes (area 17) immediately adjacent to the calcarine fissure. The visual association or cortical projection areas (areas 18 and 19) surround the primary visual area and extend into the parietal and temporal lobes anteriorly. The function of the lateral surface of the occipital lobe is closely integrated with and anatomically inseparable from the posterior portions of the parietal and temporal lobes.

A tumor involving the medial aspect of the occipital lobe or the occipital pole frequently produces a contralateral, inferior homonymous quadrantanopia, which progresses to a homonymous hemianopia. The macula is spared, unless the lateral geniculate body or optic tract is destroyed.

Damage to the visual association areas (areas 18 and 19) produces visual object agnosia, agnosia for colors, and inability to recall the appearance of familiar objects. The patient may be unable to turn the eyes toward the side of the lesion owing to involvement of the "center" for following eye movements.

Tumors growing on the lateral aspect of the occipital lobe sometimes reach considerable size without symptoms. Extension into the occipital lobe may result in partial seizures with ill-defined visual symptoms described as colored lights or "Christmas tree" or "kaleidoscope" type of photopsias. When the dominant hemisphere is involved, tumor spread into the posterior part of the temporal lobe may produce a receptive, nominal, or jargon dysphasia.

Temporal Lobe Tumors

Involvement of the Uncus. The temporal lobe has a low threshold for epileptic activity. Tumors exerting pressure on or growing in the uncus produce characteristic partial epileptic seizures (uncinate fits, see p. 353). These seizures can occur many times in a single day and usually begin with an intense hallucination of smell or taste. In 80 per cent of the patients an unpleasant odor of burnt flesh or blood is described as the first sensation. There may be a hallucinatory sense of taste (gustatory aura). The other 20 per cent describe pleasant hallucinations of smelling flowers or perfume. The seizure may spread to adjacent parts of the temporal lobe, with a clouding of consciousness, feelings of familiarity sometimes accompanied by smacking of the lips and tongue, and repetitive complex motor behavior such as palpating or unbuttoning clothing. Occasionally the seizure becomes generalized, but it usually ceases at the stage of focal discharge.

Involvement of the Temporal Lobe and Insula. Partial seizures believed to arise in this area are characterized by psychomotor, psychosensory, visceral, and automatic components of the so-called psychomotor seizure (p. 351). The initial symptoms are often followed by clouding of consciousness and automatic purposeful motor movements. Patients may walk, run, drive cars, undress, and perform a variety of well-coordinated actions during this phase of the seizure (rarely are these actions aggressive or antisocial) although they are not fully conscious, and these actions are essentially purposeless and stereotyped. Posterior temporal lobe tumors tend to produce partial seizures beginning with visual symptoms. There are frequently elementary flashes or balls of light, but some patients may experience visual hallucinations of complex scenes, which are repeated with each seizure. Macropsia or micropsia may also occur. Midtemporal tumors of the dominant hemisphere may be associated with elementary auditory hallucinations, such as whistling or hissing sounds or the sound of bells. A tumor involving the insula may give rise to partial seizures, with visceral symptoms including epigastric pain or fluttering sensations in the epigastrium or thorax. Many temporal lobe lesions are associated with partial seizures that commence with an intense sensation of familiarity with the surroundings *(déjà vu).* The opposite sensation of a feeling of strangeness in familiar surroundings *(jamais vu)* may also occur.

Severe dysphasia with both sensory and motor elements may be present in tumors involving the midtemporal portion of the dominant hemisphere. Extension of a tumor into the substance of the temporal lobe may lead to pressure on the fibers of the optic radiation that loop into the temporal lobe (Meyer's loop), resulting in a superior homonymous quadrantanopia. Deep temporal lobe tumors may involve the corticospinal tracts directly or by producing edema with consequent contralateral hemiparesis.

Tumors arising in the medial aspect of the temporal lobe or in the insula may extend into the basal ganglia, with the development of unilateral dystonia, choreoathetosis, or parkinsonian tremor. Although temporal lobe tumors frequently present with focal signs at an early stage, a tumor arising in or producing pressure on the anterolateral aspect of the temporal lobe may attain considerable size without symptoms. Others may produce progressive dementia similar to frontal lobe tumors or may be detected because of the development of headache and raised intracranial pressure rather than focal neurologic deficits.

Tumors of the Internal Capsule and Basal Ganglia

Deep-seated tumors arising in the thalamus or basal ganglia often present with headache, seizures, and progressive hemiparesis owing to early spread into the internal capsule. Disturbances of mentation with impaired memory, affective difficulties, and alteration in behavior may occur.[127] Thalamic tumors may also produce spontaneous pain and paresthesia (thalamic syndrome). Signs of increased intracranial pressure are often present by the time the patient seeks medical advice. There are hemiparesis, homonymous hemianopia, and involuntary movements in some cases with contralateral dystonia, choreoathetosis, or parkinsonian tremor.

Tumors of the Corpus Callosum

Tumors confined to the corpus callosum are often asymptomatic but may cause generalized seizures as they increase in size.[177] Extension of the tumor into the cerebral hemispheres produces additional signs due to destruction and hydrocephalus. There is often a severe progressive dementia due to involvement of the crossed and longitudinal projections of the frontal lobe, and grasp and sucking reflexes are present bilaterally. In the early stages, posteriorly located tumors produce alexia in the nondominant (usually left) visual field with inability to name colors in the nondominant field. Anteriorly located tumors of the corpus callosum are associated with agraphia and dyspraxia of the nondominant (usually left) hand.[91] Involvement of the corticospinal tracts usually produces hemiparesis on one side followed

by bilateral hemiparesis or quadriparesis with generalized increase in the deep tendon reflexes and bilateral extensor plantar responses. Extension of the tumor into the area of the basal ganglia may produce dystonia, choreoathetosis, rigidity, and tremor resembling parkinsonism.

Tumors of the Fornix

Tumors of the fornix interrupt the main efferent pathway from the hippocampus and should theoretically be associated with severe disturbance of recent memory. This symptom has been described in some cases, but there are also reports of destruction of the fornix without neurologic symptoms.[189]

Tumors of the Third Ventricle

Tumors occurring in the third ventricle are often pedunculated (such as colloid cyst). By moving like a ball valve they may produce intermittent obstruction of the flow of cerebrospinal fluid. The chief complaints may be of paroxysmal headache, vomiting, and blurred vision, which is made worse by lying supine and relieved when the head is in the prone position. Children with third-ventricular tumors frequently sleep in the prone position. A 2- to 3-cps bobbing tremor of the head and trunk has been observed in children with large cysts of the third ventricle and hydrocephalus (bobble head doll syndrome).[13] Hydrocephalus results in progressive dementia and gait disturbances in adults.[102] Invasive tumors arising in the third ventricle may extend into the thalamus, with the production of thalamic pain, or into the midbrain, with brainstem signs. Extension into the frontal lobes may produce a progressive dementia. Extension into the hypothalamus will result in symptoms of hypothalamic dysfunction such as diabetes insipidus, narcolepsy,[163] cataplexy,[4] and precocious puberty in children.[51]

Tumors of the Fourth Ventricle

Tumors of the fourth ventricle may originate within the ventricle, such as papillomas of the choroid plexus. They may also originate from its lining and from within the ventricular wall, such as the ependymomas, hemangioblastomas, and mixed gliomas. They may spread from the cerebellum, such as the astrocytomas, medulloblastomas, and meningiomas.

These tumors compress or invade the brainstem and cerebellum and produce early obstruction to the circulation of cerebrospinal fluid. The development of hydrocephalus leads to the early appearance of symptoms of increased intracranial pressure.[140, 161] Invasion of the brainstem results in bilateral involvement of cranial nerves and corticospinal and sensory tracts. Infiltration of the cerebellum produces signs of cerebellar dysfunction. Herniation of one or both cerebellar tonsils may occur through the foramen magnum, causing severe headache, nuchal rigidity, and head retraction.

Tumors of the Pineal Gland

The pineal gland is a midline structure lying beneath the splenium of the corpus callosum and anterior to the superior colliculus of the midbrain. The most common tumor of the pineal gland is the pinealoma, but teratomas, dermoids, astrocytomas, ependymomas, and simple cysts have also been described.[147] Any of these tumors may produce symptoms due to pressure on the midbrain. Pressure on the anteromedial aspect of both superior colliculi produces a loss of upward conjugate gaze (Parinaud's syndrome, p. 27). Pressure on the pretectal area of the midbrain results in lid retraction and Argyll Robertson pupils. Displacement of the brainstem or direct compression by the tumor leads to obstruction of the aqueduct, hydrocephalus, and symptoms of increased intracranial pressure.[35] The cerebral peduncles may be pressed against the clivus, with the development of bilateral corticospinal tract signs. Pinealomas may occasionally metastasize to the spinal cord or infiltrate along the floor of the third ventricle, damaging the hypothalamus.

Tumors of the Hypothalamus

Almost all cases of hypothalamic tumor (Table 10–4) develop signs of increased intracranial pressure.

TABLE 10–4

Tumors Affecting the Hypothalamus

1. Gliomas of the hypothalamus, third ventricle, and optic chiasm
2. Hamartomas of the hypothalamus
3. Extrasellar extension of chromophobe adenomas and suprasellar craniopharyngiomas
4. Intracranial metastases
5. Malignant lymphomas
6. Suprasellar meningiomas
7. Aneurysms of the terminal portion of the carotid artery
8. Ectopic pinealomas in the chiasmal region

sure due to occlusion of the foramen of Monro. In addition, hypothalamic function may be affected directly or be caused by disturbances of hypothalamic pathways which regulate pituitary function.

Disturbances of Sexual Function Secondary to Hypothalamic Tumor. Precocious sexual development in children may result from hypothalamic tumors owing to premature release of pituitary gonadotropins. The primary fault is probably an excess secretion of luteinizing hormone–releasing hormone and follicle stimulating–releasing hormone from the hypothalamus into the hypothalamic pituitary portal venous system.[148]

Impairment of sexual function is a symptom of impaired hypothalamic and pituitary function. In children it is manifested by a delay or failure of puberty; in adult women by dysmenorrhea or amenorrhea; and in adult men by impotence and aspermia. A rare combination of amenorrhea and galactorrhea has also been described in adult women with pituitary tumors. Hypothyroidism occurs in hypothalamic-pituitary insufficiency but is seldom overt. The complaint is usually of loss of energy and dry or sparse hair. An elevated blood cholesterol, low serum protein-bound iodine, and postural hypotension are indicative of a hypothalamic-pituitary dysfunction.

Impairment of ACTH Secretion. There is an inadequate response to stress when there is impairment of ACTH secretion resulting in hypotension when the appropriate response would be hypertension and tachycardia. In patients at or near addisonian crisis owing to inadequate ACTH secretion and bradycardia, supplementary steroid therapy is indicated, particularly during medical or surgical stress (i.e., during diagnostic procedures or surgery).

Deficiency of Growth Hormone. Deficiency of growth hormone may result in dwarfism, small stature, and loss of weight in children and adolescents.

Deficiency of Antidiuretic Hormone (ADH). A lack of antidiuretic hormone causes diabetes insipidus, characterized by polyuria, polydipsia, and low specific gravity of the urine. It occurs spontaneously with hypothalamic and pituitary tumors and following traumatic diencephalic injuries including surgical removal of diencephalic and pituitary tumors and metastatic pinealomas (so-called ectopic pinealomas).

Disturbances of Fluid and Electrolyte Balance. Damage to the osmoreceptors within the hypothalamic mechanism may produce neurogenic hypernatremia and hyperchloremia. The opposite metabolic condition, referred to as "cerebral salt wasting," has been described and is believed to be related to reduced corticosteroid secretion secondary to inadequate ACTH secretion. In such cases addisonian crisis with hyponatremic shock may result.

Disturbances of Appetite. Hyperphagia and anorexia both may result from hypothalamic lesions and produce either obesity or inanition. Some children show anorexia, progressive weight loss, and apathy (diencephalic syndrome or failure to thrive).[140]

Disturbances of Body Temperature Control. Impairment of temperature control is a relatively common sign of hypothalamic injury, particularly in children, and is due to dysfunction of the temperature-regulating mechanisms in the hypothalamus. Body temperatures may exceed 106° to 108°F, and, unlike septic fevers, the skin feels cool, appears pale, and little sweating occurs. Apart from invasion by diencephalic tumors, hyperthermia may result from traumatic injury of the diencephalon during the surgical removal of tumors and following hemorrhage into the third ventricle. Disturbances of pulse rate and blood pressure also occur following inappropriate inhibition or excitation of the diencephalic sympathetic control.

Seizures. Diencephalic autonomic seizures (p. 357) have been reported in patients with hypothalamic tumors. These are characterized by piloerection and sudden changes in blood pressure and pulse rate with tonic posturing of the limbs. Narcolepsy sometimes occurs.

Tumors of the Basiocciput

Tumors arising in basiocciput are relatively rare and include chordomas and meningiomas.[29] The region may be involved also by direct extension of nasopharyngeal carcinomas, lymphoepitheliomas, and glomus jugulare tumors. Resulting symptoms arise from involvement of the lower cranial nerves and compression of the brainstem.

Involvement of the lower cranial nerves by metastatic tumor deposits growing in the subarachnoid space (meningeal carcinomatosis) is highly characteristic from a clinical point of view and usually begins with involvement of the ninth, tenth, and twelfth cranial nerves. This may start unilaterally and segmentally, but bilateral involvement occurs sooner or later, with progressive paralysis of the cranial nerves up to and including pontine and midbrain levels. Compression of the brainstem usually produces damage to both corticospinal tracts, with signs of spasticity, increased reflexes, and extensor plantar responses.

Tumors Involving the Gasserian Ganglion

The gasserian ganglion may be compressed or directly invaded by a meningioma involving the tip of the petrous temporal bone or medial portion of the sphenoid wing. The proximal portion of the trigeminal nerve may itself be the site of a neurilemmoma or be compressed by an acoustic neurilemmoma. Extension of a nasopharyngeal carcinoma along the base of the skull and through the foramen ovale may also compress the gasserian ganglion and trigeminal nerve.

The initial symptoms may be paroxysmal and lancinating pains, indistinguishable from those characteristic of tic douloureux (p. 674). Occasionally, pressure on the ganglion produces other atypical forms of facial pain. Extension of the tumor into the posterior fossa below the tentorium ("dumbbell tumor") produces loss of facial sensation, facial weakness, hearing loss, nystagmus, and vertigo.[53]

Tumors Involving the Optic Chiasm

The optic chiasm is occasionally the site of a primary glioma (astrocytoma) but is more commonly compressed by a variety of lesions, including pituitary adenomas, craniopharyngiomas, parasellar meningiomas, chordomas, and suprasellar aneurysms of the terminal portion of the internal carotid artery. Resulting symptoms are highly characteristic and are usually produced by pressure that interferes with the blood supply of the optic chiasm arising from branches of the anterior cerebral arteries. Occasionally, pressure atrophy may occur in the upper part of the chiasm if it is pushed upward against the anterior cerebral arteries.

The initial symptom is often a field defect or hemianopia for colors or an upper temporal quadrantic field defect in one eye (monocular, temporal, quadrantic defect). A field defect in the upper temporal quadrant of the other eye (upper bitemporal quadrantanopia) usually develops within a short period of time. Further progression produces a bitemporal hemianopia. Some degree of optic atrophy with pallor of one or both optic nerves will usually result. Tumors in this area may also produce symptoms of hypothalamic dysfunction by interfering with the blood supply or by a direct invasion of the hypothalamus (p. 623). Later the tumor may invade the frontal lobes lying immediately above, producing progressive dementia and other signs of frontal lobe involvement (p. 618).

Midbrain Tumors

Tumors of the midbrain usually produce early stenosis or occlusion of the aqueduct with increased intracranial pressure. Small tumors only a few millimeters in diameter may be fatal if located near or in the aqueduct. Because there is a concentration of important structures in the midbrain, tumors arising in this area may be expected to produce a broad spectrum of symptoms. Increased intracranial pressure usually occurs early, with involvement of the superior colliculi, which produces loss of conjugate upward gaze (Parinaud's syndrome). Destruction of both inferior colliculi or of both medial geniculate bodies is a rare cause of cerebral deafness.

A tumor arising in the pretectal area and involving the pretecto-oculomotor pathways may rarely produce loss of the pupillary reaction to light with preservation of reaction to near vision (Argyll Robertson pupils). Involvement of the nucleus of fibers of the third nerve in the brainstem causes ipsilateral ptosis, external strabismus, and diplopia, with ipsilateral dilatation of the pupil, which no longer reacts to light.

A suitably placed tumor of the cerebral peduncle will produce a contralateral hemiparesis with ipsilateral third-nerve palsy (Weber's syndrome), and more centrally placed lesions may involve the red nucleus or the cerebello-rubrothalamic fibers. Involvement of rubral connections will result in a contralateral rubral tremor (proximal, flapping tremor of the arms). Ipsilateral or contralateral cerebellar signs may occur, according to the site of the lesion. Involvement of the third nerve together with the red nucleus results in the syndrome of ipsilateral third-nerve palsy with contralateral ataxia and flapping tremor (Benedict's syndrome). Rarely, destruction of the sub-

stantia nigra by tumor has been reported to produce a contralateral parkinsonian tremor. Extensive involvement of the central periaqueductal gray matter and reticular formation may produce a state of akinetic mutism ("coma vigil") owing to destruction of the reticular activating mechanism. Patients with this curious condition are mute, swallow food placed in their mouths, turn in bed, and follow objects with their eyes but are otherwise immobile and unresponsive. It has been said that "they gaze but do not recognize."

Pontine Tumors

Tumors arising within the pons are not infrequent. They are usually infiltrating gliomas that may grow to considerable size before producing symptoms of increased intracranial pressure (Table 10–5). The signs are usually those of ipsilateral cranial nerve palsies and contralateral hemiparesis.

Chronic vomiting, anorexia, and failure to gain weight leading to emaciation (failure to thrive) have been reported in children with pontine gliomas.[111] Tumors involving the ventral pons bilaterally may cause a "locked-in" syndrome.[30]

Tumors of the Cerebellopontine Angle

Tumors of the cerebellopontine angle may arise from the eighth nerve (acoustic neuroma or neurilemmoma) or from surrounding structures (meningiomas, gliomas, dermoids, and vascular tumors). The acoustic neurilemmoma produces early involvement of the auditory division of the eighth nerve, while other tumors may not involve this nerve initially.[173] The development of symptoms (Table 10–6) is predictable in the acoustic neurilemmoma as the tumor increases in size and extends out of the cerebellopontine angle.[123]

Bilateral acoustic neuromas, which usually occur in von Recklinghausen's disease, may be large yet behave in a different manner, often producing little or no hearing loss.[99]

Tumors of the Medulla

These are usually gliomas, chordomas, or metastatic tumors such as bronchial carcinomas. Increased intracranial pressure occurs late in tumors arising within the medulla. In a manner comparable to pontine tumors, crossed syndromes are frequent, with symptoms and signs of ipsilateral cranial nerve involvement and contralateral hemiparesis. Destruction of the ninth and tenth nuclei or their nerves in their course through the medulla

TABLE 10–5

Clinical Features of Pontine Tumors

Symptoms and Signs, in Order of Frequency	Involved Structure
Symptoms[181]	
Gait disturbance	Corticospinal tracts, cerebellar connections, 75%
Diplopia	Sixth cranial nerve, 70%
Weakness in one or more extremity	Corticospinal tracts
Headache	Raised intracranial pressure
Dysarthria, dysphagia	Ninth and tenth cranial nerves, corticospinal tracts, cerebellar connections, lateral spinothalamic tract, vestibulovagal connections
Numbness, one half of body	
Vomiting	
Hearing loss, tinnitus, vertigo	Eighth cranial nerve (auditory and vestibular)
Failure to thrive	?Tumor involving floor of fourth ventricle
Locked-in syndrome	Ventral pons bilaterally
Signs	
Motor weakness, hyperreflexia, extensor plantar response	Corticospinal tract
Cranial nerve involvement	Seventh, fifth, ninth, tenth, eighth, and sixth cranial nerves, in order of frequency
Nystagmus and cerebellar ataxia	Cerebellar connections
Sensory loss, one half of body	Lateral spinothalamic tract
Papilledema	Raised intracranial pressures
Spastic facial contracture[159a]	Seventh cranial nerve (rare)

TABLE 10–6

Clinical Features of Tumors of The Cerebellopontine Angle

Symptoms and Signs, in Order of Frequency	Involved Structure
Symptoms	
Hearing loss and tinnitus	Auditory division of eighth cranial nerve
Balance disturbance	Vestibular division of eighth cranial nerve
Unsteadiness of gait	Medullocerebellar connections
Facial numbness or pain	Fifth cranial nerve
Facial weakness	Seventh cranial nerve
Dysphagia, dysarthria	Ninth and tenth cranial nerves
Signs	
Hearing loss	Auditory division of eighth cranial nerve, 100%
Facial weakness and impaired taste	Seventh cranial nerve, 50%
Corneal reflex depressed, hypalgesia of face	Fifth cranial nerve, 50%
Gait disturbance	Medullocerebellar connections, 45%
Nystagmus	Vestibulocerebellar connections
Finger-to-nose ataxia	Medullocerebellar connections
Asymmetry of deep tendon reflexes	Corticospinal tracts
Extensor plantar response	Corticospinal tracts
Romberg test positive	Medial lemniscus
Papilledema	Raised intracranial pressure (distortion of brainstem)
Paresis of palate, pharynx, vocal cords	Ninth and tenth cranial nerves
Diplopia	Sixth cranial nerve (due to increased intracranial pressure)
Weakness of sternocleidomastoids	Eleventh cranial nerve
Weakness of tongue	Twelfth cranial nerve

results in dysarthria and dysphagia. Involvement of the twelfth nerve or its nucleus leads to progressive wasting and weakness of the tongue with fasciculations beginning on the side of the tumor. Irritation of the vomiting center in the region of the tenth-nerve nucleus by tumor or edema results in pernicious hiccupping and vomiting, which are particularly pronounced in children. Eventually, infiltration of the inferior cerebellar peduncle produces ipsilateral cerebellar signs. Medullary tumors commonly invade the ipsilateral corticospinal tract rostral to the decussation of the pyramids with contralateral hemiparesis.

Tumors of the Cerebellum

Signs and symptoms of the cerebellar tumors vary according to the site of the lesion, but certain symptoms are usually common to all cerebellar tumors. Patients with cerebellar tumors often present with a disturbance of gait. Increased intracranial pressure with papilledema tends to occur early,[65] with accompanying complaints of nausea, vomiting, and headache.[59]

The headache tends to be occipital, is usually accompanied by pain radiating down the neck, and increases when there is herniation of the cerebellar tonsils. The head is retracted and rotated with the occiput to the side opposite the lesion, and there is nuchal rigidity with spasm of cervical muscles ("cerebellar tilt of the head" or "tonsillar tilt"). Vomiting may be severe, particularly in children.

Flocculonodular Lobe Tumors. Tumors in this location have certain characteristic features. There is truncal ataxia with marked unsteadiness of gait and little evidence of ataxia on performing the heel-to-knee test. On sitting up, the patient tends to fall to one side.

When the lesion is asymmetric, the head becomes rotated, with the occiput directed to the side opposite the tumor. There is a coarse horizontal nystagmus, which is maximal toward the side of the lesion.

Midline Tumors of the Anterior Lobe. The characteristic sign of anterior lobe involvement is marked ataxia. The patient walks with a wide-based, stiff-legged gait and staggers to both sides ("drunken sailor gait"). Hypotonia is mild or absent, and finger-to-nose dysmetria, incoordination of the upper extremities, and nystagmus are also absent. Intermittent attacks of decerebrate rigidity ("cerebellar fits") tend to occur in far-advanced cases.

Tumors of the Posterior Lobe. These cerebellar tumors usually provide the classic picture of unilateral cerebellar involvement. The child or adolescent often presents with unsteadiness of gait, headache, and vomiting. There is a coarse nystagmus, which is maximal on looking toward the affected side; however, positional nystagmus (nystagmus occurring only in the right or left lateral position) may be the first sign of tumor, particularly medulloblastoma.[64] There is homolateral hypotonia involving the trunk and extremities with a pendular knee jerk. There is dysmetria when reaching for objects, and there is past pointing with the eyes open or closed. The affected limbs show some muscle weakness (asthenia), and the hand grip is jerky and irregularly sustained.

There is slowness in checking movements; hence, the patient may overfling and strike himself when the examiner suddenly releases the grip of a patient pulling his hand toward himself. Decomposition of movement results in dysmetria on finger-to-nose or heel-to-shin testing and adiadochokinesis on attempting rapid alternating movements. Finger-to-nose testing reveals a terminal intention tremor. The speech is dysarthric owing to poor coordination of articulation, phonation, and respiration. There is a tendency to fall toward the side of the lesion on walking.

Tumors of the Sphenoid Ridge

Meningiomas are by far the most common tumors that arise in the vicinity of the sphenoid ridge. They frequently produce hyperostosis and thickening of the ridge and of the wings of the sphenoid.[39, 62] The tumors are so situated that they may grow into either the anterior or middle fossa.

Tumors located medially may extend into the optic foramen, press on the optic nerve, and result in monocular amblyopia and optic atrophy. As the tumor increases in size, there may be increased intracranial pressure with contralateral papilledema (Foster Kennedy syndrome, see p. 619). Occasionally, the tumor presses on the optic chiasm or optic tract rather than the optic nerve with the development of a contralateral, homonymous quadrantic field defect or incomplete homonymous hemianopia. Unilateral exophthalmos results if there is obstruction to the venous return from the orbit.[164] Extension of a sphenoid ridge meningioma into the orbit produces papilledema, sometimes called "disk edema." This condition is associated with unilateral visual loss, edema of the disk, and prominence of anastomotic optociliary veins at the disk margin and is due to interference with venous flow through the optic nerve.

Pressure on the structures passing through the superior orbital fissure (third, fourth, and sixth nerves and ophthalmic division of the fifth nerve) results in progressive homolateral ophthalmoplegia with loss of sensation over the forehead and anterior portion of the scalp. Extension into the frontal lobe may produce dementia, and there may be an ipsilateral loss of smell owing to pressure on the olfactory nerve. Compression of the deeper structures in the hemisphere may result in progressive contralateral hemiparesis or, rarely, unilateral akinetic rigidity and involuntary movements similar to those of Parkinson's disease, owing to pressure on the basal ganglia.

Tumors arising from the middle third of the sphenoid wing may become quite large before giving rise to symptoms. Increased intracranial pressure usually gives rise to the first symptoms before tumor infiltration causes focal signs such as minimal contralateral hemiparesis, slight increase in deep tendon reflexes, and dysphasia when there is involvement of the dominant hemisphere. Extension into the frontal lobe produces dementia with signs of intellectual deterioration (p. 617), and involvement of the medial aspect of the temporal lobe (uncus) may result in partial seizures with olfactory hallucinations (uncinate fits).

Meningiomas commonly arise from the outer third of the sphenoid ridge, usually as a flat tumor ("en plaque") that tends to produce marked hyperostosis. Hyperostosis may become manifest externally as a painless mass in the temporal bone, sometimes accompanied by progressive exophthalmos on the same side. Tumor growth is exceedingly slow in the majority of cases, so that symptoms of increased intracranial pressure tend to occur late. Eventually, extension of the tumor or hyperostosis may produce pressure on the optic nerve and the structures passing through the superior orbital fissure.

The Gliomas, or Tumors of Glial Origin

Approximately 50 per cent of brain tumors and 25 per cent of tumors within the spinal canal are of glial origin. Numerous attempts have been made to classify these tumors according to their histogenetic origin, but recently, classification has been simplified. Evidence to support earlier views that they are derived from primitive cell rests is flimsy, and the current view is that they arise by dedifferentiation from preexisting adult forms of glial cells. This more modern view eliminates the use of such fanciful terms as "spongioblastoma," "astroblastoma," or "glioblastoma multiforme." The glial cell type of origin is used for classification together with an estimate of the grade of the malignancy based on the degree of cellular anaplasia, vascular proliferation, and mitotic activity.

The glial tumors can usually be graded into four categories of malignancy, with the most highly differentiated (or relatively benign) tumors placed in grade 1 and the highly malignant or anaplastic placed in grade 4. This grading has practical clinical usefulness as well as being a means of pathologic classification, because, in general, the grading bears direct relation to prognosis and life expectancy. A practical classification of the gliomas is given in Table 10–7. It can be argued that the neuroastrocytomas are not truly glial tumors. Despite controversy over the origin of these tumors, it is generally conceded that they contain neoplastic glial elements; and this fact permits their inclusion with the gliomas.

Astrocytomas

Astrocytomas are not only the most common type of tumor arising within the central nervous system, but they are also the most common tumor arising in nearly every area of the cerebral hemispheres. Astrocytomas account for the most frequent type of tumor and cause aqueductal stenosis, hydrocephalus, and early death. The occurrence of metastasis by seeding along the cerebrospinal fluid pathways is not unusual in grade 4 astrocytomas.[21] Cerebellar astrocytomas are the most common brain tumors of childhood. These tumors are usually cystic, of low-grade malig-

TABLE 10–7

Classification of Gliomas

1. Astrocytomas, grades 1–4
2. Ependymomas, grades 1–4
3. Oligodendrogliomas
4. Medulloblastomas
5. Neuroastrocytomas

nancy (grade 1 or 2), and carry a favorable prognosis.[63] More malignant forms tend to occur in this location in early adult life.

Astrocytomas of the brainstem are usually seen in childhood and adolescence.[70] Although the midbrain and medulla may be involved, a pontine location is by far the most common. These lesions are usually grade 2 astrocytomas and produce a symmetric enlargement of the pons referred to by older pathologists as "diffuse hypertrophy" of the pons. Occasionally, higher-grade astrocytomas develop in the brainstem and produce hydrocephalus at an early stage and death within one year. Pontine or medullary astrocytomas are sometimes restricted to one half of the brainstem. Astrocytomas of the spinal cord are rarer than the cerebral variety, are usually more benign, and the patient survives longer.

Pathologic Considerations. Several histologic types of astrocyte have been recognized. Descriptive terms are often used in an attempt to classify tumors having one predominant cell type. However, the majority of tumors contain astrocytes of more than one type, and such descriptive terms are therefore of limited value. Four astrocytic cell types may be mentioned.

PROTOPLASMIC ASTROCYTES. These are cells with abundant eosinophilic cytoplasm, eccentric nuclei, and short glial fibers. They are also known as gemistocytic astrocytes (from the German *gemastete,* meaning bloated or swollen).

FIBRILLARY ASTROCYTES. These are elongated cells with little visible cytoplasm and long glial fibers that may extend for some distance through the tumor.

PILOCYTIC ASTROCYTES. These are bipolar fibrillary astrocytes that tend to form parallel rows or trabeculae, probably owing to infiltration of and extension along nerve tracts. Pilocytic astrocytes are seen most commonly in tumors of the brainstem.

ANAPLASTIC ASTROCYTES. In high-grade astrocytomas, it is often impossible to recognize the cell types described above. Bizarre giant and multinucleated cells are common. Shape and size vary greatly, and mitotic activity may be high.

Astrocytomas, Grades 1 and 2. GROSS APPEARANCE. These astrocytomas may be difficult to detect because there is no line of demarcation between tumor and normal brain tissue. They have a grayish, white appearance and usually feel firmer than the surrounding tissue. About 70 per cent of grade 1 astrocytomas occur in the cerebellum in children as cystic tumors with a mural nodule. Cystic change is rare in the cerebral hemisphere.

MICROSCOPIC APPEARANCE. Microscopically, grade 1 tumors consist of increased numbers of astrocytes of normal or near-normal appearance. In grade 2 astrocytomas, the nuclei are somewhat enlarged and hyperchromatic, but pleomorphism is not marked. Protoplasmic astrocytes are sometimes prominent; blood vessels only rarely show slight endothelial thickening.

Astrocytomas, Grades 3 and 4 (Glioblastoma Multiforme). The more malignant astrocytomas are usually seen in adults and constitute about 90 per cent of gliomas that occur after the age of 60 years (Fig. 10–2). Higher grades are uncommon in the cerebellum and spinal cord but compose the most common type of glioma of the pons. The incidence of grade 3 and 4 astrocytomas in the cerebral hemispheres is highest in the frontal lobes, followed by temporal and parietal lobes, basal ganglia, and occipital lobes in decreasing order of frequency. Tumors occurring in one frontal lobe frequently extend into the opposite frontal lobe through the corpus callosum, resulting in dementia and other symptoms of diffuse frontal lobe dysfunction.

GROSS APPEARANCE. There is usually an easily defined line of demarcation between high-grade astrocytomas and the surrounding tissue, although microscopic examination reveals diffuse infiltration (Fig. 10–3). Necrosis and hemorrhage are common, particularly in grade 4 astrocytomas.

MICROSCOPIC APPEARANCE. Grade 3 astrocytomas contain few normal-appearing astrocytes and are composed of cells showing varying degrees of anaplasia. The cells show considerable variation in size, with hyperchromatic nuclei and shortened glial processes. Multinucleated giant cells and a few mitotic figures may occur. There are numerous blood vessels which show adventitial and endothelial proliferation and occasional thrombosis. Areas of necrosis may surround obliterated vessels, and these in turn are surrounded by a palisaded layer of spindled astrocytes.

Grade 4 astrocytomas differ from grade 3 astrocytomas in having a more pleomorphic cell pat-

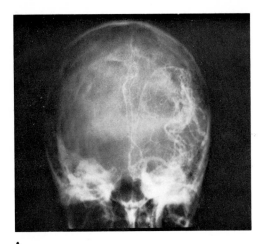 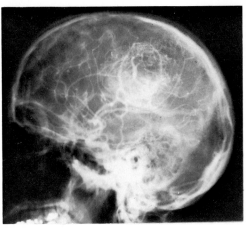

A   B

FIGURE 10–2. A left carotid arteriogram to show neovascularity and early venous drainage (tumor stain) in a grade 3 astrocytoma of the left frontoparietal region. *A.* Anteroposterior view. *B.* Lateral view.

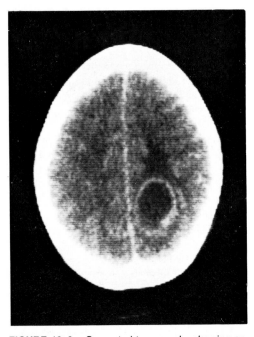

FIGURE 10–3. Computed tomography showing an area of decreased density in the right parieto-occipital area surrounded by a rim of increased density that appeared after injection of iodinated contrast material. This is an example of a diffusely infiltrating grade 3 astrocytoma, and the rim of increased density represents increased vascularity; there was no identifiable boundary to this tumor.

tern with many giant and multinucleated cells and high mitotic activity. Necrosis and vascular proliferation are also more pronounced.

In a few cases, the proliferation of the vascular endothelial cells is so pronounced that the tissue has the appearance of a sarcoma. These highly malignant tumors have been termed gliosarcoma.[117]

Ependymomas

Although ependymomas are the second most common type of glioma in the central nervous system, they are relatively infrequent when compared to the incidence of astrocytomas. The abnormal cells are derived from the ependymal cells lining the ventricles and the central canal of the spinal cord. Ectopic collections of ependymal cells are frequently found extending from the ventricles or central canal into the substance of the brain or spinal cord, and ependymomas may also arise from these cells. This presumably accounts for the occasional occurrence of ependymomas deep within the substance of the brain or spinal cord, but the majority lie in relation to and arise from the ependymal-lined cavities.

The highest incidence of ependymomas is seen in children and adolescents. Ependymomas constitute 60 per cent of gliomas arising within the spinal cord with the majority arising in the lumbosacral segments. Intracranial ependymomas are less frequent. They are predominantly infratentorial tumors, occurring in the roof or floor of the fourth ventricle and occasionally extending into the cerebellopontine angle or down the dorsal surface of the medulla through the foramen magnum onto the surface of the cervical cord.[93] Supratentorial ependymomas usually arise from the lateral or third ventricles, although they may arise elsewhere in the cerebral hemispheres. Ependymomas may be graded from 1 to 4 in much the same way as astrocytomas.

Gross Appearance. The majority of ependymomas arising in the cerebral hemispheres are large before they produce symptoms. In contrast, because of their critical location and liability to produce hydrocephalus, symptomatic infratentorial ependymomas are usually small tumors. Ependymomas of the spinal cord are not encapsulated, but those arising in the filum terminale are often easily shelled out by the neurosurgeon. Unfortunately, some grow in a diffuse manner between the nerve roots, into the cauda equina, and later invade the spinal cord substance itself.

The majority of ependymomas are solid tumors. Necrosis and hemorrhage are rare, but cyst formation is not uncommon in cerebral ependymomas. Seeding into the subarachnoid space with meningeal implants is not as common as with astrocytomas or medulloblastomas.

Microscopic Appearance. There are three histologic types of ependymomas: epithelial, papillary, and cellular.

EPITHELIAL EPENDYMOMA. The cells in this tumor resemble ependymal cells and are concentrically arranged around small spaces (ependymal rosettes), somewhat similar to the appearance of the central canal of the spinal cord.

PAPILLARY EPENDYMOMA. This tumor is composed of one or several layers of ependymal-type cells arranged on vascular connective tissue stalks in typical papillary arrangement. The connective tissue of the stalk may closely resemble that of the normal choroid plexus. This type is seen in the cauda equina.

CELLULAR EPENDYMOMA. This is by far the most common type. The cells are spindled and tend to group around the blood vessel to which their long fibrillary root processes are attached. Low-grade lesions are easy to diagnose, but it is frequently impossible to differentiate

high-grade ependymomas from high-grade astrocytomas.

A fourth type of ependymoma, papilloma of the choroid plexus, has been described, but there is controversy as to whether it is a distinct lesion or merely a low-grade papillary ependymoma. It arises from and closely duplicates the choroid plexus.

All epithelial and most papillary ependymomas are grade 1 or 2. Cellular ependymomas are also more commonly low grade, but a minority can be classified as grade 3 or 4 on the same basis as astrocytomas (p. 628).

Oligodendrogliomas

Relatively uncommon, these tumors constitute less than 10 per cent of all gliomas. They are usually found in the fourth and fifth decades of life and are predominantly supratentorial, with more than 50 per cent occurring in the frontal lobes of the brain.

Gross Appearance. Oligodendrogliomas grow slowly and arise within the white matter of the central nervous system. As they grow larger, they produce symptoms that may result from compression rather than from destruction of brain tissue. However, they are occasionally the site of massive hemorrhage with apoplectic symptoms. They are often sharply demarcated tumors, firm in consistency, with cystic areas, and calcification is common. Calcium deposits are large enough to be seen on plain roentgenograms of the skull in about 70 per cent of patients.[141] Calcium is usually related to the age of the oligodendrioglioma, with older tumors containing larger amounts of calcium. These tumors rarely cause meningeal gliomatosis.

Microscopic Appearance. The cells are characterized by round, regular, central nuclei surrounded by clear cytoplasm. They form clusters surrounded by vascular connective tissue septa. The cell membrane is often very distinct, so that the tumor has a honeycomb appearance. Calcium appears initially in the walls of the blood vessels and later forms larger plaques which are visible on roentgenography. Mitotic figures are rarely seen in these tumors. "Mixed gliomas" containing oligodendroglial cells and ependymal cells or astrocytes rarely occur. However, the appearance of atypical cells in an oligodendroglioma may account for reports of sudden explosive growth in these tumors after they have been apparently growing very slowly for many years.[152]

Medulloblastomas

The medulloblastoma is often said to be the most frequent tumor occurring in the posterior fossa in children; but, fortunately, it is less common than the more benign astrocytoma of the cerebellum. Medulloblastomas account for less than 30 per cent of gliomas in children. The tumor is almost exclusively seen in children and usually arises in the midline of the cerebellum and occasionally in the cerebellar hemispheres.

Gross Appearance. Because these tumors are soft, they may attain a considerable size before producing symptoms; inevitably, extension into the fourth ventricle occurs with development of hydrocephalus. Tumor extension into the cerebellopontine angles or over the surface of the brainstem or cerebellum is common (sugar coating). Spread through the subarachnoid space is not uncommon and gives rise to implants anywhere over the surface of the brain or spinal cord. These secondary tumors rarely cause symptoms.

Remote extracranial metastasis in bone lymph nodes or soft tissues have been described in long-surviving patients.[41] In some cases these metastatic cells have spread through a ventriculoperitoneal shunt inserted to relieve hydrocephalus in patients with medulloblastoma.[75]

Microscopic Appearance. The medulloblastoma is a highly cellular tumor consisting of small cells with elongated hyperchromatic nuclei and scanty cytoplasm. The cells tend to form incomplete rosettes similar to those seen in neuroblastomas and retinoblastomas. Histologically, neuroblastoma, small cell undifferentiated carcinoma of the lung, and medulloblastoma are difficult to differentiate.

Neuroastrocytomas

Probably, most tumors described as neuroastrocytomas or gangliogliomas in the central nervous system are really astrocytomas that have engulfed preexisting neurons. A few lesions may represent a mixed tumor of astrocytic and neuronal origin. They usually occur in children and young adults and may be located anywhere in the cerebral hemispheres and spinal cord. The most common site is the medial aspect of the temporal lobe or

the floor of the third ventricle, and signs of hypothalamic or pituitary insufficiency result.

Gross Appearance. Neuroastrocytomas are usually firm tumors, which may be quite small if located in the third ventricle. The larger examples in the cerebral hemispheres may be cystic or contain areas of calcification.

Microscopic Appearance. These tumors contain cells of apparently neuronal origin, which vary in shape and size. Nissl substance and neurofibrils are present in the cells, and the tumor contains a meshwork that appears to consist of axis cylinders. The neuronal elements are surrounded by a glial stroma, which shows the cellular features of a grade 1 or 2 astrocytoma (p. 629).

Neurilemmomas (Neurofibromas)

Incidence. Neurilemmomas are the most common type of tumor in the spinal canal (30 per cent) and rank third in frequency of all intracranial tumors. They are also the most common tumor of nerve trunks and can arise in any nerve where Schwann cells occur.[182] They are rare in children, occasionally occur in adolescents, but are usually encountered during and after the fourth decade of life.

Etiology. There is some controversy about whether these tumors are mesodermal (fibroblasts) or ectodermal (Schwann cells) in origin. At the present time, it is generally conceded that they are derived from the Schwann cell rather than from the fibroblasts of the nerve sheath.

Distribution. Almost all intracranial neurilemmomas are found attached to the eighth cranial nerve. Occasional involvement of other cranial nerves has been described, particularly in von Recklinghausen's disease, in which case multiple tumors have occurred on the fifth, ninth, and tenth nerves.

In the spinal canal, neurilemmomas occur as solitary tumors arising from the posterior nerve roots at any level but predominantly in the thoracic area.

Gross Appearance. The acoustic neurilemmoma appears in the cerebellopontine angle as a spheric or ovoid tumor that displaces the brainstem, cerebellum, and fourth ventricle. The fifth, seventh, ninth, and tenth cranial nerves may also be stretched over the surface or incorporated within the tumor mass. The tumor usually arises within the internal auditory meatus, which is enlarged; and in some cases, there is erosion of the tip of the petrous temporal bone. The cut surface varies from white to yellow depending on the lipid content.

In the spinal canal the tumors occur as small, ovoid masses displacing the spinal cord or cauda equina. They may enlarge and grow through the intravertebral foramen and attain considerable size outside the spinal column, producing a "dumbbell" or hourglass tumor.

Microscopic Appearance. The appearance of the neurilemmoma is quite characteristic. Elongated or spindle cells resembling fibroblasts form interlacing bundles. Nuclei are palisaded and somewhat resemble a picket fence. This arrangement has been eponymically described as Antoni type A tissue. Other areas (Antoni type B) consist of loose connective tissue containing many foam cells and, frequently, depositions of hemosideric pigment.

Tumors of Mesenchymal Origin and Vascular Tumors

Capillary Telangiectasia

Small collections of dilated capillaries are frequently discovered within the central nervous system at autopsy. They may be located anywhere in the central nervous system but are most common in the pons, thalamus, and midbrain regions. In nearly all cases they are incidental findings that were not associated with recognized clinical symptoms during life. Small capillary telangiectasia in the pons (telangiectasia pontis) is a rare cause of fatal pontine hemorrhage with sudden onset of pontine symptoms.

Capillary telangiectasia of the central nervous system is not a feature of multiple familial telangiectasia (Osler's disease).

Sturge-Weber Disease

The capillary-venous angiomatous malformation associated with this disease is described under Developmental Defects (p. 69).

Arteriovenous Malformations

These angiomatous malformations constitute about 3 per cent of "tumors" involving the central nervous system. They are a frequent cause of subarachnoid hemorrhage and seizures (p. 581).

Gross Appearance. Arteriovenous malformations may be found over any part of the cerebral cortex, brainstem, or cerebellum but are rare in the spinal canal. There is involvement of the leptomeninges and underlying tissue by a mass of tortuous vessels, which are supplied by one or more large abnormal arteries and drained by a series of abnormal veins. Arteriovenous fistulas are common, and large aneurysmal dilatations are frequent. The most common site is the parietal cortex in the distribution of the middle cerebral artery, but any of the major intracranial vessels may be involved. Shunting of blood through the arteriovenous malformation may rarely lead to the development of enlarged collateral vessels over the scalp, retina, or orbit. There may be abnormal vascular grooving noted in skull roentgenograms.

Microscopic Appearance. Arteriovenous malformations consist of a tangle of thin-walled blood vessels of widely differing caliber. Some show a resemblance to arteries, while others resemble veins in structure. The walls often consist of endothelium and a thin, collagenous layer with few muscle or elastic fibers. Such vessels are dilated and tortuous. There may be considerable surrounding gliosis and deposition of hemosiderin pigment indicative of prior extravasation of blood.

Venous Malformation

This form of vascular tumor much more frequently involves the vessels supplying the spinal cord (p. 542) than those to the brain. Those described in the brain are usually centrally located and drain into the great cerebral vein of Galen.

Computed Tomography. The CT scan demonstrates an area of increased density without surrounding edema. The injection of contrast material produces marked enhancement of the mass with demonstration of draining veins.[116]

Hemangioblastoma (Benign Capillary Hemangioblastoma)

These tumors are usually located in the cerebellum but occasionally arise in the medulla. Slightly more than 7 per cent of primary tumors of the posterior fossa are reported to be of this type. Hemangioblastomas of the spinal cord are infrequent and are usually associated with the formation of a syrinx. Cerebral location of these tumors is rare.[190]

The occasional association of hemangioblastoma of the brain or spinal cord with cysts of the pancreas and kidney and benign tumors of the kidney is known as Lindau's syndrome (or disease). The association of angiomatosis retinae (von Hippel's disease) with a hemangioblastoma of the central nervous system or with one or more of the other changes of Lindau's syndrome is often referred to as von Hippel-Lindau disease.

Gross Appearance. Hemangioblastomas are often cystic tumors into which projects a solid, hemorrhagic mural nodule of tumor. The cyst contents are usually xanthochromic, and there may be hemorrhage in the surrounding cerebellum. The overlying pia-arachnoid frequently contains dilated blood vessels.

Microscopic Appearance. These tumors consist of irregular capillaries lined by flattened or swollen endothelial cells. The supporting stroma contains polygonal cells whose cytoplasm contains a varying amount of lipid which gives it a foamy appearance.

Glomus Jugulare Tumors

Most pathologists consider that these tumors are derived from receptor nerve cells or paraganglionic cells of the ganglion nodosum of the vagus nerve.

Gross Appearance. These tumors are frequently seen as a red or blue mass when viewed through the tympanic membrane or as bluish pulsating tumors in the external auditory canal, where they may produce bleeding or a hemorrhagic discharge.

Microscopic Appearance. Glomus jugulare tumors are highly cellular tumors with nests of epithelial cells separated by a fine connective tissue stroma. Numerous arteriovenous communications exist throughout the tumor mass.

Clinical Features. The majority of tumors arise in the middle ear and produce progressive loss in auditory acuity. Examination may show a pulsating tumor in the external canal or a mass behind the tympanic membrane.

Extension of the growth through the petrous temporal bone causes paralysis of the third to sixth cranial nerves. Invasion of the posterior fossa results in involvement of the lower cranial nerves. Development of the tumor in the mastoid area may produce ipsilateral facial paralysis.

Diagnostic Procedures. These are as follows:

1. CT scans may show destruction of the base of the skull in the region of the jugular foramen with tumor mass.
2. Audiometric tests will show marked hearing loss, and caloric stimulation will show lack of labyrinthine response on the side of the tumor.
3. The diagnosis may be confirmed by biopsy if the tumor is present in the external auditory canal.
4. Roentgenograms may reveal clouding of the mastoid air cells, destruction of the petrous temporal bone or the base of the skull, and enlargement of the jugular foramen.[82]
5. Vertebral and carotid arteriograms with subtraction may reveal a tumor "stain" in the region of the jugular foramen. Jugular venograms may show obstruction of the jugular vein at the jugular foramen (Fig. 10–4).

Treatment. Small tumors may be treated by surgical excision. Larger tumors show some response to irradiation. Ligation of the afferent arteries or the external carotid artery has little effect owing to the rich collateral circulation around the base of the skull. Inoperable tumors can also be treated by the introduction of emboli through arterial catheters placed in the feeding vessels.[73]

Meningiomas

Incidence. Meningiomas are the second most common tumors arising in both the brain and spinal cord and account for 17 per cent of tumors of the central nervous system. They can occur at any age. They are more common in females, with a peak incidence during the fifth and sixth decades, and, occasionally, have been reported to occur in families.

Most meningiomas in children are supratentorial. They grow rapidly, are often large, and undergo sarcomatous change.[38]

Etiology. These tumors are usually attached to the meninges. A rather rare exception is a meningioma occurring in the third ventricle, which may have arisen from connective tissue of the choroid plexus. There has been some disagreement about the origin of meningiomas, but it is

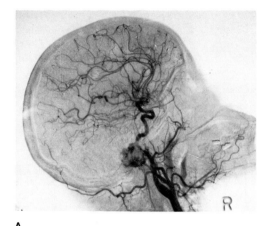

A

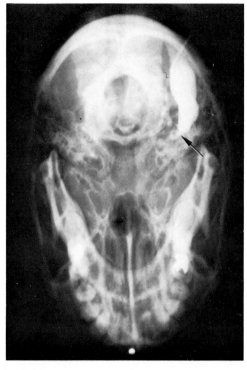

B

FIGURE 10–4. *A.* Right carotid arteriogram. The subtraction film shows the characteristic circumscribed vascular stain of a glomus jugulare tumor. The external occipital and superficial temporal branches of the external carotid artery supply blood to the tumor, which is compressing the intrapetrosal portion of the internal carotid artery. The vascular stain was difficult to visualize without the subtraction film. *B.* Right jugular venogram. Complete obstruction to the retrograde flow of contrast material is noted at the level of the right jugular foramen. The contrast material usually flows through the jugular foramen without difficulty into the petrosal and sigmoid sinuses.

now generally conceded that they are derived from the arachnoid "cap" cells found around the arachnoid villi. Lesser concentrations of these "cap" cells are also seen near the cortical veins, accounting for tumors unrelated to major venous sinuses that occur over the surface of the hemispheres. In the spinal cord, the cap cells are concentrated at the junction of the arachnoid and dura over the nerve roots.

Distribution. Supratentorial meningiomas are most common in the parasagittal region. Other common locations of meningiomas noted in order of frequency are: plaquelike tumors or round masses compressing the convexity of the brain, the sphenoid ridge, the parasellar region, and the ba-

sofrontal area (mainly in the olfactory groove) (Fig. 10–5).

The most common site for infratentorial meningiomas is on the inferior aspect of the petrous temporal bone at the cerebellopontine angle; less common sites are the margins of the transverse sinus and the foramen magnum.

Meningiomas within the spinal canal, or spinal cord meningiomas, almost invariably arise from the nerve roots and are most frequent in the thoracic area, particularly from T_4 to T_{10} (see Fig. 10–12). Occasionally, retro-orbital meningiomas may arise from the arachnoid sheath surrounding the optic nerve as it enters the orbit.

An inclusion of arachnoid "cap" cells persisting in the glabella during fusion of the frontal bones

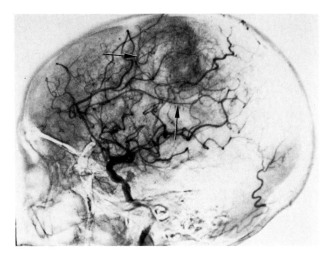

A

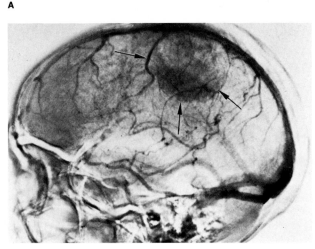

B

FIGURE 10–5. Left carotid angiogram with subtraction. There is displacement of vessels in the arterial phase *(A)* and venous phase *(B)*, which outline an oval meningioma lying over the superior aspect of the convexity of the left hemisphere.

may give rise to midline frontal meningioma in later life (ectopic meningioma).

Gross Appearance. Meningiomas are usually spheric or ovoid in shape. They are generously encapsulated and easily separated from the brain or spinal cord. The cut surface varies from pink to grayish-white and appears fibrous. A gritty sensation on cutting is due to the presence of calcified spherules, or "psammoma bodies," so-called because they look like grains of sand. Hemorrhage and cyst formation are not uncommon. Some meningiomas develop as a thin, flat plate of tumor closely applied to and following the contours of the bone (so-called meningioma "en plaque"). This type is particularly prone to invade the bone and produce hyperostosis.

Ventricular meningiomas are rare; they are usually spheric and distort the ventricular cavities. Remnants of the choroid plexus may be discernible and are stretched over the surface of the tumor.

Microscopic Appearance. There have been many subclassifications of meningiomas based on cell type or degenerative phenomena, but three basic types are now generally recognized by neuropathologists. These are (1) meningothelial, (2) psammomatous, and (3) fibroblastic meningioma.

MENINGOTHELIAL MENINGIOMA. The majority of meningiomas are of this type. The cells are indistinguishable from arachnoid "cap" cells and vary from polygonal to spindled in shape. Cell borders are indistinct and the nuclei usually oval and regular although some giant forms can occur. The cells lie in small whorls and may mimic the appearance of squamous carcinoma. There is a varying amount of collagenous stroma containing an abundance of blood vessels.

PSAMMOMATOUS MENINGIOMAS. These are meningothelial meningiomas in which formation of whorls is pronounced. The center of the whorl often contains a small blood vessel that is surrounded by hyalinized and calcified cells forming psammoma (sandlike) bodies.

FIBROBLASTIC MENINGIOMA. This is a rarer type of meningioma probably derived from the fibrous stroma of the arachnoid although islands of meningothelial cells may be found. The microscopic appearance is of interlacing bundles of fibrous tissue containing elongated spindle-shaped cells. The cells are arranged in parallel fashion, and whorls are not a feature of this type of tumor.

Any type of meningioma may undergo malignant change, although this is rare. Local recurrence of meningiomas is not uncommon but is due to incomplete removal or persistence of tumor cells in the overlying bone flap replaced after surgery. However, recurrence itself does not indicate malignancy. Malignancy should be suspected when there is marked invasion and destruction of bone rather than hyperostosis. From a clinical point of view, the absence of a definite capsule at surgery and invasion of surrounding brain tissue are the most important features of malignancy.

Under the microscope, malignant meningiomas show increased cellularity, pleomorphism, giant cells, and mitotic figures. This malignant change may be apparent when a recurrent tumor is compared to the original biopsy specimen, but the cellular variation seen in some benign meningiomas makes it extremely difficult to predict that any given tumor will behave in a malignant fashion. Intracranial or extracranial metastases are rare in all varieties of meningioma.

The hemangiopericytoma is a rare tumor of the meninges that may compress either the brain or spinal cord and may be confused with a sarcoma. It is derived from pericytes (the contractile cells lying next to capillaries), is extremely vascular, and presents considerable technical difficulty during surgical removal.

Reticulum Cell Sarcoma

Reticulum cell sarcoma of the brain is a rare tumor occurring predominantly in adolescents and young adults. The tumor has been described in patients receiving immunosuppressive therapy after an organ transplant. The increasing number and greater survival of transplant patients heighten the probability that there will be a greater frequency of reticulum cell sarcoma of the brain.[103]

Distribution. Reticulum cell sarcomas are often multiple tumors that occur in any part of the brain and rarely in the spinal cord.

Gross Appearance. The tumors are usually gray or tan with diffuse, ill-defined borders and a granular surface showing areas of hemorrhage and necrosis.[74]

Microscopic Appearance. The cells of the reticulum cell sarcoma are usually small, round, or oval with a slightly twisted nucleus. The tumor may contain large multinucleated reticulum cells in some areas. The cells often stream out from the edge of the tumor into the surrounding brain.[2]

Primary Leptomeningeal Sarcomatosis

This rare tumor occurs at any age from infancy to senescence. Leptomeningeal sarcomatosis spreads rapidly producing diffuse infiltration of the cerebral and spinal meninges and perivascular infiltration of the brain or spinal cord. There are three forms of clinical presentation:

1. Multiple cranial and spinal nerve root involvement by the tumor.
2. Cerebral with signs of a rapidly developing tumor.
3. Spinal cord compression.

The cerebrospinal fluid shows a mononuclear pleocytosis, low glucose, elevated protein, and the presence of malignant cells.[24]

Tumors of Developmental Origin and Colloid Cysts of the Third Ventricle

Paraphyseal Cysts

The paraphysis is a glandular structure located in the anterior part of the third ventricle during the early period of embryonic development. The structure usually disappears, but remnants may persist and develop into cystic structures in adult life. It is not certain that all colloid cysts of the third ventricle are derived from paraphyseal remnants. Some may develop from the choroid plexus or ependyma[158] or may be derived from epidermoid or dermoid cysts (see below), which would account for their occurrence in the lateral ventricles.

Gross Appearance. A small colloid cyst may be an incidental finding at autopsy; others become large enough to obstruct the foramina of Monro and produce acute attacks of hydrocephalus. In either case they are smooth, spheric, pedunculated structures attached to the roof or walls of the third ventricle and contain semisolid, grayish-white material originating from secretion or desquamation of the lining cells.

Microscopic Appearance. The walls of the cyst consist of a thin layer of connective tissue and an inner layer of low cuboidal epithelium.

Chordoma

Notochordal remnants occasionally give rise to tumors that may be found anywhere from the base of the skull through the spinal canal to the sacral area. The majority of chordomas are located in the sacral area. The rarer upper clivus chordoma may extend forward through the middle cranial fossa and into the sphenoid sinus. Lower clivus chordomas tend to involve the lower cranial nerves and grow into the posterior fossa or upper cervical canal.[42]

Gross Appearance. The majority of chordomas are hard tumors that extend through the dura to exert pressure on the brain, spinal cord, or cauda equina. Presacral extension of chordomas is common.

Microscopic Appearance. The cellular appearance of the chordoma is characteristic, with lobules of foamy, vacuolated cells containing glycogen and surrounded by a mucinous matrix. There is more than a superficial resemblance to a chondroma or chondrosarcoma.

Dermoid Cysts

Dermoid cysts are a relatively rare form of midline inclusion most commonly located in the lumbosacral area of the spinal canal. Sometimes they are found in the posterior fossa in the vermis of the cerebellum or floor of the fourth ventricle. Occasional examples have been described in the midline of the anterior fossa. Dermoid cysts may be associated with other congenital abnormalities and hydrocephalus.

Gross Appearance. The cysts are usually spheric structures that often communicate with the exterior through a midline dermal sinus. Such sinuses are frequently present in the lumbosacral area and are occasionally found in the occipital region in relation to a cerebellar dermoid. The sinus tracts may give rise to repeated pyogenic infections of the cyst, which may extend to the meninges causing recurrent meningitis (p. 467). Dermoid cysts contain thick sebaceous material and hair. This material is highly irritating if it escapes into the subarachnoid space and can produce a severe and often fatal granulomatous meningitis.

Microscopic Appearance. The cyst lining consists of squamous epithelium, and the lumen contains desquamated keratin. The supporting dermal tissue contains epidermal appendages such as sweat glands, hair follicles, and sebaceous glands.

Epidermoid Cysts

Unlike dermoid cysts, epidermoid cysts are not confined to the midline and are widely distributed in the cranial cavity and spinal canal.[174] The most common sites in the cranial cavity are:

1. The apex of the petrous temporal bone or cerebellopontine angle
2. The suprasellar region
3. The cerebral hemispheres or lateral ventricles
4. The fourth ventricle or cerebellum

Gross Appearance. The cysts have an irregular surface with areas of pearly white or metallic luster, hence the name "pearly tumors." The contents are white and pastelike.

Microscopic Appearance. The outer collagenous capsule is lined by a layer of stratified squamous epithelium. The lumen contains laminated keratin derived from the desquamation of lining cells.

Tumors of the Pineal Gland

This is a relatively rare but extraordinarily interesting group of tumors, which includes the pinealomas, teratomas, gliomas, and simple dermoid and epidermoid cysts. Small cysts may be asymptomatic, but larger cysts and tumors produce symptoms owing to pressure on the midbrain and posterior hypothalamus. The majority of symptomatic tumors occur in males.

Microscopic Appearance. Teratomas contain elements derived from all three germ layers and may include squamous and columnar epithelium, cartilage, bone, and smooth muscle. Occasional examples resemble choriocarcinoma or seminoma. Pinealomas have also been called atypical teratomas and consist of collections of epithelial cells lying in a loose stroma containing numerous small lymphocytic-like cells.

The gliomatous group consists of ependymomatous and astrocytomatous tumors that apparently arise within the pineal gland. Simple cysts lined by pineal tissue and dermoid or epidermoid cysts (p. 638) may also occur within the pineal gland.

Diagnostic Procedures for Intracranial Tumors

An outline for diagnostic investigation of cases of suspected brain tumor is given in Table 10–8. The order cited has evolved and proved useful in the Department of Neurology of Wayne State University over the past several years. The initial choice of relatively simple and harmless procedures can reveal the cause of symptoms to be something other than brain tumor, e.g., granulomatous meningitis or meningovascular syphilis. The necessity for further investigation is obviated. An analysis of the data also influences the selection of a major procedure, such as arteriography or ventriculography.

Roentgenograms of the Skull

Some 10 per cent of intracranial tumors are calcified sufficiently to be recognized by roentge-

TABLE 10–8

Investigation of the Brain Tumor Suspect

After the history and physical examination, the investigation begins with those procedures that are least traumatic to the patient. This allows selection of the appropriate major procedure, e.g., arteriography, pneumoencephalography, or ventriculography, on the basis of the results of the earlier studies.

1. *Roentgenograms of the skull.* This may reveal
   a. Intracranial calcification
   b. Displacement of calcified pineal gland
   c. Signs of increased intracranial pressure
   d. New bone formation
   e. Destruction of bone
   f. Air in the ventricles

Note: Laminograms of the internal auditory meatus should be obtained in all cases of suspected acoustic neurilemmoma.

2. *Roentgenograms of the chest.* Many metastatic brain tumors are associated with primary or metastatic lesions in the lung

3. *Computed tomography*

4. *Auditory evoked potentials:* tests of central auditory function

5. *Lumbar puncture.* The procedure requires caution in cases of increased intracranial pressure; in other cases, pressure, cell count, serologic tests for syphilis, glucose, protein, and malignant cell block should be obtained.

6. *Electroencephalography*

7. *Radioactive brain scan*

8. *Echoencephalography*

9. *Arteriography*

10. *Pneumoencephalography*

11. *Ventriculography*

12. *Additional studies*
    a. Blood count may reveal polycythemia in hemangioblastoma.
    b. Gonadotropins, urinary and serum steroid levels: thyroid function may be low in tumors of the third ventricle or hypothalamus.
    c. Audiometry and studies of vestibular functions are useful in suspected cases of acoustic neurilemmoma.

nograms of the skull. The highest incidence of calcification occurs in the craniopharyngioma and oligodendroglioma.[179] Although the presence of calcification is suggestive of intracranial tumor, it must be differentiated from other causes of intracranial calcification. The pineal gland is frequently calcified in adults and is a midline structure that should not be displaced laterally more than 3 mm in the anteroposterior view. Displacement of more than 3 mm is usually indicative of a space-occupying lesion on the side opposite the displacement or atrophy on the same side.

The earliest sign of increased intracranial pressure is decalcification of the posterior clinoid processes, followed by similar changes in the floor of the dorsum sellae. In long-standing increased intracranial pressure there may be enlargement of the sella, which may lead to erroneous diagnosis of pituitary tumor.

The presence of increased digital markings (hammer-beaten skull) is an unreliable sign of increased intracranial pressure in children, unless pronounced but is always a significant sign in adults.

Separation of the sutures is seen almost exclusively in children and is a reliable sign of increased intracranial pressure.

New bone formation (hyperostosis) is usually associated with meningiomas[39, 62] and may take the form of a localized density at the site of the tumor or more diffuse hyperostosis when associated with meningioma en plaque or an osteoma.

Enlargement of the internal auditory meatus occurs in acoustic neurilemmoma, and widening of the optic foramen is seen in gliomas of the optic nerve.[31] Epidermoid cysts may produce areas of bone destruction anywhere in the calvarium. Meningiomas, which have some roentgenographic abnormality in approximately 60 per cent of cases,[62, 134] are rarely associated with bone destruction even if they have undergone sarcomatous change.

Chronic increase in intracranial pressure occasionally produces cerebrospinal fluid rhinorrhea (p. 506), which is occasionally associated with roentgenographic evidence of air in the ventricles.

Roentgenograms of the Chest

Many pulmonary conditions are associated with intracranial space-occupying lesions; consequently, a chest roentgenogram should be a routine part of any neurologic investigation. This is particularly important in suspected cases of brain

tumor because intracranial metastases are associated with many primary or metastatic pulmonary tumors.

Computed Tomography

Computed tomography (CT) of the brain is now the most important study available for the diagnosis of brain tumors. CT has the capability of demonstrating the normal anatomy of the brain and abnormal pathologic processes with a clarity approaching a neuropathologic section.[80] The development of CT has radically changed the diagnostic evaluation of a patient with a suspected brain tumor. The CT scan is in fact an ideal diagnostic tool for the neurologist who has the ability to base interpretation on clinical symptoms and signs and correlate these with a knowledge of neuropathology. The following criteria should be observed if a CT scanner is available.

1. The CT scan should be obtained before any invasive tests are considered, i.e., before lumbar puncture, arteriography, or pneumoencephalography.
2. The CT scan should be performed with intravenous contrast enhancement in cases of suspected brain tumor, despite the small but definite risk in the use of contrast material.[44]

Tests of Central Auditory Function

Tests of central auditory function employ the more traditional behavioral speech audiometric techniques and newer electrophysiologic tests.[61, 107] These tests include monaural low-pass filtered speech discrimination, binaural resynthesis of segmented speech, simultaneous binaural and competing message discrimination (dichotic) tests, and measurement of auditory click evoked potentials from the auditory pathways of the brainstem. The latter is a relatively simple electrophysiologic procedure that detects and localizes brainstem disorders.

The routine audiogram and undistorted speech discrimination tests are not affected by lesions of the central auditory pathways but are useful in the assessment of peripheral auditory disorders including acoustic neurilemmoma.

Patients with temporal lobe lesions often have abnormal monaural and dichotic speech discrimination tests in the ear contralateral to the affected hemisphere. Deep parietal lobe lesions involving the interhemispheric auditory pathways that pass through the corpus callosum show abnormal dichotic speech discrimination scores in the ear ipsilateral to the dominant hemisphere for speech and language regardless of the hemisphere primarily involved. Auditory evoked potentials and binaural resynthesis of segmented speech are abnormal in patients with intra-axial or extra-axial lesions involving the auditory pathways of the pons and midbrain.[162, 166, 167] Tests of central auditory function, including auditory evoked potentials, are useful in monitoring the posttreatment course of patients with progressive and reversible lesions.[60, 106]

Lumbar Puncture

Although the need for diagnostic lumbar puncture has decreased following the introduction of computed tomography, lumbar puncture is still required in cases of suspected meningeal carcinomatosis, seeding of brain tumors in the subarachnoid space,[21] chronic granulomas, or in any case of suspected brain tumor with a negative CT scan. Brain tumors can occasionally present as an aseptic meningitis due to spillage of products of tumor necrosis or malignant cells into the cerebrospinal fluid.[14]

In all other cases, the following information is routinely recorded: the measurements of opening and closing pressure, the color and appearance of the fluid compared to water, the cell count, the differential cell count, serologic test for syphilis, glucose and protein content. Appropriate bacterial studies should be ordered if meningitis is suspected. In suspected cases of involvement by gliomas or metastatic tumors, the glucose content of the fluid is low.[36, 49, 90, 98, 170] The use of a membrane filter is recommended in such cases in an attempt to identify tumor cells in the cerebrospinal fluid.[181]

Electroencephalography

A great deal has been written about the diagnostic value of electroencephalography in brain tumor, and there is no doubt that the electroencephalogram should be a part of the total evaluation. The procedure is harmless but is not, of itself, diagnostic and rarely may appear normal when brain tumor is present. Tumors located within the cerebral hemispheres commonly produce localized EEG abnormalities, particularly if they are cortical or subcortical in location. Tumors at the base of the skull may give rise to periodic, poorly defined EEG abnormalities. Tumors of the posterior fossa may show no EEG

abnormality or the presence of bifrontal bursts of bilaterally synchronous, high-amplitude, rhythmic slow activity ranging from 2 to 4 cps.[49] Occasionally, contralateral frontal slowing and ipsilateral posterior theta activity occur.[18] These abnormalities may be falsely interpreted as a tumor located in the cerebral hemisphere.

Tumors of the cerebral hemispheres correlate with appropriate focal EEG abnormalities in about 80 per cent of patients. High-voltage delta activity is often localized in the area of the tumor; focal theta activity may be localized to the area of the tumor; loss of background activity will be found over rapidly growing tumors; alpha asymmetry with reduction of amplitude is often seen on the side of the tumor, particularly in posteriorly placed tumors. Spike, sharp wave, or spike and wave activity are often localized to the areas surrounding the tumor, particularly in persons with a history of seizures.[55, 110]

Frontal lobe and temporal lobe gliomas tend to produce high-voltage delta discharges localized to the site of tumor growth, although the background activity may be well preserved in other areas. Parietal and occipital lobe tumors tend to give rise to more diffuse delta activity, which is usually irregular but continuous and of moderate voltage and often shows preponderance on the side of the tumor where the background activity is disturbed.

In general, the more benign or slowly growing the tumor, the less the EEG abnormality and the better the preservation of background activity. On the other hand, the more malignant and rapidly growing the tumor, the more severe the abnormality and loss of background activity. Metastatic tumors are often multiple and hence tend to produce more diffuse changes in the electroencephalogram.

Radioactive Brain Scan

The CT scan has superseded the radionuclide scan as a diagnostic procedure in a suspected case of brain tumor. Nevertheless, the radionuclide scan is a sensitive study and is positive in more than 80 per cent of gliomas, meningiomas, and acoustic neurilemmomas and, therefore, remains a valuable study when a CT scan is not available.

Echoencephalography

This is a relatively simple and harmless procedure that may be used to demonstrate displacement of certain structures from the midline by a mass lesion in one hemisphere. The ultrasonic waves tend to be reflected from interfaces such as the pineal gland, septum pellucidum, and the ventricular walls of the third ventricle and temporal horns, so that ventricular displacement and the degree of hydrocephalus can be recognized. Echoencephalography is useful as a means of lateralizing a possible hemispheric brain tumor and may also, occasionally, detect enlargement of the ventricles when the tumor has caused hydrocephalus.

Arteriography

The CT scan has superseded arteriography as the definitive study of choice in the diagnosis of a brain tumor. However, many neurosurgeons still prefer to obtain arteriography as well as a CT scan before operation. The arteriogram gives an added dimension to the brain tumor, and serial arteriograms with magnification help to define the blood supply. This information is invaluable to the neurosurgeon in planning the operative approach to the tumor (Fig. 10–6).

Arteriography is also extremely useful in suspected cases of posterior fossa tumor, particularly a small brainstem tumor or an isodense acoustic neurilemmoma that may not be seen on the CT scan.[58] The use of magnification subtraction and

the study of venous patterns make the arteriogram particularly useful in the diagnosis of pontine gliomas, metastatic tumors, acoustic neurilemmomas, and cerebellar tumors in children.[185]

Pneumoencephalography

Pneumoencephalography is rarely required in the diagnosis of brain tumor. The study improves the definition of suspected intraventricular tumors or cysts and is still useful in the diagnosis of small intrasellar or parasellar lesions that are not seen by CT scan.[96]

Ventriculography

The indications for ventriculography are much the same as those given for pneumoencephalography, but the former becomes the procedure of choice when there is markedly increased intracranial pressure in order to obviate the danger of herniation.

Additional Diagnostic Studies

Diagnosis of the type and location of a brain tumor may be facilitated by certain ancillary laboratory measurements. Estimation of total blood count and blood volume may reveal polycythemia in the presence of hemangioblastoma.[176] Precisely why polycythemia should occur with some hem-

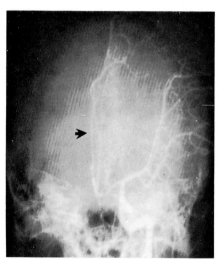

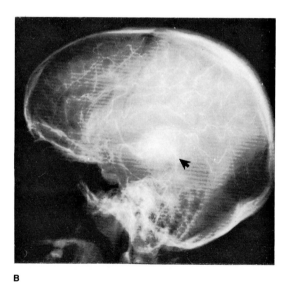

A   **B**

FIGURE 10–6. Carotid arteriograms in a case of grade 4 astrocytoma of the left temporal lobe. In *A* the arrow points to the displaced anterior cerebral arteries under the falx. In *B* the arrow points to tumor stain where the main tumor mass was found at surgery.

angioblastomas of the posterior fossa is not clear, but possibly the tumor secretes an erythropoietic hormone. Evidence of pituitary dysfunction will result when the diencephalon is involved by tumors. Measurements will reveal lowered or absent gonadotropins, and tests of adrenal and thyroid function will show depression of these target glands. This is frequently seen in tumors of the third ventricle or hypothalamus and occasionally in long-standing hydrocephalus. Audiometry may define unilateral loss of higher tones with preservation of lower tones, which is said to be characteristic of the type of nerve deafness associated with acoustic neurilemmoma. Abnormalities in visual evoked responses may be useful in the early diagnosis of suspected optic nerve gliomas.

Treatment of Intracranial Tumors

Surgery

At the present time surgical removal of brain tumors is recommended as the standard treatment because this method has the greatest likelihood of complete cure. Other forms of therapy, such as radiotherapy and chemotherapy, should be considered where attempts at surgical excision are not possible or have proved unsuccessful.

The effectiveness of surgical treatment depends on the type and site of the tumor, but the advent of microsurgery has increased the scope and lowered the mortality rate in surgically treated cases.[76, 97] Certain tumors, such as those located within the brainstems, are inaccessible. Others are noncapsulated and infiltrating, and the necessity of wide excision for their removal limits the effectiveness of surgical treatment, particularly if the tumor is invading the dominant hemisphere. Nevertheless, surgical exploration is recommended almost without exception for the following reasons:

1. Survival is favored by complete removal over partial removal and partial removal over simple biopsy.[186]
2. The only way a tissue diagnosis can be obtained is by biopsy.
3. Surgical decompression can be performed either as a palliative measure or as prophylaxis against a subsequent increase in intracranial pressure.
4. A ventriculoatrial shunt may be performed in cases of hydrocephalus caused by tumors obstructing the third ventricle, aqueduct, or fourth ventricle.

Radiation and Steroid Therapy

A permanent cure is rarely effected by radiation therapy alone, although there are many examples of prolonged remission of several years' duration following such treatment of both primary and metastatic tumors. In the majority of patients, adequate treatment may result in increased survival, particularly in cases of low-grade astrocytoma, oligodendroglioma, and ependymoma.[112, 157, 160] However, radiation therapy is the most important factor in short-term survival of grade 3 and grade 4 astrocytomas.[178]

The hazards of edema and a rapid increase in intracranial pressure, which used to be frequent complications of radiotherapy, are now rare if concomitant treatment is given with high doses of corticosteroids. Steroids should be started before irradiation and continued throughout the course. Because the period of treatment is relatively short, the drug may be given in daily or more frequent doses, but the use of a single large dose (80 to 100 mg of methylprednisolone) once every 48 hours seems to be equally effective and minimizes the side effects. The steroids may be repeated with each course of radiation therapy. Treatment with steroids alone appears to reduce the edema associated with brain tumors of almost all types, and temporary remissions with lifesaving reduction of increased intracranial pressure have been seen to result. Steroids are also advised prior to, during, and after attempts at neurosurgical removal of all types of brain tumor since the morbidity and operative mortality seem to be benefited with concurrent use of steroids.

Chemotherapy

At the present time, chemotherapy of intracranial tumors, particularly gliomas, is in the early stages of development and should be restricted to severe, inoperable, or terminal cases. Drugs may be administered systemically (mithramycin, vincristine sulfate, BCNU) or intra-arterially by continuous infusion using a polyethylene catheter in the carotid artery (nitrogen mustard, methotrexate, vinca alkaloids, bromuridine, thio-TEPA, and 5-fluorouracil). Three drugs (methotrexate, 8-azaquanine, and thio-TEPA) can be administered intrathecally.

At the present time BCNU appears to be the most effective single agent in the chemotherapy of brain tumors.[188] The use of drug combinations[187] or combined chemotherapy and radiation therapy is under active investigation.[155] Focal diffusion of chemotherapeutic agents directly into brain tumors through implanted semipermeable membranes is a future possibility.[184]

Therapeutic Considerations of the Gliomas

Successful removal of a glioma is uncommon unless it is of low-grade malignancy. If situated in the tips of the frontal, temporal, or occipital poles, it can be removed by a partial lobectomy.[15] Cystic astrocytomas of the cerebellum in children are particularly amenable to surgery. Excellent results are obtained by removal of one cerebellar hemisphere containing the tumor.[23] Although cerebellar dysfunction may be quite severe in the immediate postoperative period, remarkably good compensation can be expected with only minimal residual symptoms in most cases.

In contrast, the medulloblastoma is a rapidly growing and invasive cerebellar tumor, which is usually treated by incomplete removal, decompression, and radiotherapy.[125] The entire spinal canal and head should be irradiated, and, although the recurrence rate is high, further irradiation can be carried out.[83] Survival is higher in cerebellar hemisphere medulloblastomas.[28] Between 12 and 25 per cent of patients are alive at ten years.[28]

Gliomas of the brainstem cannot be removed surgically but should be explored because of the possibility of evacuating a neoplastic cyst.[48] Treatment consists of radiation therapy and steroids, which may prolong life from months to years.

About 25 per cent of gliomas of the optic nerve and chiasm can be treated successfully by surgery. If the tumor is confined to the optic nerve on microscopic examination, irradiation is unnecessary. All other cases should receive radiation therapy.[108]

The location of ependymomas within and adjacent to the ventricles frequently makes surgical extirpation impossible. Palliative treatment with radiation therapy and steroids usually offers six months to two years of survival after surgical exploration. Tumors of the third or fourth ventricle causing hydrocephalus should be treated by ventriculoatrial shunt to relieve hydrocephalus prior to radiation therapy.[56]

Oligodendrogliomas are more slow-growing and less malignant than the other gliomas and offer the best chance for total surgical removal. There is some evidence that the survival time is

longer in patients whose tumors were treated by partial resection and radiation therapy than in those treated by radiation therapy alone.

Therapeutic Considerations of the Meningiomas

The majority of meningiomas can be removed surgically; the recurrence rate is low, and the prognosis is good. When the tumor is located in the falx cerebri or in the retrochiasmatic suprasellar area, only partial removal is possible, and further surgery may be required if recurrence occurs after a period of years.[68] Recurrence of superficially located meningiomas may result if a bone flap containing tumor cells is replaced. There may be a tendency for malignant change to result following serial removal of a recurrent meningioma. Meningiomas are generally resistant to radiotherapy.

Therapeutic Considerations of the Neurilemmomas

The majority of these tumors arise from the acoustic nerve and are best treated by total removal. Sometimes the facial nerve can be spared, although usually it has to be sacrificed because it is stretched over the tumor. An acoustic neurilemmoma is always larger than the symptoms indicate. Delay of surgery until the development of papilledema and ataxia increases mortality and morbidity.[37, 123]

Therapeutic Considerations of Hemangioblastomas

Cystic hemangioblastomas of the cerebellum can often be excised completely with little permanent neurologic deficit. The solid hemangioblastoma is much more difficult to treat, and the mortality rate is higher due to frequent involvement of the brainstem, postoperative edema, or postoperative hemorrhage.[124]

Therapeutic Considerations of Paraphyseal Cysts

These cysts may be removed successfully with little risk of recurrence. The surgical approach is usually through the right lateral ventricle followed by removal of the cyst by suction and traction.

Therapeutic Considerations of Chordomas

Total removal of intracranial chordomas located in the parasellar region or over the clivus is usually not feasible owing to involvement of the cranial nerves and proximity of the brainstem. A combination of surgical decompression followed by radiation therapy offers the best results. The tumors are slow-growing, and survival is usually prolonged for many years.

Therapeutic Considerations of Dermoid and Epidermoid Tumors

The majority of these tumors can be diagnosed by CT scan before operation. They present as a low-density area with heterogenous consistency on CT scan, and peripheral calcification can be seen in some cases. A unique fat–cerebrospinal fluid interface has been described in intraventricular epidermoid tumors.[52]

The majority of these tumors occur in the cerebellopontine angle, suprasellar chiasmatic or parasellar sylvian region, or floor of the posterior fossa and can be removed successfully. Care is necessary to avoid contamination of the subarachnoid space by the contents during removal because this produces a severe chemical meningitis. If the epithelial lining is not completely removed, recurrence is possible within several years.

Therapeutic Considerations of Tumors of the Pineal Gland

Most pineal tumors cannot be resected although many neurosurgeons perform craniotomy for biopsy and tissue diagnosis. The major disturbance caused by these tumors is hydrocephalus, which can be treated by a ventriculoatrial shunt. The majority of pineal tumors are radiosensitive, and prolonged survival is not unusual following radiotherapy.

Tumors of the Pituitary Gland and Infundibulum

The reported incidence of tumors arising from the pituitary gland and infundibulum varies considerably in different medical centers, but these lesions usually constitute about 10 per cent of intracranial tumors. Because they may be associated with endocrinologic as well as neurologic effects, they require special consideration. Almost all tumors arising from the pituitary gland originate from cells of the anterior lobe, and tumors (gliomas) of the neurophysis (posterior lobe) are rare. The only tumor arising in relationship to the infundibulum, the craniopharyngioma, is be-

lieved to be derived either from metaplasia of epithelial cells or from epithelial cell rests.

Tumors of the pituitary gland are not alone in causing alteration of pituitary or hypothalamic function. A list of tumors and other lesions that affect the hypothalamopituitary axis is given in Table 10–9.

The release of hormones by the pituitary gland is controlled by specialized secretory neurons located in the ventral hypothalamus. The axons of these tuberoinfundibular neurons terminate directly on capillaries of the pituitary portal system and secrete hypothalamic-regulating factors that enter the portal blood and are transported to the anterior lobe of the pituitary. The synthesis of hypothalamic regulatory factors is influenced by the activity of other areas of the brain, particularly the limbic system, and by the level of circulating hormones secreted by target organs. High levels of circulating hormone in the blood lead to supression of hypothalamic activity, which in turn limits pituitary secretion (Fig. 10–7). Conversely, atrophy, necrosis, or failure of the target organ will result in low levels of its circulating hormone and produce excessive hypothalamic stimulation of the pituitary.

In the presence of such a system of control,

TABLE 10–9

Classification of Tumors and Lesions Affecting Pituitary and Hypothalamic Function

Tumors of the anterior lobe of the pituitary
Chromophobe adenoma
Eosinophilic adenoma
Basophilic adenoma

Tumors of the infundibulum
Craniopharyngioma

Parapituitary tumors
Gliomas of the third ventricle and hypothalamus
Hamartomas of the hypothalamus
Metastatic tumors
Parasellar meningiomas
Dermoid and epidermoid cysts
Chordomas
Pineal tumors

Other conditions producing hypopituitarism
Unruptured aneurysm of internal carotid artery
Granulomas, particularly sarcoidosis, and tuberculosis
Chronic hydrocephalus
Postpartum hemorrhage or infarction with necrosis of pituitary
Arachnoiditis and the "empty sella syndrome"

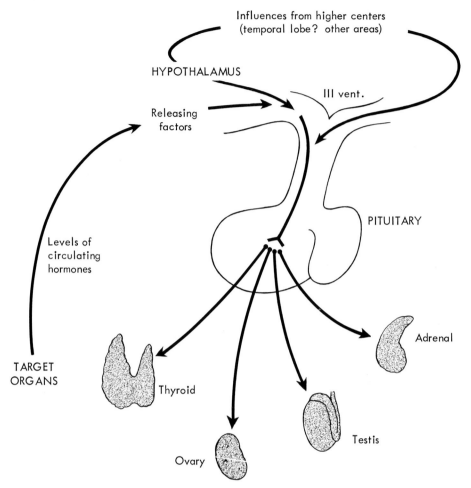

FIGURE 10–7. Control of pituitary function.

it is possible that pituitary tumors may arise as independent neoplasms within the pituitary or result from excessive stimulation by hypothalamic secretions. This stimulation may result from excessive hypothalamic response to normal fluctuations in circulating hormone levels from the target organs or from failure of target organs with persistently low levels of their hormones, either of which results in excessive hypothalamic stimulation of the pituitary.

Chromophobe Adenoma

Almost 90 per cent of pituitary tumors are chromophobe or predominantly chromophobe adenomas.

Gross Appearance

There is considerable variation in the size of these tumors. Small chromophobe adenomas

within the gland may be an incidental finding at autopsy without symptoms during life, whereas large nodular tumors passing up into the base of the brain and distorting the normal pituitary tissue may cause prolonged symptoms and death. Erosion of the floor of the sella by these tumors produces the characteristic "ballooned" sella, recognized in lateral roentgenograms of the skull. Occasionally, a tumor may destroy the floor of the sella and extend into the sphenoid sinus and nasopharynx.

Microscopic Appearance

These tumors are cellular, and chromophobe cells are preponderant. These cells are small and uniform, the nucleus is centrally placed, and cytoplasmic borders are often indefinite. Cytoplasmic granules are ambophilic. Careful examination of the edges of almost all chromophobe adenomas will reveal compressed normal cells from the unaffected anterior lobe. A number of microscopic patterns have been described. The diffuse type of tumor has little stroma between the cells, while the sinusoidal type contains strands of connective tissue and blood vessels, which divide the cells into compartments somewhat resembling the normal structure of the anterior lobe of the pituitary. A papillary variety also occurs. As with tumors of most endocrine organs (except the thyroid gland), it is virtually impossible to classify any given lesion as benign or malignant on the basis of histology. Adenocarcinoma arising in the pituitary is extremely rare, however, and therefore is seldom a diagnostic problem.

Clinical Features

Expansion of a chromophobe adenoma produces symptoms due to compression atrophy of residual pituitary tissue (panhypopituitarism) or to pressure exerted on the structures at the base of the brain (Fig. 10–8). Most commonly, expansion leads to compression of the optic chiasm, optic nerve, or less frequently the optic tract with the development of visual field defects (p. 19). Optic atrophy and blindness can result in untreated cases.

Headache is a common symptom in pituitary adenomas, particularly in the early stages of intrasellar growth when there is increasing pressure on the diaphragm sellae. The headache is usually bifrontal or bitemporal and is often accompanied by a boring pain behind the eyes.

Large tumors can involve the basal portion of both frontal lobes, producing signs of frontal lobe disturbance, or extend into the third ventricle, producing hydrocephalus.

Upward expansion compresses the anterior hypothalamus, resulting in panhypopituitarism. This is usually manifested by reduced secretion of gonadotropins, causing amenorrhea in the female, impotence in the male, and loss of secondary sex characteristics in both sexes. Axillary and pubic hair are lost, shaving of the beard becomes less necessary in the male, and the skin of the face has a soft appearance. Affected children fail to grow and infrequently become obese and somnolent, while temperature regulation may fail. Involvement of the supraopticoneurohypophyseal pathway in the hypothalamus or infundibulum may produce diabetes insipidus. Pressure on the posterior hypothalamus in children may result in sexual precosity.

Chromophobe adenomas are not necessarily

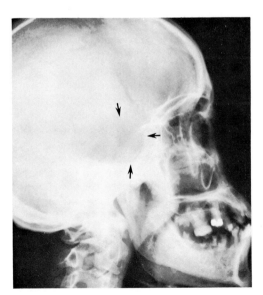

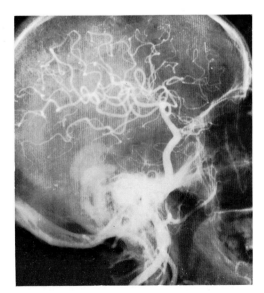

A   B

FIGURE 10–8. *A.* Plain skull roentgenograms in a case of chromophobe adenoma of the pituitary gland. *B.* Carotid arteriogram in the same case as *A;* the pituitary chromophobe adenoma has elevated the middle and anterior cerebral arteries.

nonfunctioning. A number may be classified as "mixed tumors" because they contain small numbers of eosinophilic or basophilic cells, but tumors that appear to consist entirely of chromophobe cells may also have active hormonal function. Some 10 per cent of chromophobe adenomas may secrete ACTH and cause symptoms of Cushing's syndrome. Acromegaly has also been reported in association with chromophobe tumors.

Chromophobe adenomas are occasionally prolactin-secreting tumors and may present with galactorrhea in the female and occasionally in the male. This event often occurs during the early development of the adenoma, and the prolactin-secreting tumor may be small (pituitary microadenoma). Invasive pituitary adenomas, which produce considerable bone destruction and invade the bones of the base of the skull, are often prolactin-producing tumors.[105] Hemorrhage into a pituitary adenoma may produce sudden blindness or coma with a transient lymphocytic pleocytosis in the cerebrospinal fluid.[142] This is one cause of so-called "pituitary apoplexy"; the other cause is acute infarction of the hyperplastic pituitary gland during the last trimester of pregnancy.

Eosinophilic Adenoma

Gross Appearance

About 10 per cent of pituitary tumors contain a preponderance of eosinophilic cells. They are chromophobe adenomas macroscopically and are identified microscopically but do not reach the large size of some chromophobe tumors.

Microscopic Appearance

Eosinophilic adenomas differ from chromophobe adenomas only in the somewhat larger size of the cells and the pressure of eosinophilic cytoplasmic granules. Compressed normal pituitary tissue may form a thin crescent or rim around the tumor.

Clinical Features

The endrocrine secretions of the tumor produce gigantism in children and adolescents and acromegaly in adults. In unusually large tumors, there may also be pressure effects on the optic nerve, optic chiasm, frontal lobes, and hypothalamus. The appearance of symptoms similar to those described under chromophobe adenoma will then be superimposed on the gigantism or acromegaly.

Basophilic Adenomas

Basophilic adenomas are rare, and those which secrete ACTH in amounts sufficient to cause Cushing's syndrome are even more rare. The majority of basophilic adenomas are small, asymptomatic tumors found incidentally at autopsy. Cushing's syndrome is usually caused by hyperplasia or tumor in the cortex of one or both adrenal glands rather than "pituitary basophilism," although it may occasionally occur in association with chromophobe adenomas containing basophilic cells.

Tumor of the Infundibulum: Craniopharyngioma

There is considerable variation in the reported incidence of craniopharyngiomas, but they probably account for about 5 per cent of intracranial tumors in children. At least half of the craniopharyngiomas are discovered in individuals before the age of 20 years.

Etiology

The anterior lobe of the pituitary develops as an outgrowth of the primitive stomodeum, which may result in squamous cell rests within the infundibulum either above or below the diaphragm sellae. Craniopharyngiomas may arise in such rests, but this is by no means certain. Squamous rests are found with greatest incidence in elderly individuals, while craniopharyngioma is a tumor of youth. It has therefore been suggested that these tumors may arise from chromophobe cells on the basis of metaplasia to less-differentiated squamous epithelium.

Gross Appearance

These tumors vary considerably in size, but the majority are large enough to involve the base of the brain, compressing the optic chiasm and hypothalamus and occasionally extending into the third ventricle. They are an admixture of cystic and solid areas, predominantly yellow-brown in color. Areas of calcification are present in over 70 per cent and may be recognized in roentgenograms of the skull. The cysts contain an oily, yellow, or brownish fluid of high cholesterol content.

Microscopic Appearance

The microscopic appearance is characteristic and resembles that of the adamantinoma or ameloblastoma of the jaw. Nests of stellate reticulum are bounded by a single row of tall columnar epithelial cells. Similar cells line the cystic spaces that may be formed by degeneration of the stellate reticulum. Foci of calcification are frequent.

Clinical Features

Craniopharyngiomas produce symptoms of failing vision, headache, vomiting, and behavior changes in both children and adults.[12, 76] Some 25 per cent of children and 50 per cent of adults have an endocrine abnormality. Growth in children and adolescents may be stunted, and secondary sex characteristics may not develop. Hypothalamic symptoms of polyuria and somnolence can occur. Compression of the optic chiasm produces bitemporal field defects. These are usually incongruous, beginning in one eye and involving the other eye at a later stage. Examination may reveal optic atrophy, and papilledema is uncommon. Cranial nerve palsies occur in about one third of patients. Extension into the third ventricle is rare but can cause hydrocephalus.[26]

Diagnosis of Pituitary, Infundibular, and Parapituitary Tumors

1. Roentgenograms of the skull may show calcification of intrasellar or extrasellar structures. Calcification of the internal carotid artery, petroclinoid ligaments, and interclinoid ligaments are not infrequent and must be differentiated from abnormal states. Suprasellar calcification is seen in more than 70 per cent of craniopharyngiomas in children and 40 per cent of those in adults. Approximately one third of meningiomas are calcified but calcification is rare in pituitary adenomas.[94]

   Pituitary adenomas and craniopharyngiomas usually produce enlargement of the sella turcica. However, enlargement also occurs in chronic increased intracranial pressure, primary hypothyroidism, internal carotid aneurysm, extension of an extrasellar tumor into the sella, and by extension of the subarachnoid space through a defective diaphragma sellae (empty sella syndrome).[180]

2. Pituitary and parapituitary tumors usually produce visual field defects.[77]

   a. The classic bitemporal hemianopia is produced by tumor pressure on the anterior aspect of the optic chiasm. The deficit often begins as a superior temporal defect on one side, becomes bilateral, and then progresses inward and downward to become a complete bitemporal hemianopia.

   b. Tumors impinging on the posterior aspect of the chiasm often produce bilateral scotomata which lie just to the temporal side of the macula. The scotomata progress laterally increasing the bitemporal field defects. Visual evoked potentials may be abnormal in the early stages of temporal scotomata (Fig. 10–9).

   c. Tumor pressure on the chiasm and one optic nerve produces blindness in one eye and a superior temporal field defect on the other side.

   d. An eccentric tumor may exert pressure on the optic chiasm and the optic tract producing a homonymous hemianopia.

3. Tests of olfaction may show loss of the sense of smell on one side if a pituitary or parapituitary tumor presses on the olfactory tract.

4. Large tumors can compress the oculomotor nerve as it enters the superior orbital fissure, producing diplopia, ptosis, and occasionally pupillary dilatation on the affected side.

5. Lateral extension of a large tumor into the

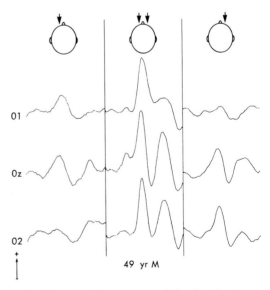

FIGURE 10–9. Pattern reversal visual evoked potentials recorded in a patient with a pituitary adenoma and a bitemporal hemianopia. Stimulation of the right eye produces a low-voltage response in the left occipital area. Similarly, stimulation of the left eye produces a low-voltage response. Stimulation of both eyes produces a much higher voltage response.

medial temporal lobe can produce complex partial seizures with olfactory symptoms (uncinate fits).

6. Pressure on the hypothalamus causes disorders of food intake; water balance (diabetes insipidus or inappropriate secretion of antidiuretic hormone); or temperature regulation. There are abnormal sleep, emotional disturbances, cardiac arrhythmias, and diencephalic seizures.

7. Endocrine studies may reveal abnormalities in some or all of the following tests.
   a. Serum thyroxine.
   b. Plasma follicle-stimulating hormone (FSH) and luteinizing hormone (LH).
   c. 24-hour urinary gonadotropins.
   d. Plasma contrast levels estimated on specimens drawn in the morning and evening.
   e. Serum thyroid-stimulating hormone levels.
   f. Plasma cortisol response to the intravenous administration of ACTH.
   g. Serum prolactin levels should be obtained in all cases of galactorrhea before and after intravenous injection of thyrotropin-releasing hormone.[89]
   h. Elevated cerebrospinal fluid levels of pituitary hormones are a sensitive indicator of suprasellar extension of a pituitary tumor.[84]

8. Computed tomography. Computed tomography is an extremely valuable and accurate procedure in the diagnosis of pituitary and parapituitary lesions. The nonenhanced scan will demonstrate enlargement of the sella and the presence of thinning or destruction of surrounding bone. Tumors usually present as an abnormal density in the intrasellar or suprasellar region with some enhancement following intravenous injection of contrast material.[19, 32] There is obliteration of the suprasellar cistern or third ventricle when the mass extends out of the sella in a vertical direction. Lateral extension of a tumor is usually well demonstrated by a CT scan.

9. Arteriography will show elevation of the proximal anterior cerebral arteries if there is anterior suprasellar extension of a tumor.

10. Pneumoencephalography remains a valuable study in a suspected case of intrasellar tumor that is not well demonstrated by a CT scan. The diagnosis of empty sella syndrome is usually confirmed by pneumoencephalography.[22, 85]

11. The presence of small intrasellar tumors can be confirmed by transnasal aspiration biopsy.

Treatment of Pituitary and Infundibular Tumors

Treatment may consist of surgical removal of the tumor followed by irradiation therapy or radiotherapy alone. There are definite indications for each form of therapy.[72, 90, 136, 165]

Indications for Surgery Followed by Irradiation

1. Progressive impairment of vision.
2. Rapid enlargement of the tumor due to hemorrhage or other cause.
3. Progressive dementia or other symptoms of an enlarging intracerebral mass.

Indications for Irradiation Alone

1. Irradiation is indicated for pituitary tumors with endocrine disturbances only.
2. Irradiation is probably a better method of treatment for invasive pituitary adenomas.

Other Considerations

The operative mortality is less than 10 per cent when tumors are removed surgically. The mortality is higher when tumors are large because of complications such as intracranial postoperative cerebral edema, brainstem damage, pituitary insufficiency, and rarely meningitis.

The recurrence rate after surgical treatment is about 7 per cent, usually within five years of treatment. The use of replacement steroid therapy before, during, and after operation has reduced the operative mortality rate. Irradiation therapy carries the risk of inducing arteritis in the circle of Willis or its major branches and, hence, cerebral infarction.

Immediate decompression of the optic nerves and chiasm, by transfrontal craniotomy or transsphenoidal neurosurgical technique, is required in cases with sudden blindness owing to pituitary apoplexy.[27a, 142, 193]

Craniopharyngiomas in children are removed totally if the tumor is small with a rounded dome.[87] Inoperable cases can be treated by stereotaxic injection of technetium-90 into the cysts followed by decompression of the cysts if symptoms do not improve.[8] Other methods of treatment include surgical decompression or palliative ventriculoatrial shunting followed by radiotherapy[156] or transsphenoidal resection under televised radiofluoroscopic control using a surgical microscope and microsurgical techniques of dissection.[9, 72]

Arachnoid Cysts

Arachnoid cysts occur in various locations in the cranial cavity and present as chronic space-occupying structures.

Etiology and Pathology

There are three broad categories of arachnoid cyst.[101]

1. Congenital
   a. Associated with congenital abnormalities of the brain surface with deficient areas of the brain replaced by a cyst.
   b. Diverticulae from ventricular surfaces that lose communication with the ventricle and gradually expand because of secretion of a CSF-like fluid.
   c. Failure of breakdown of trabeculae during formation of the subarachnoid space with the development of a cystic pocket gradually expanding due to the pulsatile force of the CSF.
   d. Splitting of the arachnoid with gradual accumulation of fluid between the split layers.
2. Traumatic. Cysts form near the site of head trauma due to local bleeding and subsequent arachnoid adhesions or splitting of the dura and herniation of the arachnoid with cyst formation.
3. Inflammatory. Inflammation of the arachnoid from any cause produces arachnoid adhesions followed by the development of diverticulae and eventual cyst formation.

   The arachnoid cyst is a thin-walled structure containing fluid resembling CSF. There is no demonstrable communication with the subarachnoid space.[67] Microscopically the cyst wall consists of arachnoid and occasionally contains choroid plexus–like structures.[143]

Clinical Features

Arachnoid cysts present as:

1. A chronically expanding intracranial mass.
2. Hydrocephalus due to cyst obstruction of CSF flow.

The cysts may occur over the surface of a congenitally abnormal hemisphere, in the suprasellar region mimicking a parasellar tumor, near the quadrigeminal plate producing hydrocephalus and signs resembling a pineal tumor, in the posterior fossa presenting as a cerebellar lesion, in the cerebellopontine angle, or in the interpeduncular fossa (paramesencephalic cyst).

Diagnostic Procedures

1. Roentgenograms of the skull may reveal enlargement of the cranial vault and thinning of bone overlying the cyst.
2. The CT scan shows a sharply defined lucent area indenting the brain and displacing midline structures (Fig. 10–10). Hydrocephalus may be present.[48]

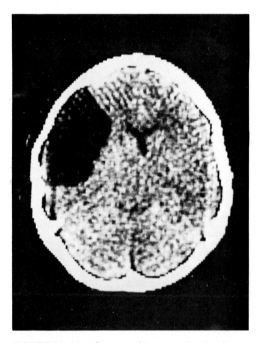

FIGURE 10–10. Computed tomography showing an area of low density in the left frontotemporal area with well-defined borders. The patient had a large arachnoid cyst.

3. Arteriography may demonstrate an avascular area with displacement of vessels around the cyst.

Treatment

Arachnoid cysts should be excised whenever possible and free communication established through the subarachnoid space.

Tumors of the Spinal Cord and Spinal Canal

Tumors of this region constitute about 20 per cent of tumors affecting the central nervous system. They are commonly classified as extradural, intradural, extramedullary, and intramedullary tumors, but the division is largely artificial from a clinical standpoint.

There is an approximately even distribution of the incidence of tumors throughout the spinal canal; but because of the varying lengths of the different anatomic parts of the spinal cord, there is some difference in the percentage of tumors related to each major division. Approximately 50 per cent occur in relation to the thoracic cord, 25 per cent to the lumbar cord, 20 per cent to the cervical cord, and 5 per cent to the cauda equina.

Tumors of the spinal canal occur equally in the two sexes and are more common in adults, in whom 60 per cent are benign lesions, mainly neurilemmomas and meningiomas. In children there is a higher incidence (40 per cent) of gliomas and sarcomas. In general, prognosis is better following surgical treatment of spinal tumors than intracranial tumors in both adults and children.

The unusual occurrence of raised intracranial pressure and papilledema has been reported in patients with thoracic and lumbar gliomas.[137] This may be due to decreased absorption of cerebrospinal fluid secondary to elevation in protein content. There may be other contributory mechanisms such as the presence of abnormal proteins due to tumor breakdown; obstruction of the spinal sites of cerebrospinal fluid absorption; and inflammatory reaction in the meninges or intercostal paralysis, with a hypoventilation syndrome and papilledema due to retention of carbon dioxide.

An increased association of syringomyelia with intramedullary tumor has been reported at autopsy. The symptoms of syringomyelia often have antedated those of the tumor for many years. In view of the theory that some instances of syringomyelia represent cavitation in a low-grade glioma (p. 221), this association may indicate one process rather than a coincidental association of two distinct diseases.[54, 119]

Extradural Tumors

Tumors arising in the extradural space eventually produce symptoms of rapidly developing compression of the spinal cord when the limited space provided by the spinal canal is used up. Extradural tumors commonly develop in surrounding bone and produce destruction of vertebral bodies, laminae, or pedicles. The following comprise the principal types:

Metastatic Tumors

These tumors are the most common of extradural tumors. The primary tumor is frequently found in the breast, prostate, lung, thyroid, or gastrointestinal tract, but primary tumors may be found in almost any other site in the body, and occasionally the primary remains undiscovered.

Primary Tumors of the Bone and Bone Marrow

The extradural space is frequently involved by multiple myeloma, malignant lymphoma, and in Hodgkin's disease. Much less commonly, osteogenic sarcomas, lipomas, chordomas, fibromas, angiomas, and rare benign lesions may compromise the space.

Extradural Cysts

These cysts are usually found in the thoracic area and may be congenital anomalies or represent diverticulae from the subarachnoid space. Unlike many other extradural tumors, they develop slowly, producing erosion of pedicles or scalloping of vertebral bodies and symptoms of a chronic compression of the spinal cord.

Epidermoids and Dermoids

These tumors comprise about 2 per cent of tumors of the spinal canal and arise in the lower thoracic and lumbosacral regions. An associated epithelial fistula occurs in the sacrococcygeal area in about half of the cases.[16] Others are believed to arise from embryonic cell rests or traumatic implantation of cells following repeated lumbar puncture, using needles without stylets in infants.[10, 149]

Intradural Extramedullary Tumors

The most common site for spinal canal tumors is within the dura but outside the cord itself. The majority are benign and can readily be removed surgically.

Neurilemmomas

Neurilemmomas arising from spinal nerve roots are identical in structure to the neurilemmomas arising from the eighth cranial nerve. They constitute the most common neoplasm (30 per cent) in the spinal canal. Although the majority of neurilemmomas arise on the nerve root between the spinal cord and the dura, a number may be found extradurally and about 20 per cent are located both intra- and extradurally. Neurilemmomas may be multiple, particularly in von Recklinghausen's disease. More commonly, however, the lesion in the latter condition is somewhat different and is better classified as a plexiform neurofibroma. Neurilemmomas may grow through the intravertebral foramen into the thoracic or abdominal cavities, where they expand, producing a typical dumbbell or hourglass tumor.

Meningiomas

Meningiomas are the second most common intraspinal tumor (25 per cent) and in relation to all tumors are relatively more frequent than meningiomas within the cranium. They are found in the thoracic region eight times more frequently than in the cervical region and are rare in the lumbar area.[145]

Arteriovenous Malformations

This type of vascular malformation constitutes about 4 per cent of intraspinal "tumors" and consists of a single enlarged varicose vein or, more commonly, a group of these vessels lying on the surface of the spinal cord. The anomaly is usually found in the thoracic segment of the cord but may extend into the cervical and occasionally into the lumbar regions.[6] There is usually some penetration of the substance of the cord by enlarged branches derived from the malformations, and these vessels are subject to thrombosis leading to cord infarction and secondary gliosis. This in turn causes symptoms of intermittent or progressive degeneration of ascending and descending tracts of the spinal cord below midthoracic levels. The thin-walled vessels may also rupture, usually in response to relatively mild trauma, with the production of severe back pain, paraparesis, and subarachnoid hemorrhage. Repeated episodes of hemorrhage may occur, each resulting in further damage to the spinal cord.

Intramedullary Tumors

The most common intramedullary tumors of the spinal cord are gliomas. Excluding the conus medullaris and filum terminale, where ependymo-

mas predominate, the incidence of astrocytomas and ependymomas is approximately equal. Considering the entire cord, ependymomas are twice as common as astrocytomas owing to the frequency with which they arise in the conus medullaris and filum terminale.[27] The cellular variety of ependymoma is most common overall except at the lower end of the spinal canal, where papillary forms predominate. Oligodendrogliomas are rare.

Some ependymomas of the filum terminale may appear encapsulated, but others grow between the nerves of the cauda equina and may seed along the length of the cord. This is a relatively slow process, and patients may live for many years with relatively little discomfort and slow progression of disability.

Clinical Features of Spinal Cord Tumors

It is often difficult to distinguish between extramedullary and intramedullary tumors on clinical grounds, but certain symptoms seem to be associated more frequently with tumors in one or the other of these locations.[139]

Symptoms of Extramedullary Tumors of the Spinal Cord

The earliest symptoms are often pains due to radicular (nerve root) irritation with paresthesias in the distribution of the affected dermatome. The muscles supplied by the affected nerve develop weakness and wasting. Pressure on the cord produces spastic weakness below the level of the lesion, with increased deep tendon reflexes and bilateral extensor plantar responses. Pressure on inhibitory fibers descending to the sacral area that lie superficially in the cord results in frequency and urgency of micturition, which progresses to urinary incontinence. Loss of anal sphincter control tends to occur later.

There is sensory loss below the level of the lesion, which, if unilateral, often begins with loss of pain and temperature sensation on the opposite side of the body to the tumor and, thus, may mimic syringomyelia. Laterally placed tumors may produce a Brown-Séquard syndrome (p. 516). Severe back pain and tenderness to percussion may occur over the site of the tumor. In advanced cases with complete destruction of the spinal cord by the tumor, there are a paraplegia in flexion, intermittent mass reflexes, and complete loss of sensation below the level of the lesion.

Symptoms of Intramedullary Tumors of the Spinal Cord

Radicular pains are less common in intramedullary tumors, although the symptoms described with extramedullary tumors may be encountered.

An intramedullary tumor may resemble syringomyelia (and may be associated with syringomyelia in some patients). There is a progressive spastic paraparesis with increased deep tendon reflexes below the level of the tumor and bilateral extensor plantar responses. Destruction of the anterior horn cells at the level of the lesion produces wasting and fasciculations in segmental muscles. A typical dissociated sensory loss may be present below this level with sparing of the sacral segments in the perianal area.

Symptoms According to the Level of the Intraspinal Tumor

Tumors Affecting the Region of the Foramen Magnum. The majority of tumors arising near the foramen magnum are extramedullary and tend to spread along the lateral aspect of the medulla and cervical cord. There is paralysis of the cranial nerves beginning with the twelfth and progressively involving the nerves of the medulla and pons on the side of the tumor.

Pressure on the cervical cord produces a progressive spastic quadriparesis, with increased deep tendon reflexes, usually more prominent on one side, and bilateral extensor plantar responses. There may be loss of pain and temperature over the face on the same side as the tumor owing to involvement of the spinal tract of the trigeminal nerve. Pain and temperature sensation is lost on the opposite side of the body. Persistent pain in the lower occiput and stiffness of the neck may be present. Signs of increased intracranial pressure may develop at any time.

Tumors Affecting the Cervical Region of the Spinal Cord. There are paralysis, loss of tone, wasting, and fasciculations of the muscles supplied by the anterior horn cells at the level of the tumor. Table 10–10 correlates cervical segmental lesions with resulting paralysis of muscles.

Cervical spinal cord tumors regularly produce progressive spasticity of all four limbs, with increased reflexes below the level of the tumor and extensor plantar responses. There may be diffuse pain in the cervical area and localized tenderness

TABLE 10–10

Correlation of Cervical Segmental Lesions with Paralysis of Muscles

Level	Muscles Involved
C_3, C_4	Diaphragm
C_5	Deltoid, biceps, infraspinatus, supraspinatus, rhomboids
C_6	Triceps, extensors of wrist
C_7	Flexors of wrist, long flexors of fingers
C_8	Small muscles of hand

to percussion at the level of the tumor. Extramedullary tumors produce radicular pains due to pressure on the cervical nerve roots. Pressure on the cord at levels above C_4 may produce facial pain or loss of pain and temperature over the face owing to involvement of the spinal tract of the trigeminal nerve. Sensation is impaired below the level of the tumor, with the development of a sensory level. There are progressive urgency and frequency of micturition leading eventually to urinary incontinence.

Tumors Affecting the Upper Thoracic Region of the Spinal Cord. Involvement of the anterior horn cells at the level of T_1 by tumor produces wasting of the hypothenar muscles. Sensory loss occurs in the first thoracic dermatome and develops below the level of the lesion with further extension of the tumor. Horner's syndrome is not uncommon when tumors arise at the lower cervical or upper thoracic levels. There is progressive spastic paraparesis, with increased reflexes and bilateral extensor plantar responses below the level of the lesion. Bladder and eventually bowel function is progressively impaired.

Tumors Affecting the Midthoracic Region of the Spinal Cord. Tumors arising in this area frequently present with paraparesis and radicular pains. There is progressive spastic paraparesis below the level of the lesion. Bladder function shows progressive impairment. There is a sensory loss below the level of the lesion, with a narrow band of hyperesthesia separating the hypoesthetic area from the area of normal sensation above the involved level.

Tumors Affecting the Lower Thoracic Region of the Spinal Cord. Pressure on the lower thoracic cord produces paralysis of the lower rectus abdominis muscles. The umbilicus will appear to move upward when the patient attempts to flex the neck or sit up owing to contraction of the upper portion of this muscle and paralysis of the lower portion of the muscle (positive Beevor's sign). The other signs are similar to those described under the midthoracic region.

Tumors Affecting the Lumbar Region of the Spinal Cord. Compression of the motor nerve roots or anterior horn cells results in weakness and wasting of the muscles of the lower limb. The segmental pattern of muscular involvement summarized in Table 10–11 permits accurate localization of the lesion.

Compression of the corticospinal tracts at this level results in hyperactive ankle jerks with bilateral extensor plantar responses. Lesions not extending below the level of L_1 and L_2 will also produce increased knee jerks. There will be sensory loss below the level of the lesion, and tumors of the lumbar cord usually produce severe sphincter paralysis.

Tumors of the Epiconus of the Spinal Cord (L_4, L_5, S_1, S_2). The presenting symptom is usually pain in the distribution of the lumbar of sacral dermatomes followed by numbness and sensory loss in the involved dermatomes.[139] Usually, after some months, muscular weakness occurs in the muscles supplied by these lumbosacral segments with flaccid paralysis of the lower limbs and of the sphincters. The paralysis is usually more severe in the distal portion of the limbs with a characteristic mixture of waddling and foot-drop gait.

Tumors of the Conus Medullaris $(S_{3-5}$ *and Coccygeal Nerves*). The first symptom is usually radicular pain occurring in the distribution of the affected sacral nerves. Impairment of sphincter control and impotence are early symptoms. Sensory loss and muscular weakness occur at a later stage. The sensory loss produces a characteristic

TABLE 10–11

Segmental Pattern of Muscular Involvement

Level	Muscles Involved
L_1, L_2, L_3	Psoas
L_3, L_4	Adductors of thigh
L_2, L_3, L_4	Quadriceps femoris

"saddle" anesthesia over the buttocks and pudendal and perianal areas. Muscular weakness is minimal because the involved segments lie below the main motor innervation of the lower limbs.

Tumors of the Cauda Equina. As in tumors of the lumbosacral cord, from which they must be distinguished by the absence of signs of corticospinal tract involvement, pain is usually the initial symptom of tumors affecting the cauda equina and may precede the development of other symptoms by many months. The pattern of motor and sensory disturbance depends on the nerve roots involved, but early manifestations may be unilateral. Sphincteric paralysis is usually late in appearance.

Diagnostic Procedures for Tumors of the Spinal Cord

Roentgenograms of the Spine

Metastatic tumors usually produce destruction or ossification (prostatic tumor) of the affected vertebral bodies or pedicles. Several or many vertebrae may be involved by certain metastatic tumors such as those originating in the breast or prostate. Benign tumors may produce erosion of the vertebral bodies or pedicles or enlargement of the intravertebral foramina (e.g., "hourglass" type of neurilemmoma).

Lumbar Puncture

Lumbar puncture may show evidence of partial or complete block during the Queckenstedt procedure. When both jugular veins are compressed in the neck, the spinal fluid pressure measured in the manometer should promptly rise. If obstruction of the subarachnoid space by the tumor is complete, there will be no rise (complete block). If the obstruction is partial, the rise in pressure will be slow and decreased. In the case of a complete block, the fluid may be xanthochromic and may clot spontaneously (Froin's syndrome). If the tumor is in the cervical region, extension, flexion, or rotation of the neck may demonstrate a block not evident with the head in the neutral position (Foster Kennedy maneuver). The protein content is usually elevated in the presence of spinal cord tumor.

Electromyography

Electromyography may be helpful in locating the segmental level of the tumor. Pressure on the

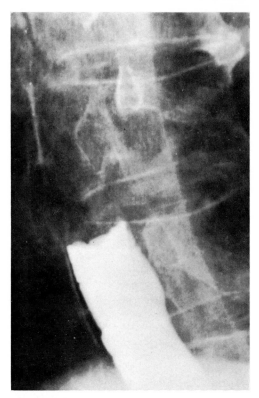

FIGURE 10–11. Myelogram showing complete block due to a meningioma at the T_{11}–T_{12} level. The Queckenstedt test also showed a complete block.

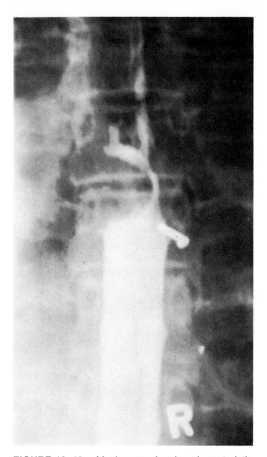

FIGURE 10–12. Myelogram showing characteristic "punched-out" defect of the isophendylate (Pantopaque) contrast media due to a meningioma at the T_4–T_5 level. The patient presented with a spastic paraparesis and lower thoracic sensory level.

spinal cord or motor nerve roots by an intraspinal tumor may produce fibrillations and a poor interference pattern, which is confined to the muscles supplied by the involved segments.

Myelography

The myelogram is the established diagnostic test for the localization of spinal cord tumors (Figs. 10–11 and 10–12). Passage of the radiopaque material may be completely obstructed at the level of the intraspinal tumor. When blockage is incomplete, extramedullary tumors tend to produce indentation of the dye column with a defect convex toward the cord, while intramedullary tumors produce thinning of the column due to widening of the spinal cord with a defect concave toward the cord.

Computed Tomography

The diagnosis of many diseases affecting the spinal cord or spinal canal has been facilitated by the introduction of the total body scanner.

CT scanning is particularly useful in the demonstration of intraspinal or paraspinal neoplasms and spinal cord arteriovenous malformations.[47] Widening of the spinal cord is well demonstrated in intraspinal tumors, and tumor calcification is readily identified by CT scans. Enlargement of intervertebral foramina and indentation of the spinal canal can be seen in extramedullary lesions.[118] The CT scan can be augmented by the injection of water-soluble contrast material into the subarachnoid space.[33] This is useful in the diagnosis of intramedullary gliomas.

Angiography

Transaortic catheterization with injection of dye at the level of the lesion may be used to fill the collateral vessels to the spinal cord in cases of vascular malformation and highly vascular tumors of the cord.[173a]

Treatment of Spinal Cord Tumors

Benign extramedullary tumors such as neurilemmomas and meningiomas are readily removed by laminectomy and excision of the tumor.[43] "Hourglass" tumors require a two-stage operation, with laminectomy preceding exploration of the mediastinum or abdomen, as removal of the portion of the tumor outside the canal during the first stage may produce damage to the spinal cord by interference with the blood supply.

Pressure on the spinal cord by extramedullary metastatic tumors or by tumors of retriculoendothelial origin requires laminectomy and decompression followed by irradiation rather than excision. The relief of pressure spares motor and sphincter function, and the combined therapy carries a relatively good prognosis in many cases.[69] The use of corticosteroids (dexamethasone, 4 mg every six hours) may have a dramatic effect in relieving spinal cord pressure temporarily.[132] Solitary plasmacytomas have been excised in some cases with apparent complete cure. Extradural cysts should be drained and the sac excised.

Intramedullary tumors are usually infiltrating gliomas, which cannot be removed surgically without severely compromising spinal cord function. Laminectomy and decompression should be performed to relieve pressure on the spinal cord in such patients. The area of involvement by tumor in the cord can be explored with a needle to drain any cysts that may be present in the tumor. If a solid tumor is felt with the exploring needle, an attempt may be made at removal through a midline incision. The chances of removing an intramedullary tumor may be increased by the development of microsurgical techniques.[57, 191] In the case of soft infiltrating gliomas, the dura should be closed without tension and the dentate ligaments sectioned at the site of cord swelling. Such decompression provides improvement in symptoms that may last for many years. Radiotherapy should be used after surgical decompression.[20, 46] Infiltrating ependymomas of the cauda equina should be treated conservatively with surgical removal of as much tumor as possible, sparing involved nerve roots, followed by radiotherapy.[154]

Prognosis of Spinal Cord Tumors

In general, intraspinal tumors carry a much better prognosis than intracranial tumors. This is partly due to the fact that more intraspinal tumors are benign. In addition, however, intramedullary gliomas tend to be less aggressive than cerebral gliomas. Intramedullary tumors thus tend to have slower growth, and laminectomy, decompression, and irradiation of spinal cord gliomas usually provide many years of useful functional activity.

Metastatic Tumors of the Brain

Approximately 20 per cent of cerebral tumors are metastatic, and symptoms owing to cerebral involvement occasionally offer the first sign of disseminated carcinoma. The highest incidence of metastatic tumors of the brain occurs just after the fifth decade of life.

Pathology

Emboli composed of tumor cells may reach the central nervous system by two possible routes. Cells originating in or filtering through the lungs pass through the heart and reach the brain through the systemic arterial system. Tumors arising in the abdominal and pelvic organs may invade the pelvic veins and pass into the vertebral system of veins (Batson's plexus). The cells ascend to the intracranial venous sinuses and the cerebral or cerebellar venous system. Tumors arising from the cranium and its structures may extend directly through the skull into the brain (tumors of the orbit, paranasal sinuses, parotid gland, pharynx, and mucous membranes).

Metastatic carcinoma is much more frequent than metastatic sarcoma, presumably because sarcomas are relatively rare lesions. Approximately 50 per cent of metastatic tumors of the brain arise from bronchial carcinomas, followed in descending incidence by carcinoma of the breast, kidney, gastrointestinal tract, prostate, and thyroid. Two relatively uncommon tumors, choriocarcinoma and malignant melanoma, also have a high incidence of cerebral metastasis.

About 70 per cent of metastases occur in the cerebral hemispheres (Fig. 10–13) and 30 per cent in the cerebellum. In at least 70 per cent of cases, metastases are multiple, although small lesions are often overlooked in the presence of a large, apparently single lesion. The incidence of metastases is approximately equal in the two hemispheres. However, metastases in the parietal and occipital lobes tend to occur at the parieto-occipital junction, the so-called "watershed area" be-

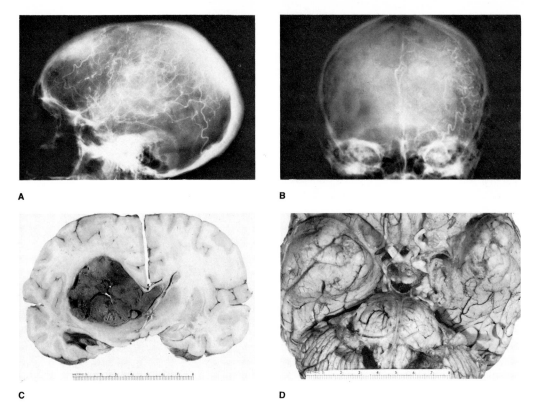

FIGURE 10–13. *A, B.* Left carotid arteriogram in a patient with a metastatic tumor involving the deep frontoparietal area of the left hemisphere. The neovascularity is apparent in the anteroposterior and lateral views. The size of the tumor and the extension into the corpus callosum are illustrated in the coronal section of the brain *(C).* Uncal herniation with necrosis of the medial aspect of the left temporal lobe occurred as a terminal event *(D).*

twεen the internal carotid and vertebral basilar circulations.

Gross Appearance. The majority of metastases are located at the junction of gray and white matter and are well-circumscribed, spheric tumors. On section they are usually firm and yellowish or white, except in areas where hemorrhage and necrosis have occurred. The surrounding brain is edematous and moist, and it is not uncommon to find a small solitary metastatic lesion associated with edema of the entire white matter of the hemisphere in which it is located.

Microscopic Appearance. The histologic appearance depends entirely on the site of the primary lesion. Anaplastic tumors may rarely be difficult to differentiate from a highly cellular glioma, particularly on a frozen section.

Diagnostic Procedures

Contrast-enhanced CT is the most sensitive study available for the detection of brain metastases and should be used in all suspected cases of cerebral metastases unless contraindicated by a history of sensitivity to iodine.[11] Patients with lung carcinoma who do not have neurologic abnormalities should have enhanced CT examinations prior to thoracic surgery, since this study may reveal unsuspected metastases in a significant number of cases.[81]

Treatment

There are reports of successful removal of solitary cerebral metastasis with up to one third of cases of bronchial carcinoma alive after one year and a 20 per cent survival rate at seven years.[113, 135]

A combination of surgical excision followed by radiation therapy may give better results.[109] Multiple metastases should be treated with radiation therapy and corticosteroids, which may produce remarkable improvement by destruction of radiosensitive tumors and reduction of cerebral edema. Improvement occurs in 80 per cent of cases following irradiation of cerebral metastasis, and 20 per cent survive for one year or more.[45, 120] Repeated courses of irradiation and steroids may provide further remission from recurrent neurologic deficit in some patients. The regression and subsequent course of cerebral metastases can be followed by serial CT scanning.[25, 44] Cerebral metastases seem to have a low sensitivity to chemotherapeutic agents except metastases from breast cancer.[133]

Neoplastic Angioendotheliosis

This rare and unusual manifestation of neoplasia may affect the central nervous system and present as a multi-infarct dementia.[138]

Etiology and Pathology

Many organs are affected, including the brain, each showing vascular endothelial proliferation within the blood vessels. The proliferated endothelial cells show all signs of malignancy, including hyperchromia and mitoses. They frequently occlude the lumen of smaller vessels or promote thrombus formation producing scattered areas of infarction.[169]

Clinical Features

The clinical course is that of progressive dementia associated with sudden and fluctuating focal neurologic deficits such as dysphasia and hemiparesis. Recurrent skin lesions and fever occur periodically during the course of the illness.

Diagnostic Procedures

1. Progressive impairment of renal function produces elevation of BUN and serum creatinine levels.
2. Renal angiography confirms the renal involvement and may suggest glomerulonephritis.
3. The diagnosis may be established by brain biopsy.

Treatment

Temporary and dramatic improvement has been reported in response to corticosteroids.

Diffuse Meningeal Carcinomatosis

Metastatic tumor cells may occasionally spread through the subarachnoid space, particularly around the base of the brain and the brainstem. There is a mild inflammatory response in the meninges to the tumor cells, and thrombosis of the penetrating arteries of the brain or brainstem may result. Proliferation of tumor cells in the subarachnoid space blocks the circulation of cerebrospinal fluid, and intracranial pressure rises progressively. The cells proliferate around the cranial nerves at the base of the brain and compress them.

Clinical Features

The signs are due to meningitis, increased intracranial pressure, and cranial nerve and brainstem involvement. The meningeal reaction produces headache and stiffness of the neck. The increased intracranial pressure results in headache, vomiting, and eventually papilledema. There is usually progressive involvement of the lower cranial nerves. Small infarcts in the brainstem produce signs of involvement of the corticospinal and cerebellar tracts.

The possibility of meningeal carcinomatosis should be considered in any patient with a primary tumor who develops signs of a subacute meningitis and in individuals presenting with meningeal signs and progressive paralysis of cranial nerves. In the latter situation, the symptoms may develop before detection of a primary lesion and the differential diagnosis must be made between tuberculous and other granulomatous meningitides.

Diagnostic Procedures

The cerebrospinal fluid is usually under increased pressure and may be clear or turbid. The cell count seldom exceeds 500 per cubic millimeter; protein content is generally elevated and glucose level depressed, often to less than 40 mg per cent. These cerebrospinal fluid abnormalities are similar to those seen in tuberculous meningitis or mycotic infections of the brain and in sarcoidosis of the central nervous system. Cytologic examination of the fluid may reveal malignant cells, and the yield of positive results has increased with the development of millipore filtration techniques.

Treatment

The condition is ultimately fatal, but remissions may result from radiotherapy. It is probable that intrathecal chemotherapy with suitable antimetabolites or cytotoxic agents may be helpful in the future as this form of therapy is successful in leukemic involvement of the meninges in children.

Tumors of the Peripheral Nerves

Nonneoplastic Tumors; Posttraumatic or Amputation Neuroma

These lesions usually result from surgical or traumatic section of a peripheral nerve followed by attempts at repair by proliferation of Schwann cells and fibroblasts. Similar lesions may result from injection of inflammatory substances into a nerve (such as into the sciatic nerve when administering intramuscular injections of penicillin and paraldehyde). A tangled mass of nerve fibers and connective tissue is formed, and the mass may become adherent to regional scar tissue. These neuromas are often painful and in an amputation stump may give rise to annoying sensations referable to "a phantom limb." This term refers to sensations felt in an amputated extremity despite the fact that the limb is missing; hence the term "phantom limb." Irritation of the nerve stump at the neuroma is responsible for these sensations and relief is usually afforded by excision of the neuroma.

Tumors Derived from Schwann Cells

Neurilemmoma

This tumor, which has been described in the section dealing with intracranial tumors, is not an infrequent lesion of peripheral nerves and may be seen in virtually any location. Sarcomatous change is rare.

Neurofibromatosis (von Recklinghausen's Disease)

The condition is characterized by the development of multiple neurofibromas and is inherited as an autosomal dominant with a high mutation rate since there appears to be a reduction in fertility in this disease.[40] Solitary neurofibromas also occur and from the pathologic standpoint are identical to the multiple variety. The prognosis is, of course, much better provided removal is technically feasible.

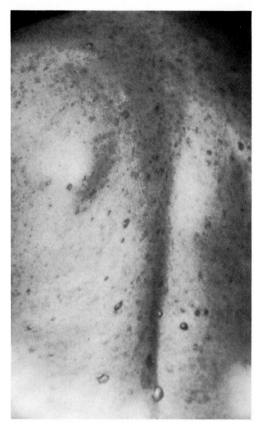

FIGURE 10–14.   Typical appearance of the skin of the back in neurofibromatosis (von Recklinghausen's disease), showing the pedunculated and sessile neurofibroma. This patient also had a neurofibroma compressing the cervical cord at C_2.

Clinical Features.   *Café-au-lait spots* are noted on the skin and consist of areas in which the cells in the basal layer of the epidermis contain excess melanin. Such areas vary in color from light to dark brown, hence the name "café-au-lait spots." They may be single or multiple. A person with six or more areas of skin pigmentation of this type (exceeding 1 to 5 cm in broadest diameter) may be presumed to have von Recklinghausen's disease, even in the absence of a family history of this disorder.

Neurofibromas are visible and palpable in the skin. They may be cutaneous or subcutaneous and are soft and mobile. They vary in number from a single lesion to many thousands in one individual (Fig. 10–14). Most of the cutaneous tumors are cone-shaped or pedunculated, but some are flat. They have a violaceous color, which tends to fade with age. Subcutaneous tumors arising in peripheral nerves may attain considerable size and have been described as "plexiform neurofibromas" or "elephantiasis neurofibromatosa." They are soft but frequently produce marked deformity in the affected area. A retrobulbar neurofibroma may produce pressure on the optic nerve and blindness.

Neurilemmoma may give rise to neurologic signs. These tumors occur on both *cranial and spinal nerves.*[40] The eighth cranial nerve is the most common cranial nerve that is involved. Neurilemmomas of the eighth nerve may be bilateral in this disease. Occasional examples involving all the other cranial nerves from the third to the twelfth have been described.

Sarcomatous change is much more frequent in plexiform neurofibroma than in neurilemmoma. The tumor that develops is probably best termed a neurofibrosarcoma or malignant schwannoma.

Osseous involvement by growth of a neurofibroma within a bone may produce a rarefied area resembling a bone cyst or hyperostosis or erosion of the bone surface. Scoliosis due to involvement of vertebral bodies is sometimes seen in advanced von Recklinghausen's disease. Congenital bowing of the tibia and fibula with pseudoarthrosis may occur.

Symptoms Referable to the Central Nervous System. There may be some association of mental retardation with von Recklinghausen's disease, but this has not been related to any structural abnormalities in the brain.

There is a significant increase in gliomas, meningiomas, and multiple tumors of the central nervous system in neurofibromatosis.[168]

Tumors of Sympathetic Ganglion Cells. These also occur in von Recklinghausen's disease. The rare association of neurofibromatosis with pheochromocytoma has also been established.

Gross Appearance. The plexiform neurofibroma resembles a tangled mass of white worms varying in diameter from threadlike to approximately 1 cm. Unlike a neurilemmoma, it is not encapsulated but infiltrates adjacent structures, making complete removal most difficult. Depending on the degree of edema, it may be rubbery, gelatinous, or mucinous.

Microscopic Appearance. The tumor is composed of tortuous, interlacing nerve bundles, each

surrounded by a fibrous capsule. Spindle cells lie in an edematous matrix, which occasionally becomes more fibrous. There is no palisading and no histiocytic infiltrate such as is seen in a neurilemmoma.

Treatment. Since removal of all the neurofibromas would be impossible in severe cases, treatment is palliative. Surgery is reserved for tumors producing pain or pressure on vital structures. Any rapid increase in growth of cutaneous tumors may indicate malignancy and is an indication for prompt removal and irradiation.[183]

Tumors Arising from Sympathetic Ganglion Cells

Ganglioneuroma

This rare, slow-growing benign tumor arising in the sympathetic ganglion is usually seen in the posterior mediastinum and retroperitoneum but may occur anywhere ganglia are located. It is usually detected in roentgenograms of the chest or is found incidentally during removal of an abdominal tumor. Occasionally, it may extend through the intravertebral foramina to compress the spinal cord or cauda equina.

Sympatheticoblastoma (Neuroblastoma)

These tumors arise from primitive sympathetic neuroblasts of the neural crests and can occur at any site where there are elements of the sympathetic nervous system. About two thirds of neuroblastomas arise from the adrenal medulla or nearby sympathetic ganglia.[131]

Clinical Features

Initial symptoms are vague and consist of fever, lymphadenopathy, diarrhea, failure to thrive, and bone pain. The mother may discover an abdominal mass while bathing the child. Further progression is associated with periorbital ecchymoses, proptosis owing to orbital metastases, and optic, oculomotor, and auditory nerve involvement. Primary cranial neuroblastoma may arise in the ciliary, sphenopalatine or submaxillary ganglia and, rarely, in the nasopharynx, producing unilateral nasal obstruction.

These tumors may also present as masses in the neck or posterior mediastinum with radicular pain and spinal cord compression, causing paraplegia if the tumor is of the "dumbbell" type. Metastases from abdominal neuroblastomas usually spread to the liver (Pepper type) or orbit (Hutchinson type).

Diagnostic Procedures

1. Roentgenograms show calcification in about half of the primary abdominal neuroblastomas.
2. Skull roentgenograms may show osteolytic defects, 0.1 to 0.5 cm in diameter, owing to metastases.
3. Similar metastases may be seen in roentgenograms of the long bones. Pathologic fractures occur in some cases.
4. The cerebrospinal fluid may be xanthochromic, with increased protein content when there is spinal cord compression by tumor.

Treatment

Neuroblastomas are highly radiosensitive and show good response to x-ray therapy or chemotherapy in many cases.[192] There is some evidence that survival is associated with maturation of a primitive neuroblastoma to a benign mature ganglioneuroma.[114]

Tumors of Paraganglia

Paraganglionic cells are found in both the sympathetic and parasympathetic ganglia. They are of two types: chromaffin and nonchromaffin. The former contain chromaffin granules in their cytoplasm, are prominent particularly in the adrenal medulla, and probably are active in the production of epinephrine and norepinephrine. The tumor arising from the chromaffin cells is the pheochromocytoma, usually located in the adrenal medulla but occasionally found in other sympathetic ganglia. Since the effect of the tumor on the central nervous system is indirect, i.e., by paroxysmal or sustained hypertension, it will not be discussed in detail. The nonchromaffin cells are believed by some to give rise to the chemodectoma most commonly located in the carotid body. The tumor of the glomus jugulare is also derived from nonchromaffin cells and has been described elsewhere (see p. 634).

Cited References

1. Actari, A. N., and Colover, J. Posterior fossa tumors with pathological laughter. *J.A.M.A.*, **235:**1469–71, 1976.
2. Adams, J. H. The classification of microgliomatosis with particular reference to diffuse microgliomatosis. *Acta Neuropathol.* (Berl.), suppl 6:119–23, 1975.
3. Aicardi, J.; Praud, E.; Barncaud, J.; Mises, J.; and Chevre, J. J. Clinical primary epilepsy and cerebral tumors in the child. *Arch. Franc. Pediat.*, **27:**1041–55, 1970.
4. Anderson, M., and Salmon, M. V. Symptomatic cataplexy. *J. Neurol. Neurosurg. Psychiat.*, **40:**186–91, 1977.
5. Andrew, V. C., and Petkov, I. Skin manifestations associated with tumors. *Br. J. Dermatol.*, **92:**675–78, 1975.
6. Antoni, N. Spinal vascular malformations (angiomas) and myelomalacia. *Neurology* (Minneap.), **12:**795–804, 1962.
7. Avery, T. L. Seven cases of frontal tumor with psychiatric presentation. *Br. J. Psychiat.*, **119:**19–23, 1971.
8. Backland, E.-O. Studies on craniopharyngiomas. III. Stereotaxic treatment with intracystic YHrum-90. *Acta Chir. Scand.*, **139:**237–47, 1973.
9. Backlund, E. O. Stereotaxic treatment of craniopharyngiomas. *Acta Neurochirurg.*, suppl 21:177–83, 1974.
10. Bailey, I. C. Dermoid tumors of the spinal cord. *J. Neurosurg.*, **33:**676–81, 1970.
11. Bardfield, P. A.; Passalaqua, A. M.; et al. A comparison of radionuclide scanning and computed tomography in metastatic lesions of the brain. *J. Computer Assisted Tomogr.*, **1:**315–18, 1977.
12. Barlette, J. R. Craniopharyngiomas. Summary of 85 cases. *J. Neurol. Neurosurg. Psychiat.*, **34:**37–41, 1971.
13. Benton, J. W.; Neuhaus, G.; Huttenlocher, P. R.; Ojemann, R. G.; and Dodge, P. R. The bobble head doll syndrome: report of a unique truncal tremor associated with third ventricular cyst and hydrocephalus in children. *Neurology* (Minneap.), **16:**725–29, 1966.
14. Bernat, J. L. Glioblastoma multiforme and the meningeal syndrome. *Neurology* (Minneap.), **26:**1071–74, 1976.
15. Betty, M. J. Quality of survival in treated patients with supratentorial gliomata. *J. Neurol. Neurosurg. Psychiat.*, **27:**556–61, 1964.
16. Bischof, W., and Nittner, K. Epidermoid and dermoid of the spinal canal. *Zentralbl. Neurochir.*, **30:**101–18, 1969.
17. Bogdanowicz, W. M., and Sach, E. The possible role of radiation in oncogenesis of meningioma. *Surg. Neurol.*, **2:**379–83, 1974.
18. Boller, F. C., and Sherwin, I. Electroencephalography and brain scan in the diagnosis of posterior fossa lesions. *Dis. Nerv. Syst.*, **31:**490–93, 1970.
19. Brennan, T. G.; Rao, C. V. G. K.; et al. Tandem lesions: Chromophobe adenoma and meningioma. *J. Computer Assisted Tomogr.*, **1:**517–20, 1977.
20. Bruni, J.; Bilbao, J. M.; and Gray, T. Primary intramedullary malignant lymphoma of the spinal cord. *Neurology* (Minneap.), **27:**896–98, 1977.
21. Bryan, P. CSF seeding of intracranial tumors: A study of 96 cases. *Clin. Radiol.*, **25:**355–60, 1974.
22. Buckman, M. T.; Husain, M.; et al. Primary

105. Lundberg, P. O.; Drettner, B.; et al. The invasive pituitary adenoma. *Arch. Neurol.,* **34:**742–49, 1977.

106. Lynn, G. E., and Gilroy, J. Neuroaudiological abnormalities in patients with temporal lobe tumors. *J. Neurol. Sci.,* **17:**167–84, 1972.

107. Lynn, G. E., and Gilroy, J. Evaluation of central auditory dysfunction in patients with neurological disorders. In Keith, Robert W. (ed.). *Central Auditory Dysfunction.* Grune & Stratton, New York, 1977, pp. 177–221.

108. MacCarty, C. S.; Boyd, A. S., Jr.; and Childs, D. S. Tumors of the optic nerve and optic chiasm. *J. Neurosurg.,* **33:**439–44, 1970.

109. Magilligan, D. J., Jr.; Rogers, J. S.; et al. Pulmonary neoplasm with solitary cerebral metastasis: Results of combined excision. *J. Thorac. Cardiovasc. Surg.,* **72:**690–98, 1976.

110. Magnus, O.; Storm Van Leeuwen, W.; and Cobb, W. A. Electroencephalography and cerebral tumors. *Electroenceph. Clin. Neurophysiol.,* suppl. **19:** 1961.

111. Maroon, J. C., and Albright, L. "Failure to thrive" due to pontine glioma. *Arch. Neurol.,* **34:**295–97, 1977.

112. Mayer, E. G.; Boone, M. L. M.; et al. Role of radiation therapy in the management of neoplasms of the central nervous system. *Adv. Neurol.,* **15:**201–20, 1976.

113. McGee, E. E. Surgical treatment of cerebral metastasis from lung cancer: Effect on quality and duration of survival. *J. Neurosurg.,* **35:**416–20, 1971.

114. McLaughlin, J. E., and Urich, H. Maturing neuroblastoma and ganglionendoblastoma: A study of 4 cases with long survival. *J. Pathol.,* **121:**19–26, 1977.

115. McNealy, D. E., and Plum, F. Brain stem dysfunction with supratentorial mass lesions. *Arch. Neurol.,* **7:**10–32, 1962.

116. Michels, L. G.; Bentson, J. R.; and Winter, J. Computed tomography of cerebral venous angiomas. *J. Computer Assisted Tomogr.,* **1:**149–54, 1977.

117. Morantz, R. A.; Feigin, I.; et al. Clinical and pathological study of 24 cases of gliosarcoma. *J. Neurosurg.,* **45:**398–408, 1976.

118. Nakagawa, H.; Huang, Y. P.; et al. Computed tomography of intraspinal and paraspinal neoplasms. *J. Computer Assisted Tomogr.* **1:**377–90, 1977.

119. Nassar, S. I.; Correll, J. W.; and Housepian, E. M. Intramedullary cystic lesions of the conus medullaris. *J. Neurol. Neurosurg. Psychiat.,* **31:**106–109, 1968.

120. Nisie, L. Z.; Hilaris, B. J.; and Chin, F. C. H. Review of experience with irradiation of brain metastasis. *Am. J. Roentgenol.,* **111:**329–33, 1971.

121. Northfield, D. W. C. Surgical treatment of acoustic neurinoma. *Proc. Roy. Soc. Med.,* **63:**769–75, 1970.

122. Ohaegbutam, S. C. Sudden death from an asymptomatic sphenoid ridge meningioma. *J. Neurol.,* **215:**291–94, 1977.

123. Ojemann, R. G.; Montgomery, W. W.; and Weiss, A. D. Evaluation and surgical treatment of acoustic neuroma. *N. Engl. J. Med.,* **287:**845–99, 1972.

124. Okawara, S.-H. Solid cerebellar hemangioblastoma. *J. Neurosurg.,* **39:**514–18, 1973.

125. Ottoni, S. P. Clinical and surgical aspects of medulloblastomas: Review of 102 cases. *Senra Med. Neurocher.* (Sao Paulo), **1:**331–42, 1973.

126. Page, L. K.; Lambrose, C. T.; and Matson, D. D. Childhood epilepsy with late detection of cerebral glioma. *J. Neurosurg.,* **31:**253–61, 1969.

127. Paillas, J. E.; Legre, J.; Alliez, B.; and Donfour, M. Diagnosis and treatment of tumors of the basal ganglions. Anatomicoclinical data from 50 cases. *Neuro-Chir.,* **16:**89–115, 1970.

128. Palgrom von Metz, I.; Bots, G. Th A. M.; and Eratz, L. J. Astrocytoma in three sisters. *Neurology* (Minneap.), **27:**1038–41, 1977.

129. Percy, A. K.; Elueback, L. R.; Okuzaki, H.; and Kurland, L. T. Neoplasms of the central nervous system: Epidemiologic considerations. *Neurology* (Minneap.), **22:**40–48, 1972.

130. Plum, F., and Posner, J. B. *The Diagnosis of Stupor and Coma.* Contemporary Neurology Series, Vol. 10. Davis, Philadelphia, 1972.

131. Pochedly, C. The broad clinical spectrum of neuroblastoma. *Postgrad. Med.,* **51:**79–85, 1972.

132. Posner, J. B.; Howieson, J.; and Cuitkovic, E. "Disappearing" spinal cord compression. Oncolytic effect of glucocorticosteroids (and other chemotherapeutic agents) on epidural metastases. *Ann. Neurol.,* **2:**409–13, 1977.

133. Pouillant, P.; Mathe, G.; et al. Trial of treatment of glioblastoma in the adult and cerebral metastases with a combination of adriamycin, WM26, and CCNU: Results of type II trial. *Nouv. Presse Med.,* **5:**1571–76, 1976.

134. Raaf, J., and Parsons, W. R. Intracranial meningiomas. *Arch. Surg.,* **102:**380–84, 1971.

135. Raskind, R., Weiss, S. R.; and Wermuth, R. E. Single metastatic brain tumors. Treatment and followup of 41 cases. *Am. J. Roentgenol.,* **11:**323–28, 1971.

136. Ray, B. S., and Patterson, R. H., Jr. Surgical experience with chromophobe adenoma of the pituitary gland. *J. Neurosurg.,* **34:**726–29, 1971.

137. Raynor, R. B. Papilledema associated with tumors of spinal cord. *Neurology* (Minneap.), **19:**700–704, 1969.

138. Reinglass, J. L.; Muller, J.; et al. Central nervous system angioendotheliosis. A treatable multiple infarct dementa. *Stroke,* **8:**218–21, 1977.

139. Rewcastle, N. B., and Berry, K. Neoplasms of the lower spinal cord. *Neurology* (Minneap.), **14:**608–15, 1964.

140. Roberson, C., and Till, K. Hypothalamus gliomas in children. *J. Neurol. Neurosurg. Psychiat.,* **37:**1047–52, 1974.

141. Roberts, M., and German, W. J. Long term study of patients with oligodendrogliomas: Follow-up of 50 cases including Dr. Harvey Cushing's series. *J. Neurosurg.,* **24:**697–700, 1966.

142. Robinson, J. L. Sudden blindness with pituitary tumors: Report of three cases. *J. Neurosurg.,* **36:**83–85, 1972.

143. Rosich-Pla, A.; Smith, B. H.; and Sil, R. Congenital arachnoid cysts with unusual clinical radiological findings. *Ann. Neurol.*, **2**:443–46, 1977.

144. Rovit, R. L.; Schlecter, M. M.; and Chodroft, P. Choroid plexus papilloma. Observation on radiologic diagnosis. *Am. J. Roentgenol.*, **110**:608–17, 1970.

145. Rupp, N. Differentiation of spinal tumors. *Fortschr. Geb. Rongenstra. Nuklearmed.*, **112**:174–82, 1970.

146. Rush, J. L.; Everett, B. A.; et al. Paroxysmal atrial tachycardia and frontal lobe tumor. *Arch. Neurol.*, **34**:578–80, 1977.

147. Sano, K. Diagnosis and treatment of tumors in the pineal region. *Acta Neurochir.*, **34**:153–57, 1976.

148. Schally, A. V.; Arimura, A.; and Kostin, A. J. Hypothalamic regulatory hormones. *Science*, **179**:341–50, 1973.

149. Shaywitz, B. A. Epidermoid spinal cord tumors and previous lumbar punctures. *J. Pediatr.*, **80**:638–40, 1972.

150. Schoenberg, B. S.; Christine, B. W.; et al. Nervous system neoplasms and primary malignancies of other sites. *Neurology* (Minneap.), **25**:705–12, 1975.

151. Schoenberg, B. S.; Christine, B. W.; et al. The descriptive epidemiology of primary intracranial neoplasms: The Connecticut experience. *Am. J. Epidemiol.*, **104**:499–510, 1976.

152. Schuier, F. Is there an anaplastic type of oligodendrioglioma? A case report. *J. Neurol.*, **213**:263–68, 1976.

153. Schurr, P. H. Aberrations of the sense of smell in head injury and cerebral tumors. *Proc. Roy. Soc. Med.*, **68**:470–72, 1975.

154. Scott, M. Infiltrating ependymomas of the cauda equina: Treatment by conservative surgery plus radiotherapy. *J. Neurosurg.*, **41**:446–48, 1974.

155. Shapiro, W. R., and Young, D. F. Treatment of malignant glioma. A controlled study of chemotherapy and irradiation. *Arch. Neurol.*, **33**:494–500, 1976.

156. Sharma, U.; Tandou, P. N.; et al. Craniopharyngiomas treated by combination of surgery and radiotherapy. *Clin. Radiol.*, **25**:13–17, 1974.

157. Sheline, G. E. Radiation therapy of brain tumors. *Cancer*, **39**:873–81, 1977.

158. Shuangshoti, S., and Netsky, M. G. Neuroepithelial colloid cysts of the nervous system; further observations on pathogenesis, location, incidence and histochemistry. *Neurology* (Minneap.), **16**:887–903, 1966.

159. Smith, K. O.; Newman, J. T.; et al. Viruses and brain tumors. *Clin. Neurosurg.*, **21**:362–83, 1973.

159a. Sogg, R.; Hoyt, W.; and Boldey, E. Spastic paretic facial contractures. A rare sign of brain stem tumors. *Neurology* (Minneap.), **13**:607–12, 1963. (Minneap.) *Clin. Neurosurg.*, 362–83, 1974.

160. Stage, W. S., and Stein, J. J. Treatment of malignant astrocytomas. *Am. J. Roentgenol. Rad. Ther. Nucl. Med.*, **120**:7–18, 1974.

161. Stanley, P. Papilloma of the choroid plexus. *Br. J. Radiol.*, **41**:848–57, 1968.

162. Starr, A., and Achor, L. J. Auditory brain-stem responses in neurological disease. *Arch. Neurol.*, **32**:761–68, 1975.

163. Stein, B. M.; Fraser, R. A. R.; and Tenner, M. S. Radiologic characteristics and surgical management of third ventricular tumors in children. *Acta Neurol. Latinen*, **17**:131–40, 1971.

164. Stern, W. E. Meningiomas in the cranio-orbital junction. *J. Neurosurg.*, **38**:428–37, 1973.

165. Stern, W. E., and Batzdorf, U. Intracranial removal of pituitary adenomas. Evaluation of varying degrees of excision from partial to total. *J. Neurosurg.*, **33**:564–73, 1970.

166. Stockard, J., and Rossiter, V. S. Clinical and pathologic correlates of brain-stem auditory response abnormalities. *Neurology* (Minneap.), **27**:316–25, 1977.

167. Stockard, J. J.; Stockard, J. E.; and Sharbrough, F. W. Detection and localization of occult lesions with brain-stem auditory responses. *Mayo Clin. Proc.*, **52**:761–69, 1977.

168. Strong, A. J.; Symon, L.; et al. Coincidental meningioma and glioma. Report of two cases. *J. Neurol.*, **45**:455–58, 1976.

169. Strough, J. C.; Donahue, S.; Ross, A.; et al. Neoplastic and angioendotheliosis. *Neurology* (Minneap.), **15**:644–48, 1965.

170. Sumi, S. M., and Leftman, H. Primary intracranial leptomeningeal glioma with persistent hypoglycorrhachia. *J. Neurol. Neurosurg. Psychiat.*, **31**:190–94, 1968.

171. Swenberg, J. A. Chemical induction of brain tumors. *Adv. Neurol.*, **15**:85–99, 1976.

172. Thomas, M.; Adams, J. H.; and Doyle, D. Neuroectodermal tumors in the cerebellum in two sisters. *J. Neurol. Neurosurg. Psychiat.*, **40**:886–89, 1977.

173. Thomsen, J. Cerebellopontine angle tumors other than acoustic neuromas: Report of 34 cases—Presentation of 7 bilateral acoustic neuromas. *Acta Otolaryngol.*, **82**:106–11, 1976.

173a. Tobin, W., and Layton, D. The diagnosis and natural history of spinal cord arteriovenous malformations. *Mayo Clin. Proc.*, **51**:637–46, 1976.

174. Toglia, J. U.; Netsky, M. G.; and Alexander, E., Jr. Epithelial (epidermoid) tumors of the cranium; their common nature and pathogenesis. *J. Neurosurg.*, **23**:384–93, 1965.

175. VanCreuel, H. Absence of papilloedema in cerebral tumors. *J. Neurol. Neurosurg. Psychiat.*, **38**:931–33, 1975.

176. Waldmann, T. A.; Levin, E. H.; and Baldwin, M. Association of polycythemia with a cerebellar hemangioblastoma. *Am. J. Med.*, **31**:318–24, 1961.

177. Wallace, D. Lipoma of the corpus callosum. *J. Neurol. Neurosurg. Psychiat.*, **39**:1179–85, 1976.

178. Weir, B. Relative significance of factors affecting postoperative survival in astrocytomas grades 3 and 4. *J. Neurosurg.*, **38**:448–52, 1973.

179. Weir, B., and Elridge, A. R. Oligodendrogliomas: Analysis of 63 cases. *J. Neurosurg.*, **29**:500–505, 1968.

180. Weisberg, L. A.; Zimmerman, E. A.; and Frantz,

A. G. Diagnosis and evaluation of patients with an enlarged sella tursica. *Am. J. Med.,* **61:**590–96, 1976.

181. Werlake, P. T.; Murkovits, B. A.; and Stellar, S. Cytologic evaluation of cerebrospinal fluid with clinical and histologic correlation. *Acta Cytol.,* **16:**224–39, 1972.

182. Whitaker, W. G., and Droulias, C. Benign encapsulated neurolemmoma: Report of 76 cases. *Am. Surg.,* **42:**675–78, 1976.

183. White, H. R., Jr. Survival in malignant schwannoma: An 18 year study. *Cancer,* **27:**720–29, 1971.

184. Wilkinson, H. A.; Kornblith, P.; et al. Focal chemotherapy of brain tumors using semipermeable membranes. *J. Neurol. Neurosurg. Psychiat.,* **40:**389–394, 1977.

185. Wilner, H. I.; Crockett, J.; and Gilroy, J. The galenic venous system: A selective radiographic study. *Am. J. Roentgenol.,* **115:**1–13, 1972.

186. Wilson, C. B. Glioblastoma multiforme: Present status. *Arch. Neurol.,* **11:**562–68, 1964.

187. Wilson, C. B. Chemotherapy of brain tumors. *Adv. Neurol.,* **15:**361–67, 1976.

188. Wilson, C. B.; Gutin, P.; et al. Single agent chemotherapy of brain tumors. *Arch. Neurol.,* **33:739–44, 1976.**

189. Woolsey, R. M., and Nelson, J. S. Asymptomatic destruction of the fornix in man. *Arch. Neurol.,* **32:**566–68, 1975.

190. Wyhe, I. G.; Heffreys, R. V.; and Maslaine, G. N. Cerebral hemangioblastoma. *Br. J. Radiol.,* **46:**472–76, 1973.

191. Yasargil, M. G.; Antia, J.; et al. Microsurgical removal of intramedullary spinal hemangioblastomas: Report of 12 cases and review of the literature. *Surg. Neurol.,* **4:**614–48, 1976.

192. Young, L. W.; Rubin, P.; and Hanson, R. E. The extra adrenal neuroblastoma: High radio curability and diagnostic accuracy. *Am. J. Roentgenol. Radium Ther. Nucl. Med.,* **108:**75–91, 1970.

193. Zervas, N. T., and Mendelson, G. Treatment of acute hemorrhage of pituitary tumors. *Lancet,* **1:**604–605, 1975.

194. Ziegler, D. K.; Kaufman, A.; and Marshall, H. E. Abrupt memory loss associated with thalamic tumor. *Arch. Neurol.,* **34:**545–48, 1977.

195. Zülch, K. J., and Minnel, H. O. New aspects of brain tumor research. *J. Neurol.,* **214:**241–50, 1977.

CHAPTER 11 DISEASES OF THE PERIPHERAL AND CRANIAL NERVES

Disorders of the Second Cranial (Optic) Nerve

Optic Atrophy in Childhood

Abnormalities of the optic nerve, including papilledema, optic neuritis, and optic atrophy, have been discussed already in Chapter 1. Two conditions, congenital coloboma of the optic disk and optic disk hypoplasia, are sometimes confused with optic atrophy. Congenital coloboma of the disk is recognized by factitious enlargement of the disk due to involvement of the retina by the colobomatous defect. Vision is usually not seriously impaired unless there is marked involvement of the fundus. Hypoplasia of the optic nerve presents as a small gray or white optic nerve head and occurs as an isolated condition or as one of the anomalies of septo-optic dysplasia (Chap. 2).

In children, optic atrophy is frequently associated with mental retardation, hydrocephalus, and degenerative conditions of the central nervous system in which primary or secondary optic atrophy is part of widespread disease of the nervous system. Some children may have suffered head injury and injury to the optic nerve with subsequent optic atrophy. Others develop optic atrophy after meningitis. All children with optic atrophy should have a serologic test for syphilis to exclude congenital syphilis. Other lesions causing optic atrophy in children include gliomas of the optic nerve and chiasm or orbital tumors. These tumors are usually demonstrated by computed tomography. Occasionally craniopharyngiomas or gliomas of the third ventricle compress the optic chiasm and cause optic atrophy. An acute dilatation of the third ventricle as a result of a posterior fossa tumor can also compress the optic chiasm and result in optic atrophy. Diseases of the bone that compress the optic nerve and cause optic atrophy include fibrosis, dysplasia, and osteopetrosis.

There are, however, a group of children who present with optic atrophy but without other signs of neurologic deficit. They are usually referred to the neurologist because of complaints of impairment of vision and/or strabismus and nystagmus which are noted by parents or teachers in school. Some of these children represent early examples of Leber's optic atrophy (see Chap. 4), a condition that appears to be a hereditary disorder of cyanide metabolism which may respond to treatment with hydroxycobalamin.[2, 20, 22, 161, 162] Unless there is a positive family history of Leber's disease, this condition cannot be established in the remainder. Some cases are examples of inherited optic atrophy which occurs as an autosomal dominant or autosomal recessive trait.[167] The dominant form of optic atrophy is readily recognized from the family history. This condition occurs in an infantile form, which is severe with complete or almost complete loss of vision, and in a childhood form, which is insidious and where the visual loss is rarely severe. In the recessive form of inherited optic atrophy, both parents are carriers and are apparently healthy. The diagnosis is often established when there is similar involvement of other siblings.

In addition to Leber's optic atrophy and inherited optic atrophy, there are several other forms of familial optic atrophy associated with Friedreich's ataxia, other spinocerebellar degenerations, Refsum's syndrome, the Laurence-Moon-Biedl syndrome, and the diabetes insipidus–diabetes mellitus–optic atrophy–deafness (DIDMOAD) syndrome.[132]

Diagnostic Procedures

1. All children with optic atrophy should have serologic tests to exclude syphilis.
2. Pattern-reversal visual evoked potentials are abnormal at an early stage in optic atrophy. As visual acuity declines, the VEP shows a parallel progression of VEP latency and can be used as an accurate assessment of progression of the atrophic process.[42, 114]
3. Computed tomography of the brain and orbit should be performed in all cases of optic atrophy. The optic nerve is well visualized if sections are taken parallel to the infraorbital meatal line.[21]

Optic Neuritis in the Adult

Although optic neuritis in the adult is commonly a part of multiple sclerosis, there are causes of adult recurrent optic neuritis unassociated with evidence of demyelination elsewhere in the nervous system. The abrupt onset of decreased visual acuity in the affected eye with pain on movement and other clinical findings have been described in Chapter 1. Adult cases other than multiple sclerosis probably have an infectious, toxic, or autoimmune etiology.[13, 84, 160]

An ischemic optic neuropathy has been described in which there is infarction of the anterior portion of the optic nerve. This condition is commonly due to temporal arteritis, but other cases are due to atherosclerosis of the ophthalmic artery often in the presence of chronic hypertension, diabetes mellitus, and extracranial vascular disease. Patients present with visual field defects, and there is swelling of the optic disk in the acute stage of the disease.

Diagnostic Procedures

1. The visual acuity is decreased, and visual field testing frequently shows a centrocecal or paracentral scotoma.
2. Pattern shift visual evoked responses are abnormal in optic neuritis and are particularly useful in confirming the presence of suspected optic neuritis in multiple sclerosis.[139]
3. Abnormalities in auditory evoked potentials and somatosensory evoked potentials may be useful in detecting potential cases of multiple sclerosis when a patient presents with optic neuritis.
4. Delayed visual perception[129] and impaired temporal resolution of vision[59] are also useful tests in the detection of unsuspected optic neuritis in multiple sclerosis.[58]

Treatment

Steroid therapy such as methylprednisolone, 80 to 120 mg every other day, should be instituted for two weeks (thereafter gradually reduced and withdrawn) in order to decrease the inflammatory edema of the optic nerves. There does not appear to be any advantage in the retro-orbital injection of corticosteroids in the treatment of optic neuritis.[65]

Disorders of the Third, Fourth, and Sixth Cranial Nerves

The Tonic Pupil (Reye-Holmes-Adie Syndrome)

The tonic pupillary syndrome consists of mydriasis, a poor or absent light reflex, slow and long-lasting pupillary constriction to near vision, and often some disturbance of accommodation.[95] The syndrome is commonly referred to as Adie's syndrome, although this hardly gives credit to the many individuals who described the syndrome at a much earlier date.

Etiology and Pathology

The tonic pupillary syndrome can occur after trauma to the eye or orbit, and following a number of infectious conditions, but there is often no known cause and the patient is apparently healthy at the time of onset. The lesion causing pupillotonia produces neuronal loss in the ciliary ganglion.[123] However, the ciliary ganglion contains about 30 times as many neurons that supply the ciliary muscles as compared to those that supply the iris. This means that surviving neurons or regenerated axons are likely to serve accommodation. However, surviving axons sprout collaterals that reinnervate both the ciliary muscle and the iris, and pupillary constriction may occur when the patient looks at a near object.

Clinical Features

The syndrome is seen in both sexes and at all ages but occurs most commonly in women aged 20 to 40 years. The pupillary dilatation is usually unilateral and rarely bilateral. In the bilateral condition the eyes may be involved together or as two separate events months or years apart. Accommodation may be normal, impaired, tonic, or may be lost at first and regained later. The deep tendon reflexes, particularly the knee jerks, are absent, diminished, or asymmetric.

It is most unusual for there to be any symptoms, and the pupillary dilatation is frequently discovered incidentally during medical examinations. Rarely, there are complaints of photophobia or blurring of vision when performing fine work. The dilatation of the pupil usually exceeds 5 mm but varies in size during the day. There may be slight irregularity of the pupil. There is slow constriction in response to light as well as tardy dilatation in darkness, and the tonic pupil may be slightly smaller than the normal pupil in darkness. Constriction on convergence is usually more rapid, with some response occurring within 20 seconds. However, when the eye is relaxed following convergence, the pupil fails to dilate promptly. Dilatation of the pupil is also slow in response to emotional or painful stimuli such as pinching the neck. The pupil is hypersensitive to concentrations of cholinergic drugs that do not affect the

normal pupil, and there is contraction when two drops of 2.5 per cent mecholyl are instilled into the conjunctival sac.

Other abnormalities may be found on neurologic examination. There may be reduction in the corneal reflex on the side of the pupillary dilatation, patchy hypalgesia, and impaired sudomotor responses[120] over the face and trunk on the affected side.

Treatment

The patient and relatives should be reassured that the condition is benign[77] and that there is no need for extensive investigations or treatment.

Palsies of the Extraocular Muscles

Numerous conditions may cause paralysis of one or more of the ocular motor nerves. Common etiologic factors are listed in Table 11–1. In this table an attempt has been made to correlate the cause with the anatomic site of the lesion. Discussion of many of these conditions will be found in other sections of this book. The majority of lesions of the brainstem cause paralysis because of involvement of the nuclei or the cranial nerves within the bulb itself. In such cases the signs are not usually limited to extraocular muscles, since other brainstem structures are almost invariably

TABLE 11–1

Paralysis of the Third, Fourth, and Sixth Cranial Nerves

Level	
Brainstem	Hereditary (Möbius) encephalitis, syphilis, tumor, infarction, multiple sclerosis, spinocerebellar degenerations
Intracranial	Meningitis, polyneuritis, diabetes, tumor, raised intracranial pressure
Intracavernous	Aneurysm, persistent trigeminal artery, ophthalmoplegic migraine, tumor of trigeminal nerve, pituitary and parapituitary tumor
Superior orbital fissure	Tumor, Paget's disease, superior orbital fissure syndrome
Orbit	Trauma, tumor, abscess, temporal arteritis, exophthalmic ophthalmoplegia, myasthenia gravis
Others	Cyclic oculomotor paralysis, benign paralysis of infants

involved and produce signs relating to disorders of the long-tracts or the vestibulocerebellar pathways.[10]

Impairment of the third, fourth, or sixth nerves in their intracranial course prior to entering the cavernous sinus may occur in meningitis, tumor, or postinfectious polyneuritis. These nerves are particularly susceptible to stretching if the brainstem is compressed downward by a supratentorial mass. The third nerve may be compressed against the free edge of the tentorium by herniation of the medial aspect of the temporal lobe following an increase in supratentorial pressure. Pressure on the third nerve causes unilateral dilatation of the pupil followed by paralysis of the extraocular muscles supplied by the third nerve and ptosis, in that order of appearance. This sequence of events following compression of the third nerve is due to the coaxial distribution pattern of the fibers within the nerve. Those fibers serving pupillary constriction lie on the outside, while fibers concerned with extraocular movements form the central core. In diabetic neuropathy due to vascular occlusion of the nutrient artery to third nerve, the central fibers are affected and the peripheral fibers are frequently spared. This produces a ptosis, with paralysis of eye movements except abduction of the affected eye (fourth and sixth nerves) and sparing of the pupil (so-called "diabetic third-nerve palsy").

The third nerve is more susceptible to the effects of pressure than other nerves that pass through the cavernous sinus. The most common cause at this level is pressure resulting from an aneurysm arising at the origin of the posterior communicating artery or in the terminal portion of the internal carotid artery.[33] The signs are those of compression, that is, dilatation of the pupil followed by abduction of the affected eye with paralysis of those eye movements supplied by the third nerve and ptosis. Other causes of compression of the third nerve in the cavernous sinus include a persistent trigeminal artery. This is a congenital anomaly in which the anastomosis between the carotid and basilar arteries persists as a large vessel. In so-called "ophthalmoplegic migraine" the third nerve may be transiently compressed. The latter condition may be the result of dilatation of the posterior communicating artery in the later stages of migraine with compression of the third nerve or it may be due to a migraine syndrome caused by an aneurysm. Isolated involvement of the sixth nerve in the cavernous sinus is rare but

has been reported in cases with aneurysm of the terminal portion of the internal carotid artery and in trigeminal schwannoma.[170]

Pituitary and parapituitary lesions usually produce early visual loss, visual field defects, and optic atrophy. However, paralysis of the third, fourth, and sixth nerves is by no means uncommon in cases of pituitary adenoma,[166] parasellar meningioma, clival chordoma, nasopharyngeal carcinoma, and sphenoidal myeloma.[145]

Transient paralysis of the third, fourth, and sixth nerves may occur due to granulomatous inflammatory tissue causing swelling and edema in the vicinity of the superior orbital fissue, termed the superior orbital fissure syndrome. This is a rare inflammation of unknown cause, and the diagnosis is made by exclusion. Roentgenograms may show narrowing of the superior orbital fissure. More persistent forms of compression at this site can occur from Paget's disease and from tumors arising at the margin of the superior orbital fissure.

The extraocular nerves are susceptible to injury in fractures of the orbit.[107] The nerves are also vulnerable to pressure from tumors or abscesses in the orbit or may be stretched in exophthalmic ophthalmoplegia. Temporal arteritis involving the orbital branches of the carotid artery can produce ischemic changes in nerves and extraocular muscles causing ophthalmoplegia.[9]

When there is paralysis of eye movements, myasthenia gravis should always be considered and the edrophonium (Tensilon) test should be performed as part of the diagnostic evaluation.

A group of benign conditions have also been described with transient paralysis of the third, fourth, or sixth nerves of unknown etiology. Spontaneous, transient paralysis of the sixth nerve is not uncommon in infants and young children. Prochlorperazine (Compazine) may induce transient sixth-nerve paralysis in predisposed children. Rarely, there may be cyclic ocular motor paralysis. This is an interesting phenomenon occasionally seen in both children and adults, consisting of unilateral ocular motor paralysis with complete ptosis lasting from several seconds to minutes in duration. Attacks are induced by volitional eye movements or occur spontaneously at irregular intervals.

In adults with diabetes, hypertension, or arteriosclerosis there may be transient and isolated palsies of the third and sixth cranial arteries, the cause of which may not be discovered despite intensive investigation including arteriography. These cases are presumed to be due to thrombosis or ischemia of the vasa nervorum and spontaneously recover after four to six weeks.

Neurologic Manifestations of Paget's Disease

Paget's disease of the skull and spine, which becomes increasingly frequent after age 40 years, may lead to multiple compression neuropathies of the cranial and spinal nerves at their foramina of exit as well as compression of the brainstem by basilar invagination and of the spinal cord owing to narrowing of the spinal canal. Thus, anosmia, optic atrophy with impaired vision, extraocular palsies, trigeminal neuralgia, hemifacial spasm, tinnitus, and deafness, have all been described as a result of Paget's disease that caused narrowing of the foramina of exit. Lesions of the lower four cranial nerves and brainstem with dysarthria, dysphagia, ataxia, and spasticity may indicate basilar invagination.[137] This condition also causes hydrocephalus with dementia and seizures.[44] Likewise, quadriplegia and paraplegia may result from spinal cord compression. Compression of the lumbosacral roots is also common in Paget's disease, with root pain, weakness, and fasciculations of the muscles of the lower extremities.

Diagnostic Procedures

1. Roentgenograms of the involved bones show the characteristic "fluffy" rarefaction, thickening, enlargement, deformity, and zones of bone resorption (Fig. 11–1) with encroachment on neural foramina.
2. Basilar invagination can be demonstrated by computed tomography of the craniovertebral junction.[8]
3. Alkaline phosphatase levels are elevated, and bone isozyme studies confirm this to be due to Paget's disease rather than prostatic malignancy.

Treatment

Medical treatment usually begins with the symptomatic use of salicylates for pain. Later oral phosphate, 1 to 2 gm per day, and intravenous calcitonin have been reported to ameliorate or arrest the course of the disease.[140, 164]

Intermittent administration of intravenous mithramycin may result in clinical improvement with relief of incapacitating root pain and compression and may reduce the alkaline phosphatase levels toward normal. Presumably this antimetabolic drug has selective inhibitory action on osteoclastic activity.[30, 134]

Disodium edetate in daily oral doses of 20 mg/kg body weight appears to reduce the excessive bone metabolism in Paget's disease.[142] It may

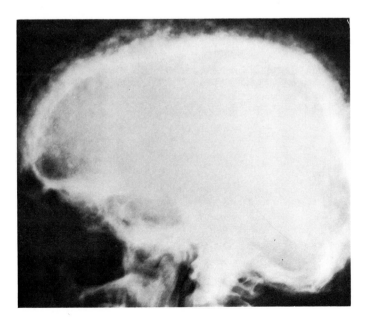

FIGURE 11–1. Lateral roentgenogram of the skull in a patient with Paget's disease and neurologic manifestations, including deafness, hemifacial spasm, and progressive spastic paraparesis.

be of benefit in the treatment of this disease and has the advantage of oral administration and lower toxicity than mithramycin. A.P.D. (3-amino-1-hydroxy-propylidine)-1, 1-biphosphonate given orally also returns bone formation to normal and relieves symptoms in 6 months.[56a]

Disorders of the Fifth Cranial (Trigeminal) Nerve

Trigeminal Neuralgia (Tic Douloureux)

The pain of trigeminal neuralgia is probably one of the most distressing complaints encountered in neurologic practice. Patients with trigeminal neuralgia are often reduced to a state of misery and depression either during or in anticipation of further attacks of this sudden and severe lancinating pain. It is fortunate that both effective medical and surgical therapy have recently become available to treat this condition.

Etiology and Pathology

The paroxysmal nature of the pain in trigeminal neuralgia has suggested to most observers that the abnormality arises as a sudden discharge of neurons subserving pain sensation in the trigeminal pathway. Theoretically, a discharge of this type could occur at three sites: in the trigeminal ganglion (gasserian ganglion), in the spinal nucleus of the trigeminal nerve, or as a result of irritation of the trigeminal nerve.

Abnormalities have been described in biopsies of the trigeminal root from many cases of trigeminal neuralgia. Many cases have aberrant arteries impinging upon the root, or there may be pressure from tumors or other masses.[94] A few younger patients with multiple sclerosis have demyelination of the most proximal portion of the trigeminal nerve.

Degenerative changes in biopsies of the trigeminal ganglion in cases with trigeminal neuralgia are now well documented. Studies of the ganglion cells by electron microscopy have shown irregular vacuolation, as well as areas of demyelination or abnormal myelination of nerve fibers within the ganglion.[11] The axis cylinders have been reported to show hypertrophy and to be excessively tortuous. Such changes appeared to be the result of arteriosclerosis involving the small blood vessels supplying the ganglion or of direct pressure from dilated and arteriosclerotic carotid arteries lying immediately beneath the ganglion. Another possible cause is demineralization of the base of the skull in the elderly with upward tilting of the petrous pyramid and angulation of the nerve root over the petrous bone. Similarly it has been postulated that mechanical stretching of the nerve root in the elderly results from a downward descent of the contents of the posterior fossa toward the foramen magnum.

The concept that paroxysmal activity arises in the neurons of the spinal nucleus of the trigeminal nerve in man as a cause of trigeminal neuralgia is largely theoretic. The majority of patients respond satisfactorily to carbamazepine (Tegretol) and diphenylhydantoin (Dilantin) therapy. Both of these drugs are anticonvulsants. Since these drugs delay synaptic transmission, their beneficial effect cannot be cited as evidence for central discharges as the origin of the trigeminal pain because they also act effectively in peripheral transmission of the nerve. Furthermore, the large number of patients formerly treated by rhizotomy with permanent relief suggest that the pain is peripheral, rather than central, in origin.[86]

It is quite possible that trigeminal neuralgia can arise when the trigeminal nerve is damaged at any of a number of different locations; so the pathology may vary but the pathophysiologic effect is stereotyped. There must be a generation of repetitive stimuli, probably originating in large myelinated fibers at the site of damage to the nerve, but spreading to smaller A, delta, and C fibers and giving rise to the paroxysms of pain so characteristic of trigeminal neuralgia.[23, 80]

Clinical Features

Trigeminal neuralgia is primarily a disease of the middle-aged and elderly. It is rare before the age of 40 years, and multiple sclerosis or tumor should always be considered in patients younger than 40. The incidence is higher in females and the neuralgia is more common on the right side of the face.

The pain is sudden, sharp, lancinating in quality, and described as occurring superficially in the skin and lasting for a few seconds to about a minute. It strikes with dramatic suddenness and may cause an involuntary exclamation, cessation of speech, or a flinching movement of the face and head. The pain is frequently associated with watering of the eye and contraction of the face on the affected side.

The pain is usually limited to one division of

the trigeminal nerve, the second or third division being involved in 95 per cent of cases. Occasionally, pain occurs in both divisions but is rarely experienced in the ophthalmic division of the nerve. Some 10 per cent of patients may experience typical attacks bilaterally but they do not occur on the two sides simultaneously.[106]

The pain may be precipitated by acts of chewing, talking, or smiling, and by touching the face, particularly within and around the mouth including the teeth or immediately below the nostrils. Patients learn to avoid touching or stimulating the trigger areas, which are often highly specific for each individual. Actions such as shaving or chewing or sudden movements of the face may initiate pain in some patients, while others are sensitive to a current of cold air blowing across the face, eating ice cream, or drinking hot beverages.

In the early stages there are long remissions between attacks. During remissions the trigger areas become insensitive, but after a period of weeks, months, or in some cases years, further attacks occur. With the passage of time the period of remission shortens, the attacks become more frequent and severe, and the patient may be reduced to a state of extreme anxiety with his whole attention focused on the dread of the next attack. Under the false belief that the pain is caused by bad teeth, these patients have often had many or all teeth removed. To avoid attacks patients may forego eating, drinking, brushing the teeth, washing the face, or shaving; consequently they lose weight, become withdrawn and seclusive, and appear almost as caricatures of ill health.

The neurologic examination, other than for the trigger area, is usually normal in patients with trigeminal neuralgia, although the evidence of arteriosclerosis and hypertension is somewhat higher than average. Examination of function of the trigeminal nerve does not reveal any deficit in motor or sensory components other than sensitivity at the trigger points.

Diagnostic Procedures

Patients with trigeminal neuralgia should have a roentgenogram of the skull with visualization of the base of the skull and the foramen ovale. Abnormal enlargement of the foramen ovale, intracranial calcification, or erosion of bone in these regions or in the adjacent petrous temporal bone suggests the possibility of a calcified aneurysm or the presence of a tumor.[99] Further investigations in such cases include computed tomography of the base of the skull using a wide window.[70] The results of this type of study are superior to conventional tomography.[12]

Treatment

Medical Therapy. In the early stages of the disease there are long intervals of freedom from pain, and surgical treatment or alcohol injection of the affected nerve or the ganglion is premature at this stage. A number of drugs may be tried in mild cases on the empiric basis that if there is no improvement with one, another may be substituted or added and may prove effective.

Diphenylhydantoin should be used initially in mild cases. The dose of diphenylhydantoin should be adjusted to give a serum level of 15 to 20 μg/ml, and the drug may be given in a single dose once a day or at 12-hour intervals. Diphenylhydantoin rarely produces serious side effects, and about 50 per cent of patients may be pain-free or suffer fewer attacks.[133]

Carbamazepine (Tegretol) is the drug of choice and has proved to be highly effective in the severe forms. However, side effects including aplastic anemia, agranulocytosis, and thrombocytopenia have rarely been reported during treatment with carbamazepine. The drug is contraindicated in patients known to be sensitive to tricyclic compounds such as imipramine and should not be given to patients who are receiving monoamine oxidase inhibitors unless the latter drug is discontinued. Carbamazepine should not be prescribed during the first trimester of pregnancy because of possible teratogenic effects, nor should it be given to nursing mothers. It has a mild anticholinergic action, and patients with increased intraocular pressure due to glaucoma require careful observation during therapy. Care should be exercised in using the drug in patients with heart disease, liver disease, or renal disease, and it should be withdrawn at the first sign of adverse effects. Despite this impressive list of possible complications, carbamazepine is regarded as a safe drug if correctly prescribed and monitored[93] and is used extensively in neurologic practice.

In view of the possibility of side effects all patients should have a complete blood count, platelet count, blood urea nitrogen, and liver function tests before the decision is made to begin therapy. The complete blood count and platelet count should be repeated every two weeks for the first three months, then at monthly intervals.

Carbamazepine is administered in doses of one-half tablet or 100 mg twice daily with meals. The dose should be increased gradually by 100-mg increments until the patient is free from pain. The effective daily dose varies between 200 and 1600 mg, and there is no reason to increase the dose beyond this level if relief has not been obtained. Once control is achieved, the dose may be reduced to a maintenance level that is sufficient to keep the patient pain-free.

There is evidence that clonazepam is effective in controlling trigeminal neuralgia beginning with 1.0 mg every 12 hours and gradually increasing to 6 to 8 mg over a period of ten days.[31] Side effects, which include drowsiness and ataxia, are not uncommon, and clonazepam can be considered a second choice in the treatment after failure with carbamazepine.

Surgical Therapy. Surgical therapy is indicated only when medical treatment has proven ineffective. When the pain of trigeminal neuralgia is limited to one division of the nerve, a mandibular, infraorbital, or supraorbital neurectomy can be performed. Both the infraorbital and supraorbital nerves can be injected with alcohol without difficulty instead of performing neurectomy, if this is desired. In either case, regeneration of the nerve occurs after a period of several months with the possibility of recurrence of pain.

When the second and third divisions of the trigeminal nerve are involved, the ganglion may be destroyed by injecting alcohol. The placement of the needle for injecting the ganglion with alcohol can be controlled radiologically with a high degree of accuracy resulting in a permanent loss of pain. There are a number of drawbacks to injection of alcohol into the ganglion. The most distressing is the occurrence of permanent anesthesia in the regions supplied by the division destroyed by injection. This may include the three divisions of the nerve, with loss of the corneal sensation and subsequent damage to the eye. Many patients complain bitterly about the lack of sensation in the appropriate region following alcohol injection or surgery, and it is important to make sure that each patient understands that he is exchanging relief from pain for anesthesia before any surgical procedure is contemplated. The patient is less likely to regret his decision to have surgical treatment if the matter is fully discussed before operation but may be disgruntled and resentful if he feels that he was not given an adequate explanation of the aftereffects.

The most commonly used surgical procedures in the treatment of trigeminal neuralgia are gangliolysis, suboccipital craniectomy, and decompression of the trigeminal nerve and trigeminal tractotomy. Percutaneous radiofrequency trigeminal gangliolysis is a safe and reliable procedure with an 80 per cent one-year cure rate. The procedure is performed under local anesthesia supplemented by brief periods of general anesthesia and is therefore particularly valuable in elderly or debilitated patients.[79, 152] Suboccipital craniectomy with decompression of the trigeminal nerve is a more extensive surgical procedure but is unique in that it provides relief of pain without sensory loss. The operation is based on the observation that trigeminal neuralgia may be caused by mechanical distortion of the posterior root of the trigeminal nerve. The offending object such as an aberrant blood vessel neoplasm or bony abnormality is identified using an operating microscope, and a small nonabsorbable sponge is placed between the nerve and the object. The immediate and long-term results of this procedure are reported to be excellent.[82]

Trigeminal tractotomy with incision of the descending trigeminal tract in the brainstem at the cervicomedullary junction should be reserved for patients in whom gangliolysis or decompression of the trigeminal nerve has failed.

Disorders of the Seventh Cranial (Facial) Nerve

Facial Paralysis

Paralysis of the facial nerve is one of the most common neurologic signs encountered in practice. It may arise from lesions occurring at a number of sites in the central nervous system and its peripheral course, yet the level of involvement may be identified on clinical grounds with great accuracy if there is some understanding of the anatomy and physiology of this nerve and its central connections (see Chap. 1).[105]

Supranuclear Paralysis

Involvement of the corticopontine pathway to the facial nerve nucleus in the pons is characterized by paralysis of the lower facial muscles with sparing of the upper. The upper face is spared because the facial nerve nucleus receives impulses from both hemispheres serving movement of the muscles to that area. The lower facial movements are served mainly by corticopontine fibers from the contralateral hemisphere. This type of facial paralysis is commonly seen in patients with a stroke resulting in damage to the hemispheric, diencephalic, or mesencephalic connections of the nerve. Emotional facial movements such as smiling are said to be retained in some cases with purely supranuclear types of facial paralysis.

Pontine Lesions

The facial nerve passes dorsally from the facial nerve nucleus and is closely related to the sixth-nerve (abducens) nucleus immediately below the floor of the fourth ventricle. It then turns and runs ventrally through the pons to emerge in the cerebellopontine angle. Dorsal lesions in the pons produce a combination of sixth- and seventh-nerve paralysis, with complete facial paralysis, while midpontine lesions may produce a combination of seventh-nerve paralysis and involvement of the spinal tract of the fifth nerve on the same side. The nerve is occasionally involved in multiple sclerosis with a peripheral type of facial paralysis owing to the development of a plaque in the pons. Taste is usually spared since the taste fibers leave the facial nerve on entering the pons and pass into the tractus solitarius.

The Cerebellopontine Angle

The seventh nerve is intimately related to the eighth cranial nerve in the cerebellopontine angle and has a short intracranial course before it enters the internal auditory meatus. Space-occupying lesions in this area including neurilemmoma, meningioma, dermoid cysts, chordoma, and aneurysms tend to produce facial paralysis and eighth-nerve involvement with loss of auditory acuity or deafness. The fifth, ninth, and tenth cranial nerves, which arise from the pons and medulla near the cerebellopontine angle, are involved at an early stage in such expanding lesions.

Bilateral involvement of the facial nerve is not unusual in postinfectious polyneuropathy (Guillain-Barré syndrome) and results from demyelination of the facial nerves just beyond the point of emergence from the brainstem.

Involvement in the Facial Canal

The nerve may be compressed by a neurilemmoma in the proximal portion of the facial canal. Infection of the neurons in the geniculate ganglion by herpes zoster virus (geniculate herpes) produces a "Ramsay Hunt syndrome." This consists of pain and the appearance of vesicles or blebs within the external auditory meatus and on the tympanic membrane associated with facial paralysis on the same side (Fig. 11–2). The rather sparse sensory component of the seventh nerve is derived from the tympanic plexus, which supplies part of the external auditory meatus and the tympanic membrane. These are the sites of the vesicles of herpes zoster when there is infection of the geniculate ganglion.

Lesions involving the facial nerve in the facial canal include otitis media, mastoiditis, cholesteatoma, and fractures of the temporal bone. Traumatic lesions have a relatively good prognosis and recovery usually occurs unless there has been severe tearing of the nerve in major fractures of the middle cranial fossa.

Some unusual causes of total (peripheral) facial paralysis include invasion and compression by leukemic deposits in the facial canal and also by sarcoidosis. The latter usually produces bilateral involvement with granulomas in both facial canals.

Bell's Palsy

The use of this term should be restricted to those cases with isolated facial paralysis of peripheral type that occurs acutely without evidence of other neurologic abnormalities. In general, it is not used in peripheral facial palsy of known etiology, e.g., following otitis media, in leukemia, or in sarcoidosis. Cases of unknown etiology are common and are believed to be viral in nature. In Bell's palsy due to herpes zoster infection (Ramsay Hunt syndrome), there is reactivation of a varicella–herpes zoster virus and a latent infection of the geniculate ganglion.[91] Some cases of Bell's palsy could also be due to herpes zoster virus without an obvious cutaneous lesion.[97, 169]

Etiology and Pathology

There is good evidence that Bell's palsy is the result of edema of the facial nerve in the facial canal. It is possible that the edema is an inflammatory response to a viral infection. However, only a small number of patients show serologic evidence of a herpes zoster or herpes simplex infection, and serologic studies do not implicate other viruses.[14] This does not exclude a local virus infection of the nerve that is not accessible to antibody-forming cells, and there is indirect evidence

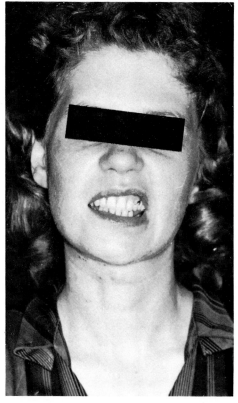
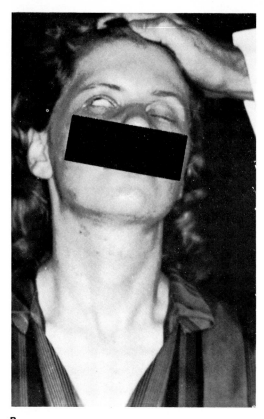

A   B

FIGURE 11–2. Thirty-year-old woman with Bell's palsy due to herpes zoster infection of the right geniculate ganglia (Ramsay Hunt syndrome). She awoke with peripheral type of paralysis on the right side of the face and skin eruption over the right side of the neck. On examination, there were herpetic vesicles in the external auditory canal. She recovered completely.

 A. Right facial weakness and skin lesions.

 B. Bell's phenomenon on attempting to close the eyes.

to support this contention. There is an increased incidence of Bell's palsy in cold weather, and occasional minor epidemics of Bell's palsy have occasionally been encountered in the practice of most experienced neurologists. As a result of inflammation, edema of the nerve occurs in the limited space of the bony facial canal, which produces pressure on the nerve with paralysis of function and wallerian degeneration involving various numbers of fibers. Since recovery is the rule, there is a gradual return of function in surviving fibers as the edema subsides and other fibers regenerate.

Clinical Features

The facial paralysis may be preceded by pain or discomfort for 24 to 48 hours in the region of the stylomastoid foramen, immediately posterior to the angle of the mandible. This is followed by an acute facial paralysis or paresis, with sagging of the face and corner of the mouth and inability to close the eye. Food accumulates in the cheek owing to paralysis of the buccinator, and there is watering of the eye owing to lack of movement of secretions across the cornea by closure of the lids. The edema extends proximally in about 10 per cent of cases to involve the chorda tympani, with loss of taste on the affected side of the tongue. Involvement of the nerve to the stapedius results in loss of the dampening effect of the stapedius muscle and apparent hyperacusis.

Recovery occurs in about 85 per cent of cases over a period of several weeks. The presence of signs of voluntary movement five days after the onset is indicative of complete functional recovery. About 15 per cent of cases have permanent, incomplete, usually loss of function, with the development of contractures, facial spasms, and ectropion. A few show the symptoms of "crocodile tears" when eating owing to the misguided migration into the lacrimal gland of regenerating fibers intended for the salivary glands.

Diagnostic Procedures

The facial nerve is stimulated as it emerges from the stylomastoid foramen, and the evoked potential is recorded using surface electrodes. Needle electrodes should be used if the response is poor. Any convenient facial muscle can be used to record the evoked potential. The two sides are compared with regard to threshold stimulus, amplitude of the evoked response, and distal motor latency. Distal motor latency of more than 4.0 milliseconds is considered abnormal. Threshold voltage two or more times that required on the normal side with a stimulus duration of 0.1 millisecond is significantly abnormal. Wallerian degeneration begins four days after the onset of Bell's palsy, and an increase in threshold and decrease in amplitude of the evoked muscle action potential will be noted. The presence of marked facial weakness but a good evoked response on stimulation of the facial nerve, seven days after the onset, indicates a significant conduction block, proximal to the point of stimulation. The prognosis is good in these patients. Loss of excitability by the seventh day indicates a poor prognosis. There is no good correlation between the distal motor latency and speed of recovery. Similarly, the degree of fibrillations alone is not useful in determining the outcome.

Treatment

1. There are both positive[163] and negative[103] prospective studies on the use of oral corticosteroids in the treatment of Bell's palsy. It is possible that oral steroids (e.g., methylprednisolone, 96 to 128 mg in a single dose once every 48 hours for ten days) are of some benefit in moderately severe or severe cases who do not have any condition that may be exacerbated by steroids.
2. Methylcellulose eyedrops should be applied to the eye on the affected side every four hours during the day, and the eye should be protected by a patch until eyelid function is adequate.

Peripheral Lesions of the Facial Nerve

The facial nerve may be damaged in the neck by penetrating wounds or pressure from enlarged lymph nodes or tumors. The branches are subject to pressure within the parotid gland by tumors, abscess, or sarcoidosis. The facial nerve is occasionally damaged during surgical procedures near the stylomastoid foramen or involving the parotid gland.

Melkersson's Syndrome

Paresis of the facial muscles may be associated with recurrent swelling of the face and lips. The condition is known as Melkersson's syndrome. The term "Melkersson-Rosenthal syndrome" is applied when lingua plicata (geographic tongue) due to atrophy of the papilla is an added feature. This disorder affects males and females equally, usually beginning in childhood and running a relapsing course. Infection and exposure to cold have been implicated as precipitating factors of attacks. There is frequently a familial occurrence. Headache and migraine are frequently associated with attacks. The swelling of the face, particularly the lips, eyelids, and cheeks, lasts for a few hours to several weeks and after repeated attacks may be permanent. There may be nonpitting induration and red-brown pigmentation of the face and atrophy of the papillae of the tongue. There are two types of this condition according to histologic findings of biopsied tissue: the sarcoid type and the lymphedematous type. Allergy, vasomotor neural disturbances, tuberculous infection, and sarcoid have been considered as the cause. Medical treatment with steroids should be considered, and plastic surgery may be recommended in advanced cases.

Myokymia and Facial Contraction

This curious, infrequent, but interesting, condition is quite different from hemifacial spasm or palatal nystagmus and is usually benign but has rarely been associated with multiple sclerosis.[151]

Etiology and Pathology

Facial myokymia occurs in normal people with severe fatigue and after excessive alcohol ingestion; however, if an organic lesion is responsible, it is likely to occur in the pons, particularly in the region of the facial nerve nucleus.

In addition to multiple sclerosis, myokymia and facial contraction have been described in pontine glioma, pontine metastasis, and tuberculoma of the pons.[17] The pathologic changes are always intra-axial suggesting that the myokymia and facial contraction are the result of interception of inhibitory supranuclear pathways to the facial nerve nucleus.

Clinical Features

The usual complaint is of a stiff and swollen face, and some patients may notice spontaneous flickering movements when looking in a mirror. There is slight contraction of the muscles on the affected side with narrowing of the palpebral fissure and drawing up of the angle of the mouth. Continuous flickering of all the facial muscles can be seen from the frontalis to the platysma. When the condition is due to multiple sclerosis, it subsides spontaneously in a variable period ranging from three weeks to six months.[102]

Diagnostic Procedures

1. Electromyographic recording shows a pattern of continuous potentials indistinguishable from those of normal motor units. The discharges may occasionally assume a rhythmic pattern, with motor units firing in short bursts followed by brief periods of quiescence.
2. Computed tomography will show enlargement of the pons and obliteration of the prepontine cistern in pontine glioma or other intra-axial masses.

Treatment

There is no specific treatment for facial myokymia, and patients with multiple sclerosis should be told that the condition will resolve spontaneously. Pontine tumors should be treated with radiation therapy.

Hemifacial Spasm

This condition must be distinguished from facial tics or habit spasms, which are repetitive stereotyped movements involving the muscles of the face.

Etiology and Pathology

Hemifacial spasm may be considered as a condition comparable to trigeminal neuralgia but occurring in the facial nerve. The lesion is usually peripheral. The most common causes are persistent hyperexcitability of the nerve, possibly because of partial demyelination; viral inflammation; or stretching due to an arteriosclerotic dilatation or aneurysm of the vertebrobasilar arterial system[97a] or tumor or inflammation of the cerebellopontine angle.[112] Hemifacial spasm is usually unilateral, rarely bilateral.

Clinical Features

The spasms occur at irregular intervals, often beginning in the orbicularis oculi and then spreading to involve all the facial muscles on one side. The movements are irregular in force and duration, lasting from a few seconds to several minutes, followed by a varying period of relaxation. They are involuntary and may be precipitated by an emotional upset or by startling the patient. The neurologic examination is otherwise normal in hemifacial spasm. When the condition is bilateral, differential diagnosis between blepharospasm (Chap. 4) may be difficult.

Diagnostic Procedures

1. The electromyogram shows irregular clusters of normal motor unit potentials without evidence of fasciculations. The seventh-nerve conduction velocity is not impaired.
2. Intractable cases should have vertebrobasilar arteriography to demonstrate possible compression of the facial nerve by an abnormal vertebral or basilar artery.

Treatment

The primary cause should be treated when possible, e.g., by removal of a tumor. Drug therapy using diphenylhydantoin (Dilantin) or carbamazepine (Tegretol) as described under the treatment for trigeminal neuralgia may be tried but is seldom effective. Surgical treatment includes decompression of the nerve if it is compressed by a tortuous vertebral or basilar artery as it emerges from the brainstem.[54a] Decompression of the nerve in its course through the facial canal at the base of the skull and selective section of peripheral filaments may be successful. Alcohol injection of one or more branches of the facial nerve may be effective if the spasm is confined to one area of the face.

Loss of Taste

Involvement of the chorda tympani in Bell's palsy is a well-recognized cause of loss of taste. Ageusia or dysgeusia (bad or disordered taste) with possible dysfunction of the chorda tympani has been described after an influenza-like infection[75] and with D-penicillamine, griseofulvin, phenylbutazone, oxyphedrine, and carbamazepine. In addition, an idiopathic loss of taste of unknown etiology is occasionally encountered.

Patients with this condition present with loss of taste of acute onset but do not have evidence of any abnormality on general physical or neurologic examination. Many give a history of a recent upper respiratory tract infection. The etiology is unknown but decreased blood zinc concentrations have been described in some cases.[76]

Treatment with oral zinc preparations may possibly help to alleviate this unusual but unpleasant condition.

Disorders of the Eighth Cranial Nerve

Hereditary Eighth-Nerve Deafness

This is a rare familial disorder, characterized by progressive nerve deafness beginning in adolescence and sometimes progressing to permanent deafness. The cause is presumed to be a familial degenerative disorder involving the cochlear division of the eighth nerve. In some families this may be associated with myoclonus (see Chap. 6) and in others with sensory peripheral neuropathy.

Toxic Eighth-Nerve Deafness Due to Antibiotics

The aminoglycoside antibiotics have a peculiar capacity to damage the eighth nerve. Streptomycin and gentamicin attack mainly the vestibular branch of the nerve and neomycin and kanamycin the auditory branch. These antibiotics should be used with caution, particularly in those patients with poor renal function. The greatest risk occurs after the administration of neomycin, since deafness is a more severe handicap than vestibular dysfunction and because toxic effects may be produced by a smaller total dose of neomycin. Since kanamycin has similar therapeutic effects and is less ototoxic, parenteral administration of neomycin has virtually been abandoned. It is still extensively used as a cream for local application to the skin. Deafness due to toxic neuropathy of the eighth nerve may result from absorption after such topical application.[39]

Disorders of the Ninth Cranial (Glossopharyngeal) Nerve

Glossopharyngeal Neuralgia

This rare, but distressing, form of neuralgia shows many similarities to trigeminal neuralgia and should be regarded as a similar condition but involving the glossopharyngeal and vagus nerves. The cause is often obscure, and, although there is no pathologic abnormality clinically demonstrable in most cases, a number show some evidence of pressure or displacement of the glossopharyngeal or vagus nerve. The condition has been described in cerebellopontine angle tumors; arachnoiditis; neoplastic conditions involving the jugular foramen, base of the skull, nasopharynx, and tonsils; peritonsillar abscesses; aneurysms of the vertebral basilar junction; compression by a vertebral artery;[109] ossification of the stylohyoid ligament; and ischemia due to external carotid artery stenosis.[4] A number of cases have apparently followed acute infections of the throat.[26]

Clinical Features

The paroxysmal pain of glossopharyngeal neuralgia may occur in any area with sensory supply by the ninth and tenth cranial nerves. The pain is lancinating or lightning-like and may be precipitated by swallowing, chewing, talking, coughing, sneezing, touching the tragus of the ear, or turning the head suddenly toward the affected side. Attacks may last from a few seconds to two minutes and many attacks may be experienced in one day in severe cases. Remissions are common but tend to become shorter in duration, with recurring attacks of pain in the same area lasting relatively longer as time passes. The affected areas include the base of the tongue, walls of the pharynx, tonsils, deep in the ear, behind the angle of the jaw, deep in the upper cervical area, or deep in the throat. There is no evidence of sensory loss in the affected zones, and the neurologic examination is negative in cases presumed to be inflammatory in nature or of unknown cause.

Manifestations other than pain include parotid hypersecretion, bradycardia, cardiac arrhythmias, hypotension, and syncope[150] due to retrograde stimulation of the vagal nuclei in the brainstem during a painful paroxysm.[81]

Diagnostic Procedures

Roentgenograms of the skull should be obtained, including adequate views of the base. Computed tomography of the base of the skull and posterior fossa should be obtained in all cases who show any abnormality or neurologic examination.

Treatment

Treatment with diphenylhydantoin or carbamazepine is successful in most cases.[49] Patients who show recurrence of symptoms during treatment with carbamazepine or who cannot tolerate carbamazepine may obtain relief by intracranial section of the glossopharyngeal nerve and the upper two rootlets of the vagus nerve on the affected side. This procedure is not without complications and has been followed by acute hypotension and cardiac arrhythmias.[110] Spinal tractotomy at the level of the first cervical segment in the area dorsal to the spinal tract of the trigeminal nerve between this tract and the posterior column has also been successfully employed in some patients. This area apparently carries the descending sensory fibers from the ninth and tenth nerves, which run in a discrete bundle in immediate dorsal relationship to the descending sensory fibers of the trigeminal nerve.[89]

Other Disorders Causing Facial Pain or Paralysis

Geniculate Neuralgia

It is difficult to separate cases of geniculate neuralgia from glossopharyngeal neuralgia, but there is some evidence that a distinct neuralgia of the nervus intermedius does occur. This nerve probably carries pain fibers arising from neurons in the geniculate ganglion which enter the spinal tract of the trigeminal nerve. The peripheral distribution is variable and includes the pinna, external auditory canal, deep structures of the face, and hard palate.

Clinical Features

Attacks of lancinating pain of increasing frequency and severity occur in the region of the pinna and external auditory canal. The pain may radiate into the orbit, face, jaw, or throat.

Treatment

Treatment with diphenylhydantoin or carbamazepine may be effective. Refractory cases require surgical excision of the geniculate ganglion for relief of pain.[122]

Superior Laryngeal Nerve Neuralgia

Neuralgic pain due to involvement of pain fibers in the superior laryngeal nerve has been described. This is a rare form of neuralgia in which paroxysms of pain occur over the side of the neck anteriorly. The pain may radiate into the mandible and behind or anterior to the ear as high as the zygoma. Occasionally, it extends down to the anterior chest wall or shoulder. Attacks may be provoked by stroking or touching the skin over the internal branch of the superior laryngeal nerve as it pierces the hyothyroid membrane.

There is usually a good response to carbamazepine. Those who do not respond to drug therapy can obtain relief by section of the nerve at the hyothyroid membrane. Examination of the larynx may disclose another trigger point where the nerve lies in the plica of mucous membrane at the upper edge of the pyriform sinus. Injection of a local anesthetic into either of these two areas will stop attacks temporarily.

Geniculate Herpes Zoster (Ramsay Hunt Syndrome)

As mentioned earlier in the discussion of Bell's palsy and illustrated in Figure 11–2, infection of the neurons in the geniculate ganglion by herpes zoster virus is followed by the appearance of cutaneous vesicles in the peripheral sensory distribution of the nervus intermedius. The inflammatory swelling of the ganglion produces pressure on the facial nerve in the facial canal and a peripheral facial paralysis.

Clinical Features

The initial complaint of pain over the pinna in the external auditory meatus deep in the ear or throat is followed by the development of typical herpetiform vesicles in the painful areas. At the same time there is a facial paralysis of a peripheral type with loss of taste of the anterior two thirds of the tongue on the affected side and ipsilateral hyperacusis.

Treatment

The patient should be given adequate analgesics to control the pain and a broad-spectrum antibiotic to prevent secondary infection in the external auditory canal. The facial palsy resolves as the swelling of the ganglion decreases, relieving the pressure on the facial nerve.

Postherpetic Facial Pain

A number of elderly people experience persistent and often severe debilitating pain following an attack of herpes zoster. This can occur after an attack at any site but is particularly disturbing following ophthalmic herpes zoster.

Etiology and Pathology

It is apparent from the limited autopsy reports available that the neuronal damage caused by herpes zoster virus occurs in other sites in addition to the posterior root ganglia. Neuronal changes have been described in the gray matter of the spinal cord near the segments showing the cutaneous eruption. Neuronal loss can also occur at higher levels in the cord, brainstem, thalamus, and cerebral cortex.

Clinical Features

A few patients experience persistent burning pain and hyperesthesia in the area of the cutaneous eruption for many months after the acute episode. In patients who have had ophthalmic herpes zoster the pain arises in the orbit and radiates up over the forehead toward the vertex. It is a constant burning pain with stabbing overtones and there is a marked hyperesthesia in the affected area, which shows the cutaneous scarring of the previous herpes vesicles and often shows excessive sweating over the same area with depigmentation of the skin.

Treatment

The wide variety of medical and surgical procedures advocated for the treatment of postherpetic neuralgia testifies to the difficulties encountered in obtaining relief. Limited experience suggests that carbamazepine (Tegretol) may prove to be effective. Phenothiazine drugs such as chlorpromazine are also helpful. Surgical procedures including avulsion of the affected nerve or undercutting of a skin flap over the forehead may be effective in patients who do not respond to medical therapy. They should be tried before more extensive procedures such as retrogasserian rhizotomy or trigeminal tractotomy are contemplated. Many patients experience a gradual lessening of symptoms with the passage of time, and while most admit to discomfort, few have severe pain after two years.

Disorders of the Eleventh (Accessory) Cranial Nerve

The accessory nerve may be injured in trauma or minor surgery to the posterior triangle of the neck or compressed by tumors or lymphadenopathy in the same area.

Clinical Features

The patient complains of pain in the neck and shoulders and is unable to elevate the arm above the horizontal plane without external rotation. Abduction of the arm produces prominent scapula displacement. The trapezius muscle is wasted.[117]

Treatment

A nerve graft should be performed if the accessory nerve is damaged or cannot be spared during surgery on the posterior triangle of the neck. In chronic cases the shoulder pain can be relieved by wearing an arm sling.

Vocal Cord Paralysis Due to Endotracheal Intubation

Occasionally after surgical anesthesia and endotracheal intubation, unilateral vocal cord paralysis with dysphonia is a temporary or permanent complication.[69] It is believed that asymmetric inflation or overinflation of the endotracheal cuff balloon just below the vocal cords causes ischemia of the recurrent laryngeal nerve. Prevention of this complication may be achieved by frequent inspection of endotracheal tubes for asymmetric filling of the cuff and avoidance of overinflation.

Hereditary Neuropathies

The hereditary neuropathies include:

1. Chronic interstitial hypertrophic polyneuropathy of Dejerine-Sottas (relatively rare)
2. Refsum's disease or heredopathia atactica polyneuritiformis (rare)
3. Tangier disease or familial alpha-lipoprotein deficiency (rare)
4. Bassen-Kornzweig disease or hypo-beta-lipoprotein deficiency (rare)
5. Hereditary sensory radicular neuropathy (rare)
6. Familial amyloid neuropathy (rare)
7. Acute intermittent porphyria (not uncommon, vide infra)
8. Peroneal muscular atrophy (not uncommon, see Chap. 4)
9. Whipple's disease (rare, vide infra)
10. Hereditary nerve deafness (relatively rare, vide infra)
11. Hereditary optic atrophy (relatively rare, vide infra)

Other familial neuropathies are considered to be primary, degenerative, toxic, or metabolic disorders of the nervous system and are discussed in the chapters devoted to those subjects.

Chronic Interstitial Hypertrophic Polyneuropathy

This is one of a number of conditions associated with hypertrophy of peripheral nerves. It is usually familial, although sporadic cases do occur, and it is possible that it may be caused by several agents rather than being the result of a single metabolic defect.

Etiology and Pathology

Familial cases are inherited as an autosomal dominant trait. The occurrence of sporadic cases and the recognition of identical histologic changes in the peripheral nerves in heredopathia atactica polyneuritiformis (Refsum's disease), in acromegaly, and as a rare sequel to postinfectious polyneuropathy suggest that chronic interstitial hypertrophic polyneuropathy may be a syndrome in which there is an abnormal response in the peripheral nerve to a number of inflammatory or immune stimuli.[159]

There appears to be an abnormality in pyruvate metabolism in some cases of chronic interstitial hypertrophic polyneuropathy and a delay in the conversion of lactate to pyruvate. It is not clear if this represents the result of poor dietary intake of thiamine in some patients or an abnormality of thiamine utilization at the cellular level.

The pathologic changes are characterized by hypertrophy of the peripheral nerves in any part of the body but are usually more marked in the limbs and neck. The histologic changes consist of a marked proliferation of the endoneurium or Schwann cells. This produces concentric rings of tissue around the axon separated by a mucin-like material. There are degenerative changes in the axons and a gradual axonal loss over many years.

Clinical Features

The disease is chronic and often runs an intermittent course with exacerbations and remissions.[41] During an exacerbation there may be pains in the limbs with weakness and ataxia. This may be followed by a period of partial recovery and further deterioration after an interval of months or years. Exacerbations tend to be precipitated by pregnancy or infection.

The established case shows a wide-based steppage gain with bilateral foot drop. The Romberg sign is positive. There is wasting of the muscles of the hands, forearms, legs, and lower thighs. The deep tendon reflexes are absent, and there is a distal sensory loss to all modalities in all four limbs. Atrophic changes and brittle nails may occur in the hands and feet. The affected nerves are enlarged, nodular, and often tender during a period of exacerbation.[61, 63] There have been occasional reports of hypertrophic neuropathy presenting as a mononeuropathy usually involving the radial nerve.[71]

Diagnostic Procedures

1. Nerve conduction velocities are considerably slowed.
2. The typical changes of chronic interstitial hypertrophic neuropathy may be seen on nerve biopsy.

Treatment

The exacerbation may be shortened and recovery promoted by daily injections of thiamine, 100 mg intramuscularly. There have been encouraging results from intermittent steroid therapy (methylprednisolone, 80 mg in a single dose, every 48 hours) given for three or four weeks during periods of exacerbation.

Refsum's Disease (Heredopathia Atactica Polyneuritiformis)

The association between a genetically determined metabolic abnormality and a familial peripheral neuropathy has been clearly established in Refsum's disease. The condition was first described in 1945 under the term "heredopathia atactica polyneuritiformis" but the eponym Refsum's disease is frequently used.[127, 128]

Etiology and Pathology

Refsum's disease is inherited as an autosomal recessive trait in which there is a deficit in the degradation of branched-chain fatty acids, with the accumulation of 3, 7, 11, 15 tetramethyl hexadecanoic acid in the tissues. This is called phytanic acid and is derived from chlorophyll- and phytol-containing substances. The metabolic abnormality produces major deficits in the peripheral nerves with less extensive but varied involvement of other organs.[50, 51]

The brain is normal in weight and appearance with some fat-laden macrophages in the meninges. Mild degenerative changes have been described in the neurons of the olivary and other nuclei of the brainstem, and there is variable demyelination of the posterior columns, medial lemnisci, cerebellar peduncles, and rubrospinal and olivocerebellar tracts. There are atrophy of the retina, loss of ganglion cells, and degenerative changes in the nuclear layer. The most obvious abnormalities are found in the peripheral nerves, which are enlarged in irregular fashion similar to the changes seen in chronic interstitial hypertrophic neuropathy. The enlargement is due to concentric layers of hypertrophied fibroblasts or Schwann cells that surround the axon. There is, in addition, considerable loss of axons, and the hypertrophied sheaths may be separated by a mucin-like material. Changes in other organs include heavy deposition of neutral fat and phytanic acid in the liver, kidneys, and myocardium.[3]

Clinical Features

The majority of patients experience night blindness and poor peripheral vision for some years prior to the development of other symptoms. A number develop a progressive deterioration in hearing of cochlear type. The earliest symptoms of peripheral neuropathy usually occur in the lower limbs, with progressive distal weakness and ataxia. Similar changes eventually develop in the upper limbs. The course is one of relapse and remissions with eventual wasting of the distal muscles and bilateral foot drop. Sensory symptoms of numbness and paresthesias in the distal portion of the extremities are prominent during exacerbations.

Examination of patients with Refsum's disease reveals atypical retinitis pigmentosa and constriction of the visual fields. The pupils may react sluggishly to light, and a number of patients develop posterior polar cataracts. Apart from variable involvement of the eighth nerve with decreased hearing, the other cranial nerves are usually intact. The motor system shows distal weakness and wasting in all four limbs with foot drop in some patients. Cerebellar ataxia is mild in most cases. There is a variable sensory loss involving touch, pinprick, vibration, and position sense in all four limbs. Deep tendon reflexes are sluggish or absent and the plantar responses equivocal owing to the presence of peripheral palsy. Other abnormalities include skeletal malformations (such as hypo- or hyperplasia of metacarpal and metatarsal bones), a high arched palate, pes cavus, and icthyosis but these are inconsistent findings in this disease.

There is a tendency to exacerbations and remissions in many cases, with deterioration precipi-

tated by pregnancy or infection. Death may occur from renal or heart failure.

Diagnostic Procedures

Early defects in visual fields can be detected by perimetry, and the audiogram will reveal deafness of the cochlear type before this is apparent to the patient. The electrocardiogram is frequently abnormal in more chronic cases, indicating the presence of myocardial involvement. There is usually a considerable elevation in the protein content in the cerebrospinal fluid.

An excess of 3, 7, 11, 15 tetramethyl hexadecanoic acid (phytanic acid) can be demonstrated in the serum of patients by gas-liquid chromatography. This substance has also been detected in the serum of heterozygote carriers of the disease.

There is slowing of motor and sensory conduction velocities. It may be impossible to obtain sensory nerve action potentials in some patients.

A skin biopsy will show the presence of lipid-containing vacuoles in the epidermis in patients who have ichthyosis.[35]

Treatment

The serum phytanic acid can be reduced to normal by a diet low in phytol- and chlorophyll-containing substances, which appears to prevent further exacerbations and deterioration in this disease. Exacerbations may also be minimized or prevented by prompt attention to infections. The more advanced cases may benefit from physical therapy and the use of splints to correct lower limb weakness and foot drop. Plasma exchange is useful in severe cases.[59a]

Neuropathy in Familial Alpha-Lipoprotein Deficiency (Tangier Disease)

A relatively mild recurrent neuropathy may occur in patients suffering from familial alpha-lipoprotein deficiency (Tangier disease).

Etiology and Pathology

There is almost complete absence of normal high-density lipoproteins in the serum. Storage of cholesterol esters occurs in many tissues in the body.[74] The disease is inherited as an autosomal recessive trait.

Clinical Features

Children may present with unduly large tonsils that contain cholesterol esters. Other cases have presented with hepatomegaly, splenomegaly, and enlarged lymph nodes. The peripheral neuropathy is mild and relapsing, consisting of a fluctuating sensory loss and motor weakness in the limbs.[53]

Diagnostic Procedures

1. There is an absence of high-density lipoproteins in the serum.
2. The serum cholesterol levels are low.
3. Abnormal foam cells may be seen on bone marrow biopsy.
4. Lipid deposits may be demonstrated in macrophages or rectal biopsy.
5. The motor conduction velocity is normal. The electromyogram shows evidence of denervation. These findings suggest axonal degeneration. Fibrosis of the intramuscular nerve twigs has been observed. The sural nerve biopsy is normal.

Treatment

There is no effective treatment for this condition.

Hypo-Beta-Lipoproteinemia (Bassen-Kornzweig Disease)

Although peripheral neuropathy is only one feature of this rare condition, it is best classified with the familial neuropathies.

Etiology and Pathology

Hypo-beta-lipoproteinemia is a genetically determined condition inherited as an autosomal recessive trait associated with the absence of beta-lipoprotein in the serum. The metabolic fault is unclear, but there appears to be adequate absorption of triglycerides from the intestine into the mucosal cells with failure to transport triglyceride into the serum.[98]

The changes in the nervous system are essentially an extensive demyelination involving the posterolateral columns, spinocerebellar tracts, and peripheral nerves. There is, in addition, a peculiar crenation of circulating red cells (acanthocytosis) and retinitis pigmentosa.[138]

Clinical Features

1. The condition may present as a steatorrhea in infancy and childhood owing to malabsorption of triglycerides. This shows spontaneous improvement later in childhood.
2. The demyelination of the posterolateral columns, spinocerebellar tracts, and peripheral nerves produces progressive ataxia and weakness leading to profound disability.
3. The retinitis pigmentosa is associated with visual failure beginning with constriction of the visual fields and progressing to amaurosis.

Diagnostic Procedures

1. The plasma beta-lipoproteins and cholesterol levels are abnormally low.
2. Wet preparations of red cells show the unusual crenations (acanthocytosis). There are accelerated hemolysis and an increased reticulocyte count.

Treatment

There is no specific treatment for this condition but the use of fat-soluble vitamins parenterally may delay the neurologic defects in these patients.

Hereditary Sensory Radicular Neuropathy—Type I

This uncommon condition is inherited as an autosomal dominant trait and is characterized by primary degeneration of cells in the posterior root ganglia. The result is atrophy and axonal loss in the peripheral portion of sensory nerves, in the posterior nerve roots, and, to a lesser extent, in the posterior columns.

Clinical Features

Symptoms usually begin after the age of 20 years with the onset of lightning pains in the lower extremities. This is followed by the development of hyperkeratosis of the soles of the feet and the formation of painless ulcers over the heads of the metatarsal bones. Examination reveals sensory loss involving the feet and extending for a variable distance proximally in the legs below the knees. The area of pain and temperature loss is usually greater than that of touch. With the passage of time the ulceration produces destruction of the metatarsal bones and deformity of the feet, and patients are frequently subjected to various surgical procedures to excise infected bone or tissue. Some cases later develop a similar sensory loss involving the upper limbs with painless injuries and burns of the fingers. Distal wasting of muscles of the extremities resembling peroneal muscular atrophy has been described in some patients. Others have developed progressive nerve deafness.

Treatment

Patients should be advised to wear special shoes, to avoid trauma to the extremities, and to seek advice at the first sign of infection. Ulcers heal spontaneously with rest of the affected part, cleansing of the wound, and the use of antibiotics.

Hereditary Sensory Neuropathy—Type II

Hereditary sensory neuropathy—type II is inherited as an autosomal recessive trait and is present at birth with very slow progression. There are no lightning pains, ulceration of the feet, or bone destruction, and examination shows the presence of atonic pupils in some cases. The sensory loss affects touch, vibration, position sense, and pressure more than pain and temperature.[108, 118]

Treatment

There is no specific treatment for this condition.

Hereditary Amyloid Neuropathy

Amyloidosis may be classified into hereditary and nonhereditary types. Two types of hereditary amyloidosis associated with peripheral neuropathy have been recognized.

Etiology and Pathology

In all forms of amyloidosis there is deposition of an abnormal type of protein material in the tissues. This results in axonal degeneration due to either a toxic metabolic process affecting the axons or compression of axons by amyloid deposits.

Clinical Features

Hereditary Amyloidosis with Lower Limb Neuropathy. This condition has been recognized as a familial disorder occurring in adults of both sexes in northern Portugal.[29] There are liver dysfunction, splenomegaly, scleroderma, progressive weakness of the lower limbs with gastrointestinal symptoms, orthostatic hypotension, loss of libido, and sphincter disturbances. A chronic peripheral neuropathy affects the lower limbs with weakness, dissociated sensory loss, and trophic ulcers. Death usually occurs within ten years from generalized amyloidosis.[7]

Hereditary Amyloidosis with Upper Extremity Involvement. A familial form of amyloidosis has been described in northern Sweden[6] and in a family of Swedish extraction living in the United States. The initial symptoms suggest a carpal tunnel syndrome with evidence of peripheral neuropathy appearing some years later. Generalized amyloidosis occurs over a period of 20 or 30 years with the usual complications of that disorder, including hepatomegaly, liver dysfunction, splenomegaly, scleroderma, cardiomegaly, hypertension, cardiovascular complications, and vitreous opacities.

Diagnostic Procedures

1. There are no specific abnormalities in serum globulin levels but they may show an increase in alpha-2-globulins.
2. Cerebrospinal fluid protein may be elevated to 50 to 100 mg/100 ml.
3. The nerve conduction velocities are consistent with axonal degeneration, being normal or mildly slowed. In some patients it may not be possible to obtain sensory nerve action potentials. Electromyogram of the involved muscles shows evidence of denervation.
4. Pain and temperature sensation are lost early in amyloid neuropathy, producing a dissociated type of sensory loss. Autonomic involvement is also seen frequently. Stimulation of the fascicular biopsy of the sural nerve in vitro shows absence or considerable decrease of the C fiber potential in the compound action potential. There is a virtual absence of unmyelinated fibers and great reduction in the number of small myelinated fibers.[45]
5. Rectal biopsy is the most reliable method in the diagnosis of amyloidosis.

Treatment

Treatment is symptomatic.

Hyperlipidemic Peripheral Neuropathy

There have been occasional reports of the association of hyperlipidemia and peripheral neuropathy, and there is evidence for the existence of a distinct neuropathy causally related to elevated blood lipid levels.[101] Many of the cases have evidence of diabetes mellitus, which suggests that the neuropathy is probably an example of the more common diabetic neuropathy.[55] However, peripheral neuropathy occurs occasionally in patients with hyperlipidemia without diabetes mellitus and is reported to improve with lowering of serum lipid levels.[28, 135]

Etiology and Pathology

The metabolism of myelin is disturbed in serum lipid disorders, and hyperlipidemic peripheral neuropathy is probably a demyelination of peripheral nerves.[98, 136]

Clinical Features

The condition presents as a chronic, mild, predominantly sensory peripheral neuropathy involving the lower extremities and spreading later to the hands. There are hypalgesia of "glove and stocking" type and absence of deep tendon reflexes.

Diagnostic Procedures

1. There is hyperlipidemia with elevation of both cholesterol and triglycerides associated with elevation of lipoproteins.
2. Both motor and sensory nerve conduction velocities are prolonged.

Treatment

1. The patient should be treated with a low-fat diet, and the plasma lipid levels should be monitored regularly.
2. The dietary regimen can be supplemented by clofibrate (Atromid S), 500 mg four times a day, where dietary treatment fails to lower plasma lipid levels.

Neuropathies Due to Viral or Presumed Autoimmune Mechanisms

Postinfectious Polyneuritis (Landry-Guillain-Barré Syndrome)

A number of synonyms have been applied to this condition, but the term "postinfectious polyneuritis" is the most satisfactory since in the majority of cases a definite history of a preceding infectious illness of a viral type is elicited and the essential change is an inflammatory response in the peripheral nerves.

Etiology, Pathogenesis, and Pathology

The inflammation of the nerves appears to be a hypersensitivity or autoimmune response with cell-mediated immunity directed against peripheral myelin.[1] This reaction appears to be diffuse rather than localized to nerve roots.[87] It is possible that an antecedent virus infection or exposure to other unknown agents leads to the production of antibodies that produce demyelination of peripheral nerves. However, the mechanism may be more complex and require some antecedent transient partial immunosuppression to trigger the autoimmune response in the peripheral nervous system.[92] The involvement of the proximal portion of the peripheral nerve within the dural sheath results in the passage of serum proteins into the subarachnoid space and cerebrospinal fluid, which produces the characteristic rise in protein in the CSF described in this condition. It is also possible that the inflammation produces hyperemia and dilatation of blood vessels of the pia in the nerve sheath, which would be an additional source for the leaking of protein into the cerebrospinal fluid.

The Guillain-Barré syndrome is known to be associated with many different types of viral infections including Coxsackie and ECHO virus,[5] cytomegalovirus, Epstein-Barr virus,[43] viral exanthemata,[38] and influenza immunization.

Further clarification of the exact role of viral infections, altered cell-mediated immunity, and the production of autoimmune antibodies in the Guillain-Barré syndrome is needed.

The pathologic changes consist of a patchy demyelination of the peripheral nerves with proliferation of Schwann cells and a perivascular, usually perivenular, infiltration of lymphocytes.

Clinical Features

The disease occurs at any age from infancy to the ninth decade, with a slight preponderance in males. Cases have been classified as primary (without preceding illness) or secondary (occurring after an obvious infection), but this division contributes little because patients may develop symptoms after a subclinical or undiagnosed infection. The disease frequently develops after an upper respiratory infection, influenza, tonsillitis, the exanthemas of childhood, and pneumonia. It has also been described following infectious mononucleosis, hepatitis, and numerous viral infections including encephalitis. The latent period between the infection and the neurologic signs varies from 1 to 28 days with a mean of nine days. A history of preceding infection can be obtained in at least 60 per cent of cases.[72, 119] The syndrome may also occur in the partially immunosuppressed and has been reported in Hodgkin's disease, in systemic lupus erythematosus, and in renal transplant recipients.

The majority of patients complain of paresthesias of the lower extremities initially, but at least one third describe muscle weakness as the first symptom. The muscle weakness is followed rapidly by a flaccid paralysis of peripheral muscles of the limbs. This is symmetric, beginning in the lower limbs and ascending to involve the trunk and upper extremities. Cranial nerve involvement occurs in 50 per cent of cases and in some cases is limited to this (cranial polyneuritis). The seventh cranial nerve is the most frequently involved, often bilaterally, and facial myokymia[155] and lid lag[85] are not at all uncommon in the early stages of the Guillain-Barré syndrome. Other cranial nerves, including the third, fourth, sixth, fifth, then ninth, tenth, eleventh, and twelfth, are involved in decreasing order of frequency. The eighth nerve is spared. Papilledema has been reported in a few cases. The cause is not known,[144] and it is unlikely that papilledema results from obstruction to the arachnoid villi because of elevated cerebrospinal fluid protein content as has been suggested in the past.

Autonomic disturbances are seen in about 25 per cent of patients. Retention of urine with distention of the bladder may occasionally occur as an early symptom and is presumably due to involvement of autonomic fibers passing through the sacral nerve roots. Postural hypotension has occasionally been recorded owing to involvement of the preganglionic sympathetic fibers in the thoracic nerve roots. Persistent hypertension is a rare complication and may be due to lesions affecting central vasomotor control or peripheral sympathetic ganglia.[34]

Sensory disturbances are always less severe than motor symptoms and usually consist of paresthesias in the lower limbs with occasional involvement of the upper extremities. Some 30 per cent of patients exhibit hypalgesia, hypesthesia, and impaired vibration and position sense, usually in the lower extremities. The condition is not always painless and about 10 per cent of patients complain of troublesome myalgia early in the course of the illness.[104]

Respiratory impairment is the major complication, which may be fatal if untreated. Some 33 per cent of patients develop respiratory insufficiency, which requires tracheotomy and assisted respiration.

The diagnosis of postinfectious polyneuritis can be made in cases that fulfill at least five of six criteria.[126]

1. Diffuse symmetric flaccid paralysis often associated with bilateral facial paralysis.

2. Subjective sensory symptoms with objective sensory findings less remarkable than the motor paralysis.
3. Complete remission within six months, which occurs in almost all cases.
4. Progressive elevation of protein levels in the cerebrospinal fluid beginning in the second week of paralysis, with no or relatively mild pleocytosis (albuminocytologic dissociation).
5. An afebrile course or only slight elevation of temperature during the development of paralysis.
6. A normal blood white cell count or lymphocytosis with little or no elevation of sedimentation rate.

Once paralysis has appeared there may be progression for the next ten days, reaching a maximum within three weeks and a mean of 12 days. Patients who develop respiratory failure show the most rapid progression of symptoms. When the symptoms have reached maximum development, the condition may remain unchanged for about 14 days before recovery begins. Recovery is a slow process, usually taking some three to six months, although some patients have shown objective improvement of muscle strength for as long as two years.

Incomplete recovery has been reported in 10 to 25 per cent of cases. These cases tend to show a longer period of maximum weakness before start of improvement. A period of more than 18 days from maximum weakness to some improvement in strength probably indicates a subsequent incomplete recovery.[46] Relapses have been described but are rare.

Diagnostic Procedures

1. The white blood count and sedimentation rate are normal unless they have been elevated by the effects of the preceding illness.
2. During lumbar puncture the cerebrospinal fluid may be under increased pressure. The most characteristic finding is an increase in protein content, which usually does not begin until after the tenth day of the neurologic illness. The cell count is within normal range or slightly elevated but usually remains below 50 cells per cubic millimeter. The cells are predominantly or entirely mononuclear (lymphocytes).
3. Measurement of respiratory function daily will indicate whether there is insufficiency.

4. Since the Guillain-Barré syndrome is characterized by a demyelinating type of peripheral neuropathy, nerve conduction studies are useful in establishing the diagnosis. There is diffuse slowing of the fastest conducting fibers in about 60 per cent of patients. The slowing of conduction may be confined only to the distal segment in some patients, as evidenced by prolonged distal motor latency and increased duration of the evoked muscle action potential. However, conduction velocities are usually reduced to a similar extent in both proximal and distal segments, suggesting a diffuse demyelinating process.[88] Stimulation at several points along the course of the nerves may reveal more than one site where conduction is blocked or delayed. The slowing of conduction may be restricted to sites where the nerve is usually subjected to compression. Sensory nerve action potentials may be difficult to obtain in some patients.

Nerve conduction and electromyographic studies are valuable in predicting the prognosis in the Guillain-Barré syndrome. Patients with abnormal nerve conduction velocities but absence of fibrillation potentials during the course of their illness recover rapidly. Affected individuals with or without nerve conduction abnormalities who show profuse fibrillations within four weeks of the onset of the disease show poor recovery with pronounced residual deficits.[48, 125]

Treatment

All patients require good nursing care with frequent turning to prevent bed sores and to drain dependent parts of the lungs. Many patients are incapacitated for long periods, and particular care should be given to pressure points and minor skin irritation. Retention of urine or incontinence requires the use of an indwelling catheter, which should be removed as soon as possible. A suitable urinary antibiotic or irrigation with antibiotic solution (p. 594) should be used.

Patients who show signs of respiratory insufficiency require endotracheal intubation and respiratory assistance with a mechanical respirator and should be treated in an intensive care unit.

Steroid therapy has been advocated on the basis that postinfectious polyneuritis is an autoimmune condition that may be suppressed by steroids. Results have been equivocal with reports of beneficial effects[73] and absence of effect[64] on the course

of the illness. It is possible that corticosteroids reduce the time from onset of illness to recovery but not the initial severity of the illness.[149]

Physical therapy should be started at an early stage while the patient is still in bed and a graded program should be designed to suit the patient's needs. This should be continued for a period of many months, if necessary.

Anatomic Considerations of the Neuropathies

Neuropathies of the Cervical Plexus

The pattern of neurologic symptoms resulting from injury to the cervical plexus depends on the anatomic arrangements of the nerves involved. The cervical plexus is formed by looped connections between the anterior primary rami of C_1, C_2, C_3, C_4, and C_5 (Fig. 11–3). It lies in the neck in front of the origins of the levator scapulae and scalenus medius muscles. It supplies muscular branches to the prevertebral muscles, the sternocleidomastoid (C_2), and the levator scapulae (C_3 and C_4), but the most important motor branch is the phrenic nerve C_3, C_4, C_5, which supplies the diaphragm. The main sensory branches include the greater occipital (C_2), lesser occipital (C_2), and greater auricular nerves (C_2, C_3), which supply the posterior part of the scalp, and the transverse cervical (C_2, C_3) and supraclavicular nerves (C_3, C_4), which supply the skin over the lower neck, shoulder, and anterior chest wall.

Occipital Neuralgia

Occipital neuralgia is a condition characterized by pain in the cutaneous distribution of the greater occipital nerve (C_2). It is occasionally encountered in neurologic practice.

Etiology and Pathology. The most common causes of occipital neuralgia are cervical spondylosis, acute contusion to the nerve resulting from a "whiplash injury" to the neck, and sleeping with a hard object beneath the head and the neck acutely flexed. In any event, the nerve root becomes compressed as it passes through the intervertebral foramen.

Clinical Features. The usual complaint is of a constant dull or burning pain, which varies in intensity, in the occipital area just to the right or left of the midline. The nerve is usually tender

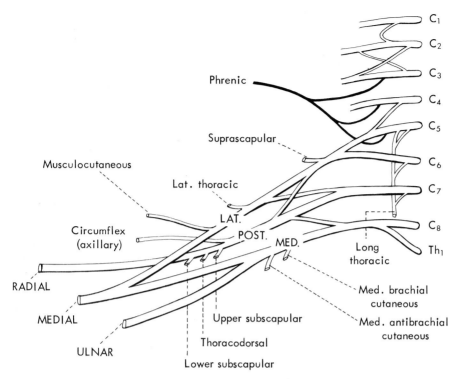

C_1
C_2
C_3
C_4
C_5
C_6
C_7
C_8
Th_1

Phrenic

Suprascapular

Musculocutaneous

Lat. thoracic

LAT.

Circumflex
(axillary)

POST.

MED.

Long
thoracic

RADIAL

Med. brachial
cutaneous

MEDIAL

Upper subscapular

Med. antibrachial
cutaneous

ULNAR

Thoracodorsal

Lower subscapular

FIGURE 11–3. Cervical-brachial plexus.

to palpation and the pain is abolished by injection of a local anesthetic over the point of maximal tenderness.

Treatment. In acute cases following whiplash injury to the neck there may be relief with analgesics and the use of a plastic cervical collar. When the pain persists, injection of 40 mg of methylprednisolone in a local anesthetic into the nerve as it passes over the occipital bone may help in some cases. The great majority of patients obtain relief from conservative measures and assurance that recovery will occur. When occipital neuralgia occurs in cervical spondylosis, the condition is often advanced and occipital neuralgia is only one of a number of neurologic complications occurring in this condition. The treatment of cervical spondylosis is discussed in Chapter 4. Occasionally, severe cases require posterior radiculotomy.

The lesser occipital nerve and greater auricular nerves (C_2, C_3) are rarely involved by neuralgia. The diagnosis can be confirmed by the injection of a local anesthetic into the affected nerve with relief of symptoms. The treatment outlined for neuralgia involving the greater occipital nerve is also applicable to these conditions.

Conditions Affecting the Phrenic Nerve

The phrenic nerve arises from the anterior primary rami of C_3, C_4, and C_5 and passes downward over the scalenus anticus muscle to enter the thorax, where it is intimately related to the mediastinum. Both phrenic nerves pass in front of the root of the lung and descend to supply the diaphragm. This is a mixed nerve with both motor and sensory fibers. Lesions involving the nerve produce a unilateral paralysis of the diaphragm. This can occur with involvement of the anterior primary rami of C_3, C_4, and C_5 in chronic meningitis, arachnoiditis, fractures and dislocations of the vertebrae, extramedullary tumors in the spinal canal, and cervical spondylosis.

The nerve is particularly susceptible to trauma in its course through the neck and may be injured by stabbing or gunshot wounds. In addition, it can be compressed by tumors, aneurysms, and enlarged lymph nodes. The main cause of phrenic paralysis in the mediastinal area is compression by enlarged lymph nodes and infiltration by bronchial carcinoma. An aortic aneurysm can also stretch or compress either phrenic nerve.

Viral infections and diphtheria may be responsible for acute phrenic paralysis, and the condition has been described after pneumonia, although the mechanism is not clear. Alcohol and lead are occasional causes of phrenic nerve paralysis.

Stimulation of the sensory fibers produces pain in the shoulder on the appropriate side. This is common in cholecystitis, pancreatic carcinoma, peritonitis, and subphrenic abscess. Localized pleurisy or peritonitis sometimes leads to peripheral irritation with persistent singultus (hiccough).

Neuropathies of the Brachial Plexus

In order to understand the patterns of neurologic symptoms arising from injuries to the brachial plexus, certain anatomic considerations must be understood. This important plexus is formed from the anterior primary rami of C_5, C_6, C_7, C_8, and T_1, with some small contribution from C_4 and T_2 (Fig. 11–3).

The fifth and sixth cervical nerves unite to form the upper trunk of the plexus, while the eighth cervical and first thoracic nerves unite to form the lower trunk. The seventh cervical nerve lies between these two trunks and constitutes the middle trunk of the plexus. The trunks lie in close relationship to the third portion of the subclavian artery and pass with this vessel toward the apex of the axilla. As they lie in the supraclavicular triangle, each trunk divides into an anterior and posterior division, which reunite to form the cords of the brachial plexus in the axilla. The three posterior divisions form the posterior cord; the anterior divisions of the upper and middle trunk unite to form the lateral cord; while the anterior division of the lower trunk continues as the medial cord. The cords of the plexus are closely related to the second part of the axillary artery in the axilla, the medial cord crossing behind the artery to the medial side, the posterior cord running behind it, and the lateral cord lying along the lateral side of the artery.

Four branches are given off before the formation of the cords: the nerve to the rhomboids from the anterior primary ramus of C_5, the nerve to the subclavius from the anterior primary rami of C_5 and C_6, and the nerve to serratus anterior (long thoracic nerve) from the anterior primary rami of C_5, C_6, and C_7. The suprascapular nerve (C_5, C_6) arises from the upper trunk of the plexus.

The lateral cord of the plexus gives off the lateral pectoral nerve, the musculocutaneous nerve, and the lateral root of the median nerve. The posterior cord gives origin to the two subscapular nerves, the nerve to latissimus dorsi, the radial nerve, and the circumflex nerve. The medial cord of the plexus gives off the medial pectoral nerve, the medial brachial cutaneous nerve, the ulnar nerve, the medial antebrachial cutaneous nerve, and the medial root of the median nerve.

Injuries to the Brachial Plexus Occurring at Birth

The roots of the brachial plexus may be injured or avulsed during birth by excessive traction on the head with the shoulder in a relatively fixed position or by traction on the limbs during breech extraction. The commonest injury involves the roots of C_5 and C_6 (Erb's paralysis), but three types of injury can occur: (a) upper C_5, C_6 Erb type, (b) lower C_8, T_1 Klumpke type, and (c) wholearm Erb-Duchenne-Klumpke type.[153]

Erb's paralysis is characterized by atrophy and loss of function involving the deltoid, biceps, brachialis, brachioradialis, infraspinatus, and occasionally the subscapularis muscles. It may be suspected in the newborn who does not show active movement of one upper limb. The typical posture of adduction, internal rotation, and extension of the limb with extreme pronation of the hand does not develop for some months after birth. Sensory loss is usually minimal and consists of a small area of hypalgesia on the upper lateral aspect of the arm. Since this condition is uniformly complicated by contractures and deformities if untreated, all children with suspected Erb's paralysis should receive prompt therapy. The arm should be carried through a full range of passive movements twice daily to prevent contractures. Bracing and splinting should be avoided. If it is apparent that recovery will not occur, orthopedic measures should be considered. These include partial section of the pectoralis major or subscapularis muscles, section of the pronator teres, and possibly tendon transplantation. Despite active treatment beginning immediately after birth, many cases develop some deformity at the elbow joint.

The lower type (Klumpke) of brachial plexus paralysis is much rarer. The tearing of the roots of C_8 and T_1 results in weakness and atrophy of the flexors of the wrist with wasting of the small muscles of the hand. The hand may have the appearance of a clawhand with sensory loss along the ulnar border of the hand and forearm. There may be an associated Horner's syndrome.

Diseases of the Brachial Plexus

The brachial plexus may be damaged by stabbing, by gunshot wounds, or as a complication of other forms of trauma to the shoulder, which are often severe enough to produce fractures of the clavicle or upper humerus.

The shoulder and brachial plexus are particularly vulnerable to injury in motorcycle accidents and competitive sports. A headlong fall onto the point of the shoulder with the head and neck flexed in the opposite direction produces stretching and avulsion of the roots of C_5, C_6 as they emerge through the intervertebral foramina. There may be associated damage to the suprascapular nerve or more extensive avulsion of the nerve roots and complete brachial plexus involvement in severe cases. This latter situation is fortunately rare, and the more common avulsion of the roots of C_5, C_6 produces loss of abduction at the shoulder owing to paralysis of the deltoid and spinati.

When the force of the fall is applied toward the front of the shoulder, the inferior cord of the brachial plexus is compressed between the clavicle and the first rib. This produces pain down the medial aspect of the upper limb and troublesome paresthesias or sensory loss in the dermatomes of C_8 and T_1.

A blow in the angle between the shoulder and neck may be followed by weakness in shoulder movements owing to damage to the suprascapular nerve or the upper cord of the brachial plexus. The accessory nerve is also vulnerable to injury in this area by similar mechanisms, with paralysis of the trapezius muscle resulting in loss of ability to shrug the shoulder and move the scapula through normal range of motion. Paralysis of the deltoid sometimes follows blows to the lateral aspect of the shoulder with crushing of the circumflex nerve.

The contents of the anterior axilla are prone to injury by blows to the front of the shoulder. This is likely to occur, for example, when the anterior part of the shoulder is struck by a football helmet. Injury to the axillary (circumflex) nerve results in weakness of abduction of the arm, which may recover within a few days if the nerve is only contused. Persistent weakness and wasting of the deltoid indicate more severe injury to the nerve, which may require surgical exploration of the brachial plexus. The musculocutaneous nerve also lies in front of the shoulder and may be injured by similar mechanisms. This results in weakness of the biceps with numbness extending down the lateral aspect of the forearm to the base of the thumb.

The contents of the axilla are also vulnerable to injury by an upward force directed into the axilla when the arm is abducted. This tends to produce a large hematoma in the region of the quadrilateral space with compression of the posterior cord of the brachial plexus. The degree of injury varies. Complete paralysis of the nerves arising from the posterior cord results in medial rotation of the arm at the shoulder, poor abduction of the arm due to weakness of the deltoid, and paralysis of the triceps and dorsiflexors of the wrist. Commonly, the injury is confined to weakness of the deltoid and triceps.

Dislocation of the shoulder may be complicated by damage to the axillary or circumflex nerve with weakness of the deltoid.

Another type of injury to the brachial plexus has been described in conditions producing forcible wrenching by a sudden increase in the angle between the head and shoulder. While this may occur in automobile, motorcycle, and football injuries, it has also resulted from carrying heavy weights with the arm abducted (pallbearer's palsy). There is damage to the nerve roots of C_5 to C_8 with weakness involving the shoulder, biceps, triceps, and forearm muscles and a sensory loss usually confined to the hand in the dermatomes of C_6, C_7, and C_8.

Gunshot and mortar wounds frequently involve the entire plexus, thus being particularly common in battle casualties resulting in a severe disability with paralysis and wasting of all the muscles in the affected upper limb and sensory loss extending up to the shoulder. Recovery occurs in those cases where a bullet wound passes close to the plexus with temporary paralysis owing to contusion and hemorrhage about the nerves.

Neoplastic involvement of the brachial plexus is not uncommon, is usually painful, and may be the first symptom of carcinoma of the breast and lung. This usually occurs by direct invasion of the plexus from bronchial carcinoma. The neoplasm infiltrates the lower roots of the cords producing pain down the medial aspect of the arm (C_8, T_1), wasting of the small muscles of the hand, and a Horner's syndrome (Pancoast's syndrome). The plexus can also be involved by metastases, particularly by lymphatic infiltration through the apex of the axilla. This is usually the method of spread in carcinoma of breast. As stated, the condition is usually painful, but since any portion of the plexus may be involved, the pain may occur in any distribution of the innervation of the plexus to the upper limb and shoulder girdle. The situation can present some difficulties in diagnosis since a similar condition sometimes occurs from irradiation of the axilla following radical resection of carcinoma of the breast. Irradiation produces a progressive neuropathy resulting from perineural fibrosis and obliteration of the vasa nervorum, which may occur 5 to 20 years following therapy. Direct damage to the nerves seldom follows radiotherapy since the nerves themselves are relatively radioresistant. In irradiation neuropathy, there is progressive weakness and pain in the upper limb on the affected side, with atrophy of the muscles of the shoulder girdle, biceps, triceps, and forearm. The deep tendon reflexes are depressed, and sensory loss is less marked and usually occurs in the hand.

Brachial Neuritis

The sudden onset of a painful paralysis of the brachial plexus rarely occurs and is most commonly an infectious or toxic neuritis involving the roots, trunks, or nerves of the brachial plexus. It frequently results following the injection into the affected limb of immunizing agents, including tetanus toxoid and antitoxin, and it may occasionally occur in diabetes mellitus.

Etiology and Pathology. Apart from toxic causes, the condition is probably due to an autoimmune disorder or a viral infection. Both herpes zoster and the Epstein-Barr virus have been implicated.[156] The pathologic changes are unknown.

Clinical Features. The disorder frequently follows exercise of the affected limb, an infectious illness, and/or immunization. It may accompany serum sickness, hence is common in young males and females. The onset is sudden with severe pain in the root of the neck or shoulder radiating into the upper limb and often requiring narcotics for relief. In cases due to herpes zoster, the herpetic lesions of the skin are in the distribution of the plexus. This is followed by muscle weakness, wasting, and sensory loss in the shoulder or limb, which depends on the roots or nerves involved. The neurologic examination is otherwise normal and the spinal fluid is clear without increase in cell count or abnormalities in protein count. Other more common causes of neurologic disorder in the affected area such as cervical disk and cervical spondylosis should be excluded.

Diagnostic Procedures. These are as follows:

1. The electromyogram shows evidence of denervation, such as fibrillation and reduction in the number of motor unit potentials.
2. The spinal fluid usually shows elevation of the gamma globulin fraction.

Treatment. The prognosis is good and nearly all cases show full recovery. This should be aided by physical therapy to strengthen the affected limb and prevent joint stiffness.

Thoracic Outlet Syndrome

The literature was replete with numerous reports of this condition over a 25-year period ending in 1950. It was described under various synonyms including thoracic inlet syndrome, scalenus anticus syndrome, costoclavicular syndrome, and cervical rib syndrome and was believed, at one time, to be a common cause of brachial neuropathy. The recognition of other causes of brachial neuropathy including prolapsed cervical disk, cervical spondylosis, and the carpal tunnel syndrome has reduced the frequency of diagnosis of the thoracic outlet syndrome, and actually it is now a relatively infrequent diagnosis in modern neurologic practice.[60] Review of the literature suggests that many cases included as examples of the thoracic outlet syndrome were probably suffering from the conditions mentioned above. Nevertheless, there are verified cases of this condition.

Etiology and Pathology. Pressure on the lower roots or cord of the brachial plexus may occur as they pass over the cervical rib or through the thoracic outlet between the first rib and the scalenus anticus.[90] There is close association between the brachial plexus and the subclavian blood vessels at this point, and some cases of thoracic outlet syndrome may result from compression of these vessels with an ischemic brachial neuropathy rather than direct pressure on nerves. Intermittent pressure on the subclavian artery also damages the endothelium, resulting in thrombosis of the subclavian artery with periodic embolization in the small arteries of the fingers and hands. Aneurysm dilatation of the subclavian artery and subclavian venous thrombosis have been reported in some cases.[62, 141]

Clinical Features. This is primarily a disease of young and middle-aged females ranging in age from 20 years to the early forties. This is the period of life so frequently associated with rearing of children and lifting and carrying, which apparently accelerate the normal gradual descent of the shoulder girdle in the adult. This accentuates neurovascular compression at the thoracic outlet. There is a history of an automobile accident with a typical "whiplash injury" to the neck immediately preceding the onset of symptoms in a significant number of patients.[25, 165]

The main symptom is deep, aching pain affecting the hands and forearms and occasionally radiating upward to the shoulder girdle and root of the neck. The pain is ill-defined and is usually precipitated by carrying objects in the hands or housework involving repetitive movements of the upper limbs and shoulder girdles. It may be troublesome at night and awaken the patient and is usually provoked by working with the arms elevated above the head.

Intermittent numbness and paresthesias of the fingers result, and some patients complain that they are awakened to find the entire limb completely numb. This is usually due to the habit of sleeping with the hands elevated above the head. Many patients experience weakness and clumsiness of the hands without objective signs of muscular weakness or wasting. Sensory loss is minimal or patchy and occurs over the palmar surfaces of the fingers.

Intermittent cyanosis and blanching of the hands and fingers (Raynaud's phenomenon) with loss of sensation occur in many patients particularly after exposure to cold. Recovery is accompanied by severe pain in the hands. Recurrent cyanosis of single fingers associated with pain, discrete areas of tenderness, and ulceration are indicative of emboli lodging in the small arteries. Recurrent paronychia, brittle nails, and dryness of the skin with painful fissuring occur in many cases.

Diagnostic Procedures. The radial pulse can be obliterated in certain positions of the head and neck. This usually occurs when the arm is abducted above the head or when the arm is abducted and the head rotated to the opposite side. There is a measurable fall in blood pressure in the limb during these maneuvers as well as reduction or obliteration of the pulse. The presence of a soft murmur on auscultation of the neck over the subclavian artery must be interpreted with caution since this is a common finding in healthy young women. The murmur may be indicative of compression of the subclavian artery if it becomes loud, coarse, and accentuated in certain positions of the head and arm that also produce the neurologic symptoms of which the patient complains.

Definitive demonstration of compression of the subclavian artery can be obtained by retrograde brachial arteriography. The procedure should be performed with the arm and head placed in the position that previous testing has shown to cause ischemia.

Treatment. The majority of patients respond to rest, analgesics, and a change in work habits. The patient should be instructed to avoid sleeping with the hands elevated above the head and to avoid exposure to cold weather. Instruction in posture, with the shoulders thrown back, physical therapy, local heat treatment to the shoulder and neck muscles, and vasodilator drugs are usually helpful. Heavy lifting should be avoided as well as working with the hands above the head. The affected arm should be supported by a sling during the day for a period of several weeks during an acute exacerbation. Surgical treatment should be reserved for patients with incapacitating symptoms, embolization to the hands, or demonstrated occlusion of the subclavian artery.[100] The surgical procedure varies from case to case but usually includes resection of a cervical rib or fascial bands[143] that are compressing the subclavian artery or brachial plexus. Patients with marked symptoms of Raynaud's phenomenon are often relieved by a cervical sympathectomy alone.

Lesions of Individual Nerves Arising from the Brachial Plexus

The Nerve to the Rhomboids (C_5). This supplies the rhomboids and partially innervates the levator scapulae, which is also supplied by C_3 and C_4. Lesions of this nerve result from carrying unusual loads on the shoulder, such as recruits marching with heavy rifles slung over the shoulder. Paralysis of the affected muscles results in downward displacement of the angle of the scapula and inability to draw the scapulae together in bracing back the shoulders.

The Nerve to the Serratus Anterior (Long Thoracic Nerve). The roots of C_5, C_6, C_7 may be injured by direct trauma including blows, gunshot wounds, and stab wounds of the axilla. They are also subject to pressure by shoulder braces used on the operating table during surgical operations. Rarely, they may be affected by an acute infectious neuritis. The nerve is sometimes cut inadvertently during radical mastectomy. Paralysis of the serratus anterior produces winging on the scapula, which is best demonstrated when the arm is thrust forward against resistance. The muscle also serves to keep the scapula in contact with the chest wall, and paralysis results in impairment of abduction of the arm with displacement and prominence of the angle of the scapula.

The Suprascapular Nerve (C_4, C_5, C_6). This nerve is subject to injury from blows to the angle between the shoulder and the root of the neck. This results in weakness of the first 15 degrees of abduction and weakness of external rotation of the shoulder with atrophy of the supra- and infraspinatus.

The Axillary Nerve (C_5, C_6). This nerve may be injured by blows to the anterior aspect of the shoulder or to the axilla. It is sometimes injured in dislocations of the shoulder and may be paralyzed in an acute infectious neuritis. The nerve supplies the deltoid and teres minor, and paralysis of these muscles results in inability to abduct the arm. There is a small area of sensory loss over the lateral aspect of the upper arm and atrophy of the deltoid muscle with loss of the normal contour of the shoulder.

The Musculocutaneous Nerve (C_5, C_6). This nerve supplies the brachialis, biceps, and coracobrachialis. The nerve is occasionally damaged by blows to the anterior aspect of the shoulder. This produces weakness of flexion at the elbow, with atrophy of the flexor muscles of the upper arm. Sensory loss occurs over the lateral aspect of the upper arm.

The Radial Nerve (C_5, C_6, C_7, C_8). This nerve arises as a continuation of the posterior cord of the brachial plexus. It supplies the triceps, anconeus, brachioradialis, and extensor carpi radialis longus. The nerve arises in the axilla and terminates just above the lateral condyle of the humerus, where it divides into a superficial branch and into the posterior interosseous nerve. The sensory supply via the posterior brachial cutaneous nerve, the dorsal antebrachial cutaneous nerve, and the superficial branch of the radial nerve innervates the posterior aspect of the arm and forearm and the dorsal aspect of the hand including the thumb but excluding the distal two phalanges of the fingers.

The radial nerve is usually injured in the axilla by stab wounds, by dislocation of the shoulder, and sometimes by the use of crutches that are too long for the patient. The radial nerve is also vulnerable to injury following fracture of the humerus and by pressure when the arm is hung over the arm of a chair during sleep (Saturday night paralysis). The nerve can also be damaged by incompetent injection of medications into the posterior aspect of the upper arm. It is occasionally involved by infectious neuritis.

The symptoms of radial nerve paralysis will depend on the level of the lesion. A proximal lesion produces wrist drop owing to paralysis of the extensors of the wrist, paralysis of the extension of the fingers and thumb; inability to extend the elbow (triceps paralysis); weakness of elbow flexion (brachioradialis paralysis); and weakness of supination due to paralysis of the supinator. If the radial nerve is damaged in the upper arm just above the brachioradialis, the triceps muscle is spared and extension of the elbow remains intact. Sensory loss is variable in radial nerve palsies owing to the overlap of sensory fibers from the median and ulnar nerves. It usually consists of impairment of sensation over the posterior surface of the forearm and hand but is often confined to the dorsal surface of the hand.

The Anterior Interosseous Nerve. Anterior interosseous nerve syndromes are rare and have been reported after trauma such as penetrating injuries, lacerations, fractures, and contusions of the upper forearm. Other causes include exercise and pressure from a plaster cast or sleeping on the forearm.

The symptoms of anterior interosseous nerve compression are characteristic and include pain in the region of the elbow with weakness of the flexor pollicis longus and flexor digitorum profundus. This presents as weakness of terminal metacarpal flexion of the thumb and fingers.[56] There is no sensory loss. Nerve conduction velocities studies show abnormal latencies from the elbow to the pronator quadratus and prolonged duration of the action potential.[111]

Most cases respond to rest, and surgical exploration is only necessary in penetrating wounds or when there is electrodiagnostic evidence of significant entrapment.

The Posterior Interosseous Nerve. The radial nerve terminates immediately above the lateral condyle of the humerus by dividing into a superficial branch and the posterior interosseous nerve. The posterior interosseous nerve winds around the lateral aspect of the radius, enters the dorsal aspect of the forearm, and lies between the superficial and deep muscles, and then passes onto the interosseous membrane. It supplies all the muscles in this region with the exception of the brachioradialis, extensor carpi longus, and anconeus, which are supplied by the radial nerve.

Lesions involving the posterior interosseous nerve are usually due to injuries involving the elbow joint. Other causes are pressure by lipomas or fibromas near the elbow. Severe involvement of the elbow joint in rheumatoid arthritis can produce traction and inflammation of the posterior interosseous nerve with paralysis.

Since the brachioradialis and extensor carpi radialis longus are spared, there is no wrist drop. The clinical picture is characterized by diminution or loss of extension of the fingers and thumb (due to paralysis of the metacarpophalangeal joints and the abductor pollicis longus).

The Median Nerve. This nerve arises from both the outer and inner cords of the brachial plexus and carries fibers from the nerve roots of C_6, C_7, C_8, and T_1. It supplies all the flexor muscles of the forearm with the exception of the flexor carpi ulnaris and the medial half of the flexor digitorum profundus. The pronator teres, pronator quadratus in the forearm, the abductor pollicis brevis, flexor pollicis brevis, opponens pollicis, and the first and second lumbricals of the hand are also supplied by this nerve. The sensory supply includes the skin over the radial side of the palm and the thumb, index, middle, and radial half of the ring finger. An anatomic variation is, however, not uncommon with an "all-median" hand, which means that the sensory supply to all fingers and most of the palm is from the median nerve.

The nerve may be injured by wounds of the upper arm or fractures of the humerus. It is also subject to injuries immediately above the wrist,

particularly from lacerations in attempted suicide. When the nerve is injured above the elbow, there is loss of ability to flex the second phalanges of all fingers and paralysis of flexion of the terminal phalanges of the index and middle fingers. The muscles of the thenar eminence with the exception of the adductor pollicis are all paralyzed, and there is inability to fully pronate the forearm. Atrophy of the muscles of the thenar eminence with extension of the thumb produces a flat hand. When the lesion lies in the forearm immediately above the wrist, the motor paralysis is confined to the hand.

CARPAL TUNNEL SYNDROME. The median nerve may be compressed as it passes beneath the flexor retinaculum to enter the palm of the hand, producing sensory symptoms and sometimes motor weakness of the thumb. The recognition of the "carpal tunnel syndrome" is important because treatment is simple and effective. Unfortunately, many cases were incorrectly diagnosed as "thoracic outlet syndrome" or "nerve root compression" in the past.

Etiology and Pathology. The carpal tunnel is a cylindric structure formed by the concavity of the carpal bones and covered by the flexor retinaculum. This latter structure extends from the scaphoid and trapezoid bones laterally to the pisiform and hook of hamate medially and extends approximately 3 cm into the palm from the distal volar crease. The carpal tunnel contains the tendon of the flexor pollicis longus, the tendons of the long flexors of the fingers, and the median nerve.

The space within the carpal tunnel is limited, and the median nerve will be compressed by any swelling of the structures within it, including swelling of the nerve itself.

The initial lesion is anoxic and is caused by obstruction of venous return from the nerve as a result of increased pressure in the carpal tunnel. This is followed by edema, increased pressure within the nerve leading to ischemia, and destruction of nerve fibers.[54, 147] The main causes of the carpal tunnel syndrome are listed in Table 11–2. The most common causes are those due to occupational trauma. The other causes are unusual.[32]

Clinical Features. The symptoms consist of numbness, pain, and paresthesias of the flexor surface of the finger. The numbness involves the thumb, index, middle, and lateral half of the ring finger in most cases, with occasional involvement

TABLE 11–2

Carpal Tunnel Syndrome

1. Occupational causes: Using machinery with repetitive blows to the wrist and using machinery with repetitive flexion and extension of the wrist (pneumatic drill paralysis)
2. Trauma: Sprains, dislocations, fractures involving the carpal bones and blows causing hematomas
3. Endocrine disturbances: Myxedema, acromegaly, pregnancy, ovariectomy, and diabetes mellitus
4. Neoplastic causes: Ganglion, lipoma, and multiple myeloma
5. Infections: Chronic tenosynovitis, tuberculosis
6. Metabolic disorders: Gout, amyloidosis, mucopolysaccharidosis,[24] chronic interstitial hypertrophic neuropathy
7. Degenerative: Osteoarthritis
8. Vascular: Systemic lupus erythematosus, dermatomyositis, scleroderma, rheumatoid arthritis
9. Surgical: After insertion of vascular shunts in the forearm in patients treated by hemodialysis, after radial artery puncture or catheterization.
10. Iatrogenic: Hematoma during anticoagulant therapy

of the little finger in the "all-median" hand. The pain is intermittent involving the same fingers but frequently radiating proximally as high as the elbow or shoulder, which may simulate the pain of a herniated disk. It is usually described as a dull ache and is exacerbated by using the fingers or working with the hands above the head, which simulates the pain of the thoracic outlet syndrome. The pain is also worse at night and may wake the patient. Relief may be obtained by hanging the hand over the side of the bed or getting up and "walking the bedroom floor" while massaging the fingers. The pain is often accompanied and followed by annoying paresthesias in the fingers.

Examination of the hand reveals surprisingly little muscular atrophy, which is restricted to the thenar eminence. Fasciculations are occasionally seen in the area of wasting. There may be some demonstrable weakness in the muscles of the thenar eminence and the lateral two lumbricals, but the strength is normal in those muscles supplied by the ulnar nerve. Sensation, including light touch and pinprick, is usually diminished over the affected fingers and pain may be elicited by percussion over the median nerve under the flexor retinaculum (deep transverse carpal ligament) (Tinel's sign). The neurologic examination does not reveal evidence of any other abnormalities.

Diagnostic Procedures. A number of cases show fibrillations confined to the thenar muscles by electromyographic examination. The motor conduction velocity from elbow to wrist may be normal, but the distal latency is usually abnormally prolonged. The distal sensory latency may be prolonged before slowing of the distal motor latency. About 25 per cent of cases have an anomalous median to ulnar nerve communication in the forearm and have an initial positive deflection when the median nerve is stimulated at the elbow and the muscle action potential is recorded at the thenar eminence. This initial positive deflection is due to the recording of the muscle action potential from the first dorsal interosseous muscle, which is generated before that from the thenar muscles because of the crossed innervation from median to ulnar nerves in the forearm. This finding indicates a delay in conduction of axons through the carpal tunnel and when present is a useful sign of carpal tunnel syndrome.[68]

Treatment. If the carpal tunnel syndrome is associated with any known cause, e.g., myxedema, the patient should receive appropriate treatment for the primary condition. Symptoms of the carpal tunnel syndrome are not unusual during pregnancy, but few patients require treatment and the majority of cases show remission before or just after delivery.[66]

Many patients with mild or early symptoms of a short duration respond to rest, oral analgesics, and splinting of the wrist. If symptoms persist, the area around the nerve beneath the flexor retinaculum should be infiltrated with 40 mg of methylprednisolone in 3 ml of 1 per cent lidocaine. This usually produces immediate and permanent relief of symptoms, although a number of patients may have a relapse after several months. This can be treated with another injection of corticosteroid in most cases. In those patients who fail to show persistent improvement following injection, particularly where there is obvious wasting of the thenar muscles, surgical incision of the deep transverse carpal ligament with relief of pressure on the median curve usually produces permanent cure.

The Ulnar Nerve. This arises from the inner cord of the brachial plexus and carries fibers from C_8 and T_1 nerve roots. It accompanies the brachial artery in the upper arm as far as the insertion of the coracobrachialis, where it inclines backward and medially to pass behind the medial epicondyle at the elbow. The nerve then passes along the medial aspect of the elbow joint and between the two heads of the flexor carpi ulnaris to continue through the forearm as far as the wrist under cover of that muscle. The distal portion of the nerve enters the palm by crossing the flexor retinaculum and divides into a superficial and deep terminal branch.

The ulnar nerve supplies the flexor carpi ulnaris and the medial half of the flexor digitorum profundus in the forearm as well as the hypothenar muscles, adductor pollicis, all the dorsal and palmar interossei, and the medial two lumbricals in the hand.

ULNAR NERVE PALSY. Ulnar nerve palsy is a common complication of fractures in the region of the elbow joint.

Etiology and Pathology. The nerve may be torn during a fracture of the medial epicondyle, producing immediate symptoms of nerve injury. In some cases nerve involvement is long delayed until after healing of the fracture when stretching or exposure of the nerve may result owing to callus formation. A late or tardy ulnar palsy, which occurs many years after a fracture, is usually associated with a progressive valgus deformity of the joint following a fracture of the lateral epicondyle (Fig. 11–4). This produces a gradual stretching of the nerve in the ulnar groove behind the medial epicondyle. A similar type of tardy ulnar nerve palsy occurs in patients with congenital shallowness of the ulnar groove, which permits repeated trauma to the nerve at the elbow. Such tardy ulnar nerve palsies may occur in certain occupations where there is repetitive trauma to the elbows, or where there is pressure over the joints for relatively long periods. An engineer on a railroad, for example, leaning with one elbow on a steel armrest in the cabin of his locomotive developed an ulnar nerve palsy.

Peripheral ulnar nerve palsy occurs at the wrist by trauma related to industrial occupations and

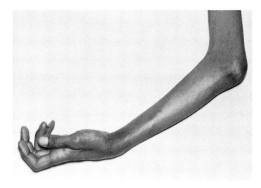

FIGURE 11–4. Appearance of the hand in a severe case of tardy ulnar nerve palsy with injury at the ulnar groove. The hand has a "clawhand" appearance. There are extension of the proximal phalanges (owing to unopposed action of the extensor digitorum) and flexion of middle and distal phalanges.

from fractures of the carpal bones or radius. It has also been described in tumors of the ulnar nerve, ganglion of the wrist, arteritis of the ulnar artery, hemorrhage secondary to hemophilia, and from prolonged compression in motorcycle and long-distance bicycle riders.[47]

Clinical Features. Examination reveals a clawhand type of deformity with extension at the metacarpophalangeal joints and flexion at the interphalangeal joints, which are particularly marked in the ring and little finger. This is due to the unopposed action of the extensor group of muscles at the metacarpophalangeal joints and paralysis of the third and fourth lumbricals, which act as flexors at these joints and as extensors of the interphalangeal joints.

There is flattening of the hypothenar eminence because of atrophy of the palmaris brevis and small muscles of the little finger. The little finger tends to be abducted from the ring finger because of paralysis of the fourth palmar interosseous muscle. There is marked atrophy of the interossei on examination of the dorsal surface of the hand with grooving between the extensor tendons. Both abduction and adduction movements of the fingers are impaired and the patient is unable to hold a piece of paper between the adducted and outstretched fingers.

When the patient attempts to make a fist, there is failure to flex the distal and interphalangeal joints of the fourth and fifth fingers. Attempted opposition of the thumb and little finger is impaired due to paralysis of the opponens digiti minimi. Paralysis of the flexor carpi ulnaris produces a tendency for radial deviation of the hand on flexion of the wrist, and the examiner is not able to feel the tendon of the flexor carpi ulnaris contract when the patient attempts to abduct the little finger against resistance.

Sensory loss is variable but there is usually hypalgesia and hypesthesia involving the little finger and the ulnar aspect of the ring finger with extension along the ulnar aspect of the palm as far as the wrist. The sensory loss usually extends on the dorsal surface of the hand to involve the middle and distal phalanges of the fourth and fifth fingers. There is no sensory loss when the deep terminal branch of the ulnar nerve is compressed at the wrist.

Diagnostic Procedures

1. Compression at the elbow can be demonstrated by stimulation of the nerve above and below the elbow joint and recording a delay in conduction around the elbow.
2. There is an impairment of distal latency to the abductor digiti quinti or the first dorsal interosseus muscle when the deep terminal branch of the ulnar nerve is compressed at the wrist.

Treatment. The clawhand deformity should be prevented or, if present, treated by splinting and physical therapy. If the condition appears to be due to repeated trauma to the ulnar nerve in the ulnar groove, the nerve can be transplanted to the anterior aspect of the elbow or medial epicondylectomy may be performed.[113] The results of treatment are good, with complete restoration of function in the majority.[96]

Neuropathies of the Lumbar and Sacral Plexuses

Anatomy of the Lumbar Plexus

The lumbar plexus (Fig. 11–5) is formed within the substance of the psoas muscle by the junction of the anterior primary rami of the upper four lumbar nerves. The first lumbar nerve gives origin to the ilioinguinal and iliohypogastric nerves, which supply the skin over the lower anterior abdominal wall. The genitofemoral nerve arises from the first, second, and third lumbar nerves and passes downward on the surface of the psoas muscle to divide into a genital branch and femoral branch, which supply the skin immediately below

the middle part of the inguinal ligament. The lateral femoral cutaneous nerve arises from the second and third lumbar nerves and runs across the iliacus muscle toward the anterior superior iliac spine. It passes beneath the inguinal ligament just medial to the anterior superior iliac spine into the subcutaneous tissue of the thigh via a foramen in the fascia lata and supplies the skin over the anterolateral and posterolateral aspects of the thigh as far as the knee.

The femoral nerve arises from the posterior branches of the second, third, and fourth lumbar nerves and supplies the iliacus muscle and enters the thigh beneath the inguinal ligament on the lateral side of the femoral artery. It divides into a number of branches in the femoral triangle immediately below the inguinal ligament and supplies the pectineus, sartorius, and the quadriceps femoris muscles. The sensory components supply the anterior and medial aspects of the thigh through the intermediate and medial cutaneous nerves of the thigh and the medial side of the leg and foot through the saphenous nerve.

The obturator nerve arises from the anterior branches of the second, third, and fourth lumbar nerves and runs down the medial aspect of the psoas muscle to enter the thigh through the obturator foramen. It supplies the muscles in the medial compartment of the thigh including the adductor magnus and gives sensory innervation to the upper part of the medial aspect of the thigh.

Anatomy of the Sacral Plexus

The sacral plexus is formed by the union of the nerve roots of L_4, L_5, S_1, S_2, S_3, and S_4. It lies in the wall of the pelvis on the anterior surface of the pyriformis muscle where it divides into its major branches. These include the superior gluteal nerve (L_4, L_5, S_1), supplying the gluteus medius, gluteus minimus, and tensor fascia lata; the inferior gluteal nerve (L_5, S_1, S_2), supplying the gluteus maximus; and the nerves to the quadratus femoris (L_4, L_5, S_1) and obturator internus (L_5, S_1, S_2), supplying these two muscles.

The posterior cutaneous nerve of the thigh (S_1, S_2, S_3) passes through the greater sciatic foramen to enter the gluteal region. It supplies sensation to a variable area on the lower part of the buttock, the lateral perineum, and the posterior thigh.

The pudendal nerve (S_2, S_3, S_4) also enters the gluteal region through the greater sciatic foramen and then bends through the lesser sciatic foramen to enter the ischiorectal fossa and the

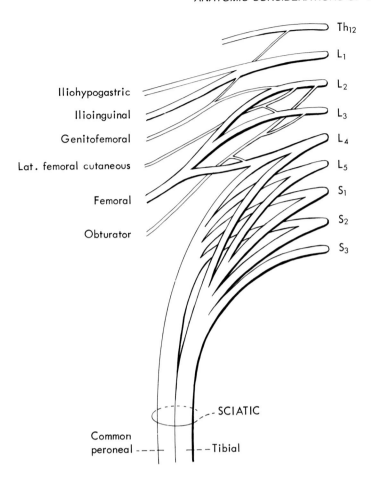

Th$_{12}$
L$_1$
Iliohypogastric
L$_2$
Ilioinguinal
L$_3$
Genitofemoral
L$_4$
Lat. femoral cutaneous
L$_5$
S$_1$
Femoral
S$_2$
Obturator
S$_3$

SCIATIC

Common peroneal ---- Tibial

FIGURE 11–5. Lumbosacral plexus.

pudendal canal. It supplies the external anal sphincter, the skin around the anus, and the perineal muscles. The mucous membrane of the urethra, the external sphincter of the bladder, and the skin of the perineum, scrotum, and penis are also supplied by the pudendal nerve.

The sciatic nerve arises from the nerve roots of L$_4$, L$_5$, S$_1$, S$_2$, and S$_3$ and passes through the greater sciatic foramen as a single trunk into the gluteal region. It then descends under cover of the gluteus maximus into the posterior aspect of the thigh to divide into the tibial and common peroneal nerves at a variable distance above the popiteal fossa.

The tibial nerve descends through the middle of the popliteal fossa to the upper level of the soleus muscle. It supplies the gastrocnemius, plantaris, soleus, popliteus, and tibialis posterior. It also has an anastomotic branch that joins the peroneal anastomotic nerve to form the sural nerve.

The posterior tibial nerve is a direct continuation of the tibial nerve arising at the level of the fibrous arch of the soleus muscle. It passes down the posterior aspect of the calf and beneath the flexor retinaculum, where it divides into the medial and lateral plantar nerves. It supplies the soleus, tibialis posterior, flexor digitorum longus, and flexor hallucis longus. It also supplies sensation to a small area over the medial aspect of the heel.

The medial and lateral plantar nerves are the terminal branches of the posterior tibial nerve supplying the small muscles on the plantar surface of the foot and sensation to the sole and the plantar surface of the toes.

The common peroneal nerve (L$_4$, L$_5$, S$_1$, S$_2$) has a short course in the popliteal fossa from its origin at the division of the sciatic nerve along the lateral border of the fossa to the head of fibula. It then winds around the neck of the fibula in a shallow groove and divides into the superficial and deep peroneal nerves. The common peroneal nerve has two branches: the lateral cutaneous nerve of the calf, which supplies sensation to the upper lateral aspect of the leg, and the peroneal anastomotic nerve, which joins the anastomotic branch of the tibial nerve to form the sural nerve.

The superficial peroneal nerve arises at or just beyond the neck of the fibula from the common peroneal nerve. It descends in front of the fibula to supply the peronei and extensor digitorum longus. The terminal branches supply sensation to the front and lateral aspect of the lower two thirds of the leg and the lateral half of the dorsal surface of the foot.

The deep peroneal nerve is the second terminal branch of the common peroneal nerve. It passes medially from the neck of the fibula to the interosseous membrane supplying the tibialis anterior, extensor digitorum longus, and extensor hallucis longus and then descends to pass beneath the superior extensor retinaculum to the dorsal surface of the foot. It supplies sensation to the medial side of the second toe and the lateral side of the great toe.

The sural nerve arises from the common peroneal and tibial nerves by anastomotic branches. It supplies the skin over the calf and posterior aspect of the lower leg and then passes behind the lateral malleolus to supply the lateral aspect of the heel, foot, and little toe.

Sciatic Pain

While by far the majority of cases of sciatic pain are due to prolapsed intervertebral disks between L_4 and L_5 or L_5 and S_1, with radiating pain due to irritation of these nerve roots, there are other causes of sciatica (Table 11–3). The emphasis on the surgical treatment of prolapsed intervertebral disks may have been overdone in the last 20 years, but depreciation of this condition as a cause of sciatic pain is not supported by practical clinical experience.

Experienced neurologists recognize other causes of sciatic pain but recognize that such cases are, for the most part, uncommon.

Clinical Features. Irritation of the lumbosacral nerve roots or sciatic nerve is characterized by pain in the lower gluteal region and back of the thigh occasionally radiating down the back of the calf or down the lateral aspect of the leg. It is usually a dull ache with irregular shooting pains and may be sufficiently severe to require the use of narcotics to obtain relief. The pain is exacerbated by flexion movements of the trunk or thigh that tend to stretch the sciatic nerve. Examination shows tenderness on palpation over the sciatic nerve in the thigh; limitation of straight leg raising (Lasègue's sign); hypesthesia in the L_5 or S_1 dermatome usually on the lateral aspect of the leg above the ankle; and diminution of the ankle jerk. Additional signs, such as loss of lumbar lordosis, scoliosis, and muscular weakness in the hamstrings, calf muscles, or extensors of the foot, depend on the type of lesions causing the sciatic pain.

Diagnostic Procedures

1. Roentgenograms of the lumbosacral spine may show osteoarthritic changes or signs of vertebral disease including bony metastasis.
2. Selective blocking of spinal nerves in the intervertebral foramina with 1 per cent xylocaine can be used to identify the site of compression of a lumbosacral nerve root.[75]
3. Nerve conduction velocity studies can be used to compare conduction velocities between right

TABLE 11–3

Sciatic Pain

---

1. Lesions in the spinal canal: Pachymeningitis due to syphilis, intrathecal injection of drugs, herpes zoster, trauma, tumors of the cauda equina, subarachnoid hemorrhage
2. Diseases of the vertebrae: Tuberculosis, trauma, metastases, Paget's disease
3. Lesions at the intervertebral foramina: Prolapsed intervertebral disk, spondylosis
4. Pelvic disease: Trauma due to fractures, pregnancy; enlarged lymph nodes; pelvic and psoas abscess; carcinoma of bowel, prostate, and other metastases; aneurysm of the pelvic arteries
5. Lesions in the gluteal area: Fractures of the femur, dislocation of the hip, hematomas, gluteal wounds, tuberculosis, echinococcal cysts—pyriformis syndrome, aneurysm of the inferior gluteal artery
6. Lesions in the thigh: Injection of drugs into the nerve (penicillin, paraldehyde), sciatic nerve entrapment
7. Vasculitis: Polyarteritis nodosa
8. All causes of neuropathy

---

and left sciatic nerves and demonstrate sciatic nerve entrapment in the thigh.[76]

Acute Injuries to the Sciatic Nerve

The nerve may be injured by gunshot wounds, particularly in wartime. When incomplete, rather than total, transection of the nerve occurs. For some reason, the lateral or peroneal portion of the sciatic nerve appears to be more susceptible to the effects of trauma and contusions than the medial portion of the nerve. Other causes of acute injury to the nerve include fracture of the femur, posterior dislocation of the hip, and the inadvertent injection of drugs (particularly penicillin and paraldehyde), which often produce permanent paralysis into the substance of the nerve.

Clinical Features. Total transection of the sciatic nerve produces paralysis involving flexion and extension of the toes, inversion and eversion of the foot, and flexion and extension of the ankle joint. The foot assumes a position of talipes equinus. Flexion is impaired at the knee owing to paralysis of the hamstrings, although some flexion is possible through the action of the sartorius (femoral nerve) and gracilis (obturator nerve). Extension of the knee and flexion of the hip are intact, but there may be some slight weakness in extension of the hip. Sensation is lost below the knee except in the area innervated by the saphenous nerve on the medial aspect of the leg and ankle. Atrophy of the denervated muscles produces marked wasting below the knee, and although the patient can stand, he flexes the hip when walking and "throws" the lower limb forward to compensate for the foot drop.

The tibial and common peroneal components of the sciatic nerve are usually interrupted, with preservation of the nerve supply to the hamstrings in wounds of the middle and posterior aspects of the thigh. The clinical signs are much the same as in transection of the nerve at a higher level except that flexion of the knee is unimpaired.

Treatment. All wounds should be explored, with removal of dead tissue and suturing of transected nerves in the absence of sepsis. Chronic cases may require the use of nerve grafts. Damage to the sciatic nerve by injection of irritative substances such as penicillin and paraldehyde is often followed by fibrosis. Some return of function may occur following surgical exploration and neurolysis with removal of scar tissue and restoration of continuity with or without a nerve graft.

Acute Injuries to the Posterior Cutaneous Nerve of the Thigh

This nerve is sometimes injured with the sciatic nerve in gunshot wounds involving the posterior aspect of the leg. This produces a sensory loss over the posterior aspect of the thigh from the buttock to the popliteal fossa and extending into the lateral part of the perineum.

Conditions Affecting the Superior Gluteal and the Inferior Gluteal Nerves

These nerves are occasionally involved in fractures of the pelvis and by metastatic spread of carcinoma within the pelvis. There are paralysis and wasting of the gluteus maximus, medius, and minimus, with atrophy of the buttock and inability to extend the thigh.

Meralgia Paresthetica

Compression of the lateral femoral cutaneous nerve produces a highly characteristic neuralgia, which usually responds dramatically to treatment.

Etiology and Pathology. The nerve may be kinked as it enters the thigh or compressed by tight garments such as a garter belt or truss. Symptoms tend to occur in obese individuals or in those who have recently lost weight who begin exercising the lower limbs after a period of inactivity. Occasionally cases of proximal compression by a pelvic tumor or degenerated disk are encountered.

Clinical Features. The neuralgia is characterized by a dull ache in the cutaneous distribution of the nerve associated with paresthesias, formication, and occasional sharp stabbing pains. There is hypalgesia to pinprick in the affected area, but the neurologic examination is normal in all other aspects. The nerve is usually tender over the point of emergence into the thigh just below the inguinal ligament.

Treatment. Many patients experience immediate and permanent relief after injection of the nerve at the point of entrance into the thigh with 40 mg of an aqueous suspension of methylprednisolone acetate (Depo-Medrol) in 3 ml of 1 per cent lidocaine. The injection may be repeated if there is a recurrence of symptoms. If this treatment fails, neurectomy should be considered, but a search should be made for a proximal compressive lesion including a pelvic tumor or a herniated lumbosacral disk.

Conditions Affecting the Femoral Nerve

The femoral nerve is formed within the psoas muscle and may be compressed by hematoma formation within the muscle. Hematomas may arise from injury, from spinal manipulation, or spontaneously in patients receiving anticoagulants,[27, 168] or in bleeding disorders such as hemophilia, leukemia, or consumption coagulopathy.[40] The femoral nerve can also be compressed by a tumor or aneurysm as it emerges at the lateral border of the psoas muscle.[154] Other causes of femoral neuropathy include diabetes mellitus, sarcoidosis, herpes zoster, and psoas abscess.[158]

Clinical Features.   There is pain over the anterior aspect of the thigh starting at the groin and radiating down the front of the thigh. The left knee and hip are held in a flexed position, and there are weakness of the quadriceps and absence of the knee jerk.

Treatment.   If anticoagulants are being given, they should be stopped immediately and the patient should be given the appropriate antagonist (protamine sulfate or vitamin K). Adequate analgesics including morphine may be required to control pain. The application of heat and supporting the affected lower limb on pillows help to relieve discomfort.

Conditions Affecting the Deep Peroneal Nerve

This nerve is susceptible to injury as it lies in a superficial position at its origin on the lateral side of the neck of the fibula. Injury can occur by direct bruising of the nerve, from injury associated with a fracture of the neck of fibula, or by pressure from a plaster cast. It is occasionally seen in individuals, particularly women, who sit for long periods with their knees crossed. The nerve is also affected in diabetic neuropathy and polyarteritis nodosa.

Deep peroneal nerve palsy leads to foot drop due to paralysis of the extensors of the foot and toes. When the condition results from crossing the knees, there is usually a dimpling of the skin and subcutaneous tissues over the neck of fibula ("dimple" sign). The patient walks with a typical high-steppage gait. In some cases, the dropped foot may be everted when the superficial peroneal nerve is spared. In long-standing cases there is wasting of the muscles in the anterior compartment of the leg, with prominence of the tibia. The sensory loss is confined to the area between the first and second toes.

Conditions Affecting the Superficial Peroneal Nerve

This nerve is affected by many of the conditions producing a deep peroneal nerve palsy. When the superficial peroneal nerve is paralyzed, the peroneal muscles are weak and there is loss of eversion of the foot, which also tends to invert on dorsiflexion. Sensory loss occurs over the lower lateral portion of the leg and dorsum of the foot.

Conditions Affecting the Common Peroneal Nerve

This nerve can be injured by wounds in the popliteal fossa, fractures of the tibia, fibula, or femur, acute inversion of the ankle, and fracture dislocation of the hip. A few cases occur without apparent cause.[16] The symptoms of common peroneal nerve paralysis are a combination of superficial and deep peroneal nerve paralysis. There is a foot drop with a tendency to inversion due to unopposed action of the tibialis posterior. The patient has a typical high-steppage gait on the affected side, with sensory loss over the lower lateral surface of the leg and dorsum of the foot.

Conditions Affecting the Tibial Nerve

This nerve is susceptible to injury by contusion or gunshot wounds. It is also subject to the usual conditions producing neuropathies. The paralysis involves the calf muscles and all the muscles of the foot, resulting in loss of plantar flexion of the foot and toes. There is complete sensory loss over the plantar surface of the foot. In chronic cases atrophy of the small muscles of the foot produces pes cavus.

Tarsal Tunnel Syndrome

Pressure on the medial plantar nerve (and occasionally the lateral plantar nerve) as they lie beneath the flexor retinaculum of the foot may produce intermittent pain and parethesias along the sole of the foot. The diagnosis may be confirmed by demonstrating prolonged distal motor latency in the medial plantar nerves.[67] The condition is comparable to the more common carpal tunnel syndrome and may be relieved by section of the flexor retinaculum with relief of pressure on the nerves.

General Considerations of the Neuropathies

Peripheral Neuropathy

The term "peripheral neuropathy" is used to describe a disorder characterized by symmetric impairment of function in peripheral nerves. "Peripheral neuropathy" is more satisfactory than "peripheral neuritis," which is often used synonymously but implies an inflammation of the nerves. Since many of the conditions described under peripheral neuropathy are noninflammatory, the term "neuritis" is less satisfactory than neuropathy. Conditions affecting single peripheral nerves (mononeuropathy) or nonsymmetric involvement of a number of peripheral nerves (polymononeuropathy) will be discussed separately.

Etiology and Pathology

The peripheral nerve trunk is surrounded by a connective tissue sheath, the epineurium. Nerve fibers lying within the epineurium are divided into bundles or fascicles by further layers of connective tissue, called the perineurium, while each nerve fiber itself is invested by a third sheath called the endoneurium.

The nerve fiber consists of a central axon surrounded by a myelin sheath. This sheath is laid down by the Schwann cells in concentric layers around the axon. The myelin sheath is divided into segments by constrictions or nodes of Ranvier, and the myelin in each internode is derived from one Schwann cell. Nutrient arteries or vasa nervorum enter the nerve at irregular intervals along its whole length.

A mixed peripheral nerve contains fibers of varying diameter, and there is some variation in the development of the myelin sheath. The larger the diameter, the faster the conduction velocity, and vice versa. The so-called unmyelinated fibers have the smallest diameter and have a single layer of myelin covering them. The motor fibers comprise a good portion of the large fibers in the mixed peripheral and cranial nerve and are the axons of the anterior horn cells in the spinal cord and corresponding motor neurons of the cranial nerve nuclei. The sensory fibers are derived from bipolar cells in the posterior root ganglia and corresponding sensory ganglia of the cranial nerves.

Peripheral neuropathy can occur under the following conditions:

1. An inflammatory condition affecting the peripheral nerve or a true "polyneuritis"
2. Secondary to an axonal neuronal degeneration with symmetric "dying back" of axons
3. Demyelination of the nerve
4. Changes in interstitial tissues surrounding the nerve
5. A combination of two or more of the above

Common conditions known to cause peripheral neuropathy are listed in Table 11–4. There are

TABLE 11–4

Classification of Peripheral Neuropathies

1. Hereditary neuropathies: Tangier, Bassen-Kornzweig, Refsum, Déjerine-Sottas
   Hereditary sensory neuropathy—type 1 and type 11
2. Infectious conditions:
   Viral—measles, mumps, infectious mononucleosis, infectious hepatitis, etc.
   Bacterial—diphtheria, brucellosis, typhoid, tuberculosis, leprosy, botulism, Whipple's disease
3. Postinfectious ("allergic") neuropathies: Guillain-Barré, serum sickness, vaccination
4. Nutritional deficiencies: Avitaminosis B_1, B_6, B_{12}, folic acid, pantothenic acid deficiency, sprue, malabsorption syndromes; gastrointestinal shunts
5. Metabolic abnormalities: Diabetes mellitus, hypoglycemia, hyperlipidemia, Addison's disease, uremia, amyloidosis, porphyria, alcohol, hypothyroidism, macrocryoglobulinemia, chronic hepatic failure
6. Remote effects of neoplasia: Carcinoma, multiple myeloma, macroglobulinemia
7. Toxic conditions: Ethyl and methyl alcohol, lead, arsenic, mercury, gold, thallium, insecticides, tricresyl phosphate, dinitrophenol, acrylamide, uremia, *n*-hexane (glue sniffing), methyl ethyl ketone, methyl *n*-butyl ketone, gasoline, nitrous oxide
8. Drugs: Barbiturates, sulfonamides, emetine, isonicotinic acid, griseofulvin, vincristine, dapsone, metronidazole, clioquinol, perhexiline, disulfiram
9. Vascular: Polyarteritis nodosa, lupus erythematosus, sarcoidosis, chronic ischemia due to atherosclerosis, diabetes mellitus

many more rare etiologic factors, and there is a continued increase in the number of new chemical or toxic agents causing peripheral neuropathy, which has resulted from the introduction of more complex chemical compounds in medicine and industry.[18] The majority of these conditions have been discussed in various sections of this book. This table lists only conditions that frequently cause peripheral neuropathy or that have been the subject of recent comment in the medical literature.

Despite the verification of numerous and diverse causes for peripheral neuropathy, a certain percentage of cases remain undiagnosed. These cases probably represent a reaction to undefined toxic metabolic or infectious agents in most cases.

Clinical Features

Peripheral neuropathy can present with disturbances involving sensory, motor, or autonomic functions. Many are selective with predominantly sensory or predominantly motor forms, which is important in considering differential diagnosis, although chronic mixed types also occur.

Diabetic peripheral neuropathy is one of the most common forms of this type of neurologic disorder seen in practice and presents with predominantly sensory symptoms in the early stages (for a more detailed discussion of the neurologic complications of diabetes mellitus, see Chap. 5). These include burning, paresthesias, and pain in the lower extremities due to axonal degeneration of small myelinated fibers.[19] Motor symptoms occur later and consist of distal weakness and wasting. Early symptoms of oculomotor paralysis are not uncommon. Advanced cases show severe sensory loss in the extremities. Autonomic involvement results in painless distention of the bladder, with retention and rarely overflow incontinence, and postural hypotension. Sensory neuropathy leads to severe ataxia and areflexia (diabetic pseudotabes).

Other common forms of predominantly sensory peripheral neuropathy occur in nutritional deficiencies, in alcoholics, and as a nonmetastatic complication of carcinoma.

Postinfectious polyneuritis (Guillain-Barré syndrome) presents as a predominantly motor neuropathy with symmetric paralysis of the lower extremities in the early stages. There is little or no demonstrable sensory loss. Other forms of predominantly motor neuropathy include diphtheria and porphyria.

The majority of polyneuropathies present with signs of motor and sensory involvement. There is usually a symmetric sensory loss involving all sensory modalities in all four limbs, often described as a "glove-and-stocking" sensory loss. Motor involvement produces distal weakness, flaccidity, and wasting of muscle, but fasciculations are rare.

Diagnostic Procedures

The investigation of a fresh case of peripheral neuropathy should include a total blood count, a sedimentation rate, serum cholesterol, phospholipids, and a five-hour glucose tolerance test to exclude mild diabetes mellitus, which may be complicated by severe peripheral nerve degeneration. Serum electrophoresis may show elevation of the globulin fractions, suggesting a collagen disease or macroglobulins in macroglobulinemia and multiple myeloma. Cell preparations for lupus cells in the peripheral blood should be performed to exclude lupus erythematosus. The urine should be tested for porphobilinogen to exclude porphyria. Serum and urine determinations of heavy metals are indicated in suspected industrial exposure to toxins. Electromyography and motor and sensory nerve conduction velocities are helpful in determining the type of peripheral neuropathy and in contributing to the differential diagnosis. Examination of the cerebrospinal fluid may show elevation of cells in infectious types and elevation of protein in some conditions such as postinfectious polyneuritis. The diagnosis may depend on nerve and muscle biopsy. Nerve biopsy should be performed on the sural nerve if possible, since the sacrifice of this nerve produces only a minor sensory deficit. Definitive diagnosis from a nerve biopsy is possible in conditions such as amyloidosis, metachromatic leukodystrophy, and polyarteritis nodosa.

Treatment

Therapy depends on the correct diagnosis. In cases due to toxic causes, the toxic agent should be removed. In cases due to ischemia associated with atherosclerosis, surgical procedures such as iliofemoral bypass graft will result in recovery.

Diabetic neuropathy may improve or the discomfort may decrease with strict control of the diabetes. A combination of fluphenazine, 1 mg every eight hours, and amitryptyline, 50 to 75 mg at bedtime, is reported to reduce or abolish pain in painful diabetic neuropathy.[36] This regimen could also be used in other types of painful neuropathies.

Where correct diagnosis cannot be established, patients should be given adequate diet, vitamin B complex supplements, physical therapy, and bracing or orthopedic measures to prevent deformities and maintain maximum function.

Peripheral Neuropathy and Polyarteritis Nodosa

Peripheral neuropathy may occur in the collagen diseases, such as disseminated lupus and, more commonly, polyarteritis nodosa. The disease presents as a "mononeuropathy multiplex" (see below) owing to serial infarction of cranial and peripheral nerves. The seventh cranial nerve and the peroneal nerves are commonly affected. Diagnosis is supported by elevation of the sedimentation rate, the presence of antinuclear antibodies in the serum, and the characteristic LE cells in preparations of the blood. The electromyogram shows denervation changes, and the motor and sensory nerve conduction velocities are prolonged. The diagnosis is established by tissue biopsy of the muscle, skin, or affected nerves. Treatment with steroids such as methylprednisolone prolongs survival and hastens recovery.[57] Peripheral neuropathy may be associated with rheumatoid arthritis and in severe forms appears to be caused by a vasculitis of the vasa nervorum similar to that of polyarteritis nodosa.

Mononeuropathy

Disorders of single nerves (mononeuropathy) or a number of nerves (polymononeuropathy) are not as common as polyneuropathy. Many of the causes have been discussed under individual nerves in this section and elsewhere in this book, but a number of other conditions of unusual interest will be described. Familial recurrent nerve palsies, which are frequently brachial in location, have been described (heredofamilial mononeuritis multiplex). The condition is inherited as an autosomal dominant trait and is often precipitated by pregnancy.[116]

The majority of causes of mononeuropathy are traumatic and have been mentioned, but peripheral nerves may be involved in immersion foot and in Volkmann's ischemic contracture. Mononeuropathy may also result from severe arteriosclerosis of the distal vessels of the leg and from iliofemoral disease.

Leprosy is the classic example of a bacterial infection producing mononeuropathy. Herpes zoster may involve any peripheral nerve. Sarcoidosis and diphtheria sometimes produce isolated lesions of peripheral neuropathy.

Mononeuropathies can occur as a complication of immunization. They have usually been described with serum sickness following injection of horse serum. The mononeuropathy often occurs in the limb receiving the injection, although there is clearly no evidence of damage to the nerve at the time of injection. The condition has also been described following injection of tetanus toxoid, although it is a rare complication of this form of immunization.

Isolated mononeuropathies can occur in the alcoholic (see Chap. 5) but are probably due to pressure and trauma on the nerves. This, then, may become superimposed on the cranial and symmetric peripheral neuropathies.

The most common cause of multiple mononeuropathy is diabetes mellitus. This is due to infarction of the nerves and may result in painful polymononeuropathies.[124] Isolated cranial and peripheral nerve involvement are also not unusual in this disease.

Painful mononeuropathy has also been reported to occur as a remote effect of carcinoma, although this condition is most uncommon and peripheral neuropathy is much more characteristic of this condition.

Isolated mononeuropathy and polymononeuropathy also occur in polyarteritis nodosa due to involvement of the vasa nervorum and infarction of the nerve.

Treatment

1. Treatment should be directed toward removal or control of the causative agent whenever possible.
2. Diphenylhydantoin or carbamazepine is sometimes effective in controlling painful neuropathies.
3. A combination of fluphenazine, 1 mg every eight hours, and amitryptyline, 75 mg at bedtime, may reduce pain.
4. Electrical stimulation to affected peripheral nerves using low-threshold stimulation and subcutaneous electrodes is reported to relieve pain in peripheral nerve lesion. The surgical implanting of electrodes around the nerve can be performed if long-term treatment is necessary.[148]

Herpes Zoster or Shingles

Herpes zoster or shingles is one of the most common neurotropic viral infections in man. It is an infectious condition in which the virus has a predilection for the posterior root ganglion and is characterized by pain and a vesicular skin eruption in the sensory distribution of the affected nerve.

Etiology and Pathology

Herpes zoster and varicella are caused by the same virus, and it is believed that varicella represents a primary infection by this virus, whereas herpes zoster is a recrudescence of infection in a person with residual antibodies from previous varicella. An alternate hypothesis is that herpes zoster is a reactivation of a latent infection by the virus in a partly immune subject. Pathologic changes are usually limited to the dorsal root or cranial nerve ganglia where there is intense inflammation with hemorrhagic necrosis and death of neurons. The hemorrhagic area is surrounded by an intense lymphocytic infiltration in which neurons show varying degrees of degeneration and neuronophagia. The inflammatory response usually extends into the posterior nerve root and occasionally involves the spinal cord with changes in the neurons of the posterior horn and, less commonly, in the anterior horn. Inflammatory changes in the anterior nerve root have also been described in some cases, and rarely there is involvement of the cranial nerve ganglia and even some inflammatory response in the brainstem. The skin changes consist of collections of fluid beneath the epithelium with polymorphonuclear infiltration of the dermis. Some of the epithelial cells contain type A intranuclear inclusions, and the fluid within the vesicles contains elementary bodies. Herpes zoster virus has been identified by electron microscopy and culture from the fluid in the vesicles.

Clinical Features

Herpes zoster affects either sex at any age, although it is rare in children. The disease occurs most commonly in adults, and there is an increased incidence in persons suffering from debilitating diseases, particularly in Hodgkin's disease, chronic leukemia, and malignancy.[130]

The incubation period is unknown. There may be a prodromal period with fever and severe pain in the distribution of the dermatome of the affected nerve. This is followed by the appearance of vesicles in the same area within 12 to 24 hours. The vesicles contain a clear fluid, although secondary infection may produce pustules. There is usually marked regional lymphadenopathy. The course varies from one to three weeks, with the development of crusts which separate, leaving small areas of irregular pigmentation of the skin. Occasionally, scars are left, particularly when secondary infection has been severe. The pain of herpes zoster is most severe and is described as burning with stabbing overtones, and there is frequently a pruritic element. This usually subsides in about four days from the onset but in some cases persists for weeks or even months. Some degree of motor weakness occurs in about 5 per cent of cases[115] probably due to an inflammatory reaction of the anterior nerve root. However, other causes of motor weakness include involvement of the anterior horn cells, encephalomyelitis, or postinfectious polyneuritis of the Guillain-Barré type. Herpes zoster affecting the sacral nerves can produce paralysis of the bladder and loss of anal sphincter control.[83]

The condition may present with cranial nerve involvement. The ophthalmic division of the fifth cranial nerve is the most frequently involved with the development of vesicles above the orbit in the distribution of the supraoptic nerve and associated corneal ulceration. Secondary infection may produce severe damage to the affected eye. Hemiplegia may occur a few weeks after and contralateral to herpes zoster ophthalmicus as a result of an arteritis affecting the intracranial vessels.[121] A similar mechanism can produce a delayed retinal thrombophlebitis.[78] Involvement of the geniculate ganglion sometimes results in a vesicular eruption involving the external auditory meatus and drum with the subsequent development of the peripheral type of facial paralysis (Ramsay Hunt syndrome).

Diagnostic Procedures

The diagnosis of herpes zoster does not usually present any difficulty. About 50 per cent of patients show a lymphocytic pleocytosis in the cerebrospinal fluid, even though there is no evidence of encephalomyelitis clinically.

Treatment

Patients usually benefit from a short period of bed rest, which diminishes irritation of the affected area by contact with clothing. Pruritic lesions may be treated by application of calamine lotion or by painting the area with collodion. The pain requires adequate use of analgesics such as aspirin and codeine or dextropropoxyphene (Darvon). A short course of corticosteroids such as methylprednisolone, 64 mg daily for seven days, may produce dramatic relief from pain in severe cases. Topical application of a solution of 5 per cent idoxuridine in 100 per cent dimethylsulfoxide is reported to reduce herpetic pain and shorten the vesicular phase and healing time. The solution is applied every four hours for four days.[37] Persistent neuralgia can be a troublesome, and debilitating, condition, but it slowly subsides over a period of time. Some cases can be controlled with the use of propoxyphene and a phenothiazine. Diphenylhydantoin, carbamazepine (Tegretol), and methylprednisolone may be helpful in those with protracted pain.

Causalgia

This is, fortunately, an uncommon complication of peripheral nerve injuries and consists of severe burning pain occurring in the cutaneous distribution of an injured nerve. The pain is subject to exacerbations and remissions. The pain is intensified by a variety of stimuli such as surface stimulation, heat, noise, emotional excitement, or even the thought of being touched.[131]

Etiology and Pathology

The majority of cases of causalgia have been reported following injury to a peripheral nerve by a high-velocity missile. Causalgia is hence much more common in battle casualties although it can also follow otherwise trivial penetrating wounds.

The essential features appear to be the following:

1. Involvement of a nerve with a large sensory fiber component.
2. The closer the lesion to the spinal ganglia, the more severe the reaction.
3. The severity of the causalgia increases with the severity of the injury.

Causalgia is probably due to the spread of axonal damage to the central nervous system resulting in a reaction in the neurons of the dorsal horns and the creation of a hyperactive focus of abnormal activity in the spinal cord.[146] These hyperactive neurons could in turn initiate a chain reaction involving sensory neurons along transmission pathways to the cerebral cortex.

Clinical Features

1. There is a history of wounding, usually by a high-velocity missile. The median and sciatic nerves are the most frequently involved. Ulnar nerve causalgia is relatively uncommon.
2. The typical burning pain may begin shortly after the injury. The majority of cases resolve within two or three months.
3. The pain is described as a distressing, burning sensation in the cutaneous distribution of the injured nerve. It may be exacerbated by use of the limbs, examination of the affected area, exertion, emotion, noise, vibration, or sudden jerking or movement of the trunk.

Treatment

Sympathectomy is an effective and permanent method of treatment, producing immediate relief from pain.[15] The reason for the effectiveness of sympathectomy is unknown but it probably results in the alteration of some central factor contributing to the hyperactivity of neurons in the dorsal horns of the spinal cord.

Cited References

1. Abramsky, O.; Webb, C.; et al. Cell mediated immunity to neural antigens in idiopathic polyneuritis and myeloradiculitis. *Neurology* (Minneap.), **25**:1154–59, 1975.
2. Adams, J. H.; Blackwood, W.; and Wilson, J. Further clinical and pathological observations on Leber's optic atrophy. *Brain*, **89**:15–25, 1966.
3. Allen, I. V.; Swallow, M.; et al. Clinicopathological study of Refsum's disease with particular reference to fatal complications. *J. Neurol. Neurosurg. Psychiat.*, **41**:323–32, 1978.
4. Alpert, J. N.; Armbrust, C. A.; et al. Glossopharyngeal neuralgia asystole and seizures. *Arch. Neurol.*, **34**:233–35, 1977.
5. Alvarez, M. R.; Bressudo L.; and Sabin, A. B. Paralytic syndromes associated with noninflammatory cytoplasmic or nuclear neuropathy. *J.A.M.A.*, **207**:1481–92, 1969.
6. Andersson, R. Familial amyloidosis with polyneuropathy. A clinical study based on patients living in Northern Sweden. *Acta Med. Scand.*, suppl. 590, 1976.
7. Andrade, C. Peculiar form of peripheral neuropathy; familiar atypical generalized amyloidosis with special involvement of peripheral nerves. *Brain*, **75**:408–27, 1952.
8. Baleriaux, D.; Mortelmans, L. L.; et al. Computed tomography for lesions of the craniovertebral region. *Neuroradiology*, **13**:59–61, 1977.

9. Barricks, M. E.; Traviesa, D. B.; et al. Ophthalmoplegia in cranial arteritis. *Brain,* **100:**209–21, 1977.

10. Bastlaensen, L. A. K.; Jaspar, H. H. J.; et al. Chronic progressive external ophthalmoplegia in a heredo-ataxia. Neurogenic or myogenic? *Acta Neurol. Scand.,* **56:**483–507, 1977.

11. Beaver, D. L.; Moses, H. L.; and Ganote, C. E. Electron microscopy of trigeminal ganglion; III trigeminal neuralgia. *Arch. Pathol.,* **79:**571–82, 1965.

12. Becker, H.; Grau, H.; et al. The base of skull: A comparison of computed and conventional tomography. *J. Computer Assisted Tomogr.,* **2:**113–18, 1978.

13. Behan, P. O.; Lessell, S.; and Roche, M. Optic neuritis in the Landry-Guillain-Barré-Strohl syndrome. *Br. J. Ophthalmol.,* **60:**58, 1976.

14. Berg, R.; Forsgren, M.; and Schiratzki, H. Acute facial palsy. Some clinical and virological observations. *Acta Otolaryngol.,* **81:**462–67, 1976.

15. Bergan, J. J.; and Conn, J. Sympathectomy for pain relief. *Med. Clin. North Am.,* **52:**147–59, 1968.

16. Berry, H.; and Richardson, P. M. Common peroneal nerve palsy: A clinical and electrophysiological review. *J. Neurol. Neurosurg. Psychiat.,* **39:**1162–71, 1976.

17. Boghen, D.; Filiatrault, R.; and Descaries, L. Myokymia and facial contractures in brain stem tuberculosis. *Neurology* (Minneap.), **27:**270–72, 1977.

17a. Boghen, D. R.; and Glaser, J. S. Ischemic optic neuropathy. The clinical profile and natural history. *Brain,* **98:**689–708, 1975.

18. Bradley, W. G.; Lassman, L. P.; Pearce, G. W.; and Walton, J. N. The neuromyopathy of vincristine in man. Clinical, electrophysiological and pathological studies. *J. Neurol. Sci.,* **10:**107–31, 1970.

19. Brown, M. J.; Martin, J. R.; and Asbury, A. K. Painful diabetic neuropathy: Morphometric study. *Arch. Neurol.,* **33:**164–71, 1976.

20. Bruyn, G. W.; and Went, L. N. A sex-linked heredo-degenerative neurological disorder, associated with Leber's optic atrophy. Part 1. Clinical studies. *J. Neurol. Sci.,* **1:**59–80, 1964.

21. Cabanis, E. A.; Salvolini, U.; et al. Computed tomography of the optic nerve. Part 11. Size and shape modifications in papilledema. *J. Computer Assisted Tomogr.,* **2:**150–55, 1978.

22. Caldwell, J. B. H.; Howard, R. O.; and Riggs, L. A. Dominant juvenile optic atrophy. A study in two families and review of hereditary disease in childhood. *Arch. Ophthalmol.,* **85:**133–47, 1971.

23. Calvin, W. H.; Loeser, J. D.; and Howe, J. F. A neurophysiological theory for the pain mechanism of tic douloureux. *Pain,* **3:**147–54, 1977.

24. Campbell, A. M. G.; and Hoffman, H. L. Sensory radicular neuropathy associated with muscle wasting in two cases. *Brain,* **87:**67–74, 1964.

25. Capistrant, T. D. Thoracic outlet syndrome in whiplash injury. *Ann. Surg.,* **185:**175–78, 1977.

26. Chawla, J. C.; and Falconer, M. A. Glossopharyngeal and vagal neuralgia. *Br. Med. J.,* **3:**529–31, 1967.

27. Chiu, W. S. The syndrome of retroperitoneal hemorrhage and lumbar plexus neuropathy during anticoagulant therapy. *South. M. J.,* **69:**595–99, 1976.

28. Christensen, S.; Dollerup, E.; and Jensen, S. E. Idiopathic hyperlipaemia, latent diabetes mellitus and severe neuropathy. *Acta Med. Scand.,* **161:**57–68, 1958.

29. Cohen, A. S., and Benson, M. D. Amyloid neuropathy. In Dyck, P. J.; Thomas, P. K.; and Lambert, E. H. (eds.). *Peripheral Neuropathy,* Vol. 11. Saunders, Philadelphia, 1975, pp. 1067–91.

30. Condon, J. R.; Reith, S. B. M.; Nassim, J. R.; Millard, F. J. C.; Hilb, A.; and Stainthorpe, E. M. Treatment of Paget's disease of bone with mithramycin. *Br. Med. J.,* **1:**421–23, 1971.

31. Court, J. E., and Kase, C. S. Treatment of tic douloureux with a new anticonvulsant (clonezepam). *J. Neurol. Neurosurg. Psychiat.,* **39:**297–99, 1976.

32. Cracchiolo, A.; and Marmor, L. Peripheral entrapment neuropathies. *J.A.M.A.,* **204:**431–34, 1968.

33. Crompton, J. L.; and Keith, C. G. Giant intracavernous aneurysm. Rare cause of isolated sixth cranial nerve palsy in a child. *Med. J. Aust.,* **2:**342–43, 1976.

34. Davidson, D. L. W.; and Jellinek, E. H. Hypertension and papilledema in the Guillain-Barré syndrome. *J. Neurol. Neurosurg. Psychiat.,* **40:**144–48, 1977.

35. Davies, M. G.; Marks, R.; et al. Epidermal abnormalities in Refsum's disease. *Br. J. Dermatol.,* **97:**401–406, 1977.

36. Davis, J. L.; Lewis, S. B.; et al. Peripheral diabetic neuropathy treated with amitriptyline and fluphenazine. *J.A.M.A.,* **238:**2291–92, 1977.

37. Dawker, R. P. R. Development and therapeutic uses of topical 5 per cent idoxuridine (IDU). *Scott. Med. J.,* **22:**310–13, 1977.

38. Dayan, A. D.; Ogul, E.; and Graveson, G. S. Polyneuritis and herpes zoster. *J. Neurol. Neurosurg. Psychiat.,* **35:**170–75, 1972.

39. Deafness after topical neomycin. Editorial. *Br. Med. J.,* **4:**181–82, 1969.

40. Dhaliwal, G. S.; Schlagenhauff, R. E.; and Megahed, S. M. Acute femoral neuropathy induced by oral anticoagulation. *Dis. Nerv. Syst.,* **37:**539–41, 1976.

41. Dolman, C. L.; and Allan, B. M. Relapsing hypertrophic neuritis. *Arch. Neurol.,* **28:**351–53, 1973.

42. Dorfman, L. J.; Nickoskelainen, E.; et al. Visual evoked potentials in Leber's hereditary optic atrophy. *Ann. Neurol.,* **1:**565–68, 1977.

43. Dowling, P.; and Cook, S. Epstein-Barr virus (EBU) antibodies in Guillain-Barré syndrome (GBS). *Clin. Res.,* **22:**440, 1974.

44. Duara, R.; Heathfield, K. W. G.; and Stewart, I. E. T. Epilepsy in Paget's disease of the skull. *Br. Med. J.,* **1:**214–15, 1978.

45. Dyke, P. J.; and Lambert, E. H. Dissociated sensation in amyloidosis: compound action potentials, quantitative histologic and teased-fiber and electron microscopic studies of sural nerve biopsies. *Arch. Neurol.,* **20:**490–507, 1969.

46. Eberle, E.; Brink, J.; et al. Early predictors of

incomplete recovery in children with Guillain-Barré polyneuritis. *J. Pediatr.,* **86:**356–59, 1975.

47. Eckman, P. B.; Perlstein, G.; and Altrocchi, P. H. Ulnar neuropathy in bicycle riders. *Arch. Neurol.,* **32:**130–31, 1975.

48. Eisen, A.; and Humphrey, P. Guillain-Barré syndrome: Clinical and electrodiagnostic study of 25 cases. *Arch. Neurol.,* **30:**438–43, 1974.

49. Ekbom, K. A.; and Westerberg, C. E. Carbamazepine in glossopharyngeal neuralgia. *Arch. Neurol.,* **14:**595–96, 1966.

50. Eldjarn, L.; Try, K.; Ackman, R. G.; and Hooper, S. N. Different ratios of the LDD and DDD diastereoisomers of phytanic acid in patients with Refsum's disease. *Biochim. Biophys. Acta,* **164:**94–100, 1968.

51. Eldjarn, L.; Try, K.; and Stokke, O. Studies on the biochemical defect in heredopathia atactica polyneuritiformis (Refsum's disease). *Pathol. Eur.,* **3:**459–67, 1968.

52. Ellenberg, M. Diabetic neuropathy of the upper extremities. *J. Mount Sinai Hosp.,* **35:**134–48, 1968.

53. Engel, W. K.; Dorman, J. D.; Levy, R. I.; and Fredrickson, D. S. Neuropathy in Tangier disease; x-lipoprotein deficiency manifesting as familial recurrent neuropathy and intestinal lipid storage. *Arch. Neurol.,* **17:**1–9, 1967.

54. Eversmann, W. W., Jr.; and Ritsick, J. A. Intraoperative changes in motor nerve conduction latency in carpal tunnel syndrome. *J. Hand Surg.,* **3:**77–81, 1978.

54a. Fabinyi, G. C. A., and Adams, C. B. T. Hemifacial spasm: Treatment by posterior fossa surgery. *J. Neurol. Neurosurg. Psychiatry,* **41:**829–33, 1978.

55. Fessel, W. J. Fat disorders and peripheral neuropathy. *Brain,* **94:**531–40, 1971.

56. Finelli, P. F. Anterior interosseus nerve syndrome following cutdown catheterization. *Ann. Neurol.,* 205–206, 1977.

56a. Fejlink, W. B.; Bijroet, O. L.; et al. Treatment of Paget's disease with (3 amino-1-hydroxy propylidene)-1,-biphosphonate (A.P.D.). *Lancet,* **1:**799–803, 1979.

57. Frohnert, P. P.; and Sheps, S. G. Long-term follow-up of periarteritis nodosa. *Am. J. Med.,* **43:**8–14, 1967.

58. Galvin, R. J.; Heron, J. R.; and Regan, D. Subclinical optic neuropathy in multiple sclerosis. *Arch. Neurol.,* **34:**666–70, 1977.

59. Galvin, R. J.; Regan, D.; and Heron, J. R. Impaired temporal resolution of vision after acute retrobulbar neuritis. *Brain,* **99:**255–68, 1976.

59a. Gibberd, F. B.; Billimoria, J. D.; et al. Heredopathia atactica polyneuritiformis (Refsum's disease) treated by diet and plasma exchange. *Lancet,* **1:**575–78, 1979.

60. Gilleatt, R. W. Thoracic outlet compression syndrome. *Br. Med. J.,* **1:**1274, 1976.

61. Gilroy, J.; Meyer, J. S.; Bauer, R. B.; Vulpe, M.; and Greenwood, D. Clinical biochemical and neurophysiological studies of chronic interstitial hypertrophic polyneuropathy. *Am. J. Med.,* **40:**368–83, 1966.

62. Gjores, J. E.; Svendler, C. A.; and Todoreskov, R. Thrombosis of the subclavian vein—a feature of the thoracic outlet syndrome. *Acta Clin. Scand.* (suppl.), **465:**78–79, 1976.

63. Gold, G. N.; and Hogenhuis, L. A. H. Hypertrophic interstitial neuropathy and cataracts. *Neurology* (Minneap.), **18:**526–33, 1968.

64. Goodall, J. A. D.; Kosmidis, J. C.; and Geddes, A. M. Effect of corticosteroids on course of Guillain-Barré syndrome. *Lancet,* **1:**524–26, 1974.

65. Gould, E. S.; Bird, A. C.; et al. Treatment of optic neuritis by retrobulbar injection of triamcinolone. *Br. Med. J.,* **1:**1495–97, 1977.

66. Gould, J. S.; and Wissinger, H. A. Carpal tunnel syndrome in pregnancy. *South. Med. J.,* **71:**144–45, 1978.

67. Guiloff, R. J.; and Sherratt, R. M. Sensory conduction in medial planter nerve, normal values, clinical applications and a comparison with the sural and upper limb sensory nerve action potentials in peripheral neuropathy. *J. Neurol. Neurosurg. Psychiat.,* **40:**1168–81, 1977.

68. Gutmann, L. Median ulnar nerve communications and carpal tunnel syndrome. *J. Neurol. Neurosurg. Psychiat.,* **40:**982–86, 1977.

69. Hahn, F. W.; Martin, J. T.; and Lillie, J. C. Vocal-cord paralysis with endotracheal intubation. *Arch. Otolaryngol.,* **92:**226–29, 1970.

70. Hammerschlag, S. B.; Wolpert, S. M.; and Carter, B. L. Computed tomography of the skull base. *J. Computer Assisted Tomogr.,* **1:**75–80, 1977.

71. Hawkes, C. H.; Jefferson, J. M.; et al. Hypertrophic mononeuropathy. *J. Neurol. Neurosurg. Psychiat.,* **37:**76–81, 1974.

72. Haymaker, W.; and Kernohan, J. W. The Landry-Guillain-Barré syndrome; clinicopathologic report of 50 fatal cases and critique of literature. *Medicine,* **28:**59–141, 1959.

73. Heller, G. L.; and DeJong, R. N. Treatment of the Guillain-Barré syndrome. Use of corticotropin and glucocorticoids. *Arch. Neurol.,* **8:**179–93, 1963.

74. Henderson, L. D.; Herbert, P. N.; et al. Abnormal concentration and anomalous distribution of apolipoprotein A-1 in Tangier disease. *Metabolism,* **27:**165–73, 1978.

75. Henken, R. I.; Larson, A. L.; and Powell, R. D. Hypogeusia, dysgeusia, hyposmia and dysosmia following influenza-like infection. *Ann. Otol. Rhinol. Laryngol.,* **84:**672–82, 1975.

76. Henken, R. I.; and Patten, B. M. A syndrome of acute zinc loss, cerebellar dysfunction, mental changes, anorexia and taste and smell dysfunction. *Arch. Neurol.,* **32:**745–51, 1975.

77. Hepler, R. S. Adie's tonic pupil. *Trans. Am. Acad. Ophthalmol. Otolaryngol.,* **83:**843–46, 1977.

78. Hesse, R. J. Herpes zoster ophthalmicus associated with delayed retinal thrombophlebitis. *Am. J. Ophthalmol.,* **84:**329–31, 1977.

79. Howe, J. F.; Loeser, J. D.; and Black, R. G. Percutaneous radiofrequency trigeminal gangliolysis in the treatment of tic douloureux. *West J. Med.,* **124:**351–56, 1976.

80. Howe, J. F.; Loeser, J. D.; and Calvin, W. H.

Impulses reflected from the dorsal root ganglia and focal nerve injuries. *Brain Res.*, **116**:139–44, 1976.

81. Jamshedi, A.; and Masroor, M. Glossopharyngeal neuralgia with cardiac syncope. *Arch. Intern. Med.*, **136**:843–45, 1976.

82. Janetta, P. J. Microsurgical approach to the trigeminal nerve for tic doloureux. *Prog. Neurol. Surg.*, **7**:180–200, 1975.

83. Jellenek, E. H.; and Tulloch, W. S. Herpes zoster with dysfunction of bladder and anus. *Lancet*, **2**:1219–22, 1976.

84. Johnson, B. L.; and Wisotzkey, H. M. Neuroretinitis associated with herpes simplex encephalitis in an adult. *Am. J. Ophthalmol.*, **83**:481–89, 1977.

85. Keane, J. R. Lid lag in the Guillain-Barré syndrome. *Arch. Neurol.*, **32**:478–79, 1975.

86. Kemble, K. Electrodiagnosis of the carpal tunnel syndrome. *J. Neurol. Neurosurg. Psychiat.*, **31**:23–27, 1968.

87. Kimura, J. Proximal versus distal slowing of motor nerve conduction velocity in the Guillain-Barré syndrome. *Ann. Neurol.*, **3**:344–50, 1978.

88. King, D.; and Asby, P. Conduction velocity in the proximal segments of a motor nerve in the Guillain-Barré syndrome. *J. Neurol. Neurosurg. Psychiat.*, **39**:538–44, 1976.

89. Kunc, Z. Treatment of essential neuralgia of the 9th nerve by selective tractotomy. *J. Neurosurg.*, **23**:494–500, 1965.

90. Lasselles, R. G.; Mohr, P. D.; et al. The thoracic outlet syndrome. *Brain*, **100**:601–12, 1977.

91. Leeming, R. Varicella-zoster virus and facial palsy. *J. Laryngol. Otol.*, **90**:365–71, 1976.

92. Lisak, R. P.; Mitchell, M.; et al. Guillain-Barré syndrome and Hodgkin's disease. Three cases with immunological studies. *Ann. Neurol.*, **1**:72–78, 1977.

93. Loeser, J. D. What to do about tic doloureux. *J.A.M.A.*, **239**:1153–55, 1978.

94. Loeser, J. D.; Calvin, W. H.; and Howe, J. F. Pathophysiology of trigeminal neuralgia. *Clin. Neurosur.*, **24**:527–37, 1976.

95. Loewenfeld, I. E.; and Thompson, H. S. The tonic pupil: A re-evaluation. *Am. J. Ophthalmol.*, **63**:46–87, 1967.

96. Lugnegard, H.; Walheim, G.; and Wennberg, A. Operative treatment of ulnar nerve neuropathy in the elbow region. *Acta Orthop. Scand.*, **48**:168–76, 1977.

97. Mair, I. W. S.; and Flugsrud, L. B. Peripheral facial palsy and herpes zoster infection. *J. Laryngol. Otol.*, **90**:373–79, 1976.

97a. Maroon, J. C.; Lunsford, L. D.; and Deeb, Z. L. Hemifacial spasm due to aneurysmal compression of the facial nerve. *Arch. Neurol.*, **35**:545–46, 1978.

98. Mars, H.; Lewis, L. A.; Robertson, A. L., Jr.; Batkus, A.; and Williams, G. H., Jr. Familial hypo-beta-lipoproteinemia: A genetic disorder of lipid metabolism with nervous system involvement. *Am. J. Med.*, **46**:886–900, 1969.

99. Marshall, P. C.; and Rosman, N. P. Symptomatic trigeminal neuralgia in a 5 year old child. *Pediatrics*, **60**:331–33, 1977.

100. Martin, J.; Gaspeird, D. J.; et al. Vascular manifes-

101. Mathew, N. T.; Meyer, J. S.; et al. Hyperlipidemic neuropathy and dementia. *Eur. Neurol.*, **14**:370–82, 1976.

102. Mathews, W. B. Facial myokymia. *J. Neurol. Neurosurg. Psychiat.*, **29**:35–39, 1966.

103. May, M.; Wette, R.; et al. The use of steroids in Bell's palsy. A prospective controlled study. *Laryngoscope*, **86**:1111–12, 1976.

104. McFarland, H. R.; and Heller, G. L. Guillain-Barré disease complex. A statement of diagnostic criteria and analysis of 100 cases. *Arch. Neurol.*, **14**:196–201, 1966.

105. Miller, H. Facial paralysis. *Br. Med. J.*, **3**:815–19, 1967.

106. Miller, H. Pain in the face. *Br. Med. J.*, **2**:577–80, 1968.

107. Miller, N. R. Solitary oculomotor nerve palsy in childhood. *Am. J. Ophthalmol.*, **83**:106–11, 1977.

108. Miller, R. G.; Nielsen, S. L.; and Sumner, A. J. Hereditary sensory neuropathy and tonic pupils. *Neurology* (Minneap.), **26**:931–35, 1976.

109. Morales, F.; Albert, P.; et al. Glossopharyngeal and vagal neuralgia secondary to vascular compression of the nerves. *Surg. Neurol.*, **8**:431–33, 1977.

110. Nagashina, C.; Sakaguchi, A.; et al. Cardiovascular complications on upper vagal rootlet section for glossopharyngeal neuralgia. *J. Neurosurg.*, **44**:248–53, 1976.

111. Nakano, K. K.; Lundergan, C.; and Okohiro, M. M. Anterior interosseous nerve syndromes. *Arch. Neurol.*, **34**:477–80, 1977.

112. Neagoy, D. R.; and Dohn, D. F. Hemifacial spasm secondary to vascular. *Cleveland Clin. Quart.*, **41**:205–14, 1974.

113. Neblett, C.; and Ehni, G. Medical epicondylectomy for ulnar palsy. *J. Neurosurg.*, **32**:55–62, 1970.

114. Nikoshelainen, E.; Sogg, R. L.; et al. The early phase in Leber's hereditary optic atrophy. *Arch. Ophthalmol.*, **95**:969–78, 1977.

115. Nord, E.; Weinberger, A.; et al. Motor paralysis complicating herpes zoster. *Dermatologia*, **154**:301–304, 1977.

116. Novak, D. J.; and Johnson, K. P. Relapsing idiopathic polyneuritis during pregnancy. Immunologic aspects and literature review. *Arch. Neurol.*, **28**:219–23, 1973.

117. Olarte, M.; and Adams, D. Accessory nerve palsy. *J. Neurol. Neurosurg. Psychiat.*, **40**:1113–16, 1977.

118. Olta, M.; Ellefson, R. D.; et al. Hereditary sensory neuropathy type II. *Arch. Neurol.*, **29**:23–37, 1973.

119. Osler, L. D.; and Sidell, A. D. The Guillain-Barré syndrome; the need for exact diagnostic criteria. *N. Engl. J. Med.*, **262**:964–69, 1960.

120. Petajan, J. H.; Danforth, R. C.; D'Allesio, D.; and Lucas, G. J. Progressive sudomotor denervation and Adie's syndrome. *Neurology* (Minneap.) **15**:172–76, 1965.

121. Prateri, R.; Freeman, F. R.; and Lowery, J. L. Herpes zoster ophthalmicus with contralateral hemiplegia. *Arch. Neurol.*, **34**:640–41, 1977.

122. Pulec, J. L. Geniculate neuralgia: Diagnosis and

tations of the thoracic outlet syndrome. *Arch. Surg.*, **111**:779–82, 1976.

surgical management. *Laryngoscope*, **86**:955–64, 1976.

123. Purcell, J. J.; Krachmer, J. H.; and Thompson, H. S. Corneal sensation in Adie's syndrome. *Am. J. Ophthalmol.*, **84**:496–500, 1977.

124. Raff, M. C.; Sangalang, V.; and Asbury, A. K. Ischemic mononeuropathy multiplex associated with diabetes mellitus. *Arch. Neurol.*, **18**:487–99, 1968.

125. Raman, P. T.; and Taori, G. M. Prognostic significance of electrodiagnostic studies in the Guillain-Barré syndrome. *J. Neurol. Neurosurg. Psychiat.*, **39**:163–70, 1976.

126. Rava, H. The Landry-Guillain-Barré syndrome; survey and a clinical report of 127 cases. *Acta Neurol. Scand.* **43**:Suppl. 30, 1947.

127. Refsum, S. Heredopathia atactica polyneuritiformis. *Saertrykk av Tiddsskrift laegeforening*, **5**:445–50, 1967.

128. Refsum, A.; and Eldjarn, L. Heredopathia atactica polyneuritiformis—an inborn defect in the metabolism of branched-chain fatty acids. *Zukunst du Neurologie*, 36–45. George Thieme, Stuttgart, 1967.

129. Regan, D.; Milner, B. A.; and Heron, J. R. Delayed visual perception and delayed visual evoked potentials in the spinal form of multiple sclerosis and in retrobulbar neuritis. *Brain*, **99**:43–66, 1976.

130. Rhodes, A. R. Herpes zoster and neoplastic disease. *J.A.M.A.*, **236**:2174–75, 1976.

131. Richards, R. L. Causalgia. *Arch. Neurol.*, **16**:339–50, 1967.

132. Richardson, J. E.; and Hamilton, W. Diabetes insipidus, diabetes mellitus, optic atrophy and deafness. 3 cases of "DIDMOAD" syndrome. *Dis. Child.*, **52**:796–98, 1977.

133. Rockliff, B. W.; and Davis, E. H. Controlled sequential trials of carbamazepine in trigeminal neuralgia. *Arch. Neurol.*, **15**:129–36, 1966.

134. Ryan, W. G.; Schwartz, T. B.; and Northrop, G. Experiences in the treatment of Paget's disease of bone with mithramycin. *J.A.M.A.*, **213**:1153–57, 1970.

135. Sandbank, U.; Bechar, M.; and Bornstein, B. Hyperlipemic polyneuropathy. *Acta Neuropath. (Berl.)*, **19**:290–300, 1971.

136. Sandbank, U.; and Bubis, J. J. Hyperlipaemic neuropathy. Experimental study. *Brain*, **96**:355–58, 1973.

137. Schmidek, H. H. Neurologic and neurosurgical sequelae of Paget's disease of bone. *Clin. Orthop.*, **127**:70–77, 1977.

138. Schwartz, J. F.; Rowland, L. P.; Eder, H.; Marks, P. A.; Osserman, E. F.; Hirschberg, E.; and Anderson, H. Bassen-Kornzweig syndrome; deficiency of serum x-lipoprotein. *Arch. Neurol.*, **8**:438–54, 1963.

139. Shahrokhi, F.; Chiappa, K. H.; and Young, R. R. Pattern shift visual evoked responses. Two hundred patients with optic neuritis and/or multiple sclerosis. *Arch. Neurol.*, **35**:65–71, 1978.

140. Shai, F.; Baker, R. K.; and Wallach, S. The clinical and metabolic effects of porcine calcium on Paget's disease of bone. *J. Clin. Invest.*, **50**:1927–40, 1971.

141. Simon, H.; Gryska, P. F.; and Carlson, D. H. The thoracic outlet syndrome as a cause of aneurysm formation. *South. Med. J.*, **70**:1282–84, 1977.

142. Smith, R.; Russell, R. G. G.; and Bishop, M. Diphosphorates and Paget's disease of bone. *Lancet*, **1**:945–47, 1971.

143. Stallworth, J. M.; Quinn, G. J.; and Acken, A. F. Is rib resection necessary for relief of thoracic outlet syndrome. *Ann. Surg.*, **185**:8581–92, 1977.

144. Sullivan, R. L., and Reeves, A. G. Normal cerebrospinal fluid protein, increased intracranial pressure and the Guillain-Barré syndrome. *Ann. Neurol.*, **1**:108–109, 1977.

145. Sundaresan, N.; Noroha, A.; et al. Oculomotor palsy as initial manifestation of myeloma. *J.A.M.A.*, **238**:2052–53, 1977.

146. Sunderland, S. Pain mechanisms in causalgia. *J. Neurol. Neurosurg. Psychiat.*, **39**:471–80, 1976.

147. Sunderland, S. Nerve lesion in the carpal tunnel syndrome. *J. Neurol. Neurosurg. Psychiat.*, **39**:615–26, 1976.

148. Sweet, W. H. Control of pain by direct electrical stimulation of peripheral nerves. *Clin. Neurosurg.*, **23**:103–11, 1975.

149. Swick, H. M.; and McQuillen, M. P. The use of steroids in the treatment of idiopathic polyneuritis. *Neurology* (Minneap.), **26**:205–12, 1976.

150. Taylor, P. H.; Gray, K.; et al. Glossopharyngeal neuralgia with syncope. *J. Laryngol. Otol.*, **91**:859–68, 1977.

151. Tenser, R. B. Myokymia and facial contraction in multiple sclerosis. *Arch. Intern. Med.*, **136**:81–83, 1976.

152. Tew, J. M., Jr.; Lockwood, P.; and Mayfield, F. H. Treatment of trigeminal neuralgia in the aged by a simplified surgical approach (percutaneous electrocoagulation). *J. Am. Geriatr. Soc.*, **23**:426–30, 1975.

153. Vassalos, E.; Prevedourakis, C.; and Parachopoulou-Prevedouvaki, P. Brachial plexus paralysis in the newborn. *Am. J. Obstet. Gynecol.*, **101**:554–56, 1968.

154. Waldiman, I., and Brain, A. I. Femoral neuropathy secondary to iliac artery aneurysm. *South. Med. J.*, **70**:1243–44, 1977.

155. Wassenstrom, W. R.; and Starr, A. Facial myokymia in the Guillain-Barré syndrome. *Arch. Neurol.*, **34**:576–77, 1977.

156. Watson, P.; and Ashby, P. Brachial plexus neuropathy associated with infectious mononucleosis. *Can. Med. Assoc. J.*, **114**:758–59, 1976.

157. Weikers, N. J.; and Mattson, R. H. Acute paralytic brachial neuritis. *Neurology* (Minneap.)., **19**:1153–58, 1969.

158. Wells, J.; and Templeton, J. Femoral neuropathy associated with anticoagulant therapy. *Clin. Orthop.*, **124**:155–59, 1977.

159. Whitaker, J. N.; Sciabbarrusi, J.; et al. Serum immunoglobulin and complement C3 levels: Study in adults with idiopathic chronic polyneuropathies and motor neuron disease. *Neurology* (Minneap.), **23**:1164–73, 1973.

160. Willerson, D., Jr.; Aaberg, T.; et al. Unusual presentation of acute toxoplasmosis. *Br. J. Ophthalmol.*, **61**:693–98, 1977.

161. Wilson, J. Leber's hereditary optic atrophy some

clinical and aetiological considerations. *Brain,* **86:**347–62, 1963.

162. Wilson, J. Skeletal manifestations in Leber's hereditary optic atrophy. A possible disorder of cyanide metabolism. *Ann. Phys. Med.,* **8:**91–95, 1965–66.

163. Wold, S. M.; Wagner, J. H.; et al. Treatment of Bell's palsy with prednisone: A prospective, randomized study. *Neurology* (Minneap.), **28:**158–61, 1978.

163a. Wolf, S. M.; Wagner, J. H.; et al. Treatment of Bell's palsy with prednisone: a prospective randomized study. *Neurology* (Minneap.), **28:**158–61, 1978.

164. Woodhouse, N. J. Y.; Reiner, M.; Bordier, Ph.; Kalu, D. N.; Fisher, M.; Foster, G. V.; Joplin, G. F.; and MacIntyre, I. Human calcitonin in the treatment of Paget's bone disease. *Lancet,* **1:**1139–43, 1971.

165. Woods, W. W. Thoracic outlet syndrome. *West. J. Med.,* **128:**9–12, 1978.

166. Wray, S. H. Neuro-ophthalmologic manifestations of pituitary and parasellar lesions. *Clin. Neurosurg.,* **24:**86–117, 1976.

167. Wybar, K. Optic atrophy in childhood. *Proc. Roy. Soc. Med.,* **69:**451–59, 1976.

168. Wynne-Stewart, E. G. Iatrogenic femoral neuropathy. *Br. Med. J.,* **1:**263, 1976.

169. Yalaburgi, S. B.; and Mistry, P. K. Bell's palsy—varicella zoster, and meningitis. *J. Laryngol. Otol.,* **91:**1073–75, 1977.

170. Yamashita, J.; Asato, R.; et al. Abducens nerve palsy as initial symptom of trigeminal schwannoma. *J. Neurol. Neurosurg. Psychiat.,* **40:**1190–97, 1977.

12 MUSCLE DISEASES

This chapter is concerned with diseases that affect voluntary muscles and the neuromuscular junction. The term "myopathy" is used to describe many of these conditions and may be defined as a disorder characterized by abnormal function of muscle in which there is no evidence of denervation on clinical, histologic, or electrical studies. The abnormality, whether biochemical, pathologic, or electrophysiologic, is presumed to be in the muscle fiber or the surrounding interstitial tissue.

Some Considerations in the Diagnosis of Weakness and Wasting of Muscle

Both myopathic and neurogenic diseases show common symptoms of weakness and wasting of muscle. The weakness and wasting are usually proximal in distribution in myopathic conditions

and generalized or distal in neurogenic conditions, although there are rare exceptions to this statement.

In upper motor neuron lesions weakness is not accompanied by wasting. The affected muscles show an increase in tone with increased stretch reflexes and the occasional presence of clonus and extensor plantar responses.

Destruction of anterior horn cells (lower motor neurons) results in weakness, wasting, and fasciculations. The stretch reflexes are depressed in pure anterior horn cell disease (e.g., spinal muscular atrophy), but the stretch reflexes are increased if there is a concomitant upper motor neuron lesion (e.g., amyotrophic lateral sclerosis).

Damage to a single motor nerve root produces weakness, wasting, and, occasionally, fasciculations in the corresponding myotome with depression of the stretch reflex elicited in the involved muscles (e.g., pressure on a C_5 nerve root by a herniated disk results in weakness and wasting of the deltoid, supraspinatus, infraspinatus, biceps, and brachioradialis muscles with depression of the brachioradialis and biceps reflexes). If the sensory nerve root is involved, there will be sensory loss in the corresponding dermatome.

In predominantly motor types of peripheral neuropathy there are muscle weakness, flaccidity, and loss of stretch reflexes, followed by muscle wasting and relatively little sensory loss.

Diseases of the neuromuscular junction or muscle are associated with weakness, which may be:

1. Nonepisodic weakness.
2. Episodic weakness.

Nonepisodic weakness is usually progressive, is often seen in proximal muscles, and is not associated with recognizable precipitating factors. Nonepisodic weakness occurs in:

a. Myopathies in which there is an abnormality in the function of muscle fibers
b. Muscular dystrophies that are inherited progressive myopathies

Episodic weakness is transitory, lasting from a few hours to a few days, is often associated with identifiable precipitating factors, and is seen in the following conditions:

a. Primary and secondary periodic paralysis
b. Myasthenia gravis
c. Acute rhabdomyolysis
d. Paramyotonia congenita

In the majority of cases, a careful history and detailed physical examination will permit an accurate diagnosis. Further laboratory testing is usually a confirmatory procedure and includes biochemical procedures, electromyography, electrocardiography, and muscle biopsy.

Biochemical Procedures

A number of serum enzymes are increased in muscle diseases. These enzymes include serum aldolase, serum glutamic oxaloacetic transaminase, serum glutamic pyruvic transaminase, lactic dehydrogenase, and creatine phosphokinase. The elevated levels in the serum are usually due to leakage of the enzymes through defective muscle cell membranes. Elevated enzyme levels are found in the Duchenne type of muscular dystrophy, inflammatory myopathies, and acute rhabdomyolysis but may be normal or only slightly elevated

in the facioscapulohumeral and limb girdle types of muscular dystrophy. Serum creatine phosphokinase levels are by far the most sensitive of the tests of enzyme activity and are generally available in most clinical laboratories. Elevated serum creatine phosphokinase levels have also been reported in some cases of amyotrophic lateral sclerosis, spinomuscular atrophies, myasthenia gravis, and occasionally after exercise or intramuscular injection. However, serum creatine phosphokinase levels are usually at least 100 times normal values in the muscular dystrophies, while the levels do not usually exceed ten times normal values in other conditions. If a series of serum enzyme levels are measured and there is an associated elevation of SGOT and LDH, the disease process is almost certainly myopathic and not neurogenic.

Electromyography

In the early stages of a myopathic process, the motor unit potentials are of low amplitude and brief duration with abundant recruitment on minimal contraction. There are a moderate number of short-duration polyphasic motor unit potentials. These changes are indicative of diminished size or number of muscle fibers per motor unit. Fibrillations, although frequently seen in neurogenic atrophy, are also present in some patients with myopathies. In a progressive myopathic process, the patient has an increased difficulty in sustained voluntary contraction with the generation of few low-voltage potentials. Some areas may be electrically silent, and multiple sampling may be necessary to record a few potentials.

Electrocardiography

Evidence of heart disease has been found in a number of muscle diseases including myotonic dystrophy, Duchenne dystrophy, limb girdle dystrophy, and facioscapulohumeral dystrophy.[198] An electrocardiogram should be obtained on all cases during the initial evaluation of a myopathy.

Muscle Biopsy

Muscle biopsy is a relatively simple procedure used to provide a definitive diagnosis in patients with persistent muscle weakness. However, this is not the only indication for muscle biopsy. It may give information in systemic diseases without muscle weakness such as polyarteritis nodosa or sarcoidosis.

It is only possible to obtain maximum benefit from muscle biopsy if there is correct selection of muscles for biopsy. Two criteria should be followed:

1. The muscle biopsy should be taken from the muscle showing the most weakness when the condition has been present for a short time.
2. In chronic muscle weakness and wasting the least affected muscle should be selected for biopsy.

Muscle biopsies are usually performed under local anesthesia, using 1 per cent lidocaine or xylocaine without epinephrine as the anesthetic agent. Local anesthesia should be confined to the skin over the muscle and the muscle should not be infiltrated by the local anesthetic. The muscle specimen should be at least 2 cm by 2 cm in size, and the fibers should be arranged in parallel fashion. The specimen should be mounted in tragacanth gum and frozen within half an hour of obtaining the biopsy. Freezing is accomplished with liquid nitrogen at −160°C, which is extremely rapid and reduces the chances of artefact. The specimen is then transferred to a cryostat for sectioning.

Many histochemical stains have been used on muscle biopsy sections but most laboratories prefer hematoxylin and eosin, modified trichrome, ATPase, and other oxidative enzyme stains.

Information obtained by histochemical processes includes:

1. The ready identification of type 1 and type 2 fibers (Fig. 12–1).
2. Evidence of terminal nerve sprouting (reinnervation) by the presence of groupings of type 1 and type 2 fibers (Fig. 12–2).
3. Abnormal mitochondria can be stained to appear as "ragged red" fibers on light microscopy.
4. The absence of specific enzymes such as phosphorylase can be demonstrated.
5. Many specific muscle fiber–type diseases can be identified. Type 1 fibers are predominantly involved in myotonic dystrophy and type 2 fibers in myasthenia gravis.

Abnormal muscle biopsies are of three main types: neurogenic biopsies, myopathic biopsies, and biopsies with specific identifiable abnormalities.

1. Neurogenic abnormalities are seen in the spinal muscular atrophies such as infantile spinal

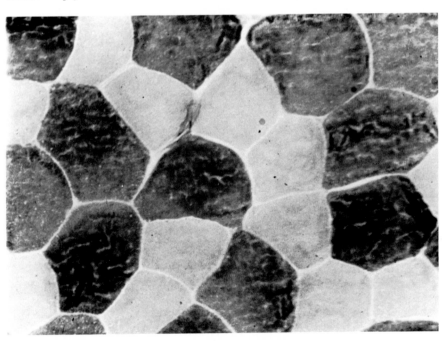

FIGURE 12–1.   Muscle biopsy of normal muscle showing two types of muscle fibers on staining by ATPase reaction at pH 9.4. Type I fibers show a lighter stain, while the darker-staining fibers are type II fibers. Normal mosaic pattern.

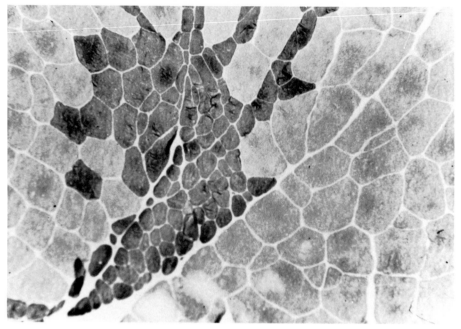

FIGURE 12-2. A muscle biopsy stained with ATPase reaction at pH 9.4 showing fiber type grouping. The normal mosaic pattern has been altered, and there is clumping of type I and type II fibers. This abnormality is seen after denervation when reinervation has taken place.

muscular atrophy (Werdnig-Hoffmann, familial spinal muscular atrophy of Kugelberg and Welander, motor neuron disease, and chronic neuropathies). Abnormal changes include the presence of angular fibers, pyknotic nuclear clumps, target fibers, type grouping (which suggests reinnervation), and type 1 fiber smallness with type 2 fiber hypertrophy.

2. Myopathic abnormalities are seen in Duchenne muscular dystrophy, facioscapulohumeral dystrophy, limb girdle dystrophy, and myotonic dystrophy. Myopathic changes also occur in polymyositis. The changes in myopathic biopsies include variations in fiber diameter, presence of many internal nuclei, degeneration of muscle fibers with phagocytosis by mononuclear cells, and poor differentiation of fiber types. There is a marked increase in endomysial and perimysial connective tissue. Myotonic dystrophy is characterized by type 1 muscle fiber atrophy, extensive proliferation of internal nuclei, and the presence of "ring benden" muscle fibers and "moth-eaten" fibers.

3. Biopsies with specific identifiable abnormalities

include myasthenia gravis which shows type 2 fiber atrophy and the presence of lymphorrhages, and periodic paralysis, which shows fiber atrophy and the presence of vacuoles in type 1 and type 2 fibers. The muscle in myophosphorylase deficiency (McArdle's disease) shows a negative histochemical reaction for phosphorylase. Many rare myopathies such as central core disease or nemaline myopathy show specific changes on muscle biopsy, which correspond to the name of the disease.

The Muscular Dystrophies

It is difficult to classify the muscular dystrophies because the pathogenesis is unknown. Any classification must, therefore, depend chiefly or solely on clinical history and observation.[92] The proposed classification outlined in Table 12-1 is based on that which has been generally accepted for the last two decades.[271, 283]

Duchenne Type of Muscular Dystrophy

The type of muscular dystrophy originally described by Duchenne is the most common form

TABLE 12–1

The Muscular Dystrophies

Type	Synonym or Eponym	Inheritance
A. *Without myotonia*		
1. Duchenne type of muscular dystrophy	Pseudohypertrophic muscular dystrophy	Sex-linked recessive or autosomal recessive
2. Benign X-linked muscular dystrophy	Becker type of muscular dystrophy	Sex-linked recessive
3. Facioscapulohumeral muscular dystrophy	Progressive atrophic myopathy of Landouzy and Dejerine	Autosomal dominant
4. Scapular peroneal muscular dystrophy	None	Autosomal dominant
5. Limb girdle muscular dystrophy	Erb	Autosomal recessive
6. Distal form of progressive muscular dystrophy	Distal form of Gowers'	Autosomal dominant
7. Ocular form of progressive muscular dystrophy	Ocular myopathy (Kiloh and Nevin)	Autosomal dominant
8. Oculopharyngeal muscular dystrophy	None	Autosomal dominant
B. *Associated with myotonia*		
9. Myotonia congenita	Thomsen's disease	Autosomal dominant
10. Paramyotonia congenita	None	Autosomal dominant
11. Myotonic dystrophy	None	Autosomal dominant

of progressive muscular dystrophy. It occurs predominantly in young males. Rare female cases have been described and in these cases the dystrophy tends to be less severe.[195, 286] The preponderance in young males indicates that inheritance is sex-linked recessive in type. However, there appears to be a number of sporadic cases, suggesting that there is a high mutation rate.

The occurrence of female cases of the Duchenne type of dystrophy may be explained by the Lyon hypothesis.[159] This suggests that a female carrier may develop inactive Barr bodies containing the normal X chromosome material, leaving the X chromosome carrying the dystrophic gene as the active chromosome in that cell.[103] Abiotrophy of the cells carrying the dystrophic gene might then occur, with the production of a slowly progressive dystrophy of muscles in the female.

Pathogenesis

The pathogenesis of the muscular dystrophies remains elusive but there are currently three hypotheses under active consideration at this time.[211]

1. The vascular theory postulates that an inadequate blood supply accounts for the degenerative changes in dystrophic muscle. An abnormal accumulation of catecholamines has been proposed in the intrafibrillar substance of muscle in muscular dystrophy. Such an accumulation would lead to vasoconstriction of capillaries and microinfarction of muscle fibers, which are subsequently replaced by collagen.[83]

2. The neurogenic theory is based on reports that the number of surviving motor units is decreased in muscular dystrophy. Since motor units are the basic elements of neural control of muscle fibers, the decrease in motor units implies a decrease in anterior horn cells, which are the motor neurons of the motor units.[171] The neurogenic theory suggests that muscular dystrophies are diseases of "sick" motor neurons.

3. The membrane theory suggests that there is a genetically determined abnormality in the surface membrane of the muscle fiber in the muscular dystrophies. The theory is supported by the leakage of muscle enzymes from the sarcoplasm through the muscle membrane into the serum in the muscular dystrophies.[241] The leakage of substances through the membrane appears to be selective and, since it is genetically determined, the membrane abnormality is present in known carriers. The membrane

abnormality is also present in erythrocytes in patients with muscular dystrophy.[158, 178]

Pathology

The muscle fibers of dystrophic muscle show marked variation in size. Many fibers show splitting and loss of cross-striations. Characteristically there is migration of sarcolemmal nuclei from their normal location at the periphery to the center of the fiber. Atrophy of muscle fibers appears to be haphazard in the affected muscles, and atrophic fibers eventually become replaced by fibrous tissue and fat. Necrosis of individual muscle fibers and abortive attempts at regeneration are now known to be more prominent than was thought in earlier descriptions of the histology of the disease. Necrotic fibers show bright eosinophilia with fragmentation of the sarcoplasm, which subsequently becomes infiltrated by histiocytes. Regenerating fibers are seen which show basophilia of cytoplasm as well as numerous enlarged central nuclei with prominent nucleoli. These changes are pronounced in early stages of the disease but become successively less so as the disease progresses and the muscle is replaced by fibrosis. Such changes may be expected to be absent in advanced atrophy of muscle. The heart is also involved in muscular dystrophy with atrophy of cardiac muscle and replacement by fibrous tissue. The histologic changes in the heart are similar to the changes seen in skeletal muscle.

Incidence, Prevalence, and Mutation Rate

The incidence of Duchenne type of progressive muscular dystrophy is 150 to 250 per million live births. The prevalence is 50 per million population, and the disease occurs in all races. About one third of the cases occur in families with similarly affected boys.

Clinical Features

The Duchenne type of progressive muscular dystrophy is the most severe form of muscular dystrophy and usually begins before the age of five years. The disease is usually not detected by the parents until the child begins to walk, and at this time the usual disability noted is "clumsiness" and "falling easily." The child then develops a characteristic type of waddling gait and, when placed prone on a carpet or floor, tends to "climb up himself" in order to assume the erect posture. These symptoms are evidence of the fact that the weakness begins in the muscles of the pelvic gir-

dle. The arm muscles are affected later, and weakness of the facial muscles may be seen in a very late stage of the disease.

Some 80 per cent of these children will show pseudohypertrophy of the muscles, particularly those of the calf. Unfortunately, there is relentless progression of muscular weakness, and most of these children become confined to a wheelchair by the age of ten. At this stage the respiratory reserve becomes decreased owing to weakness of the intercostal muscles and diaphragm.[27] The patient thereby becomes susceptible to repeated attacks of pneumonia. Cardiac involvement is almost invariably present, and, by the age of 20, heart failure and sudden death occur in 80 per cent of patients.[71] The remaining patients become severely disabled and usually die in their twenties. Rarely, cerebral embolism and anoxia from dystrophic heart disease may mimic a primary cerebral disorder and tend to confuse the diagnosis unless the cause is recognized.

The diagnosis of Duchenne type of muscular dystrophy is not difficult in the later stages but may present some problems in the young child. A characteristic feature of this condition is the pattern of muscle involvement. The initial weakness is found in the axial and proximal limb girdle muscles, with later involvement of the distal muscles. Characteristically, the pectorals, biceps, and brachioradialis muscles are weak, while the deltoids remain strong initially and become weaker at a later stage.

Mental Retardation. In recent years studies have indicated that boys with Duchenne muscular dystrophy have a mean IQ level that is lower than that of normal boys.[4] However, there does not seem to be any relation between the severity of the disease and the intelligence quotient.

Diagnostic Procedures

1. There is a marked elevation of serum muscle enzymes in the early stages of Duchenne muscular dystrophy. The abnormalities involve serum aldolase, serum glutamic oxaloacetic transaminase, serum glutamic pyruvic transaminase, lactic dehydrogenase, pyruvatekinase, and creatine phosphokinase.
2. There are electromyographic abnormalities in the affected muscle (p. 716).
3. The electrocardiogram shows a persistent tachycardia with a rate between 100 and 120 per minute in the majority of patients. The

R waves are of abnormally high voltage early in the disease. Later there is development of incomplete bundle branch block with high-voltage R waves. With progression of the disease, the high R waves tend to disappear, but incomplete bundle branch block persists. The Q waves have an abnormal appearance, and there is deviation of the S-T segment in severely disabled patients.[100]

4. Tests of pulmonary function show progressive deterioration in advanced cases.

Treatment

Numerous types of drugs have been subjected to therapeutic trials in patients with progressive muscular dystrophy without significant or reproducible success. There is no *specific* drug therapy for the muscular dystrophies at this time. However, supportive treatment should be directed as follows: the patient should be kept ambulatory as long as possible and treated at regular intervals in a well-organized physical therapy program. Bracing and orthopedic procedures may be used to prevent deformities.

When the patient becomes confined to a wheelchair, pulmonary and cardiac reserve is usually impaired. Many develop obesity owing to inactivity and excessive feeding beyond the normal caloric requirements. Respiratory tract infections should be actively treated with antibiotics. If pneumonia occurs, antibiotics, postural drainage, and oxygen should be administered and tracheotomy should be performed if there is any difficulty in handling secretions. Congestive heart failure should be treated with digitalization, diuretics, and low-salt diet. Fecal impaction may be a problem at this stage, and rectal examination should be performed at least once every three days in the severely debilitated patient to treat and prevent this complication.

Genetic Counseling

There have been some studies of mothers, sisters, and aunts of affected males who are carriers of Duchenne dystrophy. In any female carrier one X chromosome carries the abnormality for muscular dystrophy, but its activity is inhibited by the normal genetic influence exerted in the other X chromosome. In genetic counseling the following categories are used:[258]

1. Definite carrier: woman who has a son with Duchenne muscular dystrophy and also has an affected brother or maternal uncle, or has a sister whose son has the disease, or there are other male relatives in the female line of inheritance.
2. Probable carrier: mother who has two or more affected sons but has no other affected relatives.
3. Possible carrier: (a) mother of isolated case of Duchenne muscular dystrophy or (b) sister or other female relative of affected male with this disease.

Female carriers are usually unaffected clinically, but some of them have evidence on examination of minimal muscle weakness, and a few have been reported to show pseudohypertrophy. The majority of female carriers show significant elevation of serum pyruvate-kinase (PK) and creatine phosphokinase (CPK). The determination of elevated PK or CPK seems to be the most accurate biochemical study available at this time for the detection of carriers.[229a] Minimal muscle involvement may also be demonstrated by electromyography and muscle biopsy in some female carriers.

When a woman is a definite carrier, or when there are abnormal results on serum enzyme determinations, electromyography, or muscle biopsy, genetic counseling should be given and the family should be informed in simple terms that the condition has a sex-linked recessive form of inheritance.[70a] Theoretically, in any pregnancy, 50 per cent of the male offspring will probably develop the disease and 50 per cent of the female offspring will probably be carriers.

Becker Type of Muscular Dystrophy

This condition is a relatively benign form of muscular dystrophy that is inherited as a sex-linked recessive trait. The clinical features are somewhat similar to those seen in the Duchenne type of muscular dystrophy, but the progression of the disease is slower. The first signs occur after the age of five years, and the patient is still walking at the age of ten years. He may not lose the ability to walk for 25 years or more after the onset.[12] The weakness occurs predominantly in the muscles of the pelvic girdle with later involvement of the pectoral group of muscles. There is absence of or minimal cardiac involvement in most cases. Since the condition is fairly progressive with the possibility of very nearly normal activity until adult life, it may be transmitted by affected males through carrier daughters to their grandsons.

Facioscapulohumeral Muscular Dystrophy

This form of muscular dystrophy is inherited as an autosomal dominant trait. It occurs with equal frequency in males and females. It is a relatively benign form of muscular dystrophy, although moderately severe or severe forms do occur, and there is considerable variation in degree of involvement even among affected members of a family. The severe form may produce considerable disability in later life, but, in general, the condition is compatible with a normal life-span.

Etiology and Pathology

The etiology is unknown. Histopathologic changes in the affected muscles are similar to those described in the Duchenne type of muscular dystrophy (see p. 720), except that fatty replacement is rare and moderate fibrosis of muscle is more common.

Clinical Features

The disease usually begins with involvement of the lower facial muscles with inability to purse the lips or whistle, followed by involvement of the trapezius and of the sternal head of the pectoralis major. As the disease progresses, weakness and wasting of the muscles of the shoulder girdle become apparent, followed by an increase in lumbar lordosis and involvement of the spinal muscles. Finally, the pelvic muscles may be involved and there may be some weakness in the quadriceps. This leads to a "dromedary" or camel-backed type of gait due to the protrusion of the buttocks. Involvement of the face and girdle muscles is in sharp contrast to the normal appearance and strength of the distal muscles of the limbs. The disease usually begins in the second decade of life and slowly progresses, but spontaneous arrest of progression may occur at any time. In general, the prognosis for a useful life is good, although there is some variation in resulting disability.

Diagnostic Procedures

The involved muscles show electromyographic changes similar to those described in the Duchenne type of progressive muscular dystrophy. Electrocardiographic changes do not usually occur, respiratory function is normal or little reduced, and the serum enzymes pyruvate-kinase and creatine-phosphokinase are elevated in about 50 per cent of cases.[284a] A muscle biopsy should be obtained from an involved muscle.

Treatment

There is no specific treatment for this type of muscular dystrophy, but fortunately the disease rarely interferes with activity during the productive years. Patients usually have a normal life-span and the disability is rarely severe. A program of physical therapy will maintain muscle strength and limit disability.

Scapuloperoneal Muscular Dystrophy

The weakness and atrophy of scapuloperoneal distribution are part of a syndromic condition, which may be myopathic or neurogenic in origin. It has been described as a form of muscular dystrophy and appears to be inherited as an autosomal dominant or sex-linked recessive trait.[257] All types appear to run a benign course with onset in early childhood and slowly progressive muscular weakness and wasting, involving the proximal muscles of the upper limbs and shoulder girdle and distal muscles of the lower limbs.[280] Cardiac involvement may occur in adult life.[169] Electromyography and muscle biopsy will differentiate a neurogenic from a myopathic process.

Limb Girdle Type of Muscular Dystrophy (Juvenile Form of Erb)

This type of muscular dystrophy is inherited as an autosomal recessive trait. Some female cases described as having the Duchenne type of progressive muscular dystrophy may belong to this group.

Pathology

The typical changes of muscular dystrophy are apparent in the affected muscles (see p. 720).

Clinical Features

The onset is usually in the second or third decade of life. The initial complaint is weakness, which affects either the pelvic or shoulder girdle. Both areas are eventually affected, but the disease process may be confined to one or the other girdle for many years. When the pelvic girdle is involved, a typical waddling gait is seen. Wasting of the girdle muscles is striking when compared to the normal appearance and strength of the distal muscles of the limbs.

The disease usually begins in the second decade

of life and is slowly progressive, but spontaneous arrest may occur at any time. There may be involvement of the proximal lower limb muscles in the later stages of the disease, and the patient may complain of difficulty in rising from a sitting position. In a very advanced case there is weakness of the paraspinal muscles with a gradually increasing lordosis.

Diagnostic Procedures

Electromyography shows the characteristic findings seen in progressive muscular dystrophy when affected muscles are examined. Electrocardiographic abnormalities and cardiac symptoms have also been reported. The electrocardiogram may show the following changes:

1. A disturbance in rhythm and conduction with prolonged QRS complexes, first-degree heart block, and a right ventricular conduction defect.
2. Abnormal Q waves and T wave alteration.[197]

Elevation of serum enzymes occurs early in the disease.

Treatment

Treatment should be directed toward maintaining ambulation as long as possible. Physical therapy, orthopedic measures, and bracing may be necessary. If the patient becomes confined to a wheelchair, precautions (as outlined under the Duchenne type) should be followed, particularly in the prevention of respiratory infections and cardiac failure.

Distal Form of Progressive Muscular Dystrophy

This condition is relatively rare and appears to be inherited as an autosomal dominant trait, although many cases appear to be sporadic.

Pathology

The typical changes of muscular dystrophy are seen in the distally affected muscles of all four limbs.

Clinical Features

The disease occurs in adults and consists of chronic progressive wasting of the distal muscles of both upper and lower limbs. The hands may eventually become completely wasted and useless,

but the proximal muscles and the facial muscles are spared initially, although they may become involved later in the disease.

Diagnostic Procedures

Electromyographic changes compatible with muscular dystrophy are found in the affected muscle. Electrocardiographic and serum enzyme studies are within normal limits. Biopsy of the distal limb muscles shows changes characteristic of muscular dystrophy.

Prognosis

This is a relatively benign form of dystrophy and most patients are able to work in a sedentary occupation and complete a normal life-span.

Oculopharyngeal Myopathy

This condition is inherited as an autosomal dominant trait and presents with muscle weakness and wasting in the fourth or fifth decade. The earliest sign may be weakness and wasting of the fingers or feet, but some cases have presented with ptosis followed by facial weakness. There is progressive involvement of the masseters and bulbar muscles, fingers, hands, feet, and legs, and the patient ceases walking because of a bilateral foot drop.[221] The pathologic changes are those of a muscular dystrophy.

Ocular Form of Progressive Muscular Dystrophy

It is doubtful that an ocular form of muscular dystrophy or "ocular myopathy" exists as a distinct clinical entity. Ocular paresis may precede the appearance of abnormal clinical signs elsewhere and present as a spurious isolated ocular muscle disease, but the later appearance of additional features permits a more precise diagnosis in most cases.[48] The causes of ophthalmoplegia are listed in Table 12–2.

Myotonic Disorders: General Considerations

Myotonia is a clinical phenomenon characterized by sustained contraction of muscle following voluntary contraction, mechanical percussion by a hammer or similar instrument, or electrical stimulation of the muscle. Myotonia is commonly seen in:

TABLE 12–2

Causes of Ophthalmoplegia

1. *Hereditary and congenital*
   a. Congenital ptosis
   b. Congenital opthalmoplegias
2. *Neuronal ophthalmoplegias*
   a. Progressive supranuclear palsy (Steele-Richardson-Olszewski)
   b. Olivopontocerebellar degeneration (p. 206)
   c. Alzheimer's disease (p. 176)
   d. Dystonia musculorum deformans (p. 197)
   e. α-β-lipoproteinemia (p. 686)
   f. Werdnig-Hoffmann (p. 128)
   g. Kugelberg-Welander (p. 214)
   h. Ophthalmoplegia, retinitis, cardiopathy, and neuronal disorders (Kearns-Sayre syndrome)
   i. Möbius syndrome (p. 72)
3. *Peripheral neuropathies*
4. *Disorders of neuromuscular junction*
   a. Myasthenia gravis (p. 749)
   b. Botulism (p. 758)
5. *Myopathic ophthalmoplegias*
   a. Ocular muscular dystrophy
   b. Oculopharyngeal muscular dystrophy (p. 723)
   c. Myotonic dystrophy (p. 725)
   d. Chronic benign congenital myopathies (p. 728)
   e. Ophthalmoplegia in thyroid disease (p. 739)
   f. Ophthalmoplegia in glycogen storage and abnormal mitochondria (oculocraniosomatic disease with ragged red fibers)

1. Myotonia congenita
2. Paramytonia congenita
3. Myotonic dystrophy
4. Hyperkalemic periodic paralysis

Myotonia is believed to be the result of an abnormality in the membrane of the muscle fiber. In myotonic dystrophy the muscle fibers contain almost twice the normal concentration of sodium ions, suggesting that there is an increased permeability to sodium.[125] Drugs that tend to modify the passage of ions through the cell membrane, such as diphenylhydantoin, procainamide, and quinine, will modify or abolish myotonia.

Myotonia Congenita (Thomsen's Disease)

This condition may be conveniently classified with the muscular dystrophies although there is no evidence of muscle wasting. There is chronic hypertrophy in many cases. The pedigree of most families studied suggests an autosomal dominant and occasionally an autosomal recessive mode of inheritance.[114]

Etiology and Pathology

The etiology is a genetically determined abnormality of the membrane of the muscle fiber. Muscle biopsy shows atrophic fibers, increased internal nuclei, and fiber hypertrophy. The percentage of type 1 fibers is normal, but there is a complete absence of type 2B muscle fibers.[47]

Clinical Features

Disability usually begins in infancy or childhood, and there is usually some delay in the motor milestones of development. Symptoms increase through adolescence but tend to remain much the same during adult life. The patients show myotonia, poor relaxation of muscle, and sustained contraction of varying severity. These phenomena affect only the skeletal muscles. The patient often has difficulty in walking upstairs or performing a particular muscle movement. The myotonia decreases with exercise. There is a spurious appearance of dystonia because of cramps during muscular contraction. There is some difficulty in initiating walking; however, if the patient persists, the gait tends to become more normal. Nevertheless, a sudden reflex movement to maintain balance may throw the muscles into severe spasm and the patient may fall. The chief complaints are muscular stiffness, clumsiness, and frequent falls. A rapid movement may induce a generalized spasm. Some patients show spasm of the orbicularis oculi during eye blinking, involvement of the facial muscles, and myotonia of the tongue. Another one of the characteristic signs of myotonia is the inability to release the grip for as long as 60 seconds following a handshake. Examination of the patient usually shows marked hypertrophy of the muscles of the pelvic and shoulder girdles, proximal limb muscles, and calves, which have been termed "herculean" in appearance. Percussion of an affected muscle with a percussion hammer produces immediate contraction and dimpling beneath the site of the blow, which may persist for some time and then slowly relax ("percussion myotonia"). A variant with rolling-muscle contractions produced by tapping the muscle and local swelling of muscle (myedema) on percussion of the muscle has been described.[259]

Diagnostic Procedures

Electromyography. The irritability of the muscle is found to be markedly increased after insertion of the needle electrode. Movement of the needle, percussion of the muscle, and voluntary contraction produce a series of potentials varying in frequency and amplitude. When the patient is asked to relax the muscle following voluntary contraction, an intense discharge of high-amplitude potentials is seen. This is followed by potentials of smaller amplitude.[145] These two events combine to give rise to a characteristic sound heard over the loudspeaker, the so-called "dive-bomber" sound. Motor unit potential changes indicative of myopathy are not seen.

Treatment

The myotonia may be relieved successfully by the use of diphenylhydantoin, 100 mg three times daily, or procainamide in oral doses of up to 4 to 6 gm daily. Quinine, 0.3 to 0.6 gm two or three times daily, is also effective. If quinine is used, visual and audiometric tests should be performed at regular intervals because of the danger of toxic optic or otic neuritis caused by quinine in certain sensitive individuals. Corticosteroids are also effective in reducing myotonia but are of less value in the long-term treatment of patients because of side effects. Acetazolamide may reduce myotonia in some cases and can be used if patients are unresponsive or intolerant to other forms of therapy.[105a]

Paramyotonia Congenita

In this condition, which is inherited as an autosomal dominant trait,[58] the patient shows myotonia that becomes worse with repeated effort (paradoxic myotonia).[32]

Clinical Features

The condition is worse in cold weather. The myotonia appears during exercise and involves the tongue, lips, extensors of the forearms, the calf muscles, and the lateral portion of the quadriceps femoris. The appearance of myotonia is followed by progressive muscular weakness on further effort. The weakness may be extensive, and episodes of flaccid quadriparesis have occasionally been reported.[31] Affected children may be unable to write when attending school in cold weather or may develop paresis when swimming in cold water. Adults experience myotonia and loss of strength when performing manual labor and tend to seek employment in sedentary occupations. Paramyotonia congenita is often worse in females during menstruation, and the muscular weakness may be exacerbated by acetazolamide.[207]

Treatment

Treatment in this condition is symptomatic, and the patient should be advised to avoid exposure to cold temperatures.

Myotonic Dystrophy (Dystrophia Myotonica)

This condition is the most common form of the myotonic dystrophies and is inherited as an autosomal dominant trait. The pedigree in myotonic dystrophy is interesting because of certain other associated genetically determined defects. These include polar cataracts, retinal degeneration, frontal baldness, and testicular atrophy, which frequently develop in patients with myotonia and muscle wasting. Some family members may develop the frontal baldness and cataract formation without wasting of muscle or muscular symptoms. The condition has appeared in neonates but may be delayed until the fifth decade of life.[14, 263]

Etiology and Pathology

There seems to be little doubt that the major defect in myotonic dystrophy is a genetically determined abnormality in the muscle membrane. A functional membrane defect has been demonstrated in the erythrocytes in myotonic dystrophy,[209] suggesting that there may be diffuse membrane involvement in this disease. Abnormalities in membrane systems could lead to secondary muscle fiber degeneration and could account for the reported abnormalities in the central and peripheral nervous system.[51, 52, 137, 201] There is no evidence that muscle wasting in myotonic dystrophy is a "neurogenic" process since muscle fiber innervation is normal.[61] As determined by muscle biopsy, there is variation in the size of muscle fibers with an increase in the number of internal nuclei. Signs of degeneration, which include necrosis, loss of striation, and phagocytosis, occur. The endomysial connective tissue is increased in the later stages of the disease. The presence of ring fibers, which seem to encircle normal muscle fibers, and sarcoplasmic masses is said to be characteristic of myotonic dystrophy. Histochemical examination shows atrophy of type I muscle fibers and some increase in size of type II fibers, which is believed to be a relatively specific finding in myotonic dystrophy[23] (Fig. 12–3). The heart muscle is severely involved at autopsy with thinning of the myocardium and diffuse fibrosis.

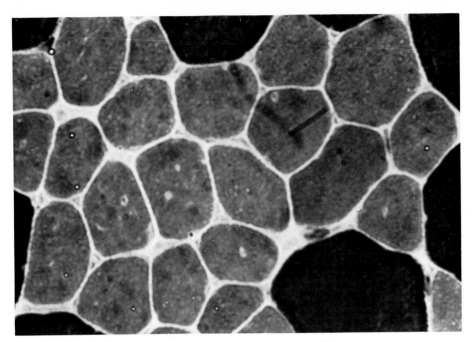

FIGURE 12–3. Muscle biopsy stained with ATPase reaction at pH 9.4 showing selective type I fiber atrophy. This abnormality is seen in myotonic dystrophy.

Clinical Features

Myotonia and Myopathy. Myotonic dystrophy usually presents with myotonia, which may precede the development of muscle wasting by several years. In some cases, however, the patients state that the two conditions occurred at or about the same time. Myotonia is first noted in the hands, and when the myotonia is fully developed, it interferes with simple activities such as grasping objects. When the muscles of the lower limbs develop myotonia, it may result in loss of balance and unexpected falls. Muscle wasting in myotonic dystrophy involves both proximal and distal muscle groups. However, the onset of wasting is usually in the hands. There is a characteristic pattern of wasting in fully developed cases involving the facial muscles, the muscles of mastication, the sternocleidomastoids, the flexors and extensors of the forearms, the quadriceps, and the dorsiflexor muscles of the feet. The combination of myotonia and wasting of the masseters may produce difficulty in chewing, and late involvement of pharyngeal muscles results in choking and difficulty in swallowing. There is a typical facial appearance owing to bilateral ptosis, wasting of the facial, temporalis, masseters, and neck muscles, which

has been described as "hatchet face" (Fig. 12–4).

Cardiac Abnormalities. Cardiac involvement is found in approximately 85 per cent of cases.[42] The following electrocardiographic abnormalities have been described:

1. A prolonged P-R interval
2. Atrial flutter and atrial fibrillation[56, 246]
3. An intraventricular conduction defect with Stokes-Adams attacks and congestive heart failure, both of which are rare complications in this disease[8]

In some cases the cardiac arrhythmias may be due to familial mitral valve prolapse, which is known to occur in myotonic dystrophy.[277]

Ophthalmic Signs. Bilateral ptosis is a classic feature of this disease, and other manifestations of ocular motor weakness are occasionally seen. In the early stages, slit-lamp examination often reveals posterior cortical cataracts, which may enlarge later, producing impairment of vision. Occasional blepharitis, conjunctivitis, and keratitis may occur, and pigmentation near the macula

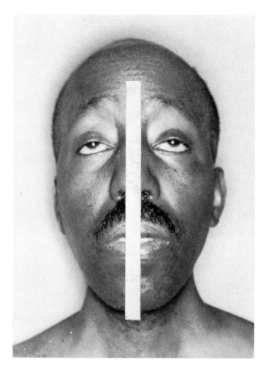

FIGURE 12–4. Typical facies of a patient with myotonic dystrophy (dystrophia myotonica). Note the corrugation of the forehead, the ptosis, and the frontal baldness.

owing to proliferation of retinal pigment epithelium has been described in some cases.[15, 30, 168]

Respiratory Abnormalities. Aspiration pneumonia and acute respiratory failure are not uncommon in advanced cases of myotonic dystrophy. Myotonia of the intercostal muscles and the diaphragm makes artificial respiration difficult. Recovery is delayed by the respiratory problems and by impairment of swallowing.[282]

Endocrine Dysfunction. The endocrine abnormalities are as follows:

1. Frontal balding is highly characteristic in this disease.
2. Gonadal atrophy or primary gonadal failure occurs in both sexes. Male patients show testicular atrophy with impotence and loss of libido. The levels of serum follicle-stimulating hormone are increased.
3. Carbohydrate metabolism is abnormal with occasional diabetic glucose tolerance curves and high serum insulin levels owing to an ab-normality in the activity of endogenous insulin.[50, 128]
4. The basal metabolic rate is low, but thyroid function appears to be normal.

Skeletal Abnormalities. There is thickening of the bones in the vault of the skull with hyperostosis frontalis interna and an unusually small sella turcica. The paranasal sinuses may be unusually large.

Smooth Muscle Involvement. Difficulty in swallowing and choking are definite threats in the terminal stages of this disease. Impaired motility of the esophagus, gastrointestinal dilatation, dilatation of the colon, and abnormal peristalsis have also been demonstrated in some cases.[101, 204]

Abnormalities of Immunoglobulins. An accelerated breakdown of immunoglobulin G has been described.[279]

The course is one of steady deterioration, and few patients live beyond the age of 60 years. The mean duration of the disease seems to be about 25 years, and death occurs from heart failure or pulmonary infection.

Diagnostic Procedures

1. If myotonia is not obvious, it will be exacerbated by exposure to cold.
2. "Myotonia discharges," which are determined by electromyography, have been described in the discussion of myotonia congenita. In addition, several motor unit potentials of low amplitude and short duration are seen even on minimal contraction. There is an increase in polyphasic motor unit potentials. These changes, indicative of a myopathy, and the myotonic discharges constitute the electromyographic changes in myotonic dystrophy.
3. Since the onset of symptoms in myotonic dystrophy is often delayed beyond the age of 30 years, it is possible for a carrier to transmit the genes for this condition while still in apparent good health.[29] A number of tests may be useful in detecting heterozygotes before they become symptomatic. These include slit-lamp examination for posterior cortical cataracts, electromyography, and estimation of serum immunoglobulin levels. Of these three tests, slit-lamp examination and electromyographic demonstration of myotonia are the most fre-

quently abnormal findings in the very early stages of this condition. The detection of abnormally low IgG levels may be of further help in detecting a heterozygote but in itself is not diagnostic. These examinations should be recommended to the offspring of patients with myotonic dystrophy as a prelude to genetic counseling following the detection of neurologically intact heterozygotes.

4. The diagnosis may be established by muscle biopsy (p. 716).

5. Electrocardiographic abnormalities occur in a high percentage of cases.

Treatment

The myotonia usually responds to diphenylhydantoin or procainamide (see Treatment of Myotonia Congenita, p. 725). Cardiac arrhythmias and heart failure should be treated promptly. Upper respiratory tract infections may lead to aspiration pneumonia and should be treated with antibiotics at an early stage in advanced cases of myotonic dystrophy. Patients with acute respiratory insufficiency or respiratory failure require skilled care in an intensive care unit.

Congenital Myotonic Dystrophy

Mothers with late-onset myotonia dystrophy occasionally give birth to infants who show symptoms immediately after birth. Many of the affected neonates have respiratory distress and appear to be weak and hypotonic with paresis of the muscles controlling sucking and swallowing. There is restriction of movement at the joints with evidence of arthrogryposis in some cases. The facial appearance is abnormal with a "tented" upper lip. Many cases show mental retardation in later life.[67, 219]

The condition is probably due in part to poor respiratory function and anoxic encephalopathy at birth, combined with maturation arrest of developing fetal muscle in severely affected infants.[220]

Chronic Benign Congenital Myopathies

There are a number of rare inherited muscular diseases which usually present with symptoms of weakness at birth or in early childhood. The weakness may be of a nonprogressive type, or there may be progression and gradual deterioration in some cases.[200] There has been some suggestion that these disorders may be due to a dysfunction of the motor neuron rather than a true myopathic process.[81]

Pathology

The benign congenital myopathies show histologic changes compatible with an active myopathic process. There are muscle fiber breakdown, scattered necrotic fibers, variations in fiber size, increased internal nuclei, atrophic and hypertrophic fibers, fiber loss, and replacement with connective tissue and fat. Some conditions such as central core disease show destructive abnormalities on light microscopy but the majority of these myopathies show abnormalities only on electron microscopy. It is likely that further improvement in electron microscopy and histochemical techniques will result in the description of additional rare myopathies.

At the present time the benign congenital myopathies include central core disease,[85, 235, 275] nemaline myopathy,[121, 243, 245] multicore disease,[76] myotubular myopathy,[244] congenital megaconial and pleoconial myopathy,[234] type 1 fiber hypotrophy and central nuclei,[86] centronuclear myopathy,[232] familial myopathy with lysis of myofibrils in type 1 fibers,[35] reducing body myopathy,[25] sarcotubular myopathy,[104] and fingerprint body myopathy.[104]

Clinical Features

There may be evidence of myopathy at birth in some cases who present as "floppy babies" with slow motor development, hypotonia, and weakness that may improve with the passage of time. The maximal involvement is of "myopathic" distribution with proximal muscle weakness and wasting producing difficulty in climbing stairs, difficulty in getting out of a chair, and easy fatigue when reaching for objects above the head. Strength in the wrists, fingers, ankles, and feet is often normal. Serum muscle enzyme levels are usually normal or only slightly elevated.

Treatment

There is no specific treatment for any of the benign congenital myopathies. Once the diagnosis is made, parents may be assured that the affected child will eventually walk. Patients may be helped by physical therapy and mechanical aids if weakness becomes severe.

Ophthalmoplegia, Retinitis, Cardiopathy, and Neural Disorder (Kearns-Sayre Syndrome)

This rare sporadic condition begins before the age of 20 years and is characterized by progressive

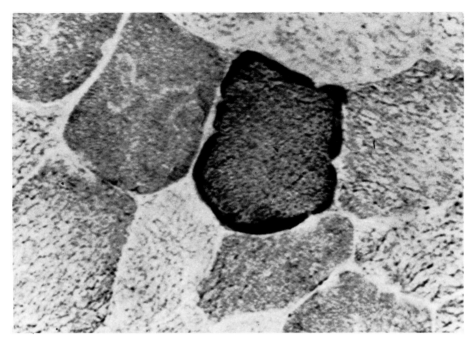

FIGURE 12–5. SDH (succinodehydrogenase) stain showing densely staining abnormal mitochondria in the subsarcolemmal zone of a muscle fiber. This densely staining zone stains red with modified trichoma stains. This appearance has given rise to the term "ragged red fibers."

external ophthalmoplegia, atypical pigmentary degeneration of the retina, and heart block. It is believed to be induced by persistent viral infection that produces widespread damage to neurons and muscles. Spongioform encephalopathy and cardiopathy have been described at autopsy, and the skeletal muscle shows mitochondrial abnormalities that appear as "ragged red fibers" (Fig. 12–5).

Patients present with progressive ophthalmoplegia followed by the gradual development of widespread neurologic deficits involving cerebellar and brainstem functions. There may be intellectual deterioration and corticospinal tract abnormalities, short stature, endocrine abnormalities, and delayed sexual maturation.[126a] The cerebrospinal fluid protein content is elevated. Signs of cardiopathy may be delayed for many years.[20]

Oculocraniosomatic Neuromuscular Disease with "Ragged Red" Fibers

Although progressive external ophthalmoplegia is a nonspecific clinical sign that occurs in many conditions (Table 12–2), it is possible to identify some cases occurring in adolescence and adult life that show abnormalities in muscle mitochondria.[180a] This syndrome may be familial[129, 252] in some cases but is usually sporadic,[180] and affected individuals show progressive external ophthalmoplegia and occasional mild weakness of the proximal limb girdle musculature. The histochemically stained muscle biopsy shows the presence of increased staining at the fiber edge and an increased granular appearance to the muscle fiber. This appearance has been termed "ragged red" fibers and indicates the presence of abnormal mitochondria in the subsarcolemma.[189]

Myositis, or Inflammatory Disease of Muscle

This category comprises a heterogenous group of diseases of muscle which have the common characteristic of inflammatory changes. Any associated destruction of muscle fibers varies according to the nature and severity of the infection. The classification of inflammatory diseases of muscle is outlined in Table 12–3.

TABLE 12–3

Inflammatory Diseases of Muscle

Etiology	
1. Viral	Epidemic pleurodynia (epidemic myalgia, Bornholm disease)
2. Bacterial	Suppuration Clostridial Tuberculous Syphilitic Leptospiral
3. Parasitic	Trichinosis Cysticercosis Hydatid *(Echinococcus)* Toxoplasmosis Trypanosomiasis Schistosomiasis
4. Fungal	Actinomycosis
5. Unknown	Polymyositis Lupus erythematosus Polyarteritis nodosa Sarcoidosis Carcinomatosis

Viral Infection of Muscle

Epidemic Pleurodynia (Epidemic Myalgia, Bornholm Disease)

The earliest descriptions of this disease were found almost exclusively in the Scandinavian literature. In 1933, a report of an outbreak occurring on the Danish island of Bornholm led to the adoption of the term "Bornholm disease." Since then, a number of isolated epidemics have been reported from other parts of the world.

The Coxsackie B group of virus (B 1–6) has been incriminated in the majority of outbreaks with isolation of the ECHO viruses in some cases. Since the disease is benign and of short duration, muscle biopsy is seldom obtained. When a muscle biopsy is taken, it shows perivascular inflammation and necrosis of muscle fibers.

Clinical Features. Outbreaks occur during the late summer and autumn predominantly among children 5 to 15 years of age. However, all age groups and either sex may be affected. Members of a family can develop symptoms within a few days of each other, suggesting that the incubation period is relatively short.

The onset is sudden, with the development of pain in the lower chest, epigastrium, or hypogastrium, exacerbated by inspiration, coughing, or sneezing. Occasionally muscle pain and tenderness occur in the back, neck, or shoulders without associated "pleurodynia." Hiccup is not uncommon, suggesting diaphragmatic involvement. Headache and fever are usually present at the onset and a pleural friction rub occurs in about 25 per cent of cases. The pain usually subsides in a few days, but some patients experience discomfort for several weeks and relapses are not uncommon. Aseptic meningitis is an occasional complication during an epidemic. The diagnosis of epidemic pleurodynia is not difficult during an epidemic. Findings in the early or isolated case may mimic pleurisy and pneumonia or acute abdominal emergencies.

Diagnostic Procedures. Leukocytosis and, occasionally, eosinophilia are seen in the early stages. Pleocytosis, with elevation of cerebrospinal fluid protein, may occur in cases with meningitis (see p. 401). Coxsackie virus may be isolated from blood, urine, and cerebrospinal fluid and the titer of antibodies in the serum rises in the first few weeks of the illness.

Treatment. Morphine or meperidine hydrochloride may be required initially for severe pain in the muscles during the early stages, and this can be followed by codeine and aspirin, as required, to control pain. The application of heat to the affected area also affords considerable relief.

Bacterial Infection of Muscle

Clostridial Myositis

Anaerobic conditions are required for proliferation of the clostridial group of organisms. Hence, these are usually found in puncture wounds, deep lacerations, and compound fractures, particularly when associated with contamination by the soil such as occurs during military campaigns. Civilian cases are usually found among agricultural workers.

Etiology and Pathology. The infection is usually caused by *Clostridium perfringens (welchii),* which produces a potent exotoxin and muscle necrosis with breakdown of muscle glycogen resulting in the release of carbon dioxide in the tissues (gas gangrene). The muscle shows coagulation necrosis surrounded by an acute inflammatory exudate containing anaerobic gas-producing bacilli. The adjoining fibers are pale and separated by gas, which may dissect widely throughout muscle and subcutaneous tissues.

Clinical Features. The exotoxin has a profound systemic effect and patients present with high fever and tachycardia. Sudden shock often occurs due to cardiovascular involvement. The affected area is swollen, with a serosanguineous exudate at the side of the wound. Palpation reveals crepitus due to the presence of gas in the surrounding muscle and subcutaneous tissues.

Treatment. Emergency treatment must be instituted as early as possible, including incision with wide exposure, drainage, and débridement of the infected areas of muscle. Hyperbaric oxygenation is reported to be most beneficial.[13] In the average adult, at least 48 million units of aqueous penicillin should be given intravenously every 24 hours until the infection is completely eradicated and the wound cultures are sterile. Amputation may be necessary in neglected cases.

Tuberculous Myositis

Involvement of skeletal muscles occasionally occurs in generalized miliary tuberculosis. The condition is often asymptomatic and may be seen at autopsy following overwhelming infection.

Tuberculous polymyositis usually produces a picture of muscle weakness and atrophy similar to Boeck's sarcoidosis, with noncaseating areas of epithelioid cells and giant cells and lymphocytes scattered throughout the connective tissue in the muscle.[140]

Sarcoid Myopathy

In systemic sarcoidosis, the skeletal muscles may be involved by the inflammatory process (see p. 426).

Syphilitic Myositis

Gumma formation in skeletal muscle is a rare complication of tertiary syphilis.[144] The existence of diffuse syphilitic involvement of skeletal muscle (syphilitic myositis) is doubtful.

Leptospiral Myositis

Involvement of skeletal muscle with focal necrosis of muscle fibers may be found in severe or fatal cases of Weil's disease. The myositis is asymptomatic and an incidental finding in these cases.

Parasitic Infestation of Muscle

Trichinosis

Trichinosis is a disease that has been recognized for thousands of years and is responsible for certain well-known religious laws prohibiting the ingestion of pork. Although millions of people have probably been infected, the majority appear to have remained asymptomatic.

The disease is caused by the nematode *Trichinella spiralis,* and infection is due to eating partly cooked pork or pork products containing the encysted larvae. The cyst walls are digested in the intestinal tract and the liberated larvae develop into adult worms within seven days. The fertilized female then burrows through the mucosal wall and deposits larvae in the lymphatics. These enter the systemic circulation from the thoracic duct. Although they are carried in great numbers to all parts of the body, including the brain, where an acute and sometimes fatal encephalitic response may result, the larvae survive only in skeletal muscle, where they form cysts.

The young larvae invade the substance of the skeletal muscle fibers and rarely the myocardium. In the skeletal muscle they assume a spiral form as they grow. The adjacent sarcoplasm shows basophilia, and adjacent muscle fibers undergo hyaline degeneration. Initially, there is an intense inflammatory reaction of neutrophilic and eosinophilic leukocytes followed by lymphocytes, plasma cells, and mononuclear cells. At this stage some muscle fibers undergo necrosis and the parasites die. After six weeks, however, the surviving larvae develop a capsule, probably from the sarcoplasm and proliferating connective tissue cells, which becomes calcified after six months. These larvae remain viable for as long as 30 years following infection.

Clinical Features. The earliest symptom of infestation may be a mild gastroenteritis due to nematodes in the intestinal tract. Muscle involvement occurs after approximately seven days and lasts about four weeks, or the length of time during which the female produces larvae in the intestinal wall. During this period, the patient develops fever accompanied by muscle pains and tenderness. There is periorbital and conjunctival edema, with fatigue and weakness, which may be confined to certain muscles or may be generalized. Jaw, tongue, neck, eye, and facial movements may be painful and limited.[53]

There seems to be a predilection for involvement of the intercostal muscles and the diaphragm, which produces respiratory difficulties in the early stages of the disease. Myocardial symptoms due to larval embolism of the coronary vessels may produce heart failure or death in the first few weeks. Symptoms subside after a six- to eight-week period, and full recovery is usual.

Diagnostic Procedures. These demonstrate the following:

1. The white blood count shows a polymorphonucleocytosis with an eosinophilia of up to 80 per cent.
2. After two weeks, intradermal injection of *Trichina* antigen gives a positive reaction.
3. Complement-fixation, precipitin, and flocculation tests become positive after two to three weeks.
4. Muscle biopsy is positive after the muscles have been involved. The demonstration of larval forms in the muscle is diagnostic.
5. Larvae calcify and may be demonstrated by x-ray of the muscles after six months.

Treatment. Treatment is as follows:

1. Although prevention is effective, there is no known parasiticide against *Trichina spiralis* once infection occurs.
2. Bed rest in the initial stages reduces the risk of heart failure.
3. Adequate analgesics should be given for muscle pain and headache.
4. If heart failure occurs, fluid reduction, low-salt diet, diuretics, and digitalization may be necessary.
5. Steroid therapy minimizes symptoms by inhibition of antigen-antibody reactions in muscle. The recommended dosage of methylprednisolone is 96 mg in a single dose once every 48 hours for two weeks, and then gradual reduction in dosage for the next six weeks.
6. Thiabendazole, 50 mg/kg/day for seven to ten days, is effective in preventing larva reproduction and has a toxic effect on larvae present in muscle.[98]
7. Prevention is accomplished by adequate cooking of pork and government inspection of meats.[112]

Cysticercosis

Under conditions of poor preventive medicine, sanitation, and hygiene, the human being may become the intermediate host for the pork tapeworm, *Taenia solium*. The ingested eggs dissolve in the intestine, and the larvae *(Cysticercus cellulosae)* penetrate the mucosa and muscle to enter the general circulation. From here they are distributed to all parts of the body and survive in many organs, including muscle and brain.

The presence of cysticerci in muscle produces a diffuse myositis with swelling of muscle fibers, fiber atrophy, and replacement with fibrous tissue. There may be diffuse swelling of limb muscles, pain, tenderness, and weakness of all muscles except the hands and feet. The diagnosis can be made by muscle biopsy, which shows a diffuse inflammatory reaction in the muscle and the presence of numerous cysticerci.

Clinical Features. Systemic invasion by the parasites is usually accompanied by malaise, fever, headache, and muscle pains, although the patient may remain asymptomatic. Following recovery, the patient remains symptom-free until the cysts begin to calcify, which occurs about six months to a year after the infestation. At this time, focal or generalized seizures may develop and persist despite the death of the larvae. In the acute phase of illness with overwhelming infection, focal neurologic signs, seizures, bilateral papilledema, and coma followed by death rarely occur.

Diagnostic Procedures. These are as follows:

1. The white blood cell count shows eosinophilia during the early stages of infection.
2. Roentgenograms of the soft tissues or skull may show calcification of the cysts in patients with seizures secondary to cysticercosis. The occurrence of rod-shaped calcifications in muscle is highly characteristic of this condition and also helps in selecting a site for diagnostic biopsy.
3. Muscle biopsy shows the characteristic cysts containing parasites.

Treatment. Therapeutic considerations include the following:

1. There is no known chemotherapeutic agent that will kill the larvae.
2. Focal or generalized seizures can be controlled by anticonvulsants.

Echinococcus (Hydatid) Cysts of Muscle and Brain

Occasionally, man becomes the intermediate host for the dog tapeworm, *Echinococcus granulosus.* The infestation is acquired by petting or handling dogs which carry the ova in their hair. The larvae hatch in the intestinal tract and pass through the muscle wall into the bloodstream. Further development of the larvae may occur in several organs, including muscle and brain, with the formation of hydatid cysts. The cysts produce few symptoms in muscle unless they rupture. Cysts in the brain usually produce focal neurologic signs. Ruptured cysts in muscle produce an intense local myositis, with pain and tenderness, and a varying systemic reaction results due to the antigenic properties of the cyst fluid that is released into the systemic circulation. Cysts rupturing in the brain produce a meningeal reaction with spread of daughter cysts.

Diagnostic Procedures.   These are as follows:

1. The white cell count in the peripheral blood shows an eosinophilia.
2. If available, the intradermal (Casoni) skin test, with hydatid antigen, will be positive.
3. If there are intracerebral cysts, the spinal fluid shows an eosinophilic pleocytosis.

Treatment.   If possible, the cysts should be removed surgically. Contamination of the surrounding muscle by the contents of the cyst should be avoided as implantation of daughter cysts may result.

Both the local and systemic reactions that follow rupture of the cysts can be modified by steroid therapy using intravenous hydrocortisone, 100 mg initially, and oral methylprednisolone in the next three weeks in gradually decreasing doses.

Toxoplasmosis

Infestation by the protozoan *Toxoplasma gondii* usually occurs in utero but occasionally occurs in children and adults (p. 437). The parasites are widely distributed throughout the body, including the skeletal muscle, where they produce an asymptomatic myositis.

Trypanosomiasis

The South American form of trypanosomiasis, due to *Trypanosoma cruzi,* may produce a myositis in man. Infection occurs when Reduviid insects excrete the parasite, which then passes through bites in the skin, resulting in a generalized bloodborne dissemination of the trypanosome. The parasites also invade various organs, including skeletal muscle, with the development of an asymptomatic myositis. Muscle biopsy may be a valuable diagnostic procedure in the chronic form of this disease.

Schistosomal Myositis

Generalized muscular weakness and wasting have been reported in patients with schistosomiasis due to *Schistosoma mansoni* or *Schistosoma haematobium,* or both.[165] Muscle biopsies show variation in size of muscle fibers, loss of striations, granular and vacuolar degenerative changes in the fibers, increase in sarcolemmal nuclei, and infiltration with macrophages. The ova have not been demonstrated in these lesions.

Inflammatory Myopathies of Unknown Etiology

Polymyositis and Dermatomyositis

Polymyositis may be defined as an inflammatory myopathy of unknown etiology. The term "dermatomyositis" is used when there are also clinical signs of involvement of the skin, but the two conditions are essentially the same.

Etiology and Pathology.   Polymyositis is currently regarded as an autoimmune disease, which implies involvement of humoral or cellular immune mechanisms in the pathogenesis of the syndrome. Antimyosin antibodies have been demonstrated in polymyositis, but similar antibodies are present in other myopathic and neurogenic disorders and are not cytotoxic to muscle cells.[247] There is some evidence that muscle fiber damage in polymyositis may result from liberated lymphotoxins produced by sensitized lymphocytes,[55, 285] and it is possible to transfer myositis from affected rats to normal rats by thoracic duct lymphocytes.[179] However, the identification of viral particles in muscle biopsies from patients with polymyositis[93, 167] adds another dimension to the possible etiology of this syndrome, although the etiology and pathogenesis remain unclear.

The muscles show an acute inflammatory reaction in the early stages of the disease with a collection of inflammatory cells around the small blood vessels. These are mainly lymphocytes and plasma cells, with the occasional presence of polymorphonuclear leukocytes. These inflammatory changes are associated with evidence of an active myopathy; that is, the muscle fibers show the presence of degeneration, with active phagocytosis in association with active regeneration. Many of the fibers show the presence of central nuclei and are of variable diameter. It is not unusual to find that the muscle fibers in the center of the muscle fascicle have a normal appearance, while those at the periphery become progressively smaller and contain vacuoles. This change is said to be characteristic of polymyositis, but similar changes are seen in systemic lupus erythematosus and carcinomatous myopathy.[9, 24] The blood vessels show progressive changes throughout the course of polymyositis. In the early stages there is proliferation of the endothelium with narrowing of the lumen. This is often of segmental distribution, and there is irregular narrowing throughout the course of the vessel. In the later stages of the disease, the blood vessels may become thickened with complete obliteration of the lumen.

Clinical Features. There are five groups of disorders in the polymyositis/dermatomyositis syndrome:[22]

Group I.   Primary idiopathic polymyositis
Group II.   Primary idiopathic dermatomyositis
Group III. Dermatomyositis or polymyositis with neoplasia
Group IV.   Childhood dermatomyositis or polymyositis with vasculitis
Group V.   Polymyositis or dermatomyositis with associated collagen-vascular disease

GROUP I. PRIMARY IDIOPATHIC POLYMYOSITIS. The essential feature in polymyositis is the occurrence of muscle weakness. This usually begins in the muscles of the pelvic girdle, particularly the iliopsoas and quadriceps femoris muscles, followed by involvement of the shoulder girdles. Sometimes the proximal muscles of the arms are affected first. Those patients with chronic polymyositis complain of difficulty climbing stairs, getting out of a chair, and raising the arms above the shoulder. There is a waddling gait with an increased lumbar lordosis in severe cases. Similarity to the Duchenne or limb girdle type of muscular dystrophy is striking, and the two conditions may be further confused by the occurrence of pseudohypertrophy in some patients with polymyositis. However, in contrast to the muscular dystrophies, polymyositis progresses over weeks or months rather than years and shows periods of spontaneous exacerbations and remissions.[194]

Facial weakness is sometimes prominent in polymyositis, and weakness and wasting of the sternocleidomastoids may be a striking feature. Weakness of pharyngeal muscles and dysphagia may occur, and infrequently involvement of the ocular muscles produces strabismus and diplopia. Shortness of breath and dyspnea are indicative of respiratory muscle involvement of interstitial fibrosis of the lungs.[188] Myotonia is uncommon in polymyositis, but increased weakness on exertion of the myasthenic type with some response to anticholinergic drugs may occur and is termed "pseudomyasthenia." Although muscle wasting is prominent in the disease, the deep tendon reflexes are usually present or may appear to be slightly brisker than usual. Symmetric muscle tenderness on palpation is severe in some cases but absent in others, and the involved muscles have a "doughy" or firmer consistency than normal on palpation. Fasciculations are rarely seen.

In the more acute forms of polymyositis, the signs and symptoms of joint involvement may overshadow the muscular weakness. The patient then complains of generalized weakness and fatigue, but examination reveals a severe and symmetric involvement of the limb girdle and quadriceps femoris muscles. Myoglobinuria may occur in cases with rapid degeneration of muscle fibers.[270]

GROUP II. PRIMARY IDIOPATHIC DERMATOMYOSITIS. The changes in the skin in dermatomyositis vary from a fleeting erythema to a generalized weeping dermatitis. The rash has been reported to precede the signs of muscle involvement in some cases.[148] The classic changes include periorbital edema with a lilac discoloration of the upper eyelids, accompanied by erythema, scaling, dermal atrophy, and dusky red patches or linear streaks over the forehead, face, neck, elbows, knuckles, upper chest, back, knees, and medial malleoli.

Raynaud's phenomenon, possibly due to arteritis of the limb vessels,[11] may also occur. Ulceration and inflammation due to endarteritis of the mucosa of the mouth, tongue, and pharynx may produce considerable discomfort and dysphagia. As the skin lesions become chronic, they may have the appearance of scleroderma, particularly on the hands and fingers. Atrophy of the pharyngeal mucosa, pulmonary fibrosis, and involvement of the small and large bowel may occur.[248] There may be extensive calcification of the skin and subcutaneous tissues with the development of indolent ulcers.

GROUP III. DERMATOMYOSITIS AND POLYMYOSITIS WITH NEOPLASIA. The association of carcinoma and polymyositis has not been proven but the incidence ranges from 5 per cent to 25 per cent in several reported series.[59] There seems to be a higher incidence of carcinoma in dermatomyositis with a more than 50 per cent association of carcinoma and dermatomyositis in males over the age of 40 years.

GROUP IV. CHILDHOOD DERMATOMYOSITIS AND POLYMYOSITIS WITH VASCULITIS. This condition is distinguished by prominent capillary damage with capillary necrosis and capillary loss in muscle fascicles. The vascular changes may be extensive, suggesting that the muscle fiber damage is a secondary phenomenon due to progressive ischemia.[36]

The onset of the disease is frequently insidious with a period of ill-defined malaise preceding the development of muscle weakness and skin rash. There is a tendency to experience remissions and relapses and progression to chronicity in some cases with muscle contractures, joint deformities, scleroderma-like changes in the skin of the face, chest, and fingers, iridocyclitis, retinopathy, and calcinosis of the skin and subcutaneous tissues with frequent ulceration and extrusion of calcium.[91, 177]

GROUP V. POLYMYOSITIS OR DERMATOMYOSITIS WITH ASSOCIATED COLLAGEN-VASCULAR DISEASES. Polymyositis is not an uncommon occurrence during the course of a clearly defined collagen-vascular disease such as scleroderma, systemic lupus erythematosus, rheumatoid arthritis, Sjögren's syndrome, or polyarteritis nodosa. In some cases the muscle biopsy shows changes that are indistinguishable from polymyositis, but there are often sufficient destructive features characteristic of the systemic collagen-vascular disorder. Nevertheless, there seems to be an overlapping group of cases with histologic changes of polymyositis and signs such as Raynaud's phenomenon, positive antinuclear factor, and positive rheumatoid factor which are more characteristic of a collagen-vascular disease.

Diagnostic Procedures. These are as follows:

BLOOD. Anemia and purpura may occur, particularly in more chronic cases of polymyositis. A polymorphonuclear leukocytosis may occur in acute cases. The sedimentation rate is usually but not invariably elevated.

URINE. Albuminuria may occur in some cases, suggesting renal involvement. Creatinuria is a fairly consistent abnormality. Myoglobulinuria may occur in severe, acute forms of polymyositis.

SERUM PROTEINS. Low serum albumin with reversal of the albumin:globulin ratio and raised gamma globulin levels is often seen.

SERUM ENZYMES. Elevated aldolase, serum glutamic oxaloacetic transaminase, and creatine phosphokinase levels occur, particularly in the acute phase of the disease.

ROENTGENOLOGY. Calcification of subcutaneous tissues and the connective tissue in the muscles may occur, particularly in children. Chest roentgenogram may reveal a bronchial carcinoma in those cases associated with malignancy.

MYASTHENIC RESPONSE. A positive Tensilon test may be obtained in some cases of polymyositis with myasthenic features but is never as dramatic as in true myasthenia gravis.

ELECTROCARDIOGRAPHY. The most frequent changes suggest pericarditis, but conduction abnormalities with changes in wave form indicate myocardial involvement.

ELECTROMYOGRAPHY. Insertion activity may be normal or increased in a manner reminiscent of myotonia. At rest, there is usually electrical silence but fibrillations may occur in some cases owing to inflammatory involvement of the terminal nerve fibers in muscle, and occasionally positive "sawtooth" waves are recorded. During activity, polyphasic motor units of shorter duration and lower amplitude than normal are seen.

MUSCLE BIOPSY. This is the unequivocal means of diagnosis if it is positive. The pathologic changes have been described. Unfortunately, possibly due to a sampling error, the muscle biopsy may be negative in about one third of cases later proved to have polymyositis.

Treatment. S T E R O I D T H E R A P Y . The use of ACTH or corticosteroids produces dramatic improvement in the majority of patients.[266] Patients with acute disease should be given methylprednisolone, 60 mg daily, and, as soon as there is improvement, 96 mg once every 48 hours. A maintenance dose may be necessary in almost every case for at least two to three years and often longer. Dosage can eventually be progressively reduced and the drug finally withdrawn in most cases. Single-dose, alternate-day corticosteroid therapy has the advantage of a marked diminution in side effects with equal or accelerated rate of improvement.[82] The dosage should be supplemented by oral potassium, antacids, and a high-protein, low-sodium, low-carbohydrate diet. A short therapeutic trial of oral steroids is indicated in patients with symptoms of polymyositis who have a negative muscle biopsy.

Intravenous methotrexate may be beneficial in corticosteroid-resistant cases.[240] This drug should only be given if the liver function tests are normal and creatinine clearance is greater than 75 ml per minute. A test dose of 5 mg of methotrexate is given, and, if there are no side effects, the drug may be increased by 10 to 15 mg every seven days until the maximal dose of 0.8 mg/kg of body weight per week is reached. Oral cyclophosphamide, 50 mg/day, is also effective.

The complete blood count and liver function test should be done each week during treatment. Any abnormality is an indication to discontinue treatment.

T H E R A P Y F O R R E S P I R A T O R Y C O M P L I C A T I O N S . In patients with respiratory muscle involvement or interstitial lung disease, respiratory function should be recorded daily. Respiratory assistance with a positive pressure respirator may be necessary (p. 760). The debilitated patient with acute polymyositis is susceptible to pneumonia, which should be treated with postural drainage and the appropriate antibiotic after determination of the sensitivity of the organisms to antibiotics from culture of the sputum.

G E N E R A L M E A S U R E S . During the acute phase the patient requires expert nursing care, high-protein diet, and treatment of any anemia. As improvement begins, a planned program of physical therapy should be instituted.

T H E R A P Y F O R A S S O C I A T E D C A R C I -
N O M A . Treatment of the primary carcinoma in cases of polymyositis associated with malignancy can produce remission in patients free from metastatic disease. Surgical excision or irradiation should be used as indicated.

Acute polymyositis may present as a fulminating disease, with death occurring after a few days, particularly from respiratory failure or pneumonia. Steroid therapy has reduced the death rate but has not abolished it. In chronic myositis, steroid therapy produces early remission with suppression of fever and muscle weakness and is more predictable for improvement if there is no associated carcinoma. Patients with polymyositis of less than one year's duration who have no associated malignancy have a better prognosis on steroid therapy and a lower relapse rate. Those who do relapse usually show a good response to steroids. Acute cases with malignancy or scleroderma carry the poorest prognosis.

Myoglobinuria

A number of diseases are associated with the presence of myoglobin in the urine (Table 12–4), and myoglobinuria should be regarded as a nonspecific sign of muscle damage caused by a heterogeneous group of disorders. There are also cases in which paroxysmal myoglobinuria is associated with acute necrosis of muscle without apparent cause (acute rhabdomyolysis). These may be termed "idiopathic myoglobinuria" and are usually familial.

Idiopathic Myoglobinuria
Etiology and Pathology

A number of cases of idiopathic myoglobinuria have been reported in families, and the condition appears to result from a genetically determined metabolic defect. The nature of the defect is obscure. It is possible that there is a failure to utilize muscle glycogen because of a genetic defect or that there is a depletion of glycogen by exercise in a normal individual. The synthesis of adenosine triphosphate (ATP) will then depend on other metabolic pathways, especially the oxidation of fatty acids in mitochondria. Impairment of ATP production in muscle mitochondria can occur in a number of circumstances, including prolonged pressure, hypothermia, and exposure to toxic agents or certain drugs. This results in damage to the muscle membrane with passage of myoglobin into the serum and myoglobinuria.

TABLE 12–4

Myoglobinuria

1. Idiopathic myoglobinuria
2. Myoglobinuria on exertion
   a. Following unusual and prolonged exercise,[105] unusual exertion, and sickle cell trait[147]
   b. Anterior tibial syndrome[99]
   c. Status epilepticus or prolonged and recurrent seizures[60]
3. Traumatic myoglobinuria ("crush syndrome")[34]
4. Ischemic myoglobinuria (acute arterial occlusion)
5. Myoglobinuria with metabolic causes
   a. Metabolic depression
      (1) Carbon monoxide poisoning[213]
      (2) Barbiturate poisoning[233]
      (3) Hypothermia[166]
      (4) Diabetic acidosis[206]
      (5) Hypokalemia
      (6) Prolonged coma[196]
   b. Toxic agent
      (1) Licorice[230,260]
      (2) Alcohol[204]
      (3) Heroin[229]
      (4) Intravenous amphetamine administration[142]
      (5) Malayan sea snake bite poison[176]
      (6) Succinylcholine[2]
      (7) Amphotericin B[64]
      (8) Epsilon aminocaproic acid[208]
6. Myoglobinuria in association with myopathies
   a. Polymyositis
   b. Phosphorylase deficiency
   c. Phosphofructokinase deficiency
   d. Muscle carnitine polonityltransferase deficiency[122]
7. Myoglobinuria owing to heat injury
   a. Malignant hyperthermia under general anesthesia
   b. Heat stroke[265]

During an acute attack the muscle shows areas of degeneration and acute necrosis with phagocytosis. The associated interstitial inflammation is less than would be expected from the extensive muscle destruction. Biopsy specimens obtained after an attack contain areas of active regeneration.

Clinical Features

Attacks of idiopathic myoglobinuria often begin in childhood and are usually preceded by exercise of untrained muscles. Patients who have frequent episodes of myoglobinuria eventually learn to limit exercise and to avoid unusual muscular exertion. The history of exercise is not invariable, however, and attacks may occur following a mild upper respiratory tract infection or there may be no apparent cause in some cases.

The usual history is of generalized muscle weakness with pain, tenderness, swelling, and muscle cramps associated with passage of dark urine. Recovery occurs after a variable period of complete rest, sometimes several days.

In the acute phase, there may be blocking of renal tubules by precipitated myoglobin, producing oliguria or, in extreme cases, anuria and azotemia. Death occurs in about 20 per cent of cases with anuria.

Diagnostic Procedures

1. Myoglobin presents as a benzidine-positive pigment in the urine, which must be differentiated from hemoglobin. Porphyrins are benzidine-negative and hence easily distinguished. A most useful clinical test in distinguishing hemoglobulinuria from myoglobulinuria is simultaneous examination of serum and urine. The renal threshold for myoglobin is 15 mg per cent and for hemoglobin it is 130 mg per cent. A level of 15 mg per cent is insufficient to color the serum visually so that the presence of pigmented benzidine-positive urine free of erythrocytes and a clear serum strongly suggests myoglobinuria. Ultrafiltration of the urine will permit the small myoglobin molecule to pass but will retain the larger hemoglobin molecule. Definite proof of the presence of myoglobin can be attained by (a) gel electrophoresis and (b) immunoprecipitation with specific antibodies.[256]
2. There is marked elevation of serum muscle enzymes, including creatine phosphokinase, aldolase, lactic dehydrogenase, and serum glutamic oxaloacetic transaminase.
3. Renal damage and azotemia result in elevated blood urea nitrogen and serum creatinine levels, associated with variable electrolyte disturbances.
4. Profound hyperuricemia may occur during the early stages of renal failure.[146]
5. Hypercalcemia may occur during the diuretic phase of the disease.

Treatment

There is no specific treatment for idiopathic myoglobinuria. A high fluid intake and output should be maintained and an infusion of sodium bicarbonate given since myoglobin is soluble in an alkaline medium. Fluid restriction may be necessary during a period of oliguria to prevent overhydration. Dialysis may be lifesaving in the anuric patient.

Myopathy of Chronic Alcoholism

Chronic alcohol ingestion has a direct toxic effect on skeletal and cardiac muscle. Electron microscopic studies show intracellular edema, widened intrafibrillar spaces containing lipid, glycogen, dilated sarcoplasmic reticulum, and irregular and enlarged mitochondria. These morphologic changes are accompanied by decreased ATPase activity, decreased transport of calcium to the sarcoplasmic reticulum, impaired muscle glycogen metabolism, and decreased contractility of actomyosin.[215]

Acute Myopathy in Chronic Alcoholism

This condition occurs in chronic alcoholics following a long bout of drinking.[199] The patient develops generalized muscle weakness associated with muscle tenderness and painful cramps, which resolve rapidly over the next few weeks.[120] In addition to the weakness, tenderness, and spontaneous cramps, these patients show myoglobinuria, elevated serum creatine phosphokinase activity, and a markedly decreased lactic acid response to ischemic exercise. The condition is believed to be due to interference with muscle phosphorylase activity and may in this respect have some resemblance to hereditary phosphorylase deficiency in muscle (McArdle's disease).

Acute Hypokalemic Myopathy in Alcoholism

Severe muscle weakness without muscle cramping, tenderness, or pain may occur in chronic alcoholics after an acute increase in alcohol consumption.[214] This condition is associated with marked hypokalemia, elevated creatine phosphokinase, and electrocardiographic changes compatible with hypokalemia and a vacuolar myopathy.[143] There is a rapid response to potassium replacement therapy.

Myopathy Associated with Renal Damage and Hyperpotassemia

This condition may occur during particularly heavy alcoholic consumption in chronic alcoholics. There are pain and tenderness of involved muscle which may be generalized or regionally located. There is usually edema of the affected muscle groups. The majority of patients show evidence of renal damage, with hyperpotassemia and myoglobinuria. Muscle biopsy demonstrates necrosis of muscle fibers in the affected muscles. Death may occur from a fatal myoglobinuria nephrosis, but the majority of patients recover from renal and muscle disease.

Chronic Myopathy in Chronic Alcoholism

Chronic myopathy in chronic alcoholism is an insidious development of weakness of the proximal muscles of the limb girdle followed by atrophy.[69]

The condition is symmetric, involving pelvic and shoulder girdles and the proximal muscles of the limbs. The weakness and atrophy are painless. Serum enzyme studies show elevation of serum glutamic oxyloacetic transaminase, serum glutamic pyruvic transaminase, serum aldolase, and creatine phosphokinase. After withdrawal from alcohol, muscle power slowly improves within a few months.

Diagnostic Procedures

1. All types show elevation of serum enzymes compatible with myopathy.[242]
2. Muscle biopsy reveals necrosis and phagocytosis of scattered muscle fibers.
3. In the acute alcoholic myopathies, serum lactic acid levels show abnormally low elevations with ischemic exercise, and muscle phosphorylase activity is depressed.

Treatment

Under the assumption that these three types of myopathy are caused by the toxic effects of alcohol, treatment should be directed as follows:

1. Withdrawal of alcohol.
2. Adequate dosage of supplementary vitamins, particularly of the B complex group.
3. A high-protein diet.
4. Suitable treatment of any associated complications of alcoholism such as hepatic cirrhosis.
5. In acute forms of the disease early stages of impaired renal function and oliguria can be treated by mannitol-induced diuresis. More severe forms of renal failure in which there are anuria, azotemia, and hyperkalemia may require dialysis.

Thyrotoxic Myopathy

A number of muscle disorders are associated with thyrotoxic cases:

1. Acute thyrotoxic myopathy
2. Chronic thyrotoxic myopathy
3. Exophthalmic ophthalmoplegia
4. Myasthenia gravis
5. Myasthenic syndrome (Lambert-Eaton)[181]
6. Periodic paralysis

Acute thyrotoxic myopathy with bulbar palsy and severe generalized muscular weakness may occur as one of the manifestations of severe acute thyrotoxicosis or "thyroid crisis."

A number of patients with thyrotoxicosis develop chronic thyrotoxic myopathy, which is characterized by pronounced muscular weakness and proximal muscle atrophy. The condition is more frequent in males (3:1) and has a tendency to occur in elderly patients with nodular goiter. However, chronic thyrotoxic myopathy has been described in childhood and adolescence.[210]

It is not unusual to find some impairment of ocular motility in patients with hyperthyroidism, and severe impairment of eye movement is an occasional but rare occurrence in chronic thyrotoxic myopathy. Severe ophthalmoplegia without exophthalmos in a patient with thyrotoxicosis is usually due to myasthenia gravis, which can be diagnosed by appropriate diagnostic tests (p. 752).

Ophthalmoplegia with exophthalmos (exophthalmic ophthalmoplegia) in which the severity of the ophthalmoplegia parallels the degree of exophthalmos is a rare complication of thyrotoxicosis. Exophthalmic ophthalmoplegia is probably due to excess secretion of an anterior pituitary factor rather than a response to the effects of thyrotropic hormone or thyroid hormones. There is an ocular myositis with infiltration of round cells, degeneration of muscle fibers, and fibrosis. Exophthalmic ophthalmoplegia presents with progressive loss of eye movement associated with swelling of the eyelids and conjunctiva. The eyelids may fail to cover the cornea, which subsequently becomes dry and ulcerated.

The frequent association of thyrotoxicosis with myasthenia gravis and periodic paralysis has been discussed elsewhere.

Diagnostic Procedures

Electromyography. Motor unit potentials of decreased amplitude and duration are found in 80 per cent of patients with chronic thyrotoxic myopathy.

Muscle Biopsy. In spite of clinical signs of muscle weakness in chronic thyrotoxic myopathy,

changes in the muscle are usually minimal with atrophy of both type I and type II muscle fibers.

Treatment

The improvement following restoration of a euthyroid state is usually quite marked in patients with thyrotoxic myopathy. Many patients show little residual weakness when tested several months after therapy, provided the euthyroid state has been maintained.

Exophthalmic ophthalmoplegia may fail to improve following treatment for thyrotoxicosis. There may in fact be an increase in exophthalmos following thyroidectomy. Treatment with corticosteroids is effective in some cases, while others require orbital decompression as the exophthalmos increases following treatment with thyrosuppressive drugs. There is apparently an increase in the secretion of the "exophthalmic factor" by the anterior pituitary after hyperthyroidism is brought under control. Prior to the introduction of steroids orbital decompression was the only method available to prevent progressive exophthalmos and blindness.

Hypothyroid Myopathy

Myopathies have been described in both congenital hypothyroidism (Kocher-Debré-Semlaigne syndrome) and myxedema (Hoffmann syndrome). They are not separate clinical entities but apparently represent variants of hypothyroid myopathy.[185] Both the syndromes have been described in children with hypothyroidism and in adult patients with myxedema.

Etiology and Pathology

The myopathy is clearly related to the hypothyroid state and is associated with a disturbance of glycogenolysis in skeletal muscle.[172] It may be spontaneous or follow treatment of hyperthyroidism by radioactive iodine, thyroidectomy, or antithyroid drugs. Biopsy of involved muscles has shown nonspecific changes in the few cases examined. Mucoid degeneration with the presence of periodic acid Schiff (PAS)–positive material in some muscle fibers has been reported.

Clinical Features

There is progressive weakness in the proximal muscles of the lower limbs with inability to step up from a chair or rise from a squatting position without using the arms. In some cases, the weak-

TABLE 12–5

Endocrine Disorders and Myopathy

Endocrine Disorder	Associated Muscle Disorder
Acromegaly	More than 50 per cent have muscle weakness and easy fatigability; biopsy negative
Cushing's syndrome	Severe wasting of the limb girdle muscles
Panhypopituitarism	Rapid generalized wasting of muscles and creatinuria
Addison's disease	Weakness and stiffness of the lower extremities with flexion contractures
Steroid and ACTH myopathy	Proximal weakness and wasting of the limb girdle muscles, similar to the wasting in Cushing's syndrome and aldosteronism[119]
Primary aldosteronism	Episodic muscular weakness, particularly of lower extremities, with flaccid paralysis; resembles hypokalemic periodic paralysis
Hypoaldosteronism	Muscle weakness due to hyperkalemia
Hyperparathyroidism	Generalized muscle weakness, hypotonicity, and hyporeflexia[90]

ness may spread to the distal muscles of the lower limbs, and there may be some involvement of the proximal muscles in the upper limbs.[7] The affected muscles may be unusually bulky (pseudo-hypertrophy),[205] and a slowness of both contraction and relaxation (pseudomyotonia)[49] may be a feature in some cases. This latter symptom is usually associated with painful muscle cramps. There are no fasciculations.

Diagnostic Procedures

1. There are the usual clinical and laboratory findings of hypothyroidism with decreased protein-bound iodine in the serum and an abnormally low uptake of radioactive iodine.
2. Elevated levels of the serum muscle enzymes, creatine phosphokinase, lactic dehydrogenase, and serum glutamic oxaloacetic transaminase have been reported in some cases.[124]
3. Electromyographic changes are less conspicuous than in thyrotoxic myopathy. Myotonia-like discharges and low-amplitude, short-duration motor unit potentials are reported to occur in different parts of the involved muscle.
4. The delay in contraction and relaxation of muscle in hypothyroidism is reflected in the tendon reflexes and may be recorded graphically from the ankle jerk. Supramaximal stimulation of a motor nerve occasionally produces a decremental response in muscle-evoked potentials resembling the response seen in myasthenia gravis.[40]

Treatment

The myopathy shows a good response to treatment of the hypothyroid state with disappearance of weakness, cramps, pseudomyotonia, and decrease in muscle bulk over a period of several months. The maintenance of a euthyroid state with adequate substitution therapy will prevent recurrence of the myopathy.

Drug-Induced Myopathies

Chloroquine Myopathy

Aminoquinoline derivatives, including chloroquine, are effective antimalarial and amebicidal agents and are used widely in tropical areas for these conditions. A number of side effects have been described from the long-term use of chloroquine, including reversible haziness of the cornea and irreversible damage to the macular area of the retina. Chloroquine myopathy presents as a proximal muscular weakness affecting the limb girdle muscles of both upper and lower extremities. Muscle biopsy in some cases has shown a marked vacuolation of muscle fibers with almost complete replacement of the sarcoplasm.[68] A similar change described in muscle in certain cases of lupus erythematosus may have been due to treatment with chloroquine rather than to the myopathy of lupus.

Other Drugs

Chronic exposure to a number of other drugs may result in a myopathy. These include corticosteroids, meperidine,[1] emetine,[65] pentazocine,[33] and epsilon-aminocaproic acid.[19] Acute muscle weakness and tenderness have been noted in uremic patients treated with clofibrate[202] and in intravenous heroin users.[190]

Myopathy in Glycogen Storage Diseases

Three of the recognized glycogen storage diseases (types 2, 4, and 5) are associated with deposition of glycogen in skeletal muscle. Type 3 (limit dextrinosis), which is due to the absence of the debranching enzyme amylo-1,6-glucosidase, is very rare and is associated with hepatomegaly, retarded motor development, and occasional mild hypoglycemic episodes. There is an accumulation of limit dextrin and abnormal glycogen in the liver and muscles.

The other two types of glycogen storage disease, which involve skeletal muscle, will be discussed in more detail.

Myopathy of Type 2 Glycogen Storage Disease (Acid Maltase Deficiency)

In this disease, glycogen deposits are found in a number of organs including skeletal muscles, motor neurons, and the myocardium. Formerly, the term "generalized glycogenosis" was used. The condition is due to a lack of the enzyme alpha-1,4-glucosidase (acid maltase) and is inherited as an autosomal recessive trait.

Pathology

At autopsy, excessive glycogen is found in a number of sites, including the parenchymal cells of the liver, muscle fibers, myocardium, and scattered neurons in the brain and spinal cord.

Clinical Features

There are three genetically distinct forms of this disease.[175] The first occurs in infancy with progressive enlargement of the heart and congestive heart failure followed by death within the first year of life. The second form is seen in older children who are normal at birth but show delay in motor development.[250] There is progressive muscular weakness with severe involvement of the neck muscles, pharynx, and limb girdle muscle. The bladder is distended in the later stages, and the anal sphincter is patulous. The heart is not involved, and death occurs at about ten years of age from intercurrent infection.[238] A more chronic form of acid maltase deficiency has been described in adults.[74, 127] These patients are often diagnosed as having muscular dystrophy with onset of weakness in the proximal muscles in the third decade of life. The disease usually runs a benign course, but involvement of the respiratory muscles and respiratory difficulty have been reported.[154]

Diagnostic Procedures

The diagnosis can be established by demonstration of a marked decrease in excretion of acid maltase in the urine.[174] Muscle biopsy shows gross vacuolar myopathy and the demonstration of a complete lack of alpha-1,4-glucosidase activity. Fasting blood sugar is usually normal, and hypoglycemic episodes are not seen in this condition.

Electromyographic examination of the clinically weak muscles shows motor unit potentials of small amplitude and short duration. There is an increase in short-duration polyphasic potentials. Fibrillations, positive waves, and bizarre high-frequency discharges may be seen. Myotonic discharges are sometimes seen, especially in the paraspinal muscles.

Treatment

There is no specific treatment. Prompt treatment of upper respiratory infections may delay the development of fatal bronchopneumonia. A low-carbohydrate diet may be beneficial in the adult form of the disease.

Myophosphorylase Deficiency (McArdle's Disease)

Another example of a glycogen storage disease is due to absence of muscle phosphorylase. The condition has been described as an autosomal dominant[41] and an autosomal recessive trait.[44] Myophosphorylase deficiency is believed to occur in two different forms. There may be an absence of muscle phosphorylase, or the disease may exist in a form in which there is an adequate amount of apparently defective phosphorylase.[88]

Etiology and Pathology

The inherited deficiency of muscle phosphorylase results in a failure of glycogen metabolism in muscle. There is an accumulation of glycogen beneath the sarcolemmal membrane, which can be demonstrated on muscle biopsy.

Clinical Features

Symptoms usually begin during childhood with limitation of exercise due to painful muscle contractions, which may last for several minutes.[107] Some patients develop myoglobinuria after exercise.[87] The condition persists throughout life and may possibly be associated with some muscle weakness in the adult. Death has been reported from acute renal failure following acute myoglobinuria.[108]

Diagnostic Procedures

Ischemic Work Test. The circulation to the arm is occluded by a blood pressure cuff placed around the upper arm and inflated to 200 mm Hg. The circulation from the hand is excluded by a second cuff inflated at the wrist. The patient is asked to exercise for one minute by rhythmically squeezing a rubber bulb. In many cases the flexor muscles of the forearm contract and become firm and painful.[212] Blood samples are drawn immediately before and after exercise and analyzed for lactate content. Normal subjects show a threefold increase in lactic acid after ischemic exercise. The response is absent in subjects with total lack of myophosphorylase but may be reduced in those who have a partial deficiency of the enzyme. Patients with a deficiency of phosphofructokinase,[254] phosphohexoseisomerase, or amylo-1, 6-glucosidase also have no lactic acid increase after exercise.

Electromyography. Recordings from the hypothenar muscles are normal, but there is a decrement in the amplitude of the evoked potential of 50 per cent or more on repetitive ulnar nerve stimulation.[66] If the electromyogram is carried out during ischemic exercise of the forearm muscle, the muscles may be seen to go into contraction and in this state they are electrically silent.

Muscle Biopsy. There is occasional necrosis of fibers and very minimal increase in connective tissue. There are two special features: (1) subsarcolemmal vacuoles containing glycogen and (2) absence of phosphorylase in all muscle fibers with appropriate histochemical stains.[161]

Serum Enzymes. The levels of serum muscle enzymes (aldolase, CPK, SGOT, SGPT, and LDH) are raised, indicating damage to the muscle cell membrane.

Treatment

Ingestion of glucose or sugar-containing food before exercise is often effective in preventing symptoms.

Phosphofructokinase Deficiency

A myopathy with symptoms similar to those seen in muscle phosphorylase deficiency, in which there is an absence of the enzyme phosphofructokinase, has been described.[149, 255] Diagnosis is established by the demonstration of lack of phosphofructokinase activity in muscle.

Muscle Wasting in Hypoglycemia

Distal muscle wasting, particularly in the hands, has been described in patients who have suffered severe hypoglycemia due to hyperinsulinism.[277] The muscle wasting is not due to peripheral neuropathy, and motor nerve conduction velocities are normal. There may be damage to anterior horn cells during hypoglycemia, and recovery is associated with the appearance of large-amplitude motor unit potentials, suggesting reinnervation of muscle fibers by collateral axon sprouting.

Hereditary Carnitine Deficiency

Carnitine (α-amino-β-hydroxybutyrate trimethylbetaine) is involved in the transport of long-chain fatty acids into mitochondria. Carnitine deficiency may occur in two forms:

1. A myopathic form in which there is a defect in carnitine activity in skeletal muscle.
2. A systemic form in which there is a failure of carnitine synthesis resulting in myopathy, cardiomyopathy, and hepatic insufficiency.[139]

Etiology and Pathology

Carnitine deficiency may be inherited as an autosomal recessive trait.[262] The muscle shows predominantly type I fiber atrophy and numerous large round spaces filled with sudanophilic lipid material[6] in the myopathic form of the disease. Similar changes in skeletal muscle have been described in the systemic form of the disease where the cardiac muscle shows separation of myofibrils by large aggregates of mitochondria without lipid accumulation.[116]

Clinical Features

The myopathic form of carnitine deficiency presents with progressive weakness of limb girdle, truncal, and neck musculature beginning in childhood and is usually diagnosed as "muscular dystrophy." The systemic form of the disease presents with similar symptoms of myopathy and recurrent episodes of hepatic insufficiency and hepatic encephalopathy. Children show evidence of cardiac involvement with tachycardia, cardiac enlargement, and occasionally cardiac failure and death.[116]

Diagnostic Procedures

1. Serum creatine phosphokinase (CPK), lactic dehydrogenase (LDH), and glutamic oxaloacetic transaminase (SGOT) levels are elevated.
2. Serum carnitine levels are usually normal or slightly decreased but muscle carnitine levels are depressed.[132]
3. The muscle biopsy shows the presence of type I fiber atrophy and vacuoles filled with sudanophilic lipid material.
4. The electrocardiogram is abnormal in the systemic form of the disease with tachycardia, increased P-R interval, prominent Q waves, and tall R waves. Cardiac abnormalities can be demonstrated by ultrasound examination.

Treatment

Oral replacement therapy with DL carnitine, 2 gm/day, produces steady improvement in muscle strength in some cases.

Myokymia

Myokymia consists of spontaneous localized or widespread constant subcutaneous fascicular movement of muscle. Unlike fasciculations, which are brief, single, isolated contractions, myokymia is slower and more repetitive and resembles a tetanic contraction.

The condition may be seen in some cases of thyrotoxicosis. Facial myokymia is usually a benign disorder and tends to occur around the eye. Rarely, it may be secondary to multiple sclerosis[5] and pontine glioma.[239] A condition of myokymia, myotonia, muscle wasting, and increased perspiration has also been described.[96]

Benign Myokymia

This condition is often familial and may be present throughout life, although it is often not noticed until adolescence. An irregular twitching of muscle fibers, with a somewhat undulating appearance, affects the majority of muscles, but is not associated with atrophy or loss of power. There are occasional painful cramps in the calf muscles. Their chief importance is that they may be mistaken for the diffuse fasciculations of amyotrophic lateral sclerosis, which has a much more serious prognosis. If doubt exists, the electromyographic findings are distinctive and consist of short bursts of action potentials, in contrast to the single high-voltage discharges of fasciculations.

Muscle Cramps

Muscle cramps are a common symptom of neurologic disease and occur in many conditions. Table 12–6 lists certain diseases in which muscle cramps are a prominent feature and which may be encountered in neurologic practice. The majority have been discussed elsewhere in this book.

Muscle cramps do not necessarily denote a disease state since they are frequently encountered under physiologic conditions. They may occur during or immediately after exercise, particularly strenuous exercise, such as swimming or running. They may be due to sudden changes in the blood supply to muscles with alteration of ionic relationships or accumulation of acid metabolites possibly causing cramps. Cramps are also not unusual in the lower limbs during the final months of pregnancy, if the fetal head causes pressure on the pelvic veins or the lumbosacral nerves. "Heat cramps" are well known to workers who toil in excessively hot atmospheres or who are exposed for prolonged periods to tropical environments. The main factor in such cases seems to be salt depletion due to excessive sweating and fluid replacement without salt.

Writer's Cramp

This condition should not be regarded as a disease since it is almost certainly syndromic. The usual complaint is stiffening and cramping of the fingers and hand when picking up a pen to write. There may be an associated feeling of anxiety or tension. The degree of disability varies, but in extreme cases, the patient is completely unable to write. In the milder form, symptoms appear during writing, and as stiffening and cramping increase, the patient is forced to cease. Many cases are examples of a conversion reaction due to anxiety neurosis. Others are due to conditions that cause rigidity and dystonia of the hand and wrist

TABLE 12–6

Muscle Cramps

1. Physiologic—after exercise
2. Pregnancy
3. Sodium depletion with water ingestion
4. Benign myokymia
5. Writer's cramp
6. Acute and chronic tetanus (p. 744)
7. Stiff-man syndrome
8. Syndrome of continuous muscle fiber activity (Isaacs)
9. Recurrent muscle spasms of central origin (Satayoshi and Yamada)
10. Adolescent familial cramps
11. McArdle's disease (p. 741)
12. Tetany (p. 257)
13. Adynamia episodica hereditaria (Gamstorp) (p. 747)
14. Myotonia congenita (p. 724)
15. Paramyotonia congenita (p. 725)
16. Dystrophia myotonica (p. 725)
17. Dystonia musculorum deformans (p. 197)
18. Wilson's disease (p. 296)
19. Parkinson's disease (p. 187)
20. Amyotrophic lateral sclerosis (p. 209)
21. Myxedema myopathy (p. 739)
22. Toxic polyneuropathy—uremia, thallium (p. 287)
23. Multiple sclerosis
24. Cervical cord compression
25. Polymyositis
26. Paramyoclonus multiplex

and include Parkinson's disease, dystonia musculorum deformans, Wilson's disease, and tetany. Writer's cramp is often the first symptom of Parkinson's disease, and the authors have seen a case of Wilson's disease in a 12-year-old girl whose first complaint was writer's cramp. Apart from history taking and the usual neurologic examination, it is important to observe the act of attempted writing. In hysteria the act of writing may be lost only under unusual circumstances such as signing the name or signing a check. The attempts to write are bizarre and dramatic. In writer's cramp due to the other named organic causes, the dystonia and bradykinesia are apparent, and micrographia and tremor can be noted. Patients require full neurologic evaluation and therapy directed toward the cause, including psychotherapy in those believed to have manifestations of a conversion reaction.

Acute and Chronic Tetanus

Acute tetanus (p. 429) produces severe muscle spasms and is usually diagnosed without difficulty. Chronic tetanus is a rare condition but has been reported to follow trauma and inadequate therapy of a puncture wound or incomplete prophylaxis against tetanus. Symptoms occur some weeks or months after injury usually when the wound has healed but may be related to a second injury or manipulation of the original wound. Patients develop trismus, painful cramps involving the abdominal and lumbar muscles, and, later, increasing stiffness, rigidity, and cramping of the limb muscles.[276] Treatment consists of administration of large doses of antitoxin and penicillin.

Stiff-Man (Stiff-Person) Syndrome

The etiology is unknown, but it is almost certain that the condition is neurogenic rather than myogenic and represents a continuous overactivity of the alpha motor neurons in the spinal cord. There is excessive secretion of urinary metabolites of norepinephrine suggesting abnormal metabolism of norepinephrine in the central nervous system.[225] This may indicate the presence of an imbalance between an inhibitory gamma aminobutyric acid system and an excitatory norepinephrine system producing net excitatory effects on the alpha motor neurons.[109] The disease usually begins with several weeks or months of aching in the axial and limb girdle muscles. This is followed by symmetric tightening of muscles of the abdomen, limbs, trunk, and neck, which become boardlike in consistency. There is limited voluntary movement, and the patient has a markedly rigid posture and walks slowly with the body flexed. The muscles are firmly contracted or in spasm on examination and the patient is unable to relax them. The abdomen is often stoney hard, reminiscent of an "acute surgical abdomen," but there is no peritoneal reflex spasm. Painful cramps become superimposed on this background of rigidity and may be provoked by stimuli such as sudden stretching or active and passive movement of a limb, talking, swallowing, chewing, and painful or emotional stimuli. The patient frequently cries out in distress during these muscle cramps, and narcotics may be required for relief. The rigidity and cramps disappear during sleep. The facial muscles and muscles of the tongue and pharynx are usually spared. Involvement of respiratory muscles may reduce the vital capacity, resulting in dyspnea and weak phonation. The intellect and remaining examination are within normal limits.

The electromyogram shows persistent firing of muscle fibers even at rest with superimposed bursts of action potentials corresponding to spasms.[162] The action potentials are, however, of normal appearance and continue after voluntary activity despite attempts to relax.

The condition responds to diazepam (Valium) or Clonazepam with dramatic improvement, manifested by loss of rigidity and disappearance of painful cramps. Diazepam is known to act on the central nervous system (possibly reticulospinal systems) rather than muscle and provides strong support of the neurologic nature of the condition.

Syndrome of Continuous Muscle Fiber Activity (Isaacs)

A rare condition has been described with some superficial resemblance to stiff-man syndrome, but which represents a separate clinical entity. The disease presents as a progressive stiffness and rigidity of muscles, including those of the trunk, extremities, tongue, ocular, and respiratory muscles. Examination shows a generalized state of muscle contraction with fasciculations, but no painful muscle cramps.[130]

The muscle biopsy shows variation in muscle fiber size, aggregation of muscle cell nuclei, and grouping of muscle fiber types on histochemical study. The motor nerve terminals show excessive branching with multiple innervation of single muscle fibers. Electron microscopy demonstrates atrophy of the postsynaptic area and widening of synaptic clefts.[158a] There is an excellent response to treatment with diphenylhydantoin or carbamazepine.[131]

Recurrent Muscle Spasms of Central Origin (Satayoshi and Yamada)

Another rare condition has been described in which there are muscle cramps but absence of muscle rigidity, which is so characteristic of the stiff-man syndrome. The essential features are the presence of muscle cramps beginning in the lower extremities, and, later, involving the trunk and limb girdle muscles, progressing to the upper extremities and, finally, the facial muscles and muscles of mastication. The cramps vary from one to several hundred attacks daily and occur on a background of hypotonia and last for several minutes before subsiding. The course is progressive and death occurs from 5 to 18 years after onset.[224a]

Electromyography shows normal insertion activity, absence of spontaneous activity at rest, and a normal interference pattern on voluntary contraction. During spasm, a 50-per-second, 5-μv discharge of action potentials may be recorded, which gradually subsides.

The etiology of this condition is also unknown. However, it is believed to be due to excessive discharge of alpha motor neurons in the spinal cord and brainstem, which in turn is possibly caused by periodic loss of the inhibitory action of the Renshaw cells.[224]

Treatment

A combination of diphenylhydantoin, quinine sulfate, and chlorpromazine has been found to be most effective in the abolition of the muscle spasm.

Adolescent Familial Cramps

A familial condition of muscle cramps that occur in adolescents during vigorous exercise has been described as an autosomal dominant trait. The muscles are normal in appearance and the electromyogram is normal at rest and during exercise. There is a marked increase in creatinine phosphokinase levels after exercise in affected individuals.

Episodic Muscle Weakness

There are a number of conditions in which an affected individual of normal strength may experience episodic, sudden weakness of variable intensity. They can be classified as follows:

1. Metabolic abnormalities of the muscle fiber
   a. Hypokalemic, periodic paralysis
   b. Hyperkalemic, periodic paralysis
   c. Thyrotoxic, periodic paralysis
2. Neuromuscular transmission defects
   a. Myasthenia gravis
   b. Myasthenic syndrome
   c. Botulism
   d. Tick paralysis
3. Peripheral nerve diseases
   a. Porphyria
   b. Postinfectious polyneuritis

Periodic Paralysis

This condition is characterized by recurrent episodes of flaccid paralysis, which may be localized or generalized. Periodic paralysis can be divided into three forms:

1. Hypokalemic periodic paralysis
2. Hyperkalemic periodic paralysis
3. Thyrotoxic periodic paralysis

Hypokalemic Periodic Paralysis

This is the most common form of this syndrome and is usually inherited as an autosomal dominant trait. About 20 per cent of cases are sporadic. The disease occurs predominantly in the male.

Etiology and Pathology

Attacks of muscular weakness are preceded by the passage of potassium ions into muscle cells.[269] This leads to serum hypokalemia, and presumably the muscle membrane becomes hyperpolarized, which blocks neuromuscular transmission. This may not be the primary abnormality in the disease, since there is some evidence of a deficiency in carbohydrate metabolism[223] in the muscle cell and an increase in cell membrane permeability to sodium and chloride ions during episodes of weakness.[80] Many of these ionic changes are compatible with intermittent hypersecretion of adrenocorticotropin or excess liberation of mineralocorticoids by the adrenal gland, and attacks may be prevented by administration of drugs such as spironolactone which suppress adrenal activity. However, elevated serum levels of mineralocorticoids have not been demonstrated consistently in this disease.

Muscle Biopsy. Muscle fibers show central vacuoles, which electron microscopy has demonstrated to be the result of dilatation of sarcoplasmic reticulum.[193] These findings are seen during the attack but do not correlate with the degree of weakness.

Clinical Features

The first attack of periodic paralysis usually occurs between the ages of 10 and 25 years in familial cases. Attacks tend to diminish in intensity with increasing age and may cease in some cases. A number of factors known to induce attacks in susceptible individuals include stress owing to traumatic injuries or surgical procedures, severe muscular exercise, exposure to cold, and emotional disturbances. Some patients experience an attack after a period of rest following exertion and usually develop symptoms on awaking in the early morning. Another important factor appears to be a high-carbohydrate meal,[106] which may precipitate an episode of weakness. Certain drugs,

including thyroid, insulin, epinephrine, corticotropin, corticosteroids, thiazides, and licorice, may induce attacks.

A number of patients experience prodromal symptoms, including muscle aching and severe thirst, before the onset of weakness. Attacks usually begin during the night, and the patient awakens with weakness in the lower limbs followed by involvement of the upper limbs, trunk, and neck and sparing of the facial muscles, pharynx, larynx, and diaphragm. Involvement of the respiratory muscles is rare but has been reported and may cause asphyxia and death. On examination, the muscles are often firm and tender to palpation during the attack, with hyporeflexia or absence of reflexes. Sensation is intact. Eyelid myotonia has been observed in some cases of hypokalemic periodic paralysis, and the presence of myotonia is not a reliable sign in distinguishing various types of periodic paralysis.

Occasional signs of myocardial involvement have been reported, with tachycardia, cardiac dilatation, and transient murmurs.

Episodes of weakness usually last from 6 to 24 hours, with extremes of one hour to three days. The frequency varies from one per week to a single episode during life. Abortive attacks with localized weakness in one limb or a group of muscles may occur and are usually of short duration.

Recovery is heralded by profuse diaphoresis followed by a gain in strength beginning in those muscles first involved. The recovery period may take as long as three hours.

Diagnostic Procedures

1. There may be some leukocytosis during an attack.
2. Urinalysis reveals slight proteinuria and glycosuria in some cases.
3. Electrocardiographic changes are compatible with hypokalemia.
4. Serum electrolyte studies show hypokalemia. The blood cholesterol level is elevated.
5. The cerebrospinal fluid is normal.
6. Between attacks the electromyogram is normal. During attacks there is (a) decrease in amplitude and duration of motor unit potentials[95] and (b) increase in number of polyphasic potentials. The completely paralyzed muscle is electrically silent. Nerve conduction studies are normal.
7. Attacks of paralysis may be induced by glucose loading. The patient receives 50 gm of glucose

dissolved in 150 ml water every hour until paralysis occurs or for a maximum period of 15 hours. Once definite paralysis is observed, it should be terminated by the intravenous infusion of a solution containing 51 mEq potassium and 103 mEq sodium/liter of water. Patients must be closely observed because of the slight risk of respiratory paralysis, although this has not been reported during induction of paralysis.[136]

8. It is possible to distinguish between hypokalemic periodic paralysis and thyrotoxic periodic paralysis using an epinephrine infusion test. This is performed by the intra-arterial injection of epinephrine into the brachial artery at the rate of 2 μg/minute for five minutes. Evoked action potentials are recorded with surface electrodes from small muscles of the hand, before infusion, during infusion, and for 30 minutes after the infusion. There is an initial increase with a rapid fall within four minutes after the infusion in the amplitude of the evoked action potentials in patients with hypokalemic periodic paralysis. The depression of the evoked action potentials is not seen in thyrotoxic periodic paralysis.

Treatment

The attack can be terminated by:

1. Oral administration of 5 to 15 gm of potassium chloride.[46]
2. Intravenous infusion of 500 mg acetazolamide.[268]

Acetazolamide, 250 mg every four to six hours, is the drug of choice in the prophylactic treatment of hypokalemic periodic paralysis.[134] The metabolic acidosis induced by acetazolamide prevents the episodic muscular weakness in this disease.[267] Diuretic drugs of the benzothiadizide group should be avoided.

Hyperkalemic Periodic Paralysis (Adynamia Episodica Hereditaria) (Gamstorp's Syndrome)

This type of periodic paralysis is rare and is inherited as an autosomal dominant trait. Attacks usually begin before the age of ten years[150] and are usually induced by hunger, a period of rest after exposure to cold, damp conditions, or after unusual exertion.[28] Accidental administration of potassium salts or drinking beer in excess (beer contains potassium) may also produce weakness. The episodes are milder than the attacks seen in the hypokalemic type (page 746) and usually last less than one hour. They tend to occur during daily activities rather than after a night's rest. The condition is reported to be more severe in males.

There is marked individual variation in the frequency of attacks. Some patients experience weakness daily from 30 minutes to three hours, although occasionally a patient may be paralyzed for one or two days. There is often a sensation of stiffness or numbness in the lower limbs before the onset of weakness, which usually involves the proximal muscles of the lower extremities with lesser involvement of the proximal muscles in the upper extremities. More generalized involvement, including difficulty with swallowing and respiration, is extremely rare. The frequency and severity of the episodes tend to decrease in adolescents and may disappear entirely in the adult. Examination during an attack shows hypotonia and decreased or absent reflexes. It may be possible to demonstrate a mild percussion myotonia involving the tongue or the thenar muscles, which can be accentuated by local cooling with ice water. A few patients in certain families have developed persistent proximal muscular weakness and diminished reflexes after several years of severe attacks of paralysis.

Diagnostic Procedures

Laboratory Findings. These are as follows:

1. Potassium ions move from the muscle fiber into the extracellular space during an attack of weakness, and there is an elevation of serum potassium levels. This is not consistent, however, and some attacks may not be accompanied by hyperkalemia (so-called "normokalemic" periodic paralysis).
2. Serum creatinine phosphokinase levels are elevated after an attack of weakness and reach a peak in about 96 hours.

Electromyography. Two main features of hyperkalemic periodic paralysis are a transient block of electrical activity in many muscle fibers and increased excitability in others. During the stage of paresis, fibrillations, regular series of positive waves, and myotonic discharges may be recorded. The motor unit potentials are decreased in duration and number. The hyperexcitability of the

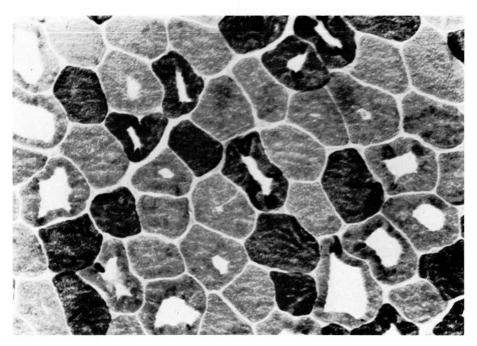

FIGURE 12–6. Muscle biopsy stained with ATPase reaction at pH 9.4 showing vacuoles in both type I and type II fibers. This abnormality is seen in hypokalemic periodic paralysis.

muscle fibers may persist even after the attacks subside.

Muscle Biopsy. There is a large variation in the size of the muscle fibers, many showing the presence of vacuoles in type I and type II fibers (Fig. 12–6). Electron microscopic studies have shown prominent vacuoles in the midportion of the muscle fibers with mitrochondrial degeneration.[160]

Treatment

Attacks may be prevented by avoiding severe exertions, exposure to cold conditions, and undue fatigue. Catecholamines alleviate hyperkalemic episodes by stimulating cellular uptake of potassium, and inhalations of salbutamol appear to be an effective form of treatment in many cases.[272] Acetazolamide, 250 mg once or twice a day, is also effective in preventing attacks.[170]

Thyrotoxic Periodic Paralysis

The majority of cases of thyrotoxic periodic paralysis has been described in people of Japanese descent.[222] However, it is known to occur in other races.[3] This condition is rare and closely resembles hypokalemic periodic paralysis. The clinical features are similar. There is accentuation by exercise, ingestion of carbohydrates, and hypokalemia. Nevertheless, there are differences between the two conditions which suggest that the hyperthyroid form of periodic paralysis is not the hypokalemic variety potentiated by hyperthyroidism.[73] In fact, the hypokalemic form of periodic paralysis is usually improved by the administration of thyroid hormones.[185]

Clinical Features

The attacks of periodic paralysis are similar to those described under hypokalemic periodic paralysis.

Treatment

This condition can be cured by adequate treatment of the hyperthyroid state, and attacks no longer occur when the patient is euthyroid.

Neuromuscular Transmission Defects: Myasthenia Gravis, Myasthenic Syndrome, Botulism, Tick Paralysis

Understanding of the etiology and rational therapy of diseases of the neuromuscular junction (particularly myasthenia gravis) requires knowledge of the anatomy and physiology of this important functional unit. A great deal has been learned from electron microscopy, histochemical techniques, and microelectrode recording. It is now possible to describe the normal neuromuscular junction in anatomic and physiologic terms since its structure and function have now been well defined. There is less certainty, however, in dealing with disorders of this region, and diseases such as myasthenia gravis are undergoing further study to identify the specific defects involving the neuromuscular junction.

Normal Histology and Physiology of the Neuromuscular Junction

The muscle fiber shows an accumulation of sarcoplasm beneath the muscle membrane (postsynaptic membrane) at the neuromuscular junction. This area differs in structure from the rest of the fiber in that it is without myofibrils but contains several large nuclei (the "sole plate nuclei") and a rich concentration of mitochondria. The terminal portion of the motor axon loses its myelin sheath and breaks into a number of branches, which are partly embedded in the depressions of the muscle membrane called synaptic gutters. There is, however, a minute space between the axon and the muscle membrane in which there is no direct contact. The surface of the gutters is covered by a thin teloglial sheath derived from the terminal Schwann cell, and the axon lies between this and the muscle membrane lining the synaptic gutter. The membranes are folded in regular lamellar fashion rather like the folds of mucosa in the jejunum.

The terminal branches of the motor axon contain numerous globular structures or "synaptic vesicles," each containing a "quantum" of approximately 10,000 molecules of acetylcholine.[117] The vesicles are particularly numerous near the terminal axon membrane (presynaptic membrane), and a small number are released spontaneously into the synaptic space producing a local depolarization termed the miniature end plate potential. Many vesicles are released when the presynaptic membrane is depolarized by a nerve impulse and a small number of the released acetylcholine molecules traverse the synaptic space to interact with acetylcholine receptors. The interaction of acetylcholine and the acetylcholine receptor results in an immediate alteration in permeability of the muscle membrane with a rapid influx of sodium ions producing a larger depolarization or end plate potential. This potential initiates an action potential that is propagated along the muscle membrane and activates the various processes that produce muscle contraction. The acetylcholine is removed by diffusion or is hydrolyzed by acetylcholinesterase that is present in the postsynaptic membrane.[141] There are between 30 and 40 million acetylcholine receptors in a neuromuscular junction, but relatively few are activated by acetylcholine after a single nerve impulse. However, although the interaction of acetylcholine and receptor is a matter of probability, the number of interactions is more than is necessary to generate an action potential. Any process that produces a reduction in the excess of interaction between acetylcholine and receptor may ultimately lead to failure of neuromuscular transmission.[62]

Myasthenia Gravis

This condition is characterized by weakness or paralysis of voluntary muscles after activity, followed by recovery of strength after a rest period varying from several minutes to several hours.

Etiology and Pathology

There is a definite link between myasthenia gravis and a number of diseases that are known or believed to be associated with disturbances of immunology. Thyroid disease in the form of thyrotoxicosis and nodular goiter, myxedema, or Hashimoto's thyroiditis occurs in about 9 per cent of males and 18 per cent of females with myasthenia gravis. There is a significant association between diabetes mellitus and myasthenia gravis, and rheumatoid arthritis is not uncommon in myasthenia. The association of systemic lupus erythematosus and myasthenia gravis shows a significant relationship to sarcoidosis, Sjögren's syndrome, pemphigus vulgaris, and ulcerative colitis.[184, 236] Additional support for an abnormal autoimmune mechanism in myasthenia gravis is provided by the demonstration of circulating antibodies to skeletal muscle, thyroid cells, and gastric parietal cells, and the presence of antinuclear factor in the serum of myasthenic patients. This work on autoimmune concomitants has culminated in the demonstration of serum antibodies that bind to acetylcholine receptors in patients with myasthenia gravis.

The immunologic basis for myasthenia gravis is further supported by the demonstration of muscular weakness and a decremental electromyographic response in animals repeatedly immunized with acetylcholine receptor extracted from the electric organ of the eel, *Electrophorus electricus,*[191] or *Torpedo california.*[70, 217]

Study of the action of the specific binding toxin from *Bungarus multicintus* (α bungarotoxin) shows that the toxin binds to acetylcholine receptor. This has led to the development of methods to demonstrate receptor sites at the neuromuscular junction.[16-18] However, the action of α bungarotoxin in animals is blocked by circulating antibodies in the serum of patients with myasthenia gravis, and it is possible to measure antibody titers to acetylcholine receptor based on this blocking effect.[155] There is a good correlation between titers of antibody and the clinical severity of myasthenia gravis. It is also possible that acetylcholine receptor antibodies destroy receptors in addition to blocking receptor sites, since there appears to be a reduction in immune complexes in patients with severe myasthenia gravis.[78]

The role of the thymus gland in myasthenia gravis remains unclear. Approximately 10 per cent of myasthenics have thymic tumors, and the thymus is histologically abnormal in a high percentage of patients with myasthenia gravis. This suggests that antibody blocking of acetylcholine receptors may be mediated by T lymphocytes. However, lymphocytes found in thymuses of myasthenia gravis patients are no different from normal thymic lymphocytes.[21] In addition, thymectomy carried out in rats with experimental autoimmune myasthenia gravis with demonstrated antibodies to acetylcholine receptor has no significant effect on the experimental myasthenia gravis,[153] although there is a marked reduction in the T cell population in peripheral blood after thymectomy in myasthenia gravis.[216] However, the thymus gland contains a number of cell types in addition to lymphocytes. One cell type, the "myoid" cell, shows cross-reaction with antimuscle antibody. Myoid cells or closely related structures obtained from the human thymus appear as typical skeletal muscle cells on tissue culture and appear to have surface acetylcholine receptors.[138] These cells may be more susceptible to autoimmune processes, possibly by some alteration in the normal thymic function that would initiate the autoimmune process and later incorporate the acetylcholine receptor at the neuromuscular junction.

Pathophysiology of Myasthenia Gravis

The muscular weakness of myasthenia gravis and the increasing weakness on exertion are due to the decreased number of acetylcholine receptors available at the neuromuscular junction,[69a] which reduces the probability of interaction between acetylcholine and the receptor.[156a] There is a normal decline in acetylcholine release on repetitive stimulation of motor nerve,[10] and the number of contacts falls below the critical threshold necessary for the generation of an end plate potential in patients with myasthenia gravis. This results in a steady decline in the muscles of functioning neuromuscular units, in a muscle during exercise, and the increasing weakness seen in myasthenia gravis.[63]

Clinical Features

Myasthenia gravis is relatively uncommon. There are probably 20,000 cases in the United States with an incidence of 1 in 10,000.[227, 228] However, it is apparent that many mild cases go unrecognized, and the true number is probably higher. It is a sporadic disease but familial occurrence has been reported.[123]

It is more common in women, with a ratio of 2:1, but appears to occur with equal frequency in all races. There is, however, some difference in the age of onset when related to sex. The maximum incidence occurs between 20 and 30 years of age in women and between 60 and 70 years of age in men, although myasthenia gravis may occur at any age, including the neonatal period.[43]

There is marked variation in the clinical features of this disease. Symptoms vary from slight localized weakness, which is apparently stable, to the severe fulminating, often fatal type of generalized weakness. Approximately 33 per cent of patients present with ocular symptoms only, while another 33 per cent of patients have ocular symptoms with other weakness. Extremity weakness without ocular muscle involvement is less frequent and occurs in some 15 per cent of cases. Approximately 20 per cent of patients have difficulty in chewing and swallowing.

The classic history of a patient with ocular myasthenia is that the first symptoms of diplopia appear in the afternoon or early evening and tend to disappear by the following morning. There is a gradual increase in duration of diplopia followed by the development of ptosis, which has a definite relationship to fatigue. If the patient is seen at this time, the extraocular movements are restricted.

Diplopia and often ptosis can be produced by sustained upward gaze. The ptosis is compensated to some degree by backward tilting of the head and wrinkling of the frontalis muscle.

If the bulbar muscles are involved, the voice has a nasal quality, which tends to fluctuate but gets worse as conversation continues, with an increasing lingual dysarthria. Temporary aphonia may result in severe cases. There is progressive weakness of the jaw on chewing. This improves with rest, but the patient frequently supports the lower jaw with the hand while sitting. Others experience increasing dysphagia and nasal regurgitation of food during a meal.

The peripheral muscle weakness of myasthenia gravis can affect any muscle group, with characteristic deterioration during exercise and improvement following rest.

Physical examination of the patient with myasthenia gravis shows that the abnormality is confined to muscles. A number of objective tests can be used to assess the degree of muscle involvement. A series of tests carried out each time the patient is examined permits quantitative assessment of the effectiveness of therapy. These are as follows:

1. Measurement of the palpebral fissures.
2. Assessment of extraocular movements in all directions.
3. Timed ability to sustain upward gaze.
4. Timed ability to sustain biting on a tongue blade.
5. The time taken during reading or counting to develop a nasal tone or dysarthria.
6. The number of times one leg can be crossed over the other before fatigue.
7. The number of times the patient can stand up on the toes before fatigue.
8. The number of times the patient can sit up from a supine position before fatigue.
9. Dynamometry and ergography are objective measurements of progressive alteration in muscle strength. The hand grip with a dynamometer is usually recorded at the first, fifth, and tenth pressures. The ergograph permits comparison of the strength during a standard number of hand grips. The test can be repeated over a period of time in an objective and graphic form, which is ideal for comparison before and after various types of treatment and also for evaluation of progress of the disease.

Classification. To assess prognosis and treatment, myasthenia gravis patients are generally classified into four groups:

GROUP I: OCULAR MYASTHENIA. In this group there is involvement of one or more

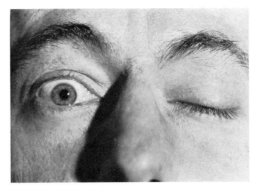

FIGURE 12–7. Patient with unilateral ptosis due to myasthenia gravis. The patient had been asked to open the eyelids as widely as possible. There is a normal response on the right side with failure due to complete ptosis and paralysis on the left side. Unilateral ptosis with normal pupillary reaction is usually due to myasthenia gravis.

ocular muscles, which produces ptosis and diplopia. The ptosis is often unilateral (Fig. 12–7). This form is usually mild but is often relatively resistant to treatment. If progression of myasthenia occurs, it usually occurs within two years of the onset of symptoms.

GROUP II: MILD GENERALIZED MYASTHENIA. These patients experience gradual onset of myasthenia beginning with ocular symptoms, which spread to involve the face (Fig. 12–8), limb, and bulbar muscles. Respiratory muscles are usually not involved. Progression to group III disability, if it occurs, does so within the first two years of the disease.

GROUP III: SEVERE GENERALIZED MYASTHENIA. In these cases the onset is usually rapid, with generalized involvement of ocular, limb, and respiratory muscles. The response to anticholinesterase therapy is good in only about 50 per cent of cases. Those with poor response to therapy are in danger of developing myasthenic or cholinergic crisis.

GROUP IV: CRISIS. Occasionally there is development of severe generalized muscle weakness with paralysis of respiratory muscles in myasthenia gravis, and this is a medical emergency. Myasthenic crises occur in patients from group III who have become refractory to anticholinesterase drugs during an intercurrent infection. Others develop paralysis due to overmedication, which is the so-called "cholinergic crisis."

A number of factors affect the course of the disease. Many patients are weaker during a febrile

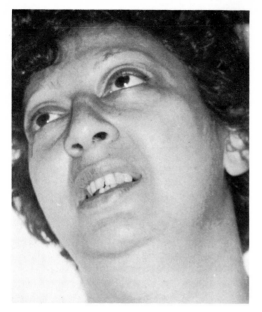

FIGURE 12–8. Characteristic facies of myasthenia gravis. The patient has a "myasthenic snarl or sneer" due to weakness of facial muscles. There is also ptosis.

illness, and group III patients commonly develop myasthenic crisis during an upper respiratory tract infection. The effect of pregnancy varies but there tends to be an exacerbation of symptoms during the postpartum period. The majority of women report that there is some increased weakness during menstruation.

Differential Diagnosis

A number of infrequent and rare conditions have been described that are associated with a myasthenia-like picture.

1. Thyrotoxicosis. The muscular weakness of thyrotoxicosis may be due to associated myasthenia gravis and is improved with neostigmine or is due to thyroid myopathy, which shows no response to anticholinesterase drugs. Some cases show an intermediate picture or pseudomyasthenia.

2. Exophthalmic Ophthalmoplegia. A similar situation exists in this condition. Weakness may be due to thyrotoxic myopathy or fatty infiltration of the orbit and extraocular muscles. Neither type shows any response to neostigmine. Patients who show partial improvement probably have associated myasthenia gravis.

3. Lupus Erythematosus. Any improvement in strength in lupus erythematosus following the use of neostigmine is probably due to the association of two diseases, lupus erythematosus and myasthenia gravis.

4. Polymyositis. There is no doubt that occasionally, patients with polymyositis show improvement and gain in strength with neostigmine. The majority of cases, however, prove to have associated carcinoma (carcinomatous myopathy). These cases with bronchial carcinoma represent the commonest form of myasthenic syndrome.

5. Myasthenic Syndrome (Lambert Eaton Syndrome). See discussion on page 757.

6. Myasthenic Syndrome with End Plate Acetylcholinesterase Deficiency. This rare condition is associated with muscular weakness beginning at an early age. There is a dual neuromuscular transmission defect with reduced release of acetylcholine and absence of acetylcholinesterase. There is an absence of response to anticholinesterase drugs and quinidine with some improvement in strength after using corticosteroids.[77]

Diagnostic Procedures

The diagnosis of severe or moderately severe cases of myasthenia gravis is seldom difficult and can be made on the basis of history and clinical examination. The correct diagnosis is frequently missed or delayed in mild and atypical cases, however, when signs are unstable and transitory. The following procedures are recommended:

Pharmacologic Tests. Confirmation of the diagnosis of myasthenia gravis is made by observing the response to the rapid intravenous injection of the anticholinesterase-like drug edrophonium (Tensilon). The Tensilon test is performed by observing the change in strength in some weak muscle group, e.g., the degree of ptosis, timed ability to bite a tongue blade, or improvement in extraocular movements. An excellent method is to record the weakness of repetitive hand grips on an ergograph and repeat the record after Tensilon. Whatever muscle group is used, the patient is tested and the baseline performance established. A preliminary intravenous injection of 2 mg of edrophonium is given and the patient observed for 20 seconds. If the patient shows no side effects (tachycardia, sweating, salivation), a further 8 mg is injected. After 20 to 30 seconds, the response is recorded once again. Improvement in strength following injection indicates a positive response to edrophonium (positive Tensilon test) and confirms the diagnosis of myasthenia gravis.

The curare provocative test (provoking an attack with a small dose of curare) is dangerous, since it may provoke a myasthenic crisis, and is not recommended.

Electrodiagnostic Tests. The diagnosis of myasthenia gravis is usually made by obtaining a careful history from the patient, which is often quite characteristic in this condition. The physical examination and pharmacologic testing then confirm the impression already obtained from the history. There are, however, a small number of patients in whom the diagnosis remains uncertain, and in this group studies of neuromuscular transmission prove to be most helpful.

The amplitude of muscle action potential to a single supramaximal stimulus is recorded. The muscle action potential is normal in amplitude in most patients with myasthenia gravis. In severe cases it may be reduced. On repetitive stimulation at slow rates, e.g., 2 per second, the amplitude of the evoked muscle action potential successively declines during the first few impulses. This defect is corrected by a short period of tetanus. A short period (10 to 30 seconds) of maximal voluntary contraction will also correct the defect. If the repetitive stimulation is continued at a rate of 2 per second, the defect reappears in 10 to 30 seconds. It is always at its worst some two to four minutes after cessation of exercise, the posttetanic exhaustion.

Several groups of muscles of proximal and distal distribution may have to be tested to demonstrate the effect of myasthenia gravis.

The electromyogram shows a moment-to-moment variation in the amplitude of the motor unit potential on sustained minimal voluntary contraction. The "end plate noise" may be decreased. On sustained maximal voluntary contraction, there is a gradual reduction in the amplitude of the interference pattern, which is finally lost. The electromyogram can be restored to normal after administration of intravenous edrophonium.

Other Tests. These include the following:
1. Roentgenographs of the chest may reveal enlargement of the thymus. All patients should have a chest film with laminograms (tomo-grams) of the mediastinum to exclude possible thymoma.
2. Thyroid function should be evaluated in all cases by determination of the levels of protein-bound iodine in the serum or triiodothyronine levels. Radioactive iodine uptake studies should also be made in any patient considered to have thyroid dysfunction.
3. Associated lupus erythematosus can be excluded by examination of blood smears for lupus erythematosus cells, determination of levels of antinuclear factor, and electrophoresis of the serum proteins.
4. All patients in groups III and IV should have daily respiratory function tests to detect any weakness in respiratory muscles. If respiratory function is severely depressed, the use of a mechanical respirator should be considered.
5. Muscle biopsy is frequently abnormal. Some cases show discrete collections of lymphocytes (lymphorrhages) lying between normal muscle fibers. Histochemical staining shows type II fiber atrophy in about 40 per cent of cases of myasthenia gravis (Fig. 12–9).

Treatment

Anticholinesterase Drugs. The anticholinesterase drugs continue to be the primary mode of treatment for many patients with myasthenia gravis. However, chronic administration of these drugs may produce damage to the postsynaptic membrane[79, 274] and a decrease in acetylcholine receptor sites. Consequently, the physician should consider corticosteroid therapy unless the response to anticholinesterase drugs is absolutely satisfactory with restoration of full activity and a minimum of side effects. Only patients with mild myasthenia gravis (groups I and II) should receive initial treatment in the office or clinic. During the period of regulation of anticholinesterase drugs, group III and IV patients require admission to the hospital for investigation and optimum control of the disease.

Group I or II patients may be given 15 mg of neostigmine every three hours or 60 mg of pyridostigmine every four hours since the peak concentration of pyridostigmine in the serum occurs two hours after oral administration.[45] The dose may be increased if the patient reports an increase in strength and if the intravenous Tensilon test is positive immediately before each additional dose of the oral preparation. It is important to recognize that excellent results from anticholi-

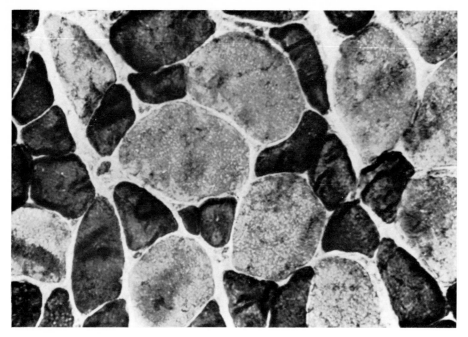

FIGURE 12–9. Muscle biopsy in myasthenia gravis stained with ATPase reaction at pH 9.4. There is type II fiber atrophy. This abnormality occurs in approximately 40 per cent of cases of myasthenia gravis.

nesterase drugs can be expected in only about 50 per cent of cases. The gradual increase in dosage without the use of intravenous Tensilon tests is dangerous and may lead to a cholinergic crisis.[112] If there is no response to intravenous Tensilon, there will not be further improvement with oral anticholinesterase agents and the dose should not be increased further. Mild cases of myasthenia treated as outpatients should also periodically receive an intravenous Tensilon test just before their next oral dose of the anticholinesterase preparation to test the adequacy of dosage.

If the patient is receiving the optimum dose of neostigmine or pyridostigmine, further improvement may result by substituting ambenomium (Mytelase) or adding ephedrine sulfate, 25 mg three times a day, and potassium chloride, 0.5 gm three times a day. The pharmacologic action of these adjuvants in myasthenia gravis is unknown, but they appear to improve strength in some cases. There is a marked individual variation in the development of cholinergic side effects to anticholinesterase drugs. However, some patients will have abdominal colic and intermittent diarrhea with optimal therapeutic doses. The side

effects may be alleviated using atropine, 0.1 mg three to four times daily.

Although patients with milder forms of myasthenia are able to maintain good function on a drug schedule that remains unchanged for many years, an increase in dosage is frequently required during a febrile illness, particularly during upper respiratory tract infections. The patient should be informed of this and should not increase the dosage without first seeking medical advice. The idea that an intelligent patient with myasthenia gravis can be given a box of anticholinesterase tablets and can then "manage" his illness without medical supervision is dangerous. Every patient with myasthenia must be supervised closely since this is a potentially fatal disease. Even the mildest cases require periodic reassessment and advice, particularly when they suffer from intercurrent illness.

Severe generalized myasthenia gravis requires emergency hospitalization for treatment. A slow, intravenous infusion of 5 per cent dextrose of 0.2 N saline should be started to permit the frequent Tensilon testing. At first the patient should be started on neostigmine orally every three hours or pyridostigmine bromide tablets (60 mg) every four hours. The Tensilon test should be performed immediately before each dose of medication is given. If the test is strongly positive, the dose can be increased; if it is negative, the medication should be withheld and the Tensilon test repeated every hour until positive. A weakly positive reaction indicates that the patient is receiving the optimum amount of anticholinesterase medication since the last dose. Tensilon tests establish the maximum amount of oral medication for the optimal time period for that particular patient. At the same time the potential danger of cholinergic crisis is avoided.

Many patients still have myasthenic weakness when the Tensilon test indicates that optimum dosage of anticholinesterase has been achieved. Ephedrine sulfate and potassium chloride may now be added. If there is thyroid dysfunction, this should be corrected, as further strength may be expected when the patient is euthyroid.[94, 183] This will require the use of thyroid-suppressive drugs or radioactive iodine in hyperthyroidism or oral thyroid replacement therapy to correct hypothyroidism.[237] The patients who are resistant to any form of treatment may be benefited by alternate steroid therapy.

Corticosteroids. Oral corticosteroids have replaced the use of adrenocorticotropic hormone (ACTH) in the treatment of myasthenia gravis. There may be some increase in weakness early in treatment if the patient is receiving anticholinesterase drugs,[84] but this can be minimized by initially using small doses of oral corticosteroids. However, patients with severe generalized myasthenia should be treated in an intensive care unit for the first few days of therapy with oral corticosteroids to reduce the risk of respiratory insufficiency.

The possibility of unacceptable side effects limited the use of corticosteroids for many years to cases of myasthenia gravis that failed to show satisfactory response to anticholinesterase drugs. However, experience has shown that oral corticosteroids given once every two days can be used for long periods without appreciable side effects if administration is kept to a minimal effective dose.[164] The patient should be placed on a small dose such as 24 mg of methylprednisolone on alternate days in the morning. The dose can be gradually increased up to 100 mg of methylprednisolone on alternate days.[231] When the patient shows improvement in strength, the dose should

TABLE 12–7

Drug Therapy in Myasthenia Gravis

Group	Drug	Preparation	Equivalent Dose (mg)	Duration of Activity (Hours)
Anticholinesterase	Neostigmine methyl sulfate (Prostigmin) (parenteral)	0.25–0.5 1.0 mg/ml	1.0	2
	Neostigmine bromide (Prostigmin) (oral)	15-mg tablets	15	3
	Pyridostigmine bromide (Mestinon) (oral)	60-mg tablets	60	4
	Pyridostigmine bromide (Mestinon timespan) (oral)	180-mg tablets	60	8
	Ambenonium chloride (Mytelase) (oral)	10 mg 25-mg tablets	5	8
Sympathomimetic	Ephedrine sulfate	25 mg	—	—
Electrolyte	Potassium chloride	0.5-gm tablets	—	—
Anticholinergic	Atropine	0.5-mg tablets	—	—
Corticosteroids	Many preparations (e.g., methylprednisolone, 4- or 16-mg tablets)			

be lowered gradually to the minimal level compatible with maintenance of strength and kept at that level. This usually varies between 16 and 32 mg of methylprednisolone on alternate days. Minor episodes of weakness may require supplementation by small doses of an anticholinesterase drug in some cases. Treatment may be necessary for many years, and the dosage of methylprednisolone should be lowered periodically to see if signs of myasthenia gravis reappear.

Alternate-day corticosteroid therapy is particularly effective in ocular myasthenia gravis, which often fails to respond to anticholinesterase drugs.[89] Corticosteroid therapy is also effective in children with myasthenia gravis, but long-term therapy may not be desirable because of possible growth retardation and side effects.[218]

Thymectomy

Although the risk of thymectomy has been reduced to a considerable degree by modern surgical and nursing techniques, the role of thymectomy in myasthenia gravis remains debatable. It is generally agreed that all patients who have a thymoma should have the tumor removed immediately or following irradiation[281] because of the risk of local metastases to the lungs. The surgical procedure should be followed by corticosteroid therapy to control the myasthenia.[102] However, there is no general agreement on the use of thymectomy in myasthenia gravis when thymoma is not present.[173] Some centers reserve thymectomy for patients who fail to respond to corticosteroid therapy while others advise thymectomy in all cases of generalized myasthenia.[126, 163] The claim that thymectomy benefits females more than males has been challenged,[72] and the increased benefit of thymectomy performed early after the onset of the disease is not substantiated.[97]

Myasthenic Crisis

Myasthenic crisis is a medical emergency because death from respiratory failure may occur if treatment is not instituted immediately. There are three causes of myasthenic crisis:

1. The patient may have sudden onset of severe myasthenia gravis because the diagnosis was not established prior to involvement of the respiratory muscles.
2. Some patients with known myasthenia gravis respond poorly to anticholinesterase drugs and then become refractory to the drug. This is usually precipitated by intercurrent infection.
3. The patient with severe myasthenia gravis may respond poorly to anticholinesterase drugs that are steadily increased in dosage without adequate control by Tensilon testing. This results in excessive anticholinesterase therapy, with the development of a cholinergic crisis.

Although much has been said of the difference in the clinical picture of "myasthenic" crisis and "cholinergic" crisis, the difference is academic and far from clear-cut. Myasthenic and cholinergic crises require prompt treatment, which is basically the same whatever their nature. Respiratory paralysis may occur with alarming speed. All patients in group III who have infections and increasing weakness should be treated as potential cases of myasthenic crisis and admitted to an intensive care unit.

Treatment of Myasthenic and Cholinergic Crises. Treatment is as follows:

1. The patient should be treated in an intensive care unit under constant and expert supervision. All medications should be discontinued.
2. A low-pressure endotracheal tube should be inserted.
3. The cuffed tube should be inflated and attached to a positive-pressure respirator (such as a volume-limited respirator) in such a manner that the patient's own respiratory efforts trigger the machine if possible. If respiratory paralysis occurs, the machine should be arranged to cycle automatically.
4. Myasthenic crisis is often precipitated by infection, which requires appropriate antibiotic therapy. Roentgenograms of the chest should be obtained as soon as possible to rule out pneumonia or atelectasis, and the chest should be examined at least once every day for signs of infection or atelectasis. Any suspicion of pulmonary complications should be followed by active treatment and repeated chest film.
5. The patient should be instructed in how to suction his own secretions from the mouth and pharynx using a soft, sterile plastic catheter. If he is unable to do so, the attending and nursing staff should perform the suction at frequent intervals. The catheter should be discarded after use. This will prevent the introduction of infection, which will result if the

catheter is unsterile. Pulmonary infection may be fatal in myasthenic crisis.

6. On admission, an intravenous infusion of 5 per cent dextrose in 0.2 N saline will provide adequate fluid intake. Once intravenous fluids are given, accurate intake-and-output records should be logged daily and serum electrolyte determinations should be made.

7. The patient should be turned every two hours to improve pulmonary function and prevent pressure ulcers of the skin.

8. A nasogastric tube should be passed, and 250 ml of a fluid or blender diet should be given every three hours. The intravenous fluids are then reduced.

9. The use of high doses of corticosteroids has been recommended in myasthenic crisis. The drug is given in doses of 80 mg of methylprednisolone daily or an equivalent amount for other corticosteroids. The tablets may be crushed and given through a nasogastric tube if the patient is unable to swallow. This is supplemented by antacid therapy, with careful scrutiny of electrolyte imbalance and occult diabetes mellitus during the period of therapy. There may be an increase in myasthenic weakness, beginning on the second or third day of therapy and reaching a maximum effect on the sixth or seventh day of therapy, with some recovery by the tenth day. In general, the greater the degree of weakness during corticosteroid therapy, the more striking the improvement following cessation of therapy at ten days. The response to anticholinesterase drugs is usually markedly improved after termination of corticosteroid therapy. This may last from a few weeks up to six months, when increased weakness may herald the onset of further crisis. In view of this, prolongation of effect may be obtained by the use of the minimal effective dose of oral corticosteroids or an alternate-day basis as described on page 755.

The dosage of corticosteroids should be reduced as soon as the patient shows a satisfactory increase in strength and the schedule gradually changed until the patient is receiving the minimum effective amount of corticosteroid in a single dose once every two days.

This method permits the use of corticosteroids for many months in refractory cases.

10. Plasma exchange transfusion, which is effective in lowering the level of circulating acetylcholine receptor antibodies, may result in remission in refractory cases of myasthenic crisis who show delayed response to corticosteroid therapy.[54]

11. When the patient begins to show improvement in respiratory function, the use of the respirator is reduced. Trial periods of voluntary respiration should be short at first but gradually increased until the use of the respirator can be entirely discontinued. Without the respirator a decision can be made to continue the use of corticosteroids alone or to add anticholinesterase drugs.

12. The Tensilon test should be strongly positive before introducing treatment with anticholinesterase drugs if the physician elects to resume this mode of therapy. Treatment can be started with intramuscular neostigmine, 1 mg every three hours, if the patient is unable to swallow the oral preparations. The Tensilon test should be performed immediately before each injection.

13. The intramuscular neostigmine may be increased up to 2 mg every three hours if the Tensilon test remains positive.

14. The medication should be changed from intramuscular neostigmine every three hours to one of the oral anticholinesterase drugs as soon as possible. An equivalent amount of the drug should be given at six-hour intervals (1.0 mg of intramuscular neostigmine is equal to 15 mg of oral neostigmine and 60 mg of oral pyridostigmine).

15. The patient should now be treated as a severe case of myasthenia gravis.

Myasthenic Syndrome

Eaton Lambert syndrome is another syndrome in which there is a defect of neuromuscular transmission. It is sometimes seen in association with oat cell carcinoma of the lung and has also been described as a complication of other neoplastic conditions. The defect in neuromuscular transmission, the clinical symptoms and signs, and the response to therapy clearly distinguish this condition from myasthenia gravis.[151, 152]

Etiology and Pathology

The etiology of this condition is not known, but there is a defect in the release of acetylcholine at the presynaptic membrane. It usually develops in the presence of a neoplasm, particularly in bronchial carcinoma. An extract of cancer tissue from a patient with oat cell carcinoma and myasthenic syndrome reduces acetylcholine release from motor nerve endings.[133] The development of the Eaton Lambert syndrome in patients with hypothyroidism, pernicious anemia, thyroiditis, Sjögren's syndrome, and hyperthyroidism suggests the possibility of an autoimmune mechanism in this condition.[110]

Degenerative changes have been described in the distal motor nerves and motor end points,[253, 278] and there are prominent proliferative changes in the secondary synaptic clefts of the postsynaptic membrane.[92]

Clinical Features

This condition presents with proximal muscle weakness and easy fatigability, which may be enhanced by impairment of acetylcholine release at the neuromuscular junction by administration of magnesium salts.[249] Patients frequently experience dryness of the mouth, impotence, and paresthesias of the thighs. The muscles supplied by the cranial nerves are involved in only about one third of the patients, and the involvement is much less severe than that seen in myasthenia gravis. The deep tendon reflexes are absent or diminished.

Diagnostic Procedures

The technique employed to demonstrate the defect of neuromuscular transmission is the same as has been described under myasthenia gravis. The amplitude of the evoked muscle action potential on supramaximal stimulation of the nerve is significantly decreased. The poor response of a well-rested muscle to a supramaximal stimulus is one of the characteristic features of this condition. Repetitive stimulation at a rate of 2 per second shows a decrement in the response. However, at repetitive stimulation at rates faster than 10 per second there is a marked increase in the amplitude of the muscle action potential. A short period (ten seconds) of maximal voluntary contraction, followed by 2-per-second repetitive stimulation, also elicits the same phenomenon. The pronounced posttetanic facilitation is another characteristic feature of this disorder.

Electromyography reveals a moment-to-moment variation in the amplitude of the motor unit potential on minimal sustained voluntary contraction. This variation is more marked than is seen in myasthenia gravis and is easier to demonstrate since it is most pronounced after a period of rest.

If the minimal contraction is maintained for a while, the amplitude of the motor unit potential is seen to increase.

Treatment

1. An effort should be made to remove the neoplasm. If this cannot be done, irradiation should be carried out.
2. The muscle weakness shows little response to anticholinesterase drugs and corticosteroids. There may be improvement with guanidine hydrochloride, beginning with 125 mg a day (tabs 25 mg, two or three times a day) and gradually increasing the dosage to the highest tolerated level, which may reach 35 mg/kg of body weight per day. Side effects include nausea, abdominal colic, and paresthesias.

Botulism

Botulism is a serious and sometimes fatal disease. It is caused by an anaerobic bacillus, *Clostridium botulinum,* whose exotoxin is one of the most potent toxins known.

Etiology and Pathology

Clostridium botulinum normally inhabits the intestinal tract of animals. The spores are highly resistant to heat and will survive in inadequately sterilized canned foods, particularly in home-prepared canned products, which have usually been incriminated as the cause of outbreaks of botulism.[37] Symptoms occur following the ingestion of food containing the exotoxin. However, botulism can also occur from wound infection by *Clostridium botulinum,* although this event is rare.[273] Human infection is usually caused by *Clostridium botulinum* type A, less frequently by type B, and rarely by type E. The exotoxin produces muscle weakness and paralysis by blocking the release of acetylcholine at the terminal axons of the neuromuscular junctions.[111]

Clinical Features

Symptoms appear some 18 to 36 hours after ingestion of the contaminated food. Gastrointestinal symptoms are mild or absent. The initial complaints are usually dryness of the mouth, difficulty focusing, ptosis, pupillary abnormalities, and diplopia, followed by weakness of the muscles supplied by other cranial nerves, resulting in dysphagia, dysphonia, and inability to handle pharyngeal secretions. This is followed by descending paralysis and dyspnea, and respiratory paralysis occurs in 50 per cent of cases usually within 12 hours after the onset of neurologic symptoms.[255] Recovery of muscle strength is a slow process and may take many months with residual ocular paralysis in some cases.

Diagnostic Procedures

1. The suspected canned food should be sent for culture and identification of the organism.
2. Electrophysiologic studies with repetitive nerve stimulation show a pattern resembling that seen in the myasthenic syndrome.[186] On supramaximal nerve stimulation at 50 Hz the muscle action potential shows a gradual increase in amplitude in mild cases but this response is absent in severe cases.[37] There is a marked increase in amplitude response after treatment with guanidine hydrochloride. Repetitive nerve stimulation may be normal in mild cases of botulism, however. Single-fiber electromyography will demonstrate abnormal neuromuscular function in such cases.[224b]

Treatment

1. A serum sensitivity test should be given to all patients suspected of having been poisoned and, if negative, 10,000 to 50,000 units of polyvalent botulinum antitoxin should be administered intravenously.
2. A cuffed endotracheal tube should be passed if pharyngeal paralysis occurs and secretions should be aspirated regularly.
3. If respiratory failure occurs, mechanical respiration should be immediately instituted (as for myasthenic crisis, see p. 760).
4. During the stage of pharyngeal paralysis, nutritional, fluid, and electrolyte balance should be maintained by nasogastric feeding.
5. Guanidine, a drug known to be of benefit in the myasthenic syndrome, is also effective in botulism.[38, 39] It acts by increasing the amount of acetylcholine released at the nerve terminals.[187] It should be given through a nasogastric tube in doses of 15 mg/kg body weight per day in divided doses, gradually increasing to 50 mg/kg/day if necessary.

Tick Paralysis

Tick paralysis is a rare but interesting condition that has been described in many parts of the world. It is unusual in that it may terminate fatally unless the tick is removed before respiratory paralysis occurs.

Etiology and Pathology

The toxic substance responsible for this condition is liberated by the adult pregnant female tick, which attaches itself to the skin of the victim. The tick toxin prevents depolarization of motor nerves with a reduction in amplitude of evoked muscle action potentials.[251] The wood tick, *Dermacentor andersoni,* and the dog tick, *Dermacentor variabilis,* have been responsible for most of the cases reported in North America.

Clinical Features

The onset is rapid. The patient develops a mild, generalized illness with anorexia, followed by ataxia of the lower limbs. A flaccid, symmetric paralysis then appears within 12 to 36 hours, ascending symmetrically through the lower extremities to the upper extremities and the bulbar muscles, and finally involving the respiratory muscles. Death occurs from respiratory paralysis.[57, 226]

Diagnostic Procedures

There are no abnormal laboratory findings in tick paralysis.

Treatment

Patients show rapid recovery following removal of the tick, which can be accomplished with a few drops of alcohol, gasoline, kerosene, ether, ethyl chloride, or petroleum jelly. The condition resembles poliomyelitis and postinfectious polyneuropathy, and the correct diagnosis may be missed for several days unless consideration is given to tick paralysis. Consequently, in patients who have a rapidly ascending flaccid paralysis a diligent search should be made for the presence of ticks, particularly in the long hair of the scalp, where discovery may be difficult.

Use of Artificial Respiration in Myasthenic Crisis, Botulism, Porphyria, and Other Conditions Producing Respiratory Paralysis or Insufficiency

Acute Respiratory Failure

Immediate efforts to maintain respiration by mouth-to-mouth or mouth-to-nose resuscitation are usually lifesaving. These should be continued until a bag and mask are available. At this point an oral pharyngeal airway should be inserted and respiration continued through the mask with regular (20-per-minute) compression of the bag. If transportation by ambulance is necessary, nasotracheal or orotracheal intubation should be instituted.

Use of the Mechanical Respirator

Acute cases of respiratory failure have an emergency need for a mechanical respirator, but because there are no well-established guidelines, the decision to employ this type of mechanical assistance for patients with subacute or chronic respiratory failure is often delayed. The respiratory insufficiency itself may cause coma, neurologic signs, confusion, and anxiety, which eventually create a vicious cycle by further interfering with respirations.

Patients with suspected respiratory insufficiency should have serial measurements of arterial P_{O_2}, pH, and P_{CO_2}. If the P_{CO_2} rises above 50 mm, and the airways are unobstructed, the patient requires assistance in respiration. The pH measurement will define the degree of compensation by the alkali reserve. On the other hand, if the P_{O_2} falls below 50 mm and the P_{CO_2} is normal, the patient may be treated by oxygen only with a nasal catheter or oxygen tent. It should be remembered that if there is a state of carbon dioxide retention (CO_2 narcosis, hypoventilation syndrome, see p. 246), the respiratory center has become refractory to the usual CO_2 stimuli and is now driven by the hypoxic stimulus, so that administration of oxygen may produce apnea and death.

A progressive decline in vital capacity is also a useful index in assessing the need for intubation or tracheotomy and assisted respiration. Intubation with an intermittent, low-pressure, cuffed endotracheal tube is indicated if the vital capacity declines to one third of predicted normal. A further fall requires use of a mechanical respirator.

Frequent analysis of arterial blood samples is necessary during mechanical respiration to maintain optimum respiratory function and to assess adjustment and removal of assisted respiration. Arterial samples of P_{CO_2} and P_{O_2} should be obtained daily. The P_{CO_2} levels are most important in the measurement of adequacy of alveolar ventilation and should be maintained at normal or near-normal levels (40 mm Hg). If the arterial P_{CO_2} is low owing to hyperventilation, cerebral blood flow becomes reduced and confusion may result. The minute volume measurement is a useful index of respiratory function and can be obtained while the respirator is operating, using special instrumentation with consultation from the pulmonary function laboratory or the inhalation therapy department. Elevated P_{CO_2} levels are an indication for resetting the respirator to increase minute volume. Estimations of compliance are also useful.

A decrease in compliance may be the first indication of pneumonia, pulmonary edema, atelectasis, or airway obstruction. Serial measurements of vital capacity give a good indication of therapeutic progress and when gradual withdrawal from assisted mechanical respiration can begin. Usually, withdrawal of the respirator can be instituted when the vital capacity exceeds one third of the normal predicted values.

Many types of mechanical respirators are available. In general, the tank or Drinker-type respirator has been replaced by the smaller, more efficient volume-limited respirators. However, satisfactory operation of any machine depends on familiarity with its use and suitable maintenance. These are important factors in the successful operation of all mechanical respirators. Since the procedure is frequently lifesaving, the equipment should be well maintained, easily available, and manned by suitably trained personnel.

Cited References

1. Aberfeld, D. C.; Brenenstock, H.; Shapiro, M. S.; Namba, T.; and Grob, D. Diffuse myopathy related to meperidine addiction in a mother and daughter. *Arch. Neurol.*, **19**:384–88, 1968.
2. Airaksimen, M. M.; and Tammisto, T. Myoglobinuria after intermittent administration of succinylcholine during halothane anesthesia. *Clin. Pharmacol. Ther.*, **7**:583–87, 1966.
3. Ali, K. Hypokalemic periodic paralysis complicating thyrotoxicosis. *Br. Med. J.*, **2**:503–504, 1975.
4. Allen, J. E.; and Rodgin, D. W. Mental retardation in association with progressive muscular dystrophy. *Am. J. Dis. Child.*, **100**:208–11, 1960.
5. Andermann, F.; Cosgrove, J. B. R.; Lloyd-Smith, D. L.; Gloor, P.; and McNaughton, F. L. Facial myokymia in multiple sclerosis. *Brain*, **84**:31–44, 1961.
6. Angelini, C.; Lucke, S.; and Cantarutti, F. Carnitine deficiency of skeletal muscle: Report of a treated case. *Neurology* (Minneap.), **26**:633–37, 1976.
7. Astrom, K.-E.; Kugelberg, E.; and Muller, R. Hypothyroid myopathy. *Arch. Neurol.*, **5**:472–82, 1961.
8. Bache, R. J.; and Sarosi, G. A. Myotonia atrophica. Diagnosis of patients with complete heart

block and Stokes–Adams syncope. *Arch. Intern. Med.,* **121:**369–72, 1968.

9. Banker, B. Q. Dermatomyositis of childhood. *Trans. Am. Neurol. Assoc.,* **87:**11–15, 1962.

10. Barrett, E. F.; and Magleby, K. L. *Physiology of Cholinergic Transmission, Biology of Cholinergic Function.* In Goldber, E. M. and Hanin, I. (eds.): *The Biology of Cholinergic Function.* Raven Press, New York, 1976, pp. 29–100.

11. Barwick, D. D.; and Walton, J. N. Polymyositis. *Am. J. Med.,* **35:**647–60, 1963.

12. Becker, P. E. Two new families of benign sex-linked recessive muscular dystrophy. *Rev. Can. Biol.,* **21:**551–66, 1962.

13. Behke, A. R., and Satlzman, H. A. Hyperbaric oxygenation (concluded). *N. Engl. J. Med.,* **276:**1478–84, 1967.

14. Bell, D. B., and Smith, D. W. Myotonic dystrophy in the neonates. *J. Pediatr.,* **81:**83–86, 1972.

15. Bellen, M. C.; Bilchik, R. C.; and Smith, M. E. Pigmentary retinopathy of myotonic dystrophy. *Am. J. Ophthalmol.,* **72:**720–23, 1971.

16. Bender, A. N.; Rengel, S. P.; et al. Myasthenia gravis: A serum factor blocking acetylcholine receptors of the human neuromuscular junction. *Lancet,* **1:**607–609, 1975.

17. Bender, A. N.; Ringel, S. P.; and Engel, W. K. The acetylcholine receptor in normal and pathologic states. Immunoperoxidase visualization of alpha-bungarotoxin at a light and electron-microscopic level. *Neurology* (Minneap.), **26:**477–83, 1975.

18. Bender, A. N.; Ringel, S. P.; Engel, W. K.; et al. Immunoperoxidase localization of alpha-bungarotoxin: A new approach to myasthenia gravis. *Ann. N.Y. Acad. Sci.,* **274:**20–30, 1976.

19. Bennett, J. R. Myopathy from episodic aminocaproic acid: A second case. *Postgrad. Med.,* **48:**440–42, 1972.

20. Berenberg, R. A.; Pellock, J. M.; et al. Lumping or splitting? "Ophthalmoplegia-plus" or Kearns-Sayre syndrome. *Ann. Neurol.,* **1:**37–54, 1977.

21. Birnbaum, G., and Isairis, P. Thymic lymphocytes in myasthenia gravis. *Ann. Neurol.,* **1:**331, 1977.

22. Bohan, A., and Peter, J. B. Polymyositis and dermatomyositis. *N. Engl. J. Med.,* **292:**344–47, 403–407, 1975.

23. Brooke, M. H., and Engel, W. K. The histographic analysis of human muscle biopsies with regard to fiber types. 3. Myotonies, myasthenia gravis and hypokalemic periodic paralysis. *Neurology* (Minneap.), **19:**469–77, 1969.

24. Brooke, M. H., and Kaplan, H. Muscle pathology in rheumatoid arthritis, polymyalgia, rheumatism and polymyositis: A histochemical study. *Arch. Pathol.,* **94:**101–18, 1972.

25. Brooke, M. H., and Neville, H. E. Reducing body myopathy. *Neurology* (Minneap.), **22:**829–40, 1972.

26. Brooks, M. H., and Neville, H. E. Reducing body myopathy. *Neurology* (Minneap.), **22:**829–40, 1972.

27. Buchsbaum, H. W.; Martin, W. A.; Turino, G. M.; and Rowland, L. P. Chronic alveolar hypoventilation due to muscular dystrophy. *Neurology* (Minneap.), **18:**319–27, 1968.

28. Buchthal, F.; Engback, L.; and Gamstrop, I. Paresis and hyperexcitability in adynamic episodic hereditaria. *Neurology* (Minneap.), **8:**347–51, 1958.

29. Bundey, S.; Carter, C. O.; and Soothill, J. F. Early recognition of heterozygote for the gene for dystrophia myotonica. *J. Neurol. Neurosurg. Psychiat.,* **33:**279–93, 1970.

30. Burian, H. M., and Burns, C. A. Ocular changes in myotonic dystrophy. *Am. J. Ophthalmol.,* **63:**22–34, 1967.

31. Burke, D.; Skuse, N. F.; and Lethlean, A. K. A neurophysiological analysis of paramyotonia congenita. *Proc. Aust. Assoc. Neurol.,* **11:**161–65, 1974.

32. Burke, D.; Skuse, N. F.; and Lethlean, A. K. An analysis of myotonia in paramyotonia congenita. *J. Neurol. Neurosurg. Psychiat.,* **37:**900–907, 1974.

33. Burnham, H. A. Pentazocine-induced fibrous myopathy. *J.A.M.A.,* **234:**913, 1975.

34. Bywater, E. G. L., and Beall, D. Crush injuries with impairment of renal function. *Br. Med. J.,* **1:**427–32, 1941.

35. Cancella, P. A.; Kalyanaraman, K.; Verity, M. A.; Tunsat, T.; and Pearson, C. M. Familial myopathy with probable types of myofibrosis in type I fibers. *Neurology* (Minneap.), **21:**579–85, 1971.

36. Carpenter, S.; Karpati, G.; et al. The childhood type of dermatomyositis. *Neurology* (Minneap.), **26:**952–62, 1976.

37. Cherington, M. Botulism. *Arch. Neurol.,* **30:**432–37, 1974.

38. Cherington, M., and Ryan, D. W. Botulism and guanidine. *N. Engl. J. Med.,* **218:**431–33, 1968.

39. Cherington, M., and Ryan, D. W. Treatment of botulism with guanidine. Early neurophysiologic studies. *N. Engl. J. Med.,* **282:**195–97, 1970.

40. Chokroverty, S. Myxedema, myopathy and myasthenia. *Trans. Am. Neurol. Assoc.,* **101:**226–29, 1976.

41. Chui, L., and Munsat, T. L. Dominant inheritance of McArdle's syndrome. *Arch. Neurol.,* **33:**636–41, 1976.

42. Church, S. The heart in myotonia atrophica. *Arch. Intern. Med.,* **119:**176–81, 1967.

43. Clarke, R. R., and Van der Velde, R. L. Congenital myasthenia gravis. A case report with thymectomy and electron microscopic study of resected thymus. *Am. J. Dis. Child.,* **122:**356–61, 1971.

44. Cochrane, P.; Hughes, R. R.; Buxton, P. H.; and Yorke, R. A. Myophospharylase deficiency (McArdle's disease) in two interrelated females. *J. Neurol. Neurosurg. Psychiat.,* **36:**217–24, 1973.

45. Cohan, S. L.; Pohlmann, J. L. W.; et al. The pharmacokinetics of pyridostigmine. *Neurology* (Minneap.), **26:**536–39, 1976.

46. Corbett, V. A., and Muttall, F. O. Familial hypokalemic periodic paralysis in blacks. *Ann. Int. Med.,* **83:**63–65, 1975.

47. Crews, J.; Kaiser, K. K.; and Brooke, M. H. Muscle pathology of myotonia congenita. *J. Neurol. Sci.,* **28:**449–57, 1976.

48. Croft, P. B.; Cutting, J. C.; et al. Ocular myopathy (progressive external ophthalmoplegia) with neu-

ropathic complications. *Acta Neurol. Scand.,* **55:**169–97, 1977.

49. Cronstedt, J.; Carling, L.; and Ostberg, H. Hypothyroidism with subacute pseudomyotonia—an early form of Hoffman's syndrome? *Acta Med. Scand.,* **198:**137–39, 1975.

50. Cudworth, A. G., and Walker, B. A. Carbohydrate metabolism in dystrophia myotonica. *J. Med. Genet.,* **12:**157–61, 1975.

51. Culebras, A.; Podolsky, S.; and Leopold, N. A. Absence of sleep-related growth hormone elevations in myotonic dystrophy. *Neurology* (Minneap.), **27:**165–67, 1977.

52. Culebras, A.; Feldman, R. G.; and Merk, F. B. Cytoplasmic inclusion bodies within neurons of thalamus in myotonic dystrophy: Light and electron microscopic study. *J. Neurol. Sci.,* **19:**319–29, 1973.

53. Davis, M. J.; Cilo, M.; et al. Trichinosis: Severe myopathic involvement with recovery. *Neurology* (Minneap.), **26:**37–40, 1976.

54. Davis, J. N.; Pinching, A. J.; et al. Myasthenia gravis (M.G.) treated by plasma exchange alone or with immunosuppression. Amsterdam 11th World Congress of Neurology. *Excerpta Medica,* p. 278, 1977.

55. Dawkins, R. L., and Mastaglia, F. L. Cell-mediated cytotoxicity to muscle in polymyositis. *N. Engl. J. Med.,* **288:**434–38, 1973.

56. deBacher, M.; Bergmann, P.; et al. Respiratory failure and cardiac disturbances in myotonic dystrophy. *Eur. J. Intensive Care Med.,* **2:**63–67, 1976.

57. DeBush, F. L., and O'Connor, S. Tick toxicosis. *Pediatrics,* **50:**328–29, 1972.

58. DeJong, J. G. Y.; Shoof, J. L.; and Vander Eerden, A. A. J. J. A family with paramyotonic congenita with the report of an autopsy. *Acta Neurol. Scand.,* **49:**480–94, 1973.

59. DeVere, R., and Bradley, W. G. Polymyositis: Its presentation, morbidity and mortality. *Brain,* **98:**637–66, 1975.

60. Diamond, I., and Aquino, T. I. Myoglobinuria following unilateral status epilepticus and ipsilateral rhahdomyolysis. *N. Engl. J. Med.,* **272:**834–37, 1965.

61. Drachman, D. B., and Fambrough, D. M. Are muscle fibers denervated in myotonic dystrophy? *Arch. Neurol.,* **33:**485–88, 1976.

62. Drachman, D. B. Myasthenia gravis. *N. Engl. J. Med.,* **298:**136–42, 1978.

63. Drachman, D. B. Myasthenia gravis. *N. Engl. J. Med.,* **298:**186–93, 1978.

64. Drutz, D. J.; Fan, J. H.; Tai, T. Y.; Cheng, J. T.; and Hsich, W. C. Hypokalemic rhabdomyolysis and myoglobinuria following amphotericin B therapy. *J.A.M.A.,* **211:**824–26, 1970.

65. Duanne, D. D., and Engel, A. G. Emetine myopathy. *Neurology* (Minneap.), **20:**733–39, 1970.

66. Dyken, M. L.; Smith, D. M.; and Peake, R. L. An electromyographic diagnostic screening test in McArdle's disease and a case report. *Neurology* (Minneap.), **17:**45–50, 1967.

67. Dyken, P. R., and Harper, P. S. Congenital dystrophia myotonica. *Neurology* (Minneap.), **23:**465–73, 1973.

68. Eadie, M. J., and Ferrier, T. M. Chloroquine myopathy. *J. Neurol. Neurosurg. Psychiat.,* **29:**331–37, 1966.

69. Ekbom, K.; Hed, R.; Kirstein, L.; and Astrom, K. E. Muscular affections in chronic alcoholism. *Arch. Neurol.,* **10:**449–58, 1964.

69a. Elias, S. B., and Appel, S. H. Acetylcholine receptor in myasthenia gravis: Increased affinity for α bungarotoxin. *Ann. Neurol.,* **4:**250–52, 1978.

70. Elmquist, D.; Mattson, C.; et al. Acetylcholine receptor protein. Neuromuscular transmission in immunized rabbits. *Arch. Neurol.,* **34:**7–11, 1977.

70a. Emery, A., and Walton, J. The genetics of muscular dystrophy. *Prog. Med. Genet.,* **5:**116–45, 1967.

71. Emery, A. E. H. Abnormalities of the electrocardiogram in hereditary myopathies. *J. Med. Genet.,* **9:**8–12, 1972.

72. Emeryk, B., and Strugalska, M. H. Evaluation of results of thymectomy in myasthenia gravis. *J. Neurol.,* **211:**155–68, 1976.

73. Engel, A. G. Thyroid function and periodic paralysis. *Am. J. Med.,* **30:**327–33, 1961.

74. Engel, A. G. Acid maltase deficiency in adults: Studies in four cases of a syndrone which may mimic muscular dystrophy or other myopathies. *Brain,* **93:**599–616, 1970.

75. Engel, A. G.; Angelini, C.; and Gomez, M. R. Fingerprint body myopathy, a newly recognized congenital muscle disease. *Mayo Clinic Proc.,* **47:**377–88, 1972.

76. Engel, A. G.; Gomez, M. R.; and Groover, R. Y. Multicore disease. A recently recognized congenital myopathy associated with multifocal degeneration of muscle fibers. *Mayo Clin. Proc.,* **46:**666–81, 1971.

77. Engel, A. G.; Lambert, E. H.; and Gomez, M. R. A new myasthenic syndrome with end-plate acetylcholinesterase deficiency, small nerve terminals and reduced acetylcholine release. *Ann. Neurol.,* **1:**315–30, 1977.

78. Engel, A. G.; Lambert, E. H.; and Howard, F. M. Immune complexes (LgG and C3) at the motor end plate in myasthenia gravis. Ultrastructural and light microscopic localization and electrophysiologic correlations. *Mayo Clin. Proc.,* **52:**267–80, 1977.

79. Engel, A. G.; Lambert, E. H.; and Santa, T. Study of long-term anticholinesterase transmission therapy: Effects on neuromuscular transmission and on motor end-plate fine structure. *Neurology* (Minneap.), **23:**1273–81, 1973.

80. Engel, A. G.; Rosevear, J. W.; and Potter, C. S. Studies on carbohydrate metabolism and mitochondrial respiratory activities in primary hypokalemic periodic paralysis. *Neurology* (Minneap.), **17:**329–36, 1967.

81. Engel, W. K. A critique of congenital myopathy and other disorders. *Excerpta Medica International Congress Series,* **147:**27–40, 1966.

82. Engel, W. K.; Borenstein, A.; DeVivo, D. C.; Schwartzman, R. J.; and Warmolts, Jr. High single dose alternate-day prednisone (HSDADPRED) in treatment of dermatomyositis/polymyositis complex. *Trans. Am. Neurol. Assoc.,* **97:**272–75, 1972.

83. Engel, W. K., and Derrer, E. G. Drugs blocking

the muscle damaging effects of JHT and noradrenaline in aortic-ligatured rats. *Nature,* **254:**151–52, 1975.

84. Engel, W. K.; Festoff, B. W.; et al. Myasthenia gravis. *Ann. Intern. Med.,* **81:**225–46, 1974.

85. Engel, W. K.; Foster, J. B.; Hughes, B. P.; Huxley, H. E.; and Manler, R. Central core disease: An investigation of a rare muscle cell abnormality. *Brain,* **84:**167–84, 1961.

86. Engel, E. K.; Gold, G. N.; and Karpati, G. Type 1. fiber hypotrophy and central nuclei. A rare congenital muscle abnormality with a possible experimental model. *Arch. Neurol.,* **18:**435–44, 1968.

87. Fattah, S. M.; Rubulis, A.; and Faloon, W. W. McArdle's disease. Metabolic studies in a patient and review of the syndrome. *Am. J. Med.,* **48:**693–99, 1970.

88. Feit, H., and Brooke, M. H. Myophosphorylase deficiency: Two different molecular etiologies. *Neurology* (Minneap.), **26:**963–67, 1976.

89. Fischer, K. C., and Schwartzman, R. J. Oral corticosteroids in treatment of ocular myasthenia gravis. *Neurology* (Minneap.), **24:**795–98, 1974.

90. Frame, B.; Heinze, E. G., Jr.; Block, M. A.; and Manson, G. A. Myopathy in primary hyperparathyroidism. Observation in three patients. *Ann. Intern. Med.,* **68:**1022–27, 1968.

91. Freeman, L. S.; Ragsdale, C. G.; et al. Dermatomyositis and the retina. *J. Pediatr.,* **88:**267–69, 1976.

92. Fukuhara, N.; Takamori, M.; Gutmann, L.; and Chou, S.-M. Eaton-Lambert syndrome ultrastructure study of motor end-plates. *Arch. Neurol.,* **27:**67–78, 1972.

93. Fukuyama, Y.; Ando, T.; and Yokota, J. Acute fulminant myoglobinuric polymyositis with picornavirus-like crystals. *J. Neurol. Neurosurg. Psychiat.,* **40:**775–81, 1977.

94. Gaelen, L. H., and Levitan, S. Myasthenia gravis and thyroid function. *Arch. Neurol.,* **18:**107–10, 1968.

95. Gamstorp, I. A study of transient muscle weakness. *Acta Neurol. Scand.,* **38:**3–19, 1962.

96. Gamstorp, I., and Wohlfort, G. A syndrome characterized by myokymia, myotemia, muscle wasting and increased perspiration. *Acta. Psychiat. Scand.,* **34:**181–94, 1959.

97. Genkins, G.; Papatestas, A. E.; et al. Studies in myasthenia gravis: Early thymectomy: Electrophysiologic and pathologic correlations. *Am. J. Med.,* **58:**517–24, 1975.

98. Gerwel, C.; Pawlowski, Z.; et al. Probable sterilization of Trichinella spiralis by thiabendazole. Proceedings of the Third International Conference on Trichinosis, Miami, 1972.

99. Getzen, L. C., and Carr, J. E., III. Etiology of anterior tibial compartment syndrome. *Surg. Gynecol. Obstet.,* **125:**347–50, 1967.

100. Gilroy, J.; Cahalan, J. L.; Berman, R.; and Newman, M. Cardiac and pulmonary complications in Duchenne's progressive muscular dystrophy. *Circulation,* **27:**484–93, 1963.

101. Goldberg, H. I., and Sheft, D. J. Esophageal and colon changes in myotonia dystrophica. *Gastroenterology,* **63:**134–39, 1972.

102. Goldman, A. J.; Hermann, C., Jr.; et al. Myasthenia gravis and invasive thymoma: A 20 year experience. *Neurology* (Minneap.), **25:**1021–25, 1975.

103. Gomez, M. R.; Engel, A. G.; et al. Failure of inactivation of Duchenne dystrophy X-chromosome in one of female identical twins. *Neurology* (Minneap.), **27:**537–41, 1977.

104. Gordon, A. S.; Newcastle, N. G.; et al. Chronic benign congenital myopathy fingerprint body type. *Can. J. Neurol. Sci.,* **1:**106–13, 1974.

105. Greenberg, J., and Arneson, L. Exertional rhabdomyolysis with myoglobinuria in a large group of military trainees. *Neurology* (Minneap.), **17:**216–22, 1967.

105a. Griggs, R. C.; Moxley, R. T. et al. Effect of acetazolamide on myotonia. *Ann. Neurol.,* **3:**531–37, 1978.

106. Grob, D.; Johns, R. J.; and Liljestrand, A. Potassium movement in patients with familial periodic paralysis: Relationship to the defect in muscle function. *Am. J. Med.,* **23:**356–75, 1957.

107. Gruener, R.; McArdle, B., Ryman, B. E.; and Weller, R. O. Contracture of phospharylase deficient muscle. *J. Neurol. Neurosurg. Psychiat.,* **31:**268–83, 1968.

108. Grünfeld, J.-P.; Ganeval, D.; Chavard, J.; Fardesu, M.; and Dreyfus, J.-C. Acute renal failure in McArdle's disease. Report of two cases. *N. Engl. J. Med.,* **286:**1237–41, 1972.

109. Guillaminault, C.; Sigwald, J.; and Costaigne, P. Sleep studies and therapeutic trial of L-dopa in a case of stiff-man syndrome. *Eur. Neurol.,* **10:**89–96, 1973.

110. Gutmann, L.; Crosby, T. W.; Takamori, M.; and Martin, J. D. The Eaton Lambert syndrome and autoimmune disease. *Am. J. Med.,* **53:**354–56, 1972.

111. Gutmann, L., and Pratt, L. Pathophysiologic aspects of human botulism. *Arch. Neurol.,* **33:**175–79, 1976.

112. Hall, W. J., and McCabe, W. R. Trichinosis, a report of a small outbreak with observations of thiabendozole therapy. *Arch. Intern. Med.,* **119:**65–68, 1967.

113. Hanson, P. A., and Mincy, J. E. Adolescent familial cramps. *Neurology* (Minneap.), **25:**454–58, 1975.

114. Harper, P. S., and Johnston, D. M. Recessively inherited myotonia congenita. *J. Med. Genet.,* **9:**213–15, 1972.

115. Harriman, D. G. F., and Haleem, M. A. Centronuclear myopathy in old age. *J. Pathol.* **108:**237–48, 1972.

116. Hart, Z. H.; Chang, C. H.; et al. Muscle carnitine deficiency and fatal cardiomyopathy. *Neurology* (Minneap.), **28:**147–51, 1978.

117. Hartzell, M. C.; Kieffler, S. W.; and Yoskikoma, D. The number of acetylcholine molecules in a quantum and the interaction between quanta at the subsynaptic membrane of the skeletal neuromuscular synapse. *Cold Spring Harbor Symp. Quant. Biol.,* **40:**175–86, 1976.

118. Havard, C. W. H. Progress in myasthenia gravis. *Br. Med. J.,* **3:**437–40, 1973.

119. Havard, C. W. H. Endocrine myopathies and

myasthenia gravis. *Practitioner,* **216**:400–406, 1976.

120. Hed, R.; Lundmark, C.; Fahlgren, H.; and Ovell, S. Acute muscular syndrome in chronic alcoholism. *Acta Med. Scand.,* **171**:585–99, 1962.

121. Heffernan, L. P.; Rewcastle, N. B.; and Humphrey, J. G. The spectrum of rod myopathies. *Arch. Neurol.,* **18**:529–42, 1968.

122. Herman, J., and Nadler, H. L. Recurrent myoglobinuria and muscle carnitine palmityltransferase deficiency. *J. Pediatr.,* **91**:247–50, 1977.

123. Herrman, C. J. Myasthenia gravis occurring in families. *Neurology* (Minneap.), **16**:75–85, 1966.

124. Hochberg, M. C.; Koppes, G. M.; et al. Hypothyroidism presenting as a polymyositis-like syndrome. *Arthritis Rheum.,* **19**:1363–66, 1976.

125. Hofmann, W. W., and DeNardo, G. L. Sodium flux in myotonic muscular dystrophy. *Am. J. Physiol.,* **214**:330–36, 1968.

126. Horowitz, S. H.; Gerkins, G.; et al. Electrophysiologic evaluations of thymectomy in myasthenia gravis: Preliminary findings. *Neurology* (Minneap.), **26**:615–19, 1976.

126a. Horwitz, S. J., and Roessmann, U. Kearn-Sayre syndrome with hypoparathyroidism. *Ann. Neurol.,* **3**:513–18, 1978.

127. Hudgson, P.; Gardner-Medwin, D.; Worsfold, M.; Pennington, R. J. T.; and Walton, J. N. Adult myopathy from glycogen storage disease due to acid maltase deficiency. *Brain,* **91**:435–62, 1968.

128. Huff, T. A.; Horton, E. S.; and Leboultz, H. E. Abnormal insulin secretion in myotonic dystrophy. *N. Engl. J. Med.,* **277**:837–41, 1967.

129. Iannaccone, S. T.; Griggs, R. C.; et al. Familial progressive external ophthalmoplegia and ragged red fibers. *Neurology* (Minneap.), **24**:1033–38, 1974.

130. Isaacs, H. A syndrome of continuous muscle fiber activity. *J. Neurol. Neurosurg. Psychiat.,* **24**:319–25, 1961.

131. Isaacs, H., and Frere, G. Syndrome of continuous muscle fiber activity: Histochemical nerve terminal and end-plate study of two cases. *S. Afr. Med. J.,* **48**:1601–1607, 1974.

132. Isaacs, H.; Heffron, J. J. A.; et al. Weakness associated with the pathological presence of lipid in skeletal muscle. A detailed study of a patient with carnitine deficiency. *J. Neurol. Neurosurg. Psychiat.,* **39**:1114–23, 1976.

133. Ishikawa, K.; Engelhart, J. K.; et al. A neuromuscular transmission block produced by cancer tissue extract derived from a patient with myasthenic syndrome. *Neurology* (Minneap.), **27**:140–43, 1977.

134. Jarrell, M. A.; Greer, M.; and Maren, T. H. The effect of acidosis in hypokalemic periodic paralysis. *Arch. Neurol.,* **33**:791–93, 1976.

135. Jerusalem, F.; Engel, A. G.; and Gomez, M. R. Sarcotubular myopathy. A newly recognized, benign, congenital, familial muscle disease. *Neurology* (Minneap.), **23**:897–906, 1973.

136. Johnsen, T. A new standardized and effective method of inducing paralysis without administration of exogenous hormone in patients with famil-

ial periodic paralysis. *Acta Neurol. Scand.,* **54**:167–72, 1976.

137. Kalyanaraman, K.; Smith, B. H.; and Chandra, A. L. Evidence for neuropathy in myotonic muscular dystrophy. *Bull. Los Angeles Neurol. Soc.,* **38**:188–96, 1973.

138. Kao, I., and Drachman, D. B. Thymic muscle cells bear acetylcholine receptors: Possible relation to myasthenia gravis. *Science,* **195**:74–75, 1977.

139. Karpati, G.; Carpenter, S.; et al. The syndrome of systemic carnitine deficiency. Clinical, morphologic, biochemical and pathophysiologic features. *Neurology* (Minneap.), **25**:16–24, 1975.

140. Katz, R.; Herman, M. A.; and Katz, S. Tuberculosis of muscle. *J.A.M.A.,* **190**:472–73, 1964.

141. Katz, B., and Milede, R. The binding of acetylcholine to receptors and its removal from the synaptic cleft. *J. Physiol.,* **231**:549–74, 1973.

142. Kendrick, W. C.; Hull, A. R.; et al. Rhabdomyolysis and shock after intravenous amphetamine administration. *Ann. Int. Med.,* **86**:381–87, 1977.

143. Khurana, R., and Kalyanaraman, K. Hypokalemic vacuolar myopathy of chronic alcoholism. A histological and histochemical study. *Dis. Nerv. Syst.,* **38**:287–89, 1977.

144. Kierland, R. R., and Underwood, L. J. Gumma of skeletal muscle: Report of a case. *Am. J. Syph. Gonor. Ven. Dis.,* **32**:491–93, 1948.

145. Kirby, J. K., and Kraft, G. F. Electromyographic studies in myotonia congenita. *Arch. Phys. Med. Rehab.,* **54**:47–50, 1973.

146. Koffler, A.; Friedler, R. M.; and Massry, S. G. Acute renal failure due to non-traumatic rhabdomyolysis. *Ann. Intern. Med.,* **85**:23–28, 1976.

147. Koppes, G. M.; Daly, J. J.; et al. Exertion-induced rhabdomyolysis with acute renal failure and disseminated intravascular coagulation in sickle cell trait. *Am. J. Med.,* **63**:313–17, 1977.

148. Krain, L. S. Dermatomyositis in six patients without initial muscle involvement. *Arch. Dermatol.,* **111**:241–45, 1975.

149. Layzer, R. B.; Rowland, L. P.; and Ranney, H. M. Muscle phosphofructokinase deficiency. *Arch. Neurol.,* **17**:512–23, 1967.

150. Layzer, R. B.; Lovelace, R. E.; and Rowland, L. P. Hyperkalemic periodic paralysis. *Arch. Neurol.,* **16**:455–72, 1967.

151. Lambert, E. H.; Eaton, L. M.; and Rooke, E. D. Defect of neuromuscular conduction associated with malignant neoplasma. *Am. J. Physiol.,* **187**:612–13, 1956.

152. Lambert, E. H.; Okihiro, M.; and Rooke, E. D. *Clinical Physiology of Neuromuscular Junction in Muscle.* Edited by W. M. Paul, E. E. Daniel, C. M. Kay, and G. Moukton. Pergamon Press, New York, 1965, p. 487.

153. Lennon, V. A.; Lindstrom, J. M.; and Seybold, M. E. Experimental autoimmune myasthenia gravis: Cellular and humoral immune responses. *Ann. N.Y. Acad. Sci.,* **274**:283–99, 1976.

154. Lightman, N. I., and Schooley, R. T. Adult-onset acid maltase deficiency. Case report of an adult with severe respiratory difficulty. *Chest,* **72**:250–52, 1977.

155. Lindstrom, J. M.; Lennon, V. A.; et al. Experimental autoimmune myasthenia gravis and myasthenia gravis: Biochemical and immunological aspects. *Ann. N.Y. Acad. Sci.,* **274:**254–74, 1976.

156. Lindstrom, J. M.; Seybold, M. E.; et al. Antibody to acetylcholine receptor in myasthenia gravis: Prevalence, clinical correlates and diagnostic value. *Neurology* (Minneap.), **26:**1054–59, 1976.

156a. Lindstrom, J. M., and Lambert, E. H. Content of acetylcholine receptor and antibodies bound to receptor in myasthenia gravis, experimental autoimmune myasthenia gravis and Eaton-Lambert syndrome. *Neurology* (Minneap.), **28:**130–38, 1978.

157. Luft, R.; Ikkos, D.; Palmieri, G.; Ernsker, L.; and Altzelius, B. A case of severe hypermetabolism of non-thyroid origin with a defect in the maintenance of mitochondrial respiratory control. A correlated clinical biochemical and morphological study. *J. Clin. Invest.,* **41:**1776–1804, 1962.

158. Lumb, E. M., and Emery, A. E. H. Erythrocyte deformation in Duchenne muscular dystrophy. *Br. Med. J.,* **2:**467–68, 1975.

158a. Lütschy, J.; Jerusalem, F.; et al. The syndrome of "continuous muscle fiber activity." *Arch. Neurol.,* **35:**198–205, 1978.

159. Lyon, M. F. Sex chromatin and gene action in mammalian x-chromosome. *Am. J. Hum. Genet.,* **14:**135–48, 1962.

160. Macdonald, R. D.; Rewcastle, N. B.; and Humphrey, J. G. The myopathy of hyperkalemic periodic paralysis. An electromicroscopic study. *Arch. Neurol.,* **19:**274–83, 1968.

161. Mahmud, M. Z.; Howell, R. R.; et al. Myophosphorylase deficiency: (McArdle's disease): Report of a family. *Can. J. Neurol. Sci.,* **3:**175–79, 1976.

162. Mamoli, B.; Heiss, W. D.; et al. Electrophysiological studies on the "stiff-man" syndrome. *J. Neurol.,* **217:**111–21, 1977.

163. Mann, J. D.; Johns, R.; et al. Long-term prednisone followed by thymectomy in myasthenia gravis. *Ann. N.Y. Acad. Sci.,* **274:**608–22, 1976.

164. Mann, J. D.; Johns, T. R.; and Campa, J. F. Long-term administration of corticosteroids in myasthenia gravis. *Neurology* (Minneap.), **26:**729–40, 1976.

165. Mansour, S. E. D., and Reese, H. H. A previously unreported myopathy in patients with schistosomiasis. *Neurology* (Minneap.), **14:**355–61, 1964.

166. Marshall, R. J., and McCaughey, W. T. E. Hypothermia myxodema coma with muscle damage and acute renal tubular necrosis. *Lancet,* **2:**754–57, 1956.

167. Mastaglia, F. L., and Walton, J. N. Coxsackie virus-like particles in skeletal muscle from a case of polymyositis. *J. Neurol. Sci.,* **11:**593–99, 1970.

168. Mausolf, R. A.; Burns, C. A.; and Burin, H. M. Morphological and functional retinal changes in myotonic dystrophy unrelated to quinine therapy. *Am. J. Ophthalmol.,* **74:**1141–43, 1972.

169. Mawatari, S., and Katayawa, K. Scapuloperoneal muscular atrophy with cardiopathy. An X-linked recessive trait. *Arch. Neurol.,* **28:**55–59, 1973.

170. McArdle, B. Adynamia episodica hereditaria and its treatment. *Brain,* **85:**121–48, 1962.

171. McComas, A. J.; Sica, R. E. P.; and Upton, A. R. M. Multiple muscle analyses of motor units in muscular dystrophy. *Arch. Neurol.,* **30:**249–51, 1974.

172. McDaniel, H. G.; Pittman, C. S.; et al. Carbohydrate metabolism in hypothyroid myopathy. *Metabolism,* **26:**867–73, 1977.

173. McQuillen, M. P., and Leone, M. G. A treatment carol: Thymectomy revisited. *Neurology* (Minneap.), **27:**1103–1106, 1977.

174. Mehler, M., and DiMauro, S. Late-onset acid maltase deficiency. *Arch. Neurol.,* **33:**692–95, 1976.

175. Mehler, M., and DiMauro, S. Residual acid maltase activity in late-onset and maltase deficiency. *Neurology* (Minneap.), **27:**178–84, 1977.

176. Meldrum, B. S., and Thompson, R. H. S. The action of snake venoms on the membrane permeability of brain, muscle and red blood cells. *Guys Hosp. Rep.,* **III:**87–97, 1962.

177. Miller, J. J., III Late progression in dermatomyositis in childhood. *J. Pediatr.,* **83:**543–48, 1973.

178. Miller, S. E.; Roses, A. D.; and Appel, S. H. Erythrocytes in human muscular dystrophy. *Science,* **188:**1131, 1975.

179. Morgan, G.; Peter, J. B.; and Newbould, B. B. Experimental allergic myositis in rats. *Arthritis Rheum.,* **14:**599–609, 1971.

180. Morgan-Hughes, J. A., and Mair, W. G. P. Atypical muscle mitochondria in oculoskeletal myopathy. *Brain,* **96:**215–24, 1973.

180a. Morgan-Hughes, J. A.; Darveniza, P.; et al. A mitochondrial myopathy characterized by a deficiency in reducible cytochrome b. *Brain,* **100:**617–40, 1977.

181. Mori, M., and Takamori, M. Hyperthyroidism and myasthenia gravis with features of Eaton-Lambert syndrome. *Neurology* (Minneap.), **26:**882–87, 1976.

182. Murphy, D. L.; Mendell, J. R.; and Engel, W. K. Serotonin and platelet function in Duchenne muscular dystrophy. *Arch. Neurol.,* **28:**239–41, 1973.

183. Namba, T., and Grob, D. Myasthenia gravis and hyperthyroidism occurring in two sisters. *Neurology* (Minneap.), **21:**377–82, 1971.

184. Noguchi, S., and Nishitani, H. Immunologic studies of a case of myasthenia gravis with pemphigus vulgaris after thymectomy. *Neurology* (Minneap.), **26:**1075–80, 1976.

185. Norris, F. H., Jr., and Panner, B. J. Hypothyroid myopathy: Clinical electromyographical and ultrastructural observations. *Arch. Neurol.,* **14:**574–89, 1966.

186. Oh, S. J. Botulism: Electrophysiologic studies. *Ann. Neurol.,* **1:**481–85, 1977.

187. Oh, S. J.; Halsey, J. H.; and Briggs, D. D. Guanidine in type B botulism. *Arch. Intern. Med.,* **135:**726–28, 1975.

188. Olsen, G. N., and Swenson, E. W. Polymyositis and interstitial lung disease. *Am. Rev. Resp. Dis.,* **105:**611–17, 1972.

189. Olson, W.; Engel, W. K.; et al. Oculocranioso-

matic neuromuscular disease with "ragged-red" fibers. *Arch. Neurol.,* **26**:193–211, 1972.

190. Pastan, R. S.; Silverman, S. L.; and Goldenberg, D. L. A musculoskeletal syndrome in intravenous heroin users. Associated with brown heroin. *Ann. Intern. Med.,* **87**:22–29, 1977.

191. Patnick, J., and Lindstrom, J. Autoimmune response to acetylcholine receptor and anti-acetylcholine receptor antibody. *Science,* **180**:871–72, 1973.

192. Pearson, C. M. Muscular dystrophy review and recent observations. *Am. J. Med.,* **35**:632–45, 1963.

193. Pearson, C. M. The periodic paralyses. Differential features and pathological observations in permanent myopathic weakness. *Brain,* **87**:341–54, 1964.

194. Pearson, C. M. Polymyositis and dermatomyositis, arthritis and allied conditions. 8th ed. Edited by J. L. Hollander and D. J. McCarthy, Jr., Lea & Febiger, Philadelphia, 1972, pp. 940–61.

195. Pearson, C. M.; Fowler, W. M.; and Wright, S. W. X-chromosome mosaicism in females with muscular dystrophy. *Proc. Nat. Acad. Sci.,* **50**:24–31, 1964.

196. Penn, A. S.; Roland, L. P.; and Fraser, D. W. Drug, coma, myoglobinuria. *Arch. Neurol.,* **26**:336–43, 1972.

197. Perloff, J. K. Cardiac involvement in heredofamilial neuromyopathic disease. *Cardiovasc. Clin.,* **4**:333–44, 1972.

198. Perloff, J. K.; DeLeon, A. C.; and O'Doherty, D. The cardiomyopathy of progressive muscular dystrophy. *Circulation,* **33**:625–48, 1966.

199. Perkoff, G. T.; Hardy, P.; and Velez-Garcia, E. Reversible acute musclar syndrome in chronic alcoholism. *N. Engl. J. Med.,* **274**:1277–85, 1966.

200. Peterson, D. I., and Minsit, T. L. The clinical presentation of nemaline myopathies. *Bull. Los Angeles Neurol. Soc.,* **43**:39–45, 1969.

201. Pollock, M., and Dyck, P. J. Peripheral nerve morphometry in myotonic dystrophy. *Arch. Neurol.,* **33**:33–39, 1976.

202. Prerides, A. M.; Alvarex-Ude, F.; Clofibrate-induced muscle damage in patients with chronic renal failure. *Lancet,* **2**:1279–82, 1975.

203. Prise, H. M.; Gordon, G. B.; Munsat, T. L.; and Pearson, C. M. Myopathy with atypical mitochondria in type 1 skeletal muscle fibers. *J. Neuropathol. Exp. Neurol.,* **26**:475–97, 1967.

204. Pruzanski, W. Smooth muscle involvement in primary muscle disease. Myotonic dystrophy. *Ann. Pathol.,* **83**:229–33, 1967.

205. Raga, J. The Kocher-Debre-Semlargne syndrome. A case report. *S. Afr. Med. J.,* **52**:200–202, 1977.

206. Rainey, R. L.; Estes, P. W.; Neely, C. L.; and Amick, L. D. Myoglobinuria following diabetic acidosis. *Arch. Intern. Med.,* **111**:564–71, 1963.

207. Riggs, J. E.; Griggs, R.; and Moxley, R. T., III. Acetazolamide induced weakness in paramyotonia congenita. *Ann. Intern. Med.,* **86**:169–73, 1974.

208. Rizza, R.; Solonick, S.; et al. Myoglobinuria following aminocaproic acid administration. *J.A.M.A.,* **236**:1845–46, 1976.

209. Roses, A. D.; Butterfield, A.; et al. Phenytoin with membrane fluidity in myotonic dystrophy. *Arch. Neurol.,* **32**:535–38, 1975.

210. Rosman, N. P. Neurological and muscular aspects of thyroid dysfunction in childhood. *Pediatr. Clin. North Am.,* **23**:575–94, 1976.

211. Rowland, L. P. Pathogenesis of muscular dystrophies. *Arch. Neurol.,* **33**:315–21, 1976.

212. Rowland, L. P.; Lovelace, R. E.; Schotland, D. L.; Araki, S.; and Carmel, P. The clinical diagnosis of McArdle's disease. *Neurology* (Minneap.), **16**:93–100, 1966.

213. Rowland, L. P., and Penn, A. S. Myoglobinuria. *Med. Clin. North Am.,* **56**:1233–56, 1972.

214. Rubenstein, A. E., and Wainapel, S. F. Acute hypokalemic myopathy in alcoholism. A clinical entity. *Arch. Neurol.,* **34**:553–55, 1977.

215. Rubin, E.; Katz, A. M.; et al. Muscle damage produced by chronic alcohol consumption. *Am. J. Pathol.,* **83**:499–516, 1976.

216. Russo, L.; Scoppeta, C.; and Tonati, P. Shifting of the blood T:B lymphocytes in myasthenia gravis patients after thymectomy. *Neurology* (Minneap.), **27**:642–45, 1977.

217. Sanders, D. B.; Johns, T. R.; et al. Experimental autoimmune myasthenia gravis in rats. *Arch. Neurol.,* **34**:75–79, 1977.

218. Sarnat, H. B.; McGarry, J.; and Lewis, J. E. Effective treatment of infantile myasthenia gravis by combined prednisone and thymectomy. *Neurology* (Minneap.), **27**:550–53, 1977.

219. Sarnat, H. G.; O'Connor, T.; and Byrne, P. A. Clinical effects of myotonic dystrophy on pregnancy and the neonate. *Arch. Neurol.,* **33**:459–65, 1976.

220. Sarnat, H. B., and Silbert, S. W. Maturation arrest of fetal muscle in neonatal myotonic dystrophy: A pathologic study of four cases. *Arch. Neurol.,* **33**:466–74, 1976.

221. Satayoshi, E., and Kinoshita, M. Oculopharyngodistal myopathy. *Arch. Neurol.,* **34**:89–92, 1977.

222. Satoyoshi, E.; Murakami, K.; Kowa, H.; Kinoshita, M.; and Nishiyama, Y. Periodic paralysis in hyperthyroidism. *Neurology* (Minneap.), **13**:746–52, 1963.

223. Satayoshi, E.; Suzuki, Y.; and Abe, T. Periodic paralysis: A study of carbohydrate and thiamine metabolism. *Neurology* (Minneap.), **13**:24–33, 1963.

224. Satayoshi, E., and Yamada, K. Recurrent muscle spasms of central origin. *Arch. Neurol.,* **16**:254–64, 1967.

224a. Satayoshi, E. A syndrome of progressive muscle spasm, alopecia, and diarrhea. *Neurology* (Minneap.), **28**:458–71, 1978.

224b. Schiller, H. H., and Stålberg, E. Human botulism studied with single-fiber electromyography. *Arch. Neurol.,* **35**:346–49, 1978.

225. Schmidt, R. T.; Stahl, S. M.; and Spehlman, R. Pharmacologic study of the stiff-man syndrome: Correlation of clinical symptoms with urinary 3-methyl-4-hydroxyphenyl glycol excretion. *Neurology* (Minneap.), **25**:622–26, 1975.

226. Schmitt, N.; Bowiner, E. J.; and Gregson, J. D. Tick paralysis in British Columbia. *Can. Med. Assoc. J.,* **100**:417–21, 1969.

227. Schwab, R. S. Problems in the diagnosis and treat-

ment of myasthenia gravis. *Med. Clin. North Am.,* **47:**1511–24, 1963.

228. Schwab, R. S., and Viets, H. R. Myasthenia gravis in neuromuscular disorders. Edited by R. D. Adams, L. M. Eaton, and G. M. Shy. *Res. Publ. Assoc. Nerv. Ment. Dis.,* **38:**624–43, 1958.

229. Schwatzfarb, L.; Singh, G.; and Marcus, D. Heroin-associated rhabdomyolysis with cardiac involvement. *Arch. Intern. Med.,* **137:**1255–57, 1977.

229a. Seay, A. R.; Ziter, F. A.; et al. Serum creatine phosphokinase and pyruvate kinase in neuromuscular disorders and Duchenne dystrophy carriers. *Neurology* (Minneap.), **28:**1047–50, 1978.

230. Sereviratne, B. I. B. Acute cardiomyopathy with rhabdomyolysis in chronic alcoholism. *Br. Med. J.,* **4:**378–80, 1975.

231. Seybold, M. E., and Drachman, D. B. Gradually increasing doses of prednisolone in myasthenia gravis: Reducing the hazards of treatment. *N. Engl. J. Med.,* **290:**81–84, 1974.

232. Sher, J. M.; Rimalovski, A. B.; et al. Familial centronuclear myopathy: A clinical and pathological study. *Neurology* (Minneap.), **17:**727–42, 1967.

233. Shulin, H., and Weil, M. H. Shock associated with barbiturate intoxication. *J.A.M.A.,* **215:**263–68, 1971.

234. Shy, G. M.; Gonatas, N. K.; and Perez, M. Two childhood myopathies with abnormal mitochondria. I. Megaconial myopathy. II. Pleoconial myopathy. *Brain,* **89:**133–58, 1966.

235. Shy, G. M., and Magee, K. R. A new congenital non-progressive myopathy. *Brain,* **79:**610–21, 1956.

236. Simpson, J. A. Myasthenia gravis: A personal view of pathogenesis and mechanism. Part 1. *Muscle and Nerve,* **1:**45–56, 1978.

237. Simpson, J. F.; Westerberg, M. R.; and Magee, K. R. Myasthenia gravis. *Acta Neurol. Scand.,* **23:**1–27, 1966.

238. Smith, J.; Zellweger, H.; and Atiti, A. K. Muscular form of glycogenosis type II (Pompe). Report of a case with unusual features. *Neurology* (Minneap.), **17:**537–49, 1967.

239. Sogg, R. L.; Hoyt, W. P.; and Boldey, E. Spastic paretis facial contractures. A rare sign of brain stem tumors. *Neurology* (Minneap.), **13:**607–12, 1963.

240. Sokoloff, M. C.; Goldberg, L. S.; and Pearson, C. M. Treatment of corticosteroid resistant polymyositis with methotrexate. *Lancet,* **1:**14–16, 1971.

241. Somer, H.; Donner, M.; et al. Serum isozyme study in muscular dystrophy: Particular reference to creatine kinase aspartate aminotransferase and lactic acid dehydrogenase isozymes. *Arch. Neurol.,* **29:**343–45, 1973.

242. Song, S. K., and Rubin, E. Ethanol produces muscle damage in human volunteers. *Science,* **175:**327–28, 1972.

243. Spiro, A. J., and Kennedy, C. Hereditary occurrence of nemaline myopathy. *Arch. Neurol.,* **13:**155–59, 1965.

244. Spiro, A. J.; Shy, G. M.; and Gonatas, N. K. Myotubular myopathy. Persistence of fetal muscle in an adolescent boy. *Arch. Neurol.,* **14:**1–14, 1966.

245. Spiro, A. J., and Kennedy, C. Hereditary occur-

rence of nemaline myopathy. *Arch. Neurol.,* **13:**155–59, 1965.

246. Spurny, O. M., and Wolf, J. W. Prolonged atrial flutter in myotonic dystrophy. *Am. J. Cardiol.,* **10:**886–89, 1962.

247. Stern, G. M.; Rose, A. L.; and Jacobs, K. Circulating antibodies in polymyositis. *J. Neurol. Sci.,* **5:**181–83, 1967.

248. Stinivas, V. Sclerodermatomyositis with megacolon, small bowel involvement and impaired lung function. *Proc. Roy. Soc. Med.,* **69:**263–64, 1976.

249. Streits, E. W. Adverse effects of magnesium salt cathartics in a patient with the myasthenic syndrome (Lambert-Eaton syndrome). *Ann. Neurol.,* **2:**175, 1977.

250. Swaiman, K. F.; Kennedy, W. R.; and Sauls, M. S. Late infantile acid maltase deficiency. *Arch. Neurol.,* **18:**642–48, 1968.

251. Swift, T. R., and Ignacio, O. J. Tick paralysis: Electrophysiologic studies. *Neurology* (Minneap.), **25:**1130–33, 1975.

252. Tamura, K.; Santa, T.; and Kuroiwa, Y. Familial oculocranioskeletal neuromuscular disease with abnormal muscle mitochondria. *Brain,* **97:**665–72, 1974.

253. Takamori, M. Caffeine, calcium and Eaton Lambert syndrome. *Arch. Neurol.,* **27:**285–91, 1972.

254. Tarui, S.; Okuno, G.; Ikura, Y.; Tanaka, T.; Suda, M.; and Nesbowa, M. Phosphofructokinase deficiency in skeletal muscles. A new type of glycogenosis. *Biochem. Biophys. Res. Commun.,* **19:**517–23, 1965.

255. Terranova, W.; Palumbo, J. N.; and Breman, J. B. Ocular findings in botulism type B. *J.A.M.A.,* **241:**475–77, 1979.

256. Teil, G. B. Separation and identification of myoglobin and hemoglobin. *Am. J. Clin. Pathol.,* **49:**190–95, 1968.

257. Thomas, P. K.; Culne, D. S.; and Elliott, C. F. X-linked scapuloperoneal syndrome. *J. Neurol. Neurosurg. Psychiat.,* **35:**208–15, 1972.

258. Thompson, M. W.; Murphy, E. G.; and McAlpine, P. J. An assessment of the creatine kinase test in the detection of carriers of Duchenne muscular dystrophy. *J. Pediatr.,* **71:**82–93, 1967.

259. Torbergsen, T. A family with dominant hereditary myotonia, muscular hypertrophy and increased irritability distinct from myotonia congenita Thomsen. *Acta Neurol. Scand.,* **51:**225–32, 1975.

260. Tourtelotte, G. R., and Hirst, A. E. Hypokalemia, muscle weakness and myoglobinuria due to licorice ingestion. *Calif. Med.,* **113:**51–54, 1970.

261. Toyka, K. V.; Drachman, D. B.; et al. Myasthenia gravis: A study of humoral immune mechanisms by passive transfer to mice. *N. Engl. J. Med.,* **296:**125–31, 1977.

262. Vandyke, D. H.; Griggs, R. C.; et al. Hereditary carnitine deficiency of muscle. *Neurology* (Minneap.), **25:**154–59, 1975.

263. Vanier, J. M. Dystrophic myotonia in childhood. *Br. Med. J.,* **2:**1284–88, 1960.

264. VanWijngaarden, G. K.; Frenry, P.; Bethlem, J.; and Meijer, A. E. F. H. Familial "myotubular" myopathy. *Neurology* (Minneap.), **19:**901–908, 1969.

265. Vertel, R. M., and Knockel, J. P. Acute renal failure due to heat injury: an analysis of 10 cases associated with a high incidence of myoglobinuria. *Am. J. Med.,* **43:**435–51, 1967.

266. Vignos, P. J., Jr.; Bowling, G. F.; and Watkins, M. P. Polymyositis: Effects of corticosteroids on final results. *Arch. Intern. Med.,* **114:**263–77, 1964.

267. Viskoper, R. J.; Fidel, J.; et al. On the beneficial action of acetazolamide in hypokalemic periodic paralysis. *Am. J. Med. Sci.,* **266:**125–29, 1973.

268. Viskoper, R. J.; Licht, A.; et al. Acetazolamide treatment in hypokalemic periodic paralysis. A metabolic and electromyographic study. *Am. J. Med. Sci.,* **266:**119–23, 1973.

269. Vroom, F. O.; Jarrell, M. A.; and Maren, T. H. Acetazolamide treatment of hypokalemic periodic paralysis. Probable mechanism of action. *Arch. Neurol.,* **32:**385–92, 1975.

270. Walton, J. N., and Adams, R. D. *Polymyositis.* E. & S. Livingstone, Edinburgh, 1958.

271. Walton, J. N., and Nattrass, F. J. On the classification, natural history and treatment of the myopathies. *Brain,* **77:**169–232, 1954.

272. Wang, P., and Clausen, T. Treatment of attacks in hyperkalemia familial period paralysis by inhalation of salbutamol. *Lancet,* **1:**221–23, 1976.

273. Wapen, B. D., and Gutman, L. Wound botulism. *J.A.M.A.,* **227:**1416–17, 1974.

274. Ward, M. D.; Forbes, M. S.; and Johns, T. R. Neostigmine methysulphate. Does it have a chronic effect as well as a transient one? *Arch. Neurol.,* **32:**808–14, 1975.

275. Warmolts, J. R., and Engel, W. K. A critique of the "myopathic" electromyogram. *Trans. Am. Neurol. Assoc.,* **95:**173–77, 1970.

276. Weinstein, L. Tetanus. *N. Engl. J. Med.,* **289:**1292–96, 1973.

277. Winters, S. J.; Schreiner, B.; et al. Familial mitral valve prolapse with myotonic dystrophy. *Ann. Intern. Med.,* **85:**19–22, 1976.

278. Wise, R. P. A myasthenic syndrome associated with bronchial carcinoma. *J. Neurol. Neurosurg. Psychiat.,* **25:**31–39, 1962.

279. Wochener, R. D.; Drews, G.; Strober, W.; and Waldmann, T. A. Accelerated breakdown of immunoglobulin G (IgG) in myotonic dystrophy. A hereditary error of immunoglobulin catabolism. *J. Clin. Invest.,* **45:**321–29, 1966.

280. Wohlfart, G.; Fex, J.; and Eliasson, S. Hereditary proximal spinal muscular atrophy—a clinical entry simulating progressive muscular dystrophy. *Acta. Psychiat. Neurol. Scand.,* **30:**395–406, 1955.

281. Wolfe, W. G.; Sealy, W. C.; and Young, W. G. Surgical management of myasthenia gravis. *Ann. Thorac. Surg.,* **14:**645–49, 1972.

282. Wolintz, A. H.; Sonnenblock, E. H.; and Engel, W. K. Stokes-Adams and atrial arrhythmia as presenting symptoms of myotonic dystrophy, with response to electrocardioversion. *Ann. Intern. Med.,* **65:**126–66, 1966.

283. World classification of the neuromuscular disorders. Appendix A to the minutes of the meeting of Research Group on Neuromuscular Disease held in Montreal, Canada, on 21 September, 1967. *J. Neurol. Sci.,* **6:**165–77, 1968.

284. Wright, T. L.; O'Neill, J. A.; and Olson, W. H. Abnormal intrafibrillar monoamines in sex-linked muscular dystrophy. *Neurology* (Minneap.), **23:**510–17, 1973.

284a. Zatz, M.; Shapiro, L. J.; et al. Serum pyruvate-kinase (PK) and creatine-phosphokinase (CPK) in progressive muscular dystrophies. *J. Neurol. Sci.,* **36:**349–62, 1978.

285. Ziff, M., and Johnson, R. L. Polymyositis and cell mediated immunity. *N. Engl. J. Med.,* **288:**465–66, 1973.

286. Zundel, W. W., and Tyler, F. H. The muscular dystrophies. *N. Engl. J. Med.,* **273:**537–43, 1965.

INDEX*

Abducens nerve, 20, 505, 671
Abscess, 338
  brain, 390
  cranial, epidural, 388
  spinal, epidural, 441
    intramedullary, 442
Absence, **347,** 366
Acceleration, mechanism of injury, 480
Achondroplasia, 86
Acromegaly, 261
Actinomycosis, 432
Addison's disease, 262
Adenoma, 646
Adhesive arachnoiditis, 428
Adie's syndrome, 24, **670**
Adiposogenital dystrophy, 261
Adynamia episodica hereditaria, 747
AEP. *See* Auditory evoked potentials
Agnosia, 7
  auditory, 8
  tactile, 8
  visual, 7
Akinetic mutism, 5, **625**
Alcardi's syndrome, 75
Alcohol, 272
  central pontine myelinolysis, 165, **276**
  cerebellar degeneration, 276
  dementia, 276
  injection, hemifacial spasm, 680
    trigeminal neuralgia, 676
  Korsakoff's syndrome, 6, **43**
  Marchiafava-Bignami disease, 165
  methyl poisoning, 308
  myelopathy, 277
  myopathy, 738

* Page numbers in **boldface** indicate primary discussion of topic.

neurological effects, 272
  peripheral neuropathy, 277
  seizures, 276
  Wernicke's encephalopathy, 274
Aldosteronism, 240
Alexia, 7
Allochiria, 60
Alper's disease, 127
Alzheimer's disease, 176
Amaurotic familial idiocies, 144
Amebiasis, cerebral, 439
Aminoacidurias, 90
  carnosinemia, 95
  citrullinemia, 94
  cystathioninuria, 94
  Hartnup disease, 95
  histidinemia, 95
  homocystinuria, 94
  hyperglycinemia, 95
  hyperlysinemia, 95
  hyperprolinemia, 95
  hypersarcosinemia, 95
  hypervalinemia, 94
  isovalericacidemia, 94
  maple syrup urine disease, 94
  methyl malonic aciduria, 94
  oasthouse urine disease, 94
  phenylalanemia, 94
  phenylketonuria (PKU), 68, **91**
  tyrosinosis, 94
Ammonia, metabolism, 115
Amnesia, transient global, 552
Amyloidosis, neurologic effects, 299
Amylopectinosis, 98
Amyotrophic lateral sclerosis, 209
  carcinomatous, 271
  Guam, 213
Amyotrophy, syphilitic, 421